Hypertension

A Companion to Braunwald's Heart Disease

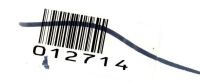

Hypertension

A Companion to Braunwald's Heart Disease

Henry R. Black, MD

Charles J. and Margaret Roberts Professor of Preventive Medicine
Professor of Internal Medicine
Rush Medical College of Rush University
at Rush University Medical Center
Chicago, Illinois

and

William J. Elliott, MD, PhD

Professor of Preventive Medicine, Internal Medicine, and Pharmacology
Rush Medical College of Rush University
at Rush University Medical Center
Chicago, Illinois

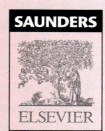

SAUNDERS

ELSEVIER

SAUNDERS
ELSEVIER

1600 John F. Kennedy Blvd.
Suite 1800
Philadelphia, PA 19103-2899

HYPERTENSION: A COMPANION TO BRAUNWALD'S
HEART DISEASE

ISBN-13: 978-1-4160-3053-9
ISBN-10: 1-4160-3053-0

Copyright © 2007 by Saunders, an imprint of Elsevier Inc.

Notice

Knowledge and best practice in this field are constantly changing. As new research and experience broaden our knowledge, changes in practice, treatment, and drug therapy may become necessary or appropriate. Readers are advised to check the most current information provided (i) on procedures featured or (ii) by the manufacturer of each product to be administered to verify the recommended dose or formula, the method and duration of administration, and contraindications. It is the responsibility of practitioners, relying on their own experience and knowledge of the patient, to make diagnoses, to determine dosages and the best treatment for each individual patient, and to take all appropriate safety precautions. To the fullest extent of the law, neither the Publisher nor the Editors assume any liability for any injury and/or damage to persons or property arising out of or related to any use of the material contained in this book.

Library of Congress Cataloging-in-Publication Data
Black, Henry R. (Henry Richard)
   Hypertension : a companion to Braunwald's heart disease / Henry R. Black,
William J. Elliott. — 1st ed.
      p. ; cm.
   Companion v. to: Braunwald's heart disease / [edited by] Douglas P. Zipes . . [et al.]. 7th ed. c2005.
   Includes index.
   ISBN 1-4160-3053-0
1. Hypertension. 2. Heart—Diseases. I. Elliott, William J., M.D. II. Braunwald's heart disease. III. Title.
   [DNLM: 1. Hypertension. WG 340 B627c 2007]
   RC685.H8B553 2007
   616.1'2—dc22   2006045231

Executive Publisher: Natasha Andjelkovic
Developmental Editor: Jerisha Parker
Publishing Services Manager: Frank Polizzano
Project Manager: Lee Ann Draud
Design Direction: Steve Stave

Printed in Canada

Last digit is the print number: 9 8 7 6 5 4 3 2 1

Henry R. Black
To my wife, Benita, the love of my life and my perfect partner, and to Dana, Matt, and Sabrina, who make it all worthwhile. To our colleagues whose work is discussed in this volume and whose contributions to understanding and treating hypertension have saved millions of lives.

William J. Elliott
To my teachers (including my parents and spouse, Melicien Tettambel, DO), my family members, and my students, although it is still unclear from whom I learned (and continue to learn) more.

Contributors

Matthew A. Allison, MD, MPH
Assistant Professor of Family and Preventive Medicine,
University of California, San Diego, School of Medicine,
La Jolla, California
Peripheral Arterial Disease in Hypertension

Craig Anderson, MBBS, PhD, FRACP
Professor of Stroke Medicine and Clinical Neuroscience,
University of Sydney Faculty of Medicine and the Institute of
Neurosciences of Royal Prince Alfred Hospital; Director,
Neurological and Mental Health Division, The George Institute
for International Health, Sydney, Australia
Cerebrovascular Disease in Hypertension

Lawrence J. Appel, MD, MPH
Professor of Medicine, Johns Hopkins University School of
Medicine, Baltimore, Maryland
Diet and Blood Pressure

Phyllis August, MD, MPH
Professor of Medicine, Medicine in Obstetrics and Gynecology,
and Public Health, and Program Director, Nephrology and
Hypertension, Weill Medical College of Cornell University;
New York–Presbyterian Hospital, New York, New York
Hypertension in Pregnancy

George L. Bakris, MD
Professor of Internal Medicine and Director of the
Hypertension Clinic in the Diabetes Institute, Pritzker
School of Medicine, University of Chicago, Chicago, Illinois
Kidney Disease in Hypertension

Robert L. Bard, MA
Research Associate, Endothelial Function Laboratory,
University of Michigan Medical Center, Ann Arbor, Michigan
Hypertension and the Perioperative Period

Jan N. Basile, MD
Professor of Medicine, Medical University of South Carolina;
Lead Physician, Primary Care Service Line, Ralph H. Johnson
Veterans Affairs Medical Center, Charleston, South Carolina
*Hypertension in the Elderly; Hypertensive Emergencies and
Urgencies*

Grzegorz Bilo, MD, PhD
Research Assistant, Department of Clinical Medicine and
Prevention, University of Milano-Bicocca, Milan, Italy; I
Cardiac Department, Jagiellonian University, Krakow, Poland
Secondary Hypertension: Sleep Apnea

Henry R. Black, MD
Charles J. and Margaret Roberts Professor of Preventive
Medicine and Professor of Internal Medicine, Rush Medical
College of Rush University at Rush University Medical
Center, Chicago, Illinois
Angiotensin Receptor Blockers

Michael J. Bloch, MD
Associate Professor of Medicine, University of Nevada School
of Medicine; Medical Director, St. Mary's Risk Reduction
Center, Reno, Nevada
Hypertension in the Elderly

Emmanuel L. Bravo, MD
Consultant, Cleveland Clinic, Cleveland, Ohio
Secondary Hypertension: Mineralocorticoid Excess States

Robert D. Brook, MD
Assistant Professor, Department of Internal Medicine,
University of Michigan Medical School, Ann Arbor,
Michigan
Hypertension and the Perioperative Period

David A. Calhoun, MD
Associate Professor of Medicine, University of Alabama
Birmingham School of Medicine, Birmingham,
Alabama
Pathophysiology of Hypertension

Barry L. Carter, PharmD
Professor, College of Pharmacy and Department of Family
Medicine, University of Iowa Roy J. and Lucille A. Carver
College of Medicine, Iowa City, Iowa
Hypertension Disease Management Services

John Chalmers, MD, PhD, FRACP
Emeritus Professor of Medicine, University of Sydney Faculty
of Medicine and Flinders University School of Medicine;
Honorary Consultant Physician, Royal Prince Alfred Hospital
and Sydney South West Area Health Service; Chairman of the
Board of Directors and Senior Director and Head of Research
Advisory Unit, The George Institute for International Health,
Sydney, Australia
Cerebrovascular Disease in Hypertension

Shalini Chandra, MD
Department of Internal Medicine, Wayne State University
School of Medicine, Detroit, Michigan
Hypertension in African Americans

Neil Chapman, BSc, MB BChir
Honorary Senior Lecturer, International Centre for Circulatory Health, Imperial College; Consultant, Cardiovascular Physician, St. Mary's Hospital, London, England
Cerebrovascular Disease in Hypertension

Kenneth L. Choi, MD
Division of Nephrology and Hypertension, Department of Internal Medicine, University of Miami School of Medicine, Miami, Florida
Kidney Disease in Hypertension

Richard S. Cooper, MD
Professor and Chair, Department of Preventive Medicine and Epidemiology, Loyola University Chicago Stritch School of Medicine, Chicago, Illinois
Genetics of Hypertension

Michael H. Criqui, MD, MPH
Professor of Medicine and Vice Chair of Family and Preventive Medicine, University of California, San Diego, School of Medicine, La Jolla, California
Peripheral Arterial Disease in Hypertension

Errol D. Crook, MD
Professor and Chairman, Department of Internal Medicine, Division of Nephrology, University of South Alabama College of Medicine, Mobile, Alabama
Hypertension in African Americans

Prakash C. Deedwania, MD, FACC, FACP, FAHA
Professor of Medicine, University of California, San Francisco, School of Medicine, San Francisco; Chief, Cardiology Section, Veterans Affairs Central California Health Care System, Fresno, California
Hypertension in South Asians

Mehul G. Desai, MD
Medical Officer, Division of Cardiovascular and Renal Products, Center for Drug Evaluation and Research, Food and Drug Administration, Silver Spring, Maryland
Antihypertensive Drug Development: A Regulatory Perspective

Kim A. Eagle, MD, FACC
Albion Walter Hewlett Professor of Internal Medicine, University of Michigan Medical School; Clinical Director, University of Michigan Cardiovascular Center, Ann Arbor, Michigan
Hypertension and the Perioperative Period

William J. Elliott, MD, PhD
Professor of Preventive Medicine, Internal Medicine, and Pharmacology, Rush Medical College of Rush University at Rush University Medical Center, Chicago, Illinois
Secondary Hypertension: Renovascular Hypertension; The Natural History of Untreated Hypertension; Angiotensin Receptor Blockers; α-Blockers

Bonita Falkner, MD
Professor of Medicine and Pediatrics, Thomas Jefferson University, Philadelphia, Pennsylvania
Hypertension in Children and Adolescents

Larry E. Fields, MD, MBA, FACP
Director, Clinical Product Development, Medco Health Solutions, Inc., Franklin Lakes, New Jersey
U.S. and Canadian Guidelines for Hypertension

John M. Flack, MD, MPH, FAHA
Professor and Associate Chair for Academic Affairs, Internal Medicine Administration; Director of Cardiovascular Epidemiology and Clinical Applications (CECA) Program, Wayne State University School of Medicine, Detroit, Michigan
Hypertension in African Americans

Veronica Franco, MD, MSPH
Instructor of Medicine, Division of Cardiovascular Disease, University of Alabama Birmingham School of Medicine, Birmingham, Alabama
Pathophysiology of Hypertension

Stanley S. Franklin, MD, FACP, FACC, FASN
Clinical Professor of Medicine and Associate Medical Director of the UCI Heart Disease Prevention Program, University of California, Irvine, School of Medicine, Irvine, California
The Special Problem of Isolated Systolic Hypertension

Ronald S. Freudenberger, MD
Associate Professor of Medicine, University of Medicine & Dentistry of New Jersey—Robert Wood Johnson Medical School; Director, Heart Failure and Transplant Cardiology, Robert Wood Johnson University Hospital, New Brunswick, New Jersey
Heart Failure in Hypertension

William H. Frishman, MD
Rosenthal Professor and Chairman of Medicine, New York Medical College; Director of Medicine, Westchester Medical Center, Valhalla, New York
β-Blockers in Hypertension

Philip B. Gorelick, MD, MHP, FACP
John S. Gavin Professor and Head, Department of Neurology and Rehabilitation, University of Illinois College of Medicine at Chicago; Chief, Neurology Service, University of Illinois at Chicago Medical Center, Chicago, Illinois
Assessment of Hypertensive Target Organ Damage

Guido Grassi, MD
Professor of Medicine, University of Milano-Bicocca, Milan; Ospedale San Gerardo, Monza, Italy
European, American, and British Guidelines: Similarities and Differences

Carlene M. Grim, MSN, SpDN
President, Shared Care Research and Education Consulting, Inc., Milwaukee, Wisconsin
Office Blood Pressure Measurement

Clarence E. Grim, MD, MS
Clinical Professor of Medicine and Professor of Epidemiology, Medical College of Wisconsin, Milwaukee, Wisconsin
Office Blood Pressure Measurement

Ehud Grossman, MD
Vice Dean of the Faculty of Medicine, Sackler School of Medicine, Tel-Aviv University, Tel-Aviv; Head of Internal Medicine and Hypertension, Chaim Sheba Medical Center, Tel-Hashomer, Israel
Rare and Unusual Forms of Hypertension

Rajeev Gupta, MD
Professor of Medicine, Mahatma Gandhi National Institute of Medical Sciences; Consultant Physician, Marilek Hospital and Research Center, Jaipur, India
Hypertension in South Asians

David J. Hyman, MD, MPH
Professor of Medicine and Family and Community Medicine, Baylor College of Medicine; Chief, General Internal Medicine, Ben Taub General Hospital, Houston, Texas
Hypertension in Hispanics

Joseph L. Izzo, Jr., MD
Professor of Medicine, Pharmacology, and Toxicology, State University of New York at Buffalo School of Medicine and Biomedical Sciences; Vice Chair, Department of Medicine, Erie County Medical Center, Buffalo, New York
Assessment of Hypertensive Target Organ Damage

Panagiotis Kokkoris, MD
Endocrinologist, Department of Endocrinology, Diabetes, and Metabolism, Hellenic Air Force General Hospital, Athens, Greece
Obesity in Hypertension

John B. Kostis, MD
John G. Detwiler Professor of Cardiology, Professor of Medicine and Pharmacology, and Chairman, Department of Medicine, University of Medicine & Dentistry of New Jersey—Robert Wood Johnson Medical School; Chief of Medical Service, Robert Wood Johnson University Hospital, New Brunswick, New Jersey
Heart Failure in Hypertension

Jane Morley Kotchen, MD, MPH
Professor of Epidemiology, Medical College of Wisconsin, Milwaukee, Wisconsin
Defining Hypertension

Theodore A. Kotchen, MD
Professor of Medicine and Epidemiology and Associate Dean for Clinical Research, Medical College of Wisconsin, Milwaukee, Wisconsin
Defining Hypertension

John C. LaRosa, MD
President and Professor of Medicine, State University of New York Downstate Medical Center, Brooklyn, New York
Dyslipidemia in Hypertension

Daniel Levy, MD
Professor, Boston University School of Medicine, Boston; Director, National Heart, Lung, and Blood Institute's Framingham Heart Study, Framingham, Massachusetts
Epidemiology of Hypertension

Philip R. Liebson, MD, FACC, FAHA
McMullan-Eybel Chair of Excellence in Clinical Cardiology, Professor of Internal Medicine, and Professor of Preventive Medicine, Rush Medical College of Rush University; Senior Attending Physician, Rush University Medical Center, Chicago, Illinois
Assessment of Hypertensive Target Organ Damage

Donald M. Lloyd-Jones, MD, ScM
Assistant Professor of Preventive Medicine and Assistant Professor of Medicine (Cardiology), Northwestern University Feinberg School of Medicine; Associate in Medicine, Northwestern Medical Faculty Foundation, Northwestern Memorial Hospital, Chicago, Illinois
Epidemiology of Hypertension

Carolina Lombardi, MD, PhD
Assistant Professor, University of Milano-Bicocca; Head of Sleep Medicine Unit, San Luca Hospital, Milan, Italy
Secondary Hypertension: Sleep Apnea

Giuseppe Mancia, MD
Professor of Medicine, University of Milano-Bicocca, Milan; Head of Internal Medicine Division, Ospedale San Gerardo, Monza, Italy
Secondary Hypertension: Sleep Apnea; European, American, and British Guidelines: Similarities and Differences

Franz H. Messerli, MD
Director, Hypertension Program, St. Luke's-Roosevelt Hospital Center, New York, New York
Rare and Unusual Forms of Hypertension

Albert Mimram, MD
Professor and Head, Medicine and Hypertension Service, University of Montpelier; Medicine and Hypertension Service, Hôpital Lapeyronie, Montpelier, France
Assessment of Hypertensive Target Organ Damage

Marvin Moser, MD, FACP
Clinical Professor of Medicine, Yale University School of Medicine, New Haven, Connecticut
Diuretic Therapy in Cardiovascular Disease

Maryann N. Mugo, MD
Department of Internal Medicine, University of Missouri–Columbia School of Medicine, Columbia, Missouri
Hypertension and Diabetes Mellitus

Samar A. Nasser, PAC, MPH
Department of Internal Medicine, Wayne State University School of Medicine, Detroit Michigan
Hypertension in African Americans

Bruce Neal, MB ChB, PhD, MRCP
Associate Professor of Medicine, University of Sydney Faculty of Medicine; Senior Director, Research and Development, The George Institute for International Health; Honorary Consultant Epidemiologist, Royal Prince Alfred Hospital, Sydney, Australia
Meta-analyses of Hypertension Trials

James D. Neaton, PhD
Professor of Biostatistics, School of Public Health, University of Minnesota, Minneapolis, Minnesota
Design of Outcome Studies

Suzanne Oparil, MD
Professor of Medicine and Physiology and Biophysics, University of Alabama Birmingham, School of Medicine; Senior Scientist, Center for Aging, and Director, Vascular Biology and Hypertension Program, University of Alabama Birmingham, Birmingham, Alabama
Pathophysiology of Hypertension

Gianfranco Parati, MD
Professor of Medicine, Department of Clinical Medicine and Prevention, University of Milano-Bicocca; Head, II Cardiology Unit, San Luca Hospital, Milan, Italy
Secondary Hypertension: Sleep Apnea

Valory N. Pavlik, PhD
Associate Professor, Department of Family and Community Medicine, Baylor College of Medicine, Houston, Texas
Hypertension in Hispanics

Thomas G. Pickering, MD, DPhil
Professor of Medicine, Columbia University College of Physicians and Surgeons; Director, Behavioral Cardiovascular Health and Hypertension Program, Columbia Presbyterian Medical Center, New York, New York
Home Monitoring of Blood Pressure

Paul Pisarik, MD, MPH
Assistant Professor, Department of Family Medicine, University of Oklahoma College of Medicine, Tulsa, Oklahoma
Hypertension in Hispanics

F. Xavier Pi-Sunyer, MD, MPH
Professor of Medicine, Columbia University College of Physicians and Surgeons; Chief, Division of Endocrinology, Diabetes, and Nutrition, St. Luke's–Roosevelt Hospital, New York, New York
Obesity in Hypertension

Tiina Podymow, MD
Associate Professor, McGill University Faculty of Medicine; Division of Nephrology, Royal Victoria Hospital, Montreal, Quebec, Canada
Hypertension in Pregnancy

James L. Pool, MD
Professor of Medicine and Pharmacology and the James L. Pool Endowed Chair in Clinical Pharmacology, Baylor College of Medicine; Director, Hypertension-Clinical Pharmacology Research Clinic, Department of Medicine, Baylor College of Medicine, Houston, Texas
α-Blockers

Jason Ramos, MD
Department of Internal Medicine, Wayne State University School of Medicine, Detroit, Michigan
Hypertension in African Americans

Priya G. Rao, DO
Department of Internal Medicine, University of Missouri–Columbia School of Medicine, Columbia, Missouri
Hypertension and Diabetes Mellitus

Shakaib U. Rehman, MD
Associate Professor of Medicine, Medical University of South Carolina; Physician Manager, Primary Care, Ralph H. Johnson Veterans Affairs Medical Center, Charleston, South Carolina
Hypertensive Emergencies and Urgencies

James J. Reidy, MD
Professor of Ophthalmology and Director of the Cornea Service, State University of New York at Buffalo School of Medicine and Biomedical Sciences; Clinical Director, Department of Ophthalmology, Erie County Medical Center, Buffalo, New York
Assessment of Hypertensive Target Organ Damage

Clive Rosendorff, MD, PhD, DScMed
Professor of Medicine, Mount Sinai School of Medicine, New York; Physician, James J. Peters Veterans Affairs Medical Center, Bronx, New York
Ischemic Heart Disease in Hypertension

John F. Setaro, MD
Associate Professor of Medicine, Section on Cardiovascular Medicine, Yale University School of Medicine, New Haven, Connecticut
Resistant Hypertension

Tariq Shafi, MD
Assistant Professor, Clinical Internal Medicine, Wayne State University School of Medicine, Detroit, Michigan
Hypertension in African Americans

Alexander M. M. Shepherd, MD, PhD
Professor and Chief, Division of Clinical Pharmacology, University of Texas Health Science Center at San Antonio, San Antonio, Texas
New and Investigational Drugs for Hypertension

Domenic A. Sica, MD
Professor of Medicine, Medical College of Virginia at Virginia Commonwealth University; Chairman, Section of Clinical Pharmacology and Hypertension, Virginia Commonwealth University Health Systems, Richmond, Virginia
Diuretic Therapy in Cardiovascular Disease; Angiotensin-Converting Enzyme Inhibitors

James R. Sowers, MD, FACE, FACP, FAHA
Associate Dean for Clinical Research and Professor of Internal Medicine, Physiology, and Pharmacology, University of Missouri–Columbia School of Medicine, Columbia, Missouri
Hypertension and Diabetes Mellitus

Norman Stockbridge, MD, PhD
Director, Division of Cardiovascular and Renal Products, Center for Drug Evaluation and Research, Food and Drug Administration, Silver Spring, Maryland
Antihypertensive Drug Development: A Regulatory Perspective

Craig S. Stump, MD, PhD
Assistant Professor of Medicine, Division of Endocrinology, University of Missouri–Columbia School of Medicine; Research Scientist, Harry S Truman Memorial Veterans Hospital, Columbia, Missouri
Hypertension and Diabetes Mellitus

Sandra J. Taler, MD
Associate Professor of Medicine, Mayo Medical School; Consultant, Department of Internal Medicine, Division of Nephrology and Hypertension, Mayo Clinic College of Medicine, Rochester, Minnesota
Transplant Hypertension

Robert Temple, MD
Associate Director for Medical Policy, Center for Drug Evaluation and Research, Food and Drug Administration, Silver Spring, Maryland
Antihypertensive Drug Development: A Regulatory Perspective

Douglas C. Throckmorton, MD
Deputy Center Director, Center for Drug Evaluation and Research, Food and Drug Administration, Silver Spring, Maryland
Antihypertensive Drug Development: A Regulatory Perspective

Fiona Turnbull, MB ChB, FAFPHM
Senior Research Fellow, The George Institute for International Health; Sydney, Australia
Meta-analyses of Hypertension Trials

Carlos Vallbona, MD
Distinguished Service Professor, Department of Family and Community Medicine, Baylor College of Medicine; Chief of Staff, Community Health Program, Harris County Hospital District, Houston, Texas
Hypertension in Hispanics

Donald G. Vidt, MD
Consultant, Department of Hypertension and Nephrology, Cleveland Clinic Foundation, Cleveland, Ohio
Hypertensive Emergencies and Urgencies

William B. White, MD
Professor of Medicine, University of Connecticut School of Medicine; Chief, Division of Hypertension and Clinical Pharmacology, Calhoun Cardiology Center, and Medical Director, Clinical Trials Unit, University of Connecticut Health Center, Farmington, Connecticut
Ambulatory Blood Pressure Monitoring in Hypertension

Peter W. F. Wilson, MD
Professor of Medicine, Department of Endocrinology, Diabetes, and Medical Genetics, Medical University of South Carolina; Program Director, General Clinical Research Center, Charleston, South Carolina
Prediction of Global Cardiovascular Risk in Hypertension

Nathan D. Wong, PhD, MPH
Professor and Director, Heart Disease Prevention Program, University of California, Irvine, School of Medicine, Irvine, California
Hypertension in East Asians and Pacific Islanders

Xiaodong Wu, PhD
Assistant Professor, Department of Preventive Medicine and Epidemiology, Loyola University Chicago Stritch School of Medicine, Chicago, Illinois
Genetics of Hypertension

William F. Young, Jr., MD, MSc
Professor of Medicine, Mayo Clinic College of Medicine; Vice-Chair, Division of Endocrinology, Diabetes, Metabolism, and Nutrition, Mayo Clinic, Rochester, Minnesota
Secondary Hypertension: Pheochromocytoma

Alberto Zanchetti, MD
Emeritus Professor of Internal Medicine, University of Milan; Scientific Director, Instituto Auxologico Italiano, Milan, Italy
Calcium Channel Blockers in Hypertension

Foreword

Hypertension has been recognized as an important cardiovascular disorder since the dawn of the 20th century, when Riva-Rocci and then Korotkoff described the sphygmomanometric method of measuring arterial pressure. Although hypertension has been studied intensively since then, this is an extraordinary time for investigators, teachers, and clinicians in the field. It is a time when hypertension is spreading to the developing world and is reaching pandemic proportions. More inclusive definitions as well as more accurate and detailed measurements of blood pressure indicate that the prevalence of hypertension is even greater in the United States and Europe than had previously been thought. Also, the health threat of hypertension in the pathogenesis of coronary heart disease, heart failure, cerebrovascular disease, peripheral vascular disease, and renal failure probably exceeds what we appreciated in the past.

At the same time, this is a time of unprecedented opportunity to deal effectively with this serious health problem. Research carried out in the last 5 years is unraveling the pathogenesis and genetics of hypertension. Simultaneously, an enormous amount has been learned about the mechanisms of action and efficacy of the numerous classes of antihypertensive agents. For the first time, rigorous comparisons among these classes have been conducted. Revised practice guidelines that synthesize much useful information for clinical practice have become available.

The goal of the Companions to *Heart Disease: A Textbook of Cardiovascular Medicine* is to provide cardiologists and trainees in this field with important additional information in critically important segments of cardiology that go beyond what is contained in the "mother book," thereby creating an extensive cardiovascular information system. *Hypertension*, brilliantly edited by Drs. Henry R. Black and William J. Elliott and superbly written by distinguished leaders in the field, clearly accomplishes this goal. We are delighted to welcome this companion into the "family."

Eugene Braunwald
Douglas P. Zipes
Peter Libby
Robert O. Bonow

Preface

Hypertension is one of the most important public health problems worldwide, and its impact is expected to increase over the next 20 years as economically developing nations improve sanitation, infant mortality, and childhood immunization rates (among other measures).[1] The prevalence of hypertension in adults is expected to grow from 26.4% (in 2000) to 29.2% in 2025, with most of the growth from 972 million to the projected 1.56 billion affected people occurring outside of North America and Europe.[1] This global "epidemic" of high blood pressure is expected to shift the burden of disease so that heart disease will become the most common cause of death worldwide by the year 2025.[2]

In the United States, hypertension is the most important and most ubiquitous risk factor for heart disease and stroke, which were the number 1 and number 3 killers in preliminary data from the year 2004,[3] regardless of whether other risk factors are present.[4] Approximately 60 million Americans have hypertension, which includes those whose blood pressure is 140 mm Hg or higher systolic or 90 mm Hg diastolic and those who are taking antihypertensive medications; an additional 5 million persons have been told twice by a health care provider that their blood pressures were elevated and are counted as "hypertensive" in some surveys.[4,5] High blood pressure was given as a primary or contributing cause of death in about 11% of the death certificates filed in 2003[4] and ranked 13th among primary causes of death in preliminary data from 2004.[3] The importance of hypertension among the living can also be ascertained from the preliminary 2004 National Ambulatory Medical Care Survey, which indicated that hypertension was the most common diagnosis for a chronic disease among all outpatients: the ICD-9 code for hypertension (401) was listed in more than 42 million medical office visits.[6]

The major reason why hypertension is so important, however, is not because of the deaths or health care provider visits that are directly attributed to it. Hypertension is the most widespread risk factor for many other diseases and illnesses, each of which carries a high morbidity and mortality rate. Coronary heart disease, still the most common killer of American men and women, has many risk factors, but one can make a persuasive case that, on a nationwide population-attributable basis, hypertension is currently more important than smoking, diabetes, or dyslipidemia.[4] Some believe that one of the major reasons for the decline in deaths from both coronary heart disease and stroke during the past 30 years is the better and more effective treatment of hypertension.[7] Hypertension is the risk factor with the highest population-attributable risk for stroke in the United States.[8] Heart failure, the most common discharge diagnosis from short-stay, acute-care hospitals for Medicare beneficiaries across the United States, is preceded in about 85% of cases by hypertension.[9]

Chronic kidney disease, an independent risk factor for cardiovascular disease, too often results in end-stage renal disease (dialysis or kidney transplantation), which has the highest annualized per-patient cost of any program supported by the Centers for Medicare and Medicaid Services. Although diabetes has typically ranked first among sole "causes" of dialysis for about 20 years, hypertension has ranked second for about the same period of time, and, when more than one cause was allowed to be cited, hypertension was either the primary or a secondary cause of end-stage renal disease in 72% of those who began dialysis in 2003.[10] Hypertension ranks second (to diabetes) as a cause of peripheral vascular disease, the most common cause of lower limb amputations in 2003.[4] Although its relationship to hypertension is often forgotten, vascular dementia ranked eighth among the top 10 causes of death in the United States in 2004[3] and second (to Alzheimer's disease) as a cause for nursing home placement.

The two major reasons for the increased prevalence of hypertension in the United States are aging and increasing weight of the population. These disproportionately affect the two ends of the age spectrum. The fastest-growing segment of the U.S. population is the "old old," that is, those aged 85 years and older.[11] The prevalence of hypertension in these individuals is thought to be more than 95%, because data from the Framingham Heart Study put the lifetime risk of hypertension (beginning at either age 55 or 65 years) at more than 90%.[12] The current nationwide epidemic of obesity and physical inactivity, particularly among children and adolescents, makes it likely that hypertension will become even more prevalent as these overweight individuals grow into adulthood.[13]

The estimated cost of hypertension and its treatment ($63.5 billion) in the United States in 2006 is but a small part of the total cost of cardiovascular disease ($403.1 billion).[4] The National Committee for Quality Assurance estimates that in 2005, if blood pressures had been better controlled, many cardiovascular events would have been prevented or delayed, between 12,000 and 32,000 deaths would have been avoided, and $328 million to $1 billion would have been saved.[14] Both direct costs of hospitalization ($6.2 billion) and nursing home care ($3.9 billion), as well as the indirect costs ($16 billion, consisting primarily of lost productivity, disability payments, and death benefits) would be considerably reduced. The major driver of the increased cost of hypertension in the United States over the last 15 years has been the cost of antihypertensive drugs, which has risen at more than seven times the inflation rate. The rate of rise will probably decrease somewhat in the near future, as most of the commonly used antihypertensive drugs will become available in generic formulations. The economics of hypertension and its treatment vary widely across nations, in part because some countries have national formularies that restrict access to expensive drugs. In some countries, even inexpensive generic formulations of antihypertensive drugs are beyond the means of many patients, which is one of the challenges in controlling hypertension worldwide.[2]

In this book, we have attempted to gather chapters that cover the most important topics in hypertension, written by world authorities in each case. We have attempted not to avoid some of the current controversies in hypertension but to allow each author to present his or her point of view, with an eye toward a balanced and objective result.

The discerning reader will recognize that several of the "hot topics" in hypertension are mentioned but not dealt with in detail, for reasons of space and because these controversies can be more effectively presented in other arenas, including the very recent medical literature. For example, the growing awareness of the necessity of assessing global risk in a hypertensive patient before embarking on treatment has been skillfully promoted[15] and adopted in most of Europe[16] but not accepted in practice in the most recent U.S. guidelines.[17] Similarly, JNC 7 recommends an initial thiazide-type diuretic for "most" patients with stage 1 hypertension and no compelling indication for a different class of drug[17]; the recent British National Institute for Health and Clinical Excellence (NICE) guidelines instead recommend either an ACE inhibitor (for young white patients) or a calcium antagonist (for black or older patients).[18] The NICE guidelines recommend a β-blocker only for fourth-line treatment of hypertension, based on their economic analyses and a recent meta-analysis[19]; the low opinion of this class of drug is shared by neither JNC 7 nor the author of this book's chapter on β-blockers. The debate about the clinical importance of incident diabetes during drug treatment of hypertension has intensified since these chapters were written,[20,21] but a brief review and salient references can be found in the appropriate chapters in this book. Whether certain classes of antihypertensive drugs have "benefits beyond blood pressure control" is still debated,[22-24] but some aspects of this controversy can be found in the chapters found within these covers.

We have attempted to edit the submitted chapters to make them as balanced, fair, and objective as possible, while trying to retain some of the opinion and flavor of the authors' points of view. We recognize, however, that errors may have crept into the text, but we hope the reader will understand that these were inadvertent and unintentional. Similarly, in a book of this scope and magnitude, there will, of necessity, be omissions of important references and shortened summaries of some individuals' opinions. We regret that it was not possible to make this book as all-encompassing as everyone would wish. The decisions to omit some aspects of hypertension-related data were those of the authors and editors, and we take full responsibility for these.

We have attempted to organize the book along classical lines. Section 1 deals with the epidemiology and pathophysiology of hypertension. Section 2 is concerned with diagnosis (including secondary hypertension) and is much longer than an analogous book would have been some 20 years ago because of the emerging data about ambulatory and home blood pressure monitoring. Risk stratification is the major theme of Section 3, whereas the usual treatment options (both lifestyle modifications and drugs) are presented in Section 4. Outcome studies are discussed, both in design and in meta-analysis, in Section 5. The various concomitant diseases that are often seen in hypertensive patients are summarized in Section 6. Hypertension has many "special populations and special situations" that are discussed in Section 7. The future of hypertension treatment is considered in Section 8, and the book ends with a discussion of hypertension guidelines (from several different points of view) in Section 9.

William J. Elliott, MD, PhD
Henry R. Black, MD

References

1. Kearney PM, Whelton M, Reynolds K, et al. Global burden of hypertension: Analysis of worldwide data. *Lancet.* 2005;**365**: 217-223.
2. Ezzati M, Lopez AD, Rodgers A, et al. Selected major risk factors and global and regional burden of disease. *Lancet.* 2002;**360**:1347-1360.
3. Miniño AM, Heron M, Smith BL. Deaths: Preliminary data for 2004. National Center for Health Statistics, Centers for Disease Control and Prevention, 2006. Found on the Internet at http://www.cdc.gov/nchs/products/pubs/pugd/hestats.prelimdeaths04/preliminarydeaths04.htm, accessed 25 JUN 06.
4. Thom T, Haase N, Rosamond W, et al. Heart disease and stroke statistics—2006 update: A report from the American Heart Association Statistics Committee and Stroke Statistics Subcommittee. *Circulation.* 2006;**113**:85-151.
5. Fields LE, Burt VL, Cutler JA, et al. The burden of adult hypertension in the United States 1999 to 2000: A rising tide. *Hypertension.* 2004;**44**:398-404.
6. Burt CW, McCaig LF, Rechtsteiner EA. Ambulatory medical care utilization estimates for 2004. National Center for Health Statistics, Centers for Disease Control and Prevention, 2006. Found on the Internet at: http://www.cdc.gov/nchs/products/pubs/pubd/hestats/estimates2004/estimates04.htm, accessed 25 JUN 06.
7. Braunwald E. Shattuck Lecture: Cardiovascular medicine at the turn of the millennium: Triumphs, concerns and opportunities. *N Engl J Med.* 1997;**337**:1360-1369.
8. Gorelick PB, Sacco RL, Smith DB, et al. Prevention of a first stroke: A review of guidelines and a multidisciplinary consensus statement from the National Stroke Association. *JAMA.* 1999; **281**:1112-1120.
9. Levy D, Larson MG, Vasan RS, et al. The progression from hypertension to congestive heart failure. *JAMA.* 1996;**275**: 1557-1562.
10. United States Renal Data System. 2003 Annual Report. Figure 2.9. Found on the Internet at: http://www.usrds.org/slides.htm. Accessed 25 JUN 06.
11. Meyer J. Age: 2000 (A Census 2000 Brief; C2KBR/01-12). US Department of Commerce: Economics and Statistics Administration: US Census Bureau, October, 2001. Found on the Internet at: http://www.census.gov/prod/2001pubs/c2kbr01-12.pdf. Accessed 15 JUN 06.
12. Vasan RS, Beiser A, Seshadri S, et al. Residual lifetime risk for developing hypertension in middle-aged women and men: The Framingham Heart Study. *JAMA.* 2002;**287**:1003-1010.
13. Ogden CL, Carroll MD, Curtin LR, et al. Prevalence of overweight and obesity in the United States, 1999-2004. *JAMA.* 2006;**295**:1549-1555.
14. National Committee for Quality Assurance. The State of Health Care Quality, 2005. Washington, DC, 2005, p. 12. Found on the Internet at www.ncqa.org/Docs/SOHCQ_2005.pdf. Accessed 25 JUN 06.
15. Jackson R, Lawes CMM, Bennett DA, et al. Treatment with drugs to lower blood pressure and blood cholesterol based on

an individual's absolute cardiovascular risk. *Lancet.* 2005;**365**: 434-441.

16. 2003 European Society of Hypertension—European Cardiology guidelines for the management of arterial hypertension. Guidelines Committee. *J Hypertension.* 2003;**21**:1011-1053.

17. Chobanian AV, Bakris GL, Black HR, et al., and the National High Blood Pressure Education Program Coordinating Committee. The Seventh Report of the Joint National Committee on Prevention, Detection, Evaluation, and Treatment of High Blood Pressure. The JNC 7 Report. *JAMA.* 2003;**289**:2560-2572.

18. National Collaborating Centre for Chronic Conditions. Hypertension: Management of hypertension in adults in primary care: partial update. London, UK: Royal College of Physicians, 2006. Found on the Internet at http://www.nice.org.uk/page.aspx?o=CG034fullguideline. Accessed 30 JUN 06.

19. Lindholm LH, Carlberg B, Samuelsson O. Should beta blockers remain first choice in the treatment of primary hypertension? A meta-analysis. *Lancet.* 2005;**366**:1545-1553.

20. Verdecchia P, Reboldi G, Angeli F, et al. Adverse prognostic significance of new diabetes in treated hypertensive subjects. *Hypertension.* 2004;**43**:963-969.

21. Kostis JB, Wilson AC, Freudenberger RS, et al. Long-term effect of diuretic-based therapy on fatal outcomes in subjects with isolated systolic hypertension with and without diabetes. *Am J Cardiol.* 2005;**95**:29-35.

22. Verdecchia P, Reboldi G, Angeli F, et al. Angiotensin-converting enzyme inhibitors and calcium channel blockers for coronary heart disease and stroke prevention. *Hypertension.* 2005;**46**: 386-392.

23. Elliott WJ, Jonsson MC, Black HR. It's NOT "Beyond the Blood Pressure," It IS the Blood Pressure. *Circulation.* 2006;**113**: 2763-2772; Response to Sever and Poulter: *Circulation.* 2006; **113**: 2773-2774.

24. Sever PS, Poulter NR. Management of hypertension: Is it the pressure or the drug? *Circulation.* 2006;**113**:2754-2763; Response to Elliott et al. *Circulation*, 2006;**113**:2773.

Acknowledgments

As with all books of this magnitude and scope, thanks are required to all chapter authors and to many others as well. Drs. Braunwald, Bonow, Libby, and Zipes allowed us to put together a volume on hypertension that we hope is worthy of being in the same bookcase as *Braunwald's Heart Disease*, for which they serve as editors. Their confidence in us to organize and compile this text was rewarding. The editors at Elsevier's Saunders branch, including Anne Lenehan, Susan Pioli, Agnes Byrne, Vera Ginsburgs, Natasha Andjelkovic, PhD, Jerisha C. Parker, Nicole Mercurio, Kimberly Hamm, Lee Ann Draud, and their several colleagues deserve credit for allowing us to proceed with manuscript preparation at a pace that was probably somewhat too slow for them. Lastly, Norma Sandoval's expert organizational skills during the process of inviting chapter authors, keeping them apprised of our progress toward our mutual goal, and collating all the manuscripts (up to the final version), were most appreciated.

William J. Elliott, MD, PhD
Henry R. Black, MD

Contents

Epidemiology and Pathophysiology

SECTION CONTENTS

Chapter 1

Epidemiology of Hypertension

Donald M. Lloyd-Jones and Daniel Levy

Systemic arterial hypertension is the condition of persistent, nonphysiologic elevation of systemic blood pressure (BP). It is currently defined as a resting systolic BP (SBP) 140 mm Hg or greater, or diastolic BP (DBP) 90 mm Hg or greater, or a condition for which a patient is receiving therapy for the indication of BP lowering.[1,2] Hypertension afflicts a substantial proportion of the adult population worldwide and a growing number of children. Numerous genetic, environmental, and behavioral factors have been shown to influence the development of hypertension. In turn, hypertension has been identified as one of the major causal risk factors for the development of cardiovascular disease (CVD) and renal disease. An understanding of the basic epidemiology of hypertension is essential for effective public health and clinical efforts to detect, treat, and control this common condition.

EPIDEMIOLOGY AND RISK FACTORS

An epidemiologic association between a proposed risk factor and a disease is likely to be causal if it fulfills the following criteria: (1) exposure to the proposed risk factor precedes the onset of disease, (2) a strong association exists between exposure and incidence of disease, (3) the association is dose dependent, (4) exposure is consistently predictive of disease in a variety of populations, (5) the association is independent of other risk factors, and (6) the association is biologically and pathogenetically plausible and is supported by animal experiments and clinical investigation.[3] Further, more definitive support for a causal association between a proposed risk factor and a disease may arise from clinical trials in which intervention to modify or abolish the risk factor (by behavioral or therapeutic interventions) is associated with a decreased incidence of the disease. As discussed later, hypertension fulfills all these criteria and represents an important target for intervention in reducing the population and individual burden of CVD and renal disease.

Several different measures are used to describe the influence of a risk factor on a disease. *Prevalence* describes the proportion of a population or group that is affected with a trait or disease at any one time and thus represents a cross-sectional measure of exposure. *Incidence* is a measure of the rate of new cases in a population or group within a defined time period. Thus, the prevalence is a function of both the incidence of disease as well as the rate at which people with the disease die or recover. In the case of hypertension, most individuals who are diagnosed with hypertension have it for the remainder of their lives.

The *relative risk* of disease is often reported in epidemiologic studies of risk factors and is defined as the ratio of disease incidence among exposed compared with nonexposed individuals. As such, relative risk measures the strength of the association between exposure and disease, but it gives no indication of the *absolute risk* of disease. Absolute risk of disease associated with a given exposure is often expressed as the rate of development of new cases of disease per unit of time (or incidence) in exposed individuals. This proportion may be compared with the proportion among unexposed subjects in a variety of ways. The *attributable risk* of a given exposure describes the proportion of the incidence of disease in a population that can be ascribed to the exposure, assuming a causal relationship exists. Attributable risk may be calculated by subtracting the incidence in unexposed individuals from the incidence in exposed individuals. However, this does not take into account the coexisting risks from other risk factors. The *population attributable risk percent* takes into account the proportion of individuals in the population who are exposed as well as the relative risk and the influence of other risk factors. Therefore, attributable risk is a useful concept in determining the public health impact of a given risk factor and in selecting risk factors that should be targeted for prevention programs.[4]

Prevalence and Secular Trends

Data from the most recent U.S. National Health and Nutrition Examination Survey (NHANES), conducted from 1999 to 2002, indicate that the prevalence of hypertension in the United States was 28.6%,[5] or more than one in four adults older than 20 years of age. In the context of the entire population, more than 65 million U.S. adults are estimated to have hypertension.[2] This number represents a substantial increase in the prevalence compared with 1988 to 1994, when there were an estimated 50 million hypertensive individuals, or 24.5% of adults.[2]

Despite the significant advances in our understanding of the risk factors, pathogenesis, and sequelae of hypertension, and multiple trials since the 1970s indicating the benefits of antihypertensive therapy, hypertension remains a significant public health problem. Although steady and significant reductions occurred from the 1970s to the early 1990s in population levels of BP and in the prevalence of hypertension in the United States,[6,7] as well as in many of the sequelae of hypertension,[8] more recent data indicate a slowing or reversal of these favorable trends. Between the late 1970s and the early 1990s, the prevalence of hypertension in the United States declined from about 32% to 25%. However, the most recent survey data indicate an increase between 1988 to 1994 and 1999 to 2002, with the current prevalence being 28.6%.[5] This proportion increases even further if one adds the people who have been told on two or more occasions by a health care provider that their BP is elevated.[2] The current pandemic of obesity and the aging of the population are likely to increase hypertension incidence and prevalence substantially over the next decades.

Table 1-1 Trends in Prevalence, Awareness, Treatment, and Control of Hypertension in the United States, from the National Health and Nutrition Examination Surveys (NHANES)

	NHANES II 1976-1980	NHANES III 1988-1991	NHANES III 1991-1994	NHANES 1999-2000
Prevalence	31.8%	25.0%	24.5%	28.7%
Awareness	51%	73%	68%	69%
Treatment	31%	55%	54%	58%
Control to <140/<90 mm Hg	10%	29%	27%	31%

African Americans, and especially African American women, have a prevalence of hypertension that is among the highest in the world. Currently, it is estimated that 38.8% of African American adults have hypertension, compared with 27.2% of non-Hispanic whites and 28.7% of Mexican Americans.[2] Asian Americans and most other ethnic groups tend to have BP levels and hypertension prevalence similar to those in whites. The prevalence of hypertension increased to a similar extent in all ethnicities during the decade of the 1990s.[7]

Substantial improvements have been made in awareness, treatment, and control of hypertension since the 1970s, but the number of hypertensive individuals who are aware of their hypertension, who are receiving treatment, or whose hypertension is treated and controlled remains far below optimal levels (Table 1-1). Data from NHANES 1999 to 2000 indicate that 68.9% of hypertensive individuals were aware of their elevated BP, and 58.4% were receiving antihypertensive therapy, but only 31.0% had controlled BP levels of <140/<90 mm Hg.[7] Extrapolating these data to the current estimate of 65 million Americans with hypertension,[2] nearly 43 million hypertensive individuals are unaware of their diagnosis or have hypertension that is untreated or treated but uncontrolled (Fig. 1-1). As

noted later, data from Europe, where clinical practice guidelines have typically recommended higher BP thresholds before initiation of drug therapy, suggest even lower rates of treatment and control of BP.[9]

Rates of awareness, treatment, and control of BP differ by age, gender, and race/ethnicity. Overall, awareness of elevated BP has not changed significantly since the early 1990s; women are slightly more likely to be aware of the problem, and Mexican Americans are the least likely to be aware of their hypertension. Women are somewhat more likely than men to receive antihypertensive drug therapy (Table 1-2). Compared with non-Hispanic whites, non-Hispanic blacks have similar overall levels of treatment, whereas Mexican Americans have substantially lower levels of treatment. Likewise, Mexican Americans have the lowest prevalence of control to BPs <140/<90 mm Hg; in only 17.3% of hypertensive Mexican-American men is BP controlled to these levels.[5]

Global Burden of Hypertension

International data indicate that hypertension is even more prevalent in countries other than the United States, including developed countries. Whereas the prevalence of hypertension in adults aged 35 to 74 years in Canada in the 1990s was similar to that of the United States (at ~28%), concurrent data from six European countries revealed an overall prevalence of 44%. Of the European countries studied, Italy had the lowest prevalence (38%), whereas Germany had the highest (55%).[10]

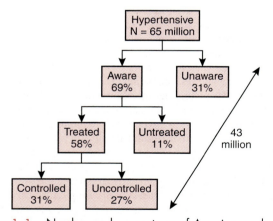

Figure 1–1   Number and percentage of Americans who are aware of their hypertension, treated, and controlled to goal levels from the National Health and Nutrition Examination Survey, 1999 to 2000. (Data from Fields LE, Burt VL, Cutler JA, et al. The burden of adult hypertension in the United States 1999 to 2000: A rising tide. *Hypertension.* 2004;**44**:398-404; Hajjar I, Kotchen TA. Trends in prevalence, awareness, treatment, and control of hypertension in the United States, 1988-2000. *JAMA.* 2003;**290**:199-206.)

Table 1-2 Awareness, Treatment, and Control of Hypertension in the United States, 1999 to 2000, by Sex and Race/Ethnicity

	Awareness	Treatment	Control to <140/<90 mm Hg
Men	66.3%	54.3%	32.6%
Women	71.2%	62.0%†	29.6%
Non-Hispanic white	69.5%	60.1%	33.4%
Non-Hispanic black	73.9%	63.0%	28.1%
Mexican American	57.8%*	40.3%‡	17.7%‡

*P < .01 compared with non-Hispanic whites.
†P < .05 compared with men.
‡P < .001 compared with non-Hispanic whites.
Data from Hajjar I, Kotchen TA. Trends in prevalence, awareness, treatment, and control of hypertension in the United States, 1988-2000. *JAMA.* 2003;**290**:199-206.

The increase in BP and in prevalence of hypertension with age was steeper in European countries than in the United States and Canada. The correlation between hypertension prevalence and stroke mortality rates was very strong ($r = 0.78$), with a stroke mortality rate of 27.6 per 100,000 in North America and 41.2 per 100,000 in European countries.[10] Furthermore, treatment rates in Europe in the 1990s were substantially lower, in association with higher BP thresholds for treatment in clinical practice guidelines promulgated in Europe and Canada. Among 35- to 64-year-old hypertensive patients, more than half (53%) were treated in the United States, compared with 36% in Canada and 25% to 32% in European countries. The associated differences in levels of BP control were dramatic; 66% of U.S., 49% of Canadian, and 23% to 38% of European hypertensive patients had BP controlled to levels of <160/<95 mm Hg, and 29%, 17%, and 10% or fewer, respectively, had BP controlled to levels of <140/<90 mm Hg.[9]

Mean SBP levels are in the 120s in North America and much of South America. In contrast, mean SBP levels are in the 130s or higher in parts of South America, in China and Russia, and in much of Europe.[11] Although these differences may seem small, they represent mean values from millions of individuals. Population SBP differences as little as 1 to 2 mm Hg can have profound differences in rates of stroke and heart attack. Few data are available regarding BP levels and prevalence of hypertension in Africa. BP levels in South Asian populations are lower, but they appear to be rising rapidly.[11]

A comparison of national surveillance data from around the world sheds interesting light on the global burden of hypertension. Kearney and associates found that the average age-standardized prevalence of hypertension was 30% or higher in countries with established market economies or former socialist economies, as well as in Latin American and the Caribbean.[12] In China, India, the Middle Eastern crescent, and sub-Saharan Africa, average prevalences were between 20% and 30%. The lowest average prevalences (<20%) were observed in other Asian and Asian island populations. Germany had the highest prevalence of any country studied, at approximately 55% for men and women. Similar age-related patterns of increasing hypertension prevalence in men and women were observed in all regional groupings.[12]

RISK FACTORS FOR HYPERTENSION

Hypertension is a complex phenotype with multiple genetic and environmental risk factors, as well as important gene-environment interactions. Age, with the concomitant changes in the vascular bed, and demographic and socioeconomic variables are among the strongest risk factors for hypertension.

Age

The prevalence of hypertension increases sharply with advancing age: whereas only 9.3% of men and 2.1% of women ages 18 to 34 years are affected, 68.1% of men and 84.0% of women age 75 and older have hypertension (Fig. 1-2). Thus, in older patients, hypertension is by far the most prevalent risk factor for CVD. About 81% of hypertensive individuals in the United States are age 45 years and older, although this group comprises only 46% of the U.S. population.[2] With the

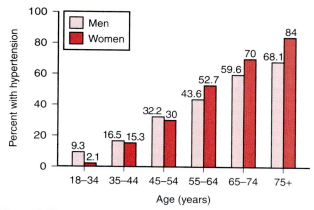

Figure 1–2 Prevalence of hypertension among men and women aged 18 years and over, from the National Health and Nutrition Examination Survey, 1999 to 2000. (Data from Fields LE, Burt VL, Cutler JA, et al. The burden of adult hypertension in the United States 1999 to 2000: A rising tide. *Hypertension.* 2004;**44**:398-404.)

aging of the population, the overall prevalence of hypertension in the population is sure to increase.

Viewed from another perspective, hypertension already affects more individuals during their life span than any other trait or disease studied to date. The concept of the *lifetime risk* of a given disease provides a useful measure of the absolute burden and the public health impact of a disease, as well as providing an average risk for an individual during his or her lifetime. Lifetime risk estimates account for the risk of developing disease during the remaining life span and the competing risk of death from other causes before developing the disease of interest. Data from the Framingham Heart Study, a long-standing study of CVD epidemiology, indicate that, for men and women free of hypertension at age 55 years, the remaining lifetime risks for development of hypertension through age 80 years are 93% and 91%, respectively. In other words, more than 9 out of 10 older adults will develop hypertension before they die. Even those who reach age 65 years free of hypertension still have a remaining lifetime risk of 90%.[13]

In Western societies, SBP tends to rise monotonically and inexorably with advancing age. Conversely, DBP levels rise until about age 50 to 55 years, after which a plateau is noted for several years, followed by a steady decline to the end of the usual life span.[10,14,15] Various factors, particularly related to changes in arterial compliance and stiffness,[16,17] contribute to the development of systolic hypertension and to decreasing DBP with age. Both these phenomena contribute to a marked increase in pulse pressure (defined as SBP minus DBP) after age 50 years. Thus, hypertension, and particularly systolic hypertension, is a nearly universal condition of aging, and few individuals escape its development. Only in societies where salt intake is low, physical activity levels are very high, and obesity is rare are age-related increases in SBP avoided.

Weight

Increasing weight is one of the major determinants of increasing BP. The current prevalence of hypertension among obese individuals, with a body mass index (BMI) greater than or equal to 30 kg/m^2, is 42.5%, compared with 27.8% for overweight individuals (25.0 to 29.9 kg/m^2), and 15.3% for individuals with a BMI lower than 25 kg/m^2.[18] Data from the Framingham Heart Study also reveal marked increases in the risk for development of hypertension with increasing BMI. Compared with adult men and women of normal weight, the multivariable-adjusted relative risks for development of hypertension in long-term follow-up were 1.48 and 1.70 for overweight men and women and 2.23 and 2.63 for obese men and women, respectively.[19]

Numerous studies have also demonstrated the important role of weight gain in BP elevation and weight reduction in BP lowering. As discussed earlier, SBP and DBP tend to rise with age beginning at around age 25 years in most adults.[14,15] However, more recent data indicate that these "age-related" increases in SBP and DBP may be avoided in young adults who maintain a stable BMI over long-term follow-up. In the Coronary Artery Risk Development in Young Adults (CARDIA) study, those who maintained a stable BMI at all six examinations over 15 years had no significant changes in SBP or DBP, whereas those who had an increase in their BMI of 2 kg/m^2 or more had substantial increases in BP.[20]

The influence of weight gain on BP and the benefits of maintaining stable weight or losing weight extend even to young children. One large birth cohort study of children examined BMI at ages 5 and 14 years and the association with SBP and DBP at age 14 years. Children who were overweight at age 5 years but who had a normal BMI at age 14 years had mean SBP and DBP similar to those children who had a normal BMI at both time points. Conversely, children who were overweight at both ages or who had a normal BMI at age 5 years and were overweight at age 14 years had higher SBP and DBP at age 14 years than those who had a normal BMI at both ages, even after adjustment for potential confounders.[21]

Other Risk Factors

As discussed earlier, gender influences the prevalence of hypertension in an age-dependent fashion. Until about the sixth decade of life, men have a higher prevalence, after which women predominate increasingly (see Fig. 1-2). Overall, more women than men are affected by hypertension, in part because of their longer life expectancy.

Race/ethnicity has also been shown to be a risk factor for hypertension. Whereas non-Hispanic white persons make up about two thirds of the U.S. adult hypertensive population, this proportion is consistent with their representation in the overall population. African Americans are disproportionately affected and have among the highest rates of hypertension in the world, with mean SBP levels approximately 5 mm Hg higher than in whites. Other race/ethnic groups in the United States, including Mexican Americans, have prevalences of hypertension that are similar to those in whites.[2,14] Education status also affects rates of hypertension; lower education levels are strongly associated with hypertension. However, much of this inverse association of education with BP appears to be explained by differences in diet and in BMI between less well educated and better educated individuals.[22]

Among dietary influences on BP level, high dietary sodium intake has consistently been related to rates of hypertension in numerous epidemiologic cohorts. Conversely, higher potassium, calcium, and magnesium intakes appear to be associated with lower rates of hypertension in various populations.[23] Patients with omnivorous diets have higher BP levels than those who are vegetarian, but the types of dietary fat do not appear to influence BP levels directly (with the possible exception of mild lowering by ω-3 fatty acids). The evidence linking heavy alcohol intake to hypertension is unequivocal. More than 50 epidemiologic studies have demonstrated an association between intake of three drinks or more per day and hypertension, although regular alcohol intake is associated with a lower risk of atherothrombotic CVD events.

Numerous studies have examined potential genetic susceptibilities for hypertension. Data consistently indicate that BP levels are heritable. Similarly, rare inherited genetic syndromes are associated with hypertension, including Liddle's syndrome and 11β-hydroxylase and 17α-hydroxylase deficiencies. Numerous large cohort genomic studies have indicated the presence of loci in discrete chromosomal regions that are linked to BP. In addition, genetic association studies have identified polymorphisms in biologically plausible candidate genes, including angiotensinogen, angiotensin-converting enzyme, α-adducin, and β-adrenergic and other receptors. However, because hypertension is a complex phenotype, and BP levels are determined by the interactions of multiple neurologic, renal, endocrinologic, cardiac, and vascular processes, no single-gene polymorphisms have been discovered that explain more than a small fraction of cases of hypertension alone or jointly in the population at large.

CLASSIFICATION OF BLOOD PRESSURE

Formal classification of BP stages by consensus panels began to take shape in the early 1970s with the first National Conference on High Blood Pressure Education. The first report of the Joint National Committee on Detection, Evaluation, and Treatment of High Blood Pressure (JNC) was published in 1977 and was followed by six subsequent reports in 1980, 1984, 1988, 1993, 1997, and 2003. The most recent report (JNC 7)[1,24] is the current clinical standard for the prevention, detection, evaluation, and treatment of hypertension in the United States. JNC 7 recognizes several important concepts that have evolved in our understanding of hypertension over the past decades. First, systolic hypertension confers at least as much risk for adverse events as diastolic hypertension, a factor that was not fully appreciated in the first four JNC reports. Thus, the JNC report recommends that for middle-aged and older hypertensive patients (who represent most hypertensive patients in the population), SBP should be the primary target for staging of BP and initiation of therapy. Second, hypertension rarely occurs in isolation and is usually present in the context of one or more other CVD risk factors. Therefore, in recommending treatment for hypertension, the JNC report recommends some consideration of global risk for CVD.

It has long been recognized that BP confers risk for CVD beginning at levels well within the clinically "normal" range, with risk increasing in a continuous, graded fashion to the highest levels, as discussed in detail later. Thus, although clinical practice guidelines impose certain thresholds for considering individuals to be hypertensive, and for initiation of therapy, this conception is an artificial construct designed to assist clinicians and patients with treatment decisions.

Table 1-3 Blood Pressure Staging System of the Seventh Report of the Joint National Committee on Prevention, Detection, Evaluation, and Treatment of High Blood Pressure (JNC 7)

JNC 7 Blood Pressure Stage	Blood Pressure Range
Normal	SBP <120 and DBP <80 mm Hg
Prehypertension	SBP 120-139 or DBP 80-89 mm Hg
Stage 1 hypertension	SBP 140-159 or DBP 90-99 mm Hg
Stage 2 hypertension	SBP ≥160 or DBP ≥100 mm Hg

DBP, diastolic blood pressure; SBP, systolic blood pressure. From Chobanian AV, Bakris GL, Black HR, et al. Seventh report of the Joint National Committee on Prevention, Detection, Evaluation, and Treatment of High Blood Pressure. *Hypertension.* 2003;**42**:1206-1252.

The current JNC 7 scheme for classifying BP stages is shown in Table 1-3. From JNC VI to JNC 7, the committee elected to change the terminology for BP levels lower than the hypertensive range. Whereas BP <120/<80 mm Hg had previously been termed "optimal," it is now termed "normal." A new category of "prehypertension" was defined, including individuals with SBP of 120 to 139 or DBP of 80 to 89 mm Hg. In addition, the earlier classification of stage 3 hypertension was dropped because of its relatively uncommon occurrence, and all individuals with SBP of 160 or higher or DBP of 100 mm Hg or higher are now classified as having stage 2 hypertension.[1]

Individuals are classified into BP stages on the basis of both SBP and DBP levels. When a disparity exists between SBP and DBP stages, patients are classified into the higher stage. Several studies[25-27] have examined this phenomenon of "upstaging" based on disparate SBP and DBP levels. In one study,[25] 3656 Framingham Heart Study participants who were not receiving therapy for hypertension were examined between 1990 and 1995, and their JNC-VI BP stages were classified on the basis of SBP alone, DBP alone, or both. In this sample, 64.6% of subjects had congruent stages of SBP and DBP, 31.6% were upstaged on the basis of SBP, and 3.8% were upstaged on the basis of DBP. Thus, among all participants, 96% were correctly classified by knowledge of their SBP alone, whereas only 68% were correctly classified by knowledge of the DBP alone. In subjects younger than 60 years of age, the numbers were 95% for SBP alone and 81% for DBP alone; in those who were more than 60 years old, they were 99% for SBP alone and 47% for DBP alone. Of 1488 subjects with high-normal BP or hypertension, who would meet criteria for recommended drug therapy, 13.0% had congruent elevations of SBP and DBP, 77.7% were upstaged on the basis of SBP, and 9.3% were upstaged on the basis of DBP; SBP alone correctly classified 91%, whereas DBP alone correctly classified only 22%. Thus, SBP elevation out of proportion to DBP is common in middle-aged and older persons, and SBP appears to play a greater role in the determination of BP stage and eligibility for therapy.[25] Similar results were also observed in data from the NHANES III sample.[27] Among younger individuals, upstaging based on DBP is somewhat more common. However, after the age of 50 years, a group that includes most hypertensive patients, upstaging based on SBP clearly occurs for an overwhelming proportion of the population and determines hypertensive status and eligibility for therapy.[27]

Isolated systolic hypertension in older people reflects progressive large artery stiffening seen with aging. In younger hypertensive patients, isolated diastolic hypertension (SBP <140 and DBP ≥90 mm Hg) and systolic-diastolic hypertension (SBP ≥140 and DBP ≥90 mm Hg) tend to predominate, whereas beyond age 50 years, isolated systolic hypertension (SBP ≥140 and DBP <90 mm Hg) predominates. Isolated systolic hypertension is the most common form of hypertension in persons older than 60 years, and it is present in more than 80% of untreated hypertensive men and women.[27]

These observations, coupled with data on the risks of systolic hypertension and the benefits of treating systolic hypertension, prompted the National High Blood Pressure Education Program's Advisory Panel to recommend a major paradigm shift in 2000 by urging that SBP become the major criterion for the diagnosis, staging, and therapeutic management of hypertension, particularly in middle-aged and older Americans.[17] This recommendation was incorporated into the staging system and treatment guidelines for JNC 7.[1,24]

SEQUELAE AND OUTCOMES WITH HYPERTENSION

Hypertension is a major risk factor for all forms of atherosclerotic and atherothrombotic CVD. Increasing BP level generally increases risk in a continuous and graded fashion for total mortality, CVD mortality, coronary heart disease (CHD) mortality, myocardial infarction (MI), heart failure (HF), left ventricular hypertrophy, atrial fibrillation, stroke or transient ischemic attack, peripheral vascular disease, and renal failure. Many of these endpoints have an effect modification by gender, with male hypertensive patients at higher risk for CVD events than female hypertensive patients (HF being a notable exception). There is also substantial effect modification by age; older hypertensive patients have a similar or higher relative risk but a much greater absolute risk than younger patients.[28] As discussed later, hypertension rarely occurs in isolation, and it confers a greater risk for CVD across the spectrum of overall risk factor burden, but with increasing importance in the setting of other risk factors.[29] As shown in Figure 1-3, absolute levels of risk for CHD are substantially elevated with increasing risk factor burden and are augmented still further by elevated BP. Thus, BP levels, and the risk they confer, must always be considered in the context of other risk factors and the patient's global risk for CVD. For example, because the combination of hypertension and diabetes is particularly dangerous, JNC 7 recommends lower goal BP levels for patients with diabetes (<130/<80 mm Hg) than for those without diabetes (<140/<90 mm Hg).[1]

Individuals with hypertension have a two- to threefold increased relative risk for CVD events compared with age-matched normotensive persons. Hypertension increases relative risks for all manifestations of CVD, but its *relative* impact is greatest for stroke and HF (Fig. 1-4). Because CHD incidence is greater than the incidence of stroke and HF, however, the *absolute* impact of hypertension on CHD is greater than for other manifestations of CVD, as demonstrated by the excess risks shown in Figure 1-4.

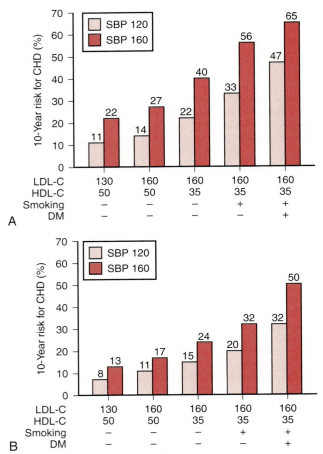

Figure 1–3 Predicted Framingham Heart Study 10-year risk for coronary heart disease (CHD) by increasing burden of risk factors and systolic blood pressure (SBP) in a 65-year-old man (**A**) and woman (**B**). DM, diabetes mellitus; HDL-C, high-density lipoprotein cholesterol; LDL-C, low-density lipoprotein cholesterol. (Data from Wilson PW, D'Agostino RB, Levy D, et al. Prediction of coronary heart disease using risk factor categories. *Circulation.* 1998;**97**:1837-1847.)

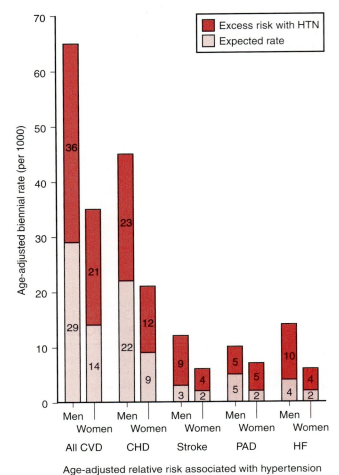

Figure 1–4 Age-adjusted biennial rates, relative risks, and absolute excess risks associated with hypertension for different cardiovascular endpoints: Framingham Heart Study, 36-year follow-up, persons aged 35 to 64 years. CHD, coronary heart disease; CVD, cardiovascular disease; HF, heart failure; HTN, hypertension; PAD, peripheral arterial disease.

To illustrate the importance of hypertension as a risk factor, let us consider the case of HF. From 75% to 91% of individuals who develop HF have antecedent hypertension.[8,30] In data from the Framingham Heart Study, hypertension conferred a hazard ratio for the development of HF of approximately 2 for men and 3 for women over the ensuing 18 years.[30] As shown in Figure 1-5, the hazard ratios for HF associated with hypertension (2 to 3) were far lower than the hazard ratios for HF associated with MI, which were greater than 6 for both men and women. However, the population prevalence of hypertension was 60%, compared with approximately 6% for MI. Therefore, the population-attributable risk of HF, that is, the fraction of HF in this population that was the result of hypertension, was 59% in women and 39% in men. The population-attributable risks for MI were 13% and 34% for women and men, respectively.[30]

Importance of Systolic Blood Pressure

Investigators have recognized for decades that elevated SBP confers at least as great and, in most groups studied, substantially greater risk for CVD as elevated DBP.[31] However, translation of this knowledge into clinical guidelines and clinical practice has been slow. In numerous studies, increasing SBP has consistently been associated with a higher risk for adverse events than increasing DBP, whether these BP variables are considered separately or together, and whether they are treated as linear covariates or in quintiles, deciles, or JNC stages. For example, in the Cardiovascular Health Study of older U.S. residents (Table 1-4), an increment of 1 standard deviation in SBP was associated with higher adjusted risk for CHD and stroke than was an increment of 1 standard deviation in DBP (or pulse pressure). In models with SBP and DBP together or with SBP and pulse pressure together, SBP consistently dominated as the greater risk factor.[32] When men who were screened for inclusion in the Multiple Risk Factor Intervention Trial (MRFIT) were stratified into quintiles of SBP or DBP, risks for each SBP quintile were the same or higher than for the corresponding quintile of DBP (Fig. 1-6A).[33] Similar findings were observed when participants in MRFIT were stratified during screening into deciles of SBP and DBP; at every level, SBP was consistently associated with higher risk for CHD mortality than the corresponding decile of DBP (Fig. 1-6B).[34] Finally, when men were stratified by JNC level of SBP and DBP, SBP was associated with greater risk for CHD mortality than DBP in each JNC BP stage.[34]

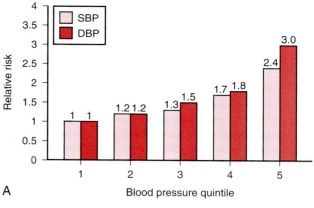

A

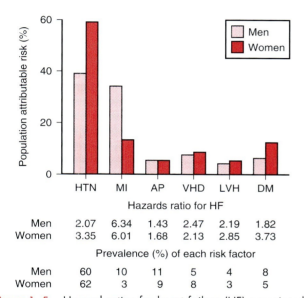

	HTN	MI	AP	VHD	LVH	DM
Hazards ratio for HF						
Men	2.07	6.34	1.43	2.47	2.19	1.82
Women	3.35	6.01	1.68	2.13	2.85	3.73
Prevalence (%) of each risk factor						
Men	60	10	11	5	4	8
Women	62	3	9	8	3	5

Figure 1–5 Hazard ratios for heart failure (HF) associated with selected risk factors, prevalence of each risk factor, and population-attributable risk for each factor in heart failure. AP, angina pectoris; DM, diabetes mellitus; HTN, hypertension; LVH, left ventricular hypertrophy; MI, myocardial infarction; VHD, valvular heart disease. (Data from Levy D, Larson MG, Vasan RS, et al. The progression from hypertension to congestive heart failure. *JAMA.* 1996;**275**:1557-1562.)

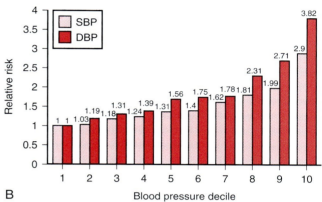

B

Figure 1–6 Relative risks for coronary heart disease mortality among men screened for the Multiple Risk Factor Intervention Trial, by quintiles (**A**) or deciles (**B**) of systolic blood pressure (SBP) and diastolic blood pressure (DBP). (Data from Neaton JD, Wentworth DN. Serum cholesterol, blood pressure, cigarette smoking, and death from coronary heart disease: Overall findings and differences by age for 316,099 white men. *Arch Intern Med.* 1992;**152**:56-64; Neaton JD, Kuller L, Stamler J, Wentworth DN. Impact of systolic and diastolic blood pressure on cardiovascular mortality. *In:* Laragh JH, Brenner BM [eds]. Hypertension: Pathophysiology, Diagnosis, and Management. New York: Raven Press, 1995, pp 127-144.)

Table 1-4 Risks for Cardiovascular Disease Associated with Different Components of Blood Pressure in the Cardiovascular Health Study

		Adjusted Hazard Ratio (95% CI)	
	1 Standard Deviation	Myocardial Infarction	Stroke
Systolic blood pressure	21.4 mm Hg	1.24 (1.15-1.35)	1.34 (1.21-1.47)
Diastolic blood pressure	11.2 mm Hg	1.13 (1.04-1.22)	1.29 (1.17-1.42)
Pulse pressure	18.5 mm Hg	1.21 (1.12-1.31)	1.21 (1.10-1.34)

CI, confidence interval.
Data from Psaty BM, Furberg CD, Kuller LH, et al. Association between blood pressure level and the risk of myocardial infarction, stroke, and total mortality. *Arch Intern Med.* 2001;**161**:1183-1192.

Table 1-5   Rates of Control to Systolic Blood Pressure Less than 140 mm Hg or Diastolic Blood Pressure Less than 90 mm Hg, among 1944 Hypertensive Framingham Heart Study Participants, 1990 to 1995

	SBP <140 mm Hg	SBP ≥140 mm Hg	Total
DBP <90 mm Hg	29.0%	53.9%	82.9%
DBP ≥90 mm Hg	3.7%	13.4%	17.1%
Total	32.7%	67.3%	100%

DBP, diastolic blood pressure; SBP, systolic blood pressure.
Data from Lloyd-Jones DM, Evans JC, Larson MG, et al. Differential control of systolic and diastolic blood pressure: Factors associated with lack of blood pressure control in the community. *Hypertension.* 2000;**36**:594-599.

In fact, when DBP is considered in the context of the SBP level, an inverse association between DBP and CHD risk has been observed. Franklin and associates demonstrated that, at any specified level of SBP, relative risks for CHD decreased with increasing DBP.[35] For example, at an SBP of 150 mm Hg, the estimated hazard ratio for CHD was 1.8 when the DBP was 70 mm Hg, but it was only approximately 1.3 when the DBP was 95 mm Hg. The higher the SBP level, the steeper was the decline in CHD risk with increasing DBP.[35] These data provide some compelling evidence for the importance of pulse pressure as a measure of risk, because pulse pressure represents the difference between SBP and DBP, and higher risk was observed in this study when the pulse pressure widened.[35] Pulse pressure is discussed in greater detail later.

The increased risks associated with SBP are clear. When it is also appreciated that systolic hypertension out of proportion to DBP elevation is by far the most common form of hypertension, as discussed earlier, it becomes clear that the population-attributable risk for CVD conferred by SBP vastly outweighs the population-attributable risk for DBP. Finally, lack of control to goal BP in the community is overwhelmingly the result of lack of SBP control to less than 140 mm Hg.[27,36,37] As shown in Table 1-5, among hypertensive participants attending examinations at the Framingham Heart Study in 1990 to 1995, 29.0% had BP controlled to the overall goal of <140/<90 mm Hg. Within this poor overall prevalence of control to goal BP, 82.9% of hypertensive individuals had DBP lower than 90 mm Hg, whereas only 32.7% had SBP controlled to less than 140 mm Hg. Similar findings were observed in the NHANES III cohort.[27]

Cross-sectional predictors of lack of SBP control (and lack of overall control to goal) in the Framingham Heart Study include older age, the presence of electrocardiographic left ventricular hypertrophy, and obesity.[36] In national samples, significant cross-sectional predictors of lack of BP control among those who are aware of their hypertension include age 65 years or older, male sex, and the lack of visits to a physician in the preceding 12 months.[37] Age and the presence of left ventricular hypertrophy likely represent a higher initial SBP before initiation of therapy and a longer duration of hypertension, both of which can contribute to greater difficulty in achieving lower BP levels. In addition, it appears likely that clinicians are reluctant to treat older hypertensive individuals to the recommended BP goals, perhaps as a result of concerns over orthostasis and the risk for falls, the effects of polypharmacy, or the controversial observation that CVD events and

mortality may increase among the oldest hypertensive patients when DBP is lowered to less than 60 or 65 mm Hg.[38]

Because of the difficulty in collecting detailed and repetitive data, few studies have examined prospective predictors of initiating antihypertensive therapy or achieving BP control. Among 1103 hypertensive Framingham Heart Study participants who were untreated at a baseline examination between 1987 and 1999, 350 (31.7%) subjects were receiving therapy at a follow-up examination 4 years later, including 25.7% of subjects with stage 1 and 51.2% of those with stage 2 or higher hypertension at baseline. Multivariate predictors of initiation of therapy included higher SBP and DBP, prevalent and interim CVD, and the presence of left ventricular hypertrophy. The presence of other cardiovascular risk factors did not predict initiation of treatment, a finding indicating that global risk may not have been considered in decisions to initiate therapy.[39] Among 2475 hypertensive participants whose BP was uncontrolled (treated or untreated) at baseline, 988 (39.9%) had controlled hypertension at follow-up. Prevalent CVD and interim initiation of therapy predicted control of BP; older age and higher baseline SBP levels predicted lack of control in this prospective analysis.[39] Thus, achievement of SBP control remains a major obstacle to achieving better rates of BP control and to lowering risks for adverse events in the population.

Risk across the Spectrum of Blood Pressure and the Importance of "Mild" Hypertension

As noted earlier, increasing BP is associated with increasing risks for CVD beginning at levels well within the so-called "normal" range. A pooling study of nearly 1,000,000 men and women in numerous large epidemiologic cohorts, and including data on more than 56,000 decedents, demonstrated that the risk for CVD death increases steadily beginning at least at levels as low as SBP of 115 mm Hg and DBP of 75 mm Hg. When considered in isolation, for each 20 mm Hg increase in SBP and each 10 mm Hg increase in DBP, the risk for death related to stroke and for death related to ischemic heart disease approximately doubles for both men and women.[28]

Similarly, the large data set of more than 347,000 men aged 35 to 57 years who were screened for MRFIT provides a precise estimate of incremental CVD risk beginning at lower BPs. The data from the MRFIT screenees, shown in Figure 1-7A,

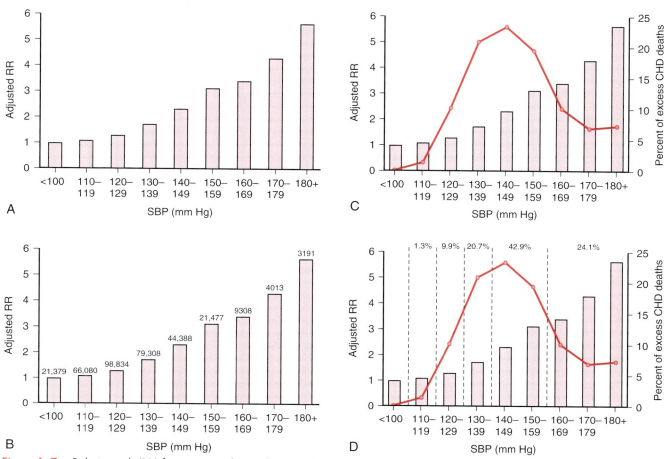

Figure 1-7 Relative risk (RR) for coronary heart disease (CHD) mortality among screenees for the Multiple Risk Factor Intervention Trial by level of systolic blood pressure (SBP) (**A**), with number of men in each stratum of SBP (**B**), distribution of excess CHD deaths by SBP stratum (**C**), and distribution of excess CHD deaths by Joint National Committee on Prevention, Detection, Evaluation, and Treatment of High Blood Pressure stage (**D**). (Data from Neaton JD, Kuller L, Stamler J, Wentworth DN. Impact of systolic and diastolic blood pressure on cardiovascular mortality. *In:* Laragh JH, Brenner BM [eds]. Hypertension: Pathophysiology, Diagnosis, and Management. New York: Raven Press, 1995, pp 127-144.)

confirm a continuous, graded influence of SBP on multivariable-adjusted relative risk for CHD mortality beginning at pressures much lower than 140 mm Hg.[40] Men with SBP of 150 to 159 mm Hg had more than three times the risk and men with SBP higher than 180 mm Hg had nearly six times the risk of men with SBP lower than 100 mm Hg. These data also make an important point about BP levels in the population in which most CVD events occur. In Figure 1-7B, the numbers above each bar indicate the number of men in that stratum of SBP at baseline. Taking into account the number of men in each stratum and the expected rates of CHD-related death, the CHD death rates observed in the MRFIT screenee cohort indicate an of excess CHD-related deaths occurring at the rates indicated by the line in Figure 1-7C. The proportions of excess CHD-related deaths by SBP stratum are indicated in Figure 1-7D. As indicated, nearly two thirds of excess CHD-related deaths occurred in men with SBP between 130 and 159 mm Hg, relatively "mild" levels of elevated BP.

Data from the Framingham Heart Study also indicate that the risk associated with BPs in the range of 130 to 139 mm Hg SBP or 85 to 89 mm Hg DBP are substantial, even though these levels are not as yet classified as hypertension. These

levels of BP are associated with a significantly elevated multivariable-adjusted relative risk for CVD of 2.5 in women and 1.6 in men.[41] Likewise, individuals with SBP between 120 and 139 mm Hg or DBP between 80 and 89 mm Hg have a high likelihood of progressing to frank hypertension over the next 4 years, especially if they are 65 years old or older.[42]

Pulse Pressure and Risks for Cardiovascular Disease

Pulse pressure is defined as SBP minus DBP. In recent years, interest in pulse pressure as a risk factor for CVD has been intense. However, various investigators have struggled with how best to "anchor" the pulse pressure. For example, a patient with a BP of 120/70 mm Hg has the same pulse pressure (50 mm Hg) as a patient with a BP of 180/130 mm Hg, although the latter patient is clearly at higher risk for adverse events. Different investigators have anchored the pulse pressure to the DBP, the mean arterial pressure, and the SBP. As discussed earlier, Franklin and colleagues demonstrated that increasing pulse pressure was associated with marked increases in hazard of CHD for subjects with the same SBP.[35]

Chae and associates also found that pulse pressure was an independent predictor of HF in an elderly cohort, even after adjustment for mean arterial pressure, prevalent CHD, and other HF risk factors.[43] In another study, Haider and colleagues observed that SBP and pulse pressure conferred similar risk for HF.[44] However, other studies have found that SBP confers greater risk than pulse pressure, when SBP and pulse pressure are considered separately or as covariates in the same multivariable model.[32] The Prospective Studies Collaboration, which pooled data from 61 large epidemiologic studies and nearly 1,000,000 men and women, found that the most informative measure of BP for prediction of CVD events was the mean of SBP and DBP, which was a better predictor than SBP or DBP alone and was much better than the pulse pressure.[28] At present, JNC 7 recommends that clinical focus should remain on the SBP in determining need for therapy and achieving goal BP.[1]

Renal Disease

Hypertension is also a major risk factor for the development of renal disease. Of the estimated 93,000 cases of incident end-stage renal disease diagnosed in 2001, it was estimated that more than 25% were the result of hypertension, and more than 40% were sequelae of diabetes.[45] However, these numbers may substantially underestimate the contribution of BP to the increasing incidence of renal disease, because these data provide only a single diagnostic cause, and hypertension is present in most patients with diabetes. African Americans have approximately four times the risk of whites of developing end-stage renal disease, in part because of their significantly higher prevalence of hypertension.[8] In addition to its contribution to end-stage renal disease, elevated BP also occurs in and exacerbates milder forms of chronic kidney disease and worsens proteinuria.

RISK FACTOR CLUSTERING

As anticipated by the JNC VI panel, hypertension occurs in isolation very infrequently. Data from 4962 Framingham Heart Study subjects who were examined between 1990 and 1995 were used to assess the cross-classification of JNC VI BP stages and risk groups (Fig. 1-8) in a middle-aged and older community-based population.[46] In this study, higher BP stages were associated with a higher mean number of risk factors and higher rates of clinical CVD and target organ damage. Overall, among those with high-normal BP or hypertension, only 2.4% had no associated risk factors, whereas 59.3% had at least one associated risk factor, and 38.2% had target organ damage, clinical CVD, or diabetes.[46]

The epidemic of obesity among Western societies has led to a greater understanding of the phenomenon of risk factor clustering and of the pathophysiologic links among hypertension, obesity, diabetes, and risk for CVD. The cluster of risk factors including central obesity, atherogenic dyslipidemia (with low high-density lipoprotein cholesterol, high triglycerides, and small, dense low-density lipoprotein cholesterol particles), impaired glucose metabolism, vascular inflammation, proatherogenic milieu, and elevated BP has been termed the *metabolic syndrome*. Visceral adiposity and insulin resistance appear to play central roles in the development

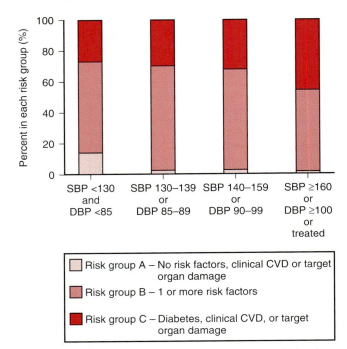

Figure 1–8   Cross-classification of risk groups and blood pressure stages among 4962 Framingham Heart Study subjects. CVD, cardiovascular disease; DBP, diastolic blood pressure; SBP, systolic blood pressure. (DBP and SBP both in mm Hg.) (Data from Lloyd-Jones DM, Evans JC, Larson MG, et al. Cross-classification of JNC VI blood pressure stages and risk groups in the Framingham Heart Study. *Arch Intern Med.* 1999;**159**:2206-2212.)

of metabolic syndrome, and elevated BP is a key diagnostic feature.[47] In some ethnicities, such as African Americans, elevated BP is the most common criterion leading to diagnosis of the metabolic syndrome. Hypertension confers increased risk for CVD in the absence of risk factors, but absolute risk increases dramatically when other risk factors are present, as shown in Figure 1-3.

HYPERTENSION IN OLDER INDIVIDUALS

Elderly persons comprise one of the fastest growing segments of the U.S. population,[48] and they also have the greatest prevalence of hypertension.[2,8] As shown in Figure 1-2, the percentage of individuals with hypertension exceeds 50% in those more than 60 years of age and exceeds 75% in those more than 75 years old.[2] Despite multiple trials demonstrating the benefits of BP lowering among older hypertensive individuals, available data suggest that rates of treatment of hypertension and BP control in older individuals are suboptimal.[7,27,36,37,39] In NHANES 1999 to 2000, 69.8% of hypertensive individuals aged 60 years old or older were aware of their hypertension, 62.7% were treated, and only 27.4% had the condition controlled to goal BP. Compared with hypertensive patients 40 to 59 years old, this represents similar rates of awareness and treatment, but substantially lower rates of control, as shown in Table 1-6.[7] However, national surveillance data are often limited to adults younger than age 75 years.[1,6,14] Data are sparse regarding current patterns of treat-

Table 1-6 Awareness, Treatment, and Control of Hypertension by Age Group in the United States, National Health and Nutrition Examination Survey 1999 to 2000

Age (yr)	Awareness	Treatment	Control
40-59	73.3%	62.9%	41.6%
≥60	69.8%	62.7%	27.4%

Data from Hajjar I, Kotchen TA. Trends in prevalence, awareness, treatment, and control of hypertension in the United States, 1988-2000. *JAMA.* 2003;**290**:199-206.

ment and control of hypertension among individuals 80 years of age and older.

Hypertension occurs in the absence of other CVD risk factors only rarely in older persons, and it is often accompanied by a clustering of other risk factors.[49,50] The prevalence of three or more coexisting risk factors is four times higher among hypertensive than among normotensive older individuals.[51]

Older hypertensive patients appear to be at risk for a somewhat different spectrum of first CVD events than younger patients. Among studied patients younger than 60 years old who had new-onset hypertension, the most common first major CVD event after 12 years of follow-up was MI or hospitalization for unstable angina. Conversely, in those with the onset of hypertension at age 60 years or older, the most common first major CVD event was a stroke, particularly among older women.[52] Whereas the risk for CHD increases steadily with increasing age, the risks for HF and atrial fibrillation increase dramatically among older compared with younger hypertensive patients.[53,54]

CONCLUSIONS

Hypertension is the most prevalent major risk factor for CVD and renal disease. Risk factors for development of hypertension are well understood, and numerous dietary and personal habits, as well as societal issues, must be addressed if we are to lower population levels of BP and to control individual patients' BP levels, particularly SBP. Major public health and clinical efforts are needed to improve prevention of hypertension, especially through better control of weight. Although the benefits of antihypertensive therapy are substantial, too few patients achieve optimal reduction in BP levels and so do not realize the potential reductions in their risk for CVD and renal disease. More widespread treatment and control-to-goal levels are needed, particularly among older hypertensive patients, who are at the highest risk for the consequences of hypertension.

References

1. Chobanian AV, Bakris GL, Black HR, et al. Seventh report of the Joint National Committee on Prevention, Detection, Evaluation, and Treatment of High Blood Pressure. *Hypertension.* 2003;**42**:1206-1252.
2. Fields LE, Burt VL, Cutler JA, et al. The burden of adult hypertension in the United States 1999 to 2000: A rising tide. *Hypertension.* 2004;**44**:398-404.
3. Hill AB. The environment and disease: Association or causation? *Proc R Soc Med.* 1965;**58**:295-300.
4. Hennekens CH, Buring JE. Epidemiology in Medicine. Boston: Little, Brown, 1987.
5. Glover MJ, Greenlund KJ, Ayala C, Croft JB. Racial/ethnic disparities in prevalence, treatment, and control of hypertension: United States, 1999-2002. *MMWR Morb Mortal Wkly Rep.* 2005;**54**:7-9.
6. Burt VL, Culter JA, Higgins M, et al. Trends in the prevalence, awareness, treatment, and control of hypertension in the adult us population: Data from the health examination surveys, 1960 to 1991. *Hypertension.* 1995;**26**:60-69.
7. Hajjar I, Kotchen TA. Trends in prevalence, awareness, treatment, and control of hypertension in the United States, 1988-2000. *JAMA.* 2003;**290**:199-206.
8. American Heart Association. Heart Disease and Stroke Statistics: 2005 update. Dallas, TX: American Heart Association, 2004.
9. Wolf-Maier K, Cooper RS, Kramer H, et al. Hypertension treatment and control in five European countries, Canada, and the United States. *Hypertension.* 2004;**43**:10-17.
10. Wolf-Maier K, Cooper RS, Banegas JR, et al. Hypertension prevalence and blood pressure levels in 6 European countries, Canada, and the United States. *JAMA.* 2003;**289**:2363-2369.
11. Mackay J, Mensah G. Atlas of Heart Disease and Stroke. Geneva, World Health Organization, 2004. Available online at http://www.who.int/cardiovascular_diseases/resources/atlas/en/print.html. Accessed May 6, 2005.
12. Kearney PM, Whelton M, Reynolds K, et al. Global burden of hypertension: Analysis of worldwide data. *Lancet.* 2005;**365**: 217-223.
13. Vasan RS, Beiser A, Seshadri S, et al. Residual lifetime risk for developing hypertension in middle-aged women and men: The Framingham Heart Study. *JAMA.* 2002;**287**:1003-1010.
14. Burt VL, Whelton P, Roccella EJ, et al. Prevalence of hypertension in the US adult population: Results from the Third National Health and Nutrition Examination Survey, 1988-1991. *Hypertension.* 1995;**25**:305-313.
15. Franklin SS, Gustin W, Wong ND, et al. Hemodynamic patterns of age-related changes in blood pressure: The Framingham Heart Study. *Circulation.* 1997;**96**:308-315.
16. Lakatta EG, Levy D. Arterial and cardiac aging: Major shareholders in cardiovascular disease enterprises. Part I. Aging arteries: A "set up" for vascular disease. *Circulation.* 2003;**107**: 139-146.
17. Izzo JL, Levy D, Black HR. Importance of systolic blood pressure in older Americans. *Hypertension.* 2000;**35**:1021-1024.
18. Wang Y, Wang QJ. The prevalence of prehypertension and hypertension among US adults according to the new Joint National Committee guidelines. *Arch Intern Med.* 2004;**164**: 2126-2134.
19. Wilson PWF, D'Agostino RB, Sullivan L, et al. Overweight and obesity as determinants of cardiovascular risk: The Framingham experience. *Arch Intern Med.* 2002;**162**:1867-1872.
20. Lloyd-Jones DM, Liu K, Colangelo LA, et al. Consistently stable body mass index and changes in risk factors associated with the metabolic syndrome: The CARDIA study [abstract]. *Circulation.* 2004;**110 (Suppl III)**:III772.
21. Mamun AA, Lawlor DA, O'Callaghan MJ, et al. Effect of body mass index changes between ages 5 and 14 on blood pressure at age 14: Findings from a birth cohort study. *Hypertension.* 2005;**45**:1083-1087.
22. Stamler J, Elliott P, Appel L, et al. Higher blood pressure in middle-aged American adults with less education-role of multiple dietary factors: The InterMAP study. *J Hum Hypertens.* 2003;**17**:655-665.
23. Stamler J, Rose G, Elliott P, et al. Findings of the international cooperative InterSALT study. *Hypertension.* 1991;**17 (Suppl 1)**: I9-I15.

24. Joint National Committee on Prevention, Detection, Evaluation, and Treatment of High Blood Pressure. The seventh report of the Joint National Committee on Prevention, Detection, Evaluation, and Treatment of High Blood Pressure. *JAMA*. 2003;**289**:2560-2571.

25. Lloyd-Jones DM, Evans JC, Larson MG, et al. Differential impact of systolic and diastolic blood pressure level on JNC-VI staging. *Hypertension*. 1999;**34**:381-385.

26. Pogue VA, Ellis C, Michel J, Francis CK. New staging system of the fifth Joint National Committee Report on The Detection, Evaluation, and Treatment of High Blood Pressure (JNC-V) alters assessment of the severity and treatment of hypertension. *Hypertension*. 1996;**28**:713-718.

27. Franklin SS, Jacobs MJ, Wong ND, et al. Predominance of isolated systolic hypertension among middle-aged and elderly US hypertensives. *Hypertension*. 2001;**37**:869-874.

28. Prospective Studies Collaboration: Age-specific relevance of usual blood pressure to vascular mortality: A meta-analysis of individual data for one million adults in 61 prospective studies. *Lancet*. 2002;**360**:1903-1913.

29. Wilson PW, D'Agostino RB, Levy D, et al. Prediction of coronary heart disease using risk factor categories. *Circulation*. 1998;**97**:1837-1847.

30. Levy D, Larson MG, Vasan RS, et al. The progression from hypertension to congestive heart failure. *JAMA*. 1996;**275**:1557-1562.

31. Kannel WB, Gordon T, Schwartz MJ. Systolic versus diastolic blood pressure and risk of coronary heart disease: The Framingham Study. *Am J Cardiol*. 1971;**27**:335-345.

32. Psaty BM, Furberg CD, Kuller LH, et al. Association between blood pressure level and the risk of myocardial infarction, stroke, and total mortality. *Arch Intern Med*. 2001;**161**:1183-1192.

33. Neaton JD, Wentworth DN. Serum cholesterol, blood pressure, cigarette smoking, and death from coronary heart disease: Overall findings and differences by age for 316,099 white men. *Arch Intern Med*. 1992;**152**:56-64.

34. Neaton JD, Kuller L, Stamler J, Wentworth DN. Impact of systolic and diastolic blood pressure on cardiovascular mortality. *In:* Laragh JH, Brenner BM (eds). Hypertension: Pathophysiology, Diagnosis, and Management. New York: Raven Press, 1995, pp 127-144.

35. Franklin SS, Khan SA, Wong ND, et al. Is pulse pressure useful in predicting risk for coronary heart disease? The Framingham Heart Study. *Circulation*. 1999;**100**:354-360.

36. Lloyd-Jones DM, Evans JC, Larson MG, et al. Differential control of systolic and diastolic blood pressure: Factors associated with lack of blood pressure control in the community. *Hypertension*. 2000;**36**:594-599.

37. Hyman DJ, Pavlik VN. Characteristics of patients with uncontrolled hypertension in the United States. *N Engl J Med*. 2001;**345**:479-486.

38. Somes GW, Pahor M, Shorr RI, et al. The role of diastolic blood pressure when treating isolated systolic hypertension. *Arch Intern Med*. 1999;**159**:2004-2009.

39. Lloyd-Jones DM, Evans JC, Larson MG, Levy D. Treatment and control of hypertension in the community: A prospective analysis. *Hypertension*. 2002;**40**:640-646.

40. Stamler J, Stamler R, Neaton JD. Blood pressure, systolic and diastolic, and cardiovascular risks: US population data. *Arch Intern Med*. 1993;**153**:598-615.

41. Vasan RS, Larson MG, Leip EP, et al. Impact of high-normal blood pressure on the risk of cardiovascular disease. *N Engl J Med*. 2001;**345**:1291-1297.

42. Vasan RS, Larson MG, Leip EP, et al. Assessment of frequency of progression to hypertension in non-hypertensive participants in the Framingham Heart Study. *Lancet*. 2001;**358**:1682-1686.

43. Chae CU, Pfeffer MA, Glynn RJ, et al. Increased pulse pressure and risk of heart failure in the elderly. *JAMA*. 1999;**281**:634-639.

44. Haider AW, Larson MG, Franklin SS, Levy D. Systolic blood pressure, diastolic blood pressure, and pulse pressure as predictors of risk for congestive heart failure in the Framingham Heart Study. *Ann Intern Med*. 2003;**138**:10-16.

45. United States Renal Data System (USRDS). USRDS 2003 Annual Data Report. Bethesda, MD: National Institute of Diabetes and Digestive and Kidney Diseases, National Institutes of Health, 2003.

46. Lloyd-Jones DM, Evans JC, Larson MG, et al. Cross-classification of JNC VI blood pressure stages and risk groups in the Framingham Heart Study. *Arch Intern Med*. 1999;**159**:2206-2212.

47. Third report of the National Cholesterol Education Program (NCEP) Expert Panel on Detection, Evaluation, and Treatment of High Blood Cholesterol in Adults (Adult Treatment Panel III): Final report. *Circulation*. 2002;**106**:3143-3421.

48. Meyer J. Age: 2000. Census 2000 Brief. Washington, DC: U.S. Department of Commerce, Economics and Statistics Administration, U.S. Census Bureau, 2001.

49. Reaven GM. Banting lecture 1988: Role of insulin resistance in human disease. *Diabetes Care*. 1988;**37**:1595-1607.

50. Reaven GM. Insulin resistance, hyperinsulinemia, and hypertriglyceridemia in the etiology and clinical course of hypertension. *Am J Med*. 1991;**90 (Suppl 2A)**:7S-12S.

51. Kannel WB, Wilson PW, Silbershatz H, D'Agostino RB. Epidemiology of risk factor clustering in elevated blood pressure. *In:* Gotto AM, L'Enfant C, Paoletti R (eds). Multiple Risk Factors in Cardiovascular Disease. New York: Kluwer Academic Publishers, 1998, pp 325-333.

52. Lloyd-Jones DM, Leip EP, Larson MG, et al. Novel approach to examining first cardiovascular events after hypertension onset. *Hypertension*. 2005;**45**:39-45.

53. Benjamin EJ, Levy D, Vaziri SM, et al. Independent risk factors for atrial fibrillation in a population-based cohort: The Framingham Heart Study. *JAMA*. 1994;**271**:840-844.

54. Ho KK, Pinsky JL, Kannel WB, Levy D. The epidemiology of heart failure: The Framingham Study. *J Am Coll Cardiol*. 1993;**22**:6A-13A.

Chapter 2

Genetics of Hypertension

Xiaodong Wu and Richard S. Cooper

A review of the genetics of hypertension first needs to be situated in the general context of hypertension research and practice. Several paradoxes are quickly apparent when one tries to integrate the discussion of genetics and blood pressure (BP) regulation into the field as a whole. Hypertension is the most common cardiovascular condition in all human populations, and it accounts for about 12% of adult mortality in the United States.[1] New knowledge about the pathogenesis of this complex disorder will therefore always be of value. At the same time, we already know a great deal about the causal risk factors that lead to the common forms of hypertension, and we have inexpensive, safe, and effective medications that can control elevated BP in virtually all patients. Nonetheless, in practice we have not been able to implement successful programs that prevent the rise of BP with age in the population, and, as implemented in the clinical setting, drug treatment is inefficient, resulting in control rates that range from 5% to 30% in most societies.[2] Considerable room for improvement therefore exists in our approach to both prevention and treatment of hypertension. It seems unlikely that the modalities currently at our disposal will close the gap between what we would hope to accomplish and what is possible.

In many areas of biology and medicine, much has been staked on the potential for molecular genetics to resolve some of the most difficult unmet clinical challenges. Although the application of molecular technology has created exciting new research opportunities, whether it will make important contributions to the diagnosis, prevention, and treatment of common illnesses is still far from certain. In a sense, attempts to apply molecular genetics to the problem of hypertension can therefore be seen as a "high-risk/high-impact" venture. Although the technology allows us to undertake a whole new class of experiments, as yet we have no clear examples in which this strategy has been shown to be effective as a widely applicable clinical tool. For the moment, it is therefore more appropriate to withhold judgment on the value of what genetics can deliver in relation to common chronic illnesses and hypertension in particular.

From this perspective, we review the basic concepts of the genetics of high BP and describe the most important new developments in molecular research. Less emphasis is placed on traditional epidemiologic findings in hypertension because that material is well described elsewhere (see Chapter 1). Because this is a rapidly changing field and many fundamental questions are still unanswered, we give particular emphasis to methodologic issues. This chapter assists the reader in evaluating the ongoing flow of new information in this field. In the final section, we return to a consideration of the implications of what is already known and the possible impact of potential new contributions to this field.

HERITABILITY AND STATISTICAL ESTIMATION OF GENETIC EFFECTS

In the absence of knowledge of the specific deoxyribonucleic acid (DNA) variants that influence a trait, the impact of genetic factors can be estimated indirectly by examining familial resemblance. Typically, studies of nuclear families (i.e., first-degree relatives) or twins have been used to quantify the magnitude of the genetic effects. Children of the same parents, on average, share 50% of their genetic material, and the degree of phenotypic resemblance should reflect half of the total impact of genes with additive effects. Height, for example, is a highly heritable trait, to which multiple genes contribute. Accurate predictions can be made for the future height of children, based on the heights of the parents.

Many phenotypes are also influenced by environmental factors, however, that are likely to be shared by members of the same family. Shared genetic components among family members can be estimated by controlling for known environmental factors or contrasting family members with varying degrees of relatedness, for example, monozygotic compared with dizygotic twins. Because monozygotic twins share 100% of their genetic material, whereas dizygotic twins share only half, the difference in the degree of resemblance between sets of these two types of twins has served as an important measure of the overall impact of genetics.[3,4] Separating out the nongenetic component shared by family members can sometimes be difficult in practice, however, and can limit the degree of confidence one can place in heritability as a summary measure of the action of genes. For example, the life patterns of twins are often atypical, and the general tendency is to overestimate the impact of genes in twin studies.

To provide more robust estimates of heritable effects and to give appropriate samples for DNA analysis, most research currently focuses on nuclear families or sibships. The statistic of interest in these analyses is "narrow sense heritability," represented by the following equation:

$$H^2 = \sigma_A^2 / \sigma_P^2$$

where H^2 is the term for heritability, σ_A^2 is the variance attributable to additive genetic effects, and σ_P^2 is the total phenotypic variance. The basic calculation involves the estimation of phenotypic covariance among relatives within families. For example, this can be approximated by doubling the simple correlation coefficient between parent and children, because this resemblance represents half of the average effect of genes. A comprehensive review of heritability based on family studies has yielded an estimate for BP in the range of 35%.[5] These estimates can be put in context by the observation that H^2 for height is generally 70% to 80%, whereas for body mass index it is approximately 45%.

Considerable confusion arises in the interpretation of heritability. The most common mistake is to assume that the magnitude of H^2 is an expression of the overall strength of the genetic effect. In fact, because it is calculated as a ratio, H^2 simply reflects the proportion of phenotypic variation that is accounted for by familial resemblance. Thus, if a trait varies little in a population, and a substantial proportion of that variation occurs within families, heritability could be high, although the genetic effect is weak in absolute terms. By the same token, in a cultural setting where large environmental effects are present at the individual level, which reduces the correlation among family members, heritability would be low. In fact, some evidence indicates that in environments such as rural Africa, where the impact of risk factors is more limited, heritability for BP may be 40% or higher, whereas in some studies of African Americans, the familial component can be less than 20%.[6]

The heritability statistic is also commonly used as a rough guide to the potential impact of individual genes. Thus, if one assumes that the genetic effect is roughly 35%, and one hypothesizes that there are 10 genes with equal effects, on average each gene will account for only 3.5% of the variation. Although it is entirely possible that in certain families individual genes may have substantially larger effects, under most assumptions specific mutations will have only a modest to very small impact on an individual's BP. The clear implication is that these effects will be difficult to identify, and once identified they will in most instances have little clinical relevance for a given patient.

OVERVIEW OF MOLECULAR TERMINOLOGY

The human genome can vary among individuals in several distinct ways. Studies of genetic epidemiology rely almost exclusively on two sources of this variation: single nucleotide polymorphisms (SNPs) and microsatellite repeats. SNPs in coding or regulatory regions of genes form the basis of functional and structural variation in phenotypes, although most SNPs across the genome are not in genes and are silent. Microsatellites are composed of long repetitive segments of nonfunctional DNA that mutate rapidly and therefore vary considerably among individuals. Microsatellites are used frequently in the first stages of gene mapping to localize segments of the genome that appear to vary in association with the trait. Because SNPs are much more common than microsatellites, they can also be used as anonymous markers to detect regions of interest. Ultimately, the goal of gene mapping, no matter which approach is taken first, is to identify the SNPs that alter function.

A series of daunting challenges is faced by genetic epidemiologists in their quest to isolate the SNPs that lead to variation in traits such as BP. The human genome consists of approximately 3 billion base pairs, with SNPs occurring at a frequency of 1 in every 800 to 1000 nucleotides. Currently, the genome is thought to include at least 7 million SNPs, and most have been deposited in computer databases such as dbSNP (http://www.ncbi.nlm.nih.gov/projects/SNP/). Because most of this genetic variation is silent or nonfunctional so far as we know now, statistical analyses must account for large numbers of false-positive associations.

Mutations with large effects on phenotypes are extremely rare, and most SNPs that influence BP are likely to have weak effects and be identified only in studies with large sample sizes. In addition, individuals inherit chromosomes, rather than genes or individual SNPs, and large blocks of chromosomes are shared in common among many families.[7] This structural property of the genome is referred to as *linkage disequilibrium* (LD) and results in a correlation among SNPs in the same genomic segments. Thus, many SNPs that appear to be in association with a trait have that relationship only because they are in LD with an undetected causal SNP.

Finally, the underlying pattern of causal SNPs for complex diseases is unknown, and we lack a theoretical model of how these variants are likely to be distributed. Unlike mendelian or single-gene disorders, variation in a number of genes can confer susceptibility to hypertension. Just how many genes may be involved, however, remains an open question. Until recently, it was widely assumed that a relatively small set of SNPs, common in the population, underlie most variations, the so-called "common disease/common variant" hypothesis.[8] More recently, it has been argued that the susceptibility alleles are likely to remain at low frequency, and therefore rare, virtually family-specific SNPs are more important. Evidence that rare SNPs influence common traits such as BP and cholesterol has, in fact, started to emerge.[9] Although each individual SNP may be infrequent, a large, diverse collection of these rare SNPs could be present in the population. The sum of their effects would determine a given individual's risk.

The pattern of distribution of SNPs has enormous implications, both for research and for future clinical applications. If common SNPs are the dominant form of causal variants, then it should ultimately be possible to characterize an individual's risk in some detail. Conversely, if most of the genetic effect is restricted to a broad range of rare SNPs, not only will they be difficult to find, but also screening individual patients will be virtually impossible. Only additional research will answer these questions.

TYPES OF STUDY DESIGN

Given the inconclusive nature of the evidence for gene effects in the common forms of hypertension, an interpretation of the current knowledge base requires an understanding of the strengths and weaknesses of the research methods. In this section, we briefly summarize the study designs that can be used to search for the relevant mutations.

An early approach to the genetic epidemiology of complex traits, known as *segregation analysis,* was based on the assumption that the inheritance could be modeled as a mixture of several distinct normal distributions, each corresponding to the effect of an influential locus. If the measured phenotype corresponded to a mixture model, it was then assumed that a major gene effect was present and was taken as justification for a search to identify the causal variants. With the development of high-throughput genotyping, this modeling phase has now become obsolete and has fallen from favor.

Because the resemblance of phenotypic traits within families reflects to some degree the action of genes, a search for the pattern of the co-occurrence of the trait and specific mutations has been the most widely used method in genetic epidemiology. When markers are placed on the 22 autosomal chromosomes, this approach is referred to as *genome-wide linkage analysis.* Coupled with efficient laboratory methods for genotyping, this approach has been used with great efficiency in studies of monogenic diseases. For complex traits such as high BP, however, in which multiple genetic and environmental factors operate, family studies have weak resolving power.

Given the extensive knowledge of physiology and the structure of the human genome, it is now possible to locate large numbers of genes involved in BP regulation. Targeted studies of the variation in and around those genes that occurs in hypertensive patients compared with normotensive persons can offer much more statistical precision. In genetic epidemiology, these case-control studies are generally called *association studies.* The success of this design will obviously depend on whether the candidate gene that has been chosen for study is, in fact, involved in hypertension. However, spurious associations can result from population stratification in association studies. This situation can occur when multiple subpopulations are mixed in what is assumed to be a relatively homogeneous population. Such stratification can represent either recent admixture or the incorrect matching of cases and controls. For example, if an association is performed in a population consisting of subpopulations with different disease prevalences, a random sample of cases and controls will contain different portion of individuals from each subpopulation. If the tested genetic marker also has different allele frequencies in the two subpopulations, a significant association will be detected, even if the genetic marker is not linked with the causal genetic variation. Empirical data show that the allele frequencies could be quite different in different human ethnic groups. Thus, it is important to match for ethnicity in the

case-control design. Family-based designs have been used to eliminate the concern that population stratification may be the cause of the association. In such studies, the comparison is between the frequencies of alleles transmitted from heterozygous parents to the affected child and those not transmitted. If association and linkage are present, the frequency of the high-risk allele is expected to be higher in the alleles transmitted than in the alleles not transmitted, and this can be statistically tested using the transmission disequilibrium test.[10] Compared with case-control studies, family-based studies require that samples derive from the intact nuclear families; these are more difficult to collect. Moreover, more samples are needed to achieve the same power for the family-based association test compared with case-control design.

In the last several years, the special demographic features of societies where large-scale recent migration has taken place have been used in a novel approach known as *admixture mapping.*[11] With intermarriage, distinct genetic patterns can be recognized, whereby individuals inherit large genomic segments that are common in one or the other of the ancestral populations. If one of the ancestral populations was enriched for mutations that conferred susceptibility at a given locus, the correlation between the presence of this segment and the occurrence of the trait should be detectable.

FINDINGS

Monogenic Forms of Hypertension

Gene mapping techniques have been most successful in identifying underlying genes for mendelian forms of hypertension. The molecular basis for a subset of these rare disorders has been established and is summarized in Table 2-1. Each of

Table 2-1 Mendelian (Monogenic) Forms of Hypertension

Syndrome	Mode of Inheritance	Mutation
Glucocorticoid remediable aldosteronism (GRA)	Dominant	Unequal crossover between steroid 11β-hydroxylase *(CYP11B1)* and steroid 18β-hydroxylase *(CYP11B2)* genes
Apparent mineralocorticoid excess (AME)	Recessive	Nonfunctional 11β-hydroxysteroid dehydrogenase (11β-HSD)
Liddle's syndrome	Dominant	Mutations in β (SCNN1B) or γ (SCNN1G) subunit of ENaC
Hypertension exacerbated in pregnancy	Dominant	Mutation in mineralocorticoid receptor
Recessive pseudohypoaldosteronism type 1 (PHA 1)	Recessive	Mutations in α (SCNN1A), β (SCNN1B), or γ (SCNN1G) subunit of ENaC
Pseudohypoaldosteronism type 2 (PHA 2)	Dominant	Mutations in *WNK1, WNK4*
Gitelman's syndrome	Recessive	Mutation in the thiazide-sensitive sodium chloride cotransporter (SLC12A3)
Bartter's syndrome	Recessive	Mutation in the barttin *(BSND)* gene or by simultaneous mutation in both the chloride channel Ka *(CLCNKA)* and chloride channel Kb *(CLCNKB)* gene
Hypertension with brachydactyly	Dominant	Mutations at 12p11.2-12.2
Peroxisome proliferator-activated receptor γ (PPARγ)	Dominant	Mutations in PPARγ

CYP11B1, cytochrome P450 11B1 isoenzyme; *CYP11B2,* cytochrome P450 11B2 isoenzyme; ENaC, epithelial sodium channel; *WNK1,* lysine-deficient protein kinase 1; *WNK4,* lysine-deficient protein kinase 4.

these syndromes involves either loss of function or gain in function for hormones related to salt and water balance. This evidence provides important support for the theory that excess sodium intake, in combination with genetic variants that alter sodium balance in more subtle ways, is a central process in nonfamilial hypertension. However, because monogenic disorders of hypertension are rare, they do not contribute directly to our understanding of the genetics of primary (or essential) hypertension, which is much more common in the population.

Family Studies

Identifying genes for BP variation and essential hypertension has been far less successful than for monogenic forms of hypertension. Currently, 27 genome-wide linkage analyses for BP or hypertension can be identified in PubMed. Individually, many of these reports have provided weak or contradictory evidence, and the most efficient way to summarize the quantitative results is through meta-analysis.

Two meta-analyses of hypertension and BP genome scans have been published.[12,13] Province and associates performed a meta-analysis for the genome scans of hypertension and BP in the Family Blood Pressure Program (FBPP).[14] This analysis included 6245 individuals, about half the total number of participants in the FBPP study, from four individual networks (Genetics Network [GenNet], Genetic Epidemiology Network of Atherosclerosis [GENOA], Hypertension Genetic Epidemiology Network [HyperGEN], and Stanford Asian Pacific Program in Hypertension and Insulin Resistance [SAPPHIRe]). Nine genome scans were first performed within four ethnic groups (white, African American, Hispanic, Chinese, and Japanese). Modified Fisher's method of combining P values was used to pool the linkage information.[15] No region reached high levels of significance (log odds >2) when all nine studies were combined, but several small peaks were identified, including chromosome 2p, in which several previous reports had found evidence of linkage to hypertension. Koivukoski and colleagues applied the genome search meta-analysis (GSMA) method to nine published genome scans of hypertension and BP from European-origin populations.[16] They found genome-wide significance or highly suggestive linkage on chromosome 3p14.1-q12.3 and 2p12-q22.1. The regions showing linkage evidence on chromosome 2 overlap in these two studies. A meta-analysis using the final data from the FBPP, which includes more than 12,000 individuals, was also completed in 2006. Suggestive linkage evidence was reported around 2p14 and 3p14.1 regions, a finding further supporting that susceptibility genes for BP and hypertension may reside in these regions.[17]

The results of these meta-analyses provide somewhat consistent results, suggesting that genomic regions harboring genes that influence BP may be found on chromosomes 2 and 3. Some important studies with large sample sizes, such as the United Kingdom's BRItish Genetics of HyperTension (UK BRIGHT) study,[18] which examined 2010 affected sibling pairs, were left out, however, and a final conclusion must be withheld. It is also not clear to what extent these results, which were obtained primarily in European-origin populations, would be replicated in other populations. For all other ethnic groups, the number of studies included in these meta-analyses is very small. Only three studies sampled African Americans, one enrolled Mexican Americans, and two Asian populations were included in the FBPP. The evidence available from genome scans must therefore be considered incomplete.

Case-Control or Association Studies

Compared with linkage studies, association studies are likely to have greater power to detect a small genetic effect.[19] The candidate gene approach is the most frequently used design in association studies. It aims to detect a correlation between the genetic variants in a preselected gene and the phenotype using statistical tests. These genes are selected based on a priori hypotheses about their etiologic role in disease. For example, the renin-angiotensin system (RAS) plays an important role in regulating BP. Thus, the most frequently studied candidate genes in hypertension association studies have involved the RAS, particularly angiotensinogen (AGT) and angiotensin I–converting enzyme (ACE). In addition, linkage studies can provide information about the genomic locations that could harbor the candidate genes.

Until recently, most genetic association studies concentrated on analyzing a small number of individual SNPs. With the availability of high-throughput genotyping technologies,[20] SNPs can be chosen for genotyping based on their function and LD structure, thus improving the power to detect an association. Although each SNP can be analyzed independently of other SNPs, it is much more informative to analyze SNPs in a region of interest simultaneously as a haplotype, formed by the combination of marker alleles on a single chromosome. Statistical analysis based on haplotypes may be more powerful, and this has been demonstrated in both simulations and empirical studies.[21] As a result, there has been considerable interest in defining the haplotype structure of the human genome, because this would be informative about local patterns of LD. The large-scale National Institutes of Health–funded project known as the HapMap is designed to describe genome-wide LD structure.[22] Haplotypes may also provide critical information on human evolution history that cannot be obtained by studying single SNPs, such as recombination.

Prioritizing SNPs for association studies can also be based on whether they are likely to affect gene function, which can be inferred from the location and type of the sequence variants in a gene. For example, a missense mutation that changes an amino acid in a protein or a nonsense mutation that results in a premature stop codon should be given the highest priority for genotyping in candidate genes. Polymorphisms in transcriptional promoters that regulate gene expression should also be given priority for genotyping. Another important consideration when selecting SNPs for genotyping in candidate genes is the LD structure in candidate genes. If complete LD exists among several SNPs, genotypes of other SNPs can be inferred, based on the genotype of one sentinel or "tagging" SNP, thereby reducing the number of genotypes to be performed.

A necessary feature of studies that seek to identify genes for complex diseases is accurate and reproducible phenotyping for the traits of interest. Unfortunately, BP is an extremely "noisy" phenotype. This diagnosis can be thought of as a synthesis of many risk factors, with intermediate phenotypes as subtotals. Genetic factors contributing to intermediate phenotypes would then generally be easier to identify, because the intermediate phenotypes are usually controlled by fewer loci and environmental factors and thus have an improved signal-to-noise ratio in the fraction of variance explained by any single factor. Concerted efforts have therefore been made to identify intermediate, heritable, quantitative traits that may connect genetic variation to the "distant phenotype" of hypertension. The RAS has been an attractive biologic system in this regard. At least two intermediate phenotypes, ACE and AGT plasma levels, can be measured directly. On the basis of the hypothesis that, over the course of a lifetime, small increases in RAS activity elevate the risk of developing hypertension in some individuals, these intermediate phenotypes could be a guide to the genetic makeup of hypertension.

Based on a bibliographic search, more than 70 genes that affect different physiologic and biochemical systems in BP regulation have been studied in various types of association studies. A partial list of candidate genes involving different physiologic pathways for BP regulation is presented in Table 2-2. The most frequently investigated genes are ACE and AGT from the RAS. Jeunemaitre and colleagues first showed a significant association for a SNP (M235T) with AGT level and BP in 1992.[22a] Since then, numerous association studies have been performed on SNPs for AGT in different human ethnic groups. An insertion/deletion polymorphism in the ACE gene has also been under intensive investigation since the mid-1990s. Studies on rare monogenic forms of hypertension, such as Liddle's syndrome, provide important information about the physiologic and biochemical pathways for developing hypertension. Genes responsible for these syndromes are good candidate genes for essential hypertension. For example, Liddle's syndrome is caused by mutations in the β subunit of the epithelial sodium channel and has implications for the regulation of this epithelial ion channel, as well as BP homeostasis. Thus, genes coding for the subunits of epithelial sodium channel (SCNN1A, SCNN1B, and SCNN1G) are logical candidate genes for hypertension.

The results of these candidate gene studies are inconsistent, and meta-analysis is needed to obtain an overall estimate. Five meta-analyses of association studies for candidate genes of hypertension and BP have been published (Table 2-3).[23-27] All these meta-analyses were performed for either ACE or AGT. Two common polymorphisms, M235T and G-6A in the AGT gene, have been the subject of intensive investigation for association with AGT levels, BP, and hypertension. The G-6A polymorphism is in the promoter region of AGT gene and is in nearly complete disequilibrium with M235T. These two polymorphisms have been investigated in several ethnic groups, including whites, blacks, and Asians. The overall result for BP is negative in all these ethnic groups, although positive results were found for hypertension in one ethnic group (see Table 2-3). The other two meta-analyses examined the potential role of the insertion/deletion polymorphism in the ACE gene, which has been investigated in numerous association studies with cardiovascular risk factors. Although significant

Table 2-2 Suggested Candidate Genes for Essential Hypertension

Renin-Angiotensin-Aldosterone System
Angiotensinogen (AGT)
Angiotensin II type 1 receptor (AGTR1)
Renin (REN)
Renin binding protein (RENBP)
Angiotensin-converting enzyme (ACE)
Steroid 18β-hydroxylase (CYP11B2)
Kallikrein 1 (KLK1)

G-Protein/Signal Transduction Pathway System
β_3 Subunit of G-protein gene 3 (GNB3)
α Subunit of the G stimulatory protein 1 (GNAS1)
Regulator of G-protein signaling 2 (RGS2)

Ion Channels
α Subunit of ENaC (SCNN1A)
β Subunit of ENaC (SCNN1B)
γ Subunit of ENaC (SCNN1G)
α-Adducin (ADD1)

Immune System and Inflammation
Nitric oxide synthase 3 (NOS3)
Interleukin-6 (IL-6)
Transforming growth factor-β_1 (TGFB1)

Sympathetic Nervous System
β_1-Adrenergic receptor (ADRB1)
β_2-Adrenergic receptor (ADRB2)
Dopamine receptor D_1 (DRD1)
Dopamine receptor D_3 (DRD3)

CYP11B2, cytochrome P450 11B2 isoenzyme; ENaC, epithelial sodium channel.

Table 2-3 Meta-analyses of Association Studies for Hypertension/Blood Pressure Candidate Genes

Authors	Polymorphism	Ethnicity	Number of Studies	Results
Sethi et al.[23]	AGT M235T	White, black, Asian	41	Nonsignificant for BP Significant for HT*
Province et al.[24]	AGT G-6A	White, black, Japanese, Chinese	9	Nonsignificant for BP
Agerholm-Larsen et al.[25]	ACE I/D	White	17	Nonsignificant for BP
Kato et al.[26]	AGT M235T	Japanese	6	Nonsignificant for HT
Staessen et al.[27]	ACE I/D	White	23	Nonsignificant for HT and BP

*Significant association with hypertension in white and Asian subjects, but not in black subjects; no significant association with blood pressure (systolic and diastolic) in any of the three ethnic groups.
ACE, angiotensin I–converting enzyme; AGT, angiotensinogen; BP, blood pressure; HT, hypertension; I/D, insertion/deletion.

association of the insertion/deletion polymorphism was found with ACE levels, both meta-analyses gave negative results for BP or hypertension.

Until recently, most genetic association studies have concentrated on one or, at most, two individual SNPs at a given locus. In the future, we would anticipate more genetic association studies using haplotype analysis, with the increased availability of tagging SNPs from the HapMap.

Admixture

As noted earlier, theoretical considerations suggest that the information generated by recent admixture of genetically distinct populations could be used to map disease-associated genes. If, for example, a disease variant and a marker allele exhibit substantially different frequencies across parental populations, strong LD between the disease variant and the marker may result, and it may be preserved for several generations in the admixed group if the disease variant and the marker are sufficiently close. Because of their history of admixture, many populations in the Americas, including African Americans and Mexican Americans, have been investigated using this approach.[28] As proof of principle, the Duffy blood group allele was mapped based on these assumptions in African Americans. This mutation confers resistance to *Falciparum vivax* malaria and occurs at a frequency of 100% in persons from endemic areas of Africa, but it is absent in other parts of the world.

Two types of admixture mapping have been proposed. In the *global approach,* one assumes that under conditions of equal environmental exposure, the phenotypic trait is more common in hypothetic population A than in population B. Individuals in the population that result from the admixture of A and B are genotyped at markers that are distinctive for one or the other of the ancestral populations. Only about 20 to 30 well-selected markers need to be used to distinguish populations that have been geographically separated for long periods of time (e.g., China versus Europe). Statistical analyses can then determine, on average, the percentage of the genome for a given individual that is derived from population A or B. If a correlation exists between the trait value and the percentage admixture, then one can infer that the contribution from the gene pool of population A contributed excess risk. So far, these methods have been tested using skin color as the phenotype in several populations.[29]

The global approach suffers from some important limitations, however. It is often difficult to remove the confounding effect of the environment. Thus, in stratified societies such as the United States, important environmental exposures are more common in one racial group than in others. If this environmental factor is the underlying cause of the increased prevalence, any genetic marker that is also more common in that population will falsely appear to be associated with the condition. This problem can only be partially eliminated by statistical methods that control for proxy measures of these environmental exposures because many are difficult to measure, and the presence of other unobserved exposures cannot be excluded. In addition, the global approach offers no indication of where in the genome the putative susceptibility genes may lie.

Locus-specific admixture, conversely, provides evidence of linkage for specific genomic locations when the appropriate populations are studied. With this approach, markers that can be designated as having arisen from one or the other of the parental populations are typed across the genome. If the variant from hypothetic population A is found more often than expected by chance in cases, then one can conclude that it is likely to represent a susceptibility locus, similar to the logic of family-based linkage studies. An initial test of this method from the FBPP demonstrated "overtransmission" among hypertensive patients of regions on chromosomes 6 and 21 (Fig. 2-1).[11] The region on chromosome 6 was identified in previous studies, thus lending credence to this observation; the significance of the finding on chromosome 21 is less clear. This study relied on a relatively sparse set of microsatellite markers, however, and had limited statistical power. A marker set is now available to provide greater information across the genome about European versus African ancestry,[30,31] and it could provide a reasonable test of the value of admixture mapping.

Pharmacogenetic Studies

Genetic technology has two potential applications in pharmacology that could be useful in hypertension and its treatment. First, considerable investment is being made in the use of molecular applications for drug discovery and development. It is hoped that information about susceptibility genes will provide novel targets, potentially even suggesting specific molecular configurations of new agents. This specialized topic is not discussed here, although it represents a potentially important application of molecular genetics technology. The second potential role of molecular genetics lies in the opportunity to tailor the choice of drug to an individual's genotype. The rationale and the conceptual difficulties of this strategy are described next.

Individual responses to antihypertensive medications vary substantially, and some of this variation is likely to result from genetics. The relative size of this source of variation associated with currently available drugs is difficult to estimate, however. Trials of antihypertensive agents routinely yield a standard deviation of systolic BP change in the range of 10 mm Hg, which usually implies that some individuals have no response whatsoever. The observed variation among individuals in such trials, however, includes substantial random noise introduced from normal fluctuations of BP that can be mistaken for true interindividual variation in drug response. What is required are data on repeated challenges of different drugs to the same individuals.

Repeated challenges with multiple drugs to the same patients have, in fact, documented correlations in change in BP of about 0.6, a finding suggesting a strong effect of factors specific to the individual. Several drug classes with different mechanisms of action, including inhibitors of the RAS, calcium channel blockers, adrenergic receptor blockers, and diuretics, are available for treatment of hypertension. However, it is difficult to predict the efficiency of response to antihypertensive medications in the individual patient. Currently, no clinically useful biomarkers for unerringly predicting individual responses to antihypertensive treatment are available. Candidate genes for regulating BP or metabolizing drugs are likely involved in the response to antihypertensive drug treatment. Hence, SNPs in these genes could be potential pharmacogenetic markers for predicting the response to a

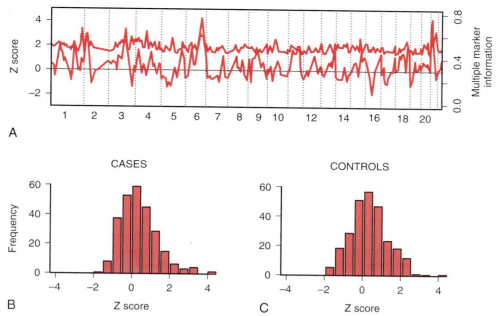

Figure 2–1   Genome-wide admixture mapping with microsatellite markers. **A**, Marker information content for admixture mapping *(upper line)* and genome-wide Z-score plot in cases *(lower line)*. Marker information content was measured by allele frequency difference in ancestry populations. For African Americans, the ancestry populations are African blacks and European whites. The Z score is a standardized measurement of excess of African ancestry at a marker location. It has an approximate standard normal distribution under the null hypothesis of no linkage. As shown, the highest Z scores are at chromosomes 6 and 21. **B**, The distribution of Z scores in cases. **C**, The distribution of Z scores in controls. The distribution of African ancestry was shifted upward in cases versus controls, a finding that suggests that some markers at the tail of distribution in **B** are linked with disease loci. (Modified from Zhu X, Luke A, Cooper RS, et al. Admixture mapping for hypertension loci with genome-scan markers. *Nat Genet.* 2005;37:177-181.)

certain drug and thus guide the selection of the optimal drug for each individual patient. By far the most extensively studied have been the genes involved in the RAS. For example, SNPs in two of the genes in the RAS, AGT and AGT type 1 receptor (AGTR1), have additive effects on BP response to a thiazide diuretic among African-American women.[32] Association studies for candidate genes in other physiologic pathways have also been reported. For example, a single SNP in another candidate gene in the G-protein/signal transduction pathway system, GNB3, has been associated with antihypertensive response to a thiazide diuretic.[33] However, no clear picture has emerged from such association studies. Thus, the potential utility of genetic characterization of predictors of response to antihypertensive drugs for individual patients has yet to be realized.

Racial or Geographic Population Effects

Differences in the prevalence of hypertension among various populations have long been considered potential evidence of genetic effects. The primary interest in this question has always focused on African Americans, who experience 50% higher rates of hypertension compared with Americans of European descent. The inferences from these epidemiologic analyses have all been indirect, however, because measurement of genetic variation at the molecular level was not feasible. In the genomic era, this topic has been revisited, thus highlighting both the challenges and the potential for genetic epidemiology.

Before racial or population differences can be studied rigorously, it is necessary to characterize what these demographic units represent and to define the average degree of genetic differentiation. Because *Homo sapiens* is a young species, regional differentiation is much lower than is found in other animal species. Depending on the set of markers chosen, 85% to 95% of the total genetic variation occurs within any large regional population, with the rest occurring among groups.[34] Furthermore, the appropriate size of each of the groups to be designated as distinct is problematic. Most analyses rely on the concept of "continental races," driven in part by the demography of the United States. Thus, groups designated as "African," "Asian," "European," "Native American," and "Pacific Islanders" are seen as primary categories.[35] However, many large regional populations, such as those in North Africa, the Middle East, Central Asia, and South Asia (India and Pakistan), are not adequately accounted for by this system. Because our species underwent most of its evolutionary development in Africa, diversity in modern African populations is more extensive than elsewhere[36]; a single reference category of "African" cannot capture that heterogeneity. Even within relatively small, isolated populations such as that of Iceland, important regional differentiation can be identified using the sophisticated methods now available.[37] The appropriate size of the population units that should be considered in a genetic analysis comparing hypertension frequency is thus far from obvious. Moreover, the mutations that influence BP in the general population are almost entirely undiscovered, and analyses of population differences are based solely on neutral or untranslated markers that have no direct consequence for the phenotype.

Quantitative statistical calculations, such as measures of heritability, do not provide insight into the overall impact of genes in various populations. Because this quantity represents the ratio of additive genetic effects to the total variance, it will be sensitive to the environmental context in which it is measured. A larger environmental effect will lead to a smaller relative genetic effect. Family studies that rely on linkage analysis also provide no information about the average impact of genes.

In fact, whether differences in hypertension among racial/ethnic populations have any basis in genetics is an unresolved question.[38] Environmental factors alone could account for the observed epidemiologic differentials between U.S. blacks and whites. Large differences in hypertension prevalence have been observed between U.S. whites and Europeans, groups that share a common genetic heritage, a finding demonstrating the possibility for environmentally induced contrasts.[39] Likewise, a gradient in prevalence exists among African-origin populations, with low rates in West Africa, moderate rates in the Caribbean, and high rates in the United States, again emphasizing the role of variation in causal exposures. Because many noncausal genetic variants occur at different frequencies in Europeans and Africans, a large potential risk for a false-positive result exists that does not take account of the confounding from environmental exposures. In effect, rigorous studies of this question can be undertaken only after the underlying genetic factors have been well characterized at the molecular level.

Direct examination of this question therefore requires knowledge of variants in specific genes. Two conditions must then be satisfied before the conclusion can be reached that genes account for differences in population risk. First, the variants must be consistently associated with hypertension in the two populations being compared. Second, the mutations themselves must be at different frequencies in each population. Even if these conditions are met, it must further be assumed that major gene-gene or gene-environment interactions are not present.

Gene-Environment Interactions

Conceptually, genes can be considered to have a *latent effect*. That is to say, the functional impact of a gene can be recognized only when it is expressed. Because organisms develop in a specific environment, it follows that the functional implications of a gene must always be considered the combination of the effects of variation in the DNA code and the conditioning influences of the external environment. Although the deleterious effect of some mutations is manifest more or less independently of the range of variation in the environment experienced by humans, for the genes that underlie the complex system regulating BP, it is more likely that gene-environment relationships are important.

Two basic sets of gene-environment relationships can be described in biologic systems. First, it is possible that the effects of alteration in one or the other parameter are simply additive. In its simplest form, for example, we may find that a specific variant has a constant proportional effect in both a low-risk and a high-risk environmental setting, and the effect

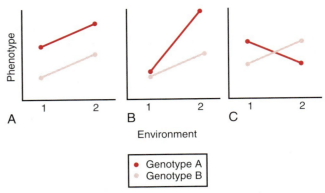

Figure 2-2   Gene-environment interaction. **A,** The differences between genotypes A and B are the same in two different environments, although the effect of genotype A is bigger than that of genotype B in both environments, a finding that indicates an absence of gene-environment interaction. **B,** Both genotypes have the same effect in environment 1, but genotype A has a much bigger effect than genotype B in environment 2, a finding that indicates gene-environment interaction. **C,** Genotype A has a bigger effect than genotype B in environment 1, but genotype B has a bigger effect than genotype A in environment 2, a finding that is a more extreme case for gene-environment interaction. (Modified from Anholt RH, Mackay TF. Quantitative genetic analyses of complex behaviours in *Drosophila. Nat Rev Genet.* 2004;5:838-849.)

of the environment is simply *additive* (Fig. 2-2A).[40] In populations with a low sodium intake, a specific mutation may therefore confer a 30% increase in lifetime risk of hypertension; the actual risk with persons carrying the genotype would still be relatively low. However, in a setting in which sodium intake is high, although the increase in risk would still be 30%, the absolute risk achieved would be higher given the greater background exposure. A second scenario posits a *multiplicative* effect (see Fig. 2-2B). Under these assumptions, the proportional increase in susceptibility in the high-risk environment in carriers relative to noncarriers would be larger than is found in the low-risk setting. If, in fact, large gene-environment interactions are present, then the potential would exist to provide patients with focused, individual-specific advice about prevention based on their genotype because the risk reduction could be quite large.

Although the interaction between genes and the environment is a well-established concept in quantitative genetics, it is difficult to apply to humans. In studies of plants, for example, it is easy to control both the genes and the environment, and the phenotypic effects may be apparent in a short time. Hypertension typically occurs after 50 years of low levels of exposure to factors that may be difficult to measure. In addition, of course, we currently lack good information about the genetic polymorphisms that influence risk.

One approach to the study of gene-environment interactions is the examination of genetically related populations or families in widely contrasting social settings. We have used this framework in studies of families of African descent in West Africa, the Caribbean, and the United States.[4] An overall additive effect of the environment is apparent from the large increase in population prevalence, which parallels increases in risk factors, as one moves from east to west. As noted earlier, some changes in heritability are also seen; however, although this reflects variation in the relative magnitude of the genetic versus environmental contributors, it does not specifically indicate the presence of interactions. Once appropriate markers have been identified, more detailed studies could attempt to characterize the molecular risk relationships.

For the moment, therefore, the goal of providing individualized risk assessment continues to elude us. Given the lifetime incidence risk of 70% to 80% in populations such as that of the United States, we know that the susceptibility genes for hypertension must be widespread in human populations. On average, it can therefore be assumed that exposure to dietary risk factors such as a high intake of sodium and low intake of fruits and vegetables interacts with common genetic variants in an additive fashion to raise BP. Whether some individuals experience a multiplicative effect on exposure is not yet known.

Implications for Research and Practice

Despite a very substantial investment since the mid-1990s, the genetics of complex diseases, including hypertension, remains an enigma. This has important potential implications for medicine in the genomic era. In this concluding section, we offer a perspective on the future of the genetic epidemiology of BP.

Contemporary research methods make the detection of deleterious mutations with a large effect that cause familial disorders a predictable and straightforward task. However, when applied to complex disorders such as hypertension, these techniques have met with very little success. If common variants with large effects were present in the population, it is likely that they would have already been detected. We can certainly anticipate that the refinement of epidemiologic and statistical approaches, and the rapid improvement in genotyping technology now occurring, will over time lead to the identification of loci with small or moderate effects. Before this can be accomplished, however, it may well be necessary first to work out in more detail whether the causal variants affect protein function or whether they moderate expression. Likewise, it will be crucial to understand whether common variants or large numbers of rare variants are involved. Currently, the most conservative prediction would suggest that both types of variants could be playing a role, thus further complicating the task.

Based on what is currently known, it is therefore difficult to argue that genetics will assume major importance in everyday medical practice related to hypertension. Of course, should major new developments occur, that prediction would become invalid. Nonetheless, within the foreseeable future, it is most reasonable to expect that the importance of genetics will be restricted to the field of research.

How can we justify the foregoing claims? It is axiomatic that genetics is most useful in conditions in which genes have a high penetrance or a large individual effect. Neither of those conditions applies to hypertension. If, in fact, multiple loci are involved, and various mutations within those genes contribute to overall risk, then the pattern found in any given individual will be a complex mosaic. Furthermore, if the sum effect of all these loci reflects important gene-gene and gene-environment interactions, then the statistical challenges will be even more daunting.

Conversely, this characterization by no means dismisses the ultimate importance of the project to unravel genetic effects, nor does it automatically imply that the challenges are any more difficult than those faced in earlier eras of biomedical research. It seems clear at this point, nonetheless, that the genomic revolution has led to excessively optimistic expectations among both researchers and practitioners. This situation creates the risk that the research agenda will be distorted by the unfounded belief that final answers can be obtained with current methods, and, contrariwise, that the small, incremental progress that is achieved will be dismissed as irrelevant.

The two most plausible clinical applications of genetics are risk stratification and drug development. The predictive value of a genetic test depends on the penetrance and the size of the effect. Because the risk markers for hypertension will be low to moderate on both those characteristics, as suggested earlier, it is difficult to see how genetic testing would be of value in the general population. Nonetheless, as has been the case in cancer, it is entirely possible that relatively uncommon variants with moderate effects will be present in high-risk families. Reliable tests that could be applied to young adults in these families would be of considerable value. In that setting, the diagnosis and treatment of prehypertension, with lifestyle interventions or drugs, would be particularly useful. Although drug treatment would still require adherence to standard guidelines, the intensity of preventive efforts could well be tailored to genotype. Further research may answer the question whether knowing the genetic makeup of an individual patient will add much to the phenotypic information we now have. In the area of drug development, many innovative applications of the available molecular tools are being used. Although the drugs currently on the market can control the BP of most patients, two or more drugs are often required, and side effects are relatively common.

Thus, while exploiting the unique strengths of genomics, the claims made about it should not be overstated, nor should they overshadow the pragmatic needs of the long-term movement toward prevention through creation of a healthier environment as the most effective means to control common diseases, including hypertension.

References

1. Cooper RS, Liao Y, Rotimi C. Is hypertension more severe among U.S. blacks, or is severe hypertension more common? *Ann Epidemiol.* 1996;**6**:173-180.
2. Wolf-Maier K, Cooper RS, Kramer H, et al. Hypertension treatment and control in five European countries, Canada, and the United States. *Hypertension.* 2004;**43**:10-17.
3. Feinleib M, Garrison RJ, Fabsitz R, et al. The NHLBI twin study of cardiovascular disease risk factors: Methodology and summary of results. *Am J Epidemiol.* 1977;**106**:284-285.
4. Zhu X, Bouzekri N, Southam L, et al. Linkage and association analysis of angiotensin I–converting enzyme (ACE)–gene polymorphisms with ACE concentration and blood pressure. *Am J Hum Genet.* 2001;**68**:1139-1148.
5. Ward R. Familial aggregation and genetic epidemiology of blood pressure. In: Laragh JH, Brenner BM (eds). Hypertension: Pathophysiology, Diagnosis and Management. New York: Raven Press, 1990, pp 81-89.

6. Thiel BA, Chakravarti A, Cooper RS, et al. A genome-wide linkage analysis investigating the determinants of blood pressure in whites and African Americans. *Am J Hypertens.* 2003;**16**:151-153.

7. Gabriel SB, Schaffner SF, Nguyen H, et al. The structure of haplotype blocks in the human genome. *Science.* 2002;**296**:2225-2229.

8. Pritchard JK, Cox NJ. The allelic architecture of human disease genes: Common disease–common variant … or not? *Hum Mol Genet.* 2002;**11**:2417-2423.

9. Cohen JC, Kiss RS, Pertsemlidis A, et al. Multiple rare alleles contribute to low plasma levels of HDL cholesterol. *Science.* 2004;**305**:869-872.

10. Spielman RS, McGinnis RE, Ewens WJ. Transmission test for linkage disequilibrium: The insulin gene region and insulin-dependent diabetes mellitus (IDDM). *Am J Hum Genet.* 1993;**52**:506-516.

11. Zhu X, Luke A, Cooper RS, et al. Admixture mapping for hypertension loci with genome-scan markers. *Nat Genet.* 2005;**37**:177-181.

12. Province MA, Kardia SL, Ranade K, et al. A meta-analysis of genome-wide linkage scans for hypertension: The National Heart, Lung and Blood Institute Family Blood Pressure Program. *Am J Hypertens.* 2003;**16**:144-147.

13. Koivukoski L, Fisher SA, Kanninen T, et al. Meta-analysis of genome-wide scans for hypertension and blood pressure in Caucasians shows evidence of susceptibility regions on chromosomes 2 and 3. *Hum Mol Genet.* 2004;**13**:2325-2332.

14. FBPP Investigators. Multi-center genetic study of hypertension: The Family Blood Pressure Program (FBPP). *Hypertension.* 2002;**39**:3-9.

15. Province MA. The significance of not finding a gene. *Am J Hum Genet.* 2001;**69**:660-663.

16. Koivukoski L, Fisher SA, Kanninen T, et al. Meta-analysis of genome-wide scans for hypertension and blood pressure in Caucasians shows evidence of susceptibility regions on chromosomes 2 and 3. *Hum Mol Genet.* 2004;1;**13**(**19**):2325-2332.

17. Wu X, Kan D, Province MA, et al. An updated meta-analysis of genome scans for hypertension and blood pressure in the NHLBI family blood pressure program (FBPP). *Am J Hypertens.* 2006;**19**:122-127.

18. Caulfield M, Munroe P, Pembroke J, et al. Genome-wide mapping of human loci for essential hypertension. *Lancet.* 2003;**361**:2118-2123.

19. Risch N, Merikangas K. The future of genetic studies of complex human diseases. *Science.* 1996;**273**:1516-1517.

20. Marziali A, Akeson M. New DNA sequencing methods. *Annu Rev Biomed Eng.* 2001;**3**:195-223.

21. Bader JS. The relative power of SNPs and haplotype as genetic markers for association tests. *Pharmacogenomics.* 2001;**2**:11-24.

22. International HapMap Consortium. The International HapMap Project. *Nature.* 2003;**426**:789-796.

22a. Jeunemaitre X, Soubrier F, Kotelevtsev YV, et al. Molecular basis of human hypertension: Role of angiotensinogen. *Cell.* 1992;**71**(**1**):169-180.

23. Sethi AA, Nordestgaard BG, Tybjaerg-Hansen A. Angiotensinogen gene polymorphism, plasma angiotensinogen, and risk of hypertension and ischemic heart disease: A meta-analysis. *Arterioscler Thromb Vasc Biol.* 2003;**23**:1269-1275.

24. Province MA, Boerwinkle E, Chakravarti A, et al. Lack of association of the angiotensinogen-6 polymorphism with blood pressure levels in the comprehensive NHLBI Family Blood Pressure Program: National Heart, Lung and Blood Institute. *J Hypertens.* 2000;**18**:867-876.

25. Agerholm-Larsen B, Nordestgaard BG, Tybjaerg-Hansen A. ACE gene polymorphism in cardiovascular disease: Meta-analyses of small and large studies in whites. *Arterioscler Thromb Vasc Biol.* 2000;**20**:484-492.

26. Kato N, Sugiyama T, Morita H, et al. Angiotensinogen gene and essential hypertension in the Japanese: Extensive association study and meta-analysis on six reported studies. *J Hypertens.* 1999;**17**:757-763.

27. Staessen JA, Wang JG, Ginocchio G, et al. The deletion/insertion polymorphism of the angiotensin converting enzyme gene and cardiovascular-renal risk. *J Hypertens.* 1997;**15**:1579-1592.

28. McKeigue PM. Prospects for admixture mapping of complex traits. *Am J Hum Genet.* 2005;**76**:1-767.

29. Parra FC, Amado RC, Lambertucci JR, et al. Color and genomic ancestry in Brazilians. *Proc Natl Acad Sci USA.* 2003;**100**:177-182.

30. Smith MW, Patterson N, Lautenberger JA, et al. A high-density admixture map for disease gene discovery in African Americans. *Am J Hum Genet.* 2004;**74**:1001-1013.

31. Patterson N, Hattangadi N, Lane B, et al. Methods for high-density admixture mapping of disease genes. *Am J Hum Genet.* 2004;**74**:979-1000.

32. Frazier L, Turner ST, Schwartz GL, et al. Multilocus effects of the renin-angiotensin-aldosterone system genes on blood pressure response to a thiazide diuretic. *Pharmacogenomics J.* 2004;**4**:17-23.

33. Turner ST, Schwartz GL, Chapman AB, Boerwinkle E. C825T polymorphism of the G protein beta(3)-subunit and antihypertensive response to a thiazide diuretic. *Hypertension.* 2001;**37**:739-743.

34. Romualdi C, Balding D, Nasidze IS, et al. Patterns of human diversity, within and among continents, inferred from biallelic DNA polymorphisms. *Genome Res.* 2002;**12**:602-612.

35. Mountain JL, Risch N. Assessing genetic contributions to phenotypic differences among "racial" and "ethnic" groups. *Nat Genet.* 2004;**36**:S48-53.

36. Jorde LB, Watkins WS, Bamshad MJ, et al. The distribution of human genetic diversity: A comparison of mitochondrial, autosomal, and Y-chromosome data. *Am J Hum Genet.* 2000;**66**:979-988.

37. Helgason A, Yngvadottir B, Hrafnkelsson B, et al. An Icelandic example of the impact of population structure on association studies. *Nat Genet.* 2005;**37**:90-95.

38. Cooper R, Rotimi C. Hypertension in populations of West African origin: Is there a genetic predisposition? *J Hypertens.* 1994;**12**:215-227.

39. Cooper RS, Wolf-Maier K, Luke A, et al. An international comparative study of blood pressure in populations of European vs. African descent. *BMC Med.* 2005;**3**:2 (available at http://www.biomedcentral.com/1741-7015/3/2. Accessed April 1, 2005).

40. Anholt RH, Mackay TF. Quantitative genetic analyses of complex behaviours in *Drosophila. Nat Rev Genet.* 2004;**5**:838-849.

Chapter 3

Pathophysiology of Hypertension

Veronica Franco, David A. Calhoun, and Suzanne Oparil

In most (>90%) of cases of human hypertension, no specific mechanism can be identified to account for blood pressure (BP) elevation or to guide preventive or therapeutic strategies. High BP tends to cluster in families and represents a collection of genetically based diseases or syndromes with resultant inherited biochemical abnormalities.[1-4] The resulting phenotypes can be modulated by various environmental factors, thereby altering the severity of BP elevation and related target organ damage, as well as the timing of onset of hypertension.

Many pathophysiologic factors have been implicated in the genesis of hypertension. These include the following: increased sympathetic nervous system activity; heightened exposure or response to psychosocial stress; overproduction of sodium (Na^+)–retaining hormones and vasoconstrictors; long-term high Na^+ intake; inadequate dietary intake of potassium (K^+) and calcium (Ca^{2+}); increased or inappropriate renin secretion with resultant increased production of angiotensin II (Ang II) and aldosterone; deficiencies of vasodilators, such as prostacyclin, nitric oxide (NO), the natriuretic peptides, and a variety of other vasodilator peptides, including the angiotensin (1-7) peptide, calcitonin gene–related peptide (CGRP), substance P, and adrenomedullin; alterations in expression of the kallikrein-kinin system that affect vascular tone and renal salt handling; abnormalities of resistance vessels, including selective lesions in the renal microvasculature; diabetes mellitus; insulin resistance; obesity; increased activity of vascular growth factors; alterations in adrenergic receptors that influence heart rate, inotropic properties of the heart, and vascular tone; and altered cellular ion transport (Fig. 3-1).[1] The novel concept that structural and functional abnormalities in the vasculature, including endothelial dysfunction (with associated overexpression of endothelin and reduced generation/availability of NO), increased oxidative stress, vascular remodeling, and decreased compliance, may antedate hypertension and contribute to its pathogenesis has gained support in recent years.

Although many factors clearly contribute to the pathogenesis and maintenance of BP elevation, renal mechanisms probably play a primary role, as hypothesized by Fahr and Borst and Borst-de Geus, systematized by Guyton, and reinforced by extensive experimental and clinical data. Other mechanisms amplify (e.g., sympathetic nervous system activity and vascular remodeling) or buffer (e.g., increased natriuretic peptide or kallikrein-kinin expression) the pressor effects of renal salt and water retention. These interacting pathways play major roles in both increasing BP and mediating related target organ damage. Understanding these complex mechanisms has important implications for the targeting of antihypertensive therapy to effect more efficient BP control and to achieve benefits beyond BP lowering.

GENETICS

Genes clearly contribute to variation in BP: analyses of BP patterns in families suggest that genetic factors account for 40% to 50% of BP variance, whereas shared environment accounts for 10% to 30% of variance.[5] See Chapter 2 for a more comprehensive discussion of this topic. Twin studies document greater concordance of BPs in monozygotic than dizygotic twins,[6] and population studies show greater similarity in BP within than among families.[7] The latter observation is not entirely attributable to a shared environment, because adoption studies demonstrate greater concordance of BP among biologic siblings than adoptive siblings living in the same household.[8] Single genes can have major effects on BP, thus accounting for the rare mendelian forms of high and low BP.[4,5] Mendelian forms of BP deviation (both increases and decreases), as reviewed by Harrap,[5] are summarized in Table 3-1. These mutations affect BP by altering renal salt handling, thereby reinforcing the hypothesis of Guyton that the development of hypertension depends on genetically determined renal dysfunction with resultant salt and water retention (Fig. 3-2).[9]

Although major mutations in these genes do not account for the burden of hypertension in the population, deoxyribonucleic acid (DNA) variants in these and other candidate genes with more subtle effects on gene expression or function may have greater impact.[5] For example, whereas Gitelman's syndrome is caused by rare homozygous mutations in the Na^+/chloride (Cl^-) cotransporter (*NCCT*) gene, which leads to loss of function and thus reduced renal tubular Na^+ reabsorption, other polymorphisms of the same gene have been associated with hypertension and an exaggerated natriuretic response to thiazide diuretic administration, a finding suggesting enhancement of function.[10] The hypertensive diathesis was seen even in persons heterozygous for these alleles, and this increases the likelihood that these genetic factors may contribute to BP elevation in some populations and may predict a favorable response to thiazide diuretic treatment. The latter prediction is biologically plausible, because the NCCT located in the distal tubule is the target of the diuretic effect of thiazides. Thus, further study of these mendelian forms of high and low BP may elucidate pathophysiologic mechanisms that predispose to more common forms of hypertension and may suggest novel therapeutic approaches.[4,5]

The best-studied monogenic cause of hypertension is Liddle's syndrome, a rare but clinically important disorder in which constitutive activation of the epithelial Na^+ channel (ENaC) predisposes to severe, treatment-resistant hypertension.[11] Constitutive ENaC activation related to mutations in the β or γ subunits of the channel causes inappropriate Na^+

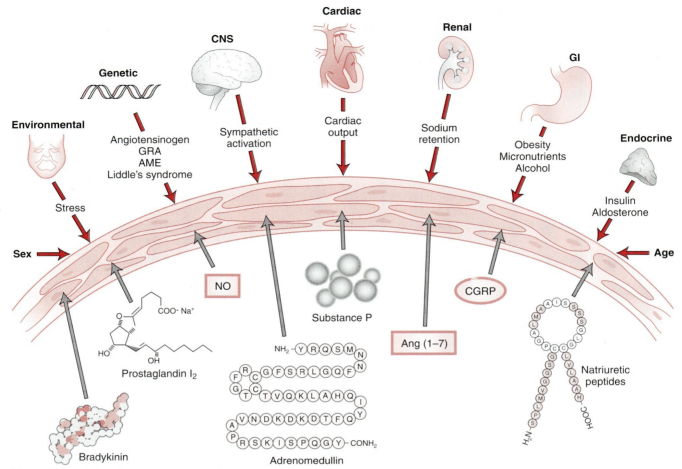

Figure 3–1 Pathophysiologic mechanisms of hypertension. *Red arrows* show hypertension-promoting mechanisms; *gray arrows* show hypertension-opposing mechanisms. AME, syndrome of apparent mineralocorticoid excess; Ang (1-7), angiotensin (1-7) peptide; CGRP, calcitonin gene–related peptide; CNS, central nervous system; GI, gastrointestinal; GRA, glucocorticoid-remediable aldosteronism; NO, nitric oxide. (Modified from Calhoun DA, Zaman A, Oparil S. Etiology and pathogenesis of systemic hypertension. *In:* Crawford MH, DiMarco JP [eds]. Cardiology. Philadelphia: Mosby, 2001, pp 1.1-1.10.)

retention at the level of the renal collecting duct. Gain-of-function mutations in short, proline-rich segments in the carboxyl termini of the ENaC subunits result in either an inability to remove active channels from the apical cell surface, thus causing them to remain constitutively active, or direct kinetic activation of the channels. This function appears to be mediated by binding of cytoskeletal proteins to the proline-rich segment of the channels. Affected patients typically present with volume-dependent, low-renin, and low-aldosterone hypertension. Renal transplantation completely corrects the disorder, a finding indicating that the defect is intrinsic to the kidney. Patients with Liddle's syndrome also respond to the administration of triamterene or amiloride, inhibitors of ENaC. Liddle's syndrome is very rare and does not contribute substantially to the prevalence of hypertension in the general population.[12]

In selected populations, however, ENaC activation may be a more common cause of hypertension. For example, ENaC activation, as evidenced by increased Na^+ conductance in peripheral lymphocytes, has been noted in 25% of patients with resistant hypertension (BP uncontrolled on ≥ three

medications) who present at our clinic.[13] In contrast, none of the tested patients with stage 1 hypertension had constitutively active ENaC. A therapeutic trial with amiloride was undertaken in this population and resulted in dramatically decreased BP in patients with constitutively activated EnaC, but modest effects in patients with refractory hypertension but normal ENaC activity. These findings exemplify the concept that genetic causes of hypertension, albeit uncommon in general hypertensive populations, may be more frequent in selected patient populations, particularly in those resistant to conventional pharmacologic therapies.

Identification of genes having relevance to disease development and progression, so-called candidate genes, is the traditional approach to the problem of finding BP-related genes. The candidate gene approach typically compares the prevalence of hypertension or the level of BP among individuals of contrasting genotypes at candidate loci in pathways known to be involved in BP regulation. The most promising findings of such studies relate to genes of the renin-angiotensin-aldosterone system (RAAS). These include the *M235T* variant in the angiotensinogen gene, which has been associated with

Table 3-1   Rare Mendelian Forms of Blood Pressure Deviation

Disease	Phenotype	Genetic Cause
Glucocorticoid-remediable hyperaldosteronism	Autosomal dominant, hypertension, variable hyperaldosteronism	Chimeric 11β-hydroxylase aldosterone synthase gene
Syndrome of apparent mineralocorticoid excess	Autosomal recessive, volume expansion, hypokalemia, low renin and aldosterone	Mutations in the 11β-hydroxysteroid dehydrogenase gene
Liddle's syndrome	Autosomal dominant, hypertension, volume expansion, hypokalemia, low renin and aldosterone	Mutation subunits of the epithelial Na+ channel SCNN1B and SCNN1G genes
Pseudohypoaldosteronism type II (Gordon's syndrome)	Autosomal dominant, hypertension, hyperkalemia, volume expansion, normal glomerular filtration rate	Linkage to chromosomes 1q31-q42 and 17p11-q21
Gitelman's syndrome	Autosomal recessive, low blood pressure, hypokalemic alkalosis, hypocalciuria	Mutations in the Na+/Cl− cotransporter NCCT gene
Bartter's syndrome	Autosomal recessive, low blood pressure, hypokalemic alkalosis, hypercalciuria	Mutations in the Na+/K+/2Cl− cotransporter NKCC2 gene or mutations in the K+ channel ROMK gene
Bartter's syndrome type III	Autosomal recessive, low blood pressure, hypokalemic alkalosis, hypercalciuria without nephrocalcinosis	Mutations in the Cl− channel CLCNKB gene
Pseudohypoaldosteronism type I: severe	Autosomal recessive, low blood pressure, renal salt wasting, hyperkalemia and metabolic acidosis, elevated aldosterone levels	Mutation subunits of the epithelial Na+ channel SCNN1B and SCNN1G genes
Pseudohypoaldosteronism type I: mild	Autosomal recessive, low blood pressure, renal salt wasting, hyperkalemia and metabolic acidosis, elevated aldosterone levels that remit with age	Mutations in mineralocorticoid receptor gene
Polycystic kidney disease	Autosomal dominant, renal cysts, hypertension and renal failure, liver cysts, cerebral aneurysms, valvular heart disease	Mutations in the PKD1 and PKD2 genes
Pheochromocytoma	Multiple endocrine neoplasia type 2A: autosomal dominant, medullary thyroid carcinoma, pheochromocytoma, hyperparathyroidism	Mutations in the RET proto-oncogene
	von Hippel–Lindau disease: autosomal dominant, retinal angiomas, hemangioblastoma of the cerebellum and spinal cord, renal cell carcinomas, adrenal pheochromocytomas	Mutations in the VHL tumor suppressor gene
	Neurofibromatosis type 1: autosomal dominant, multiple neurofibromas, café au lait spots, Lisch's nodules of the iris and pheochromocytomas	Mutations in the NF1 tumor suppressor gene
	Nonsyndromic pheochromocytomas	Mutations in RET, VHL, SDHB, SDHD genes
Hypertension exacerbated in pregnancy	Autosomal dominant, early-onset, severe hypertension with low aldosterone levels, exacerbated in pregnancy	Missense mutation resulting in substitution of leucine for serine at codon 810 (MR$_{L810}$)

Cl−, chloride; K+, potassium; Na+, sodium.

increased circulating angiotensinogen levels and BP in many distinct populations[14-16]; an insertion/deletion (I/D) polymorphism in intron 16 of the angiotensin-converting enzyme (ACE) gene associated with differences in ACE activity, which increases in codominant fashion with the D allele,[17] and in some studies with BP variation in men[18,19]; and a polymorphism (A1166C) in the 3′ untranslated region of the Ang II type 1 receptor (AT$_1$R) gene associated with hypertension, especially pregnancy-induced hypertension, myocardial infarction, lacunar infarction of the brain, and accelerated deterioration in renal function.[20] The D allele of the ACE gene has also been associated with several cardiovascular phenotypes, including higher BP levels and greater risk of target organ damage in hypertensive individuals.[21] A Gly460Trp polymorphism of the α-adducin gene has been associated with hypertension in some populations.[22,23] Carriers of one or

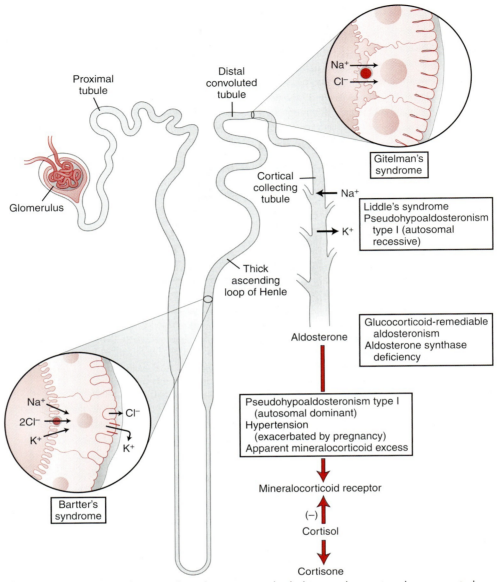

Figure 3–2   Molecular mechanisms mediating salt reabsorption in the kidney and associated monogenic hypertensive diseases. Monogenetic diseases that alter blood pressure are shown in *boxes*. (From Nabel EG. Cardiovascular disease. *N Engl J Med.* 2003;**349**:60-72.)

two copies of the variant Trp460 allele display high rates of renal tubular Na$^+$ reabsorption and a volume-expanded form of hypertension, associated with impaired natriuresis,[24] low plasma renin activity,[25] and greater BP reduction in response to a low-Na$^+$ diet.[25]

Analysis of gene variation has the potential to improve our understanding of determinants of antihypertensive drug response, to individualize drug selection (see also Chapter 2).[23] This is an important issue for the clinician, because BP responses and clinical outcomes of treatment with specific antihypertensive drugs vary greatly from patient to patient, and traditional predictors of response are of limited value in identifying the optimal drug and optimal dose for an individual. Accordingly, many of the large, randomized, controlled outcome trials of antihypertensive treatment have a

pharmacogenetic component, designed to determine whether genotype interacts with the type of antihypertensive drug treatment to modify the risk of cardiovascular disease outcomes.[26] Results of those large pharmacogenomic studies are forthcoming.

To date, differential BP responses to antihypertensive drugs have been demonstrated in association with various genotypes in small studies. For example, the BP response to diuretics has been shown to be more pronounced in persons with the variant Trp460 adducin allele than in those homozygous for the wild type in most,[27] but not all,[28] studies, particularly after adjustment for covariates, including ethnicity, gender, age, and waist-to-hip ratio. Further, in an observational, case-control study carried out in 1038 hypertensive subjects, diuretic therapy was associated with a lower risk of myocardial infarction or stroke than other antihypertensive therapies in carriers of the adducin variant.[29] Similarly, ACE genotype predicted BP response to hydrochlorothiazide in a gender-specific manner: the BP effect of hydrochlorothiazide increased progressively with the number of I alleles among women and with the number of D alleles among men.[30] In addition, the genotypes that were associated with the greatest BP responses to hydrochlorothiazide (II homozygotes in women and DD homozygotes in men) had the lowest pretreatment aldosterone excretion and the greatest increase in urinary aldosterone in response to the diuretic. However, these genotypic variants seem to affect baseline BP and antihypertensive medication responsiveness only modestly, and they lack consistency across populations. Thus, pharmacogenomic studies of antihypertensive treatment strategies remain in their infancy and have yet to affect clinical practice.

In most cases, hypertension results from a complex interaction of genetic, environmental, and demographic factors, and it is therefore unlikely that a few major genes account for the pathogenesis of this heterogeneous disorder. Improved techniques of genetic analysis, especially genome-wide linkage analysis, have enabled a search for complex sets of genes that may contribute to the development of primary hypertension in the population.[31-33] Recently, genomic mapping strategies have been combined with high-throughput differential gene expression profiling, a transcriptomic approach, in the search for novel genes that are likely to be involved in the pathogenesis of hypertension.[34] Computational methods for performing genome-wide association analysis using data from expression profiling (i.e., microarray data) that are currently under development have the potential for revealing novel coding and noncoding genomic regions that regulate the phenotypes of hypertension and related cardiovascular disease.[35]

INHERITED CARDIOVASCULAR RISK FACTORS

Cardiovascular risk factors, including hypertension, tend to co-segregate more commonly than would be expected by chance. Approximately 40% of persons with essential hypertension also have hypercholesterolemia, and genetic studies have established a clear association between hypertension and dyslipidemia.[36] Hypertension and type 2 diabetes mellitus also tend to coexist. The leading cause of death in patients with type 2 diabetes is coronary heart disease, and diabetes increases the risk for acute myocardial infarction as much as a previous myocardial infarction in a nondiabetic person.[37] Because many of the cardiovascular complications of diabetes are attributable to hypertension, diabetic patients need aggressive antihypertensive treatment, with a BP goal of less than 130/80 mm Hg,[38] as well as treatment of dyslipidemia and glucose control.

Hypertension, insulin resistance, dyslipidemia, and obesity often occur concomitantly and are frequently associated with microalbuminuria, high serum uric acid levels, hypercoagulability, and accelerated atherosclerosis.[39] This constellation of abnormalities, both genetic and environmental, referred to as the *metabolic syndrome,* increases cardiovascular disease risk. Physicians must assess and treat these risk factors individually and must recognize that many hypertensive patients have insulin resistance, dyslipidemia, or both.

SYMPATHETIC NERVOUS SYSTEM

Increased sympathetic nervous system activity is a major determinant of BP elevation. It contributes to both the development and the maintenance of hypertension through stimulation of the heart, peripheral vasculature, and kidneys, thus causing increased cardiac output, increased vascular resistance, and fluid retention.[40] Autonomic imbalance (increased sympathetic tone accompanied by reduced parasympathetic tone) has been associated with many metabolic, hemodynamic, trophic, and rheologic abnormalities that result in vascular damage and ultimately in increased cardiovascular morbidity and mortality (Fig. 3-3). Several population-based studies, such as the Coronary Artery Risk Development in Young Adults (CARDIA) study,[41] have shown a positive correlation between heart rate and the development of hypertension (elevated diastolic BP). Because in humans, sustained increases in heart rate are mainly the result of decreased parasympathetic tone, these findings support the concept that autonomic imbalance contributes to the pathogenesis of hypertension. Diastolic BP relates more closely to vascular resistance than to cardiac function per se, and these results also suggest that increased sympathetic tone may increase diastolic BP by causing vascular smooth muscle cell (VSMC) proliferation and vascular remodeling. Norepinephrine spillover studies, which provide an index of norepinephrine release from sympathoeffector nerve terminals, demonstrate that sympathetic cardiac stimulation is greater in young hypertensive patients than in normotensive controls of similar age, a finding supporting the interpretation that increased cardiac sympathetic stimulation may contribute to the development of hypertension.[42]

The mechanisms of increased sympathetic nervous system activity in hypertension are complex and involve alterations in baroreflex and chemoreflex pathways at both peripheral and central levels (Fig. 3-4). Reflex and behavioral control of BP is integrated in the rostral ventrolateral nucleus of the medulla oblongata (RVLM), sometimes referred to as the vasomotor control center.[43] Cell bodies of efferent cardiovascular stimulatory neurons of the sympathetic nervous system lie in the C_1 subregion, which also receives and sends neural projections to and from many other brain centers. The most critical RVLM input comes from the adjacent nucleus tractus solitarius (NTS), which receives afferent fibers from stretch-sensitive mechanoreceptors in the carotid sinus and aortic arch (aortocarotid baroreflexes) and the cardiac atria and ventricles (cardiopulmonary baroreflexes).[44]

Acute adjustments in BP to maintain stable perfusion pressure and blood flow to peripheral organs are accomplished via these baroreflex pathways. Stretch receptors in the walls of the aorta and carotid artery sense acute increases in arterial pressure and initiate negative afferent signals that stimulate the NTS to limit efferent sympathetic outflow.[43] Conversely, reductions in BP unload the aortocarotid baroreflexes and send positive afferent signals via the NTS to activate efferent sympathetic outflow, thus increasing BP via positive inotropic and chronotropic effects on the heart and arteriolar and venous vasoconstriction. Similarly, low-pressure stretch receptors in the heart and great veins sense acute changes in central blood volume, or cardiac preload, and trigger cardiopulmonary baroreflexes. Decreases in preload, whether caused by blood loss, salt depletion, upright posture, or

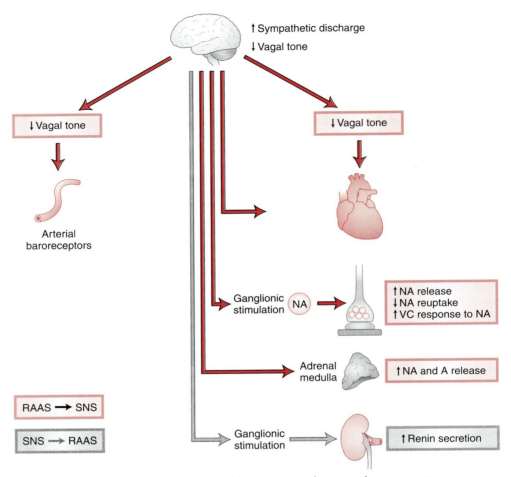

Figure 3–3 Schematic representation of the sites of possible interactions between the autonomic nervous system and the renin-angiotensin-aldosterone system (RAAS). These influences are bidirectional, meaning that the RAAS increases sympathetic tone *(red arrows)*, and, conversely, the sympathetic nervous system (SNS) activates the RAAS *(gray arrows)*. In particular, angiotensin II potentiates adrenergic cardiovascular drive at the level of both the central nervous system and peripheral nerves, where it favors sympathetic neural discharge, norepinephrine (NA [noradrenaline]) release, and norepinephrine-mediated vasoconstrictor (VC) responses and reduces norepinephrine reuptake by adrenergic nerve terminals. Angiotensin II also promotes increased norepinephrine and epinephrine (A [adrenaline]) secretion from adrenal glands. Via these proadrenergic effects, angiotensin II may participate in the development of sympathetic overactivity in the setting of essential hypertension. Angiotensin II exerts parasympatholytic effects by reducing vagal tone via both central and reflex mechanisms (arterial baroreceptor impairment). Increased adrenergic tone enhances renin release from the kidney. (Modified from Grassi G. Renin-angiotensin-sympathetic crosstalks in hypertension: Reappraising the relevance of peripheral interactions. *J Hypertens.* 2001;**19**:1713-1716.)

(experimentally) by lower body negative pressure, lead to sympathetic nervous system activation with resultant increases in muscle sympathetic nerve activity, renal vascular resistance, renal overflow of norepinephrine, plasma renin activity and Ang II levels, and reductions in forearm and splanchnic blood flow.[43,45] Conversely, extracellular fluid volume expansion, often related to dietary salt supplementation, activates the low-pressure cardiopulmonary receptors, which send negative afferent signals that stimulate the NTS to reduce sympathetic outflow.

The NTS also receives signals from stimulatory chemoreceptors in the kidneys and skeletal muscle and integrates a variety of signals from stimulatory and inhibitory centers in other brain regions, including the area postrema, which does not have a blood-brain barrier.[46] The area postrema is exquisitely sensitive to circulating Ang II, which acts to blunt the inhibitory effect of the NTS, thereby increasing RVLM-dependent sympathetic nervous system outflow. Sensory input from excitatory peripheral chemoreceptor afferent neurons in the kidney and skeletal muscle also enhances or sustains RVLM-dependent sympathetic outflow.

Studies in animal models of hypertension have clearly elucidated a role for these neuronal groups in BP control. For example, ablation of the NTS in normotensive rats causes increased sympathetic nervous system outflow and either severe BP lability or severe chronic hypertension with target organ damage, which can be abolished by simultaneous lesions of the RVLM.[43] Lesions in the area postrema lower BP

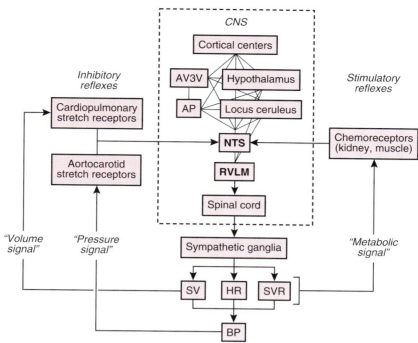

Figure 3–4   Central nervous system control of sympathetic outflow. Efferent sympathetic nervous system (SNS) output is the result of integrated actions of several central nervous system (CNS) centers, including many areas of the cortex as well as lower centers in the hypothalamus, basal ganglia (especially the locus ceruleus), and circumventricular regions, including the area postrema (AP). The critical integrator region is the nucleus tractus solitarius (NTS) in the medulla oblongata. The NTS receives inhibitory afferent signals from the baroreflexes (volume and pressure signals) and stimulatory afferent signals from renal and muscular chemoreceptors (metabolic signals). SNS outflow is ultimately dependent on stimulation of the rostral ventrolateral medulla (the RVLM or vasomotor control center), which is tonically inhibited by the adjacent NTS. Circumventricular regions such as the AP have no blood-brain barrier, and stimulation of the AP by circulating angiotensin II blunts the inhibitory effects of the NTS. RVLM stimulation sends signals via the spinal cord and sympathetic ganglia to regulate heart rate (HR), cardiac stroke volume (SV), and systemic vascular resistance (SVR), which together determine blood pressure (BP) levels. AV3V, anteroventral third ventricular area of the brain. (From Izzo JL Jr. The sympathetic nervous system in acute and chronic blood pressure elevation. In: Oparil S, Weber MA [eds]. Hypertension, 2nd ed. A Companion to Brenner & Rector's The Kidney. Philadelphia: Elsevier, 2005, pp 60-76.)

in rats with genetic and steroid-induced hypertension, whereas stimulation of the area postrema by Ang II sustains hypertension in these models.[46]

Neuronal groups within the hypothalamus integrate behavioral and cardiovascular responses to environmental stress by modulating sympathetic nervous system function.[43] The posterolateral hypothalamus mediates defense reactions such as the fight-or-flight response, which induces massive RVLM activation, associated with increased heart rate and BP and vasodilation in skeletal muscle. The median preoptic nucleus integrates water balance and thirst-sensing mechanisms with cardiovascular signals and may mediate organ-specific responses such as skeletal muscle vasodilation. It is likely that this complex interplay of central nervous system influences on sympathetic nervous system outflow, so elegantly delineated in animal models, may also play a role in BP control and in the pathogenesis of hypertension in humans. For example, Izzo and associates demonstrated that a person's hemodynamic responses to environmental stimuli vary according to his or her cognitive appraisal of the nature of the stimulus.[43,47,48] Stimuli perceived as challenging or manageable are characterized by sympathetic nervous system–mediated increases in cardiac output, whereas stimuli per-

ceived as threatening or outside the individual's range of control are associated with systemic vasoconstriction.

The hypothalamus also has chronic, sustained, regionally specific effects on BP. For example, stimulation of the posterior hypothalamus tends to elevate BP, and lesions in this region reduce BP in a variety of animal models of hypertension. In contrast, lesions of the anterior hypothalamus increase BP via adrenomedullary stimulation in normotensive animals, whereas electrical stimulation of this region causes hypotension. Ablation of the paraventricular nucleus prevents the development of hypertension in the spontaneously hypertensive rat (SHR).

Salt sensitivity of BP is mediated by activation of central and peripheral nervous systems,[49] and the mechanism of neurally mediated salt-sensitive hypertension has been elucidated in studies carried out in SHR.[50] In this model, dietary salt increases BP by reducing norepinephrine release from nerve terminals in the anterior hypothalamic area (AHA), thus reducing activation of local sympathoinhibitory neurons (Fig. 3-5). This, in turn, results in increased sympathetic outflow and higher BP. Two mechanisms contribute to this effect: (1) reduced noradrenergic input into the AHA via baroreflex pathways and (2) local inhibition of norepinephrine release in

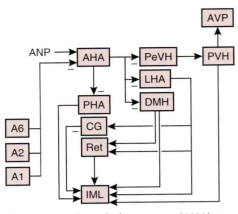

Figure 3–5　Anterior hypothalamic area (AHA) in salt-sensitive hypertension. Schematic representation of the major noradrenergic projections to the AHA and the major direct and indirect projection from the AHA to "pressor" nuclei. In spontaneously hypertensive rats (SHR), increased activity of the inhibitory neuromodulator ANP in the AHA and reduced input from baroreceptor afferents synapsing in brainstem nuclei reduce norepinephrine release in the AHA, resulting in reduced inhibitory control of sympathetic outflow. The (–) indicates synaptic inhibition. A1, A2, A6, brainstem noradrenergic nuclei; ANP, atrial natriuretic peptide; AVP, arginine vasopressin release; CG, central gray of the midbrain; DMH, dorsomedial nucleus of the hypothalamus; IML, preganglionic sympathetic nucleus; LHA, lateral hypothalamic area; PeVH, periventricular hypothalamic nucleus; PHA, posterior hypothalamic area; PVH, paraventricular hypothalamic nucleus; Ret, medullary reticular formation. (From Oparil S, Chen YF, Berecek K, et al. The role of the central nervous system in hypertension. *In:* Laragh JH, Brenner BM [eds]. Hypertension: Pathophysiology, Diagnosis, and Management. New York: Raven Press, 1995, pp 713-740.)

the AHA by the inhibitory neuromodulator atrial natriuretic peptide (ANP). Microinjection studies in which a blocking monoclonal antibody to ANP is introduced directly into the AHA and the NTS have shown that endogenous ANP in the brain is functionally active in the tonic control of BP and baroreflex sensitivity in the SHR, but it plays a lesser role in the normotensive Wistar Kyoto control animal. In the normotensive animal, excitation of NTS neurons by baroreflex afferents leads to activation of sympathoinhibitory neurons in NTS and AHA, strong inhibition of sympathetic nervous system outflow, and a decrease in BP. In SHR, brain ANP acts at the levels of the NTS and the AHA to perturb this baroreflex regulatory pathway. Endogenous ANP tonically activates sympathoinhibitory neurons in the caudal NTS of SHR, thereby restraining the rise in BP, and it tonically inhibits baroreflex responsiveness to alterations in BP. Thus, ANP appears to act at a number of sites in brain to facilitate the development and maintenance of sympathetically mediated hypertension in the SHR model.

Arterial baroreceptors are reset to a higher pressure in hypertensive persons, and this peripheral resetting may return to normal when BP is normalized.[51,52] Resuming normal baroreflex function helps to maintain reductions in BP, a beneficial regulatory mechanism that may be clinically important.[53] Central resetting of the aortic baroreflex also occurs in hypertensive subjects, thus disinhibiting sympathetic outflow after activation of aortic baroreceptor nerves.[54] This baroreflex resetting is at least partly mediated by a central action of Ang II,[55] which also amplifies the response to sympathetic stimulation by a peripheral mechanism, presynaptic facilitatory modulation of norepinephrine release.[56] Additional small molecule mediators that suppress baroreceptor activity and contribute to exaggerated sympathetic drive in hypertension include reactive oxygen species and endothelin.[57,58]

In addition to resetting, arterial baroreflex blunting, whereby the relative ability of a given increase in BP to reduce sympathetic outflow is diminished, also occurs in hypertensive subjects.[43] Arterial baroreflex blunting in hypertension has been attributed to increased arterial stiffness and reduced mechanoreceptor distensibility.[43,59] Blunting of cardiopulmonary baroreflexes has also been described in hypertension and in aging. Thus, baroreflex blunting provides an attractive unifying explanation for age-related increases in vascular stiffness, BP, and sympathetic nervous system activity.

Finally, hypertensive subjects show evidence of exaggerated chemoreflex function, leading to markedly enhanced sympathetic activation in response to stimuli such as apnea and hypoxia.[60] A clinical correlate of this phenomenon is the exaggerated increase in sympathetic nervous system activity that is sustained in the awake state and contributes to hypertension in patients with obstructive sleep apnea.[61]

Chronic sympathetic stimulation induces vascular remodeling and left ventricular hypertrophy by direct and indirect actions of norepinephrine on its own receptors, as well as on release of various trophic factors, including transforming growth factor-β, insulin-like growth factor-I, and fibroblast growth factors. Positive correlations among circulating norepinephrine levels, left ventricular mass, and reduced radial artery compliance (an index of vascular hypertrophy) have been demonstrated in clinical studies.[1] Thus, sympathetic mechanisms contribute to the development of target organ damage, as well as to the pathogenesis of hypertension.

Renal sympathetic nerve stimulation is increased in hypertensive patients. Infusion of the α-adrenergic antagonist phentolamine into the renal artery increases renal blood flow to a greater extent in hypertensive than in normotensive patients, a finding consistent with a functional role for increased sympathetic tone in controlling renal vascular resistance.[62,63] In animal models, direct renal nerve stimulation induces renal tubular Na^+ and water reabsorption and decreases urinary Na^+ and water excretion, thus resulting in intravascular volume expansion and increased BP.[64] Direct assessments of renal sympathetic nerve activity have consistently demonstrated increased activation in animal models of genetically mediated and experimentally induced hypertension, and renal denervation prevents or reverses hypertension in these models.[65] All these lines of evidence support a role for increased sympathetic activation of the kidney in the pathogenesis of hypertension. Peripheral sympathetic nervous system activity is greatly increased in patients with renal failure compared with age-matched, healthy, normotensive individuals with normal renal function.[66] This increase is not seen in patients who have undergone bilateral nephrectomy, a finding suggesting that sympathetic overactivity in patients with renal failure is caused by a neurogenic signal originating in the failing kidneys. The specific signaling mechanism involved has yet to be identified.

Centrally acting sympatholytic agents and α- and β-adrenergic antagonists are effective in reducing BP in patients with essential hypertension, thus providing indirect clinical evidence for the importance of sympathetic mechanisms in the maintenance phase of human hypertension.[67] Declining utilization of these agents in treating hypertension relates to problems with adverse effects and the absence of outcomes studies, rather than their lack of efficacy in reducing BP.

Exposure to stress increases sympathetic outflow, and repeated stress-induced vasoconstriction may result in vascular hypertrophy, leading to progressive increases in peripheral resistance and BP.[68] This may contribute to the increased incidence of hypertension in lower socioeconomic groups, because they endure greater levels of stress associated with daily living. Persons with a family history of hypertension manifest augmented vasoconstrictor and sympathetic responses to laboratory stressors, such as cold pressor testing and mental stress, that may predispose them to hypertension. This is particularly true of young African Americans.[69] Exaggerated stress responses may contribute to the increased incidence of hypertension in this racial group.

VASCULAR TONE AND REMODELING

Hypertensive patients manifest greater vasoconstrictor responses to infused norepinephrine than normotensive controls.[1] Increased circulating norepinephrine levels generally downregulate noradrenergic receptors in normotensive persons, but not in hypertensive patients, and this process results in enhanced sensitivity to norepinephrine, increased peripheral vascular resistance, and BP elevation. Vasoconstrictor responsiveness to norepinephrine is also increased in normotensive children of hypertensive parents, compared with controls without a family history of hypertension, a finding suggesting that the hypersensitivity may be inherited and may not simply be a consequence of elevated BP.

Peripheral vascular resistance is elevated in hypertension because of alterations in structure, mechanical properties, and function of small arteries. Remodeling of these vessels contributes to the development and maintenance to high BP and its associated target organ damage.[70] Peripheral resistance is determined by precapillary vessels, including the arterioles (arteries containing a single layer of smooth muscle cells) and the small arteries (lumen diameters <300 μm). The elevated resistance in hypertensive patients is related to rarefaction (decrease in number of parallel-connected vessels) and an increased wall-to-lumen ratio, resulting in narrowing of the lumen of resistance vessels. Examination of gluteal skin biopsy specimens obtained from patients with untreated essential hypertension has uniformly revealed reduced lumen areas and increased media-to-lumen ratios, without an increase in medial area in resistance vessels (inward, eutropic remodeling). That these changes are present even in persons with prehypertension suggests that vascular remodeling begins early in life, antedating the development of fixed hypertension, but further investigation of this issue is warranted.

Antihypertensive treatment with several classes of agents, including ACE inhibitors, angiotensin receptor blockers (ARBs), and calcium channel blockers (CCBs), can normalize resistance vessel structure,[71] whereas unfavorable vascular remodeling is progressive in persons with uncontrolled hypertension. In contrast, β-blocker therapy does not reverse resistance vessel remodeling, even when it effectively lowers BP.[1] Whether antihypertensive drugs that normalize resistance vessel structure are more effective in preventing target organ damage and cardiovascular events than agents that lower BP without affecting vascular remodeling remains to be determined.

Hypertension can also be reversed rapidly by acute maneuvers (e.g., unclipping the one-kidney, one-clip Goldblatt model) that do not affect vascular hypertrophy or remodeling. Further, various observations, including the dissociation between the BP lowering and structural effects of antihypertensive drugs and the ability of Ang II to induce vascular remodeling when infused at subpressor doses, indicate that the altered resistance vessel structure seen in hypertension is not strictly secondary to the BP and is not sufficient to sustain hypertension. To what extent resistance vessel tone and structure play a direct role in BP setting and in the pathogenesis of hypertension is a subject of ongoing study and controversy.

Vascular tone is regulated by myosin light chain (MLC) phosphorylation and dephosphorylation in VSMCs, as reviewed in Figure 3-6.[72] Abnormalities in contractile pathway proteins in VSMCs can alter vascular tone and cause hypertension in animal models. For example, VSMCs from mice with abnormalities in the large conductance Ca^{2+}-activated K^+ channel ($BK_{Ca^{2+}}$), an important regulator of vascular relaxation, develop abnormal vascular contraction and hypertension. $BK_{Ca^{2+}}$ is activated by cyclic guanosine monophosphate (cGMP)-dependent protein kinase (PKG) and by local Ca^{2+} sparks, resulting in hyperpolarization of the VSMC, decreased Ca^{2+} entry, and relaxation. Mouse models in which these $BK_{Ca^{2+}}$-activating processes are deranged also manifest vascular contractile dysfunction and hypertension.[72] Further, G protein–coupled receptors that affect VSMC contraction by mobilizing intracellular Ca^{2+} and activating MLC kinase also activate Rho/Rho kinase, which augments contraction by inhibiting myosin phosphatase, thereby preventing dephosphorylation of MLCs. Rho kinase has been recognized as a novel therapeutic target for antihypertensive therapy, and Rho kinase inhibitors have been shown to lower BP.[73] Fasudil, a Rho kinase inhibitor, is being tested in clinical trials for hypertension and vasospasm.

Cross-transplantation experiments with kidneys from genetically matched wild-type mice and $Agtr1a$ mice homozygous for a targeted disruption of the gene locus encoding the $AT_{1A}R$ have revealed that the absence of $AT_{1A}Rs$ in kidney and in the extrarenal organs resulted in equivalent approximately 20 mm Hg reductions in BP.[74] Thus, $AT_{1A}Rs$ in nonrenal tissues made a nonredundant contribution to BP that was similar in magnitude to that of $AT_{1A}Rs$ in the kidney. Animals lacking both renal and extrarenal $AT_{1A}Rs$ had even lower BPs, a finding supporting the independence of the mechanisms. Aldosterone-clamp experiments demonstrated that the BP effects of deleting extrarenal $AT_{1A}Rs$ could not be explained by alterations in aldosterone excretion alone. These findings support the general concept, elucidated by Mendelsohn,[72] that primary abnormalities in vascular cell function can directly cause abnormal vascular tone and disorders of BP regulation, including hypertension, and they challenge the concept that genetic causes of BP variation are restricted to the kidney. The

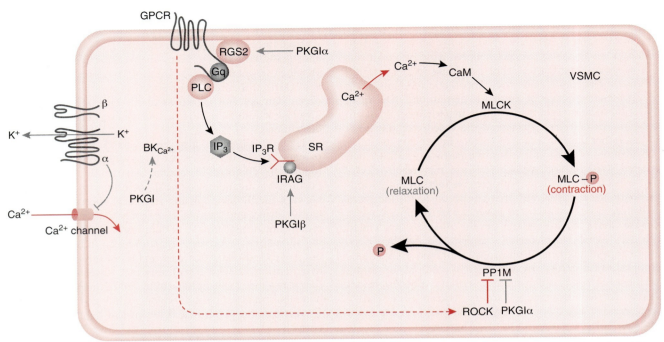

Figure 3–6 Regulation of vascular tone. Vascular tone is dynamically regulated by myosin light chain (MLC) phosphorylation and dephosphorylation in vascular smooth muscle cells (VSMCs). Increases in VSMC intracellular calcium level via receptor-activated (pharmacomechanical) or ion channel–activated (electromechanical) pathways lead to MLC kinase (MLCK) activation. MLCK phosphorylates MLCs (thus making phosphorylated myosin light chains [MLC-P]); this process activates myosin adenosine triphosphatase (ATPase) and actinomyosin cross-bridging and increases tension. PP1M dephosphorylates MLC-P, thus decreasing cell tension. PP1M is activated by the nitric oxide and nitrovasodilator effector (cyclic guanosine monophosphate–dependent protein kinase [PKGI]), which has two isoforms (PKGIα and PKGIβ). RGS2, which is essential for normal blood pressure, causes VSMC relaxation by attenuating Gq protein–coupled receptor (GPCR) activation and associated rises in intracellular calcium concentration; it too is activated by PKGI. PP1M is inhibited by Rho/Rho kinase (ROCK). The calcium-activated potassium channel, $BK_{Ca^{2+}}$, is activated by PKG and by local calcium sparks, thus hyperpolarizing the cell, decreasing calcium entry and decreasing MLCK activity. This shifts the equilibrium between MLC and MLC-P and causes relaxation. *Gray*, relaxant pathway; *red*, contractile pathway. CaM, calmodulin; IP_3R, IP_3 receptor; IRAG, IP_3R-associated cyclic guanosine monophosphate kinase substrate; PLC, phospholipase C; PP1M, protein myosin phosphatase; RGS2, regulator of G protein signaling 2; SR, sarcoplasmic reticulum. (From Mendelsohn ME. *J Clin Invest.* 2005;**115**:840-844.)

search is on for nonrenal candidate genes that influence BP in humans. Genome-wide linkage studies have identified hypertension-associated loci containing such candidate genes, including the Rho kinases (ROCK1) and the BK channel β subunit.[72] Further study is needed to establish their pathophysiologic significance in human populations.

RENAL MICROVASCULAR DISEASE: A HYPOTHETIC UNIFYING PATHOPHYSIOLOGIC MECHANISM

This hypothesis, originally proposed by Henke and Lubarsch and Goldblatt, that primary renal microvascular disease may be responsible for the development of essential hypertension, was revived by Johnson and colleagues,[75] and it has been tested in various animal models (Fig. 3-7). These authors hypothesized that the development of essential hypertension

occurs in two phases: (1) factors such as hyperactivity of the sympathetic nervous system or the RAAS or hyperuricemia resulting from diet or genetics lead to episodes of renal vasoconstriction; during this initial phase, hypertension is renin dependent and salt resistant, and the kidney is normal; and (2) as a result of chronic vasoconstriction-induced ischemia, preglomerular arteriolosclerosis eventually develops, associated with inflammation resulting from an influx of leukocytes and local generation of reactive oxygen species and Ang II. Local generation of Ang II at sites of renal injury has been invoked as a stimulus for structural alterations (renal microvascular disease) and adverse hemodynamic effects (increased vascular resistance, low ultrafiltration coefficient, and decreased Na^+ filtration) which lead to a salt-sensitive, volume-dependent, renal-dependent form of hypertension. Although this pathway ties in many of the established theories of the pathogenesis of hypertension (see Fig. 3-7), it has yet to be confirmed in human disease.

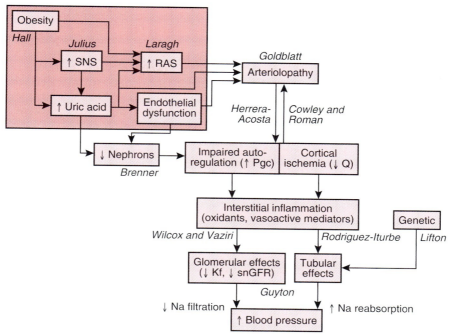

Figure 3–7 A pathway for the development of essential hypertension. In this schema, various interplaying factors lead to the development of the afferent arteriolar lesion, including obesity, a hyperactive sympathetic nervous system (SNS), activation of the renin-angiotensin system (RAS), endothelial dysfunction, and uric acid. The last two variables may have a role in causing a loss in nephron number during development. During this phase *(highlighted in dark red)*, the hypertension is salt resistant, may be associated with a low blood volume, is more likely to be renin dependent, and is relatively independent of the kidney. The arteriolar lesion then may predispose to both persistent renal vasoconstriction with ischemia and in some instances impaired autoregulation, resulting in increased glomerular pressure. These changes result in renal cortical ischemia with the infiltration of leukocytes, which generate oxidants and angiotensin II, coupled with local generation of oxidants and vasoactive factors favoring continued renal vasoconstriction. The microvascular disease may also lead to different degrees of relative renal ischemia, leading to a heterogeneous renin response. The consequence is both a reduction in sodium (Na) filtration (by reducing the cortical ultrafiltration coefficient [Kf] and single-nephron glomerular filtration rate [snGFR]) and increased tubular reabsorption of sodium, leading to increased blood pressure. As renal perfusion pressure increases, the ischemia is partially relieved, allowing sodium handling to return toward normal, but at the expense of a shift in pressure natriuresis and a rise in systemic blood pressure. The names of the investigators *(in italics)* are those whose theories about the pathophysiology of hypertension can be incorporated into this model. Pgc, glomerular capillary pressure; Q, glomerular plasma flow. (From Johnson RJ, Rodriguez-Iturbe B, Kang D-H, et al. A unifying pathway for essential hypertension. *Am J Hypertens.* 2005;**18**:431-440.)

URIC ACID: A PROPOSED PATHOPHYSIOLOGIC FACTOR IN HYPERTENSION

Hyperuricemia is associated with hypertension and cardiovascular disease in humans, but whether it is an independent risk factor with a pathogenic role in cardiovascular disease or only a marker for associated cardiovascular risk factors, such as insulin resistance, obesity, diuretic use, hypertension, and renal disease, is unclear.[76] Hyperuricemia in humans is associated with renal vasoconstriction,[77] and it is positively correlated with plasma renin activity in hypertensive patients, findings suggesting that uric acid could have adverse effects that are mediated by an activated RAAS. Further, hyperuricemia resulting from diuretic therapy has been implicated as a risk factor for cardiovascular disease events. The Systolic Hypertension in the Elderly Program (SHEP) trial found that participants who developed hyperuricemia while receiving chlorthalidone sustained cardiovascular disease events at a rate similar to those treated with placebo.[78] The Losartan

Intervention for Endpoint Reduction in Hypertension (LIFE) trial showed that baseline serum uric acid level was associated with increased risk for cardiovascular disease events in women, even after adjustment for concomitant risk factors, including use of thiazide diuretics, which was similar in both randomized arms of the trial.[79] Treatment with the uricosuric ARB losartan attenuated the time-related increase in serum uric acid in the LIFE trial, and 27% of the treatment effect on the composite cardiovascular disease endpoint could be attributed to this effect. In general, serum uric acid levels correlate with decreased glomerular filtration rate (GFR) and should be adjusted for these measures, as was done in the LIFE study. These provocative findings suggest a need for further studies of the role of uric acid in the pathogenesis of hypertension and cardiovascular disease in humans and its potential as a therapeutic target.

Uric acid has been shown in a rodent model to stimulate renal afferent arteriolopathy and tubulointerstitial disease, leading to hypertension.[80] In this model, mild hyperuricemia induced by the uricase inhibitor, oxonic acid, resulted in hypertension associated with increased expression of renin by the juxtaglomerular apparatus and decreased expression of NO synthase (NOS) in the macula densa neurons. The renal lesions and hypertension could be prevented or reversed by lowering uric acid levels and by treatment with an ACE inhibitor, the ARB losartan, or arginine, but hydrochlorothiazide did not prevent the arteriolopathy, despite controlling BP. The observations that uric acid can induce platelet-derived growth factor A-chain expression and proliferation in VSMCs,[81] and that these effects can be partially blocked by losartan, provide a mechanism to account for these findings. Whether uric acid has similar nephrotoxic and hypertension-promoting effects in humans is controversial and deserves further investigation.

ARTERIAL STIFFNESS

Systolic BP and pulse pressure (PP) increase with age, mainly because of reduced elasticity (increased stiffness) of the large conduit arteries. Arteriosclerosis in these arteries results from collagen deposition and smooth muscle cell hypertrophy, as well as thinning, fragmenting, and fracture of elastin fibers in the media.[1] In addition to these structural abnormalities, endothelial dysfunction, which develops over time from both aging and hypertension, contributes functionally to increased arterial rigidity in elderly persons with isolated systolic hypertension.

Reduced NO synthesis or release, perhaps related to the loss of endothelial function and reduction in endothelial NOS (eNOS), contributes to increased wall thickness of conduit

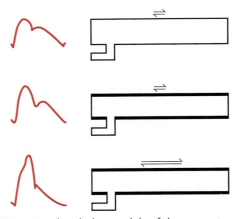

Figure 3–8 Simple tubular models of the systemic arterial system. *Top,* Normal distensibility and normal pulse-wave velocity. *Middle,* Decreased distensibility but normal pulse-wave velocity. *Bottom,* Decreased distensibility with increased pulse-wave velocity. At *left* are the amplitude and contour of pressure waves that would be generated at the origin of these models by the same ventricular ejection (flow) waves. Decreased distensibility per se increases pressure-wave amplitude, whereas increased wave velocity causes the reflected wave to return during ventricular systole. (From O'Rourke MF, Hayward CS, Lehmann ED. Arterial stiffness. In: Oparil S, Weber MA [eds]. Hypertension, 2nd ed. A Companion to Brenner & Rector's The Kidney. Philadelphia: Elsevier, 2005, pp 134-151.)

vessels. The functional importance of NO deficiency in isolated systolic hypertension is supported by the ability of NO donors, such as nitrates, to increase arterial compliance and distensibility and to reduce systolic BP without decreasing diastolic BP. Other factors that decrease central arterial compliance, including estrogen deficiency, high salt intake, tobacco use, elevated homocysteine levels, and diabetes, may operate by damaging the endothelium.

The distending pressure of conduit vessels is a major determinant of stiffness. The two-phase (elastin and collagen) content of load-bearing elements in the media is responsible for the behavior of these vessels under stress.[1] At low pressures, stress is borne almost entirely by the distensible elastin lamellae; at higher pressures, less distensible collagenous fibers are recruited and the vessel appears stiffer. Conduit vessels are relatively unaffected by neurohumoral vasodilator mechanisms; vasodilation is caused by increased distending pressure and is associated with increased stiffness. Conversely, conduit vessels do respond to vasoconstrictor stimuli, including electrical nerve stimulation and norepinephrine infusion.

Increased arterial stiffness contributes to the wide PP commonly seen in elderly hypertensive patients by causing the pulse-wave velocity to increase. With each heart beat, a pressure (pulse) wave is generated that travels from the heart to the periphery at a finite speed that depends on the elastic properties of the conduit arteries. The pulse wave is reflected at any point of discontinuity in the arterial tree and returns to the aorta and left ventricle. The timing of the wave reflection depends on the elastic properties and length of the conduit arteries.

In younger persons (Fig. 3-8, *top*), pulse-wave velocity is relatively slow (~5 m/second), and the reflected wave reaches the aortic valve after closure, thus leading to a higher diastolic BP and enhancing coronary perfusion. In older persons, particularly if they are hypertensive, pulse-wave velocity is greatly increased (approximately 20 m/second) because of central arterial stiffening, thereby causing the reflective wave to reach the aortic valve before closure and leading to a higher systolic BP, PP, and afterload and a decreased diastolic BP, potentially compromising coronary perfusion pressure (Fig. 3-8, *bottom*). Acceleration in pulse-wave velocity contributes to the increase in systolic BP and PP and the decrease in diastolic BP seen in elderly patients. This phenomenon is exaggerated in hypertensive persons. The rise in systolic BP increases cardiac metabolic requirements and predisposes to left ventricular hypertrophy and heart failure. PP is closely related to systolic BP and is linked to advanced atherosclerotic disease and cardiovascular disease events, such as myocardial infarction and stroke. In patients who are more than 50 years old, PP is generally thought to be a better predictor of cardiovascular disease risk than either systolic BP or diastolic BP.

Most antihypertensive drugs act on peripheral muscular arteries, rather than on central conduit vessels, and they reduce PP through indirect effects on the amplitude and timing of reflected pulse waves. Nitroglycerin causes marked reductions in wave reflection, central systolic BP, and left ventricular load without altering systolic or diastolic BP in the periphery. Vasodilator drugs that decrease the stiffness of peripheral arteries, including ACE inhibitors and CCBs, also reduce pulse-wave reflection and thus augmentation of the central aortic and left ventricular systolic pressure, independent of a corresponding reduction in systolic BP in the periphery. Antihypertensive drugs from several classes have been shown to reduce systolic BP and cardiovascular disease morbidity and mortality in patients with isolated systolic hypertension.

RENIN-ANGIOTENSIN-ALDOSTERONE SYSTEM

The RAAS is the most carefully studied mechanism of BP and volume regulation, and development of pharmacologic antagonists to its various components has proved useful in the treatment of hypertension and related target organ damage (Fig. 3-9). Renin is an aspartyl protease that is synthesized as an inactive precursor, prorenin, primarily in the juxtaglomerular cells surrounding the afferent arteriole of the glomerulus. Renin is activated by proteolytic cleavage of an N-terminal peptide while still in the kidney. Both prorenin and activated renin are stored in granules in the juxtaglomerular apparatus and are released in a regulated fashion in response to a variety of stimuli, including decreases in BP or renal interstitial pressure via intrinsic juxtaglomerular baroreceptors, sympathetic nervous system activation of the renal nerves, and macula densa stimulation by decreased distal tubular Na+ delivery. The primary mechanism by which the RAAS contributes to acute changes in BP and volume homeostasis is regulation of renin release into the circulation.[82] In one study, circulating renin levels, as indexed by plasma renin activity, were an independent (of BP) risk factor for myocardial infarction.[83] Although this finding has not been consistent, it does suggest the intriguing possibility that renin may have actions other than BP regulation. The recent finding of a specific receptor for the renin molecule and the active search for direct inhibitors of the catalytic action of renin are consistent with the interpretation that renin per se may have biologic importance above and beyond that of its catalytic products.

Renin reacts with angiotensinogen to produce the decapeptide, angiotensin I (Ang I), which is biologically inactive (Fig. 3-10). Ang I is cleaved by a variety of enzymes, including ACE and other proteolytic enzymes such as the serine pro-

tease, chymase, to generate Ang II, an octapeptide that is responsible for most of the known biologic activity of the system. In addition, nonrenin enzymes, including tonin and cathepsin, are capable of generating Ang II directly from angiotensinogen. ACE2, a zinc metalloprotease that shares 42% homology with the catalytic site of ACE, is expressed in endothelial cells of heart, kidney, and testis and functions as a

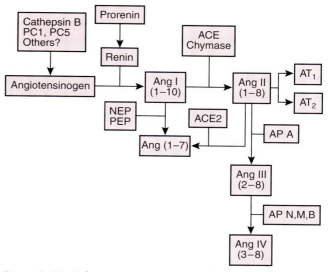

Figure 3–9 Schematic representation of the renin-angiotensin-adolsterone system. The *arrows* indicate the enzymes that catalyze the corresponding step. ACE, angiotensin-converting enzyme; Ang, angiotensin (roman numerals refer to the nomenclature for the peptide; numbers in parentheses refer to the amino acid positions in the peptide relative to Ang I, which has 10 amino acids); AP, aminopeptidase; AT1, angiotensin II type 1; AT2, angiotensin II type 2; NEP, neutral endopeptidase; PC1, prohormone convertase 1; PC5, prohormone convertase 5; PEP, prolyl endopeptidase. (From Reudelhuber TL. Renin. *In:* Oparil S, Weber MA [eds]. Hypertension, 2nd ed. A Companion to Brenner & Rector's The Kidney. Philadelphia: Elsevier, 2005, pp 89-94.)

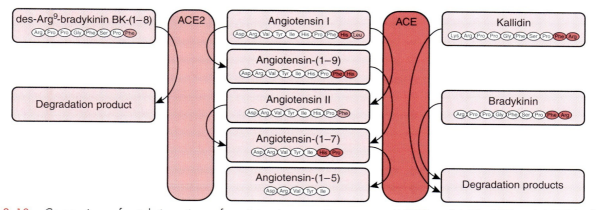

Figure 3–10 Comparison of catalytic actions of angiotensin-converting enzyme (ACE)2 and ACE. ACE and ACE2 both hydrolyze angiotensin I, but the vasoconstrictor peptide angiotensin II is generated only by ACE, because ACE2 only removes one single amino acid from the carboxyl terminus of its substrate, whereas ACE acts as a dipeptidyl carboxypeptidase. Neither bradykinin nor kallidin is metabolized by ACE2, but des-Arg9-bradykinin (the endogenous agonist of B1 kinin receptor) is. (From Fleming I, Kohlstedt K, Busse R. New fACEs to the renin-angiotensin system. *Physiology.* 2005;**20**:91-95.)

carboxypeptidase to convert Ang II to Ang (1-7) and Ang I to Ang (1-9).[84] ACE2 is insensitive to ACE inhibitors.

Ang I and Ang II are susceptible to digestion at a number of sites by angiotensinases, peptidases that remove amino acids sequentially from the amino terminus (aminopeptidases) or the carboxyl terminus (carboxypeptidases) or cleave peptide bonds in the interior of the molecule (endopeptidases). The resultant peptide fragments are found in the circulation and have functions that may be distinct from those of Ang II. For example, Ang III (the 2-8 peptide) has functions identical to those of Ang II, whereas Ang IV (the 3-8 peptide) may bind selectively to a novel receptor (AT_4R) and may stimulate release of plasminogen activator inhibitor-1, a potent antithrombolytic agent. The Ang (1-7) peptide binds to the distinct non-AT_1AT_2R AT_{1-7} to stimulate vasodilation, increases in glomerular filtration rate, inhibition of Na^+,K^+–adenosine triphosphatase (ATPase), and down-regulation of AT_1Rs.[85] Ang (1-7) can be generated from Ang I, Ang (1-9), and Ang II primarily in kidney by the carboxypeptidase ACE2 and by a variety of endopeptidases, including neprilysin, prolyl endopeptidase, and thimet oligopeptidase. ACE2 and Ang (1-7) levels have been shown in preclinical studies to increase during inhibition of the classical RAAS with an ACE inhibitor or an ARB, a finding suggesting that activation of ACE2 and generation of the downstream Ang (1-7) peptide may oppose the effects of activating the classical RAAS. The biologic significance of these novel peptides in humans has yet to be fully elucidated.

Ang II acts on two major receptors. The AT_1R, which causes vasoconstriction, aldosterone release, and other functions that tend to elevate BP and cause hypertrophy or hyperplasia of target cells, and the AT_2R, which is thought to inhibit cell growth and promote cell differentiation and apoptosis, have been cloned and characterized. The novel receptors that bind to the other Ang peptides have not yet been cloned and are not fully accepted by all investigators.

Ang II elevates BP by a variety of mechanisms, including constriction of resistance vessels, stimulation of aldosterone synthesis and release and renal tubular Na^+ reabsorption (directly and indirectly via aldosterone), stimulation of thirst and release of antidiuretic hormone, and enhancement of sympathetic outflow from the brain.[1] Ang II also induces cardiac and vascular cell hypertrophy and hyperplasia directly, via activation of the AT_1R, and indirectly by stimulating release of a number of growth factors and cytokines. Activation of the AT_1R stimulates a variety of tyrosine kinases, which, in turn, phosphorylate the tyrosine residues in a number of proteins, leading to vasoconstriction, cell growth, and proliferation (Fig. 3-11). Activation of the AT_2R subtype stimulates a phosphatase that inactivates mitogen-activated

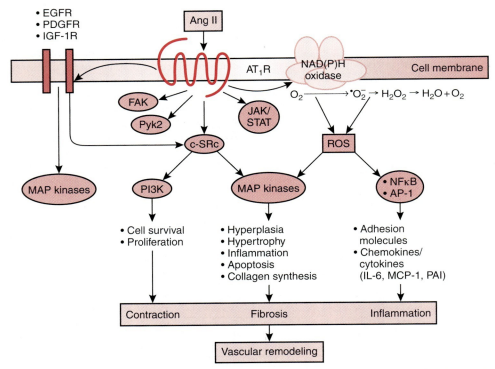

Figure 3–11   Angiotensin II (Ang II)–mediated cellular events regulating vascular structure. Ang II binds to the AT_1 receptor (AT_1R), leading to activation of tyrosine kinases, mitogen-activated protein (MAP) kinases, and nicotinamide adenine dinucleotide phosphate (NAD(P)H) oxidase. These signaling events regulate vascular smooth muscle cell function. Under pathologic conditions, increased signaling leads to altered growth, fibrosis, and inflammatory processes, which contribute to structural remodeling in hypertension. AP-1, aminopeptidase-1; EGFR, epidermal growth factor receptor; FAK, focal adhesion kinase; IGF-1R, insulin-like growth factor-1 receptor; IL, interleukin; JAK, Janus family kinase; MCP-1, monocyte chemotactic protein-1; NF-κB, nuclear factor-κB; PAI, plasminogen activator inhibitor; PDGFR, platelet-derived growth factor receptor; PI3K, phosphatidylinositol 3-kinase; Pyk2, proline-rich tyrosine kinase 2; ROS, reactive oxygen species; STAT, signal transducer and activator of transcriptase. (From Touyz RM. The role of angiotensin II in regulating vascular structural and functional changes in hypertension. *Curr Hypertens Rep.* 2003;**5**:155-164.)

protein kinase, a key enzyme involved in transducing signals from the AT_1R. Thus, activation of the AT_2R opposes the biologic effects of AT_1R activation and leads to vasodilation, growth inhibition, and cell differentiation (Fig. 3-12).[1] The physiologic role of the AT_2R in human adults is unclear, but it is thought to function under stress conditions (e.g., vascular injury, ischemia, or reperfusion). When an ARB is administered, renin is released from the kidney resulting from removal of feedback inhibition by Ang II. This leads to increased generation of Ang II, which is shunted to the AT_2R, thus favoring vasodilation and attenuation of unfavorable vascular remodeling. Expression of the AT_2R is linked to growth states and fetal development. During embryogenesis and fetal development, the AT_2R is expressed in large quantities, and expression is decreased in the postnatal period. The regulation of the AT_2R gene in adult humans is not well elucidated. Some evidence from animal models indicates that AT_2R expression is up-regulated in several pathologic conditions, such as in vascular injury, in Na^+ depletion, after myocardial infarction, and in congestive heart failure, but it is down-regulated in diabetes mellitus.

Local production of Ang II in a variety of tissues, including the blood vessels, heart, adrenals, and brain, is under the control of ACE and other enzymes, including the serine proteinase chymase. The activity of local renin-angiotensin

ANGIOTENSIN II EFFECTS AT RECEPTORS

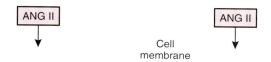

AT₁ receptor

- Vasoconstriction
- Cell growth and proliferation
- CV hypertrophy
- PAI-1 expression
- Aldosterone release
- Central sympathetic activation
- Sodium and water retention
- Inhibits renin release

AT₂ receptor

- Vasodilation
- Inhibits hypertrophy
- Antiproliferation
- Mediates NO and PGF_2 in the kidney
- Renal Na^+ excretion
- Dilates afferent arteriole
- Causes renin release

Figure 3–12 The angiotensin II (Ang II) subtype receptors have generally opposing effects. The angiotensin II subtype 1 (AT_1) receptor leads to vasoconstriction, cell growth, and cell proliferation, whereas the angiotensin II subtype 2 (AT_2) receptor has the opposite effects, leading to vasodilatation, antigrowth, and cell differentiation. The AT_1 receptor is antinatriuretic; the AT_2 receptor is natriuretic. AT_1 receptor stimulation results in free radicals; AT_2 receptor stimulation produces nitric oxide (NO), which can neutralize free radicals. The AT_1 receptor induces plasminogen activator inhibitor-1 (PAI-1) and other growth family pathways; the AT_2 receptor does not. Angiotensin receptor blockers bind to and block selectively at the AT_1 receptor, preventing stimulation of the receptor by angiotensin II. CV, cardiovascular; PGF_2, prostaglandin F_2. (From Carey RM, Siragy HM. Newly recognized components of the renin-angiotensin system: Potential roles in cardiovascular and renal regulation. *Endocr Rev.* 2003;**24**:261-271.)

systems and alternative pathways of Ang II formation may make important contributions to remodeling of resistance vessels and the development of target organ damage (including left ventricular hypertrophy, heart failure, atherosclerosis, stroke, end-stage renal disease, myocardial infarction, and arterial aneurysm) in hypertensive persons.[1]

ANGIOTENSIN II AND OXIDATIVE STRESS

Ang II increases cardiovascular risk in part by stimulating oxidant production. Hypertension associated with chronic infusion of Ang II is linked to up-regulation of vascular p22phox messenger ribonucleic acid (mRNA), a component of the oxidative enzyme nicotinamide adenine dinucleotide phosphate (NAD(P)H) oxidase.[86] Ang II receptor–dependent activation of NAD(P)H oxidase is associated with enhanced formation of the oxidant superoxide anion ($O_2 \cdot^-$), which readily reacts with NO to form the oxidant peroxynitrite ($ONOO^-$). The consequent reduction in NO bioactivity may provide an additional mechanism to explain the enhanced vasoconstrictor response to Ang II in hypertension. NAD(P)H oxidase may also play an important role in the hypertrophic response to Ang II, because stable transfection of vascular smooth muscle cells with antisense to p22phox inhibits Ang II–stimulated protein synthesis. Other vasculotoxic responses to Ang II that are triggered by activation of NAD(P)H oxidase include the oxidation of low-density lipoprotein cholesterol and increased mRNA expression for monocyte chemoattractant protein-1 (MCP-1) and vascular cell adhesion molecule-1 (VCAM-1), thus linking activation of the RAAS to the development of the atherosclerosis.[87]

ACE inhibitors and ARBs limit oxidative reactions in the vasculature by blocking the activation of NAD(P)H oxidase. These findings have led to the hypothesis that the ACE inhibitors and ARBs may have clinically important vasoprotective effects beyond BP lowering. Numerous important randomized clinical trials, discussed in Chapters 20 and 21, support that hypothesis.

ALDOSTERONE

Aldosterone is a steroid hormone synthesized primarily, if not exclusively, in the zona glomerulosa of the adrenal cortex that acts as a physiologic regulator of salt and water balance. It was originally characterized as a mineralocorticoid, a hormone promoting unidirectional transepithelial Na^+ transport.[88] More recently, aldosterone has been shown to have important physiologic and pathophysiologic effects on the heart, blood vessels, and brain that are mediated by activation of high-affinity mineralocorticoid receptors (MRs) (Fig. 3-13). These MRs are members of the steroid/thyroid/retinoid/orphan receptor family of nuclear *trans*-activating factors, closely related to the glucocorticoid, androgen, and progestin receptors. MRs act as transcription factors, binding to response elements in the promoter regions of downstream target genes, as well as to coregulators, and thus modulate gene transcription. MR-regulated genes in epithelial tissues, including ENaC and Na^+,K^+-ATPase, regulate Na^+ transport. Activated MRs in the amygdala stimulate salt appetite; in the circumventricular

New concepts of aldosterone biology

Multiple modulators of aldosterone secretion
Angiotensin II – K⁺ – ACTH – Norepinephrine – Serotonin – Endothelin – NO

↓

Aldosterone production
Adrenal gland, Brain, Heart, Blood vessels

↓

Locations of aldosterone receptors

• Previously known   • Recently discovered

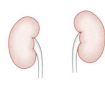 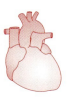 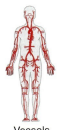

Kidneys   Brain   Heart   Vessels

Figure 3–13 New concepts of aldosterone biology. ACTH, adrenocorticotropic hormone; NO, nitric oxide. (From Lombes M, Farman N, Bonvalet JP, et al. Identification and role of aldosterone receptors in the cardiovascular system. Ann Endocrinol [Paris]. 2000;**61**: 41-46)

region of the hypothalamus, they raise BP, and in the arterial wall, they stimulate vasoconstriction. The postreceptor mechanisms involved in these functions are not yet well defined. Aldosterone has rapid nongenomic effects in VSMCs and cardiomyocytes that are mediated by the MR.[89]

MRs can bind both mineralocorticoids and glucocorticoids and contain the enzyme 11β-OH-steroid dehydrogenase II, which inactivates glucocorticoids. Activation of MRs is thought to stimulate intravascular and perivascular fibrosis and interstitial fibrosis in the heart. The nonselective aldosterone antagonist spironolactone and the novel selective aldosterone blocker eplerenone are effective in preventing or reversing vascular and cardiac inflammation and subsequent collagen deposition in experimental animals. Spironolactone treatment of patients with heart failure has also been shown to reduce circulating levels of procollagen type III aminoterminal aminopeptide, a finding indicating an antifibrotic effect. Spironolactone and the better-tolerated selective aldosterone blocker eplerenone are being utilized in the treatment of hypertension, heart failure, and acute myocardial infarction complicated by left ventricular dysfunction or heart failure because of their unique tissue protective effects.

Aldosterone excess and associated MR activation may be far more common causes or contributing factors to hypertension than previously thought. Historically, hypokalemia was thought to be a prerequisite of primary hyperaldosteronism, but it is now recognized that many patients with primary hyperaldosteronism do not manifest low serum K⁺ levels. Some studies even report normal plasma K⁺ levels in all participants ($[K^+] = 3.9 \pm 0.2$ mEq/L).[90] Accordingly, screening of hypertensive patients for hyperaldosteronism has expanded, and a higher prevalence of the disorder has been revealed. Prevalence rates between 8% and 32% have been reported, based on the patient population being screened (higher in referral practices, where the patient mix tends to be enriched with those with refractory hypertension, and lower in family practices or community databases).[91] In our own referral practice, which includes a high proportion of patients with resistant hypertension, the prevalence of aldosterone excess is 24%, and BP in these patients is strikingly responsive to spironolactone.[92] The mechanisms by which MR activation mediates resistant hypertension and target organ damage are under active investigation.

ENDOTHELIAL DYSFUNCTION

NO is a potent vasodilator, inhibitor of platelet adhesion and aggregation, and suppressor of migration and proliferation of VSMCs. It is released by normal endothelial cells in response to a variety of stimuli, including changes in BP, shear stress, and pulsatile stretch, and it plays an important role in BP regulation, thrombosis, and atherosclerosis.[1] The cardiovascular system in normotensive persons is exposed to continuous NO-dependent vasodilator tone, but this NO-related vascular relaxation is diminished in hypertensive persons. In vivo delivery of superoxide dismutase (an enzyme that reduces superoxide to hydrogen peroxide) reduces BP and restores NO bioactivity, thus providing evidence that oxidant stress contributes to the inactivation of NO and the development of endothelial dysfunction in hypertensive models. Investigators have suggested that Ang II enhances formation of the oxidant superoxide at concentrations that have a minimal effect on BP.[93] These findings suggest that increased oxidant stress and the development of endothelial dysfunction may predispose to the development of hypertension. Further, antihypertensive drugs that interrupt the RAAS, including ACE inhibitors, ARBs, and MR antagonists, are effective in reversing endothelial dysfunction in peripheral arteries,[93] as well as in the kidney, where they reduce microalbuminuria and proteinuria, an effect that has been related to prevention of cardiovascular disease events.[94] The extent to which favorable effects on the endothelium account for the cardioprotective effects of these agents remains to be determined.

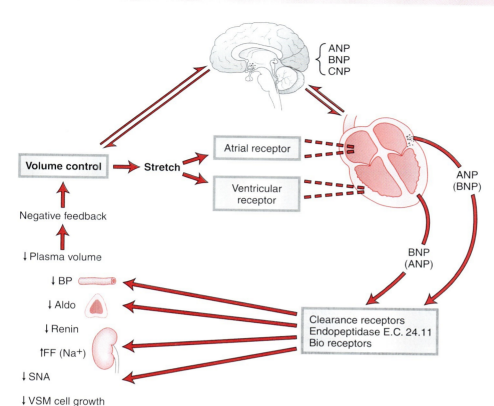

Figure 3–14 The regulation and actions of natriuretic peptides. Aldo, aldosterone; ANP, atrial natriuretic peptide; BNP, brain natriuretic peptide; BP, blood pressure; CNP, C-type natriuretic peptide; FF, filtration fraction; SNA, sympathetic nervous activity; VSM, vascular smooth muscle. (Modified from Espiner EA. Physiology of natriuretic peptides. *J Intern Med.* 1994;**235**:527-541.)

ENDOTHELIN

Endothelin is a potent vasoactive peptide produced by endothelial cells that has both vasoconstrictor and vasodilator properties. Endothelin is secreted in an abluminal direction by endothelial cells and acts in a paracrine fashion on underlying VSMCs to cause vasoconstriction and elevate BP without necessarily reaching increased levels in the systemic circulation. Endothelin also stimulates VSMC proliferation; the result is vascular remodeling, which tends to stabilize the hypertensive state. Endothelin receptor antagonists reduce BP and peripheral vascular resistance in both normotensive persons and in patients with mild to moderate essential hypertension,[95] a finding supporting the interpretation that endothelin plays a role in the pathogenesis of hypertension. Development of this drug class for systemic hypertension has been limited because of toxicity (teratogenicity, testicular atrophy, and hepatotoxicity). However, an endothelin antagonist is indicated for the treatment of pulmonary hypertension, and others may yet prove clinically useful in the therapy of other forms of renal and vascular disease.

VASODILATORS

Natriuretic Peptides

The most carefully studied of the endogenous antihypertensive mediators are the natriuretic peptides (see Fig. 3-1). The seminal observation of deBold and associates that atrial extracts have potent natriuretic and BP-lowering effects led to the discovery of a complex system of natriuretic peptides that play important roles in the integrative control of cardiovascular and renal function and in the pathogenesis of hypertension and related target organ damage. In addition to natriuresis, these peptides have a variety of other functions, including vasodilation, vascular remodeling, inhibition of cell proliferation, and modulation of sympathetic nervous system and RAAS function (Fig. 3-14). All these effects tend to lower BP and reduce related target organ damage.

Five distinct natriuretic peptides have been identified and characterized, as follows[96]:

1. ANP is a 28–amino acid peptide synthesized and secreted primarily by the cardiac atria that is an important regulator of Na⁺ balance and BP (Fig. 3-15). ANP deficiency has been associated with impaired renal Na⁺ excretion and BP elevation in animal models and humans.
2. Brain natriuretic peptide (BNP) is a 32–amino acid peptide synthesized and secreted primarily by the cardiac ventricles that resembles ANP in structure. The term "brain" is a misnomer resulting from the fact that BNP was originally isolated from brain. BNP is overexpressed in the hypertrophic ventricle and is released in response to ventricular stretch, leading to natriuresis and an acute reduction in preload. These properties have resulted in the utilization of plasma BNP assay as a diagnostic tool in heart failure and to the development of recombinant human BNP for the treatment of decompensated heart failure.
3. C-type natriuretic peptide (CNP), including a 53–amino acid precursor form and a 22–amino acid active form, is widely distributed in brain and peripheral organs, including endothelium, kidney, heart, and adrenal gland. It appears to have similar biologic properties, but lower potency than ANP or BNP.

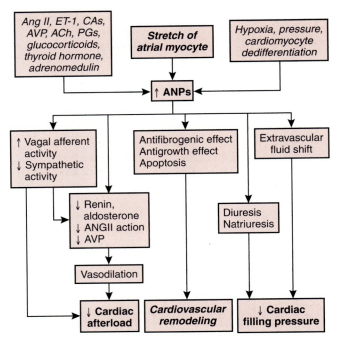

Figure 3–15   The regulation and actions of atrial natriuretic peptides (ANPs) in cardiovascular system. ACh, acetylcholine; Ang II, angiotensin II; AVP, arginine vasopressin, CAs, catecholamines; ET-1, endothelin-1; PGs, prostaglandins.

4. Dendroapis natriuretic peptide (DNP), a 38–amino acid peptide isolated from the venom of the green mamba snake, *Dendroapis augusticeps*, has natriuretic and arterial vasorelaxant activity, and DNP-like immunoreactivity has been detected in human atrial myocardium and plasma. Its function in mammals remains to be elucidated.

5. Urodilatin, a nonglycosylated 32–amino acid peptide originally isolated from human urine, shares the ANP sequence but has an additional Thr-Ala-Pro-Arg peptide at the amino terminus. Urodilatin is synthesized only in the renal tubules and is secreted into the tubular lumen. It functions as a natriuretic peptide with greater potency than ANP.

The biologic effects of the natriuretic peptides are mediated by specific natriuretic peptide receptors (NPRs), members of the guanylyl cyclase receptor family. The A and B isoforms (NPR-A and -B) have an extracellular ligand-binding domain, an intracellular guanylate cyclase domain, and a protein kinase–like domain that catalyzes the formation of cGMP from guanosine triphosphate. cGMP acts on a variety of intracellular targets, including protein kinases, gated ion channels, and cyclic nucleotide phosphodiesterases. NPR-C lacks the intracellular protein kinase–like and guanylyl cyclase domains and functions as a clearance receptor and the primary regulator of circulating natriuretic peptide levels (see Fig. 3-14).

ANP is expressed in and released from atrial myocytes in response to stretch and a variety of neurohumoral stimuli (see Fig. 3-15). By activating NPR-A, ANP has renal, hemodynamic, and neurohumoral (inhibition of sympathetic nervous system and RAAS activity) effects that reduce extracellular volume and systemic vascular resistance and thus lower BP. In addition, ANP inhibits growth and proliferation of critical cell types in the heart and vasculature and thereby prevents adverse cardiovascular remodeling and fibrosis in the setting of hypertension or excess stimulation by growth factors such as Ang II. Mice with homozygous deletion of ANP or NPR-A develop hypertension and cardiac hypertrophy, particularly when they are fed a high-salt diet. Further, we have shown exaggerated interstitial and perivascular fibrosis and early failure in hearts of ANP null mice subjected to systolic overload stress, a finding demonstrating the functional significance of ANP as a cardioprotective hormone.[97]

Relative ANP deficiency, reflected in a blunted increase or a paradoxical decrease in plasma ANP in response to high dietary salt intake, has been demonstrated in humans with salt-sensitive hypertension and in children of hypertensive parents.[96] Further, polymorphisms in the ANP gene have been associated with hypertension in some populations, particularly African Americans and Japanese, but not in others. A significant association between allelic variants of the ANP gene and aldosterone responsiveness to Ang II has been shown in patients with an aldosterone-producing adenoma. Suppressed circulating ANP levels associated with a reduced NPR-A/NPR-C ratio in adipose tissue have been demonstrated in obese hypertensive patients.[96] The latter finding suggests that overexpression of NPR-C in adipose tissue may lead to increased peripheral clearance of ANP, thus reducing its biologic activity and predisposing obese persons to salt-sensitive hypertension. The observation that NPR-C expression in adipose tissue is suppressed in rats following fasting, with resulting increased ANP activity, diuresis, and natriuresis, is consistent with this interpretation. Taken together, experimental and clinical studies suggest a role for ANP in the regulation of BP and the pathogenesis of some forms of hypertension and their associated target organ damage. Exploitation of the natriuretic peptide–signaling pathway as a therapeutic target has been suggested by the demonstration that inhibition of phosphodiesterase-5 with sildenafil reverses pressure overload–induced cardiac hypertrophy in the mouse.[98]

Kallikrein-Kinin System

The kallikrein-kinin system operates in parallel with the RAAS but has many functions (i.e., BP reduction, vasoprotection, natriuresis) that oppose the actions of Ang II and aldosterone.[99] Kinins, peptides that contain the sequence of bradykinin, are generated from protein precursors called kininogens by action of kallikrein, an enzyme that is expressed mainly in submandibular glands, pancreas, and kidney, but it is also detectable in vascular tissues, heart, and adrenal glands. Kinins are rapidly hydrolyzed and inactivated by a number of kininases, including ACE (kinase II) and neutral endopeptidase 24.11 (enkephalinase), which also inactivate other vasoactive peptides. Because of this rapid hydrolysis, the kinins circulate in very low concentrations and act mainly near their site of origin.

The kinins act via the B_2 and B_1 receptors: the B_1 receptor is expressed only in the setting of tissue injury, whereas the B_2 receptor mediates most of the functions of the kinins. B_2 receptor activation stimulates release of a variety of vasodilator/natriuretic/antitrophic mediators, which are responsible for the cardiovascular effects of the kinins. Cross-talk exists between the B_2 receptor and ACE, as well as serine proteases such as kallikrein; the results are B_2 receptor activation and potentiation of bradykinin. The B_2 receptor also forms heterodimers with the AT_1R, thus activating AT_1R signaling, and forms a complex with eNOS that inhibits NO generation. The functional consequences of these receptor-receptor interactions remain to be fully elucidated, but it is clear that the kinins mediate some of the cardiovascular and renal effects of the ACE inhibitors and ARBs, as well as some of the adverse effects of the former drug class. In addition, bradykinin appears to play an important role in mediating the counterregulatory vasoprotective effects of AT_2R activation, as well as the depressor effects of Ang (1-7).

Decreased activity of the kallikrein-kinin system has been linked to human hypertension in that low urinary kallikrein excretion was described in normotensive children of hypertensive parents, whereas high urinary kallikrein was associated with a decreased risk of essential hypertension.[99] However, animal models with genetic deletion of components of the kallikrein-kinin system do not develop hypertension, a finding suggesting that the kinins do not play a fundamental role in the pathogenesis of hypertension. They do, however, appear to play an important modulatory role in the salt sensitivity of BP, as well as in the antihypertensive and cardioprotective effects of the ACE inhibitors and ARBs.

Calcitonin Gene–Related Peptide

CGRP is a 37–amino acid neuropeptide synthesized in the central and peripheral nervous systems by tissue-specific splicing of the primary RNA transcript of the calcitonin/CGRP gene.[100] CGRP is a potent vasodilator via both direct (cyclic adenosine monophosphate on VSMCs) and indirect (NO release from endothelium) effects, and it also has positive inotropic and chronotropic actions. CGRP plays an important compensatory vasodilator role to attenuate the BP increase in rodent models of hypertension, and homozygous deletion of the α-CGRP gene in the mouse results in BP elevation, increased heart weight, and an exaggerated BP response to deoxycorticosterone-salt treatment. However, the role of CGRP in human hypertension remains unclear.

Substance P

Substance P is an 11–amino acid peptide member of the tachykinin family that mediates pain, touch, and temperature.[100] It is expressed almost exclusively in neuronal tissues, but it produces vasodilation by an endothelium-dependent mechanism involving release of both NO and endothelium-derived hyperpolarizing factor (EDHF). Substance P may act to counteract the BP increases seen in animal models of salt-dependent hypertension. Decreased levels of substance P have been reported in human hypertension, but the pathophysiologic significance of this alteration is unclear.

Adrenomedullin

Adrenomedullin is a 52–amino acid peptide member of the CGRP/amylin/calcitonin superfamily that was first isolated from human pheochromocytoma tissue.[100] Adrenomedullin was subsequently found to be expressed in highest levels in endothelial cells and to be secreted by the vascular endothelium into the circulation. Circulating adrenomedullin levels are increased in hypertension, heart failure, and renal failure

in humans and in animal models, likely as a compensatory response to BP elevation and vascular damage. Adrenomedullin delays the BP rise and protects against target organ damage in rodent models of hypertension. Available data suggest that adrenomedullin functions as a compensatory vasodilator in hypertensive states, but its mechanism of action and precise role in human hypertension are unclear.

SUMMARY

The complexity of pathophysiologic mechanisms that lead to BP elevation is such that selective, mechanistically based antihypertensive treatment is rarely possible in any given hypertensive patient. Current treatment guidelines generally recommend a generic approach to treating hypertension, with little emphasis on selecting therapy based on the underlying pathophysiology of the elevated BP. With increased recognition of specific causes, it may be possible to develop therapies selective for distinct pathophysiologic mechanisms with fewer adverse effects, resulting in more effective BP reduction. Utilization of powerful new techniques of genetics, genomics, and proteomics, integrated with systems physiology and population studies, may make more selective and effective approaches to the treatment and even prevention of hypertension possible in the coming decades.

References

1. Oparil S, Zaman A, Calhoun DA. Pathogenesis of hypertension. *Ann Intern Med.* 2003;**139**:761-776.
2. Calhoun DA, Zaman A, Oparil S. Etiology and pathogenesis of systemic hypertension. *In:* Crawford MH, DiMarco JP, Paulus WJ (eds). Cardiology, 2nd ed. Philadelphia: Mosby, 2003, pp 463-471.
3. Delgado MC, Weder AB. Pathophysiology of hypertension. *In:* Oparil S, Weber MA (eds). Hypertension, 2nd ed. A Companion to Brenner & Rector's The Kidney. Philadelphia: Elsevier, 2005, pp 29-38.
4. Lifton RP, Gharavi AG, Geller DS. Molecular mechanisms of human hypertension. *Cell.* 2001;**104**:545-556.
5. Harrap SB. Blood pressure genetics. *In:* Oparil S, Weber MA (eds). Hypertension, 2nd ed. A Companion to Brenner & Rector's The Kidney. Philadelphia: Elsevier, 2005, pp 39-59.
6. Feinleib M, Garrison RJ, Fabsitz R, et al. The NHLBI twin study of cardiovascular disease risk factors: Methodology and summary of results. *Am J Epidemiol.* 1977;**106**:284-285.
7. Longini IM, Higgins MW, Hinton PC, et al. Environmental and genetic sources of familial aggregation of blood pressure in Tecumseh, Michigan. *Am J Epidemiol.* 1984;**120**:131-144.
8. Biron P, Mongeau JG, Bertrand D. Familial aggregation of blood pressure in 558 adopted children. *Can Med Assoc J.* 1976;**115**:773-774.
9. Guyton AC. Blood pressure control: Special role of the kidneys and body fluids. *Science.* 1991;**252**:1813-1816.
10. Matsuo A, Katsuya T, Ishikawa K, et al. G2736A polymorphism of thiazide-sensitive Na-Cl cotransporter gene predisposes to hypertension in young women. *J Hypertens.* 2004;**22**: 2123-2127.
11. Shimkets RA, Warnock DG, Bositis CM, et al. Liddle's syndrome: Heritable human hypertension caused by mutations in the β-subunit of the epithelial sodium channel. *Cell.* 1994;**79**:407-414.
12. Melander O, Orho M, Fagerudd J, et al. Mutations and variants of the epithelial sodium channel gene in Liddle's

syndrome and primary hypertension. *Hypertension.* 1998;**31**:1118-1124.

13. Carter AR, Zhou ZH, Calhoun DA, Bubien JK. Hyperactive ENaC identifies hypertensive individuals amenable to amiloride therapy. *Am J Physiol.* 2001;**281**:C1413-C1421.

14. Jeunemaitre X, Soubrier F, Kotelevtsev YV, et al. Molecular basis of human hypertension: Role of angiotensinogen. *Cell.* 1992;**71**:169-180.

15. Corvol P, Persu A, Giminez-Roqueplo AP, Jeunemaitre X. Seven lessons from two candidate genes in human essential hypertension: Angiotensinogen and epithelial sodium channel. *Hypertension.* 1999;**33**:1324-1331.

16. Staessen JA, Kuznetsova T, Wang JG, et al. M235T angiotensinogen gene polymorphism and cardiovascular renal risk. *J Hypertens.* 1999:**17**:9-17.

17. Rigat B, Hubert C, Alhenc-Gelas F, et al. An insertion/deletion polymorphism in the angiotensin I–converting enzyme gene accounting for half the variance of serum enzyme levels. *J Clin Invest.* 1990;**86**:1343-1346.

18. Fornage M, Amos CI, Kardia S, et al. Variation in the region of the angiotensin-converting enzyme gene influences interindividual differences in blood pressure levels in young white males. *Circulation.* 1998;**97**:1773-1779.

19. O'Donnell CJ, Lindpaintner K, Larson MG, et al. Evidence for association and genetic linkage of the angiotensin-converting enzyme locus with hypertension and blood pressure in men but not women: The Framingham Heart Study. *Circulation.* 1998;**97**:1766-1772.

20. Spiering W, Kroon AA, Fuss-Lejeune MJ, de Leeuw PW. Genetic contribution to the acute effects of angiotensin II type 1 receptor blockade. *J Hypertens.* 2005;**23**:753-758.

21. Niu T, Chen X, Xiping X. Angiotensin converting enzyme gene insertion/deletion polymorphism and cardiovascular disease. *Drugs.* 2000;**62**:977-993.

22. Bianchi G, Ferrari P, Staessen JA. Adducin polymorphism: Detection and impact on hypertension and related disorders. *Hypertension.* 2005;**45**:331-340.

23. Turner ST, Schwartz GL. Gene markers and antihypertensive therapy. *Curr Hypertens Rep.* 2005;**7**:21-30.

24. Manunta P, Cusi D, Barlassina C, et al. Alpha-adducin polymorphisms and renal sodium handling in essential hypertensive patients. *Kidney Int.* 1998;**53**:1471-1478.

25. Grant FD, Romero JR, Jeunemaitre X, et al. Low-renin hypertension, altered sodium homeostasis, and α-adducin polymorphism. *Hypertension.* 2002;**39**:191-196.

26. Arnett DK, Boerwinkle E, Davis BR, et al. Pharmacogenetic approach to hypertension therapy: Design and rationale for the Genetics of Hypertension Associated Treatment (GenHAT) study. *Pharmacogenomics J.* 2002;**2**:309-317.

27. Cusi D, Barlassina C, Azzani T, et al. Polymorphisms of alpha-adducin and salt sensitivity in patients with essential hypertension. *Lancet.* 1997;**349**:1353-1357.

28. Turner ST, Chapman AB, Schwartz GL, Boerwinkle E. Effects of endothelial nitric oxide synthase, alpha-adducin, and other candidate gene polymorphisms on blood pressure response to hydrochlorothiazide. *Am J Hypertens.* 2003;**16**:834-839.

29. Psaty BM, Smith NL, Heckbert SR, et al. Diuretic therapy, the α-adducin gene variant, and the risk of myocardial infarction or stroke in persons with treated hypertension. *JAMA.* 2002;**287**:1680-1689.

30. Schwartz GL, Turner ST, Chapman AB, Boerwinkle E. Interacting effects of gender and genotype on blood pressure response to hydrochlorothiazide. *Kidney Int.* 2002;**62**:1718-1723.

31. Manunta P, Tripodi G. Haplotype analysis in human hypertension. *J Hypertens.* 2005;**23**:711-712.

32. International Human Genome Sequencing Consortium. Finishing the euchromatic sequence of the human genome. *Nature.* 2004;**431**:931-945.

33. Persu A, Vinck WJ, Khattabi OE, et al. Influence of the endothelial nitric oxide synthase gene on conventional and ambulatory blood pressure: Sib-pair analysis and haplotype study. *J Hypertens.* 2005;**23**:759-765.

34. Yagil C, Hubner N, Monti J, et al. Identification of hypertension-related genes through an integrated genomic-transcriptomic approach. *Circ Res.* 2005;**96**:617-625.

35. Winslow RL, Gao Z. Candidate gene discovery in cardiovascular disease [editorial]. *Circ Res.* 2005;**96**:605-606.

36. Selby JV, Newman B, Quiroga J, et al. Concordance for dyslipidemic hypertension in male twins. *JAMA.* 1991;**265**:2079-2084.

37. Haffner SM, Lehto S, Rönnemää T, et al. Mortality from coronary heart disease in subjects with type 2 diabetes and in nondiabetic subjects with and without prior myocardial infarction. *N Engl J Med.* 1998;**339**:229-234.

38. Chobanian AV, Bakris GL, Black HR, et al., and the National High Blood Pressure Education Program Committee. Seventh report on the Joint National Committee on Prevention, Detection, Evaluation, and Treatment of High Blood Pressure. The JNC 7 Report. *Hypertension.* 2003;**42**:1206-1252.

39. Reaven GM, Lithell H, Landsberg L. Hypertension and associated metabolic abnormalities: The role of insulin resistance and the sympathoadrenal system. *N Engl J Med.* 1996;**334**:374-381.

40. Brook RD, Julius S. Autonomic imbalance, hypertension and cardiovascular risk. *Am J Hypertens.* 2000;**13**:112S-122S.

41. Kim J-R, Kiefe CI, Liu K, et al. Heart rate and subsequent blood pressure in young adults: The CARDIA Study. *Hypertension.* 1999;**33**:640-646.

42. Esler M. The sympathetic system and hypertension. *Am J Hypertens.* 2000;**13**:99S-105S.

43. Izzo JL Jr. The sympathetic nervous system in acute and chronic blood pressure elevation. *In:* Oparil S, Weber MA (eds). Hypertension, 2nd ed. A Companion to Brenner & Rector's The Kidney. Philadelphia: Elsevier, 2005, pp 60-76.

44. Abboud FM. The sympathetic system in hypertension. *Hypertension.* 1982;**4**:208-225.

45. Joyner MJ, Shepherd JT, Seals DR. Sustained increases in sympathetic outflow during prolonged lower body negative pressure in humans. *J Appl Physiol.* 1990;**68**:1004-1009.

46. Fink GD, Haywood JR, Bryan WJ, et al. Central site for pressor action of blood-borne angiotensin in rat. *Am J Physiol.* 1980;**239**:R358-R361.

47. Allen K, Shykoff BE, Izzo JL Jr. Cognitive appraisal of threat or challenge predicts hemodynamic responses to mental arithmetic and speech tasks [abstract]. *Am J Hypertens.* 1998;**11** (**Suppl 1**):134A.

48. Shykoff BE, Allen K, Izzo JL Jr. Interactions of social support and family history in blood pressure reactivity to psychological stressors [abstract]. *Am J Hypertens.* 1998;**11** (**Suppl 1**):135A.

49. Oparil S, Chen YF, Berecek K, et al. The role of the central nervous system in hypertension. *In:* Laragh JH, Brenner BM (eds). Hypertension: Pathophysiology, Diagnosis and Management. New York: Raven Press, 1995, pp 713-740.

50. Oparil S, Chen YF, Peng N, et al. Anterior hypothalamic norepinephrine, atrial natriuretic peptide and hypertension. *Front Neuroendocrinol.* 1996;**17**:211-246.

51. Chapleau MW, Hajduczok G, Abboud FM. Mechanisms of resetting of arterial baroreceptors: An overview. *Am J Med Sci.* 1988;**295**:327-334.

52. Xie P, Chapleau MW, McDowell TX, et al. Mechanisms of decreased baroreceptor activity in chronic hypertensive rabbits: Role of endogenous prostanoids. *J Clin Invest.* 1990;**86**:625-630.

53. Xie P, McDowell TS, Chapleau MW, et al. Rapid baroreceptor resetting in chronic hypertension: Implications for normalization of arterial pressure. *Hypertension.* 1991;**17**:72-79.

54. Guo GB, Abboud FM. Impaired central mediation of the arterial baroreflex in chronic renal hypertension. *Am J Physiol.* 1984;**15**:H720-H727.

55. Guo GB, Abboud FM. Angiotensin II attenuates baroreflex control of heart rate and lumbar sympathetic nerve activity. *Am J Physiol.* 1984;**15**:H80-H89.

56. Abboud FM. Effects of sodium, angiotensin, and steroids on vascular reactivity in man. *Fed Proc.* 1974;**33**:143-149.

57. Li Z, Mao HZ, Abboud FM, Chapleau MW. Oxygen-derived free radicals contribute to baroreceptor dysfunction in atherosclerotic rabbits. *Circ Res.* 1996;**79**:802-811.

58. Chapleau MW, Hajduczok G, Abboud FM. Suppression of baroreceptor discharge by endothelin at high carotid sinus pressure. *Am J Physiol.* 1982;**263**:R103-R108.

59. Randall OS, Esler MD, Bulloch EG, et al. Relationship of age and blood pressure to baroreflex sensitivity and arterial compliance in man. *Clin Sci Mol Med.* 1976;**Suppl 3**: 357S-360S.

60. Somers VK, Mark AL, Abboud FM. Potentiation of sympathetic nerve responses to hypoxia in borderline hypertensive subjects. *Hypertension.* 1988;**11**:608-612.

61. Somers VK, Dyken ME, Clary MP, Abboud FM. Sympathetic neural mechanisms in obstructive sleep apnea. *J Clin Invest.* 1995;**96**:1897-1904.

62. Esler M, Jennings G, Lambert G, et al. Overflow of catecholamine neurotransmitters to the circulation: Source, fate, and functions. *Physiol Rev.* 1990;**70**:963-985.

63. Hollenberg NK, Adams DF, Solomon H, et al. Renal vascular tone in essential and secondary hypertension: Hemodynamic and angiographic responses to vasodilators. *Medicine (Baltimore).* 1975;**54**:29-44.

64. DiBona GF, Kopp UC. Neural control of renal function: Role in human hypertension. *In:* Laragh JH, Brenner BM (eds). Hypertension: Pathophysiology, Diagnosis, and Management, 2nd ed. New York: Raven Press, 1995, pp 1349-1358.

65. Thoren P, Ricksten S-E. Recordings of renal and splanchnic sympathetic nervous activity in normotensive and spontaneously hypertensive rats. *Clin Sci.* 1979;**57** (**Suppl 5**):197S-199S.

66. Converse RL Jr, Jacobsen TN, Toto RD, et al. Sympathetic overactivity in patients with chronic renal failure. *N Engl J Med.* 1992;**327**:1912-1918.

67. Frohlich ED. Other adrenergic inhibitors and the direct-acting smooth muscle vasodilators. *In:* Oparil S, Weber MA (eds). Hypertension. A Companion to Brenner and Rector's The Kidney. Philadelphia: WB Saunders, 2000, pp 637-643.

68. Light KC. Environmental and psychosocial stress in hypertension onset and progression. *In:* Oparil S, Weber MA (eds). Hypertension. A Companion to Brenner and Rector's The Kidney. Philadelphia: WB Saunders, 2000, pp 59-70.

69. Calhoun DA, Mutinga ML, Collins AS, et al. Normotensive blacks have heightened sympathetic response to cold pressor test. *Hypertension.* 1993;**22**:801-805.

70. Folkow B. Physiological aspects of primary hypertension. *Physiol Rev.* 1982;**62**:347-504.

71. Schiffrin EL. Effects of antihypertensive drugs on vascular remodeling: Do they predict outcome in response to antihypertensive therapy? *Curr Opin Nephrol Hypertens.* 2001;**10**:617-624.

72. Mendelsohn ME. In hypertension, the kidney is not always the heart of the matter. *J Clin Invest.* 2005;**115**:840-844.

73. Hirooka Y, Shimokawa H, Takeshita A. Rho-kinase, a potential therapeutic target for the treatment of hypertension. *Drug News Perspect.* 2004;**17**:523-527.

74. Crowley SD, Gurley SB, Oliverio MI, et al. Distinct roles for the kidney and systemic tissues in blood pressure regulation by the renin-angiotensin system. *J Clin Invest.* 2005;**115**: 1092-1099.

75. Johnson RJ, Rodriguez-Iturbe B, Kang D-H, et al. A unifying pathway for essential hypertension. *Am J Hypertens.* 2005;**18**:431-440.

76. Culleton BF, Larson MG, Kannel WB, Levy D. Serum uric acid and risk for cardiovascular disease and death: The Framingham Study. *Ann Intern Med.* 1999;**131**:7-13.

77. Messerli FH, Frohlich ED, Dreslinski GR, et al. Serum uric acid in essential hypertension: An indicator of renal vascular involvement. *Ann Intern Med.* 1980;**93**:817-821.

78. Franse LV, Pahor M, Di Bari M, et al. Serum uric acid, diuretic treatment and risk of cardiovascular events in the Systolic Hypertension in the Elderly Program. *J Hypertens.* 2000;**18**:1149-1154.

79. Hoieggen A, Alderman MA, Kjeldsen SE, et al., for the LIFE Study Group. The impact of serum uric acid on cardiovascular outcomes in the LIFE study. *Kidney Int.* 2004;**65**:1014-1019.

80. Mazzali M, Kanellis J, Han L, et al. Hyperuricemia induces a primary renal arteriolopathy in rats by a blood pressure–independent mechanism. *Am J Physiol Renal Physiol.* 2002;**282**:F991-F997.

81. Rao GN, Corson MA, Berk BC. Uric acid stimulates vascular smooth muscle cell proliferation by increasing platelet derived growth factor A-chain expression. *J Biol Chem.* 1991;**266**: 8604-8608.

82. Reudelhuber TL. Renin. *In:* Oparil S, Weber MA (eds). Hypertension, 2nd ed. A Companion to Brenner & Rector's The Kidney. Philadelphia: Elsevier, 2005, pp 89-94.

83. Alderman MH, Madhavan S, Ooi WL, et al. Association of the renin-sodium profile with the risk of myocardial infarction in patients with hypertension. *N Engl J Med.* 1991;**324**:1098-1104.

84. Tipnis SR, Hooper NM, Hyde R, et al. A human homolog of angiotensin-converting enzyme: Cloning and functional expression as a captopril-insensitive carboxypeptidase. *J Biol Chem.* 2000;**277**:33238-33243.

85. Tea BS, Der Sarkissian S, Touyz RM, et al. Proapoptotic and growth-inhibitory role of angiotensin II type 2 receptor in vascular smooth muscle cells of spontaneously hypertensive rats in vivo. *Hypertension.* 2000;**35**:1069-1073.

86. Carey RM, Siragy HM. Newly recognized components of the renin-angiotensin system: Potential roles in cardiovascular and renal regulation. *Endocr Rev.* 2003;**24**:261-271.

87. Fukui T, Ishizaka N, Rajagopalan S, et al. p22phox mRNA expression and NADPH oxidase activity are increased in aortas from hypertensive rats. *Circ Res.* 1997;**80**:45-51.

88. Funder JW. Aldosterone and mineralocorticoids. *In:* Oparil S, Weber MA (eds.) Hypertension, 2nd ed. A Companion to Brenner & Rector's The Kidney. Philadelphia: Elsevier, 2005, pp 117-122.

89. Mihailidou A, Mardini M, Funder JW. Rapid, nongenomic effects of aldosterone in the heart mediated by epsilon protein kinase C. *Endocrinology.* 2004;**145**:773-780.

90. Fardella CE, Mosso L, Gomez-Sanchez C, et al. Primary hyperaldosteronism in essential hypertensives: Prevalence, biochemical profile, and molecular biology. *J Clin Endocrinol Metab.* 2000;**85**:1863-1867.

91. Goodfriend TL, Calhoun DA. Resistant hypertension, obesity, sleep apnea, and aldosterone: Theory and therapy. *Hypertension.* 2004;**43**:518-524.

92. Nishizaka MK, Zaman MA, Calhoun DA. Efficacy of low-dose spironolactone in subjects with resistant hypertension. *Am J Hypertens.* 2003;**16**:925-930.

93. Nishizaka MK, Zaman MA, Green SA, et al. Impaired endothelium-dependent flow-mediated vasodilation in hypertensive subjects with hyperaldosteronism. *Circulation.* 2004;**109**:2857-2861.

94. Ibsen H, Olsen MH, Wachtell K, et al. Reduction in albuminuria translates to reduction in cardiovascular events in

hypertensive patients: Losartan Intervention For Endpoint Reduction in Hypertension study. *Hypertension.* 2005;**45**: 198-202.

95. Krum H, Viskoper RJ, Lacoucière Y, et al. The effect of an endothelin-receptor antagonist, bosentan, on blood pressure in patients with essential hypertension: Bosentan Hypertension Investigators. *N Engl J Med.* 1998;**338**:784-790.

96. Campese VM, Nadim MK. Natriuretic peptides. *In:* Oparil S, Weber MA (eds). Hypertension, 2nd ed. A Companion to Brenner & Rector's The Kidney. Philadelphia: Elsevier, 2005, pp 169-192.

97. Wang D, Oparil S, Feng JA, et al. Effects of pressure overload on extracellular matrix expression in the heart of the atrial natriuretic peptide-null mouse. *Hypertension.* 2003;**42**:88-95.

98. Takimoto E, Champion HC, Li M, et al. Chronic inhibition of cyclic GMP phosphodiesterase 5A prevents and reverses cardiac hypertrophy. *Nat Med.* 2005;**11**:214-222.

99. Carretero O, Yang XP, Rhaleb NE. The kallikrein-kinin system as a regulator of cardiovascular and renal function. *In:* Oparil S, Weber MA (eds). Hypertension, 2nd ed. A Companion to Brenner & Rector's The Kidney. Philadelphia: Elsevier, 2005, pp 203-218.

100. Watson RE, DiPette DJ, Supowit SC, et al. Vasodilator peptides: CGRP, substance P, and adrenomedullin. *In:* Oparil S, Weber MA (eds). Hypertension, 2nd ed. A Companion to Brenner & Rector's The Kidney. Philadelphia: Elsevier, 2005, pp 193-202.

Diagnosis

Defining Hypertension
Theodore A. Kotchen and Jane Morley Kotchen

OVERVIEW

The definition of hypertension has changed dramatically over time in response to better understanding of the pathophysiology, actuarial considerations of the life insurance industry, studies of blood pressure (BP) in diverse communities or groups of people, consideration of the interaction of BP levels and co-morbid conditions, landmark studies of BP-related health outcomes, and the development and evaluation of effective antihypertensive therapies. Should the "usual" BP in a population be considered normal? Should the rise of BP with age be considered pathologic? Both epidemiologic data and clinical information provide complementary approaches for arriving at a definition. Data obtained from epidemiologic studies and clinical trials provide a wealth of information relevant to the pathophysiology of cardiovascular disease and to the outcome of patients with elevated arterial pressure. In this chapter, we review some of the observations and perspectives that have "defined" hypertension. Ultimately, any definition of hypertension becomes somewhat arbitrary.

HISTORICAL PERSPECTIVE

Soon after the sphygmomanometer was introduced into medical practice, observations based on case studies documented that high levels of arterial pressure are associated with renal, vascular, and cardiac diseases.[1] Recommended upper limits of normal BP were based on arbitrary values, depending on the beliefs of individual medical practitioners. In the opinion of some eminent practitioners, high BP was considered beneficial. In an address given in 1912 before the Glasgow Southern Medical Society and entitled "High Blood Pressure: Its Associations, Advantages, and Disadvantages," Sir William Osler made the following statement about high BP associated with atherosclerosis: "In this group of cases it is well to recognize that the extra pressure is a necessity—as purely a mechanical affair as in any great irrigation system with old encrusted mains and weedy channels. Get it out of your heads, if possible, that the high pressure is the primary feature, and particularly the feature to treat."[2]

Early clinical observations that BP, particularly systolic BP (SBP), increases with age led to extensive debates about whether age-related increases in BP are part of normal aging. One approach to determining normal upper limits of SBP was to calculate an upper limit of normal SBP as "100 plus the age of the individual." Another approach to determining normal BP ranges in populations was to relate BP to the age-specific distribution of BPs in the population. This meant that normal ranges varied for different population groups. The life insurance industry was the first to relate mortality outcomes to BP levels in studies that clearly indicated strong and positive linear associations between BP levels and mortality.[3] Subsequent definitions for the upper level of normal ranges of BP for adults have evolved and have been based on epidemiologic findings relating BP levels and risks for subsequent adverse outcomes in populations or evidence from clinical trials demonstrating reduced risks of adverse outcomes with antihypertensive therapies.

SHOULD AGE BE A CONSIDERATION IN DEFINING HYPERTENSION?

In industrialized societies, both cross-sectional and longitudinal studies document an increase of arterial pressure with age.[4] This age-related BP increase occurs over the entire range of BPs, not merely in individuals with relatively higher BPs. An earlier concept of two populations, one with a definite rise of BP in middle age and another with little or no rise, has proved to be erroneous.[5]

BP is considerably lower in children than in adults and increases steadily throughout the first 2 decades of life. In children and adolescents, BP is closely associated with growth and maturation. Based in part on data derived from the National Health and Nutrition Examination Surveys (NHANES), BP standards (50th, 90th, 95th, and 99th percentiles) for children have been developed based on age, gender, and height.[6] For any given age, BP norms increase as height increases. Numerous studies document tracking of BP over time in children as well as tracking from adolescence into young adulthood.[7-16] Excessive weight gain in adolescence and a family history of hypertension increase the risk of higher BP in early adult life.[15]

In adults, several population-based samples of the United States, including NHANES III, have demonstrated that mean SBP is higher for men than for women during early adulthood, although among older individuals, the age-related rate of rise is steeper for women.[17] Consequently, among individuals age 60 and older, SBP of women is higher than that of men.[18] To some extent, this may be related to selective mortality among men with higher SBPs. Among adults, diastolic BP (DBP) also increases progressively with age until approximately age 55 years, after which DBP tends to decrease. The consequence is a widening of pulse pressure beyond age 60 years (Fig. 4-1), possibly resulting from loss of vascular elasticity.

Based on the age-related rise of BP, in a 1951 publication, increasing BP ranges were proposed for defining normal BP and hypertension in men and women.[19] For example, a proposed lower limit of hypertension increased from 140 to 145/90 mm Hg to 190/110 mm Hg between the ages of 16 and

MALES

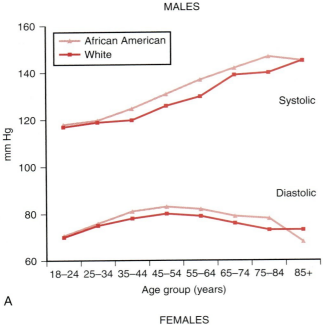

A

FEMALES

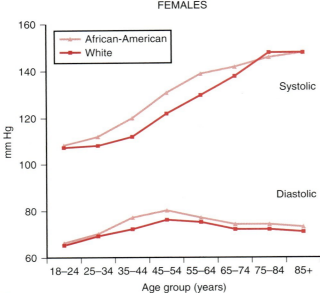

B

Figure 4–1 **A** and **B,** Impact of age on blood pressure in adults, based on cross-sectional data obtained from the third National Health and Nutrition Examination Survey. (Data from the National Center for Health Statistics, Hyattsville, MD.)

60 years. As reviewed later, subsequent epidemiologic observations and clinical trials do not support an age-based definition of hypertension in adults.

Although age-related BP trends may be similar across societies, regional variations of mean BP levels exist,[20] presumably the result of both genetic and environmental factors, including diet. A few primitive societies have been identified in which no increase of BP occurs during adulthood.[21] The absence of an age-related increase of BP is likely the result of extremely low dietary intakes of salt and other lifestyle factors.

EPIDEMIOLOGIC APPROACH TO DEFINING HYPERTENSION: BLOOD PRESSURE AND CARDIOVASCULAR DISEASE RISK

The epidemiologic approach focuses on the relationship between BP level and the risk of cardiovascular disease. Sir George Pickering clearly articulated this in 1968, when he wrote: "Arterial pressure is a quantity and its adverse effects are related numerically to it. The dividing line (between normal BP and hypertension) is nothing more than an artifact."[22]

Subsequent epidemiologic data generally support a continuous, incremental risk of cardiovascular disease, stroke, and renal disease across levels of both SBP and DBP.[23-25] Data collected by insurance companies demonstrate a quantitative relationship between arterial pressure and expectation of life, even at the lower levels of pressure. The Multiple Risk Factor Intervention Trial (MRFIT), which included more than 350,000 male participants, confirms a continuous and graded influence of both SBP and DBP on coronary heart disease mortality, extending down to SBPs of 120 mm Hg.[25,26] Data from the Framingham Heart Study indicate that cardiovascular disease risk is increased 2.5-fold in women and 1.6-fold in men with "high-normal" BPs (SBP 130 to 139 mm Hg or DBP 85 to 89 mm Hg).[23,27] SBP and, to a lesser extent, DBP are also associated with risk of death from both hemorrhagic and nonhemorrhagic stroke. MRFIT data also indicate that risk estimates for end-stage renal disease are graded for both SBP and DBP, and SBP is the stronger predictor of subsequent risk.[28]

Although early definitions of hypertension focused on levels of DBP, it is now recognized that SBP is a more powerful predictor of coronary heart disease than DBP, particularly among older individuals.[29,30] According to Framingham data, before age 50 years, DBP is a stronger predictor of coronary heart disease. However, with increasing age, there is a transition from DBP to SBP as the dominant predictor of coronary heart disease. After age 60 years, coronary heart disease is more closely related to SBP, and wide pulse pressure is also predictive of coronary heart disease. An analysis of the Framingham data indicates that at any level of SBP, the risk of coronary heart disease increases as DBP decreases; that is, higher risk is associated with an increased pulse pressure.[31,32] Similarly, a meta-analysis of several large clinical trials in the elderly indicated that although total mortality is positively correlated with SBP at entry, the association with DBP is negative.[33] This finding again highlights the importance of pulse pressure as a risk factor in the elderly. In elderly and middle-aged men and women, based on data from the Framingham Heart Study, the risk of heart failure is also greater for SBP and pulse pressure than for DBP.[34]

Several additional cohort studies also suggest that SBP and pulse pressure are better predictors of cardiovascular outcomes than DBP.[32,35] Risks of stroke, coronary heart disease, and all-cause mortality are higher in individuals with isolated systolic hypertension (SBP ≥160 mm Hg, DBP <90 mm Hg) than in individuals with diastolic hypertension (DBP ≥90 mm Hg).[25,29] In a prospective cohort of middle-aged men, over a 32-year follow-up period, isolated diastolic hypertension (DBP >90 mm Hg, SBP <140 mm Hg) was not associated with increased mortality.[36] However, a review of nine

SYSTOLIC BLOOD PRESSURE DIASTOLIC BLOOD PRESSURE

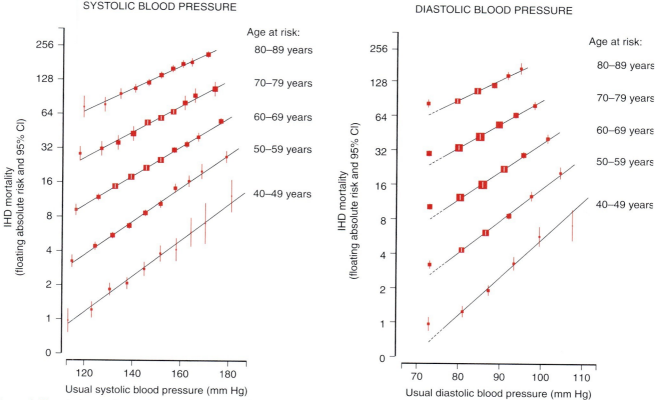

Figure 4–2   Ischemic heart disease (IHD) mortality risk in each decade of age versus usual blood pressure at the start of that decade. CI, confidence interval. (From Prospective Studies Collaboration. Age-specific relevance of usual blood pressure to vascular mortality: A meta-analysis of individual data for one million adults in 61 prospective studies. *Lancet.* 2002;**360**:1903-1913.)

prospective, observational studies documented continuous, positive, independent associations of stroke and coronary heart disease with DBPs in the range of 70 to 110 mm Hg.[37] There was no evidence of any threshold below which DBPs were not associated with lower risks.

Results of a meta-analysis of data from 61 prospective studies involving almost 1 million participants demonstrated that "usual BP" down to a level of 115/75 mm Hg is strongly and directly related to ischemic heart disease mortality, stroke mortality, and mortality from other vascular causes, without evidence of a threshold (Figs. 4-2 and 4-3).[38] Both SBP and DBP were independently predictive of stroke and coronary mortality. The contribution of pulse pressure to cardiovascular risk increased after age 55 years. Between the ages of 40 and 69 years, in both men and women, each 20 mm Hg difference of SBP or approximately 10 mm Hg DBP was associated with more than a twofold difference in stroke death rates and with a twofold difference in death rates from ischemic heart disease and other vascular causes. The relationship of BPs with cardiovascular mortality was reduced by approximately 50% at ages 80 to 89 years. Based on an overview of prospective cohort studies, in individuals aged 60 to 79 years, each 10 mm Hg lower SBP is associated with a 33% decreased risk of stroke.[39]

CLINICAL APPROACH TO DEFINING HYPERTENSION: BLOOD PRESSURE GOALS FOR ANTIHYPERTENSIVE DRUG THERAPY

From a clinical perspective, hypertension may be defined as that level of BP at which the institution of therapy reduces BP-related morbidity and mortality. In 1971, Evans and Rose defined hypertension "...in terms of a BP level above which investigation and treatment do more good than harm."[40] A closely related corollary to this definition is the determination of the target or goal BP to be achieved by antihypertensive therapy.

In the late 1960s, in placebo-controlled trials, the landmark antihypertensive therapy–related Veterans' Administration Cooperative Studies documented reductions in cardiovascular morbidity and mortality in men with DBPs in the range of 115 to 129 mm Hg and in a subsequent study in men with DBPs of 90 to 114 mm Hg.[41,42] Approximately a decade later, based on comparison of stepped care versus usual care of hypertension, results of the Hypertension Detection and Follow-up Program (HDFP) demonstrated reductions of all-cause mortality, stroke incidence, and cerebrovascular deaths

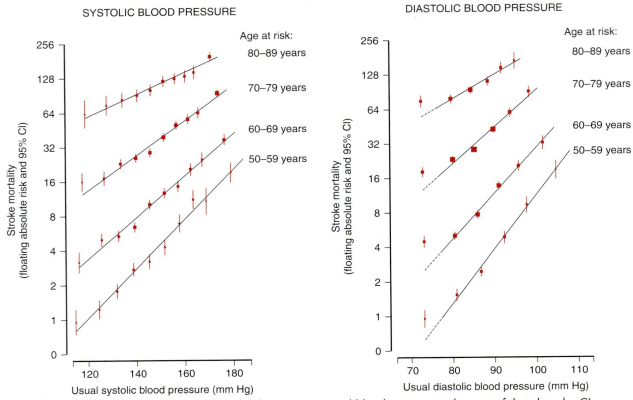

Figure 4–3 Stroke mortality risk in each decade of age versus usual blood pressure at the start of that decade. CI, confidence interval. (From Prospective Studies Collaboration. Age-specific relevance of usual blood pressure to vascular mortality: A meta-analysis of individual data for one million adults in 61 prospective studies. *Lancet.* 2002;**360**:1903-1913.)

associated with blood pressure reductions in individuals with "mild" (DBP 90 to 104 mm Hg), "moderate" (DBP 105 to 114 mm Hg), and "severe" (DBP >114 mm Hg) hypertension.[43] In 1982, a World Health Organization Committee summarized results of the HDFP, in addition to three other trials of hypertension treatment conducted about the same time (US Public Health Service study, the Australian National BP Study, and the Oslo Study).[44] These trials documented the reduction of cardiovascular complications by antihypertensive therapy. However, with follow-up periods ranging from 5 to 7 years, the four trials failed to demonstrate convincingly a reduction of coronary artery disease or nonfatal myocardial infarction. Although acknowledging the beneficial impact of the trials, the World Health Organization Committee concluded that "much knowledge is still needed before safe, effective, and economic control of high BP and its complications can be achieved…."

Since these earlier studies, numerous clinical trials have documented the benefits of antihypertensive therapy on the reduction of cardiovascular disease, including stroke, coronary artery disease, and renal disease.[39,45] Antihypertensive therapy has been associated with average reductions in incidence of stroke by 35% to 40%, myocardial infarction by 20% to 25%, and heart failure by more than 50%.[45] In general, the degree of benefit is related to the magnitude of the BP reduction. For example, a review of clinical trial data suggests that a 10 mm Hg reduction of SBP is associated with a 31% reduction in stroke risk.[39] A meta-analysis of eight trials of isolated systolic hypertension (SBP >160 mm Hg and DBP <95 mm Hg) in the elderly (a total of almost 16,000 participants) indicated that active drug treatment reduced total mortality by 13%, cardiovascular mortality by 18%, all cardiovascular complications by 26%, stroke by 30%, and coronary events by 23%.[33]

A widely cited trial, the Hypertension Optimal Treatment (HOT) trial, attempted to identify the optimum DBP goals for antihypertensive therapy.[46] The trial recruited 18,790 hypertensive subjects, aged 50 to 80 years, with DBPs of 100 to 115 mm Hg. Subjects were randomly assigned to one of three DBP goals: less than 90 mm Hg, less than 85 mm Hg, or less than 80 mm Hg. Average follow-up was 3.8 years. Most cardiovascular endpoints decreased with lower target BPs, but the overall differences were not significant, perhaps because the achieved DBP differences were only about 2 mm Hg. The maximum protection against combined cardiovascular endpoints was observed in the range of 80 to 85 mm Hg for DBP and 135 to 140 mm Hg for SBP.

EVOLVING DEFINITIONS OF HYPERTENSION

Any definition of hypertension should be based on the assumption that appropriate techniques are used for the measurement of blood pressure and that the conditions under which the measurement is obtained are described (see Chapter 5). The Joint National Committee on Prevention, Detection, Evaluation, and Treatment of High Blood Pressure

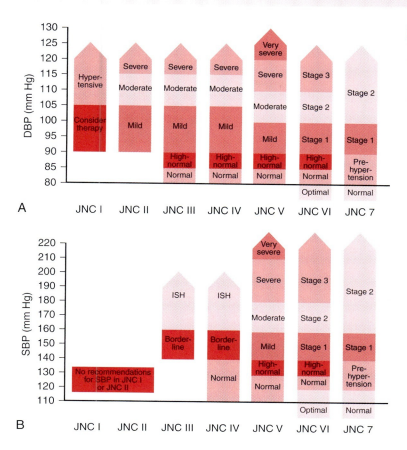

Figure 4–4   **A** and **B,** Changing Joint National Committee (JNC) blood pressure classifications over time. DBP, diastolic blood pressure; ISH, isolated systolic hypertension; SBP, systolic blood pressure. (From Giles TD. Examining therapeutic goals: Population versus individual based approaches. *Am J Hypertens.* 2003;**16**:20S-30S.)

(JNC) guidelines for the definition of hypertension are based on the average of two or more seated BP readings in each of two or more office visits.[47]

Over time, various expert panels have modified guidelines for defining hypertension and for recommending target BP goals for antihypertensive therapy, as more information has become available. In 1971, the Hypertension Study Group recommended criteria for BP screening and referral for individuals with SBP greater than 140 mm Hg or DBP greater than 90 mm Hg.[48] Drug treatment was recommended for patients with hypertension-related cardiovascular disease as well as for "most patients" with DBPs consistently between 95 and 105 mm Hg or higher. There were no recommendations regarding initiation of treatment for SBP.

In 1977, JNC I classified hypertension as DBP 105 mm Hg or higher and suggested only that consideration be given to giving therapy to patients with DBP 90 mm Hg or higher.[49] In 1980, JNC II defined hypertension as DBP 90 mm Hg or higher.[50] There were no recommendations for classifying or treating SBP in JNC I or II. Subsequent JNC reports have recommended progressively more rigorous criteria for defining and treating hypertension (Fig. 4-4).[29]

Numerous classifications for hypertension currently exist. The most recent report for the United States, JNC 7, published in 2003, defines "normal" BP as lower than 120/80 mm Hg.[47] JNC 7 further states that individuals with SBP from 120 to 139 mm Hg or DBP from 80 to 89 mm Hg should be considered "prehypertensive," and health-promoting lifestyle modifications are recommended for these persons. Individuals with SBP 140 mm Hg or higher and/or DBP 90 mm Hg or higher are considered to have hypertension, and

drug therapy is recommended to achieve a goal BP lower than 140/90 mm Hg. Isolated systolic hypertension is defined as SBP 140 mm Hg or higher and DBP lower than 90 mm Hg, whereas isolated diastolic hypertension is defined as DBP 90 mm Hg or higher and SBP lower than 140 mm Hg.

Table 4-1 compares hypertension definitions recommended in 2003 by JNC 7 and by the European Society of Hypertension/European Society of Cardiology.[47,51] The European classification has been endorsed by the World Health Organization and International Society of Hypertension.[52] Although similar, the most notable difference between JNC 7 and the European classification is the distinction between normal BP (SBP <120 mm Hg and DBP <80 mm Hg) and prehypertension (SBP 120 to 139 mm Hg or DBP 80 to 89 mm Hg) in JNC 7 and the definitions of "optimal" (SBP <120 mm Hg and DBP <80 mm Hg), "normal" (SBP <120 to 129 mm Hg or DBP 80 to 84 mm Hg), and "high normal" (SBP 130 to 139 mm Hg or DBP 85 to 89 mm Hg) BP in the European classification.

In approximately 15% to 20% of patients with stage 1 hypertension as defined by JNC 7, BP may be elevated only in the presence of a health care worker, but not when measured at home or at work.[53,54] This phenomenon is referred to as "white-coat" hypertension. A frequently used definition of white-coat hypertension is a persistently elevated average office BP of greater than 140/90 mm Hg and an average awake ambulatory reading of less than 135/85 mm Hg. Although individuals with white-coat hypertension may have less cardiovascular disease risk than individuals with raised office BP as well as raised ambulatory BP, several, but not all, studies suggest that this condition is associated with target organ

Table 4-1 Definitions and Classifications of Blood Pressure Levels

Blood Pressure Classification	Seventh Report of the Joint National Committee		
	SBP (mm Hg)		DBP (mm Hg)
Normal	<120	and	<80
Prehypertension	120-139	or	80-89
Stage 1 hypertension	140-159	or	90-99
Stage 2 hypertension	≥160	or	≥100

Blood Pressure Classification	European Society of Hypertension		
	SBP (mm Hg)		DBP (mm Hg)
Optimal	<120	and	<80
Normal	120-129	or	80-84
High normal	130-139	or	85-89
Grade 1 hypertension (mild)	140-159	or	90-99
Grade 2 hypertension (moderate)	160-179	or	100-109
Grade 3 hypertension (severe)	≥180	or	≥110
Isolated systolic hypertension	≥140	and	<90

SBP, systolic blood pressure; DBP, diastolic blood pressure.
Data from National High Blood Pressure Education Program Coordinating Committee. The Seventh Report of the Joint National Committee on Prevention, Detection, Evaluation and Treatment of High Blood Pressure. *Hypertension.* 2003;**42**:1206-1252; and Guidelines Committee. 2003 European Society of Hypertension: European Society of Cardiology guidelines for the management of arterial hypertension. *J Hypertens.* 2003;**21**:1011-1053.

damage.[51,54] Home BPs and average 24-hour ambulatory BPs are generally lower than clinic BPs, and the discrepancy increases with increasing clinic BP values.[55] Although limited, increasing evidence suggests that home BPs predict target organ damage and morbid events more reliably than do clinic measurements.[53] Several recent studies have attempted to identify the normal ranges for these measurements in two ways: (1) comparison of the BP level that best corresponds to a clinic BP of 140/90 mm Hg; and (2) relating ambulatory BPs to risk in prospective studies.[53] One large study proposed a level of 137/74 mm Hg as an acceptable upper limit for home readings, based on the observation that cardiovascular risks increase above this level.[56] An ad hoc committee of the American Society of Hypertension recommended 135/85 mm Hg as the upper limit of normal for home and ambulatory BPs.[57] Similarly, a committee of the American Heart Association Council on High Blood Pressure Research suggested values for the upper limit of normal ambulatory BPs (Table 4-2).[53]

The 2004 report of the National High Blood Pressure Education Program Working Group on High Blood Pressure in Children and Adolescents defined hypertension in children and adolescents as SBP and/or DBP consistently higher than the 95th percentile for age, gender, and height.[6] To be consistent with JNC 7, BPs between the 90th and 95th percentiles are termed "prehypertensive" and are considered an indication for lifestyle interventions.

REDEFINING HYPERTENSION FOR SELECTED GROUPS OF PATIENTS

More aggressive BP targets may be appropriate for patients with diabetes, coronary heart disease, or chronic kidney disease or patients with additional cardiovascular disease risk

Table 4-2 Suggested Values for the Upper Limit of Normal Ambulatory Blood Pressure (in mm Hg), According to a Recent Report of the Subcommittee of Professional and Public Education of the American Heart Association Council on High Blood Pressure Research

	Optimal (mm Hg)	Normal (mm Hg)	Abnormal (mm Hg)
Daytime	<130/80	<135/85	>140/90
Nighttime	<115/65	<120/70	>125/75
24-hour	<125/75	<130/80	>135/85

From Pickering TG, Hall JE, Appel L, et al. Recommendations for blood pressure measurement in humans and experimental animals. Part 1. Blood pressure measurement in humans: A statement for professionals from the Subcommittee of Professional and Public Education of the American Heart Association Council on High Blood Pressure Research. *Hypertension.* 2005;**45**:142-161.

factors.[58-60] In patients with diabetes, effective BP control reduces the risk of cardiovascular events and death, as well as the risk for microvascular disease (nephropathy, retinopathy). Risk reduction with BP control is greater in diabetic than in nondiabetic individuals. In the United Kingdom Prospective Diabetes Study (UKPDS), 1148 patients with type 2 diabetes were randomly assigned to "tight" BP control versus "less tight" control groups.[61] Mean BP was lower in the tight control group (144/82 mm Hg versus 154/87 mm Hg) during a median follow-up of 8.4 years. Compared with the less tightly controlled group, tight BP control was associated with 32% fewer deaths, 44% fewer strokes, a 56% reduction of heart failure, and a 37% reduction in microvascular endpoints. In the HOT trial, a reduction in DBP from 85 to

81 mm Hg resulted in a 50% decreased risk of cardiovascular events in patients with type 2 diabetes.[46]

Several expert panels have recommended more aggressive BP targets for patients with type 2 diabetes. JNC VI had recommended that diabetic patients with BPs higher than 130/85 mm Hg be started on antihypertensive therapy. In large part because of results of the UKPDS and HOT trials, the guidelines published by the JNC 7, the European Society of Hypertension/European Society of Cardiology, the World Health Organization/International Society of Hypertension, and the Canadian Hypertension Society all recommend less than 130/80 mm Hg as the target BP for patients with type 2 diabetes.[47,51,62] JNC 7 also recommends a goal of less than 130/80 mm Hg for patients with chronic kidney disease.

In a prospective, randomized, placebo-controlled trial of 1991 patients with angiographically documented coronary artery disease and "normal" BP (baseline average, 129/78 mm Hg), BP was decreased by 4.8/2.5 mm Hg with amlodipine therapy and by 4.9/2.4 mm Hg with enalapril.[63] Over a 24-month trial, amlodipine significantly decreased cardiovascular events by 31% compared with placebo-treated patients. A similar, but not statistically significant trend was observed in enalapril-treated patients. Although the reduction of cardiovascular events may have been related to effects of amlodipine and enalapril other than BP reduction, these results raise the possibility that current target goals for BP should be set at lower levels for patients with established coronary artery disease.

Despite theoretical concerns about decreasing cerebral, coronary, and renal blood flow by overaggressive antihypertensive therapy, evidence for a "J-curve" phenomenon is limited. Large clinical trials have found no evidence of a J-curve related to treatment.[39,64,65] Even among patients with isolated systolic hypertension, who are selected on the basis of not having an elevated DBP, further lowering of the DBP does not result in harm.

PERSPECTIVE

As a result of information obtained from both observational studies and prospective clinical trials, since the 1960s hypertension has been defined in terms of progressively lower levels of BP. Currently recommended BP targets may change as additional clinical trial data become available. Further, the definition of hypertension and the determination of BP targets based on results of clinical trials may be somewhat arbitrary because different classes of antihypertensive agents may have additional cardiovascular protective effects beyond their capacity to lower BP. Clinically, other factors in addition to the BP level should be considered when applying recommended guidelines to the care of the individual patient. Decisions about goal BP should also be based on the assessment of overall cardiovascular disease risk, patients' co-morbidities, and the availability of effective and well-tolerated drugs.

References

1. Holden E. The Sphygmograph: Its Physiological and Pathological Indications. Philadelphia, PA: Lindsay and Blakiston, 1874.
2. Osler W. High blood pressure: Its associations, advantages and disadvantages. BMJ. 1912;2:1173-1177.
3. Hunter A, Rogers OH. Mortality study of impaired lives. Actuarial Soc. 1923;24:338.
4. Rodriguez BL, Labarthe DR, Huang B, et al. Rise of blood pressure with age: New evidence of population differences. Hypertension. 1994;24:779-785.
5. Platt R. Nature of essential hypertension. Lancet. 1959;2:55-57.
6. National High Blood Pressure Education Program Working Group on High Blood Pressure in Children and Adolescents. The fourth report on the diagnosis, evaluation, and treatment of high blood pressure in children and adolescents. Pediatrics. 2004;114:555-576.
7. Becket LA, Rosner B, Roche AF, et al. Serial changes in blood pressure from adolescence into adulthood. Am J Epidemiol. 1972;135:1166-1177.
8. Yong LC, Kuller LH. Tracking of blood pressure from adolescence to middle age: The Dormont High School Study. Prev Med. 1994;23:418-426.
9. Wilsgaard T, Jacobson BK, Schirmer H, et al. Tracking of cardiovascular risk factors: The Tromso Study 1979-1995. Am J Epidemiol. 2001;154:418-426.
10. Vos LE, Oren A, Uiterwaal C, et al. Adolescent blood pressure and blood pressure tracking into young adulthood are related to subclinical atherosclerosis: The Atherosclerosis Risk in Young Adults (ARYA) Study. Am J Hypertens. 2003;16:549-555.
11. Lauer RM, Clarke WR, Beaglehole R. Level, trend, and variability of blood pressure during childhood: The Muscatine Study. Circulation. 1984;69:242-249.
12. Bao W, Threefoot S, Srinivasan S, et al. Essential hypertension predicted by tracking of elevated blood pressure from childhood to adulthood: The Bogalusa Heart Study. Am J Hypertens. 1995;8:657-665.
13. Cook N, Gillman M, Rosner B, et al. Prediction of young adult blood pressure from childhood blood pressure, height and weight. J Clin Epidemiol. 1997;50:571-579.
14. Munter P, He J, Cutler JA, et al. Trends in blood pressure among children and adolescents. JAMA. 2004;291:2107-2113.
15. Burke V, Beilin LJ, Dunbar D. Tracking of blood pressure in Australian children. J Hypertens. 2001;19:1185-1192.
16. Kotchen JM, McKean HE, Kotchen TA. Blood pressure trends with aging. Hypertension. 1982;4 (Suppl 3):128-134.
17. Hajjar IM, Kotchen TA. Trends in prevalence, awareness, treatment, and control of hypertension in the United States, 1988-2000. JAMA. 2003;290:199-206.
18. Wiinberg N, Hoegholm A, Christensen HR, et al. 24-h ambulatory blood pressure in 352 Danish subjects, related to age and gender. Am J Hypertens. 1995;8:978-986.
19. Master AM, Goldstein I, Walters MB. New and old definitions of normal blood pressure: Clinical significance of the newly established limits. Bull NY Acad Med. 1951;27:452-465.
20. Kotchen TA, Kotchen JM. Regional variations of blood pressure-environment or genes? Circulation. 1997;96:1071-1073.
21. Page LB, Damon A, Moellering RC Jr. Antecedents of cardiovascular disease in six Solomon Islands societies. Circulation. 1974;49:1132-1146.
22. Pickering G. High Blood Pressure, 2nd ed. New York: Grune & Stratton, 1968, pp 1-3.
23. Vasan RS, Larson MG, Leip EP, et al. Impact of high normal blood pressure on the risk of cardiovascular disease. N Engl J Med. 2001;345:1291-1297.
24. Qureshi AI, Suri FK, Mohammad Y, et al. Isolated and borderline systolic hypertension relative to long-term risk and type of stroke. Stroke. 2002;33:2781-2788.
25. Kannel WB, Vasan RS, Levy D. Is the relation of systolic blood pressure to risk of cardiovascular disease continuous and graded, or are there critical values? Hypertension. 2003;42:453-456.

26. Neaton JD, Kuller L, Stamler J, et al. Impact of systolic and diastolic blood pressure on cardiovascular mortality. *In:* Laragh JH, Brenner BM (eds). Hypertension: Pathophysiology, Diagnosis, and Management, 2nd ed. New York: Raven Press, 1995, pp 127-144.

27. Kannel WB. Blood pressure as a cardiovascular risk factor: Prevention and treatment. *JAMA.* 1996;**275**:1571-1576.

28. Klag MJ, Whelton PK, Randall BL, et al. Blood pressure and end stage renal disease in men. *N Engl J Med.* 1996;**334**:13-18.

29. Giles TD. Examining therapeutic goals: Population versus individual based approaches. *Am J Hypertens.* 2003;**16**:20S-30S.

30. Rutan GH, Kuller LH, Neaton JD, et al. Mortality associated with diastolic hypertension and isolated systolic hypertension among men screened for the Multiple Risk Factor Intervention Trial. *Circulation.* 1988;**77**:504-514.

31. Franklin SS, Larson MG, Kahn SA, et al. Does the relation of blood pressure to coronary heart disease risk change with aging? *Circulation.* 2001;**103**:1245-1249.

32. Black HR. Risk stratification of older patients. *Am J Hypertens.* 2002;**15**:77S-81S.

33. Staessen JA, Gasowski J, Wang JG, et al. Risks of untreated and treated isolated systolic hypertension in the elderly: Meta-analysis of outcome trials. *Lancet.* 2000;**335**:865-872.

34. Haider AW, Larson MG, Franklin SS, et al. Systolic blood pressure, diastolic blood pressure, and pulse pressures as predictors for congestive heart failure in The Framingham Heart Study. *Ann Intern Med.* 2003;**138**:10-16.

35. Borghi C, Dormi A, Ambrosioni E, et al. Relative role of systolic, diastolic and pulse pressure as risk factors for cardiovascular events in the Brisighella Heart Study. *J Hypertens.* 2002;**20**:1737-1742.

36. Strandberg TE, Salomaa VV, Vanhanen HT, et al. Isolated diastolic hypertension, pulse pressure, and mean arterial pressure as predictors of mortality during a follow-up of up to 32 years. *J Hypertens.* 2002;**20**:399-404.

37. MacMahon S, Peto R, Cutler J, et al. Blood pressure, stroke, and coronary artery disease. *Lancet.* 1990;**335**:765-774.

38. Prospective Studies Collaboration. Age-specific relevance of usual blood pressure to vascular mortality: A meta-analysis of individual data for one million adults in 61 prospective studies. *Lancet.* 2002;**360**:1903-1913.

39. Lawes CMM, Bennett DA, Feigin VL, et al. Blood pressure and stroke: An overview of published reviews. *Stroke.* 2004;**35**:1024-1033.

40. Evans, JG, Rose G. Hypertension. *Br Med Bull.* 1971;**27**:37-42.

41. Veterans Administration Cooperative Study Group on Antihypertensive Agents. Effects of treatment on morbidity in hypertension: Results in patients with diastolic blood pressure averaging 115 through 129 mm Hg. *JAMA.* 1967;**202**:1028-1034.

42. Veterans Administration Cooperative Study Group on Antihypertensive Agents. Effects of treatment on morbidity in hypertension. II. Results in patients with diastolic blood pressure averaging 90 through 114 mm Hg. *JAMA.* 1970;**213**:1143-1152.

43. Hypertension Detection and Follow-Up Program Cooperative Group. Five-year findings of the Hypertension Detection and Follow-Up Program. III. Reduction in stroke incidence among persons with high blood pressure. *JAMA.* 1982;**247**:633-638.

44. World Health Organization/International Society of Hypertension Mild Hypertension Liaison Committee. Trials of the treatment of mild hypertension: An interim analysis. *Lancet.* 1982;**319**:149-156.

45. Neal B, MacMahon S, Chapman N. Effects of ACE inhibitors, calcium antagonists, and other blood pressure lowering drugs: Results of prospectively designed overviews of randomized trials. *Lancet.* 2000;**356**:1955-1964.

46. Hansson L, Zanchetti A, Carruthers SG, et al. Effects of intensive blood-pressure lowering and low dose aspirin in patients with hypertension: Principal results of the Hypertension Optimal Treatment (HOT) randomized trial. *Lancet.* 1998;**351**:1755-1762.

47. National High Blood Pressure Education Program Coordinating Committee. The Seventh Report of the Joint National Committee on Prevention, Detection, Evaluation and Treatment of High Blood Pressure. *Hypertension.* 2003;**42**:1206-1252.

48. Wood JE, Barrow JG, Freis ED, et al. Hypertension Study Group guidelines for the detection, diagnosis and management of hypertensive population. *Circulation.* 1971;**44**:A263-A272.

49. Report of the Joint National Committee on Detection, Evaluation, and Treatment of High Blood Pressure. A cooperative study. *JAMA.* 1977;**237**:255-261.

50. Joint National Committee on Detection, Evaluation, and Treatment of High Blood Pressure. The 1980 Report of the Joint National Committee on Detection, Evaluation, and Treatment of High Blood Pressure. *Arch Intern Med.* 1980;**140**:1280-1285.

51. Guidelines Committee. 2003 European Society of Hypertension/European Society of Cardiology guidelines for the management of arterial hypertension. *J Hypertens.* 2003;**21**:1011-1053.

52. World Health Organization, International Society of Hypertension Writing Group. 2003 World Health Organization (WHO)/International Society of Hypertension (ISH) statement on management of hypertension. *J Hypertens.* 2003;**21**:1983-1992.

53. Pickering TG, Hall JE, Appel L, et al. Recommendations for blood pressure measurement in humans and experimental animals. Part 1. Blood pressure measurement in humans: A statement for professionals from the Subcommittee of Professional and Public Education of the American Heart Association Council on High Blood Pressure Research. *Hypertension.* 2005;**45**:142-161.

54. Verdecchia P, O'Brien E, Pickering T, et al. When can the practicing physician suspect white coat hypertension? Statement from the Working Group on Blood Pressure Monitoring of the European Society of Hypertension. *Am J Hypertens.* 2003;**16**:87-91.

55. Parati G, Mancia G. Hypertension staging through ambulatory blood pressure monitoring. *Hypertension.* 2002;**40**:792-794.

56. Ohkubo T, Imai Y, Tsuji I, et al. Reference values for 24-hour ambulatory blood pressure monitoring based on a prognostic criterion: The Ohasama Study. *Hypertension.* 1998;**32**:255-259.

57. Pickering T. Recommendations for the use of home blood pressure monitoring. American Society of Hypertension Ad Hoc Panel. *Am J Hypertens.* 1996;**9**:1-11.

58. Bakris G, Williams M, Dworkin L, et al. Preserving renal function in adults with hypertension and diabetes: A consensus approach. *Am J Kidney Dis.* 2000;**36**:646-661.

59. Snow V, Weiss KB, Mottur P, et al. The evidence for tight blood pressure control in the management of type 2 diabetes mellitus. *Ann Intern Med.* 2003;**138**:587-592.

60. Vijan S, Hayward R. Treatment of hypertension in type 2 diabetes mellitus: Blood pressure goals, choice of agents, and setting priorities in diabetes care. *Ann Intern Med.* 2003;**138**:593-602.

61. United Kingdom Prospective Diabetes Study Group. Tight blood pressure control and risk of macrovascular and microvascular complications in type 2 diabetes. UKPDS 38. *BMJ.* 1998;**317**:703-713.

62. Feldman RD, Campbell N, Larochelle P, et al. 1999 Canadian recommendations for the management of hypertension. *Can Med Assoc J.* 1999;**161**:S1-S17.

63. Nissen SE, Tuzcu EM, Libby P, et al. Effect of antihypertensive agents on cardiovascular events in patients with coronary disease and normal blood pressure. The CAMELOT Study: A randomized controlled trial. *JAMA.* 2004;**292**:2217-2226.

64. Cruickshank JM. J curve in antihypertensive therapy: Does it exist? A personal point of view. *Cardiovasc Drugs Ther.* 1994;**8**:757-760.

65. Farnett L, Mulrow CD, Linn WD, et al. The J-curve phenomenon and the treatment of hypertension: Is there a point beyond which pressure reduction is dangerous? *JAMA.* 1991;**265**:489-495.

Office Blood Pressure Measurement

Clarence E. Grim and Carlene M. Grim

Blood pressure (BP) ranks third (after age and tobacco use) among predictors of mortality.[1,2] Before hypertension can be properly diagnosed, and attempts made to lower BP using lifestyle modifications or drug therapy, accurate measurement of BP is essential. Unfortunately, BP measurement is hardly ever performed according to recognized guidelines, published by the American Heart Association (AHA) periodically since 1938.[3] The European Society of Hypertension recently issued a plea for manufacturers to develop an accurate and reliable BP measuring device for use in low-resource settings, because high BP is now the leading cause of death and disability in every country in the world.[4,5] We would argue that such a device currently exists—a trained health care worker using a mercury manometer and a stethoscope.

A BRIEF HISTORY OF MORE THAN A CENTURY OF BLOOD PRESSURE MEASUREMENT

In the early 1900s, with the advent of standard methods for measuring BP, it became apparent that elevated BP was an important predictor of premature death and disability in patients who reported feeling ill. Janeway coined the term *hypertensive cardiovascular disease* after following 7872 consecutive new patients in whom he measured BP by palpation from 1903 to 1912.[6] He noted that 53% of the men and 32% of the women with symptomatic hypertension died in this 9-year period, and 50% of those who died had done so in the first 5 years after being seen. Cardiac insufficiency and stroke accounted for 50% of the deaths and uremia for 30%. By 1914, the life insurance industry had learned that even in asymptomatic men, the measurement of BP was the best way (after age) to predict premature death and disability, and all insurance examiners were required to measure BP for a person to obtain a life insurance policy. In 1913, the chief medical officer of the Northwest Mutual Life Insurance Company stated, "No practitioner of medicine should be without a sphygmomanometer. This is a most valuable aid in diagnosis."[1]

Population-based studies of standardized BP measurement began in 1948 with the Framingham Heart Study. Using standardized measurement of BP according to the guidelines developed by the AHA, Framingham investigators demonstrated that cardiovascular risk increased continuously from the lowest to the highest levels of pressure and that the systolic pressure was the most predictive. At least 91% of persons who developed heart failure had high BP before they developed overt heart failure.[7] The impact of BP was even more devastating in African Americans in Evans County, GA, where 40% of all deaths in black women were attributed to high BP.[8]

These results, and the discovery of drugs that lowered BP, led to the implementation of large-scale trials in the 1960s to determine the level of pressure at which the risks of lowering high BP outweighed the risks of not lowering it. These trials required design and implementation of quality improvement strategies to ensure that all personnel at many study centers would measure BP with the highest accuracy and reliability over 5 years. Methods of training developed for these and other trials, as well as for the several population-based National Health and Nutrition Examination Surveys (NHANES), evolved into a standardized training, certification, and quality improvement program.[9] The results of these training programs need to be transferred to the day-to-day practice of medicine if the impressive benefits of these trials are to be relayed to the general population. We have modeled our video and digital video disk (DVD)–based training and certification program on their experiences.[10] Implementation of these training and certification programs for personnel working in NHANES has improved the quality of BP measurements in this important program.[11] In most large-scale hypertension trials, the difference in BP between the treated and untreated groups over 5 years was less than 10/5 mm Hg. Thus, errors of this magnitude, if falsely low, will deny the proven benefits of treatment to millions of people who truly have high BP but who will be incorrectly told that their BPs are not high enough to warrant treatment. Of course, errors that lead to a falsely increased reading will result in overdiagnosis, potentially harmful and expensive treatment, and labeling a person as being hypertensive, which can have significant economic and psychological effects.

ENVIRONMENTAL CONCERNS ABOUT ELEMENTAL MERCURY IN THE MEDICAL WORKPLACE

Since the early 1990s, regulatory authorities (including the U.S. Occupational Health and Safety Administration) have urged removal of mercury and other known toxic substances from all workplaces.[12-15] In some jurisdictions (e.g., Sweden, Minnesota) and health care systems (e.g., U.S. Department of Veterans' Affairs Medical Centers), mercury sphygmomanometers have been prohibited by executive fiat and are being replaced.[13-15] This presents both challenges and opportunities.

The obvious benefit of removal of the known toxin, elemental mercury, is that health care workers will no longer be exposed to even low levels of mercury vapor. Chronic inhalation of mercury vapor has been linked to decreased mental acuity, renal impairment, peripheral neuropathy, and death.[16] Problems have not been reported with mercury exposure from BP devices, except among individuals who repaired them many years ago. The clear concern is that the mercury sphygmomanometer will be difficult to replace, because it is the traditional, very accurate, highly reproducible, and simple method of measuring BP. It has been the "gold standard" device for measurement of office BP for more than 100 years. In fact, the design of the mercury sphygmomanometer is essentially unchanged today from what was used 50 years ago, except today's instrument is less likely to discharge liquid mercury, particularly if it is dropped. Because of the constant density of mercury at all altitudes and inhabitable environments, and its use as a "standard" in all kinds of pressure measurements, there is little difference in accuracy across brands, certainly not the case with other types of sphygmomanometers. Despite the simplicity of the mercury sphygmomanometer, it must be properly maintained and cleaned occasionally. A survey of mercury sphygmomanometers in Brazilian hospitals found that 21% of the devices had technical problems that could reduce their accuracy[17]; a similar study in England found more than 50% of mercury columns that were defective.[18] Most of the problems with these devices were related to the bladders, cuffs, and valves, not the mercury manometers themselves.

Unfortunately, no generally accepted replacement for mercury manometers currently exists, and the most recent set of guidelines from the AHA continues to recommend the use of mercury, if it is available.[19,20] Although the Seventh Report of the Joint National Committee on Prevention, Detection, Evaluation, and Treatment of High Blood Pressure (JNC 7) has not fully endorsed the use of alternatives to the mercury sphygmomanometer,[21] newer BP measurement devices (that do not contain mercury) are being adopted in many centers. Unfortunately, very few "professional" BP measurement devices have been thoroughly tested[22] and proven as reliable, accurate, and long-lived as the mercury column. Most of the inexpensive devices currently on the market are meant for home use (where they may be activated perhaps once daily). These are probably neither accurate nor durable enough to be recommended for a busy health care facility, at which BP is literally measured hundreds to thousands of times a day. Inexpensive aneroid sphygmomanometers are susceptible to damage (particularly after being dropped to the floor), thus resulting in inaccurate measurements that are not easily recognized.[17] Oscillometric devices that have been appropriately validated[23] are uncommon or expensive.[24,25]

Current recommendations from both the AHA and European Expert Committees recommend that whenever a sphygmomanometer that does not contain mercury is to be used, it should be checked regularly against a standard mercury column to ensure its accuracy.[20,26]

HOW CAN WE IMPROVE THE MEASUREMENT OF BLOOD PRESSURE IN CLINICAL PRACTICE?

We agree with the recommendation of the most recent AHA guidelines:

In view of the consequences of inaccurate measurement, including both the over-treatment and under-treatment, it is the opinion of this committee that regulatory agencies should establish standards to ensure the use of validated devices, routine calibration of equipment, and the training and retraining of manual observers. Because the use of automated devices does not eliminate all major sources of human error, the training of observers should be required even when automated devices are used.[19]

Although BP measurement is "taught" in all schools for health professionals, from office assistant to medical school, current evidence shows that correct measurement techniques, according to the AHA's guidelines,[19] are hardly ever taught and are therefore not practiced. Our research suggests that this is the result of an initial failure to master the knowledge, skills, and techniques needed to obtain an accurate BP measurement, as well as the lack of periodic retraining and reevaluation thereafter, which the AHA recommends on a semiannual basis.[19] Neither beginning medical students (who claim to have learned proper BP measurement technique) nor practicing nurses in Australia had sufficient knowledge to pass a standardized test regarding correct technique in BP measurement.[27,28]

The importance of retraining and retesting was illustrated in the British Regional Heart Study, in which simultaneous BP readings were taken by trained nurses who used a triple-headed stethoscope during training.[29] Immediately after the initial training, the interindividual variability in the field (shown on the y-axis of Fig. 5-1) was very small, but it increased progressively during the first 6 months of the study. After the preplanned retraining session at 6 months (designated by a T at the top of Fig. 5-1), the interindividual variability decreased again, nearly to baseline levels. However, because the nurses considered the training tedious and unnecessary, the second retraining session, scheduled for 12 months, was not held. At 14 months into the study, however, the systolic BPs recorded by observers 1 and 2 differed by an

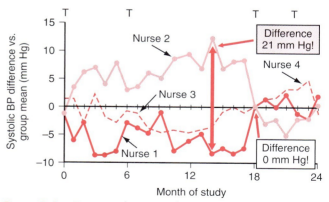

Figure 5–1 Training decreases between-observer measurement differences in blood pressure. In this 24-month British Regional Heart Study, three nurses measured blood pressure during a population survey, and their interindividual variation is plotted on the y-axis over time. After training sessions (T at the *top*), the interindividual variations decreased markedly. When the training session scheduled at 12 months was omitted, the variation hit a peak, but it dropped back to very little after the next training session at 14 months. (Modified from Bruce NG, Shaper AG, Walker M, Wannamethee G. Observer bias in blood pressure studies. *J Hypertens.* 1988;**6**:375-380.)

average of 21 mm Hg. After retraining at 18 months, the interindividual variability returned to 0 mm Hg. The authors suggested that retraining and retesting should be done every few months for research studies, but this may not be practical in routine medical practice. We disagree and have developed, tested, and published a video-tutored program that teaches the AHA guidelines and tests mastery of the knowledge, skills, and techniques required to obtain an accurate and reliable BP.[10] In our experience, 6 to 8 hours of contact time are needed, but few curricula in the medical profession devote sufficient time to practice and then test a student's mastery of this critical skill. In addition, equipment maintenance and observer quality assurance programs should be part of the curriculum.

BLOOD PRESSURE MEASUREMENT: PROPER TECHNIQUE FOR QUALITY ASSURANCE AND IMPROVEMENT

This section summarizes our curriculum that reviews, reinforces, and tests the knowledge, skills, and technique needed to obtain an accurate BP measurement.[10] It is based on all six of the AHA recommendations for BP measurement[19,30] and on many years of experience teaching these skills and certifying practitioners in research studies or clinical practice, funded by the National Institutes of Health, the pharmaceutical industry, and public and private health care delivery systems.

Critical Skills for Any Blood Pressure Observer

Any person who measures BP or who interprets the readings made by others must possess the skills, knowledge, and mastery of techniques summarized in Figure 5-2. Proper measurement of BP involves coordination hands, eyes, ears, and mind, and deficits in any one of these areas can lead to imprecise and erroneous measurements. In our testing of experienced observers, we have found persons who could not hear well enough to identify Korotkoff sounds. Other individuals could not remember the systolic pressure without writing it down during cuff deflation. Staff in every practice setting can be screened for these problems by testing with standard videotapes and multiple-earpiece stethoscope BP measurements (described later).

Manometers and Their Calibration

A mercury manometer, two aneroid gauges (one intact and one with the face removed) and an electronic BP measuring device are shown in Figures 5-3 and 5-4. The mercury

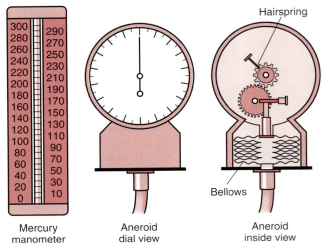

Figure 5–3 Two manometers commonly used in blood pressure measurement. The mercury column *(left)* has been the traditional "gold standard" for pressure measurement in science, industry, and medicine; the aneroid manometer with the dial *(center)* and with dial removed *(right)* are shown.

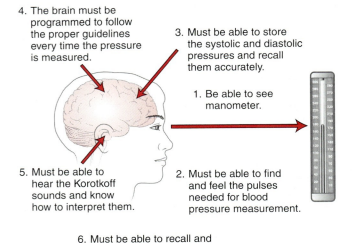

Figure 5–2 The skills needed to obtain an accurate blood pressure. High-level integration of eye, hand, ear, and brain coordination is necessary.

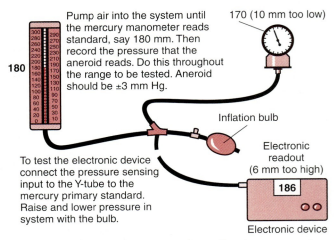

Figure 5–4 Diagrammatic setup for calibrating manometers against the "gold standard" of the mercury column. Note the use of the Y-tube to connect the devices in parallel with the mercury manometer, to allow simultaneous measurement of the pressure.

manometer is the primary (reference) standard for all pressure measurements in science, industry, and medicine. The pressure is read at the top of the liquid mercury meniscus to the nearest 2 mm Hg. All who measure BP with nonmercury devices should have at least one reference mercury device available to check other devices regularly, or they should have an electronic calibration device traceable directly to the mercury standard. The tube containing the mercury should be large enough to allow rapid increases and decreases in pressure. The 2-mm graduated markings should be on the tube itself. The standard glass tube, which can break, should be replaced with either a Mylar-wrapped glass tube or a plastic tube. The inside view of the aneroid device (see Fig. 5-3) shows that it contains a delicate system of gears and bellows that can be easily damaged by rough handling. Such devices also ultimately develop metal fatigue, which leads to inaccuracy. In a recent survey, at least 30% of aneroid devices were out of calibration, and the error was almost always too low.[10,31] To detect an inaccurate aneroid device, inspect the face for cracks and be sure the needle is at zero. If it does not read zero, it will nearly always be inaccurate and should be recalibrated before reuse. Once an aneroid device is out of calibration, it is difficult to detect the direction of the variance without calibrating it against a mercury or other reference standard. This process is uncommon, both in the United States and in England.[18,19]

Calibrating the Manometer

If a mercury device is at zero and the column is clean and rises and falls rapidly with inflation and deflation, the manometer is, by definition, accurate. To calibrate other manometers, they should be connected in parallel by Y-tubes (e.g., Fig. 5-4). Mercury or aneroid devices should be checked for leaks by wrapping the BP cuff around a book or can and inflating the cuff to 200 mm Hg. Wait 1 minute. Record the pressure. If it is lower than 170 mm Hg, there is a leak that must be found. If pinching the tubing just before the inflation bulb stops the leak, the leak is in the valve, which can be taken apart and cleaned or replaced. If the leak continues when the tubing is pinched just before the manometer, the leak is in the manometer. If this is the case, the procedure is as follows: (1) note whether the mercury column rises and falls smoothly, (2) locate and correct any leaks by replacing the appropriate part (although a leak of <2 mm/second can be tolerated, because this is the correct deflation rate), and (3) date the device to indicate when it was last inspected or repaired. Now reinflate again to 200 mm Hg. Deflate the pressure in the system slowly, and check the aneroid manometer against the mercury column at the critical decision points for BP: 180, 160, 140, 130, 120, 110, 100, 90, 80, and 70 mm Hg. The standard for reading both mercury and aneroid manometers is as follows: if the Korotkoff sound occurs or the tip of the aneroid needle is at or above the middle of the 2-mm mark, one should round up the reading to the nearest 2 mm Hg; if the reading is below the middle of the 2-mm mark, the reading is rounded down to the nearest 2 mm. With the Y-tube connecting the aneroid and mercury manometers, if the average of readings from the nonmercury device differs from that of the mercury column by more than ±3 mm Hg,[32] the nonmercury device should be either recalibrated by trained personnel or discarded.

To calibrate an electronic device, connect the electronic instrument and the mercury column using the Y-tube, and check the pressures registered on the electronic manometer as described earlier. Activate the inflation mechanism of the electronic device, and compare the pressure on the digital display with the mercury column. Occasionally, it is necessary to squeeze the rolled-up cuff to simulate a pulsating arm, to avoid an error signal and automatic deflation of the electronic monitor.

Is This Electronic Device Accurate When Used for an Individual Patient?

Now that the electronic manometer is properly calibrated, the question arises whether the specific electronic device records an accurate BP in a specific patient. Unfortunately, no standard method exists to determine this for a single patient. We recommend using the following protocol: Connect the electronic and mercury manometers in parallel with a Y-tube. Place a piece of paper over the digital readout (to avoid bias). Trigger the automatic device, and measure the BP in the usual fashion, by watching the mercury manometer and detecting Korotkoff sounds with the stethoscope (see later for more details). Immediately write down the BP reading, then uncover the digital readout and record the electronic device's reading. If working with another observer, both observers should measure the BP simultaneously, using a double-earpiece stethoscope. Take at least three readings, and compare the average to that of the electronic device. To meet the Association for the Advancement of Medical Instrumentation's current criteria for electronic monitors, the average difference must be less than 5 mm Hg (both systolic and diastolic), and the standard deviation of the difference must be less than 8 mm Hg.[32] An expert panel from the European Society of Hypertension proposed a simpler set of validation criteria that require only four simultaneous readings, and the new device is approved if both systolic and diastolic readings are within 5 mm Hg of the standard device in at least two of the four readings.[33] In our opinion, these methods of validating monitors are not detailed enough to be useful, but they do require a formal comparison of a new device with the traditional mercury column. Although electronic BP measurement devices must meet standard criteria to be marketed to the public in Great Britain, no such requirements exist in the United States. Every 90 days, the dabl Educational Trust updates their useful Web site that lists available BP monitors by type and validation status (http://www.dableducational.org/sphygmo-manometers/device_index.html).

Stethoscope

The bell, or low-frequency detector head, of the stethoscope is designed to transmit low frequency (e.g., Korotkoff) sounds more accurately and can be placed more precisely over the brachial artery than the diaphragm. We do not recommend electronic stethoscopes, because it may be difficult to adjust the amplification so the person using the electronic stethoscope hears what a standardized observer hears with the bell. The tubing connecting the bell to the earpieces should be thick and 12 to 15 inches in length. For sound transmission, earpieces should be worn tilted in the direction of the ear canal, that is, toward the nose. Numerous types of ear tips are available, and each observer should determine which type works best for sound transmission into that person's ears. One way to determine whether the skin seal with the bell over the artery is adequate is to touch the skin lightly next to the bell. If the finger touching the skin cannot be heard, then adjust the stethoscope so the bell is not open to the air, there is an air-tight skin seal around the bell, the stethoscope earpieces face forward, and finally, the earpieces fit well within the ear canals. We call this the "touch" test to document that the sound conducting system is functioning properly, from the skin over the artery to the earpieces of the stethoscope in the ears.

Application of the Most Accurate Blood Pressure Cuff

Measure the Arm Circumference at the Midbiceps

Have the subject stand and drop the arm, but flex the forearm at 90 degrees. Place the end of the tape measure at the acromioclavicular joint (tip of the shoulder), and measure to the tip of the elbow (olecranon). Divide this length in half, and place a small mark on the lateral biceps at this distance from the acromion. Let the patient's forearm hang down, and measure the circumference of the upper arm at this mark in a plane parallel to the floor. The tape should lie against the skin without indenting it. This circumference is used to select the correct size of cuff from those available. Unfortunately, no standards exist for BP cuff sizes, and different manufacturers make different-sized bladders, sold by the same name. The newest AHA guidelines[20] radically changed the cuff size recommendations, and we recommend that observers do not adopt this aspect of these recommendations (as compared with the last several guidelines[30,34]) until this dispute about cuff sizes is resolved. Table 5-1 presents bladder sizes from both the previous and current AHA guidelines; very few commercially available bladders correspond to the new guidelines.

Table 5-1   Blood Pressure Cuff Sizes and Arm Circumferences Recommended by the American Heart Association in 2001 and in 2005 (in parentheses)

Cuff Label	Arm Circumference (cm)	Width (cm)	Length (cm)
Child	16-21	8	21
Small adult	22-26	10 (12)	24 (22)
Adult	27-34	13 (16)	30 (30)
Large adult	35-44	16 (16)	38 (36)
Thigh	45-52	20 (16)	42 (42)

Data from Pickering TG, Hall JE, Appel LJ, et al. Recommendations for blood pressure measurement in humans and experimental animals. Part 1. Blood pressure measurement in humans: A Statement for Professionals from the Subcommittee of Professional and Public Education of the American Heart Association Council on High Blood Pressure Research . *Hypertension.* 2005;**45**:142-161; Perloff D, Grim C, Flack J, et al. Human blood pressure determination by sphygmomanometry. Dallas, TX: American Heart Association, 2001. (Found on the Internet at http://www.americanheart.org/presenter.jhtml?identifier=3002913. Accessed December 30, 2004.)

All guidelines agree that the width of the cuff bladder should be at least 40% of the arm circumference, and the length of the bladder must encircle at least 80% of the arm. Because of increasing obesity in the population, a cuff with a width that is at least 40% of the arm circumference[35] will exceed the distance between the axilla and the antecubital fossa in many people.[36] Some manufacturers provide markings on the BP cuff that denote the smallest and largest circumference arms for which the cuff has the appropriate size; we recommend making these marks on cuffs that do not have them provided. The correct way to mark a cuff is shown in Figure 5-5. Mark an S line for the smallest arm for this cuff and an L for the largest arm for this cuff. When positioning the BP cuff, observe where the index line falls. If it is outside the L line, use a larger cuff. If it is inside the S line, use a smaller cuff. Choosing the incorrect size of BP cuff has been the most common error in BP measurement for more than 20 years.[36,37] In a study of British hypertensive patients, 83% of the mistakes of this type resulted from choosing the smaller cuff for larger arms.[38]

Wrap the Cuff over the Upper Arm and Center the Bladder over the Brachial Artery at Heart Level (Right Atrium or Fourth Intercostal Space)

Two dimensions of the bladder require proper placement to determine an accurate BP. The center of the bladder *length* must go over the brachial artery, typically just above and medial to the antecubital fossa, just under the medial bicipital groove. The center of the *width* of the bladder should be halfway up the length of the upper arm (see earlier). Finally, the arm height must be adjusted so the center of the bladder width on the arm is at "heart level" (the fourth intercostal space). If the center of the cuff is above this line, the pressure measured will be falsely low, and vice versa. Each inch of displacement from this point will change BP by 2.5 mm Hg. A small pillow is often used to support the patient's elbow and upper arm when one measures BP in barrel-chested people

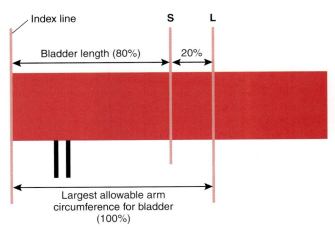

Figure 5-5   Schematic diagram for marking the blood pressure cuff to designate the lower limit of arm circumference that should be used (same as the bladder length, marked S), and the upper limit of arm circumference that should be used (20% longer than the bladder length, marked L).

who are supine, because the arm would otherwise be 5 to 8 cm below the right atrium.[19]

Preparing for an Accurate Reading

In the United States, seated BP measurements are traditional; in most of Europe, supine measurements are routine. Diastolic BP is usually higher (by ~5 mm Hg) when one is seated than when one is supine, but the differences in systolic BP are smaller.[39,40] The arm wearing the BP cuff should be supported, usually at the elbow, by an armrest or a nearby table if the patient is seated (Fig. 5-6) or by a stand or the observer if the patient is standing. Do not measure BP with the patient seated on the examining table, because the muscular work involved in sitting without back support increases the diastolic BP about 5 mm Hg.[40,41]

The purpose of preparation is to inquire about, note, and control factors that can cause changes in BP, to obtain the best-standardized estimate of BP. The observer should inquire about and note factors that could acutely affect BP: pain, recent tobacco use, distended bowel or bladder, food or caffeine ingestion, over-the-counter medications (including cold preparations and nonsteroidal anti-inflammatory drugs), or strenuous exercise during the last 30 minutes. The setting should be quiet and relaxed, because talking raises systolic BP

about 10 mm Hg, and listening about half as much. Feet should be relaxed and flat on the floor (if the patient is seated), because crossing the legs raises systolic BP about 5 mm Hg.[42] The manometer should be placed so the scale is visible at eye level of the observer. We recommend that the observer also be seated, because this is more comfortable and decreases extraneous sounds generated by observer movement when standing, leaning over the patient, and moving around the room. Extraneous sound generation can also be reduced by resting the observer's arm holding the stethoscope head on the table, as well as resting the observer's hand holding the bulb on the table. Other sources of noise (e.g., heating or air conditioning) should also be minimized.

Measuring the Blood Pressure

After a brief explanation of the need for silence, multiple readings (typically three) in short sequence, and correct posture, apply the appropriately sized BP cuff, and then leave the patient alone (and silent) for 5 minutes. If the patient is not wearing a short-sleeved shirt or blouse, provide a gown or remove the patient's arm from the sleeve, and suggest wearing a loose, short-sleeved garment at future visits.

Which Arm Should Be Used?

At the first visit, BP should be recorded in both arms. This is the only way to avoid missing a significant difference between the two arms, which can be as much as 100 mm Hg. After the first visit, the arm with the higher BP is traditionally used. The most common cause of a between-arm difference in older people is a hemodynamically significant atherosclerotic stenosis of the left subclavian artery. Such a stenosis is 10 times more likely on the left than on the right side. Most coarctations of the aorta that result in BP differences in the two arms also cause lower BP in the left arm. In the screening situation in which BP is to be measured in only one arm, unless the subject knows that one arm has a higher BP, the right arm is traditionally chosen. Recent research involving 854 normotensive and 2395 hypertensive subjects validates this recommendation, because the right arm BP was significantly higher (by 3/5 mm Hg) than the left in all six sequential BP measurements.[43]

How High Should the Cuff Be Inflated to Avoid Missing an Auscultatory Gap?

An auscultatory gap is the name given to situation in which Korotkoff sounds temporarily disappear between phase 1 and phase 4, only to reappear at a lower BP. It is more common in older people with wide pulse pressures and target organ damage.[44] To avoid missing this phenomenon, the maximum inflation level (MIL) must first be found, as follows:

1. Inflate the cuff to 60 mm Hg, then inflate by 10 mm Hg increments until the radial pulse at the wrist can no longer be felt. Inflate another 10 mm Hg, and then deflate at 2 mm Hg/second. Note where the pulse reappears as the cuff is slowly deflated. This is the palpated systolic pressure, which is very close to the true intra-arterial systolic pressure.
2. Release the pressure completely.

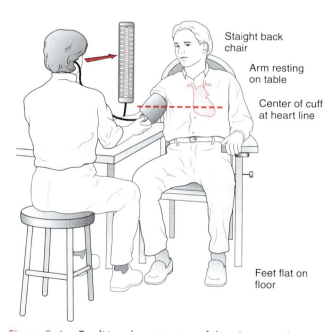

Figure 5–6   Traditional positioning of the observer, the manometer, the cuff, and the patient for a seated blood pressure measurement. Important features of the positioning include the following: the subject is comfortably seated with his back against the chair, feet flat on the floor, arm bent at the elbow, but supported by the table, with the cuff positioned at the level of the heart (fourth intercostal space) and centered at the midpoint of the humerus. The observer is comfortably seated, with the manometer at eye level, silent, and not touching the cuff with the bell of the stethoscope (the last detail is difficult to appreciate, given the resolution of the figure).

Staight back chair

Arm resting on table

Center of cuff at heart line

Feet flat on floor

3. Add 30 mm Hg to the palpated systolic pressure; this is the MIL. Inflating the cuff above this level will cause discomfort and will waste time in the office setting. For example, if the palpated systolic pressure is 100 mm Hg and the cuff is inflated to 200 mm Hg and is then deflated at 2 mm/second, it will take 50 seconds before the phase 1 Korotkoff sound is heard.

What Are the Steps for Properly Taking and Recording the Pressure?

To take the reading, the procedure is as follows:

1. Inflate the cuff quickly to the MIL.
2. Immediately begin to deflate at 2 mm/second.
3. Remember the systolic pressure at the point at which you hear the first of at least two regular or repetitive Korotkoff phase 1 sounds.
4. Repeat this number silently to yourself at each auscultated heartbeat until Korotkoff phase 5 (the diastolic pressure) is detected. This is the level at which the last regular sound is heard. Write down the reading immediately.
5. If Korotkoff sounds are heard to zero, repeat the reading and note the phase 4 Korotkoff (or muffling of sounds), and record all three sounds (e.g., 142/66/0 mm Hg).
6. Record the arm, position, cuff size used, and the systolic and diastolic pressure.
7. Wait 1 minute. Repeat the reading two more times. Some experts recommend taking a fourth reading if the difference between the second and third readings exceeds 5 mm Hg (systolic or diastolic). Many recommend discarding the first readings and averaging the last two, because this has been the protocol followed for many epidemiologic and intervention studies. The National Committee on Quality Assurance accepts the lowest single BP measurement in any position as the "blood pressure for that visit," which is why some managed care organizations require each individual reading to be recorded in the patient's chart.[45]

Where Do I Listen to Hear the Best Blood Pressure Sounds?

In general, sounds are louder closer to the brachial artery, which can be palpated just medial to and usually under the biceps tendon in the antecubital fossa. Extending the patient's arm as straight as possible with the palm up will make it easier to detect Korotkoff sounds. One way to do this is to place the observer's left clenched fist under the patient's right elbow and extend the patient's arm, as if the intent was to hyperextend and break the patient's arm backward at the elbow. The brachial artery should now be easily palpated. Place a small mark over the palpated pulse point. If a pulse cannot be felt close to the medial aspect of the biceps tendon, then palpate other areas over the crease in the bend of the elbow. If a good pulse cannot be palpated, do not use this arm to measure BP, and make a note of this fact in the patient's chart. Place the bell of the stethoscope directly over the palpated pulse to hear the best Korotkoff sounds. Be certain that you have an adequate seal with the edges of the bell and the skin. If the seal is incomplete, the Korotkoff sounds may not be audible. In the rare situation when neither brachial pulse is palpable and a radial artery can be palpated, the cuff may be placed on the forearm and the radial artery auscultated at the wrist, although this technique overestimates systolic BP.[46]

How Can the Korotkoff Sounds Be Made Louder?

One or both of two methods can be chosen. The first ("make a fist" method) uses the increased flow of blood into an arm that has been rendered transiently ischemic by exercise while the arterial circulation is shut off to the arm by the inflated BP cuff. To perform this maneuver, inflate the cuff to the MIL, and have the patient vigorously open and close the fist 10 times. Then have the patient relax the hand and measure BP in the standard fashion. If sounds are still difficult to hear, try the second technique. This technique ("raise the arm method") combines the first with "draining" the blood out of the patient's arm by holding it straight up over the patient's head for 1 minute, then inflating the cuff another 30 mm Hg above the MIL. The arm is then lowered into the usual position, and the BP is measured. If the sounds are still difficult to hear, combine both methods: raise the arm, inflate the cuff, and have the patient squeeze the fist 10 times. Then lower the arm, and record the Korotkoff sounds. In the presence of dysrhythmias, it may be difficult to estimate the BP, and many electronic devices are inaccurate in this situation. It is best to take several BP readings at one sitting, and use the average, because of the beat-to-beat variability of cardiac output in atrial fibrillation and other cardiac dysrhythmias. In extreme cases, it may be necessary to perform an intra-arterial BP measurement, particularly if the patient has a positive "Osler maneuver" (see Chapter 12).

STANDARDIZED MONITORING FOR ACCURACY, REPRODUCIBILITY, AND OBSERVER BIAS

The accuracy of BP measurement can be done with a standardized video test or a stethoscope with two or more sets of earpieces. We recommend using both methods, because Korotkoff sounds in real people are frequently more difficult to interpret than the carefully selected sounds in the videotaped examples. We developed a form to standardize the evaluation of observer accuracy under two circumstances (Fig. 5-7). For video testing, the observers being tested view a videotape consisting of 12 examples (falling mercury columns and corresponding Korotkoff sounds), and then the correct answers are provided and the differences are calculated. This same form can be used with a double stethoscope, in which the instructor or supervisor listens to live Korotkoff sounds simultaneously with the student or observer. The results are graded in the same manner. The form can also be used to assess terminal digit bias over 12 random BPs taken by an observer in different patients. Ideally, the terminal digits (0, 2, 4, 6, or 8) should be evenly distributed among the 24 readings (systolic and diastolic).

All staff members who measure BP should undergo the following on at least an annual basis: (1) they should be observed while taking seated or standing BP and have the technique critiqued and corrected if needed; (2) they should be tested with a double stethoscope for the ability to hear, interpret, and record BPs accurately; and (3) they should be

BP Measurement

GRADING BP ACCURACY AND RELIABILITY

Name _____ Date _____

View the videotape and record your answers in the spaces below.

Example number		Your answer		T	Correct answer	Difference (record sign [±] of diff.)
Example 1	Sys	1	2	8	126	+2
	Dias		5	8	62	−4
Example 2	Sys	2	2	0	220	0
	Dias	1	1	0	118	−8
Video 1	Sys					
	Dias					
Video 2	Sys					
	Dias					
Video 3	Sys					
	Dias					
Video 4	Sys					
	Dias					
Video 5	Sys					
	Dias					
Video 6	Sys					
	Dias					
Video 7	Sys					
	Dias					
Video 8	Sys					
	Dias					
Video 9	Sys					
	Dias					
Video 10	Sys					
	Dias					
Video 11	Sys					
	Dias					
Video 12	Sys					
	Dias					

BP Measurement — Quality Assessment

GRADING BP ACCURACY AND RELIABILITY ACCURACY:

Subtract the correct answer from your answer and place this difference (with sign) in the "Difference" column. Count and record the differences you have from the correct answers in the table below.

Accuracy table

Range	0	±2	±4	±6	≥±8
Count					

To be graded as accurate you should have at least 22 answers that are ±2 and only 2 can be ±4 mm Hg.

ARE YOU ACCURATE?   YES   NO

If you have answers that are ±8 or greater it is likely that you misread the manometer by about 10 mm Hg.

RELIABILITY:

Each of the examples you saw in the standardized video-test was repeated in the sequence. You should be ±2 mm Hg in all of the repeat pairs. Complete the table below to assess your reliability.

Pair	1 and 11	2 and 8	3 and 10	4 and 7	5 and 9	6 and 12
±2?						

ARE YOU RELIABLE?   YES   NO

If you are not reliable it is likely you need to read the manometer more carefully or you have a memory problem.

DIRECTION BIAS:

If you read above or below the correct answer, you have direction bias. Record the number of times your answers are above the correct answer (number of +'s) and the number of times you were below the correct answer (number of −'s) in the table below.

+'s =	Least freq. sign =	1	2	3	4	5	6	7
−'s =	Sum of +'s, −'s =	8–10	11–12	13–15	16–17	18–20	21–22	23–24

You should have about 50% +'s and −'s. Enter the sum of +'s and −'s here = _____ . If this is ≤7, you do not have direction bias. If ≥8, match your sum of +'s and −'s with the cell in the bottom row of the table above. If your least frequent sign is ≤ the value of the cell above it (in the top row) you have direction bias ($P < 0.05$). If you tend to read the systolic too low and the diastolic too high you may have a hearing problem.

TERMINAL DIGIT BIAS:

The last digit of a BP reading should end in an even number if you follow AHA guidelines. Count the number of times your answers ended in 0 and enter it into the "n" row in the table below under the 0's column. Repeat for 2's, 4's, 6's, and 8's. Any answer ending in an odd number is wrong.

End digit =	0's	2's	4's	6's	8's	odd#?
n =						
n^2 =						

Now square each "n" and enter it in the n^2-row. Now add the n^2 in this row and enter here Σn^2 = _____ . If $\Sigma n^2 \geq 161$ you have terminal digit bias ($P < 0.05$). You need to be more careful.

DO YOU HAVE TERMINAL DIGIT BIAS?   YES   NO

BETWEEN OBSERVER BIAS can be assessed by comparing your answers with others who watched the same video.

Figure 5–7   Form for testing accuracy, reproducibility, direction bias, and terminal digit bias of 12 blood pressure (BP) measurements shown on our videotape. AHA, American Heart Association. (From Grim CM, Grim CE. A curriculum for the training and certification of blood pressure measurement for health care providers. *Can J Cardiol.* 1995;**11 (Suppl H)**: 38H-42H.)

assessed with a standardized video test for accuracy, reliability, terminal digit bias, and direction bias. Those who have these errors should be counseled and retested every month until no bias exists. Individuals who cannot be certified as accurate and reliable after several training sessions should not be permitted to measure BP.

INSPECT EQUIPMENT FOR QUALITY ASSURANCE

We recommend that someone in every practice be provided with the training and responsibility to perform regular calibration and quality control so all patients' BP measurements are accurate and reliable. This process involves several steps:

1. Test the mercury manometer. At least once a year, a staff member should inspect each BP-measuring device, document the results, and initiate maintenance if needed.
2. Test the aneroid or electronic manometer. Each one of these must be calibrated against a mercury manometer, using a Y-tube. At least twice a year, a staff member should inspect each BP-measuring device, document the results, and initiate maintenance if needed.
3. Test the stethoscope. Each stethoscope should be checked periodically for wear and damage.

ASSESS KNOWLEDGE ABOUT BLOOD PRESSURE MEASUREMENT

We have found a series of questions to be useful in quickly determining which staff members should undergo more frequent retraining about BP measurement:

1. Which part of the stethoscope head should be used to best hear the low-pitched Korotkoff sounds?
2. How do you know your (or your staff's) hearing is good enough to be able to identify the Korotkoff sounds accurately?
3. How do you know the BP device you use every day is accurate?
4. What is the error caused by having my patient sit on the examining table when BP is measured?
5. Which arm should be used for the most reliable BP?
6. How do you select the correct size of cuff for your patient?
7. When placing the cuff on the arm, where does one place the center of the bladder?
8. When you seat the patient in a straight-backed chair or you take a standing pressure, where do you place the arm to avoid errors in the recorded BP caused by hydrostatic pressure effects?
9. Where do you place the bell of your stethoscope to obtain the best Korotkoff sounds?
10. How high do you inflate the pressure before you start listening?
11. How fast do you deflate the manometer (in mm Hg/second)?
12. Which Korotkoff sound do you (and your staff) use to use to define the systolic BP reading?
13. Which Korotkoff sound do you (and your staff) use to use to define the diastolic BP reading?
14. Your patient with renal disease is 75 years old and has left ventricular hypertrophy detected by the an electrocardiogram, chest radiograph, and echocardiogram. Your nurse reports that she can feel a radial and brachial pulse but cannot hear any Korotkoff sounds. She cannot pump the cuff up high enough to obliterate the pulse, even though she pumps it up to 300 mm Hg. What is the problem?
15. Your elderly patient with angina and claudication has a BP of 122/74 mm Hg in the right arm and 86/50 mm Hg in the left, but this patient has striking left ventricular hypertrophy detected on an electrocardiogram and an echocardiogram and grade IV hypertensive retinopathy. At cardiac catheterization, the aortic BP is 240/140 mm Hg. What do you suspect?
16. What are the likely problems in Table 5-2, a list of BP readings? We recommend that you cover the right part of Table 5-2 until you have made your diagnosis of the BP measurement error.
17. When was the last time you were required to test knowledge, skills, and technique for quality improvement of BP accuracy?

Incorrect or uncertain answers to any two of these questions should motivate health care professionals to update both themselves and their staff in the rationale and techniques required to obtain an accurate BP measurement, which, since 1914,[1] has been one of the simplest and most cost-effective medical procedures that can be done to predict cardiovascular event-free longevity and to improve prognosis.[30]

Table 5-2 Diagnosing Blood Pressure Measurement Errors

122/74	Only one reading. AHA and JNC 7 guidelines recommend two to three readings, to obtain an average, at each visit.
170/75, 165/70, 160/65	BP readings that end in an odd number (5). AHA guidelines indicate that BP should be measured to the nearest 2 mm Hg.
140/80, 150/90, 140/80	Terminal digit bias for 0. The likely cause is deflating too fast or rounding to the nearest "10" instead of the nearest "2."
146/84, 146/84, 146/84	Failure to take second and third BP and just re-recording the first reading as the last two. This was a major problem in several of the MONICA study sites.
188/166, 180/164, 182/162	Failure to recognize an auscultatory gap leads to a falsely high diastolic pressure.

AHA, American Heart Association; BP, blood pressure; JNC 7, seventh report of the Joint National Committee on Prevention, Detection, Evaluation and Treatment of High Blood Pressure; MONICA, Multinational Monitoring of Trends and Determinants in Cardiovascular Disease.

References

1. Fisher JW. The diagnostic value of the sphygmomanometer in examinations for life insurance. *JAMA.* 1914;**63**:1752-1754.
2. Prospective Studies Collaborative. Age-specific relevance of usual blood pressure to vascular mortality: A meta-analysis of individual data for one million adults in 61 prospective studies. *Lancet.* 2002;**360**:1903-1913.
3. McKay DW, Campbell NR, Parab A, et al. Clinical assessment of blood pressure. *J Hum Hypertens.* 1990;**4**:639-645.
4. Parati G, Mendisb S, Abegundeb D, et al. Recommendations for blood pressure measuring devices for office/clinic use in low resource settings. *Blood Press Monit.* 2005;**10**:3-10.
5. Kearney PM, Whelton M, Reynolds K, et al. Global burden of hypertension: Analysis of worldwide data. *Lancet.* 2005;**365**:217-223.
6. Janeway TC. A clinical study of hypertensive cardiovascular disease. *Arch Intern Med.* 1913;**12**:752-786.
7. Levy D, Larson MG, Vasan RS, et al. The progression from hypertension to congestive heart failure. *JAMA.* 1996;**275**:1557-1562.
8. Deubner DC, Tyroler HA, Cassel JC, et al. Attributable risk, population risk and population attributable risk fraction of death associated with hypertension in a biracial community. *Circulation.* 1975;**52**:901-908.
9. Curb JD, Labarthe DR, Cooper SP, et al. Training and certification of blood pressure observers. *Hypertension.* 1983;**5**:610-614.
10. Grim CM, Grim CE. A curriculum for the training and certification of blood pressure measurement for health care providers. *Can J Cardiol.* 1995;**11 (Suppl H)**:38H-42H.
11. Ostchega Y, Prineas RJ, Paulose-Ram R, et al. National Health and Nutrition Examination Survey 1999-2000: Effect of observer training and protocol standardization on reducing blood pressure measurement error. *J Clin Epidemiol.* 2003;**56**:768-774.
12. O'Brien E. Has conventional sphygmomanometry ended with the banning of mercury? *Blood Press Monit.* 2002;**7**:37-40.
13. O'Brien E. Replacing the mercury sphygmomanometer requires clinicians to demand better automated devices. *BMJ.* 2000;**320**:815-816.
14. Aylett M. Pressure for change: Unresolved issues in blood pressure measurement. *Br J Gen Practice.* 1999;**49**:136-139.
15. Padfield PL. The demise of the mercury sphygmomanometer. *Scott Med J.* 1998;**43**:87-88.
16. Clarkson TW, Magos L, Myers GJ. The toxicology of mercury: Current exposures and clinical manifestations. *N Engl J Med.* 2003;**349**:1731-1737.
17. Mion D, Pierin AM. How accurate are sphygmomanometers? *J Human Hypertens.* 1998;**12**:245-248.
18. Markandu ND, Whitcher F, Arnold A, Carney C. The mercury sphygmomanometer should be abandoned before it is proscribed. *J Hum Hypertens.* 2000;**14**:31-36.
19. Pickering TG, Hall JE, Appel LJ, et al. Recommendations for blood pressure measurement in humans and experimental animals. Part 1. Blood pressure measurement in humans: A Statement for Professionals from the Subcommittee of Professional and Public Education of the American Heart Association Council on High Blood Pressure Research. *Hypertension.* 2005;**45**:142-161.
20. Jones DW, Frohlich ED, Grim CM, et al. Mercury sphygmomanometers should not be abandoned: An advisory statement from the Council on High Blood Pressure Research, American Heart Association. Professional Education Committee, Council for High Blood Pressure Research. *Hypertension.* 2001;**37**:185-186.
21. Chobanian AV, Bakris GL, Black HR, et al. Seventh Report of the Joint National Committee on Prevention, Detection, Evaluation and Treatment of High Blood Pressure. National High Blood Pressure Education Program Coordinating Committee. *Hypertension.* 2003;**42**:1206-1252.
22. O'Brien E, Petric J, Littler WA, et al. The British Hypertension Society Protocol for the evaluation of automated and semi-automated blood pressure measuring devices with special reference to ambulatory systems. *J Hypertens.* 1990;**8**:607-619.
23. O'Brien E, Asmar R, Beilin L, et al. European Society of Hypertension recommendations for conventional, ambulatory, and home blood pressure measurement: European Society Working Group on Blood Pressure Monitoring. *J Hypertens.* 2003;**21**:821-848.
24. White WB, Anwar YA. Evaluation of the overall efficacy of the Omron office digital blood pressure HEM-907 monitor in adults. *Blood Press Monit.* 2001;**6**:107-110.
25. Graves JW, Tibor M, Murtagh B, et al. The Accuson Greenlight 300, the first non-automated mercury-free blood pressure measurement device to pass the International Protocol for Blood Pressure Measuring Devices in Adults. *Blood Press Monit.* 2004;**9**:13-17.
26. O'Brien E, Waeber B, Parati G, Myers MG. Blood pressure measuring devices: Recommendations of the European Society of Hypertension. *BMJ.* 2001;**322**:531-536.
27. Grim CE, Grim CM, Li J. Entering medical students who say they have been trained to take blood pressure do not follow American Heart Association guidelines [abstract]. *Am J Hypertens.* 1999;**12**:122A.
28. Armstrong RS. Nurses' knowledge of error in blood pressure measurement technique. *Int J Nurs Pract.* 2003;**8**:118-126.
29. Bruce NG, Shaper AG, Walker M, Wannamethee G. Observer bias in blood pressure studies. *J Hypertens.* 1988,**6**:375-380.
30. Perloff D, Grim CM, Flack J, et al. Recommendations for human blood pressure determination by sphygmomanometry. *Circulation.* 1993;**88**:2460-2470.
31. Gerin W, Schwartz AR, Schwartz JE, et al. Limitations of current validation protocols for home blood pressure monitors for individual patients. *Blood Press Monit.* 2002;**7**:313-318.
32. Association for the Advancement of Medical Instrumentation (AAMI). American National Standard: Electronic Sphygmomanometers. ANSI/AAMI SP10-1992. Arlington, VA: AAMI, 1993, p 40.
33. O'Brien E, Pickering T, Asmar R, et al. Working Group on Blood Pressure Monitoring of the European Society of Hypertension International Protocol for Validation of Blood Pressure Measuring Devices in Adults. *Blood Press Monit.* 2002;**7**:3-17.
34. Perloff D, Grim C, Flack J, et al. Human Blood Pressure Determination by Sphygmomanometry. Dallas, TX: American Heart Association, 2001. (Found on the Internet at http://www.americanheart.org/presenter.jhtml?identifier=30029 13. Accessed December 30, 2004.)
35. Marks LA, Groch A. Optimizing cuff width for noninvasive measurement of blood pressure. *Blood Press Monit.* 2005;**5**:153-158.
36. Graves JW, Darby CH, Bailey K, Sheps SG. The changing prevalence of arm circumference in NHANES III and NHANES 2000 and its impact on the utility of the "standard adult" blood pressure cuff. *Blood Press Monit.* 2003;**8**:223-227.
37. Maxwell MH, Waks AU, Schroth PC, et al. Error in blood-pressure measurement due to incorrect cuff size in obese patients. *Lancet.* 1982;**2**:33-36.
38. Manning DM, Kuchirka C, Kaminski J. Miscuffing: Inappropriate blood pressure cuff application. *Circulation.* 1983;**68**:763-766.
39. Netea RT, Lenders JW, Smits P, Thien T. Influence of body and arm position on blood pressure readings: An overview. *J Hypertens.* 2003;**21**:237-241.

40. Sala C, Santin E, Rescaldani M, et al. What is the accuracy of clinic blood pressure measurement? *Am J Hypertens.* 2005;**18**:244-248.

41. Cushman WC, Cooper KM, Horne RA, Meydrech EF. Effect of back support and stethoscope head on seated blood pressure. *Am J Hypertens.* 1990;**3**:240-241.

42. Peters GL, Binder SK, Campbell NR. The effect of crossing legs on blood pressure: A randomized single-blind cross-over study. *Blood Press Monit.* 1999;**4**:97-101.

43. Arnett DK, Tang W, Province MA, et al. Interarm differences in seated systolic and diastolic blood pressure: The Hypertension Genetic Epidemiology Network study. *J Hypertens.* 2005;**23**:1141-1147.

44. Cavallini MC, Roman MJ, Blank SG, et al. Association of the auscultatory gap with vascular disease in hypertensive patients. *Ann Intern Med.* 1996;**124**:877-883.

45. National Committee for Quality Assurance (NCQA). HEDIS 3.0, vol. 1. Washington, DC: NCQA, 1997.

46. Singer AJ, Kahn SR, Thode HC Jr, Hollander JE. Comparison of forearm and upper arm blood pressures. *Prehosp Emerg Care.* 1999;**3**:123-126.

Chapter 6

Home Monitoring of Blood Pressure

Thomas G. Pickering

Although the diagnosis of hypertension and the monitoring of antihypertensive treatment are usually performed using blood pressure (BP) readings made in the physician's office, and hypertension is by far the most common reason for visiting a physician, the process is neither reliable nor efficient. Thus, physician's measurements are often inaccurate as a result of poor technique, they are often unrepresentative because of the white-coat effect (WCE), and they rarely include more than three readings made at any one visit. It is often not appreciated how great the variations of clinic BP can be. In a study conducted by Armitage and Rose in 10 normotensive subjects, two readings were taken on 20 occasions over a 6-week period by a single trained observer.[1] The authors were so impressed by the spontaneous variability of BP that they concluded that, "The clinician should recognize that the patient whose diastolic pressure has fallen 25 mm Hg from the last occasion has not necessarily changed in health at all; or, if he is receiving hypotensive therapy, that there has not necessarily been any response to treatment." The practical limitation on the number of readings that can be taken at any one visit and on the number of visits means that readings taken during clinic visits will almost always have relatively low reliability.

Home BP monitoring (HBPM) avoids these limitations by enabling larger numbers of readings to be taken in a more representative setting, and it plays an increasingly important role in the diagnosis and treatment of hypertension. Its use has been endorsed by guidelines such as the Seventh Report of the Joint National Committee on Prevention, Detection, Evaluation, and Treatment of High Blood Pressure (JNC 7) and the American Heart Association in the United States,[2,3] as well as the European Society of Hypertension.[4] HBPM complements conventional clinic or office measurement and 24-hour ambulatory BP monitoring (ABPM). It is now used by about 70% of hypertensive patients in Germany, and its use in the United States is also increasing rapidly. To a large extent, this growth has been driven by direct marketing to the consumer, but physicians are now becoming more enthusiastic regarding its use. A recent survey asked 138 U.S. physicians about their attitudes to HBPM, and although 94% agreed that it could be useful, only 63% reported that they encouraged patients to use it.[5]

ADVANTAGES AND LIMITATIONS OF HOME MONITORING

The potential utility to hypertensive patients of measuring BP at home, either by using self-monitoring or by having a family member make the measurements, was first demonstrated in 1940 by Ayman and Goldshine.[6] They found that home BPs could be 30 or 40 mm Hg lower than the physicians' readings, and these differences often persisted over a period of 6

months. This finding raised the question of which set of readings was more meaningful. HBPM has the theoretical advantage of being able to overcome the two main limitations of clinic readings: the small number of readings that can be taken and the WCE. It provides a simple and cost-effective means for obtaining large number of readings, which are at least representative of the natural environment in which patients spend a major part of their day. HBPM has four practical advantages: (1) it is helpful for distinguishing sustained from white-coat hypertension, (2) it can be used to assess the response to antihypertensive medication, (3) it may improve patient adherence to treatment regimens, (4) and it may reduce costs. There is also evidence that it can predict clinical outcomes (Table 6-1).

The limitations of HBPM also need to be specified. First, readings tend to be taken in a relatively relaxed setting, so they may not reflect the BP occurring during stress; second, patients may misrepresent their readings; and third, occasional patients may become more anxious as a result of self-monitoring.

TESTING AND VALIDATION OF MONITORS

Patients should be advised to use only monitors that have been validated for accuracy and reliability according to standard international testing protocols. The original two protocols that gained the widest acceptance were developed in the United States by the Association for the Advancement of Medical Instrumentation in 1987 and the British Hypertension Society in 1990, with revisions to both in 1993. These protocols required testing of a device against two trained human observers in 85 subjects, a criterion that made validation studies difficult to perform. One consequence of this has been that many devices still on the market have never been adequately validated. More recently, an international group of experts who are members of the Working Group on Blood Pressure Monitoring of the European Society of Hypertension produced an International Protocol that should replace the two earlier versions,[7] and it is also easier to perform. Briefly, it requires comparison of the device readings (four in all) alternating with five mercury readings taken by two trained observers. Devices are recommended for approval if both systolic BP (SBP) and diastolic BP (DBP) readings taken are at least within 5 mm Hg of each other for at least 50% of readings.

When HBPM was first used, most studies relied on aneroid sphygmomanometers. In the past few years, automated electronic devices have become increasingly popular. The standard type of monitor for home use is now an oscillometric device that records BP from the brachial artery. Unfortunately,

Table 6-1 Advantages and Limitations of Home Monitoring of Blood Pressure

Advantages	Disadvantages
Elimination of white-coat effect	Possible underestimation of daytime pressure
Increased number of readings	Possible patient misreporting of readings
Assessment of response to antihypertensive treatment	Possible increase in anxiety levels
Reduced costs	
Improved adherence to therapy	
Prediction of outcomes	

Table 6-2 Home Monitoring Devices That Have Been Tested by the Protocols of the Association for the Advancement of Medical Instrumentation and the British Hypertension Society

Recommended or Questionable*	Not Recommended
AND Lifesource 631, 767, 774, 779, 787	Fortec Dr MI100
Microlife BP	Healthcheck CX-5
NuMed Stabil-O-Graph	Nissei Analogue, DS-175
Omron HEM 705, 711, 713, 722, 735, 737	Omron HEM-400C, -403C, -706
Omron M4, M5, MX-2	Philips HP
	Rossmax
	System Dr
	Visomat OZ2

*The name of the manufacturer is given first, followed by the specific model designation.

only a few devices have been subjected to proper validation tests such as the Association for the Advancement of Medical Instrumentation and British Hypertension Society protocols, and several devices have failed the tests. An up-to-date list of validated monitors is available on the dabl Educational Web site (http://www.dableducational.com). Those that have passed the protocols (classified as Recommended or Questionable) are shown in Table 6-2.

The fact that a device passed a validation test does not mean that it will provide accurate readings in all patients. In substantial numbers of individual subjects, the error is consistently greater than 5 mm Hg, even with a device that has achieved a passing grade.[8] This situation may be more likely to occur in elderly or diabetic patients.[9,10] For this reason, it is recommended that each oscillometric monitor should be validated for each patient who will use it before the readings are accepted. No formal protocol has yet been developed for this procedure, but if sequential readings are taken with a mercury sphygmomanometer and then with the device, major inaccuracies can be detected. Simultaneous measurements using a Y-tube connecting both the monitor and a mercury sphygmomanometer to the cuff are likely to be more accurate.

CHOICE OF MONITORS FOR HOME USE

Electronic devices are now available that will record BP from the upper arm, wrist, or finger. Although the use of the more distal sites may be more convenient, measurement of BP from the arm (brachial artery) has always been the standard method, and is likely to remain so for the foreseeable future. SBP and DBP vary substantially in different parts of the arterial tree. In general, the SBP increases in more distal arteries, whereas DBP decreases. Mean arterial pressure falls by only 1 to 2 mm Hg between the aorta and the peripheral arteries.[11]

Arm Monitors

Monitors that measure the BP in the brachial artery with a cuff placed on the upper arm continue to be the most reliable, and they have the additional advantage that the brachial artery pressure is the measure used in all the epidemiologic studies of high BP and its consequences. A typical device is shown in Figure 6-1.

Wrist Monitors

Wrist monitors are the most recent type to be introduced, and they have the advantage of being the most convenient to use. They are also very compact. These devices have the potential advantage that the circumference of the wrist increases relatively little in obese individuals, so there is less concern about cuff size. The smaller diameter of the wrist in comparison with the upper arm means that less battery power is needed to inflate the cuff, and these devices also cause less discomfort for the patient. A potential disadvantage is that the wrist must be held at the level of the heart when a reading is being taken, a requirement that increases the possibility of erroneous readings. Experience with wrist monitors is relatively limited at present, and few monitors have passed the validation studies (see http://www.dableducational.com). They are generally not recommended for routine clinical use.[3,4,12]

Finger Monitors

These devices incorporate a cuff encircling the finger. They are easy to use and are compact. To control for the hydrostatic effect of the difference between the level of the finger and the heart, it is recommended that the readings be taken with the finger held on the chest over the heart; even so, they are not accurate.[3,4] Their use should be discouraged.

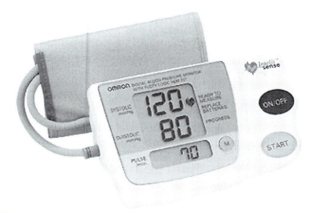

Figure 6–1   A typical home blood pressure monitor. (Courtesy of Omron Healthcare, Bannockburn, Ill.)

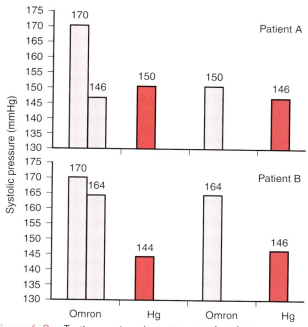

Figure 6–2   Testing patients' monitors in the clinic.

PRACTICAL ISSUES

Several practical issues need to be resolved before patients can start to monitor their BPs on a regular basis.

Is Home Monitoring Acceptable to Most Patients?

With the currently available electronic monitors, most patients can successfully monitor their own BP, because little manual dexterity is required, and adequacy of hearing is not an issue. A potential concern with the use of HBPM is that it will increase the patient's anxiety about his or her condition. In practice, this has usually been found not to be the case: in one study from 1975, 70% of patients reported that they found the technique reassuring. Nevertheless, some patients become so obsessed with their BP readings that HBPM becomes counterproductive. In a study of hypertensive patients in three family practices in England, patients were asked to rate (on a range of 1 [very little] through 7 [very strong]) the degree to which the various methods of BP measurement made them anxious.[13] The median score for HBPM was 2, compared with 4 for the clinic readings taken by physicians. These patients were also asked about the acceptability of ABPM, which they reported to cause discomfort and inconvenience, but not anxiety.

Checking Patients' Monitors

When patients acquire their own home BP monitor, it is very important to have them bring it in to the clinic to check their technique and also the accuracy of the monitor. If a Y-tube is not used to calibrate the home monitor simultaneously, the patient should be asked to take two readings with the monitor, followed by a mercury sphygmomanometer reading, a third reading with the device, and another mercury reading. Figure 6-2 shows results from two patients evaluated by this protocol. In patient A, the readings with the device overlap the mercury readings, and the device can be considered accurate in that patient. In patient B, however, the device significantly underestimates the mercury readings.

Do Patients Provide Accurate Reports of Their Readings?

Substantial discrepancies have been observed in home glucose values reported by patients and those recorded by a device that contained a memory chip (of which the patients were unaware). Extreme readings were especially underreported. The availability of oscillometric HBPM devices with memory chips such as the Omron IC (Omron, Bannockburn, Ill) has enabled the same sort of study to be done with HBPM. In two studies, patients were given home monitors, but they were not told that the devices stored the readings in on-board memory. Patients were urged to record all readings carefully, but in both studies, more than half the subjects omitted or fabricated readings.[14,15] Another study found that 20% of BP readings were reported with an error of more than 10 mm Hg, and that this was particularly likely to happen in patients with poorly controlled hypertension.[16] Devices that have memory or printouts of the readings are therefore recommended.

Does It Matter Who Takes the Readings?

Home monitoring is frequently equated with self-monitoring, but some patients, particularly those who are elderly or disabled, may find it easier to have a family member take the readings. One study compared readings taken either by the patient or a family member in 30 treated hypertensive patients and found that they were the same.[17]

What Is the Reproducibility of Home Readings?

Relatively little has been published on this issue, but it is important. In study in which my colleagues and I compared the reproducibility of home, clinic, and ambulatory readings, all measured twice separated by an interval of 2 weeks, we found that hypertensive patients had a significant decline of

SBP in the clinic over this period, but the home and ambulatory BPs showed no significant change.[18] Normotensive subjects showed no consistent change in any of the three measures of BP. In an earlier study, clinic and home BPs were measured 3 times over a 4-week interval in 17 hypertensive patients. The clinic BPs fell from 181/97 to 162/93 mm Hg, whereas the home BP showed no change (153/89 to 154/89 mm Hg). The superior reproducibility of home and ambulatory measurements may be partly explained by the greater number of readings. These findings support the notion that the fall of clinic BPs on successive visits is primarily the result of habituation to the clinic setting or regression to the mean.

A commonly used attribute of the stability of a measure is the standard deviation of the difference (SDD) between successive readings. When a measure is reproducible, this number is low. In our study, the SDD for the home readings was 5.6/4.6 mm Hg, which was similar to the SDD for ambulatory readings (5.3/5.4) and lower than for clinic reading (9.7/6.7).[18] The correlation coefficients for all three sets of measurements were very close (0.96/0.94 for home, 0.93/0.87 for ambulatory, and 0.94/0.87 for clinic readings). Another study of 133 hypertensive subjects found that home BP gave the lowest SDD for SBP and DBP (6.9/4.7 mm Hg), compared with 8.3/5.6 mm Hg for ABPM and 11.0/6.6 mm Hg for clinic BP.[19]

The studies described earlier investigated the reproducibility of home BPs over a period of weeks, and it could be expected that the reproducibility would be lower over a longer time. This is not necessarily the case, however. In Ohasama, Japan, where home BPs were extensively studied in a population-based sample, 136 untreated subjects measured home BP for 3 days on 2 occasions 1 year apart. The correlations between the two occasions were high ($r = 0.84$ and 0.83 for SBP and DBP), and there were no consistent changes over the year. In contrast, the clinic BPs declined 4/3 mm Hg over the same period and were less closely correlated ($r = 0.69$ for SBP and 0.57 for DBP). Thus, home BP appears to be relatively stable over a prolonged time period.

How Often Should Readings Be Taken?

A wide variety of schedules has been used to evaluate the home BP levels in published studies, ranging from two readings taken on a single day to six readings a day for a week or more. The frequency of BP readings can be varied according to the stage of the patient's evaluation. In the initial diagnostic period, frequent readings are desirable, but when the BP is stable and well controlled, the frequency can decrease. The first reading is typically higher than subsequent readings; therefore, multiple readings (two or three at each session) are routinely recommended. For estimating the true BP, at least 30 readings are advisable. This number can be justified in two ways. First, the maximum reduction in the SDD of home readings is obtained when there are at least 30 measurements (3 per day for 10 days).[3,4] Second, the Ohasama study, which was the first to establish the prognostic value of home BP readings, found that the prediction of the risk of stroke became stronger with more home readings, up to a maximum of 25 measurements; no evidence suggested a threshold number of readings.[20]

It is desirable to obtain readings both in the morning and in the evening, both to detect diurnal variations in BP in the untreated state and to assess the adequacy of treatment in patients who are taking medications. Readings taken in the morning before or just after taking the medication can be used as a rough measure of the "trough" effect of treatment, and those taken in the evening are a measure of the "peak" effect.

In the patients with newly diagnosed hypertension, a typical recommendation would be to take 3 consecutive readings in the morning and three in the evening on 3 days a week for at least 2 weeks (a total of ≤36 readings). This approach represents a reasonable compromise between obtaining the maximal number of readings and not overburdening the patient. It is also helpful to obtain some readings on weekend days in patients who work during the week, because these readings are often lower than those taken on weekdays. It is often convenient to provide the patient with a form on which to enter the readings. Other situations in which frequent readings are needed are when a new medication is prescribed and a change is made in the dose of an existing medication.

DEMOGRAPHIC FACTORS INFLUENCING HOME BLOOD PRESSURE LEVELS

Gender

The general consensus is that home BP is lower in women than in men, as is true for clinic and ambulatory BP. This finding has been well documented in several large epidemiologic studies.[21,22] However, the clinic-home differences are generally the same for men and women.

Age

Age also influences home BP. All studies that evaluated this factor showed an increase in older people. In the largest population study to investigate this topic, the study conducted in Ohasama, Japan, the increase with age was surprisingly small: the average home BP was 118/71 mm Hg for men aged 20 to 29 years, and it was 127/76 mm Hg for men more than 60 years of age.[23] The difference between clinic and home BP increased with age, a finding consistent with other data showing that the WCE tends to increase with age. The published results almost certainly underestimate the true changes, because subjects taking antihypertensive medications were usually excluded, and the prevalence of hypertension increases with age.

Another age-related change is the increase of BP variability, as shown by the Ohasama study. The day-to-day variability of SBP increases markedly with age in both men and women, whereas DBP is little affected, and the variability of heart rate actually decreases.[22]

ENVIRONMENTAL FACTORS INFLUENCING HOME BLOOD PRESSURE LEVELS

As with any other measure of BP, the level of pressure recorded during HBPM shows considerable variability and is likely to be influenced by a number of factors. These are summarized in the following subsections and in Table 6-3.

Table 6-3 Factors Affecting Home Blood Pressure

Increase BP	Decrease BP
Winter	Summer
Caffeine	Exercise
Cigarettes	
Stress	
Talking	

BP, blood pressure.

Season of the Year

Home BP tends to be up to 5 mm Hg higher in the winter than in the summer in temperate climates.[3,4] Similar changes are seen in clinic and ambulatory BPs.

Time of Day

In studies in which both morning and evening measurements were taken, the evening readings tended to be higher for SBP (by ~3 mm Hg), but no consistent differences were noted for DBP.[23] These differences may be more pronounced in hypertensive patients: in one study of untreated hypertensive patients, the average home BP was 147/86 mm Hg at 8 AM, 145/82 mm Hg at 1 PM, and 152/86 mm Hg at 10 PM.[24] The differences between morning and evening BPs may be higher in men and in smokers.[23]

The pattern of BP change over the day may vary considerably from one patient to another, depending on daily routines. Antihypertensive treatment may also have a major influence.[23] For these reasons, it is generally recommended that patients should take readings both in the early morning and at night.

Day of the Week

Relatively little information exists on whether home BPs recorded on nonwork days are the same as those recorded on workdays. In a 1993 study using AMBP, my colleagues and I found that the BPs at home in the evening were consistently higher if the patient had gone to work earlier in the day.

Meals

Younger subjects typically have an increase of heart rate, a decrease of DBP, and little change of SBP for up to 3 hours after a meal. Older persons may have a pronounced fall of both SBP and DBP after eating. Thus, one study compared the effects of a breakfast of two eggs, two slices of toast, and orange juice in healthy elderly subjects (mean age, 82 years) and controls (aged 35 years). The average fall of BP between 30 and 60 minutes after the meal was 16/10 mm Hg in the elderly subjects, but only 4/3 mm Hg (not significant) in the young subjects.

Alcohol

In men who drink regularly, moderate alcohol consumption (66 mL/day) decreases evening BP by 7/6 mm Hg, beginning on the first day of consumption, but it increases morning BP (5/2 mm Hg) only after consuming alcohol daily for 2 weeks.[25]

Caffeine

Drinking coffee increases BP, but not heart rate. The increase of BP begins within 15 minutes of drinking coffee, is maximal in about 1 hour, and may last for as much as 3 hours. Typical increases are 5 to 14/9 to 10 mm Hg. Drinking decaffeinated coffee produces little or no change in BP. These changes depend on the level of habitual caffeine intake: in people who do not consume it regularly, the changes are much greater than those seen in habitual caffeine users (12/10 versus 4/2 mm Hg, respectively). Older subjects show greater increases of BP than younger ones. Caffeine also has an additive effect on the BP response to mental stress: higher absolute levels of BP are achieved after caffeine, but the rise of BP during the stressor is not affected.

Smoking

Smoking a cigarette raises both heart rate and BP. In patients who smoked in their natural environment during intra-arterial ABPM, BP increased by about 11/5 mm Hg, sometimes preceded by a transient fall of BP; changes were quantitatively similar in normotensive and hypertensive subjects. The effect of smoking on BP is seen within a few minutes and lasts about 15 minutes. Coffee and cigarettes are often taken together, and they may have an interactive effect on BP. Home BPs are usually lower than clinic BPs, but this difference is less in smokers,[26] presumably because they are likely to have smoked before taking the home readings.

Talking

Talking is a potent pressor stimulus that has both physical and psychological components. Reading aloud produces an immediate increase of both SBP and DBP (by ~10/7 mm Hg in normotensive individuals) and of heart rate, with an immediate return to baseline levels once silence is resumed. Reading silently, however, does not affect BP. Speaking fast produces a bigger increase than speaking slowly. Although this is unlikely to be a factor in patients using a stethoscope to record their BP, it could be relevant when another person performs the measurements.

Stress

Emotional stress can produce marked elevations of BP that can outlast the stimulus. In a study in which people were asked to recall a situation that made them angry, BP increased by more than 20 mm Hg in some people, and it was still elevated by more than 10 mm Hg 15 minutes later.[27] In a survey of hypertensive patients who were monitoring their BP at the time of the Hanshin-Awaji earthquake in Japan in 1995, those who lived within 50 km of the epicenter showed an increase of BP of 11/6 mm Hg on the day following the quake that took a week to wear off, whereas those living further away showed no change. After the terrorist attacks on the World Trade Center in New York City on September 11, 2001, my colleagues and I observed a 30 mm Hg increase of home SBP that persisted for several days in a patient whose office was immediately opposite one of the towers.[28] In a larger series of subjects who were monitoring their BPs using a teletransmission device (described later) in the months before and after September 11, 2001, in four sites in the United States, we observed a 2 mm Hg increase of SBP.[29] This was not a seasonal effect, because comparable data were available for the same time during the previous year.

Exercise

Although BP rises markedly during physical exercise, it rapidly returns to its baseline level when the exercise is completed, and there may be a period of several hours after a bout of heavy exercise when the BP may remain lower than the pre-exercise level, a phenomenon described as *postexercise hypotension*.[30]

HOME BLOOD PRESSURE IN NORMOTENSIVE SUBJECTS

As with ambulatory BP, there is no universally agreed on upper limit of normal home BP, but several studies have compared home and office levels of BP, and others have described average levels in normotensive populations. Six large epidemiologic studies of home BP have attempted to define the normal ranges. These studies are summarized here by the names of the geographic areas in which the surveys were made.

The Tecumseh Study

In this Michigan town, 608 healthy young adults aged 18 to 41 recorded their BP for 1 week using an aneroid device.[31] The average value was 121/75 mm Hg for men and 111/70 mm Hg for women. The authors proposed an upper limit of normal of 142/92 mm Hg for men and 131/85 mm Hg for women.

The Dubendorf Study

In Switzerland, 503 subjects randomly selected from the population took morning and evening readings for 14 days with an oscillometric semiautomatic device.[21] Office readings were obtained at the beginning and end of the 14-day period. Average home readings were 123/78 mm Hg, and office readings were 130/82 mm Hg. Both sets of readings were lower in women than in men, but office-home differences were the same across genders.

The Ohasama Study

This community-based sample of 871 Japanese (7 to 98 years old) excluded subjects taking antihypertensive medications.[22] Subjects took home readings in the morning using an electronic device (the Omron HEM-401C) every day for 4 weeks (actual average number of readings, 21). There was also one pair of screening BP readings. Both home and screening BPs increased gradually with age, SBP more than DBP.

The Limbourg Study

This community-based sample of 718 Belgian subjects excluded those taking antihypertensive drugs. Five BP readings were taken in the home by trained nurses using mercury sphygmomanometers on each of two visits.[32] Ambulatory BP was also measured.

The Didima Study

This community-based sample of 694 Greek adults aged 18 or more, which included 103 treated hypertensive subjects, had two clinic visits. Subjects also monitored home BP both in the morning and in the evening on 3 working days.[33]

The PURAS Study

This survey of 1184 adults who were randomly selected from a Spanish population included 195 persons who were known to be hypertensive.[34]

All six studies found that home BPs were higher in men than in women (as has been shown for ambulatory BPs), and five of the six studies showed that home BPs increased with age (the Tecumseh Study did not evaluate this parameter).

COMPARISON OF HOME AND CLINIC PRESSURES

The original observation of Ayman and Goldshine that home BPs are usually much lower than clinic BPs has been confirmed in a number of studies,[6] including the population surveys described earlier, in which most subjects were normotensive. In the Didima study of 562 normotensive subjects, home and clinic BPs were very similar (using the second of two clinic visits): clinic SBP was 1 mm lower, and DBP was 1 mm higher.[33] Home BP was higher on day 1 of monitoring than on subsequent days. These differences may be more marked in older subjects.[34] The correlations between the clinic and home readings in the population studies were quite close, ranging from 0.73/0.64 (for SBP and DBP, respectively) in the Pressioni Arteriose Monitorate e Loro Associazioni (PAMELA) study to 0.84/0.77 in PURAS.[34]

In hypertensive subjects, the differences between clinic and home BPs are greater than in normotensive subjects, as shown in Figure 6-3. A notable exception to this was the Hypertension Optimal Treatment (HOT) trial, which included a substudy of 926 treated hypertensives who had their BP evaluated by both clinic and home measurements, using a semiautomatic device in both cases.[35] No differences were noted between the two (the average levels of BP were 137/83 mm Hg both in the clinic and at home). The reasons for this are not clear, but the authors suggested that patients with white-coat hypertension were unlikely to have been

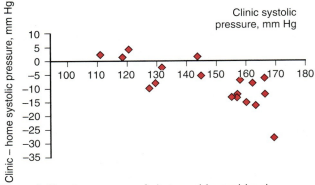

Figure 6–3 Comparison of clinic and home blood pressures in 18 studies published since 1992.

included in HOT. However, as shown in Figure 6-3, the greatest discrepancies between home and clinic BPs occur in people with higher clinic BPs.

In patients with severe hypertension, clinic BPs may be 20/10 mm Hg higher than home readings, and these clinic readings are also higher than readings taken in hospital by a nurse. The Ohasama study found that the correlations between home and clinic BPs were stronger in untreated (r = 0.57 and 0.54 for SBP and DBP) than treated hypertensive subjects (r = 0.30 and 0.38).[24]

In some cases, home BPs may show a progressive decline with repeated measurement, but this is by no means always seen.[36] Kenny and colleagues measured BP by four different techniques on three occasions, separated by intervals of 2 weeks, in 19 patients with borderline hypertension.[36] The techniques included conventional clinic measurement, basal BP (measured after lying for 30 minutes in a quiet room), daytime ambulatory BP, and self-recorded home BP. None of the four measures showed any consistent change over the 3 study days, although a nonsignificant downward trend was noted in all of them. For all 3 days, the clinic BPs were consistently higher than any of the other measures, but there were no significant differences between any of the other three measures. The average difference between clinic and home BPs was 9/4 mm Hg.

That the clinic-home difference results from the setting rather than the technique of BP measurement can be demonstrated by having patients take readings both at home and in the clinic. In the clinic, the patients' and the physicians' readings are usually very similar, and in both cases they are higher than home readings. In 30 treated hypertensive patients who were evaluated with both clinic and home readings, clinic BPs were taken either by the physician or by the patient using an electronic device, and the values were the same.[17]

Home Monitoring and the White-Coat Effect

The WCE is conceptualized as the increase of BP that occurs during a clinic visit. Although investigators agree that it should be defined as the difference between the clinic BP measured by a physician or other health care worker and some other BP, there is less agreement concerning what the measure of basal BP should be. The most widely used is the daytime ambulatory BP, mainly because this is convenient, and also because it is the best predictor of cardiovascular morbidity. Another way of measuring it would be to use the home BPs instead of ambulatory BPs. Because the home BP is usually very close to the daytime average of the ambulatory BP, it follows that the WCE will generally be similar when measured in either of these two ways. Most studies have found that home BP is not itself associated with a significant WCE. In a study of hypertensive patients in three family practices in England, Little and associates measured an average WCE of 18.9/11.4 mm Hg for ABPM and 14.3/5.0 for HBPM.[37] In another study, the correlations between home and ambulatory BP WCEs were close (r = 0.83 for SBP and 0.68 for DBP), a finding that is not surprising because they were not truly independent measurements.[38] An example of the WCE demonstrated by self-monitoring is shown in Figure 6-4; the first home readings were high, and subsequent ones were much lower than the readings taken in the clinic.

The similarity and correlations between the home and ambulatory estimates of the WCE do not necessarily imply that home BP can replace ambulatory BP for identifying individuals who have an exaggerated WCE. Stergiou and associates examined this issue in 189 hypertensive patients.[39] The average WCE was the same by both home and ambulatory criteria, and the two methods gave moderately good correlations (0.64/0.59), but on an individual basis, for the identification of an exaggerated WCE (defined as >20/10 mm Hg) the agreement was not so close. Of the 189 patients, 164 (87%) were classified the same (for systolic WCE) by both methods, whereas 25 (13%) were classified differently. Expressed another way, 13 patients (7%) had an exaggerated systolic WCE by both methods, 18 (9.5%) by ambulatory BP but not home BP, and 7 (4%) by home BP and not ambulatory BP. Although these results are disappointing, the WCE is inherently not a highly reproducible measure.

Correlations between Home and Ambulatory Pressures

The discrepancy between home and clinic BPs raises the following question: Which is closer to the patient's true BP? In practice, the best approximation to the true BP is the daytime or 24-hour average, obtained with 24-hour monitoring, because of all the available measures of BP, this gives the best prediction of risk. Several studies have compared home, clinic, and ambulatory BP levels in the same individuals. An example of this is a study that my colleagues and I performed in the early 1980s in 93 patients with a wide range of BPs. These patients took their own BPs over a 3-week period, and they also had measurements of clinic BP and 24-hour ABPM. The home BPs were closer to the 24-hour average than the clinic BPs and were more closely correlated (r = 0.69 for SBP and 0.71 for DBP) with the daytime BP than the clinic BPs. In addition, there was a progressively greater discrepancy between the clinic BP and the true BP at higher levels of clinic

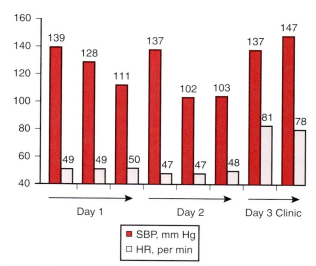

Figure 6–4 Self-monitored systolic blood pressure (SBP) and heart rate (HR) taken on 2 consecutive days preceding a clinic visit (on day 3). All measurements were made by the patient using the same monitor.

BP. Since then, several others (including the Ohasama study) have confirmed that the correlation between home and ambulatory BP is closer than for either of them with clinic BP.

What Is a Normal Home Blood Pressure?

The distribution of BP in the population is in the form of a gaussian or bell-shaped curve, which tails off at the higher end. Any division into "normal" and "high" BP is thus arbitrary, and this applies whichever measure of BP is used. In practice, the need for such a dividing line is that it can be used as a treatment threshold. One common technique used to define the upper limit of a variable such as BP, which is continuously distributed in the population, is to take the 95th percentile, which defines the upper 5% as being "abnormal." A variation of this method is to use the mean plus 2 SD, which is very similar to the 95th percentile. An obvious problem with this is that hypertension affects more than 95% of the individuals, especially at older ages; another is that hypertensive individuals are often excluded from population surveys. Thus, if in the population studies described earlier, the upper limit of normal home BP was defined as the 95th percentile, the values would range from 137/86 to 152/99 mm Hg, which are clearly too high. In a meta-analysis of 17 studies of home BPs in normotensive subjects, Thijs and associates used a number of techniques to define the upper limit of normal.[40] One was to use the 95th percentile, which gave a level of 135/86 mm Hg; the mean plus 2 SD gave 137/89 mm Hg.

An alternative method of defining the upper limit of normal home BP is to estimate the home BP equivalent to a clinic BP of 140/90 mm Hg, as has also been done for ambulatory BP. In the meta-analysis by Thijs and associates, two techniques were used to derive the home BP equivalent to 140/90 mm Hg.[40] The first was to compute the linear regression between clinic and home readings, which gave a value for the home BP of 125/79 mm Hg. The second was the percentile method, which calculated the percentile in the distribution of clinic BPs that corresponded to 140/90 mm Hg, and used the same percentile for the distribution of the home BP; this gave a value of 129/84 mm Hg. In the PAMELA study, the home BP equivalent to a clinic BP of 140/90 was 133/82 mm Hg, calculated by the linear regression method.[41] The values for some of the more important population studies are shown in Table 6-4.

In 1996, the American Society of Hypertension recommended that an appropriate level for the upper limit of normal home BP would be 135/85 mm Hg.[42] This was based on the finding that home BPs tend to be somewhat lower than clinic BPs and is in accord with the results of several studies,

as described earlier. It is also consistent with the prospective findings of the Ohasama study, in which home BPs higher than 138/83 mm Hg were found to be associated with increased mortality.[43] The same value has been adopted by JNC 7 and the American Heart Association.[2,3] As with office BP, a lower home BP goal is advisable for certain patients, including diabetic patients, pregnant women, and patients with chronic kidney disease.

Home Monitoring in Children

Increasing attention is being paid to the issue of hypertension in children, particularly because, with the epidemic of obesity, it is likely that its prevalence will increase. The phenomenon of white-coat hypertension occurs in children just as in adults,[44] so it makes sense to use out-of-office monitoring in addition to clinic measurements. So far, relatively few studies of HBPM have been conducted in children. One useful study was performed by Stergiou and associates in 55 children aged 6 to 18 years, of whom 26 were hypertensive by clinic BP criteria.[45] Strong correlations existed between clinic BP and home BP (0.73 for SBP and 0.57 for DBP) and also between home BP and ambulatory BP (0.72/0.66). In the hypertensive children, the home SBP was lower than both clinic and ambulatory BPs, whereas in normotensive children, the ambulatory BP was higher than both clinic and home BPs. The authors concluded that home BP is difficult to interpret in children. Clearly, more studies are needed in this area.

HOME BLOOD PRESSURES, TARGET ORGAN DAMAGE, AND PROGNOSIS

One of the factors that has limited the acceptance of home BPs for clinical decision making has been the lack of prognostic data, but evidence now indicates that home BP predicts cardiovascular morbidity better than clinic BPs. A larger body of evidence shows that home BP correlates more closely than clinic BP with measures of target organ damage, which can be regarded as surrogate measures for morbidity.

Home Blood Pressure and Target Organ Damage

In one of the first studies using HMBP, investigators reported that regression of left ventricular hypertrophy (LVH) evaluated by electrocardiography correlated more closely with changes of home BP than with clinic BP following the initiation of antihypertensive treatment.[46] Several studies since then have

Table 6-4 Proposed Upper Limits of Normal Home Blood Pressure from Population Studies

Study	N	Clinic BP	Home BP	Home BP Equivalent to 140/90 mm Hg in Clinic	
				Percentile	Regression
PAMELA[41]	1,438	127/82	119/74	—	132/81
Didima[33]	562	118/73	120/72	140/86	137/83
Dubendorf[21]	503	130/82	123/77	133/86	—
PURAS[34]	989	126/76	118/71	134/84	131/82

BP, blood pressure; N, number of subjects.

indicated that the correlation between echocardiographically determined LVH and BP is better for home than for clinic readings.[47] However, in one study of 84 previously untreated hypertensive patients, home SBP and clinic SBP gave similar correlations with left ventricular mass index (LVMI, $r = 0.31$ and 0.32), but they were not as close as the correlation between ABPM and LVMI ($r = 0.51$).[24] In a study of treated hypertensive patients, home BP correlated with LVMI, but clinic BP did not.[48]

Home BP has also been related to other measures of target organ damage. It has been reported to correlate more closely than clinic BP with microalbuminuria,[47] as well as with carotid artery intima-media thickness.[49]

Home Blood Pressure and Prediction of Cardiovascular Events

Two studies compared the predictive value of clinic and office measurements, and both showed that home measurements are potentially superior. In the first study, a population-based survey in the town of Ohasama, Japan, 1789 people were evaluated with home, clinic, and 24-hour BP measurements.[50] Over a 5-year follow-up, home BP predicted risk better than clinic readings. After 10 years, prediction of risk became stronger with more home readings, up to a maximum of 25 measurements; there was no evidence of a threshold number.[20] The second study of home BP and prognosis was conducted in France and recruited 4939 elderly hypertensive patients who were currently receiving treatment. The investigators found that morbid events observed over a 3.2-year follow-up period were predicted by the home BP at baseline, but not by the clinic BP.[51] One particularly interesting aspect of this study was that patients who had normal clinic BPs but high home BPs were at increased risk, a phenomenon known as *masked hypertension*. It is not known whether the variability of home BP readings is an independent predictor of events, although some evidence indicates that the variability of daytime readings measured with ABPM may be.[52]

Isolated diastolic hypertension, in which the SBP is normal and the DBP is raised, is a common finding, especially in younger hypertensive patients. There has been some controversy about its prognosis, but the only report using HBPM (the Ohasama study) concluded that the condition is benign.[53] The threshold values for defining it were a home SBP lower than

138 mm Hg and a DBP higher than 85 mm Hg. In contrast, patients with isolated systolic hypertension were at increased risk.

Home BPs have correlated with prognosis in at least two other settings. A prospective study of 77 hypertensive diabetic patients whose clinical course was followed over a 6-year period using both clinic BP and HBPM found that home BP predicted the loss of renal function (decrease of glomerular filtration rate) better than the clinic BP.[54] In the Tecumseh study of 735 healthy young adults (mean age, 32 years), home BP predicted future BP over 3 years better than clinic BP.[55] The relative advantages of clinic BP, HBPM, and ABPM are shown in Table 6-5.

HOME MONITORING FOR THE DIAGNOSIS OF HYPERTENSION

The goal of BP measurement in the initial evaluation of hypertensive patients is to obtain an estimate of the true BP, or the average over prolonged periods of time, for which any of the three measures available for clinical use (clinic BP, HBPM, and ABPM) is a surrogate measure. It is generally accepted that the best measure is the 24-hour level, on the grounds that several prospective studies found that it is the best predictor of risk. As discussed earlier, two studies also showed that home BP is predictive. Because many of the readings taken during ABPM are taken in the setting of the home, reasonably close agreement would be expected, although the self-monitored home readings tend to be taken during periods of relative inactivity. The potential advantages of home readings over clinic readings for evaluating the true BP are twofold: first, the home readings largely eliminate the WCE; and second, larger numbers of readings can be taken. Investigators have demonstrated that a better estimate of the true BP can be obtained by taking a few readings on several different occasions than by taking a larger number on a single occasion.[1]

A limitation of home BPs is that they usually represent the level of BP at the lower end of the waking range, when the patient is relatively relaxed. Thus, they do not necessarily provide a good guide to what happens to the patient's BP during the stresses of daily life, such as at work. The BP at work tends to be higher than the BP at home, and it is similar to the clinic BP, although the latter is not necessarily a good guide to the level of BP at work. In patients with mild hypertension, my colleagues and I found only a moderate correlation between home and work BPs ($r = 0.55$ for SBP and 0.65 for DBP). Although most subjects do show a higher BP at work than at home, we have encountered others whose BP is the same or even higher at home. This is particularly true of women with young children.

Diagnosis of White-Coat versus Sustained Hypertension

In the patients with newly diagnosed hypertension in the clinic setting, the first issue is whether the patient has sustained hypertension or white-coat hypertension, because antihypertensive mediation is more likely to be prescribed in the former case. White-coat hypertension is conventionally diagnosed by comparing the clinic and ambulatory (typically daytime) BPs. Whether self-monitored home BPs can be used as

Table 6-5 Value of Different Methods of Blood Pressure Measurement in Clinical Practice

Utility	Method of BP Measurement		
	Clinic	Home	Ambulatory
Predicts outcome	+	+	++
Diagnostic use	+	+	++
"Normal" limit	140/90	135/85	135/85 (day)
Evaluation of treatment	+	++	+
Improves adherence	−	+	−

BP, blood pressure; ++, well demonstrated; +, demonstrated in at least 1 study; −, not yet demonstrated.

substitutes is unresolved. Larkin and associates found that 79% of patients would be classified the same way using either ambulatory or home readings, whereas the remaining 21% would not.[56] Two other studies found that home BPs are not very reliable for diagnosing white-coat hypertension.[55,57]

Some years ago, my colleagues and I proposed an algorithm for the detection of patients with white-coat hypertension (Fig. 6-5), whereby patients with persistently elevated clinic BP and no target organ damage would undergo self-monitoring; if this showed high readings (>135/85 mm Hg), the patient would be diagnosed with sustained hypertension, but if it was lower than this level, 24-hour BP monitoring would establish which patients had white-coat hypertension. This algorithm was evaluated in 133 previously untreated hypertensives, all of whom had elevated clinic BPs on two visits and measured their home BP for 6 days.[58] All underwent ABPM, which identified 38 (28%) with white-coat hypertension. However, nearly half of these patients (39%) were not diagnosed by the algorithm, because they had high home BPs. The main finding from this study was that a high home BP does not exclude the possibility of white-coat hypertension. However, these data did support the idea that if the home BP was normal, white-coat hypertension was likely. A somewhat similar study was performed by Mansoor and White in 48 untreated patients with at least two elevated clinic BP readings who were evaluated with home BP (three readings in the morning and evening for 7 days) and ABPM.[38] These investigators studied how well a home BP of 135 mm Hg or higher predicted ambulatory hypertension (defined as a daytime SBP >135 mm Hg or DBP >85 mm Hg). The sensitivity was 41%, and the specificity was 86%. The low sensitivity is perhaps not surprising because, as discussed earlier, home readings may underestimate the daytime BP. These investigators found that the sensitivity for detecting ambulatory BP could be increased by lowering the threshold level for home BP to 125/76 mm Hg, but this of course would result in a larger number of false-positive results. Because the correlations between home and ambulatory BPs are in the region of 0.7 to 0.8, it would be unreasonable to expect a precise correspondence between any level of home BP and the establishment or exclusion of ambulatory hypertension.

HOME MONITORING FOR THE EVALUATION OF ANTIHYPERTENSIVE TREATMENT IN CLINICAL PRACTICE

When patients are having their antihypertensive medication initiated or changed, it is necessary to measure their BP on repeated occasions. HBPM is ideal for this purpose because it can obviate the need for many clinic visits. It has the additional advantage of avoiding the biases inherent in clinic BP measurements.

The validity of using home readings for monitoring the effects of antihypertensive treatment has been well established in numerous studies that compared the response to treatment evaluated by clinic, home, and ambulatory BPs. Despite the general parallel between clinic and home BPs during treatment, considerable discrepancy may exist between the two in individual patients. Thus, in a study of 816 patients treated with trandolapril, the correlation coefficient between the clinic and home BP response, although highly significant, was only 0.47 for SBP and 0.36 for DBP.[59] The slope of the line was also rather shallow and indicates that a decrease of 20 mm Hg in clinic BP is on average associated with a decrease of home BP of only 10 mm Hg. Other studies have shown that drug treatment lowers clinic BP more than home BP; in a study of 760 hypertensive patients who were treated with diltiazem 300 mg/day, the clinic BP fell by 20/13 mm Hg, and the home BP fell by 11/8 mm Hg.[60] In another study, losartan lowered clinic BP by 17/13 and home BP by 7/5 mm Hg, and trandolapril lowered clinic BP by 17/13 and home BP by 7/5 mm Hg; changes of ambulatory BP were closer to the changes of home BP.[61] It is well recognized that drug treatment also lowers ambulatory BP less than clinic BP.[62] One study looked at the effects of exercise training on clinic and home BP. Clinic BP fell by 13/8 in the experimental group and 6/1 mm Hg in the controls, whereas home BPs fell by 6/3 and 1/−1 mm Hg, respectively.[63] Examples of the different responses of clinic and home BP are shown in Figure 6-6.

An example of the potential value of HBPM for evaluating the effects of antihypertensive treatment is shown in Figure 6-7, which illustrates the results of a study in which two anti-

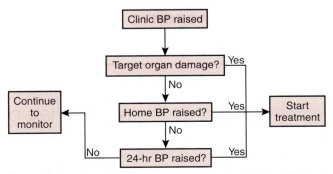

Figure 6–5 Algorithm for evaluating hypertensive patients using clinic, home, and ambulatory blood pressures (BPs).

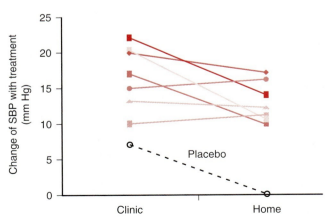

Figure 6–6 Change of clinic and home systolic blood pressures (SBPs) with antihypertensive drug treatment: results of nine recent studies, one of which included a placebo period.

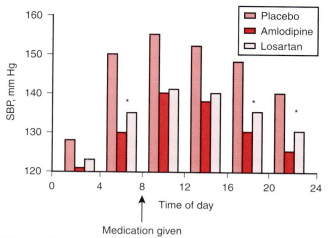

Figure 6–7 Comparison of the effects of two antihypertensive drugs (amlodipine and losartan) versus placebo evaluated by ambulatory blood pressure monitoring. *Asterisks* show where a significant BP difference was noted between the two drugs. (Data from Ishimitsu T, Minami J, Yoshii M, et al. Comparison of the effects of amlodipine and losartan on 24-hour ambulatory blood pressure in hypertensive patients. *Clin Exp Hypertens.* 2002;**24**:41-50.)

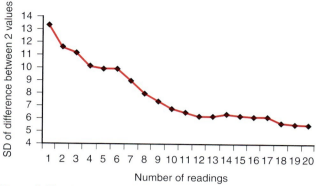

Figure 6–8 Reduction of the standard deviation (SD) of the difference between two values (means for home blood pressure) as a function of the number of readings used to define the mean values. (Modified from Chatellier G, Day M, Bobrie G, Menard J. Feasibility study of N-of-1 trials with blood pressure self-monitoring in hypertension. *Hypertension.* 1995;**25**:294-301.)

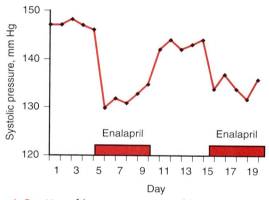

Figure 6–9 Use of home monitoring of blood pressure to evaluate the effectiveness of an antihypertensive drug (enalapril). Note the rapidity of the response. (Modified from Chatellier G, Day M, Bobrie G, Menard J. Feasibility study of N-of-1 trials with blood pressure self-monitoring in hypertension. *Hypertension.* 1995;**25**:294-301.)

hypertensive drugs (amlodipine and losartan) were compared with placebo by ABPM.[64] The medications were taken at 8 AM, and both drugs had a similar effect on lowering BP in the middle of the day (when patients are most likely to be seen in the clinic). However, in the early morning (corresponding to the trough measurement) and in the evening, the longer-acting amlodipine was clearly superior. These differences between the two drugs would be detected by HBPM.

How Many Readings Are Needed to Establish the Efficacy of Treatment?

It is helpful to know what the minimum number of home readings should be to establish a stable level when assessing the response to antihypertensive treatment, whether using medications or nonpharmacologic treatment. To determine the influence of the number of readings used to define the difference between two average BP levels (which may be before and after treatment), Chatellier and associates instructed patients to take three readings in the morning and three in the evening over a period of 3 weeks.[65] These investigators then calculated the SDD between two means derived from increasing numbers of individual readings over two 10-day periods. As shown in Figure 6-8, the SDD between the two means decreased progressively as larger numbers of individual readings were used to define each of the two means. About 80% of this reduction was obtained when 15 readings were used to define a mean, and including a larger number of readings brought little additional precision. The authors concluded that three readings taken over 5 days (preferably at the same time of day) should be sufficient to detect a drug-induced fall of BP.[65]

Identifying Optimal Treatment

The increasing number of drugs available for the treatment of hypertension has done relatively little to improve the success of controlling hypertension in the population. In part, this may be because people vary widely in the degree to which they respond to any one drug, and there is no infallible way of predicting which drug is best for which patient. It is thus largely a matter of trial and error, which has traditionally required a large number of clinic visits. One potential way of improving this situation is using home monitoring for "N-of-1" trials, in which each patient is given a number of different medications in sequence.[65] Because individual drugs vary in the time needed to achieve their full effects on BP, it is likely that a minimum of 3 weeks would be needed to test each drug, although the BP readings need be taken only for the last few days of each period. However, as shown in Figure 6-9, the response in some instances may be quite rapid.

Home Monitoring for Guiding the Intensity of Treatment

One important study examined the implications of using home readings to guide antihypertensive therapy.[66] Four hundred patients with poorly controlled hypertension were randomized to have their medication adjusted either by their home or clinic DBP, but the practitioners were blinded as to which measure was being used. If the DBP was higher than 89 mm Hg, treatment was intensified, if it was between 80 and 89 mm Hg, no adjustment was made, whereas if it was less than 80 mm Hg, the intensity of treatment was reduced. Because clinic BP readings tend to be higher than home readings, it is perhaps not surprising that more patients in the home BP group had their medications discontinued than in the clinic BP group, and conversely, those in the clinic BP group had more medications added. At the end of the study, all the measures of BP (clinic, home, and ambulatory) were higher in the home BP group. LVMI was not significantly higher in the home BP group, however. The authors concluded that the HBPM strategy could be more cost-effective, but they admitted that in the absence of large-scale prospective studies, management of hypertension based exclusively on HBPM could not be recommended.

Does Home Monitoring Improve Blood Pressure Control?

Substantial evidence indicates that HBPM can improve BP control; a recent meta-analysis of 18 randomized trials comparing home monitoring with usual care found that BP control was improved by about 4/2 mm Hg in the home monitoring groups.[67] One study randomized hypertensive African Americans to usual care, self-monitoring of BP, or "community-based monitoring," which involved having BP checked three times a week in a community health center. At 3 months, the BP had decreased the most in the self-monitoring group, with smaller changes in the community-monitored group, and no change in the controls.[68] Another study compared self-monitored BP against usual care and found a significant reduction of 24-hour BP in the former, again with no change in the control group.[69] The changes were most pronounced in African Americans, in whom mean arterial pressure decreased by 9.6 mm Hg in the monitored group, but it increased by 5.2 mm Hg in the usual care group. In a study of 622 hypertensive patients who were treated with losartan, there was a modest increase in BP control as a result of adding HBPM (66% versus 60% achieving target) that was more pronounced in women than in men.[70]

Table 6-6 Advantages of Home Blood Pressure over Clinic Blood Pressure Monitoring in Trials of Antihypertensive Treatments

Better correlation with changes of target organ damage
Smaller sample size
Evaluation of time course
No placebo effect
Estimation of the trough-to-peak ratio

HOME MONITORING FOR THE EVALUATION OF ANTIHYPERTENSIVE TREATMENT IN CLINICAL TRIALS

Most of the large clinical trials of antihypertensive treatment have used clinic-based BP measurements. It is surprising how little use has been made of HBPM in clinical trials, despite its obvious advantages, which are summarized in Table 6-6.

Better Correlation with Target Organ Damage

These studies raise the question of which measure of BP best describes the changes of the true BP. One of the strongest arguments for using HBPM to assess the response to antihypertensive treatment comes from the Italian Study on Ambulatory Monitoring of blood Pressure and Lisinopril Evaluation (SAMPLE), which used three methods of BP measurement (clinic, ambulatory, and self-monitoring) to relate the changes in BP resulting from treatment with an angiotensin-converting enzyme inhibitor to the regression of LVH.[71] The changes of clinic BP showed no significant correlation with the changes in LVMI, whereas both HBPM and ABPM did. The implication of this finding is that when a discrepancy exists between the effects of antihypertensive drug treatment on clinic and home-measured BP, the latter may be more meaningful.

Evaluation of Time Course of Treatment

HBPM is also ideal for evaluating the time course of the treatment response. As shown in Figure 6-9, for a drug with a relatively rapid onset of action such as enalapril, the maximal fall of BP is seen within 1 day of starting the drug, and the BP also returns to the pretreatment level quite promptly.[65]

Estimation of the Trough-to-Peak Ratio

An ideal antihypertensive drug regimen should lower BP smoothly throughout the day and night. This is usually evaluated by estimating the trough-to-peak (T/P) ratio. The trough is the BP reduction at the end of each dosing period, measured just before the next dose of medication is taken. The peak is the maximal BP reduction recorded after taking the medication. It is desirable to have a T/P ratio of at least 60%, but the closer it is to 100%, the smoother the BP control will be. HBPM can be a useful way of estimating the T/P ratio. Morning readings are taken just before the dose (trough), and evening readings (or midday) approximate the peak effects for many long-acting drugs. Menard and associates used this procedure to evaluate the effects of enalapril and found a T/P ratio of 77%, which is similar to estimates made using ABPM.[72]

No Placebo Effect

Another advantage of HBPM is that it is relatively immune to the placebo effects seen with clinic BP.[73] This is probably because much of the placebo effect seen with clinic BP measurement is nothing more than an attenuation of the WCE. The dotted line at the bottom of Figure 6-6 illustrates this point.

Smaller Sample Size

One of the advantages of using HBPM rather than traditional clinic measurements in trials of antihypertensive drugs is that fewer patients should be needed to show an effect. The greater statistical power inherent in the use of home recordings rather than clinic recordings for the evaluation of antihypertensive medications was well illustrated in a study by Menard and associates.[74] They used a double-blind, within-patient crossover study, with 2-week periods of three different treatments (a diuretic, a β-blocker, and both together), separated by 2-week placebo periods. They measured clinic BPs at the end of each treatment period, and patients also recorded their BPs at home using a semiautomatic machine. The effectiveness of all three treatments was similar for both measures of BP. The greater number of home readings increased the sensitivity of the study to detect a difference of BP between the different treatments. It was estimated that to detect a treatment effect of 5 mm Hg, 27 patients would be needed if clinic BPs were used for the evaluation, but only 20 patients if home BPs were used. Similar results were obtained in a different study by Imai and colleagues.[73] Using an SDD of 7.0 mm Hg for SBP and 5.1 mm Hg for DBP, 23 subjects would be needed to detect a 5 mm Hg decrease of SBP and DBP at an α of 0.05. Thus, the high reproducibility and low placebo effect of home BP mean that it is very efficient at detecting treatment changes.

COST-EFFECTIVENESS OF HOME MONITORING

Some evidence indicates that self-monitoring may be cost-effective (Table 6-7). In a randomized study conducted by the Kaiser Permanente Medical Care Program in San Francisco, 430 patients with mild hypertension, most of whom were taking antihypertensive medications, were randomized either to a usual care group or to self-monitoring.[75] The patients' technique was checked by clinic staff, and they were asked to measure their BP twice weekly and to send in a record of their readings every month. At the end of 1 year, the costs of care (which included physician visits, telephone calls, and laboratory tests) were 29% lower in the self-monitoring group, which also had slightly better BP control. Most patients and their physicians considered the self-monitoring procedure to be worthwhile. The authors estimated that the annual cost of self-monitoring was $28 per year (in 1992 dollars), which assumed a $50 monitor depreciated over 5 years, $10 for training (also depreciated), $1 for BP reporting, and $6 for

Table 6-7   Cost-Effectiveness of Home Monitoring*

Service	Home BP	Usual Care	Difference
Office visit	$54	$101	$47
Phone calls	$17	$8	–$8
Procedures	$17	$16	–$1
Total	$88	$125	$37

*Costs are reported in 1992 dollars.
Data from Soghikian K, Casper SM, Fireman BH, et al. Home blood pressure monitoring: Effect on use of medical services and medical care costs. *Med Care.* 1992;**30**:855-865.

follow-up to enhance adherence. Combining this estimate with their study results led to an estimated cost saving per patient of $20 per year. Projecting these numbers on a national level, the investigators estimated that about 15 million hypertensive patients in the United States are candidates for self-monitoring, and that 20 of the 69 million annual hypertension-related physician visits could be saved, with a cost saving of $300 million per year. These numbers seem very optimistic, but they clearly establish the potential for cost saving using home BP monitoring.

FUTURE TRENDS

It is likely that the use of self-monitoring for the routine evaluation of hypertensive patients will continue to grow in the foreseeable future. Several factors will drive this trend. They include the recognition of the inaccuracy of physicians' measurements, increasing time pressure on physicians to spend less time with patients, the cost and inconvenience of having to make an office visit for a BP check, and the increasing availability of inexpensive and accurate electronic devices. This may be viewed as part of a general movement in which patients are playing an increasingly important role in the management of their health. In the past, the paternalistic medical model assumed that only physicians knew how to take BP, and the patient's only duty was to follow orders. Medical care was centered in the hospital or clinic (Fig. 6-10,

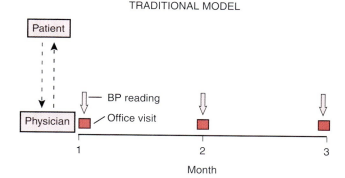

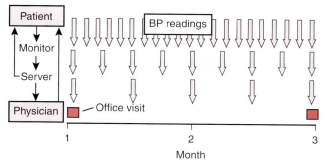

Figure 6–10   Two models of hypertension care. *Upper,* The traditional model in which blood pressure (BP) is measured only at clinic visits. *Lower,* The virtual hypertension clinic, in which patient care is home based, and BP readings are transmitted to the physician on a regular basis.

upper). This is rapidly changing. BP monitors are advertised directly to the consumer rather than to the physician, and patients are playing an ever larger role in their own management. For a condition such as hypertension, the center of care may soon be the patient's home rather than the physician's office (Fig. 6-10, *lower*).

Teletransmission of Readings

Because HBPM involves the acquisition of relatively large numbers of readings, processing of the data is also needed. Thus, a typical protocol will involve three readings twice a day on 3 days a week, which over a 2-week period would give 36 readings. Most studies have used manual data entry by the patient, which is clearly inefficient and has a potential for systematic bias (patients may disbelieve and ignore extreme readings) and error. Because the readings are taken by electronic devices, there is in principle no reason why the patient should have to write them down at all. Readings can be stored and processed in several ways. Some devices have a printer attached, which at least avoids observer bias. Others have a memory, from which the data can be downloaded (for example into the physician's computer, as in the Omron IC), transmitted by a telephone-modem link to a central computer, or connected to the patient's own personal computer if available. So far, teletransmission of home BP data has been used only for research purposes, mainly because insurance companies and Medicare have not been willing to pay the cost of the procedure. It is to be hoped that this will change in the near future.

CONCLUSIONS

The growth of the use of HBPM and of its accompanying technology raises the issue of relationships with ambulatory and clinic measurements of BP. Clearly, the clinic measurement is going to remain the cornerstone of BP measurement for the foreseeable future, but it is increasingly going to be supplemented by measurements made outside the medical environment. It is likely that roles will exist for both self-monitoring and ABPM, because the two procedures give basically different types of information. Thus, ABPM can give a representative profile of BP over the whole 24-hour period, but it is less well suited to tracking changes of BP over prolonged periods. Self-monitoring is usually only carried out during periods of relative relaxation and is therefore unlikely to be able to capture what happens during stressful periods. Similarly, it cannot be used to obtain any information about sleep-related BP changes.

References

1. Armitage P, Rose GA. The variability of measurements of casual blood pressure. I. A laboratory study. *Clin Sci.* 1966;**30**:325-335.
2. Chobanian AV, Bakris GL, Black HR, et al., and the National High Blood Pressure Education Program Coordinating Committee. The Seventh Report of the Joint National Committee on Prevention, Detection, Evaluation, and Treatment of High Blood Pressure. The JNC 7 report. *JAMA.* 2003;**289**:2560-2572.
3. Pickering TG, Hall JE, Appel LJ, et al. Recommendations for blood pressure measurement in humans and experimental animals. Part 1. Blood pressure measurement in humans: A statement for professionals from the Subcommittee of Professional and Public Education of the American Heart Association Council on High Blood Pressure Research. *Hypertension.* 2005;**45**:142-161
4. O'Brien E, Asmar R, Beilin L, et al. European Society of Hypertension recommendations for conventional, ambulatory and home blood pressure measurement. *J Hypertens.* 2003;**21**:821-848.
5. Cheng C, Studdiford JS, Diamond JJ, Chambers CV. Primary care physician beliefs regarding usefulness of self-monitoring of blood pressure. *Blood Press Monit.* 2003;**8**:249-254.
6. Ayman P, Goldshine AD. Blood pressure determinations by patients with essential hypertension. I. The difference between clinic and home readings before treatment. *Am J Med Sci.* 1940;**200**:465-474.
7. O'Brien E, Pickering T, Asmar R, et al. Working Group on Blood Pressure Monitoring of the European Society of Hypertension International Protocol for validation of blood pressure measuring devices in adults. *Blood Press Monit.* 2002;**7**:3-17.
8. Gerin W, Schwartz AR, Schwartz JE, et al. Limitations of current validation protocols for home blood pressure monitors for individual patients. *Blood Press Monit.* 2002;**7**:313-318.
9. van Popele NM, Bos WJ, de Beer NA, et al. Arterial stiffness as underlying mechanism of disagreement between an oscillometric blood pressure monitor and a sphygmomanometer. *Hypertension.* 2000;**36**:484-488.
10. van Ittersum FJ, Wijering RM, Lambert J, et al. Determinants of the limits of agreement between the sphygmomanometer and the SpaceLabs 90207 device for blood pressure measurement in health volunteers and insulin-dependent diabetic patients. *J Hypertens.* 1998;**16**:1125-1130.
11. O'Rourke MF. From theory into practice: Arterial haemodynamics in clinical hypertension. *J Hypertens.* 2002;**20**:1901-1915.
12. Parati G, Asmar R, Stergiou GS. Self blood pressure monitoring at home by wrist devices: A reliable approach? *J Hypertens.* 2002;**20**:573-578.
13. Little P, Barnett J, Barnsley L, et al. Comparison of acceptability of and preferences for different methods of measuring blood pressure in primary care. *BMJ.* 2002;**325**:258-259.
14. Mengden T, Hernandez Medina RM, et al. Reliability of reporting self-measured blood pressure values by hypertensive patients. *Am J Hypertens.* 1998;**11**:1413-1417.
15. Myers MG. Self-measurement of blood pressure at home: The potential for reporting bias. *Blood Press Monit.* 1998; **3 (Suppl 1)**:S19-S22.
16. Johnson KA, Partsch DJ, Rippole LL, McVey DM. Reliability of self-reported blood pressure measurements. *Arch Intern Med.* 1999;**159**:2689-2693.
17. Stergiou GS, Efstathiou SP, Alamara CV, et al. Home or self blood pressure measurement? What is the correct term? *J Hypertens.* 2003;**21**:2259-2264.
18. James GD, Pickering TG, Yee LS, et al. The reproducibility of average ambulatory, home, and clinic pressures. *Hypertension.* 1988;**11**:545-549.
19. Stergiou GS, Baibas NM, Gantzarou AP, et al. Reproducibility of home, ambulatory, and clinic blood pressure: Implications for the design of trials for the assessment of antihypertensive drug efficacy. *Am J Hypertens.* 2002;**15**:101-104.
20. Ohkubo T, Asayama K, Kikuya M, et al. How many times should blood pressure be measured at home for better prediction of stroke risk? Ten-year follow-up results from the Ohasama study. *J Hypertens.* 2004;**22**:1099-1104.

21. Weisser B, Grune S, Burger R, et al. The Dubendorf Study: A population-based investigation on normal values of blood pressure self-measurement. *J Hum Hypertens*. 1994;**8**:227-231.

22. Imai Y, Satoh H, Nagai K, et al. Characteristics of a community-based distribution of home blood pressure in Ohasama in northern Japan. *J Hypertens*. 1993;**11**:1441-1449.

23. Imai Y, Nishiyama A, Sekino M, et al. Characteristics of blood pressure measured at home in the morning and in the evening: The Ohasama study. *J Hypertens*. 1999;**17**:889-898.

24. Kok RH, Beltman FW, Terpstra WF, et al. Home blood pressure measurement: Reproducibility and relationship with left ventricular mass. *Blood Press Monit*. 1999;**4**:65-69.

25. Kawano Y, Pontes CS, Abe H, et al. Effects of alcohol consumption and restriction on home blood pressure in hypertensive patients: Serial changes in the morning and evening records. *Clin Exp Hypertens*. 2002;**24**:33-39.

26. Hozawa A, Ohkubo T, Nagai K, et al. Factors affecting the difference between screening and home blood pressure measurements: The Ohasama Study. *J Hypertens*. 2001;**19**:13-19.

27. Glynn LM, Christenfeld N, Gerin W. The role of rumination in recovery from reactivity: Cardiovascular consequences of emotional states. *Psychosom Med*. 2002;**64**:714-726.

28. Lipsky SI, Pickering TG, Gerin W. World Trade Center disaster effect on blood pressure. *Blood Press Monit*. 2002;**7**:249.

29. Gerin W, Chaplin W, Schwartz JE, et al. Sustained blood pressure elevation following an acute stressor: The effects of the September 11, 2001, attack on the New York City World Trade Center. *J Hypertens*. 2005;**23**:279-284.

30. MacDonald JR. Potential causes, mechanisms, and implications of post exercise hypotension. *J Hum Hypertens*. 2002;**16**:225-236.

31. Mejia AD, Julius S, Jones KA, et al. The Tecumseh Blood Pressure Study: Normative data on blood pressure self-determination. *Arch Intern Med*. 1990;**150**:1209-1213.

32. Staessen J, Bulpitt CJ, Fagard R, et al. Reference values for the ambulatory blood pressure and the blood pressure measured at home: A population study. *J Hum Hypertens*. 1991;**5**:355-361.

33. Stergiou GS, Thomopoulou GC, Skeva II, Mountokalakis TD. Home blood pressure normalcy: The Didima Study. *Am J Hypertens*. 2000;**13**:678-685.

34. Divison JA, Sanchis C, Artigao LM, et al. Home-based self-measurement of blood pressure: A proposal using new reference values (the PURAS study). *Blood Press Monit*. 2004;**9**:211-218.

35. Kjeldsen SE, Hedner T, Jamerson K, et al. Hypertension Optimal Treatment (HOT) study: Home blood pressure in treated hypertensive subjects. *Hypertension*. 1998;**31**:1014-1020.

36. Kenny RA, Brennan M, O'Malley K, O'Brien E. Blood pressure measurements in borderline hypertension. *J Hypertens*. 1987;**5 (Suppl 5)**:483-485.

37. Little P, Barnett J, Barnsley L, et al. Comparison of agreement between different measures of blood pressure in primary care and daytime ambulatory blood pressure. *BMJ*. 2002;**325**:254.

38. Mansoor GA, White WB. Self-measured home blood pressure in predicting ambulatory hypertension. *Am J Hypertens*. 2004;**17**:1017-1022.

39. Stergiou GS, Zourbaki AS, Skeva II, Mountokalakis TD. White coat effect detected using self-monitoring of blood pressure at home: Comparison with ambulatory blood pressure. *Am J Hypertens*. 1998;**11**:820-827.

40. Thijs L, Staessen JA, Celis H, et al. Reference values for self-recorded blood pressure: A meta-analysis of summary data. *Arch Intern Med*. 1998;**158**:481-488.

41. Sega R, Cesana G, Milesi C, et al. Ambulatory and home blood pressure normality in the elderly: Data from the PAMELA population. *Hypertension*. 1997;**30**:1-6.

42. Pickering T. Recommendations for the use of home (self) and ambulatory blood pressure monitoring: American Society of Hypertension Ad Hoc Panel. *Am J Hypertens*. 1996;**9**:1-11.

43. Ohkubo T, Imai Y, Tsuji I, et al. Reference values for 24-hour ambulatory blood pressure monitoring based on a prognostic criterion: The Ohasama Study. *Hypertension*. 1998;**32**:255-259.

44. Sorof JM, Poffenbarger T, Franco K, Portman R. Evaluation of white coat hypertension in children: Importance of the definitions of normal ambulatory blood pressure and the severity of casual hypertension. *Am J Hypertens*. 2001;**14**:855-860.

45. Stergiou GS, Alamara CV, Kalkana CB, et al. Out-of-office blood pressure in children and adolescents: Disparate findings by using home or ambulatory monitoring. *Am J Hypertens*. 2004;**17**:869-875.

46. Ibrahim MM, Tarazi RC, Dustan HP, Gifford RW Jr. Electrocardiogram in evaluation of resistance to antihypertensive therapy. *Arch Intern Med*. 1977;**137**:1125-1129.

47. Mule G, Caimi G, Cottone S, et al. Value of home blood pressures as predictor of target organ damage in mild arterial hypertension. *J Cardiovasc Risk*. 2002;**9**:123-129.

48. Cuspidi C, Michev I, Meani S, et al. Left ventricular hypertrophy in treated hypertensive patients with good blood pressure control outside the clinic, but poor clinic blood pressure control. *J Hypertens*. 2003;**21**:1575-1581.

49. Tachibana R, Tabara Y, Kondo I, et al. Home blood pressure is a better predictor of carotid atherosclerosis than office blood pressure in community-dwelling subjects. *Hypertens Res*. 2004;**27**:633-639.

50. Imai Y, Ohkubo T, Tsuji I, et al. Prognostic value of ambulatory and home blood pressure measurements in comparison to screening blood pressure measurements: A pilot study in Ohasama. *Blood Press Monit*. 1996;**1 (Suppl 2)**:S51-S58.

51. Bobrie G, Chatellier G, Genes N, et al. Cardiovascular prognosis of "masked hypertension" detected by blood pressure self-measurement in elderly treated hypertensive patients. *JAMA*. 2004;**291**:1342-1349.

52. Kikuya M, Hozawa A, Ohokubo T, et al. Prognostic significance of blood pressure and heart rate variabilities: The Ohasama study. *Hypertension*. 2000;**36**:901-906.

53. Hozawa A, Ohkubo T, Nagai K, et al. Prognosis of isolated systolic and isolated diastolic hypertension as assessed by self-measurement of blood pressure at home: The Ohasama study. *Arch Intern Med*. 2000;**160**:3301-3306.

54. Rave K, Bender R, Heise T, Sawicki PT. Value of blood pressure self-monitoring as a predictor of progression of diabetic nephropathy. *J Hypertens*. 1999;**17**:597-601.

55. Nesbitt SD, Amerena JV, Grant E, et al. Home blood pressure as a predictor of future blood pressure stability in borderline hypertension: The Tecumseh Study. *Am J Hypertens*. 1997;**10**:1270-1280.

56. Larkin KT, Schauss SL, Elnicki DM. Isolated clinic hypertension and normotension: False positives and false negatives in the assessment of hypertension. *Blood Press Monit*. 1998;**3**:247-254.

57. Den Hond E, Celis H, Vandenhoven G, et al. Determinants of white-coat syndrome assessed by ambulatory blood pressure or self-measured home blood pressure. *Blood Press Monit*. 2003;**8**:37-40.

58. Stergiou GS, Alamara CV, Skeva II, Mountokalakis TD. Diagnostic value of strategy for the detection of white coat hypertension based on ambulatory and home blood pressure monitoring. *J Hum Hypertens*. 2004;**18**:85-89.

59. Zannad F, Vaur L, Dutrey-Dupagne C, et al. Assessment of drug efficacy using home self-blood pressure measurement: The SMART study: Self Measurement for the Assessment of the Response to Trandolapril. *J Hum Hypertens*. 1996;**10**:341-347.

60. Leeman MJ, Lins RL, Sternon JE, et al. Effect of antihypertensive treatment on office and self-measured blood pressure: The Autodil study. *J Hum Hypertens.* 2000;**14**:525-529.

61. Ragot S, Genes N, Vaur L, Herpin D. Comparison of three blood pressure measurement methods for the evaluation of two antihypertensive drugs: Feasibility, agreement, and reproducibility of blood pressure response. *Am J Hypertens.* 2000;**13**:632-639.

62. Mancia G, Parati G. Office compared with ambulatory blood pressure in assessing response to antihypertensive treatment: A meta-analysis. *J Hypertens.* 2004;**22**:435-445.

63. Ohkubo T, Hozawa A, Nagatomi R, et al. Effects of exercise training on home blood pressure values in older adults: A randomized controlled trial. *J Hypertens.* 2001;**19**:1045-1052.

64. Ishimitsu T, Minami J, Yoshii M, et al. Comparison of the effects of amlodipine and losartan on 24-hour ambulatory blood pressure in hypertensive patients. *Clin Exp Hypertens.* 2002;**24**:41-50.

65. Chatellier G, Day M, Bobrie G, Menard J. Feasibility study of N-of-1 trials with blood pressure self-monitoring in hypertension. *Hypertension.* 1995;**25**:294-301.

66. Staessen JA, Den Hond E, Celis H, et al. Antihypertensive treatment based on blood pressure measurement at home or in the physician's office: A randomized controlled trial. *JAMA.* 2004;**291**:955-964.

67. Cappuccio FP, Kerry SM, Forbes L, Donald A. Blood pressure control by home monitoring: Meta-analysis of randomised trials. *BMJ.* 2004;**329**:145.

68. Artinian NT, Washington OG, Templin TN. Effects of home telemonitoring and community-based monitoring on blood pressure control in urban African Americans: A pilot study. *Heart Lung.* 2001;**30**:191-199.

69. Rogers MA, Small D, Buchan DA, et al. Home monitoring service improves mean arterial pressure in patients with essential hypertension: A randomized, controlled trial. *Ann Intern Med.* 2001;**134**:1024-1032.

70. Vetter W, Hess L, Brignoli R. Influence of self-measurement of blood pressure on the responder rate in hypertensive patients treated with losartan: Results of the SVATCH Study. Standard vs. Automatic Treatment Control of COSAAR in Hypertension. *J Hum Hypertens.* 2000;**14**:235-241.

71. Mancia G, Zanchetti A, Agabiti-Rosei E, et al. Ambulatory blood pressure is superior to clinic blood pressure in predicting treatment-induced regression of left ventricular hypertrophy: SAMPLE Study Group. Study on Ambulatory Monitoring of Blood Pressure and Lisinopril Evaluation. *Circulation.* 1997;**95**:1464-1470.

72. Menard J, Chatellier G, Day M, Vaur L. Self-measurement of blood pressure at home to evaluate drug effects by the trough:peak ratio. *J Hypertens.* 1994;**12 (Suppl)**:S21-S25.

73. Imai Y, Ohkubo T, Hozawa A, et al. Usefulness of home blood pressure measurements in assessing the effect of treatment in a single-blind placebo-controlled open trial. *J Hypertens.* 2001;**19**:179-185.

74. Menard J, Serrurier D, Bautier P, et al. Crossover design to test antihypertensive drugs with self-recorded blood pressure. *Hypertension.* 1988;**11**:153-159.

75. Soghikian K, Casper SM, Fireman BH, et al. Home blood pressure monitoring: Effect on use of medical services and medical care costs. *Med Care.* 1992;**30**:855-865.

Chapter 7

Ambulatory Blood Pressure Monitoring in Hypertension

William B. White

Since the 1970s, studies have supported direct and independent associations of cardiovascular risk with observed ambulatory blood pressure (BP) and inverse associations with the degree of BP reduction from day to night. The daytime and nighttime mean BPs, as well as the difference between daytime mean and nighttime mean BP derived from ambulatory BP monitoring (ABPM) data, allow the identification of high-risk patients, independent of the BP obtained in the clinic or office setting. Although ABPM is not required for the routine diagnosis of hypertension, it can identify white-coat hypertension and can evaluate the extent of BP control. Clinical trials during the past decade clearly demonstrate the importance of ABPM in the evaluation of antihypertensive drug therapy to ensure 24-hour BP control.

In the 1960s, intra-arterial recording provided the only means of following changes in BP over time during typical activities of daily living. The development and commercial availability of lighter-weight, quiet, easy-to-wear automated noninvasive BP recorders facilitated the collection of large volumes of data (~100 measurements in a 24-hour study period) while a subject pursues activities of daily living. Data derived from ABPM have made important contributions to our understanding of BP behavior and its complications, as well as the definitions of daytime and nighttime normotension, the prognostic value of ambulatory BP, and the evaluation of antihypertensive drug therapy.

CIRCADIAN VARIATION OF BLOOD PRESSURE

The circadian variation in BP and its association with cardiovascular events, including both myocardial infarction and stroke, are well established.[1] BP follows a highly reproducible pattern, characterized by a low span during sleep, an early morning, postawakening rise, and a higher sustained span during wakefulness. Evidence that the circadian periodicity of BP is synchronized with the sleep-wake cycle also comes from observations in shift workers. For example, a complete and immediate reversal of the circadian BP rhythm occurs on the first occasion of a session of night shifts.[2] As a result of the shift in work schedules, the peak BP in night workers is recorded at about 10 to 11 PM, rather than during the typical early morning period.[3]

Clinical Importance of the Nighttime Decline ("Dipping") in Blood Pressure

Nocturnal BP reductions of 10% to 30% are consistently found in the majority of people. However, about 25% to 30% of hypertensive patients do not display this decline in nocturnal BP[4]; instead, some have a blunted drop, or none at all, and others have an excessive drop in BP. The absence of a nocturnal decline in BP varies according to the patient population and is more prevalent in the elderly,[5] in African Americans,[6] and in postmenopausal women.[7] The term *nondippers* was coined by O'Brien to describe those individuals in whom the decline in nighttime BP is less than 10% of the daytime value and who also have a higher propensity for stroke.[4-8] Subsequently, other investigators showed that nondipping of both systolic BP (SBP) and diastolic BP (DBP) was associated with more severe target organ damage and a poorer prognosis.[9,10] Cardiovascular risk has been shown to be directly associated with the difference between the observed value of the 24-hour ambulatory BP and that predicted from the office BP.

The validity of an arbitrary proportional threshold to define dipping status has been questioned.[11] The reproducibility of the proportional fall in nighttime BP compared with daytime values has proved poor in some studies,[12,13] because sleep quality and the depth of sleep from one night to the next may influence the degree of dipping. Larocca and I proposed that an absolute BP value may be more appropriate to define nocturnal hypertension.[11] A consensus panel of the American Society of Hypertension originally proposed the definition of nocturnal hypertension as being a mean nighttime SBP/DBP higher than 125/80 mm Hg,[14] based on epidemiologic and cross-sectional studies that measured target organ damage. More recently, a committee organized by the American Heart Association suggested using a value of 125/75 mm Hg.[15]

When evaluated in a systematic fashion, the reproducibility of an absolute definition of nocturnal hypertension was superior to the proportional decreases used typically in the literature.[11] Twenty-four-hour BP data were extracted from recordings obtained during the placebo run-in phase of a series of clinical trials conducted in hypertensive patients diagnosed according to clinic BP. Patients with hypertension at night were identified using three different criteria: those with a less than 5% decrease in nocturnal BP compared with daytime, those with a less than 10% decrease in nocturnal BP compared with daytime, and those with a mean nocturnal BP of more than 125/80 mm Hg. Repeatability analyses confirmed that a mean nighttime BP of more than 125/80 mm Hg is more reproducible than the other two criteria. About half of the patients identified as nondippers on the basis of the first ABPM were considered nondippers based on the second assessment performed after 4 to 8 weeks.[11] The reproducibility of the dipper status also proved superior using SBP rather than DBP (Fig. 7-1). These findings suggest that the effect on

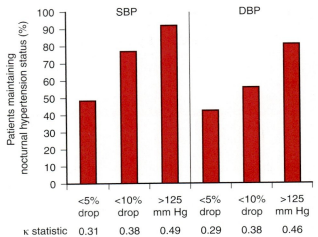

Figure 7–1 Proportion of patients maintaining nocturnal hypertension status (defined as <5% drop, <10% drop, or an absolute value of >125/80 mm Hg) after two 24-hour ambulatory blood pressure monitoring sessions 4 to 8 weeks apart. κ, the agreement between the sets of data; DBP, diastolic blood pressure; SBP, systolic blood pressure. (From White WB, Larocca GM. Improving the utility of the nocturnal hypertension definition by using absolute sleep blood pressure rather than the "dipping" proportion. *Am J Cardiol.* 2003;**92**:1439-1441.)

the absolute nocturnal BP may provide a more appropriate approach to evaluating the efficacy of antihypertensive agents.

Early Morning Blood Pressure Surge

In most individuals who sleep at night, a rapid rise in both BP and heart rate occurs during the early morning, a phenomenon termed the *early morning BP surge*. At this time of day, a corresponding increase is noted in the incidence of cardiovascular events. Studies have consistently shown that acute myocardial infarction is more prevalent between 6 AM and noon than at other times of the day or night.[16] Additionally, the incidences of subarachnoid hemorrhage,[17] ischemic stroke,[18] hemorrhagic stroke,[18,19] and transient ischemic attacks[20] are highest in the first 4 to 6 hours after awakening.

Evidence for a link between the increase in BP during the morning hours and target organ damage comes from a study conducted in elderly Japanese hypertensive patients.[21] Using ABPM, the level of the early morning BP surge was calculated by means of the difference between the average SBP during the 2 hours after awakening and the average SBP during the 1 hour that included the lowest value during sleep. The 519 patients studied were divided into two groups according to the extent of the morning surge. The highest deciles of the population had a surge of 55 mm Hg or greater (average, 69 mm Hg), and at baseline there was a 57% prevalence of silent cerebral infarcts, as opposed to only 33% in the remaining patients whose average morning surge in SBP was 29 mm Hg. During the follow-up period, which averaged 3.5 years, 19% of patients with a large early morning BP surge suffered a clinical stroke, compared with 7.3% of those with the smaller BP surge. Future research in this area needs to evaluate the impact of antihypertensive therapies to provide cerebrovascular protection.

PROGNOSTIC VALUE OF AMBULATORY BLOOD PRESSURE

Both prospective clinical and population-based studies have shown that ambulatory BP predicts cardiovascular events, even after adjustment for conventional BP in the doctor's office or clinic. The first study to evaluate ambulatory BP in a prospective fashion was by Perloff and colleagues, who established that the incidence of cardiovascular events was greater in patients with higher daytime ambulatory BP than in those with lower daytime values, independent of the office BP values.[22] Subsequently, several outcome studies showed than ambulatory BP is superior to conventional clinic BP measurements in predicting cardiovascular events.[23-31] Of these studies, two considered the prognostic value of ambulatory BP in the general population.[24,31] In both studies, after adjustment for gender, age, smoking status, baseline clinic BP, and antihypertensive treatment, ambulatory SBP proved to be a superior predictor of cardiovascular death, compared with clinic BP. Additionally, in the study by Sega and co-workers,[31] nighttime BP was the best parameter for predicting cardiovascular outcomes.

Until 2003, the ambulatory BP data used to predict cardiovascular endpoints were typically recorded in untreated subjects participating in clinical trials who were receiving placebo during the run-in phase. The prognostic value of ambulatory BP in patients with treated hypertension was reported in the Office versus Ambulatory Blood Pressure Study.[30] This study followed 1963 patients for a median of 5 years (range, 2 to 12 years), during which 157 patients had new major cardiovascular events. After adjustment for age, sex, body mass index, use of lipid-lowering drugs, and a history of cardiovascular events, the study showed that higher 24-hour mean ambulatory SBP and DBP were independent risk factors for new cardiovascular events. Even after adjusting for clinic BP, 24-hour and daytime SBP and DBP predicted outcomes. Comparison of outcomes for patients with a 24-hour mean ambulatory SBP of less than 135 mm Hg versus those with a mean value of 135 mm Hg or higher showed that those with the higher 24-hour mean SBP had a higher cardiovascular risk. This was true especially when the patients were classified according to their clinic BP (Fig. 7-2).

WHITE-COAT HYPERTENSION

Two prospective studies using ABPM established the relatively benign prognosis of white-coat hypertension.[25,29] Although the white-coat "effect" is quite common, the diagnosis of true white-coat hypertension in the untreated patient occurs in just 1 out of 10 patients reporting to the physician's office or clinic.[32]

In 1994, Verdecchia and co-workers from Italy defined white-coat hypertension as an office BP greater than 140/90 mm Hg but a daytime mean BP of 136/87 mm Hg in men and 131/86 mm Hg in women diagnosed with hypertension; the incidence of fatal and nonfatal cardiovascular events in a follow-up period of up to 7.5 years was virtually identical in normotensive and white-coat hypertensive subjects (0.47 and 0.49 events per 100 patient-years, respectively).[29] By comparison, the incidence rates of cardiovascular events in

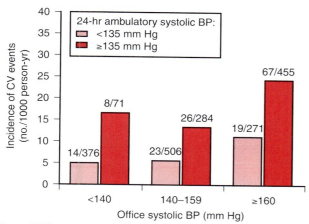

Figure 7–2 Impact of office versus ambulatory blood pressure (BP) on cardiovascular (CV) outcomes in the Office versus Ambulatory Study. (Modified from Clement DL, De Buyzere ML, De Bacquer DA, et al. Prognostic value of ambulatory blood-pressure recordings in patients with treated hypertension. *N Engl J Med.* 2003;**348**:2407-2415.)

dippers and nondippers with ambulatory hypertension were 1.79 and 4.99 per 100 patient-years, respectively.

In the United Kingdom, Khattar and co-workers used a different definition of white-coat hypertension: clinic SBP of 140 to 180 mm Hg and 24-hour mean ambulatory SBP lower than 140 mm Hg and DBP lower than 90 mm Hg, measured using intra-arterial monitoring.[25] In patients without complications at baseline, incidence rates of left ventricular hypertrophy and degrees of carotid intimal-medial hypertrophy over the 10-year follow-up period were significantly lower in the patients with white-coat hypertension than in those with sustained hypertension. The clinical relevance of this study comes into question however, because intra-arterial recordings are not routinely used in practice and often yield much different results than noninvasively derived ABPM values.

The low risk of cardiovascular events in patients with white-coat hypertension could suggest that little to no benefit may be gained by treating them. This concept was supported by observations from the Systolic Hypertension in Europe study, in which incidence rates of stroke and myocardial infarction were significantly higher in the patients with moderate sustained hypertension (by ABPM) than in those with nonsustained hypertension.[28] Active antihypertensive treatment (nitrendipine alone or in combination with a thiazide diuretic or an angiotensin-converting enzyme inhibitor) reduced the incidence of such events only in patients with moderately sustained hypertension, with the most benefit derived by patients with a daytime mean SBP of 160 mm Hg or greater.[23] In contrast, Verdecchia and colleagues performed a three-country prospective cohort analysis of the relationship between ambulatory BP and stroke outcomes in nearly 6000 patients and control subjects.[33] During the follow-up period, the adjusted hazard ratio for stroke was 1.15 (95% confidence interval, 0.61, 2.16) for the white-coat hypertensives (*P* = .66) and 2.01 (95% confidence interval, 1.31, 3.08) for the ambulatory hypertension group (*P* = .001). Nevertheless, concern regarding a possibly higher long-term risk was raised by the

investigators, because stroke rates began to increase in the white-coat hypertensive subjects, compared with the normotensive subjects, after about 8 years of observation.

A long-term controversy regarding white-coat hypertension that has not been resolved is whether this syndrome predisposes patients to sustained hypertension. A consensus from the European Working Party on Blood Pressure Measurement in 2001 recommended that further longitudinal research be conducted to clarify the transient, persistent, or progressive nature of the condition in the long term.[32] A 10-year follow-up study of newly diagnosed hypertensive patients in Denmark comprising 420 with white-coat hypertension and 344 who were confirmed as being truly hypertensive, according to baseline ABPMs, were compared with 146 normotensive subjects.[34] The incidence of events was greatest in the truly hypertensive group, but it was also significantly greater in the white-coat hypertensive compared with the normotensive group.

CLINICAL SIGNIFICANCE OF WHITE-COAT NORMOTENSION

The converse of white-coat hypertension has been termed *white-coat normotension* or masked hypertension (i.e., normal clinic BP, but elevated ambulatory BP).[35] It is likely that because most patients with white-coat normotension would tend not to be diagnosed as hypertensive, and would hence go untreated for a considerable time, they are likely to be at enhanced risk of the long-term consequences of hypertension. In fact, Liu and associates reported that, in patients with masked hypertension, left ventricular mass index and relative wall thicknesses in the heart and carotid arteries were similar to the values observed in patients with sustained hypertension.[36] The prevalences of discrete atherosclerotic plaques and increased carotid intimal-media thickness were also similar in patients with white-coat normotension and in those with sustained hypertension.[36] The prevalence of white-coat hypertension has been estimated at about 8%, and masked hypertension at values have been estimated at 5%, although this topic has been poorly studied.[1,35]

USING AMBULATORY BLOOD PRESSURE MONITORING IN THE MANAGEMENT OF HYPERTENSION

The diagnosis of hypertension and the decision to initiate drug treatment are traditionally based on office BP measurements. However, prospective cohort studies clearly show that the prognostic capabilities of office BP have been inferior to those of ABPM when the two were compared directly in many research reports.[37,38] Most notably, clinic BP measurements correlate poorly with 24-hour mean ambulatory BP, especially in men both before and during antihypertensive treatment.[38] The findings of the study by Clement and co-workers support the more extensive use of ABPM.[30]

ABPM has certain advantages in the evaluation and treatment of patients with hypertension, but its use needs to be considered in relation to the cost of the equipment and data evaluation, information gained, additional consultations required, and possible inconvenience to the patient. An

Use Of Ambulatory Blood Pressure In Hypertension Management

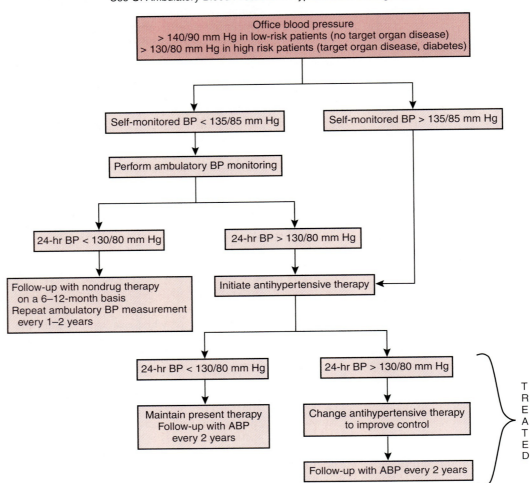

Figure 7–3 Use of ambulatory blood pressure (ABP) in hypertension management. BP, blood pressure. (Modified from White WB. Ambulatory blood-pressure monitoring in clinical practice. *N Engl J Med.* 2003;**348**:2377-2378.)

algorithm for the use of self-monitoring of BP and ABPM measurements may help to maximize the benefits of ABPM when identifying patients who would benefit from antihypertensive therapy (Fig. 7-3).[37] Self-monitoring (or home monitoring) of BP helps to restrict the use of ABPM to those patients who have a large disparity between clinic measurements and out-of-clinic values. Ideally, patients should measure their BP twice daily at home and while at work over a minimum of a 1-week period. During the past 1 to 2 years, research suggests that a normal average home BP is about 120/80 mm Hg.[15,37,39]

Impact of Ambulatory Blood Pressure Monitoring on Advances in Treatment

ABPM has been increasingly used for drug efficacy evaluation. ABPM may reveal important differences among antihypertensive agents as well as among different doses of a particular drug. This effect is most notable for determining the duration of action, because the devices are capable of obtaining numerous values over the course of a 24-hour dosing period. Not surprisingly, some commonly used once-daily antihyper-

tensive drugs have been shown to provide suboptimal control toward the end of the dosing interval.[38] As discussed later, with once-daily dosing and drug administration in the morning on arising to encourage patient adherence to therapy, incomplete BP control at the end of the dosing interval could actually coincide with the time of the greatest risk of an acute cardiovascular event.

Analyses of Ambulatory Blood Pressure Data in Antihypertensive Drug Trials

Data from ambulatory BP studies in hypertension trials may be analyzed in several ways (Table 7-1). A consensus regarding a superior, single method of analysis has not been reached, despite numerous attempts by many committees in several countries. The use of 24-hour means, daytime and nighttime means (or preferably awake and sleep values), BP loads (the proportion of values higher than a cutoff value during wakefulness (typically >140/90 mm Hg) or sleep (typically >120/80 mm Hg) divided by the total number of BP readings), area under the 24-hour BP curve, and smoothing techniques designed to remove some of the variability from

Table 7-1 Means for Assessment of Ambulatory Blood Pressure Data in Clinical Trials

24-hour averages (standard deviation is used as a measure of variability)

Hourly means (used in assessment of 24-hour curves)

Awake (daytime) and sleep (nighttime) means (requires accurate patient diaries or actigraphy)

Blood pressure loads (proportions or areas under the blood pressure-time curve)

Changes from 24-hour baseline values (placebo subtracted)

Smoothness index (a form of data reduction to take into consideration blood pressure variability)

Nocturnal blood pressure decline (dipper/nondipper)

Data smoothing techniques (cosinor analyses, Fourier transformation, modeling)

the raw BP data analysis are among the most popularly utilized methods of analysis.[40-42]

Features of any method of analysis for ambulatory BP data should include the statistical ease of calculation, the clinical relevance of the measure, and the relationship of the parameter with the hypertensive disease process. Many of these analytic methods meet all these criteria. For example, the 24-hour mean BP remains the most important parameter for evaluation in antihypertensive drug trials because it is a strong predictor of hypertensive target organ disease, is easy to calculate, utilizes all of the ambulatory BP data, and is highly reproducible in both short-term and long-term studies.[43,44]

Smoothing of ambulatory BP data may be used to aid in the identification of the peak and trough effects of an antihypertensive drug.[40,41] The variability in an individual's BP curve may be large, as a result of both mental and physical activity; thus, evaluating the peak antihypertensive effect of a short-acting or intermediate-acting drug may be difficult. Other than the benefits associated with examining pharmacodynamic effects of new antihypertensive drugs, data and curve smoothing for 24-hour BP monitoring appear to have little clinical relevance. Furthermore, editing protocols are not uniform in the literature, and missing data may alter the balance of mean values for shorter periods of time. To avoid excessive data reduction in a clinical trial, one statistical expert suggested that data smoothing should be performed on individual BP profiles rather than on group means.[45]

Utility of Ambulatory Blood Pressure Monitoring in Clinical Trials

ABPM has been helpful in comparing antihypertensive drugs, especially when assessing duration of action. Numerous examples in the literature now illustrate this benefit, including the superiority of ambulatory BP over clinic BP in assessing the trough-to-peak ratio of various agents.[40,41]

Comparisons of Drugs within the Same Class

In a multicenter study, Neutel and colleagues compared the β-blockers bisoprolol and atenolol in 606 patients by means of both clinic BPs and ABPM.[46] Following therapy, the seated BP in the clinic at the end of the dosing period was reduced 12/12 mm Hg by bisoprolol and 11/12 mm Hg by atenolol.

Although these changes were significantly different from baseline for both drugs, no significant differences occurred during comparisons across drugs. By using ABPM, it was determined that the daytime BPs (6 AM to 10 PM) and the BPs during the last 4 hours of the dosing interval (6 AM to 10 AM) were lowered significantly more by bisoprolol than by atenolol. This finding was present whether the assessment was made by examination of the overall means, area under the curve, or BP loads. These data demonstrated that despite no difference in office BP, significant differences in efficacy and duration of action were demonstrated when the drugs were assessed by 24-hour ABPM.

Comparisons of Drugs in Different Classes

Lacourcière and co-workers in Canada studied the angiotensin II receptor blocker telmisartan (at doses of 40 to 120 mg once daily) and compared it with the long-acting calcium antagonist amlodipine (5 to 10 mg once daily) in a clinical trial using 24-hour ABPM at baseline and following 12 weeks of double-blind treatment.[47] Although these agents have similar and very long plasma half-lives, they have entirely different mechanisms of action. This bears relevance because it is known that as BP and heart rate fall during sleep, plasma renin activity gradually increases. The renin-angiotensin-aldosterone system is further activated in the early morning on awakening, thus increasing the contribution of angiotensin to the postawakening surge in BP.[41]

Both amlodipine and telmisartan lowered *clinic* BP to similar values at the end of the dosing period. However, reductions in ambulatory DBP with telmisartan were greater than those with amlodipine during the nighttime, as well as during the last 4 hours of the dosing interval. In addition, the ambulatory BP control rates (24-hour DBP <85 mm Hg) were higher following telmisartan treatment (71%) than following amlodipine (55%). Thus, these data also demonstrate the improved ability of ABPM to discern pharmacodynamic changes between two drugs with relatively similar pharmacokinetic profiles.

Assessing the Effects of Chronotherapeutic Agents

In general, chronotherapeutics attempts to match the effects of a drug to the timing of the disease being treated or prevented.[48] In the case of hypertension and cardiovascular diseases, this pharmacologic concept has a great deal of clinical relevance because BP and heart rate have distinct, reproducible circadian rhythms. Additionally, most cardiovascular diseases, including myocardial infarction, angina and myocardial ischemia, and stroke, have circadian patterns with their highest incidence in the early morning.[41]

The approach for the chronotherapeutic treatment of hypertension and angina pectoris differs from conventional treatments that deliver medication to achieve a constant effect, regardless of the circadian rhythm of BP. Researchers have made attempts to alter the effects of conventional drugs by administering these agents before sleep versus on arising.[41,48,49] In one of these studies,[49] the angiotensin-converting enzyme inhibitor quinapril was given in the early morning versus at bedtime in patients with stage 2 hypertension. The study was conducted in a double-blind crossover design with quinapril given at either 8 AM or 10 PM for 4 weeks

Table 7-2 Evaluation of the Effects of Morning versus Evening Dosing of Antihypertensive Therapy to Patients with Hypertension

BP Parameter (mm Hg)	Quinapril (20 mg)		
	Baseline	AM Dosing	PM Dosing
Daytime systolic BP	154±16	138±16	137±14
Daytime diastolic BP	101±7	89±9	90±9
Nighttime systolic BP	140±15	132±20	127±18*
Nighttime diastolic BP	90±7	83±10	81±9†

*P < .001 versus morning administration.
†P < .05 versus morning administration.
BP, blood pressure.
Modified from Palatini P, Racioppa A, Raule G. Effect of timing of administration on the plasma ACE inhibitor activity and the antihypertensive effect of quinapril. *Clin Pharmacol Ther.* 1992;**52**:378-383.

in each period. As shown in Table 7-2, daytime BP was reduced similarly by both dosing regimens. In contrast, nighttime SBP and DBP were decreased to a significantly greater extent with the evening administration of quinapril. Measurement of angiotensin-converting enzyme activity showed that the evening administration of quinapril induced a more sustained decline in plasma angiotensin-converting enzyme, but not a more pronounced change. The findings in this study are of substantial interest because nocturnal BP has not been an area of focus, and in many types of hypertensive patients, BP during sleep may remain unknowingly elevated, despite seemingly normal BP in the physician's office.

Other studies showed little change in BP or heart rate in response to altering the dosing time of these long-acting agents to the nighttime.[41,50] However, many of these studies had small sample sizes and low statistical power to show changes less than 5 to 7 mm Hg in ambulatory BP. Thus, whether altering the dosing time of a long-acting antihypertensive agent truly changes the level of ambulatory BP control has not been proven with any degree of statistical confidence.

Chronotherapeutic Drug Delivery

Delivery systems have been specifically developed for the chronotherapeutic delivery of antihypertensive therapy; examples of these are the controlled-onset extended-release (COER) delivery system and the chronotherapeutic oral drug absorption system (CODAS) delivery system—both use verapamil HCl as the active agent.[41] In multicenter double-blind randomized clinical trials, these agents were shown to lower early morning BP, heart rate, and the rate-pressure product effectively when they were administered at bedtime. These findings may be of clinical importance in hypertensive patients, especially those who have increased risk of coronary disease, because epidemiologic analyses show that heart rate is an independent predictor of cardiovascular risk in patients with hypertension.[51] Furthermore, the reduction in the rate-pressure product, an index of myocardial oxygen demand, may benefit patients whose augmented rate-pressure product increases their risk for myocardial ischemia, as shown by Deedwania and Nelson.[52] The CONVINCE trial was designed

in part to understand the benefits of delivering a chronotherapeutic regimen of verapamil in the early morning.[53] This large-scale outcome study failed to show a difference in early morning events among chronotherapy, COER-verapamil, and standard of care administration of atenolol or hydrochlorothiazide. However, the reason may well have been the lack of statistical power to show differences as a result of early termination of the trial for a nonmedical and nonscientific rationale.[53]

BEFORE YOU GET STARTED: THE MONITORING DEVICES AND THEIR VALIDATION

The ABPM recorders are automated, programmable devices that utilize either an auscultatory or oscillometric method for measurement. In general terms, the auscultatory devices employ the use of a microphone to detect Korotkoff sounds and are reasonably accurate for BP measurement, especially if the Korotkoff sound is gated to the R wave of the electrocardiogram.[54,55] The oscillometric technique detects initial and maximal arterial "vibrations" in the cuff and calculates the mean arterial pressure via an algorithm developed by the manufacturer of the device. The more sensitive the algorithm, the more accurate is the device. Oscillometric BP devices lose precision with extremes of high and low BP values.[56]

The newest devices have become quite small and lightweight—most weighing 200 to 300 g—and have quiet motors capable of obtaining up to 100 BP readings in a 24-hour period. The devices are fairly simple to program for measurements at 15- to 20-minute intervals during the daytime and every 20 to 30 minutes during the night. Most of the devices have an algorithm built into their software that recognizes "erroneous" readings (excessive motion, physiologically impossible values) and will perform a repeat of the scheduled BP measurement in 1 to 2 minutes after the failed measurement. Although this is often an annoyance to patients, this feature makes the devices far more likely to obtain at least two to three valid BP readings per hour, so the entire 24-hour period can be fully evaluated.

It is practical for the staff applying the ABPM recorder to be fully trained in the handling of the equipment, to have the means to calibrate the device with a T-tube connected to a mercury column, and to become skilled in educating patients on various aspects of the recording that they are about to undertake. Anis Anwar and I have found over the years that patient education greatly enhances the potential for a successful 24-hour recording of the BP.[55] ABPM should be performed on typical working days, so the most representative values will be obtained.

Having independent clinical validation of these devices is important, because physicians need to be satisfied that ABPM devices have been evaluated according to established criteria.[57] It is highly advisable to use only ABPM devices that have been independently validated and have passed the test criteria of one of the various published standards for automated BP devices.

The Association for the Advancement of Medical Instrumentation published a standard for electronic or aneroid sphygmomanometers in 1987,[58] which included a protocol for the evaluation of the accuracy of devices, and this was followed in 1990 by the protocol of the British Hypertension Society.[59] Both protocols were revised in 1993.[60,61] These protocols had the common objective of standardization of validation procedures to establish minimum standards of accuracy and performance and to facilitate comparison of one device with another. Since their introduction, many BP measuring devices have been evaluated according to one or both protocols (see http://www.dableducational.org).

In 2002, the Working Group on Blood Pressure Monitoring of the European Society of Hypertension produced an updated protocol, named the International Protocol, which permits simplification of validation procedures without losing the merits of the much more complicated earlier protocols.[62] The International Protocol is applicable to the majority of BP measuring devices on the market, so the validation procedure has been confined to adults more than 30 years old (because this group contains the majority of subjects with hypertension), and it has no recommendations for special groups, such as children, pregnant women, and the elderly, or for special circumstances, such as exercise.

CONCLUSIONS

Results generated by ABPM have established that, even after adjustment for established risk factors, a progressive increase occurs in the risk of cardiovascular morbidity and mortality with elevated 24-hour, daytime, and nighttime BP. Studies in older Japanese patients showed the importance of the early morning BP surge on cerebrovascular target organ damage. The technique of ABPM measurements has become widely adopted to identify effective therapeutic options that provide BP control throughout the dosing interval.

In the practice setting, the contribution of ABPM to the management of hypertensive patients is increasingly acknowledged. Although in the past, this technology was considered experimental, this designation has changed recently, with improved insurance coverage for performing ABPM in specific patients and support for its use in certain subgroups of hypertensive patients both by the Seventh Report of the Joint National Committee on Prevention, Detection, Evaluation, and Treatment of High Blood Pressure[39] and by the Council on High Blood Pressure Research of the American Heart Association.[15]

References

1. White WB. Circadian variation of blood pressure: Clinical relevance and implications for cardiovascular chronotherapeutics. *Blood Press Monit.* 1997;**2**:47-51.
2. Sundberg S, Kohvakka A, Gordin A. Rapid reversal of circadian blood pressure rhythm in shift workers. *J Hypertens.* 1988;**6**:393-396.
3. Sternberg H, Rosenthal T, Shamiss A, et al. Altered circadian rhythm of blood pressure in shift workers. *J Hum Hypertens.* 1995;**9**:349-953.
4. White WB, Mansoor GA, Tendler BE, et al. Nocturnal blood pressure epidemiology, determinants, and effects of antihypertensive therapy. *Blood Press Monit.* 1998;**3**:43-51.
5. Di Iorio A, Marini E, Lupinetti M, et al. Blood pressure rhythm and prevalence of vascular events in hypertensive subjects. *Age Aging.* 1999;**28**:23-28.
6. Harshfield GA, Hwang C, Grim CE. Circadian variation of blood pressure in blacks: Influence of age, gender and activity. *J Hum Hypertens.* 1990;**4**:43-47.
7. Sherwood A, Thurston R, Steffen P, et al. Blunted nighttime blood pressure dipping in postmenopausal women. *Am J Hypertens.* 2001;**14**:749-754.
8. Rocco MB, Nabel EG, Selwyn AP. Circadian rhythms and coronary artery disease. *Am J Cardiol.* 1987;**59**:13C-17C.
9. Cuspidi C, Macca G, Sampieri L, et al. Target organ damage and non-dipping pattern defined by two sessions of ambulatory blood pressure monitoring in recently diagnosed essential hypertensive patients. *J Hypertens.* 2001;**19**:1539-1545.
10. Verdecchia P. Prognostic value of ambulatory blood pressure: Current evidence and clinical implications. *Hypertension.* 2000;**35**:844-851.
11. White WB, Larocca GM. Improving the utility of the nocturnal hypertension definition by using absolute sleep blood pressure rather than the "dipping" proportion. *Am J Cardiol.* 2003;**92**:1439-1441.
12. Mochizuki Y, Okutani M, Donfeng Y, et al. Limited reproducibility of circadian variation in blood pressure dippers and nondippers. *Am J Hypertens.* 1998;**11**:403-409.
13. Omboni S, Parati G, Palatini P, et al. Reproducibility and clinical value of nocturnal hypotension: Prospective evidence from the SAMPLE study. Study on Ambulatory Monitoring of Pressure and Lisinopril Evaluation. *J Hypertens.* 1998;**16**:733-738.
14. Pickering T, American Society of Hypertension Ad Hoc Panel. Recommendations for the use of home (self) and ambulatory blood pressure monitoring. *Am J Hypertens.* 1996;**9**:1-11.
15. Pickering TG, Hall JE, Appel LJ, et al. Recommendations for blood pressure measurement in humans and experimental animals. Part 1. Blood pressure measurement in humans. *Circulation.* 2005;**111**:697-716.
16. White WB. Cardiovascular risk and therapeutic intervention for the early morning surge in blood pressure and heart rate. *Blood Press Monit.* 2001;**6**:63-72.
17. Wroe SJ, Sandercock P, Bamford J, et al. Diurnal variation in incidence of stroke: Oxfordshire community stroke project. *BMJ.* 1992;**304**:155-157.
18. Elliott WJ. Circadian variation in the timing of stroke onset: A meta-analysis. *Stroke.* 1998;**29**:992-996.
19. Casetta I, Granieri E, Portaluppi F, et al. Circadian variability in hemorrhagic stroke. *JAMA.* 2002;**287**:1266-1267.
20. Gallerani M, Manfredini R, Ricci L, et al. Chronobiological aspects of acute cerebrovascular diseases. *Acta Neurol Scand.* 1993;**87**:482-487.
21. Kario K, Pickering TG, Umeda Y, et al. Morning surge in blood pressure as a predictor of silent and clinical cerebrovascular disease in elderly hypertensives: A prospective study. *Circulation.* 2003;**107**:1401-1406.
22. Perloff D, Sokolow M, Cowan R. The prognostic value of ambulatory blood pressure. *JAMA.* 1983;**249**:2793-2798.
23. Fagard RH, Staessen JA, Thijs L, et al. Response to antihypertensive therapy in older patients with sustained and nonsustained systolic hypertension. *Circulation.* 2000;**102**:1139-1144.
24. Imai Y, Ohkubo T, Sakuma M, et al. Predictive power of screening blood pressure, ambulatory blood pressure and blood pressure measured at home for overall and cardiovascular mortality: A prospective observation in a cohort from Ohasama, northern Japan. *Blood Press Monit.* 1996;**1**:251-254.
25. Khattar RS, Senior R, Lahiri A. Cardiovascular outcome in white-coat versus sustained mild hypertension: A 10-year follow-up study. *Circulation.* 1998;**98**:1892-1897.
26. Khattar RS, Swales JD, Banfield A, et al. Prediction of coronary and cerebrovascular morbidity and mortality by direct continuous ambulatory blood pressure monitoring in essential hypertension. *Circulation.* 1999;**100**:1760-1766.

27. Redon J, Campos C, Narciso ML, et al. Prognostic value of ambulatory blood pressure monitoring in refractory hypertension: A prospective study. *Hypertension.* 1998;**31**: 712-718.

28. Staessen JA, Thijs L, Fagard R, et al. Predicting cardiovascular risk using conventional vs ambulatory blood pressure in older patients with systolic hypertension. *JAMA.* 1999;**282**:539-546.

29. Verdecchia P, Porcellati C, Schillaci G, et al. Ambulatory blood pressure: An independent predictor of prognosis in essential hypertension. *Hypertension.* 1994;**24**:793-801.

30. Clement DL, De Buyzere ML, De Bacquer DA, et al. Prognostic value of ambulatory blood-pressure recordings in patients with treated hypertension. *N Engl J Med.* 2003;**348**:2407-2415.

31. Sega R, Facchetti R, Bombelli M, et al. Prognostic value of ambulatory and home blood pressures compared with office blood pressure in the general population. *Circulation.* 2005;**111**:1777-1783.

32. Staessen JA, Asmar R, De Buyzere M, et al. Task Force II: Blood pressure measurement and cardiovascular outcome. *Blood Press Monit.* 2001;**6**:355-370.

33. Verdecchia P, Reboldi GP, Angeli F, et al. Short- and long-term incidence of stroke in white-coat hypertension. *Hypertension.* 2005;**45**:203-208.

34. Gustavsen PH, Hoegholm A, Bang LE, et al. White coat hypertension is a cardiovascular risk factor: A 10-year follow-up study. *J Hum Hypertens.* 2003;**17**:811-817.

35. Selenta C, Hogan BE, Linden W. How often do office blood pressure measurements fail to identify true hypertension? An exploration of white-coat normotension. *Arch Fam Med.* 2000;**9**:533-540.

36. Liu JE, Roman MJ, Pini R, et al. Cardiac and arterial target organ damage in adults with elevated ambulatory and normal office blood pressure. *Ann Intern Med.* 1999;**131**:564-572.

37. White WB. Ambulatory blood-pressure monitoring in clinical practice. *N Engl J Med.* 2003;**348**:2377-2378.

38. Neutel JM. The importance of 24-h blood pressure control. *Blood Press Monit.* 2001;**6**:9-16.

39. Chobanian AV, Bakris GL, Black HR, et al., and the National High Blood Pressure Education Program Coordinating Committee. The Seventh Report of the Joint National Committee on Prevention, Detection, Evaluation, and Treatment of High Blood Pressure. The JNC 7 Report. *JAMA.* 2003;**289**:2560-2572.

40. Mansoor GA, White WB. Contribution of ambulatory blood pressure monitoring to the design and analysis of antihypertensive therapy trials. *J Cardiovasc Risk.* 1994;**1**: 136-142.

41. White WB. Advances in ambulatory blood pressure monitoring for the evaluation of antihypertensive therapy in research and practice. *In:* White WB (ed). Blood Pressure Monitoring in Cardiovascular Medicine and Therapeutics. Totowa, NJ: Humana Press, 2000, pp 273-298.

42. White WB. Usefulness of ambulatory monitoring of the blood pressure in assessing antihypertensive therapy. *Am J Cardiol.* 1989;**63**:94-98.

43. James GD, Pickering TG, Yee LS. The reproducibility of average ambulatory, home and clinic pressures. *Hypertension.* 1988;**11**:545-549.

44. Mansoor GA, McCabe EJ, White WB. Long-term reproducibility of ambulatory blood pressure. *J Hypertens.* 1994;**12**:703-708.

45. Dickson D, Hasford J. Twenty-four hour blood pressure measurement in antihypertensive drug trials: Data requirements and methods of analysis. *Stat Med.* 1992;**11**:2147-2157.

46. Neutel JM, Smith DHG, Ram CVS. Application of ambulatory blood pressure monitoring in differentiating between antihypertensive agents. *Am J Med.* 1993;**94**:181-186.

47. Lacourcière Y, Lenis J, Orchard R, et al. A comparison of the efficacies and duration of action of the angiotensin II receptor blocker telmisartan and amlodipine. *Blood Pressure Monit.* 1998;**2**:295-302.

48. White WB. A chronotherapeutic approach to the management of hypertension. *Am J Hypertens.* 1996;**10**:29s-33s.

49. Palatini P, Racioppa A, Raule G. Effect of timing of administration on the plasma ACE inhibitor activity and the antihypertensive effect of quinapril. *Clin Pharmacol Ther.* 1992;**52**:378-383.

50. White WB, Mansoor GA, Pickering TG, et al. Differential effects of morning versus evening dosing of nisoldipine ER on circadian blood pressure and heart rate. *Am J Hypertens.* 1999;**12**:806-814.

51. Gillman MW, Kannel WB, Belanger A, D'Agonstino RB. Influence of heart rate on mortality among persons with hypertension: The Framingham Study. *Am Heart J.* 1993;**125**:1148-1154.

52. Deedwania PC, Nelson JR. Pathophysiology of silent myocardial ischemia during daily life: Hemodynamic evaluation by simultaneously electrocardiographic and blood pressure monitoring. *Circulation.* 1990;**82**:1296-1304.

53. Black HR, Elliott WJ, Grandits G, et al. Principal results of the Controlled Onset Verapamil Investigation of Cardiovascular End Points (CONVINCE) trial. *JAMA.* 2003;**289**:2073-2082.

54. White WB, Schulman P, McCabe EJ, Nardone MB. Clinical validation of the Accutracker, a novel ambulatory blood pressure device using R-wave gating for Korotkoff sounds. *J Clin Hypertens.* 1987;**3**:500-509.

55. Anis Anwar Y, White WB. Ambulatory monitoring of the blood pressure: Devices, analysis, and clinical utility. *In:* White WB (ed). Blood Pressure Monitoring in Cardiovascular Medicine and Therapeutics. Totowa, NJ: Humana Press, 2000, pp 57-74.

56. Anis Anwar Y, Giacco S, McCabe EJ, et al. Evaluation of the efficacy of the Omron 737 Intellisense in adults according to the recommendations of the Association for the Advancement of Medical Instrumentation. *Blood Press Monit.* 1998;**3**:261-265.

57. O'Brien E, Waeber B, Parati G, et al., on behalf of the European Society of Hypertension Working Group on Blood Pressure Monitoring. Blood pressure measuring devices: Validated instruments *BMJ.* 2001:**322**:531-536.

58. Association for the Advancement of Medical Instrumentation (AAMI). The National Standard of Electronic or Automated Sphygmomanometers. Arlington, VA: AAMI, 1987.

59. O'Brien E, Petrie J, Littler W, et al. The British Hypertension Society Protocol for the evaluation of automated and semi-automated blood pressure measuring devices with special reference to ambulatory systems. *J Hypertens.* 1990;**8**:607-619.

60. O'Brien E, Petrie J, Littler WA, et al. The British Hypertension Society protocol for the evaluation of blood pressure measuring devices. *J Hypertens.* 1993;**11 (Suppl 2)**:S43-S63.

61. American National Standard. Electronic or Automated Sphygmomanometers. Arlington, VA: Association for the Advancement of Medical Instrumentation, 1993.

62. O'Brien E, Pickering T, Asmar R, et al., on behalf of the Working Group on Blood Pressure Monitoring of the European Society of Hypertension. International Protocol for validation of blood pressure measuring devices in adults. *Blood Press Monit.* 2002;**7**:3-17.

Secondary Hypertension: Renovascular Hypertension

William J. Elliott

In most Westernized countries, and especially among older individuals, renovascular hypertension is the most common remediable cause of elevated blood pressure (BP).[1-4] Although Goldblatt and colleagues developed the animal model that led to an understanding of the basic pathophysiology of this condition in 1934,[5] the diagnosis and management of this condition have changed substantially since the mid-1970s, in large part because of more efficient diagnostic procedures, more effective and more specific antihypertensive medications, and the results of randomized clinical trials.[6] This chapter attempts to review the more recent data that support the use of risk assessment before screening tests, the selective use of angiography, and the limitation of invasive but potentially curative procedures to those patients who are most likely to benefit from them.

DEFINITIONS

Renovascular Hypertension versus Renal Artery Stenosis

Unlike the diagnosis of most other cardiovascular and nephrologic conditions, renovascular hypertension can be diagnosed only *retrospectively,* by means of a physiologic BP response to an intervention. In this sense, renovascular hypertension is analogous to some infectious diseases, in which a firm diagnosis can be made only after acute and convalescent titers are compared. Classically, renovascular hypertension can be correctly and properly diagnosed 6 to 12 weeks *after* an intervention (see later), only if the BP is lower than it was before the intervention, with the patient taking the same or fewer antihypertensive medications.[7] The patient is said to be "cured" when the diastolic BP is less than 90 mm Hg without antihypertensive medications or "improved" if *either* the diastolic BP is less than 90 mm Hg with fewer medications than before the intervention *or* the diastolic BP is lower by 15% or more with the same or fewer medications than before the intervention.

In contrast to renovascular hypertension, which has a physiologic basis for its diagnosis, renal artery *stenosis* is a diagnosis based on anatomic criteria. Classically, renal artery stenosis was diagnosed when the patient had a greater than 75% narrowing of the diameter of a main renal artery or a more than 50% luminal narrowing with a poststenotic dilatation.[7] These criteria were based on planar images derived from renal angiograms. For various reasons, many contemporary authors use less stringent criteria; typically, a 50% luminal narrowing is the minimum in the current literature.

The distinction between renovascular hypertension and renal artery stenosis has several important ramifications. First,

as many as 32% of normotensive people (and 56% of those >60 years old) have relatively advanced renal arterial stenoses at angiography, but few have resistant hypertension.[8] This important fact has been rediscovered recently, as a result of "incidental" findings in people having angiography in other vascular beds (see later).[9,10] Second, surgical removal of a small kidney presumed to have ischemic nephropathy (from renovascular hypertension) was followed by normotension in only 25% of the patients in whom it was attempted.[11] Third, results of attempts to categorize the diagnostic performance of tests meant to assist in the identification of people with renovascular hypertension are likely to be different from similar attempts to identify renal arterial stenoses, because the latter can usually include two arteries per person, whereas the former can only be done on a per-patient basis.

Subtypes of Renovascular Disease

Fibromuscular Dysplasia

Fibromuscular dysplasia (FMD) is a noninflammatory, nonatherosclerotic vascular disease that preferentially affects small to medium-sized arteries.[12] Although described in nearly every vascular bed, it most commonly affects the renal arteries (60% to 75%, where it preferentially involves the distal two thirds of the main renal arteries), the neck and intracranial arteries (25% to 30%), the visceral arteries (10%), and the arteries of the extremities (5%). Three major pathologic types have been discerned: medial dysplasia (which is the most common type that affects the renal arteries), intimal fibroplasia (<10% of cases), and adventitial (or periarterial) fibroplasia (<1% of cases).[13] Medial dysplasia itself can be divided into three subtypes. The most common is medial fibroplasia (75% to 80% of all cases), which is recognized pathologically by alternating bands of thinned media and thickened collagen-containing fibromuscular ridges. This condition appears on an angiogram as the typical "string of beads" in which the diameter of the beads is greater than the diameter of the arterial lumen. Perimedial fibroplasia accounts for only 10% to 15% of cases, is recognized pathologically by heavy collagen deposits in the outer half of the media, and angiographically resembles medial fibroplasia, except the "beads" are smaller than the diameter of the arterial lumen. Medial hyperplasia (1% to 2% of cases) has true smooth muscle cell hyperplasia, but no fibrosis, and it appears angiographically as a smooth stenosis, without banding or beading.

The origin of FMD is uncertain, but it may be, in part, genetic. It is much more common in women, and is, by far, the most common cause of renovascular hypertension in young women (15 to 30 years of age). It has been associated with cigarette smoking, ergotamine, methysergide, α_1-antitrypsin deficiency, pheochromocytoma, type IV Ehlers-Danlos syndrome, Alport's syndrome, cystic medial necrosis, neurofibromatosis, and coarctation of the aorta (the last two especially in children).

FMD is important in renovascular hypertension for two major reasons. Unlike atherosclerotic disease, it rarely progresses to renal arterial occlusion or ischemic nephropathy. Most important, when FMD is found in the main renal arteries, patients respond *extremely* well to angioplasty without stenting. Most recent series indicate that about 40% to 55% are "cured," with another 30% to 40% "improved" after angioplasty. Because FMD occurs most commonly in young women, the prospect of saving years of expensive drug treatment by performing successful angioplasty is economically attractive.

Atherosclerotic Disease

Probably about 90% of current patients with renovascular hypertension have atherosclerotic disease as the underlying pathologic reason for the arterial stenosis. This progressive, occlusive process preferentially affects the ostium and proximal third of the main renal artery, as well as the nearby aorta. As with all other atherosclerotic vascular diseases, it is found with increasing frequency with advancing age, and it has the usual associated risk factors (diabetes, dyslipidemia, tobacco use, and prior history of cardiovascular events).

Other (Less Common) Causes of Renovascular Disease

Many additional causes (either extrinsic or intrinsic to the vessel) of renovascular hypertension have been described. On a population basis, Takayasu's arteritis may be the most important, especially in India or Japan. Renal arterial aneurysms are a common finding in patents with medial fibroplasias, but these lesions are often seen in saccular forms (as large as 2 cm) at the bifurcation of the renal artery. Case reports have been published of renovascular disease attributed to nonstenotic, but quite long, aberrant renal arteries.[14] Renal arterial stenoses can arise from emboli that are frequently generated during endovascular manipulation, which can sometimes lead to acute deterioration in renal function. In about 20% of hypertensive patients with aortic dissection, renovascular hypertension has developed, typically without dissection of the renal artery. Finally, several case reports of kidneys that move more than 7.5 cm while patients change from supine to erect posture suggest that this can result in FMD, and nephropexy is curative.

ESTIMATES OF PREVALENCE AND RISKS (IF UNTREATED)

Traditionally, the prevalence of renovascular hypertension was estimated at about 5% of all hypertensive individuals, but it varied from less than 1% to more than 50%, depending on the degree of screening in the study population. FMD is much more common among young hypertensive women; it comprised 30% to 40% of cases of renovascular hypertension at referral centers when angioplasty was just becoming estab-

lished. Today, its prevalence is diminishing (to <10%), as the general population ages and atherosclerotic renovascular disease becomes more prevalent.

Some risks of renovascular hypertension are probably independent of its underlying pathology. The risk of cardiovascular events increases exponentially with ascending levels of BP, irrespective of the cause of hypertension.[15] Renovascular hypertension tends to be resistant to the usual drug therapies, but administration of either angiotensin-converting enzyme inhibitors or angiotensin receptor blockers can provoke acute deterioration of renal function. Recurrent pulmonary edema can be a presenting symptom of renovascular hypertension, and it frequently improves or disappears after opening the artery.

Other risks of renovascular hypertension depend on the underlying disease process. Patients with FMD, for example, seldom sustain renal artery occlusion or ischemic nephropathy, which is a major risk for patients with atherosclerotic renal vascular disease. In an important series of 220 patients with atherosclerotic disease who were followed by ultrasound (US) to observe the natural history of the disease, progressive renal arterial stenosis was seen in 31% over 3 years, including 18% of originally nonstenotic arteries, with eventual occlusion in 9 of 295 arteries.[16] For those with stenoses of less than 60% originally, 28% had disease progression, as opposed to 49% in those with stenoses greater than 60%. In addition, progressive renal cortical atrophy was noted in 21% of patients when the original degree of renal arterial stenosis was more than 60%.[17] In the Cardiovascular Health Study, renovascular hypertension (detected by duplex ultrasonography) was associated with a 1.96-fold increased risk of coronary events, independent of baseline BP.[18] Ischemic nephropathy is an important (albeit often unrecognized) consequence of atherosclerotic renovascular hypertension and a common cause of end-stage renal disease,[19] and it is associated with an extremely poor prognosis, even after dialysis is instituted.[20] These important, but potentially preventable, sequelae of atherosclerotic renovascular disease have called attention to the need for better detection and treatment of this disease.

PATHOPHYSIOLOGY

Classically, the pathophysiology of renovascular hypertension involves progressive stenosis of the renal artery, that leads to hypoperfusion of the juxtaglomerular apparatus, release of renin, and increased production of angiotensin II. This process causes increases in sympathetic nerve activity, intrarenal prostaglandin synthesis, aldosterone synthesis, and nitric oxide production, and, most important for the development of hypertension, a direct *decrease* in renal sodium excretion.[21] This sequence has been well validated acutely, beginning with Goldblatt's dogs,[5] but the situation in chronic renovascular disease is somewhat more complicated. Over time, the increased plasma renin activity falls as plasma volume expands, especially when chronic kidney disease is present (most easily modeled in animal experiments by a prior contralateral nephrectomy, which has been called the one-clip, one-kidney Goldblatt model). During the chronic phase, both BP and intravascular volume can be reduced by angiotensin II antagonists or by relief of the arterial stenosis.

In some animal models, a "third phase" exists in the two-kidney, one-clip Goldblatt model, during which removal of the arterial stenosis does not result in an abrupt or complete fall in BP to that of the age-matched control animal. This finding may be important in humans, because early experience with revascularization surgery had more successes in lowering BP when hypertension had been present for less than 5 years before the operation.

DIAGNOSTIC EVALUATION

Many authorities have proposed multiple diagnostic algorithms for renovascular hypertension. Most, however, share the basic steps discussed here (and shown in Fig. 8-1):

1. An initial estimation of the absolute risk of renovascular hypertension can be based solely on clinical clues.
2. If the patient is unwilling to accept surgery (should it be required, even to repair a dissection or perforation during angioplasty), only medical management is advised.
3. A sensitive screening test can be offered to patients with an intermediate probability of renovascular hypertension. The result will dichotomize between those who need no further testing (but only medical management) and those who require a more specific test.
4. A renal angiogram can be offered to patients at high risk for renovascular hypertension.

Controversy still exists, however, regarding appropriate cutoff points for the decision points for steps 3 and 4, and especially about which screening test is most appropriate for most patients.[22-24]

Initial Risk Estimation

Since the early 1970s, many authors have identified characteristics that distinguish individuals with renovascular hypertension from those who have primary (or "essential") hypertension. Many of these were identified in the now classic study of 2442 hypertensive patients, of whom 880 had renovascular disease (35% of whom had FMD).[7] Repeatedly identified characteristics that differentiate between renovascular hypertension and primary hypertension are shown in Table 8-1. These features make it possible to estimate the absolute risk of renovascular hypertension for an individual using only clinical information (i.e., without *any* diagnostic testing).[25] It is no longer necessary to submit every hypertensive patient to an extensive workup for renovascular hypertension, because most patients fall into the very low-risk category (<15% in Fig. 8-1).

Dutch investigators proposed a "clinical prediction rule" (summarized in Table 8-2) that they derived from one cohort of patients, validated in a separate cohort,[26] and revalidated in a third cohort of patients with drug-resistant hypertension (35 with renovascular hypertension and 145 without it at angiography).[27] A nomogram (summarized in the right-hand columns of Table 8-2) provides the prior probability of renovascular disease, from a sum of the number of "points" accrued, based on that individual's history, physical examination, and simple laboratory studies. This method of identifying individuals at high risk for renovascular hypertension has been adopted by those responsible for preauthorization of renal angiograms in several managed care systems in the United States. It does not address all the risk factors for renovascular disease; the BP or serum creatinine response to a renin-angiotensin blocker would be a welcome addition.[23]

Screening Tests

Many reasonably sensitive screening tests for renovascular hypertension have been developed. Some are based on physiologic parameters (e.g., renin activity or blood flow to each kidney), some are more anatomically based (magnetic resonance angiography [MRA] and computed tomographic angiography [CTA]), and some combine aspects of each (Doppler US and captopril scintigraphy [CS] (Fig. 8-2).

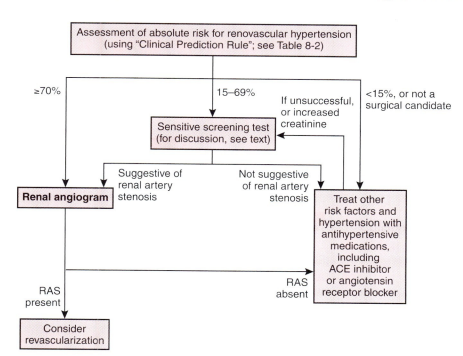

Figure 8–1 A diagnostic algorithm for renovascular hypertension. ACE, angiotensin-converting enzyme; RAS, renal artery stenosis.

Table 8-1 Clinical Clues to Renovascular Hypertension

Characteristic	Approximate Relative Risk (vs. Primary Hypertension)
Abdominal bruit (especially diastolic component)	5
Recent loss of BP control (or onset of hypertension)	2
Unilateral small kidney	2
Keith-Wagener-Barker grade III or IV fundi	2
History of "accelerated/malignant hypertension"	2
Unprovoked hypokalemia (<3.4 mEq/L)	2
Increase in serum creatinine after ACE inhibitor or ARB	1.8
No family history of hypertension	1.8
Atherosclerotic disease in another vascular bed	1.8
Elevated plasma renin activity	1.8
History of cigarette smoking	1.7
Recurrent pulmonary edema	1.5
Proteinuria	1.4
Older age (per decade of life)	1.2
Hypertension refractory to an appropriate three-drug regimen	1.2

ACE, angiotensin-converting enzyme; ARB, angiotensin receptor blocker; BP, blood pressure.

Table 8-2 Clinical Prediction Rule for Estimating the Absolute Risk of Renovascular Hypertension*

Clinical Characteristic	Never Smoked	Current or Former Smoker	Points (Sum from Left Side)	Probability of Renovascular Hypertension (95% Confidence Interval)
Age (yr)			≥20	≥90 (92–100)
20–29	0	0	19	90 (82–97)
30–39	1	4	18	89 (78–95)
40–49	2	8	17	87 (72–92)
50–59	3	5	16	80 (62–86)
60–69	4	5	15	72 (46–84)
70–79	5	6	14	62 (40–80)
Female gender	2	2	13	47 (28–65)
ASCVD*	1	1	12	37 (18–55)
History of hypertension ≤2 years	1	1	11	25 (14–40)
BMI <25 kg/m^2	2	2	10	15 (7–28)
Abdominal bruit	3	3	9	11 (5–20)
Serum creatinine			8	8 (3–12)
0.5–0.75 mg/dL	0	0	7	5 (2–10)
0.75–1.0 mg/dL	1	1	6	3 (1–8)
1.0–1.2 mg/dL	2	2	≤5	<2 (0–5)
1.2–1.65 mg/dL	3	3		
1.7–2.2 mg/dL	6	6		
≥2.3 mg/dL	9	9		
Hypercholesterolemia (>250 mg/dL, or on treatment)	1	1		

*The sum of the point score (from the second or third column, depending on the history of smoking, is found in the fourth column and correlates with the prior probability of renovascular hypertension (in the fifth column).
ASCVD, signs, symptoms, or clinical evidence of atherosclerotic cardiovascular disease; BMI, body mass index (weight in kg/[height in cm]^2).
Data from Krijnen P, van Jaarsveld BC, Steyerberg EW, et al. A clinical prediction rule for renal artery stenosis. *Ann Intern Med.* 1998;**129**:738-740.

Dutch investigators reported a selective overview of the world's literature regarding the relative performance of screening tests for renal artery *stenosis*. This endpoint was chosen because many studies (especially for MRA and CTA) report only correlations between the arterial appearance in the screening test and the angiogram (i.e., analysis per artery), rather than per patient (as should be the case if renovascular hypertension were the endpoint). In an attempt to avoid various biases that often complicate evaluations of test performance (relative to renal angiography), they included only 4 studies of the captopril challenge test, 14 reports about CS, 24 publications regarding Doppler US, 15 trials of MRA, and

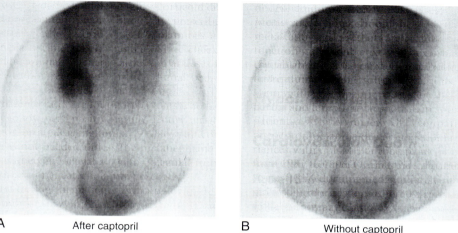

A   After captopril   B   Without captopril

Figure 8–2   Scintigrams suggestive of renovascular hypertension. **A,** One hour after captopril, 25 mg orally. **B,** Without captopril (or another angiotensin-converting enzyme inhibitor as part of his routine antihypertensive drug regimen). Note the impressive difference in the uptake in the left kidney, despite bilateral disease found subsequently (see Fig. 8-3**A**). This patient's blood pressure was reduced so much after a second angioplasty that his daily antihypertensive regimen was reduced from four drugs to one (an α-blocker he preferred to continue for its benefits on nocturia, not for blood pressure).

5 studies of CTA.[28] After comparing the area under the receiver-operator curves for each test, these investigators concluded that CTA and gadolinium-enhanced MRA were the best tests, but more experience was warranted with each. Three years later, they reported the results of a prospective, multicenter study of CTA and gadolinium-enhanced MRA compared with angiography in 356 patients and concluded that neither CTA nor MRA was sufficiently reproducible or sensitive enough to rule out renal artery stenosis in hypertensive patients[29] (Fig. 8-3).

The summary of a more inclusive literature review of the sensitivity and specificity of each of the four tests in common clinical use today to screen for renal artery stenosis is provided in Table 8-3. These data were obtained by reviewing the world's published literature from 1990 to 2004 and abstracting articles that reported the results of each test, compared with renal angiography. Case reports were excluded. The minimal diagnostic criterion for renal artery stenosis varied across studies (range, 50% to 75%). Some authors counted patients and others arteries; either was accepted, but the former was used if both were provided.

Older Tests

Many tests have been evaluated to screen the general hypertensive population for renovascular disease. Several of these

Table 8-3   Performance Characteristics (Weighted Averages of the World's Literature 1990 to 2004) and Advantages and Disadvantages of Four Commonly Used Screening Tests for Renovascular Hypertension

Screening Test	Captopril Scintigraphy	Doppler Ultrasound	Magnetic Resonance Angiogram	Computed Tomographic Angiogram
Number of publications	56	39	23	11
Number of patients/arteries	4295	3470	1788	1485
Sensitivity	0.79	0.82	0.88	0.86
Specificity	0.82	0.90	0.88	0.94
Advantages	Noninvasive; not expensive; may predict BP results after revascularization	Noninvasive; inexpensive; predicts BP results after revascularization	No contrast needed; excellent image quality	Excellent image quality
Disadvantages	Less accurate in renal impairment, bilateral disease, obstructive uropathy	Operator-dependent; less useful in obesity, bowel gas, branch lesions, FMD	Expensive; poor images with stents or distal stenoses (e.g., FMD); overcalls moderate stenoses	Expensive; time-consuming to process and interpret; not widely available; large amount of contrast sometimes needed

BP, blood pressure; FMD, fibromuscular dysplasia.

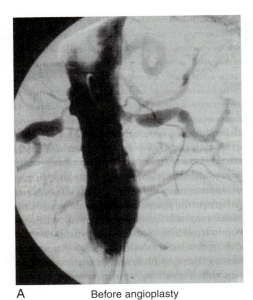
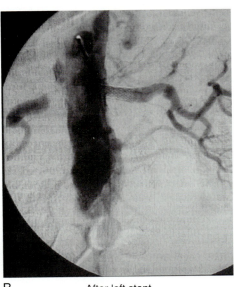

A   Before angioplasty   B   After left stent

Figure 8–3   Digital subtraction renal angiograms from the same patient as Figure 8-2. **A,** Before angioplasty. **B,** After left renal angioplasty and stent placement. Angioplasty and stent placement were first attempted on the left side because of the scintigram in Figure 8-2, which suggested this was the kidney more at risk for progressive disease or thrombosis. There was little blood pressure lowering 6 weeks after the left stent placement, so a second angioplasty was performed (with stent placement) into the right renal artery. Four years later, the patient suffered a posterior dissection of the infrarenal aorta, which was successfully repaired surgically without manipulation of the renal arteries; he died 1.5 years later of an acute myocardial infarction, with all office blood pressures lower than 140/90 mm Hg since the second stent placement.

were reported to be useful in certain patients, locales, or situations, but they have generally fallen into disuse. The original assay for plasma renin activity, which is acutely involved in the pathophysiology of renovascular hypertension, was found not to be very sensitive or specific; the newer assay may be better, as is using it in conjunction with an estimate of the 24-hour urinary excretion of sodium. The original claims for the "captopril challenge test" (of Müller and colleagues[30]) have not been verified in several other series,[31,32] although it is better than the random (or "unstimulated") plasma renin activity.[32] Plasma aldosterone concentrations can be elevated in primary or secondary hyperaldosteronism, so the test's specificity for renovascular hypertension is reduced. Several methods of comparing renin activity in blood taken from renal and other veins have been studied (renal vein renin ratios and the renal–systemic renin index, each with and without captopril stimulation), but these require an invasive procedure, usually with intravenous contrast to document the position of the catheter, and they have therefore become less widely used.

In about 1964, a rapid-sequence intravenous pyelogram became the standard screening test for renovascular hypertension, and it was once recommended for all patients with newly diagnosed hypertension. The need for intravenous contrast and its relatively poor performance characteristics (74% sensitivity, 86% specificity over the literature), however, caused this test to fall into disfavor in the late 1980s and to be displaced by CS and Doppler US. Renal scintigraphy (without captopril) avoids intravenous contrast, but it has only about 74% sensitivity and 77% specificity. It is now performed usually only after a CS scan has been interpreted as abnormal.

Captopril Scintigraphy

The performance characteristics of isotopic scans using technetium-99 diethylenetriaminepentaacetic acid (^{99}Tc-DTPA), iodine-121 hippurate, and ^{99}Tc-mercaptoacetyltriglycine (^{99}Tc-MAG$_3$, also known as ^{99}Tc-mertiatide) have all been enhanced after acute inhibition of the renin-angiotensin system by an oral dose of captopril. Using patient- and artery-weighted averages, over the entire world's literature, this test is about 79% sensitive and 82% specific, but these estimates are heavily influenced by several publications that report much worse results than the rest of the world. In fact, a proper meta-analysis of these data should not be reported, because of the high degree of inhomogeneity across the studies ($P < 10^{-8}$ by Riley-Day test). Some of the variability may be because different isotopes were used (e.g., MAG$_3$ is better for detecting bilateral disease), unusual characteristics of subjects studied (accuracy may be decreased in blacks and in patients who take calcium antagonists), or different diagnostic criteria used in different studies. The test is now widely available, relatively inexpensive, and simple to perform; criteria for interpretation have been published by a consensus panel.[33]

Disparities about the performance of CS can be highlighted in the reports with large numbers of patients. The most remarkable of these publications include the following: the report with the largest number (505 patients, 263 with renal artery stenosis: 68% sensitivity, 90% specificity), done in Holland[34]; the second-largest (380 patients, 125 with >70% stenosis, 83% sensitive, 93% specificity), done as a prospective, multicenter cooperative study in Europe[35]; the one with the highest prevalence of disease (100 patients, 54 with stenosis >70%, 92% sensitivity, 80% specificity)[32]; and the one with the worst results (140 patients, 41 with renal artery stenosis, 77% sensitivity, 44% specificity).[36] Bilateral renal arterial disease, obstructive uropathy, and an elevated serum creatinine concentration (>2.0 mg/dL) all reduce the accuracy of CS using ^{99}Tc-DTPA, the most commonly used isotope. Whether these factors account for the differences reported in these studies is unknown.

Several retrospective analyses suggest that the results of CS may correlate better with BP outcomes after angioplasty or surgery than with the results of renal angiography. In hypertensive patients with normal renal function, CS had an overall sensitivity and specificity of about 90% each for *renovascular hypertension* when results were interpreted using now-current standard techniques; the mean positive predictive value in 291 patients from 10 studies was 92%.[37] Conversely, the only prospective, randomized clinical trial to date (discussed later) showed no relationship between CS results and BP response after angioplasty.[38] A 1996 cost analysis suggested that CS, followed by angioplasty, was cost-effective only when it was performed in a population with a pretest probability greater than 30%; other screening tests available at that time were not cost-effective.[39]

Doppler Ultrasound

Duplex US provides both anatomic and physiologic information, by directly identifying renal arteries (using B-mode US) and providing hemodynamic measurements within them (Doppler flow studies). Its disadvantages (time consumed, operator dependence, and limited quality of images owing to obesity or overlying bowel gas) can be overcome by scanning fasting patients in the early morning, after a "bowel preparation" similar to that undertaken before colonoscopy.[40] Even with such precautions, however, there is little agreement in the literature about the performance characteristics of Doppler US for renal artery stenosis: 82% sensitivity (range, 0% to 98%) and 90% specificity (range, 73% to 100%). Again, one sees a high degree of inhomogeneity across the world's literature regarding Doppler US ($P < 10^{-15}$ by Riley-Day test) that no doubt reflects its operator dependence and the need for proper patient preparation. In addition, Doppler US often makes it difficult to distinguish between a 50% to 69% stenosis and a more than 70% stenosis, so most reports of Doppler US use a 50% stenosis as the lower limit of detection of a "significant stenosis."

Several studies have confirmed the value of the renal resistive index (measured during Doppler US) as a predictor of BP outcomes after angioplasty. In the original report involving 5950 patients screened with Doppler US, 131 of 138 patients with renal artery stenosis by angiogram underwent revascularization.[41] Little BP lowering after angioplasty was found in 34 of 35 with renal resistance indices of 80 mm Hg or more, but successful results were obtained in 90 of 96 with a renal resistance index of less than 80 mm Hg. The authors therefore concluded that patients with renal artery stenosis and a renal resistance index of at least 80 mm Hg are unlikely to have lower BP after revascularization, stabilization of renal function, or kidney survival. A report involving 74 patients who had renal revascularization not only confirmed these observations, but also indicated that administering captopril before Doppler US (but *not* CS) distinguished between patients who did and those who did not have a BP reduction after revascularization.[42] A cost-to-benefit analysis (based on clinical studies of 74 patients seen in Québec, Canada) suggested that Doppler US is more cost-efficient, but less sensitive than MRA.[43]

Magnetic Resonance Angiography

MRA was first reported to show excellent images of native stenotic renal arteries in 1993, and 22 subsequent publications assessed the performance characteristics of this technique (and variants, including phase-contrast and gadolinium-enhanced imaging) relative to renal angiography (see Table 8-3). Across all studies, MRA has a sensitivity of 88%, a specificity of 88%, and no significant inhomogeneity ($P = .19$). In the 2001 review of Vasbinder and associates, gadolinium-enhanced MRA and CTA had identical and nearly perfect performance characteristics,[28] but the prospective study reported by the same group in 2004 indicated that both interobserver variation and sensitivity were much poorer than expected.[29] Some of the problem may result from the high prevalence of FMD (36%) in their sample, because these stenoses are typically in the distal two thirds of the renal artery, an area not well visualized by the MRA technique.

Most of the technical challenges related to image acquisition (relative to the duration of breath holding), contrast injection, and subject positioning have now been overcome.[22] The remaining limitations to MRA of the renal arteries include its expense, contraindication in claustrophobia (said to affect ~10% of patients), a tendency to overestimate moderate stenoses (40% to 69%), the need for carefully timed intravenous injection of gadolinium, reduced accuracy in small, branch and distal renal arteries, obfuscation of signal by indwelling stents, and lack of functional information in the results. Its major advantages include the lack of nephrotoxic contrast, excellent image quality, and utility in patients with advanced renal impairment.

Only one study has so far compared outcomes after angioplasty based on MRA measurements before the procedure.[44] Although this report breaks new ground regarding criteria for a "successful angioplasty" (reduction in diastolic BP >15% or reduction in serum creatinine >20%), and it uses "normal renal volume" along with a calculated "renal flow index" as a stratifying tool, the authors reported that it had a 91% sensitivity and a 67% specificity predicting outcomes in their 23 patients. This experience bears repetition. More recently, a prospective three-way comparison of CS, captopril-enhanced Doppler US, and MRA (each versus renal angiography) in 41 patients with a 75% prevalence of renal artery stenosis showed MRA to have the best performance characteristics.[45] Furthermore, because of this, MRA as the primary screening test leads to the lowest direct costs if the prevalence of renal artery stenosis in the tested population is greater than 20%. Almost any strategy involving successful revascularization saved more lives than did medical treatment alone in their cost-utility model.[46]

Computed Tomographic Angiography

With the exception of its need for intravenous contrast and more effort involved in reconstructing images of interest, CTA is similar to MRA for screening for renal artery stenosis. CTA has not been as widely studied as other methods, but it had nearly perfect performance characteristics in the original analysis of Vasbinder and colleagues.[28] Even after the disappointing results in their prospective study, however, the overall sensitivity of CTA is 86%, with a specificity of 94%. More worrisome is the presence of significant inhomogeneity ($P < .0001$) among only 11 studies; only about 25% of this is the result of the prospective study of Vasbinder and associates.[29] Nearly all the rest is the result of three studies that report nearly perfect correlation with renal angiography.

CTA is not yet as widely available as the other screening tests and so far has not been correlated with BP-lowering outcomes after intervention. The technique requires extensive computer technology and programming expertise to track all possible nonplanar arterial segments, so the time to reconstruct and interpret images is longer than for other screening tests. Major concern exists about the volume of intravenous contrast that is necessary to obtain good images. Like MRA, CTA is not quite as accurate with small, branch, or distal renal arteries, and it can be a problem for claustrophobic patients. Indwelling stents are not a concern, as they are with MRA. Cost-effectiveness calculations have not yet been done for this modality, but it is likely that they should be similar (if a bit more expensive) than those done for MRA.

Angiography

General agreement exists across the literature that renal angiography is the "gold-standard" for the diagnosis of renal artery stenosis. Similarly, nearly all authorities agree that individuals who have a very high absolute risk of renal artery stenosis or renovascular hypertension should proceed directly to renal angiography, rather than undergo an imperfect screening test. If the result were to be read as normal, the ordering physician would likely regard it as a false-negative result and would send the patient to angiography, anyway. Renal angiography gives no functional information about the relative status of the kidneys, and it carries several risks, including anaphylactoid shock, radiocontrast-induced renal failure, and complications related to vascular access.

Intravenous Digital Subtraction Renal Angiography

This method, which was developed in the early 1980s to avoid arterial puncture and its attendant risks, involves the administration of contrast in a large bolus through a vein. With appropriate breath holding and widely available digital subtraction technology, intravenous digital subtraction renal angiography can produce images that rival those of conventional intra-arterial dye delivery. Although the intravenous angiogram cannot be followed as quickly by angioplasty (because it requires an arterial puncture that was originally avoided), its proponents point out that this allows some time for reflection by physicians regarding whether angioplasty is truly appropriate (see later).

Intra-aortic Renal Angiogram

Intra-aortic renal angiography is the traditional method of diagnosing renal artery stenosis. As with all angiograms, intra-arterial limitations to blood flow may not revealed by a two-dimensional "lumenogram."[47] Many cardiologists are now comfortable with intravascular US as a useful method of interrogating the vascular lumen for various types of obstruction; this may be more useful for FMD of the renal arteries.[48] Catheter-based measurements of gradients across renal arterial stenoses were once nearly universal, but these are seldom performed today. Most operators prefer to place a guidewire (for the following angioplasty catheter) across the stenosis, rather than a pressure-measuring catheter.

"Drive-by" Renal Angiograms

A major controversy in many hospitals and in medicine today involves the expanding role of cardiologists in the "fortuitous" diagnosis and subsequent immediate, catheter-based management of renal artery stenosis.[10] There is little doubt that cardiologists can, and often do, diagnose renal artery stenosis during routine cardiac catheterization, in 11% to 39% of patients.[9,49,50] Reported yields in patients undergoing peripheral angiography are even higher (44% to 50%). So far, only one group has reported the results of selective renal angiography done during scheduled coronary angiography, before which the patients were stratified by criteria that could put them at risk for renovascular hypertension.[9] These included (1) severe atherosclerosis, (2) severe or resistant hypertension, (3) unexplained renal impairment, and (4) history of acute pulmonary edema. These investigators found that 39% of their 837 patients had renal atherosclerosis; 14% had stenoses of 50% or greater, and 7% had stenoses of 70% or greater. The last group was more likely to be older and female and to have poorer renal function, higher BP, and carotid arterial disease. Although the report carefully avoids mention of whether any patient underwent renal angioplasty, the authors plan to follow these patients for cardiovascular and renal complications, and this will add to our knowledge of the natural (or postintervention) history of patients with fortuitously discovered renal artery stenosis.

Although injection into the main renal arteries can be done easily and selectively, with as little as 4 mL of contrast injected by hand, and is associated with few reported acute complications,[9] many clinicians have questioned why such investigations are done. Indeed, the largest reported single-center experience with stenting renal arteries comes from cardiologists; 363 arteries were stented between 1993 and 1998, with 100% procedural success and a 21% restenosis rate at an average of 16 months.[51] In some health care systems, payments for coronary angiography are higher if other vessels are injected, and they are higher still when angioplasty of another vessel is performed. At least one author has written, "routine imaging of renal arteries during coronary angiography … is not indicated."[52]

As with many controversies in medicine, few published data exist to support either position regarding routine percutaneous intervention after fortuitous discovery of a renal artery stenosis. A conservative approach is supported by two reports of its natural history. One involved a series of 68 patients with renal artery stenosis found during aortography done for other reasons at the Mayo Clinic in Rochester, Minnesota. During only medical management for 39 months, these patients had no change in BP, an increase in antihypertensive medications from 1.6 to 1.9 per patient, and only a slight increase in serum creatinine concentration (1.4 to 2.0 mg/dL).[53] More recently, among 85 patients with incidentally discovered renal artery stenosis, few required renal revascularization, and 24 of the 27 deaths during 2 years of follow-up were unrelated to the renal arteries.[54] The risks and benefits of angioplasty for incidentally discovered renal artery stenosis are cogently summarized by Textor,[49] and they require balancing the hazards of stenting (atheroemboli, dissections, thrombosis, and renal failure) with the potential benefit on BP, progressive renal disease, or recurrent pulmonary edema. One wonders whether a renal artery stenosis discovered fortuitously will have a different response to such therapy than one found after an intensive, premeditated search, based on prior probabilities.

THERAPY

For reasons discussed in detail later, controversy currently exists regarding not only which method of revascularization is better for most patients, but also whether *any* revascularization at all is warranted, thus leaving most patients simply to be treated with medications.[23,24,49,55] Table 8-4 lists some factors that help in this decision with an individual patient. There is general agreement that if BP cannot be controlled, or if a progressive decline in renal function occurs (perhaps owing, in part, to efforts to control BP), revascularization should be more strongly considered.[56]

Surgical Revascularization

Surgical revascularization for renal artery stenosis is performed less frequently than in the past probably because renal angioplasty with or without stenting has increased in popularity.[57] Some surgeons believe that angioplasty changes

Table 8-4 Factors Influencing Selection of Patients for Revascularization

Positive (Favorable) Response after Revascularization
Recurrent "flash" pulmonary edema
Refractory hypertension despite an appropriate three-drug regimen
Progressive declining renal function
Acute, reversible increase in serum creatinine after angiotensin-converting enzyme inhibitor or angiotensin receptor blocker therapy
Recent institution of dialysis in a patient suspected of ischemic nephropathy
Renal resistive index <80 mm Hg on Doppler ultrasound
Negative (or No Favorable) Response after Revascularization
Blood pressure <140/90 mm Hg on fewer than three antihypertensive drugs
Normal renal function
Unilateral small kidney (<7.5 cm length)
History or clinical evidence of cholesterol embolization
Renal resistive index ≥80 mm Hg on Doppler ultrasound
Heavy proteinuria (>1 g/day)
More than 10-year history of hypertension
Renal artery stenosis <70%

only the timing of the "definitive procedure": in case of a misadventure with angioplasty, emergency surgery is required; in other cases, angioplasty may only postpone an inevitable operation. For these reasons, it is useful and customary to arrange surgical backup when scheduling a renal angiogram with possible angioplasty. For technical and anatomic reasons, bypasses from nonaortic donor (splenic, celiac, mesenteric, or hepatic arterial) sites are now more popular than traditional aortorenal bypass and renal endarterectomies. These newer and more elaborate procedures limit manipulation of the diseased aorta and minimize atheroembolism, but at the expense of a somewhat higher perioperative mortality rate (2% to 6%). Most of the deaths are related to graft failure or other complications of widespread atherosclerotic vascular disease.

Several very experienced surgeons have reported an 80% to 90% rate of "cured" or "improved" BP after an operation. Patients with normal renal function fare better than those with renal impairment. Nine surgical series from 1987 to 1995 reported improved or stabilized renal function in 82% of 596 patients with renal impairment over an average of 35 months of follow-up (with 5% mortality), compared to 64% of 383 patients with renal impairment treated with angioplasty during the same time period (and a mean follow-up time of only 11 months).[58] One large series of 247 patients reported similar outcomes, whether open surgical or percutaneous revascularizations were performed.[59]

Angioplasty

Currently, angioplasty (alone) is the treatment of choice for fibromuscular dysplasia. Technical success rates vary between 82% and 100%, and restenosis rates vary between 5% and 11% after 1 year.[6] In seven large series, 78% of patients having primary angioplasty had either "cure" (using classic terminology) or "improvement" in BP.[58] Branch lesions or those in segmental arteries are more difficult to reach with a catheter, and therefore fewer patients with these achieve lower BPs.[12]

Angioplasty (without stenting) for atherosclerotic disease is less successful than for FMD. In a review of large series of adults undergoing renal angioplasty through 1995, only 65% of 1664 procedures resulted in "cured" or "improved" BPs.[58] About 19% were technical failures, and the restenosis rate at 1 year was about 13%. Less success was found with angioplasty of ostial lesions, sequential stenoses of a single artery, or stenoses in multiple renal arteries to the same side. This observation led to a randomized trial of angioplasty versus angioplasty *plus* stenting in 84 patients with ostial lesions.[60] At 6 months, restenosis was much less common in those receiving stents (25% versus 70%), but no differences were noted across groups in BP or deterioration in renal function. About one third of the patients had major complications related to the procedure.

The results of uncontrolled series reporting renal angioplasty to preserve renal function are difficult to interpret because of the lack of a comparable control group. Overall, most large series report little change in serum creatinine concentration or other measures of renal function after angioplasty (compared with preprocedure values), although this may well result from about the same proportion of patients who experience deteriorating renal function as those who improve.[19] One report suggests that angioplasty can stabilize or delay shrinkage of the renal cortex,[61] but this observation bears repeating with more sensitive measures of renal function in a large number of patients.

Angioplasty Plus Stenting

The addition of an expandable stent to balloon angioplasty in the renal arterial bed has many theoretical advantages, particularly in locations at high risk for restenosis. Stenting reduces or resolves complications from local dissection, prevents elastic recoil (thought to be involved in acute restenosis and thrombosis), and nearly eliminates pressure gradients across lesions after angioplasty. Because of these advantages, many operators now prefer to place a stent whenever possible in the renal arterial bed, despite the paucity of published comparative data and the relatively short time of follow-up available since its introduction.

The largest experience with renal artery stenting comes from a registry of 1058 patients followed for at least 6 months.[62] Technical success was universal; overall, there was a significant decline in BP ($168 \pm 29/84 \pm 15$ to $147 \pm 21/78 \pm 12$ mm Hg; $P < .05$), a slight decrease in antihypertensive medications per patient (2.4 to 2.0), and an improvement in renal function (from 1.7 ± 1.1 to 1.3 ± 0.8 mg/dL) in a 4-year follow-up period, during which the overall mortality was 26%. Other smaller and more recent reports show similar results, although about the same number of patients suffered deteriorating renal function as improved after the procedure.[19,51,63,64] Restenosis rates vary between 10% and 30% (depending on the length of follow-up). Stenting may have special benefits in renovascular hypertension in patients with deteriorating (as opposed to abnormal but stable) renal function.[65,66] A recent report suggests that successful angioplasty with stenting resulted in a reduced serum level of brain natriuretic peptide in 27 patients, but no control group was studied simultaneously.[67]

Medical Management

Another option for patients with renovascular disease that has taken on greater importance since the publication of recent clinical trials (see later) is intensified antihypertensive drug therapy, with additional measures to improve other atherosclerotic risk factors (e.g., aspirin, hepatic 3-methylglutaryl–coenzyme A reductase inhibitors, smoking cessation, and glycemic control). Most would agree that the latter should be widely adopted, particularly because the long-term prognosis in atherosclerotic renovascular disease (despite all available interventions) is at least as poor as seen in diabetic patients and in patients with a previous myocardial infarction. This finding would support a recommendation that the low-density lipoprotein cholesterol level for patients with renovascular hypertension should be less than 100 mg/dL, as it is for other patients at high risk for atherosclerotic cardiovascular disease.

The major concern about intensified antihypertensive drug therapy is the risk of acute deterioration in renal function that sometimes occurs when an angiotensin-converting enzyme inhibitor or an angiotensin receptor blocker is added to the regimen. These drugs are effective in reducing BP in 86% to 92% of patients with renovascular hypertension (most commonly in combination with a diuretic and a calcium antagonist) and, in the largest published experience, require discontinuation in only about 5% of patients during the first 3 months.[68] The increase in serum creatinine concentration typically reverts to baseline after stopping the angiotensin-converting enzyme inhibitor or angiotensin receptor blocker; this can be an indication for renal revascularization.

CLINICAL TRIALS AND META-ANALYSES THEREOF

Three major types of clinical trials related to therapy of renovascular hypertension have been organized, although their interpretation is complicated by crossovers, other confounders, and the continuing evolution of what is considered "state-of-the art" treatment protocols.

Surgery versus Angioplasty

One small study randomized hypertensive patients with atherosclerotic renal artery stenosis to surgery versus balloon angioplasty (before stents became popular). Surviving patients had a follow-up angiogram at 4 years. The patency of both renal arteries was higher for surgically treated patients than for those who underwent angioplasty (96% versus 75%). Otherwise, few differences were noted, including total costs of care.[69]

Surgery versus Medical Management

Fifty-two patients with atherosclerotic renal artery stenosis at risk for ischemic nephropathy were randomized to surgery or medical therapy in the mid-1990s. Mortality at 5 years of follow-up was not different between the groups; most patients died of comorbid diseases, not renal failure.[70]

Angioplasty versus Medical Management

Three studies have compared an initial angioplasty (without stenting) with medical therapy. In the French study, 49 of 76 eligible hypertensive patients with unilateral atherosclerotic renal artery stenosis of 75% or greater (or ≥60% with a positive screening test) were randomized from 1992 to 1995, and ambulatory BP monitoring at 6 months after randomization (or time of termination) was the primary endpoint.[71] Medical management was given to 26 patients; 23 had angioplasty (2 of whom had stents). During follow-up, one patient in the medical management group was withdrawn because of a BP-related hospitalization, seven were terminated early for refractory hypertension, and seven required angioplasty before 6 months. In the angioplasty group, one had a dissection of the renal artery with segmental renal infarction, five others had hematomas, and three developed restenoses requiring a repeat procedure, but all completed 6-months of follow-up. A that time, no significant differences in ambulatory BP were noted between groups, but significantly fewer medications were needed in the angioplasty group ($P = .009$). Surprisingly, office BPs measured by doctors were also significantly lower in the angioplasty group, but not when BPs were measured by an objective oscillometric device. The authors concluded that angioplasty reduces antihypertensive drug requirements, but it is associated with more complications than previous authors had noted.

In the Scottish and Newcastle Renal Artery Stenosis trial, 55 of 135 eligible hypertensive patients who were taking at least 2 antihypertensive drugs and who had a 50% or greater renal artery stenosis on angiogram were randomized, stratified by unilateral (n = 27) or bilateral disease.[72] The primary endpoints were the changes in BP and serum creatinine, at baseline and at 6 months of follow-up. Among the intervention group, there were 2 nephrectomies, 2 venous bypasses, and 21 angioplasties. Five patients in each group had angioplasties during follow-up (3 to 54 months). After 6 months of follow-up, BP differences across groups were not significant, although at the last follow-up, in the bilateral disease group, these were lower (by 26/10 mm Hg; $P < .05$) in the intervention group. No significant differences were noted in serum creatinine concentration, either before and after follow-up or across randomized groups. Regarding safety, there were no differences in major outcome events during follow-up, but 40 of 135 patients who had angioplasty suffered complications. The authors concluded that a modest improvement in BP was seen with angioplasty only in those patients with bilateral disease, at the expense of a significant complication rate.

The largest study was from the Dutch Renal Artery STenosis Intervention Cooperative (DRASTIC) group.[38] These investigators randomized 106 of 169 eligible patients: 56 to angioplasty (2 with stent) and 50 to drug therapy. All patients were either taking at least two antihypertensive drugs or had previous deterioration in renal function with an angiotensin-converting enzyme inhibitor, and they had a 50% or greater renal artery stenosis and a serum creatinine concentration lower than 2.3 mg/dL at baseline. At 3 months of follow-up, BPs were not different between the groups, although the number of antihypertensive drugs was lower in the angioplasty group (1.9 ± 0.9 versus 2.5 ± 1.0; $P = .002$). Serum creatinine, creatinine clearance (by Cockroft and Gault's formula), and the percentage of patients with an abnormal CS all favored the angioplasty group. During the next 9 months, 3 of the angioplasty group had revascularization surgery, and 22 (or 44%) of the original drug therapy group underwent angioplasty (and 2 more were lost to follow-up). Using intent-to-treat analyses, no significant differences were noted in any parameter between groups at 12 months. The authors therefore concluded that angioplasty has little advantage over antihypertensive drug therapy. However, this widely quoted study has certain controversial aspects. The categoric BP responses at 12 months are often overlooked: the angioplasty group had more improved (68% versus 38%), fewer worsened (9% versus 33%; $P = .002$), and more "cured" (7% versus 0%) patients. Within the group originally assigned to drug therapy, those who later underwent angioplasty had a significantly larger fall in BP from 3 to 12 months than those who were maintained on drug therapy alone ($P < .0001$), a finding suggesting a problem with the intent-to-treat analysis. According to expert radiologists who reviewed all angiograms after randomization, five patients in each group had stenoses of less than 50% (and did not meet this inclusion criterion). Angioplasty was technically unsuccessful in four patients (7%) randomized to that group. Renal arteriography was repeated at 12 months in 91 of the original 106 patients; 23 of 48 (48%) in the angioplasty group had restenosis of 50% or greater, compared with 35 of 43 (81%) in the drug-treatment group (including 4 occlusions); these restenosis rates are much higher than seen in previous studies.[10,58] Fully 35% of the patients had a "normal" CS, which has been reported to predict little BP response to angioplasty; this may be the reason that the baseline CS was not predictive in this cohort. Aside from the finding that only 2 of 56 patients received a stent, many unanswered questions remain after DRASTIC. Some will perhaps be answered by STents in Atherosclerotic Renovascular disease (STAR),[73] which plans to randomize 140 patients with a 50% or greater renal artery stenosis and a creatinine clearance of less than 80 mL/minute/1.73 m² to angioplasty plus stent plus medical therapy (with antihypertensive and lipid-lowering drugs) versus medical therapy alone. The primary outcome is a 20% reduction in creatinine clearance over a 2-year period, with extended follow-up to 5 years.

The three trials of angioplasty versus medical therapy were subjected to two meta-analyses.[74,75] Surprisingly, despite considering the same 210 patients, these trials had slightly different conclusions. In one, no significant differences were found in any endpoint (BP, medications, or renal function).[75] Patient-specific data were available to Ives and associates, who reported a slightly larger overall reduction in BP in the angioplasty group (6.3/3.3 mm Hg; $P = .02/.03$) versus drug treatment.[74] The change in serum creatinine concentration was just barely beyond significance ($P = .06$), but it favored the angioplasty group. The ASTRAL trial (Angioplasty and Stent for Renal Artery Lesions, comparing angioplasty with or without stent with drug therapy), proposed to the United Kingdom's Medical Research Council, may resolve the uncertainties, but only if several hundred patients are enrolled.

SUMMARY

Although many unanswered questions about renovascular hypertension remain, most authorities agree on the following: (1) the absolute risk for the disease can be estimated with reasonable accuracy, using only clinical information, thereby sparing many patients further evaluation; (2) patients with a very high absolute risk of disease should proceed to angiography if they are willing to undergo revascularization; (3) a screening test should be done for those with an intermediate absolute risk of disease; the choice of test may depend more on local expertise and cost that on a comparison of published performance characteristics; (4) angioplasty should be offered to patients with fibromuscular dysplasia; and (5) whether the current enthusiasm for angioplasty with or without stenting is warranted for atherosclerotic renovascular hypertension is still uncertain, and the topic needs further research.

References

1. Alcazar JM, Rodicio JL. European Society of Hypertension: How to handle renovascular hypertension. *J Hypertens.* 2001;**19**:2109-2111.
2. 1995 Update of the Working Group Reports on Chronic Renal Failure and Renovascular Hypertension. National High Blood Pressure Education Program Working Group. *Arch Intern Med.* 1996;**156**:1938-1947.
3. 2003 European Society of Hypertension. European cardiology guidelines for the management of arterial hypertension: Guidelines Committee. *J Hypertens.* 2003;**21**:1011-1053.
4. National High Blood Pressure Education Program Coordinating Committee. Seventh Report of the Joint National

Committee on Prevention, Detection, Evaluation and Treatment of High Blood Pressure. *Hypertension.* 2003;**42**: 1206-1252.

5. Goldblatt H, Lynch J, Hanzal RF, Summerville WW. Studies on experimental hypertension. I. The production of persistent elevation of systolic blood pressure by means of renal ischemia. *J Exp Med.* 1934;**59**:347-380.

6. Safian RD, Textor SC. Renal-artery stenosis. *N Engl J Med.* 2001;**344**:431-442.

7. Maxwell MH, Bleifer KS, Franklin SS, Varady PD. Cooperative study of renovascular hypertension: Demographic analysis of the results. *JAMA.* 1972;**220**:1195-204.

8. Eyler WR, Clark MD, Garman JE, et al. Angiography of the renal areas including a comparative study of renal arterial stenoses in patients with and without hypertension. *Radiology.* 1962;**78**:879-892.

9. Buller CE, Nogareda JG, Ramanathan K, et al. The profile of cardiac patients with renal artery stenosis. *J Am Coll Cardiol.* 2003;**43**:1606-1613.

10. Weinrauch LA, D'Elia JA. Renal artery stenosis: "Fortuitous diagnosis," problematic therapy [editorial]. *J Am Coll Cardiol.* 2003;**43**:1614-1616.

11. Smith HW. Unilateral nephrectomy in hypertensive disease. *J Urol.* 1956;**76**:685-701.

12. Begelman SM, Olin JW. Fibromuscular dysplasia. *Curr Opinion Rheumatol.* 2000;**12**:41-47.

13. Harrison EG, McCormack LJ. Pathologic classification of renal arterial disease in renovascular hypertension. *Mayo Clin Proc.* 1971;**46**:161-167.

14. Kem DC, Lyons DF, Wenzl J, et al. Renin-dependent hypertension caused by nonfocal stenotic aberrant renal arteries: Proof of a new syndrome. *Hypertension.* 2005;**46**: 380-385.

15. Prospective Studies Collaborative. Age-specific relevance of usual blood pressure to vascular mortality: A meta-analysis of individual data for one million adults in 61 prospective studies. *Lancet.* 2002;**360**:1903-1913.

16. Caps MT, Perissinotto C, Zierler RE, et al. Prospective study of atherosclerotic disease progression of the renal artery. *Circulation.* 1998;**98**:2866-2872.

17. Caps MT, Zierler RE, Polissar NL, et al. Risk of atrophy in kidneys with atherosclerotic renal artery stenosis. *Kidney Int.* 1998;**53**:735-742.

18. Edwards MS, Craven TE, Burke GL, et al. Renovascular disease and the risk of adverse coronary events in the elderly: A prospective, population-based study. *Arch Intern Med.* 2005;**165**:207-213.

19. Textor SC, Wilcox CS. Renal artery stenosis: A common, treatable cause of renal failure? *Annu Rev Med.* 2001;**52**: 421-442.

20. Fatica RA, Port FK, Young EW. Incidence trends and mortality in end-stage renal disease attributed to renovascular disease in the United States. *Am J Kidney Dis.* 2001;**37**:1184-1190.

21. Barger AC. The Goldblatt memorial lecture. Part I. Experimental renovascular hypertension. *Hypertension.* 1979;**1**:447-455.

22. Soulez G, Oliva VL, Turpin S, et al. Imaging of renovascular hypertension: Respective values of renal scintigraphy, renal Doppler US, and MR angiography. *Radiographics.* 2000;**20**:1355-1368.

23. Claus T, Schmitt R, Stabroth C, et al. Where do we stand with renovascular hypertension? *Nephrol Dial Transplant.* 2005;**20**:1495-1498.

24. Shepherd S, Cadwallader K, Jankowski TA. Does early detection of suspected atherosclerotic renovascular hypertension change outcomes? *J Family Pract.* 2005;**54**:813-816.

25. Rosner MH. Renovascular hypertension: Can we identify a population at high risk? *Southern Med J.* 2001;**94**:1058-1064.

26. Krijnen P, van Jaarsveld BC, Steyerberg EW, et al. A clinical prediction rule for renal artery stenosis. *Ann Intern Med.* 1998;**129**:738-740.

27. Krijnen P, Steyerberg EW, Postma CT, et al. Validation of a prediction rule for renal artery stenosis. *J Hypertens.* 2005;**23**:1583-1588.

28. Vasbinder GB, Nelemans PJ, Kessels AG, et al. Diagnostic tests for renal artery stenosis in patients suspected of having renovascular hypertension: A meta-analysis. *Ann Intern Med.* 2001;**135**:401-411.

29. Vasbinder GBC, Nelemans PJ, Kessels AGH, et al. Accuracy of computed tomographic angiography and magnetic resonance angiography for diagnosing renal artery stenosis: Renal Artery Diagnostic Imaging Study in Hypertension (RADISH) Study Group. *Ann Intern Med.* 2004;**141**:674-682.

30. Müller FB, Sealey JE, Case DB, et al. The captopril test for identifying renovascular disease in hypertensive patients. *Am J Med.* 1986;**80**:633-644.

31. Postma CT, van der Steen PHM, Hoefnagels WHL, et al. The captopril test in the detection of renovascular disease in hypertensive patients. *Arch Intern Med.* 1990;**150**:625-628.

32. Elliott WJ, Martin WB, Murphy MB. Comparison of two non-invasive screening tests for renovascular hypertension. *Arch Intern Med.* 1993;**153**:755-764.

33. Taylor AJ Jr, Fletcher JW, Nally JV Jr, et al. Procedure guideline for diagnosis of renovascular hypertension: Society of Nuclear Medicine. *J Nucl Med.* 1998;**39**:1297-1302.

34. van Jaarsveld BC, Krikjnen P, Derkx F, et al. The place of renal scintigraphy in the diagnosis of renal artery stenosis: Fifteen years of clinical experience. *Arch Intern Med.* 1997;**157**:1226-1234.

35. Fommei E, Ghione S, Hilson AJW, et al. Captopril radionuclide test in renovascular hypertension: A European multicentre study. *Eur J Nucl Med.* 1993;**20**:617-623.

36. Svetkey LP, R Wilkinson J, Dunnick NR, et al. Captopril renography in the diagnosis of renovascular disease. *Am J Hypertens.* 1991;**4**:711S-715S.

37. Taylor A. Renovascular hypertension: Nuclear medicine techniques. *Q J Nucl Med.* 2002;**46**:268-282.

38. van Jaarsveld BC, Krijnen P, Pieterman H, et al. The effect of balloon angioplasty on hypertension in atherosclerotic renal-artery stenosis: Dutch Renal Artery Stenosis Intervention Cooperative Study Group. *N Engl J Med.* 2000;**342**:1007-1014.

39. Blaufox MD, Middleton ML, Bongiovanni J, Davis BR. Cost efficacy of the diagnosis and therapy of renovascular hypertension. *J Nucl Med.* 1996;**37**:171-177.

40. Lee H-Y, Grant EG. Sonography in renovascular hypertension. *J Ultrasound Med.* 2002;**21**:431-441.

41. Radermacher J, Chavan J, Bleck J, et al. Use of Doppler ultrasound to predict the outcome of therapy for renal artery stenosis. *N Engl J Med.* 2001;**344**:410-417.

42. Soulez G, Therasse E, Qanadli SD, et al. Prediction of clinical response after renal angioplasty: Respective value of renal Doppler sonography and scintigraphy. *AJR Am J Roentgenol.* 2003;**181**:1029-1035.

43. Bolduc JP, Oliva VL, Therasse E, et al. Diagnosis and treatment of renovascular hypertension: A cost-benefit analysis. *AJR Am J Roentgenol.* 2005;**184**:931-937.

44. Binkert CA, Debatin JF, Schneider E, et al. Can MR measurement of renal artery flow and renal volume predict the outcome of percutaneous transluminal renal angioplasty? *Cardiovasc Intervent Radiol.* 2001;**24**:233-239.

45. Qanadli SD, Soulez G, Therasse E, et al. Detection of renal artery stenosis: Prospective comparison of captopril-enhanced Doppler sonography, captopril-enhanced scintigraphy, and MR angiography. *AJR Am J Roentgenol.* 2001;**177**:1123-1129.

46. Carlos RC, Axelroad DA, Ellis JH, et al. Incorporating patient-centered outcomes in the analysis of cost-effectiveness: Imaging

strategies for renovascular hypertension. *AJR Am J Roentgenol.* 2003;**181**:1653-1661.

47. Radermacher J, Haller H. The right diagnostic work-up: Investigating renal and renovascular disorders. *J Hypertens.* 2003;**21** (**Suppl 2**):S19-S24.

48. Gowda MS, Loeb AL, Crouse LJ, Kramer PH. Complementary roles of color-flow duplex imaging and intravascular ultrasound in the diagnosis of renal artery fibromuscular dysplasia: Should renal arteriography serve as the "gold standard?" *J Am Coll Cardiol.* 2003;**41**:1305-1311.

49. Textor SC. Managing renal arterial disease and hypertension. *Curr Opin Cardiol.* 2003;**18**:260-267.

50. Aqel RA, Zoghbi GJ, Baldwin SA, et al. Prevalence of renal artery stenosis in high-risk veterans referred to cardiac catheterization. *J Hypertens.* 2003;**21**:1157-1162.

51. Lederman RJ, Mendelsohn FO, Santos R, et al. Primary renal artery stenting: Characteristics and outcomes after 363 procedures. *Am Heart J.* 2001;**142**:314-323.

52. Haller C. Arteriosclerotic renal artery stenosis: Conservative versus interventional management. *Heart.* 2002;**88**:193-197.

53. Chàbovà V, Schirger A, Stanson AW, et al. Outcomes of atherosclerotic renal artery stenosis managed without revascularization. *Mayo Clin Proc.* 2000;**75**:437-444.

54. Pillay WR, Kan YM, Crinnion JN, et al. Prospective multicentre study of the natural history of atherosclerotic renal artery stenosis in patients with peripheral vascular disease. *Br J Surg.* 2002;**89**:737-740.

55. Plouin PF. Stable patients with atherosclerotic renal artery stenosis should be treated first with medical management. *Am J Kidney Dis.* 2003;**42**:851-857.

56. Fernando D, Garasic J. Percutaneous intervention for renovascular disease: Rationale and patient selection. *Curr Opin Cardiol.* 2004;**19**:582-588.

57. Novick AC, Ziegelbaum M, Vidt DG, et al. Trends in surgical revascularization for renal artery disease: Ten years' experience. *JAMA.* 1987;**257**:498-501.

58. Aurell M, Jensen G. Treatment of renovascular hypertension. *Nephron.* 1997;**75**:373-383.

59. Galaria II, Surowiec SM, Rhodes JM, et al. Percutaneous and open renal revascularizations have equivalent long-term functional outcomes. *Ann Vasc Surg.* 2005;**19**:218-228.

60. van de Ven PJ, Kaatee R, Beutler JJ, et al. Arterial stenting and balloon angioplasty in ostial atherosclerotic renovascular disease: A randomised trial. *Lancet.* 1999;**353**:282-286.

61. Mounier-Vehier C, Haulon S, Lions C, et al. Renal atrophy in atherosclerotic renovascular disease: Gradual changes 6 months after successful angioplasty. *J Endovasc Ther.* 2002;**9**:863-872.

62. Durros G, Jaff M, Mathiak L, et al. Multicenter Palmaz stent renal artery stenosis revascularization registry report: Four-year follow-up of 1068 successful patients. *Catheter Cardiovasc Interv.* 2002;**55**:182-188.

63. Isles CG, Robertson S, Hill D. Management of renovascular disease: A review of renal artery stenting in 10 studies. *Q J Med.* 1999;**92**:159-167.

64. Gill KS, Fowler RC. Atherosclerotic renal arterial stenosis: Clinical outcomes of stent placement for hypertension and renal failure. *Radiology.* 2003;**226**:821-826.

65. Watson PS, Hadipetrou P, Cox SV, et al. Effect of renal artery stenting on renal function and size in patients with atherosclerotic renovascular disease. *Circulation.* 2000;**102**:1671-1677.

66. Beutler JJ, van Ampting JMA, van der Ven PJG, et al. Long-term effects of arterial stenting on kidney function for patients with ostial atherosclerotic renal artery stenosis and renal insufficiency. *J Am Soc Nephrol.* 2001;**12**:1475-1481.

67. Silva JA, Chan AW, White CJ, et al. Elevated brain natriuretic peptide predicts blood pressure response after stent revascularization in patients with renal artery stenosis. *Circulation.* 2005;**111**:328-333.

68. Hollenberg NK. Medical therapy for renovascular hypertension: A review. *Am J Hypertens.* 1988;**1**:338S-343S.

69. Weibull H, Bergqvist D, Bergentz SE, et al. Percutaneous transluminal renal angioplasty versus surgical reconstruction of atherosclerotic renal artery stenosis: A prospective randomized study. *J Vasc Surg.* 1993;**18**:841-852.

70. Uzzo RG, Novick AC, Goormastic M, et al. Medical vs. surgical management of atherosclerotic renal artery stenosis. *Transplant Proc.* 2002;**34**:723-725.

71. Plouin PF, Chatellier G, Darne B, Raynaud A. Blood pressure outcome of angioplasty in atherosclerotic renal artery stenosis: A randomized trial. Essai Multicentrique Medicaments vs Angioplastie (EMMA) Study Group. *Hypertension.* 1998;**31**: 823-829.

72. Webster J, Marshall F, Abdalla M, et al. Randomised comparison of percutaneous angioplasty vs. continued medical therapy for hypertensive patients with atheromatous renal artery stenosis: Scottish and Newcastle Renal Artery Stenosis Collaborative Group. *J Hum Hypertens.* 1998;**12**:329-335.

73. Bax L, Mali WP, Buskens E, et al. The benefit of STent placement and blood pressure and lipid-lowering for the prevention of progression of renal dysfunction caused by Atherosclerotic ostial stenosis of the Renal artery: The STAR study. Rationale and study design. *J Nephrol.* 2003;**16**:807-817.

74. Ives NJ, Wheatley K, Stowe RL, et al. Continuing uncertainty about the value of percutaneous revascularization in atherosclerotic renovascular disease: A meta-analysis of randomized trials. *Nephrol Dial Transplant.* 2003;**18**:298-304.

75. Nordmann AJ, Wood K, Parkes R, Logan AG. Balloon angioplasty or medical therapy for hypertensive patients with atherosclerotic renal artery stenosis? A meta-analysis of randomized controlled trials. *Am J Med.* 2003;**114**:44-50.

Secondary Hypertension: Mineralocorticoid Excess States

Emmanuel L. Bravo

Since the mid-1970s, the number of distinct hypertensive syndromes clearly related to increased mineralocorticoid activity has grown. The list includes excessive aldosterone production (resulting from primary aldosteronism and glucocorticoid-remediable aldosteronism [GRA]), excessive deoxycorticosterone (DOC) production (resulting from congenital adrenocortical enzyme deficiency of 11β-hydroxylase or 17α-hydroxylase and glucocorticoid resistance), and activation of mineralocorticoid receptors by cortisol (resulting from incomplete conversion of cortisol to cortisone at target tissues with cortisol gaining inappropriate access to mineralocorticoid receptors). In these disorders, the underlying hormonal disturbance alters blood pressure (BP) regulation, and definitive mechanisms have been elucidated.

CLINICAL PRESENTATION

Mineralocorticoid hypertension is usually of adrenocortical origin and is associated with symptoms and signs that raise clinical suspicion of the diagnosis and help the physician in planning a rational diagnostic and therapeutic approach. The diagnostic evaluation should start with a careful history and a thorough physical examination. The clinical history should include the age of onset of hypertension, any family history of mineralocorticoid hypertension, early death of affected family members resulting from cerebrovascular accidents and development of secondary sexual characteristics, and signs and symptoms related to hypokalemia (i.e., muscle weakness, tachycardia or palpitations, and polyuria). During the physical examination, the examiner should look for signs of chronic severe elevated BP and should note the presence or absence of secondary sexual characteristics and the signs of androgen or cortisol excess. Following this, a few basic laboratory tests are indicated. Laboratory testing should include the determination of serum electrolytes, blood urea nitrogen, creatinine, plasma concentrations of aldosterone, cortisol, renin activity, and 24-hour urinary excretions of sodium, potassium, creatinine, aldosterone, and free cortisol. The types of information thus obtained are categorized into groups, each indicating either a diagnosis or a need for further testing (Table 9-1).

INITIAL EVALUATION

Assessment for mineralocorticoid hypertension is recommended under the following circumstances:

1. Patients who develop spontaneous hypokalemia
2. Patients who develop moderately severe hypokalemia (serum potassium concentration <3.0 mEq/L) with conventional doses of diuretics, even if levels normalize after diuretics are withdrawn
3. Serum potassium levels that fail to normalize after 4 to 6 weeks without diuretics
4. Angiotensin II blockade that fails to normalize serum potassium values
5. Patients with refractory hypertension with no obvious evidence for a secondary cause

In the hypokalemic patient, the initial assessment should determine whether the hypokalemia is the result of renal potassium wasting. A 24-hour urinary potassium excretion greater than 30 mEq when the serum potassium is less than 3.5 mEq/L usually reflects renal potassium wasting, whereas lower excretion rates suggest extrarenal loss (Fig. 9-1). The occurrence of hypokalemia with renal potassium wasting suggests an exaggerated exchange of sodium for potassium exchange at renal distal tubular sites. The response to spironolactone (100 mg twice daily for 5 days) during a salt load can demonstrate conclusively whether renal potassium wasting is truly mineralocorticoid dependent. An elevation in serum potassium concentration with a concomitant reduction in urinary potassium excretion with spironolactone indicates mineralocorticoid-mediated renal potassium wasting. Liddle's syndrome, a familial, non–steroid-dependent, renal potassium-wasting disorder associated with hypokalemia and hypertension, does not respond to spironolactone.[1]

HYPERTENSIVE SYNDROMES RESULTING FROM EXCESS PRODUCTION OF DEOXYCORTICOSTERONE

Adrenocortical Enzyme Deficiency

The best-defined circumstance in which DOC plays a significant role is in syndromes characterized by a deficiency of 11β- or 17α-hydroxylation of steroids (Fig. 9-2).[2,3] These disorders are usually congenital, but they may be induced by excessive production of estrogen[4] or androgens[5] from either a benign or a malignant tumor. In addition to these two hypertensive forms of congenital adrenal hyperplasia, excess DOC production occurs in a variety of disorders, including DOC-producing tumors[6] and primary glucocorticoid resistance.[7]

Table 9-1 Mineralocorticoid-Dependent Renal Potassium-Wasting Disorders with Hypertension

Condition	Plasma Humoral Characteristics		
	Cortisol	Renin	Aldosterone
Cushing's syndrome (ectopic ACTH excess)	↑	—	—
Primary aldosteronism (adenoma)*	N	↓	↑
Idiopathic aldosteronism* (hyperplasia)	N	↓	↑
Secondary aldosteronism	N	↑↑	↑↑
Dexamethasone-responsive aldosteronism	N	↓	↑↑
Excess deoxycorticosterone production*	N	↓	↑
Excess corticosterone production†	N	↓	↓
11β-hydroxylase deficiency†	↓	—	—
17α-hydroxylase deficiency†	↓	—	—

*Spironolactone responsive.
†Dexamethasone responsive.
N, normal.
ACTH, adrenocorticotropic hormone.

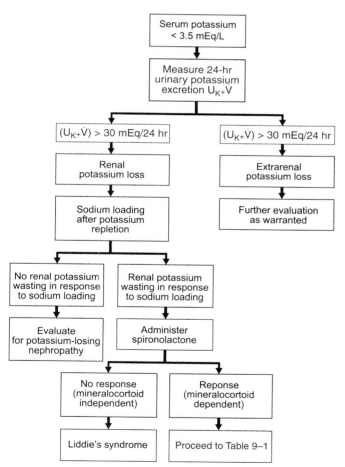

Figure 9–1   A simplified approach to determine the origin of hypokalemia in a hypertensive patient. $U_{K^+}\dot{V}$, urine potassium per 24-hr urine volume. (Modified from Bravo EL. What to do when potassium is high or low. *Diagnosis.* 1988;**10**:1-6.)

11β-Hydroxylase Deficiency

Findings on physical examination provide the most important clues to the presence of this enzymatic deficiency. Virilization in female patients or precocious puberty with advanced masculinization in male patients (caused by increased androgen production) are prominent features of 11β-hydroxylase deficiency. Deficiency of 11β-hydroxylase results in reduced production of cortisol, corticosterone, and aldosterone. Subsequent overproduction of adrenocorticotropic hormone (ACTH, also known as corticotropin) drives the zona fasciculata to increase production of DOC, which produces a type of mineralocorticoid hypertension. There is also increased formation of dehydroepiandrosterone (DHEA) and androstenedione, which produces hypergonadism. Deficiency of 11β-hydroxylase is confirmed by demonstrating increased levels of plasma 11-deoxycortisol and urinary tetrahydro-11-deoxycortisol and 17-ketosteroids.

17α-Hydroxylase Deficiency

Abnormalities in steroid production in the 17α-hydroxylase deficiency syndrome result in reduced production of 17α-hydroxyprogesterone and the distal steroids in the 17-hydroxy pathway, deoxycortisol and cortisol. Resultant overproduction of ACTH stimulates the uninvolved 17-deoxy pathway to increase the levels of progesterone, DOC, corticosterone, 18-OH DOC, and 18-hydroxycorticosterone. Because DOC causes salt and water retention, total suppression of renin synthesis and subsequent suppression of aldosterone result.

Deficiency of 17α-hydroxylase reduces production of all adrenal and gonadal androgens, including testosterone, DHEA, and androstenedione, resulting in a form of hypergonadotropic hypogonadism and abnormalities of sexual development. The hypogonadal consequence of the enzyme deficiency accounts for most of the clinical features of the disorder. Women with this syndrome have primary amenorrhea, disproportionately long limbs relative to the trunk, absent

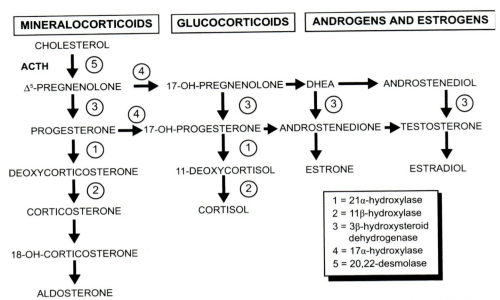

Figure 9–2   Pathways of adrenal hormone synthesis. DHEA, dehydroepiandrosterone. (From Watts NB. Congenital adrenal hyperplasia. *In:* Hurst JW [ed]. Medicine for the Practicing Physician, 4th ed. Stamford, CT: Appleton & Lange 1996, p 566.)

axillary and pubic hair, infantile breast and genital development, absent uterus, and an incomplete vagina. In men, the testes do not produce testosterone, with resulting decreased masculinization; male patients also have reduced axillary and public hair and ambiguous genitalia. Increased production of DOC and corticosterone, as well as decreased androgen secretion, establishes the diagnosis of 17α-hydroxylase deficiency.

In both 11β- and 17α-hydroxylase deficiency disorders, dexamethasone, by inhibiting ACTH release, decreases DOC production and results in normalization of arterial BP and serum potassium concentration.

Glucocorticoid Resistance

The control of cortisol synthesis is through a negative feedback loop in which cortisol feeds back on the pituitary to inhibit ACTH secretion.[8] In generalized inherited glucocorticoid resistance, cortisol secretion remains ACTH dependent, but it is reset to a higher level than normal. Affected individuals do not develop features of Cushing's syndrome, because the peripheral tissues and pituitary are equally resistant. An ACTH-dependent increase in mineralocorticoids (primarily DOC) and in adrenal androgens occurs. Because there is no peripheral resistance to these hormones, they produce clinical effects. Therefore, the clinical presentation is caused by excess adrenal androgens (virilization, precocious puberty) and by excess mineralocorticoids (hypertension, hypokalemia).

Two strategies are used to treat generalized glucocorticoid resistance. The first employs high amounts of exogenous glucocorticoid, such as dexamethasone, to suppress adrenal stimulation by ACTH. Therapy is monitored by measuring the serum concentrations of cortisol, DOC, and androgen.

Alternatively, mineralocorticoid or androgen antagonists can be used.

HYPERTENSIVE SYNDROMES RESULTING FROM ACTIVATION OF MINERALOCORTICOID RECEPTORS BY CORTISOL

11β-Hydroxysteroid Dehydrogenase Deficiency

11β-hydroxysteroid dehydrogenase deficiency syndromes result in excessive activation of mineralocorticoid receptors by a steroid dependent on ACTH, rather than by the conventional mineralocorticoid agonist. This steroid appears to be cortisol. Mineralocorticoid receptors in the distal nephron have equal affinity for their two ligands—aldosterone and cortisol—but are protected from cortisol by the presence of 11β-dehydrogenase, which inactivates cortisol by converting it to cortisone (Fig. 9-3).[9] The 11,18-hemiacetal structure of aldosterone protects it from the action of 11β-hydroxysteroid dehydrogenase so that aldosterone gains specific access to the receptors. When this mechanism is defective because of either congenital 11β-hydroxysteroid dehydrogenase deficiency or enzyme inhibition (by licorice or carbenoxolone), intrarenal levels of cortisol increase, causing inappropriate activation of mineralocorticoid receptors.[10] The resulting antinatriuresis and kaliuresis lead to hypertension and hypokalemia. Biochemically, elevations in urinary free cortisol excretion and in the ratio of the urinary metabolites of cortisol to those of cortisone, as well as prolongation of the half-life of titrated cortisol, are noted. Plasma cortisol concentrations usually are

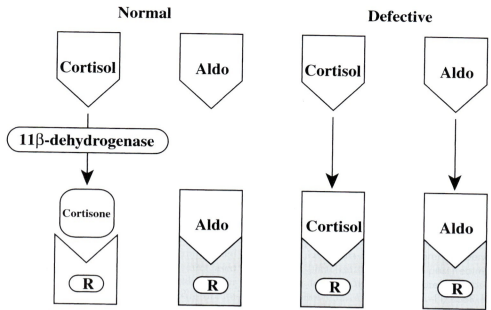

Figure 9–3 Enzyme-mediated receptor protection. Normal 11β-hydroxysteroid dehydrogenase converts cortisol to inactive cortisone, protecting mineralocorticoid receptors (R) from cortisol and allowing selective access for aldosterone (Aldo). When 11β-dehydrogenase is defective, such as in congenital deficiency or after licorice administration, cortisol gains inappropriate access to mineralocorticoid receptors, with resulting antinatriuresis and kaliuresis. (From Walker BR, Edwards CR. Licorice-induced hypertension and syndromes of apparent mineralocorticoid excess. *Endocrinol Metab Clin North Am.* 1994;**23**: 359-377.)

not elevated. The signs and symptoms are reversed by spironolactone or dexamethasone and are exacerbated by administration of physiologic doses of cortisol.

Cushing's Syndrome (Resulting from Ectopic Adrenocorticotropic Hormone Excess)

The recognizable causes of Cushing's syndrome include Cushing's disease (72%), ectopic ACTH excess (12%), adrenal adenoma (8%), carcinoma (6%), and hyperplasia (4%) (see also Chapter 12). The typical clinical presentation of Cushing's syndrome includes truncal obesity, moon facies, hypertension, plethora, muscle weakness and fatigue, hirsutism, emotional disturbances, and typical purple skin striae. Carbohydrate intolerance or diabetes, amenorrhea, loss of libido, easy bruising, and spontaneous fracture of ribs and vertebrae may also be encountered. Patients with ectopic ACTH excess may not have the typical manifestations of cortisol excess, but they may present with hyperpigmentation of the skin, severe hypertension, and marked hypokalemic alkalosis.

The incidence of hypokalemic alkalosis in the ectopic ACTH syndrome is greater than 90%, compared with only 10% in Cushing's syndrome of other causes.[11] It is widely supposed that corticosterone or 11-DOC is responsible for mineralocorticoid excess, but poor correlation exists between the levels of these steroids and the degree of hypokalemia. A better predictor of hypokalemia is the level of cortisol.[12,13] Several studies suggest that the ratio of cortisol to cortisone metabolites is increased in all forms of Cushing's syndrome.[14,15] Ulick and associates advanced the hypothesis that

excessive circulating cortisol overwhelms the enzyme, thus escaping conversion of cortisol to cortisone and gaining inappropriate access to mineralocorticoid receptors.[16] Walker and co-workers demonstrated a negative correlation between the extent of impairment of 11β-hydroxysteroid dehydrogenase and plasma potassium concentration in 26 patients with Cushing's syndrome, 9 of whom had higher cortisol-to-cortisone ratios than the 15 patients with pituitary Cushing's and the 2 patients with adrenal adenomas.[17]

The determination of the 24-hour urinary free cortisol concentration is the best available test for documenting endogenous hypercortisolism.[18] A level higher than 100 μg/24 hours suggests excessive cortisol production. There are virtually no false-negative results. False-positive results may be obtained in non-Cushing's hypercortisolemic states (e.g., stress, chronic strenuous exercise, psychiatric states, glucocorticoid resistance, and malnutrition). If differentiation between pituitary and ectopic sources of ACTH cannot be made based on plasma levels alone, pharmacologic manipulation of ACTH secretion should be performed. The overnight dexamethasone suppression test requires only a blood collection for serum cortisol the morning after the patient has taken a 1.0-mg dose of dexamethasone at 11 PM of the previous evening. In physiologically normal subjects, cortisol levels at 8 AM will be suppressed to 5.0 μg/dL or less.

When the syndrome has been diagnosed by appropriate biochemical testing, the cause must be identified. Radioimmunoassay of plasma ACTH is the procedure of choice for pinpointing the basis of hypercortisolism, but this test is not available in many hospitals. In patients with ACTH-independent Cushing's syndrome, ACTH levels have usually been suppressed to less than 5 pg/mL. In contrast, patients with the ACTH-dependent form tend to have either normal or elevated levels of ACTH, usually higher than 10 pg/mL. In patients with Cushing's disease (i.e., basophilic pituitary microadenomas), ACTH release can be inhibited only at much higher doses of dexamethasone (2 mg every 6 hours for 2 days). The established criterion for the test is that suppression of the 24-hour urine and plasma steroids to less than 50% of baseline indicates pituitary Cushing's syndrome (i.e., Cushing's disease). Failure to suppress these concentrations to less than 50% of baseline is considered consistent with an ectopic source of ACTH or ACTH-independent Cushing's syndrome. The best way to differentiate pituitary ACTH excess from the ectopic production of ACTH is with the inferior petrosal sinus procedure for ACTH concentration, which is invasive and carries its own risks.[19] The test has been characterized in the literature as having 100% specificity and 100% sensitivity. The criterion currently used after corticotropin-releasing hormone administration is that the ACTH gradient between the inferior petrosal sinus and the peripheral site will be greater than 2 if the patient has Cushing's disease.

Surgical resection of a pituitary or ectopic source of ACTH or of a cortisol-producing adrenocortical tumor is the treatment of choice for Cushing's syndrome. For pituitary Cushing's syndrome, transsphenoidal pituitary adenomectomy is the treatment of choice,[20] but total hypophysectomy may be required in patients with diffuse hyperplasia or large pituitary tumors. Bilateral adrenalectomy for Cushing's disease is universally successful in alleviating the hypercortisolemic state; however, 10% to 38% of individuals may later develop pituitary tumors and hyperpigmentation (Nelson's syndrome).[21] Radiotherapy (i.e., external pituitary irradiation, seeding the pituitary bed with yttrium or gold) has also been used, with occasionally good results.[22] The long-acting analogue SMS 201-995 (octreotide) has been used with varied success to treat ectopic ACTH syndromes[23]; some benefit has been reported in Cushing's disease and Nelson's syndrome. Cyproheptadine has had limited success in the treatment of Cushing's disease. Ketoconazole, an inhibitor of several steroid biosynthetic pathways, has been used for rapid correction of hypercortisolism in patients awaiting definitive intervention.[24] Mitotane (o,p'-DDD), an insecticide derivative, induces destruction of the zonae reticularis and fasciculata with relative sparing of the zona glomerulosa. Mitotane has been used to treat Cushing's syndrome associated with adrenal carcinoma and to suppress cortisol secretion in Cushing's disease.[25]

HYPERTENSIVE SYNDROMES RESULTING FROM EXCESSIVE ALDOSTERONE PRODUCTION

Primary Aldosteronism

Clinical Recognition

The clinical manifestations of primary aldosteronism are not distinctive. The clinical decision to initiate a laboratory assessment is based on observing one of a number of clinical characteristics described in the previous section on initial evaluation.

Screening Tests

For screening purposes, hypokalemia, whether spontaneous or provoked, provides an important clue to the presence of primary aldosteronism. However, substantial numbers of patients with primary aldosteronism do not present with hypokalemia (Fig. 9-4); the serum potassium concentration is normal in 7% to 38% of reported cases.[26-29] In addition, 10% to 12% of patients with proven tumors may not have hypokalemia during short-term salt loading (Fig. 9-5).

Plasma renin activity (PRA) of less than 1 ng/L/hour that fails to rise to more than 2 ng/mL/hour after salt and water depletion and upright posture have been used as a screening test to exclude primary aldosteronism. However, many (~35%) patients have values that rise to more than 2 ng/mL/hour in response to appropriate stimulation (Fig. 9-6). In addition, about 40% of subjects with essential hypertension have suppressed PRA, and 15% to 20% of these patients have values lower than 2 ng/mL/hour under conditions of stimulation.[26]

The plasma aldosterone to plasma renin ratio is used to define the appropriateness of PRA for the circulating concentration of aldosterone.[30] It is assumed that the volume expansion associated with the presence of an aldosterone-producing tumor suppresses the release of renin without affecting the autonomous production of aldosterone. The test has several limitations. First, the inherent variability in plasma levels of aldosterone, even in the presence of a tumor, translates into variability in the absolute value of the ratio. Second, the use of drugs that prolong stimulation of renin long after their discontinuation may alter the ratio. Third, many (~40%) patients have suppressed PRA, which gives rise to a high rate of false-positive tests.[26] In my experience, the sensitivity of the test is only 58%.

Diagnosis

The diagnosis of primary aldosteronism often can be established with relative ease. In the hypertensive patient receiving no treatment who demonstrates significant hypokalemia (<3 mEq/L) with inappropriate kaliuresis (24-hour urinary potassium >30 mEq), PRA less than 1 ng/mL/hour, and elevated plasma or urinary aldosterone values, the diagnosis is unequivocal. Often, however, the diagnosis is not obvious because of equivocal values. In such cases, multiple measurements are needed during salt loading (Table 9-2). In my experience, the single best test for identifying patients with primary aldosteronism is the measurement of 24-hour urinary aldosterone excretion during salt loading.[26] An aldosterone excretion rate greater than 14 μg/24 hours following salt loading distinguishes most patients with primary aldosteronism from those with essential hypertension; only 7% of patients with primary aldosteronism have aldosterone excretion values that fall within the range for essential hypertension (Fig. 9-7). In contrast, substantial numbers (~39%) of patients with primary aldosteronism have plasma aldosterone values that fall within the range for essential hypertension. The findings of hypokalemia and suppressed PRA provide corroborative evidence for the diagnosis of primary aldosteronism, but their absence does not preclude the diagnosis. The sensitivity of various screening and diagnostic tests for primary aldosteronism is shown in Table 9-3.

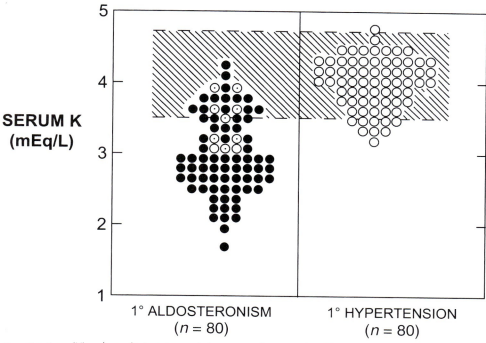

Figure 9–4   Serum potassium (K) values during normal dietary sodium intake. Each point represents the mean of at least three determinations. For patients with primary aldosteronism, solid circles represent adenomas (n = 70) and *open circles with dotted centers* represent hyperplasia (n = 10). The *crosshatched area* represents 95% confidence limits (3.5 to 4.6 mEq/L) of values obtained from 60 healthy subjects. (From Bravo EL, Tarazi RC, Dustan HP, et al. The changing clinical spectrum of primary aldosteronism. *Am J Med.* 1983;**74**:641-651.)

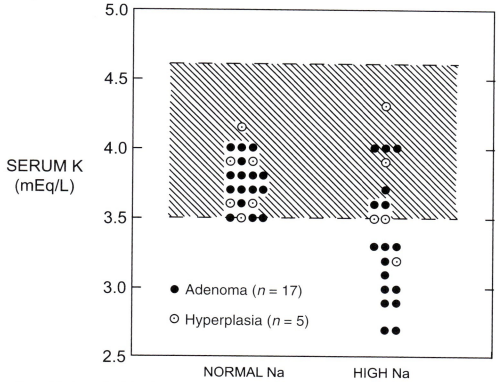

Figure 9–5   The effect of 3 days of salt loading on serum potassium (K) values in 22 patients with normal basal values. Patient identification is as in Figure 9-4. Six of 17 patients with adenoma and 4 of 5 patients with hyperplasia remained normokalemic despite salt loading. Aldosterone excretion rates and renal function were similar in those who remained normokalemic and in those who became hypokalemic. Na, sodium. (From Bravo EL, Tarazi RC, Dustan HP, et al. The changing clinical spectrum of primary aldosteronism. *Am J Med.* 1983;**74**:641-651.)

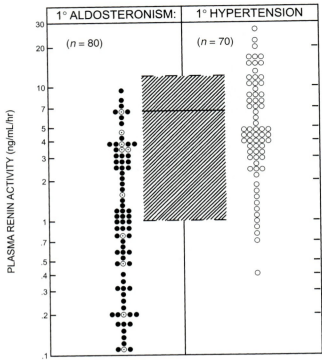

Figure 9–6 Supine plasma renin activity values the morning after 4 days of sodium deprivation. Patient identification is as in Figure 9-4. The *crosshatched area* represents the 95% confidence limits (1.06 to 12/18 ng/mL/hour) of values obtained from 47 healthy subjects. Twenty-nine patients (36%) with primary aldosterone had values higher than 2.0 ng/mL/hour; 12 patients (17%) with primary hypertension had values lower than 2.0 ng/mL/hour. (From Bravo EL, Tarazi RC, Dustan HP, et al. The changing clinical spectrum of primary aldosteronism. *Am J Med.* 1983;**74**:641-651.)

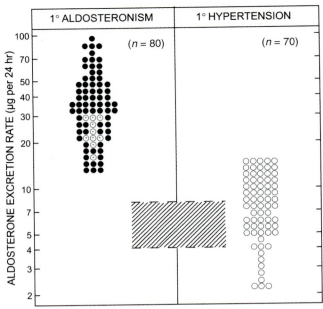

Figure 9–7 Aldosterone excretion rate after 3 days of high sodium intake. For patients with primary aldosterone, *solid circles* represent adenomas (n = 70) and *open circles* represent hyperplasia (n = 10). The *crosshatched area* represents the mean (4.0 µg/24 hour) and +2 standard deviations (8.0 µg/24 hour) of values obtained from 47 healthy subjects. No patient with primary aldosteronism had a value within the 95% normal range. Ten patients (14%) with primary hypertension had values that fell within the range obtained in patients with primary aldosteronism. Using a reference value of greater than 14 µg/24 hours after a high sodium intake for 3 days, the sensitivity and specificity of the test are 96% and 93%, respectively. (From Bravo EL, Tarazi RC, Dustan HP, et al. The changing clinical spectrum of primary aldosteronism. *Am J Med.* 1983;**74**:641-651.)

Table 9-2 Outpatient Oral Salt-Loading Protocol

Preparation
Discontinue all diuretic agents.
Raise serum potassium if it is still less than 3.5 mEq/L after 1 to 2 weeks of diuretic abstinence.
If elevated blood pressure is a concern, use calcium antagonists, α-blockers, or β-blockers.

Procedure
At baseline, draw blood for sodium, potassium, chloride, and carbon dioxide.
On days 1 to 5 inclusive, add to usual dietary intake 1 level full teaspoon of salt daily.
On days 4 and 5 of increased salt intake, collect 24-hour urine for sodium, potassium, chromium, and aldosterone.
On day 6 (the morning after the last urine collection), draw blood for sodium, potassium, chloride, carbon dioxide, plasma aldosterone, and plasma renin activity.

Biochemical Differentiation between Adenoma and Hyperplasia

The most common cause (70% to 80% of all proven cases) of primary aldosteronism is an aldosterone-producing adenoma. Approximately 20% to 30% of cases are caused by hyperplasia of the zona glomerulosa layer of the adrenal cortex (idiopathic hyperaldosteronism). Some reports suggest the rare occurrence of a syndrome intermediate between adenoma and hyperplasia.[31] The distinction between these two processes is important because surgical intervention is not effective in cases of hyperplasia. An adenoma is likely in the presence of spontaneous hypokalemia of 3.0 mEq/L or less, plasma 18-hydroxycorticosterone values greater than 100 ng/dL,[32]

Table 9-3   Sensitivity and Specificity of Various Screening and Diagnostic Tests for Primary Aldosteronism

Test	Standard	Sensitivity* (Number of Patients)	Specificity† (Number of Patients)
Serum potassium‡	Spontaneous (<3.5 mEq/L)	0.73 (58/80)	0.94 (66/70)
Serum potassium§	Provoked (<3.5 mEq/L)	0.86 (70/80)	0.96 (67/70)
Plasma renin activity¶¶	Suppressed (<2.0 ng/mL/hr)	0.64 (51/80)	0.83 (58/70)
Aldosterone excretion rate§¶	Nonsuppressible (>14 µg/24 hr)	0.96 (77/80)	0.93 (65/70)
Plasma aldosterone concentration§¶	Nonsuppressible (>22 ng/dL)	0.72 (31/43)	0.91 (31/34)

*Sensitivity: fraction of subjects with the disease who have positive results.
†Specificity: fraction of subjects without disease who have negative results.
‡Normal sodium intake for 3 to 5 days.
§High sodium intake for 3 days.
¶¶Low sodium intake for 4 days.
¶Standards for aldosterone excretion rate and plasma aldosterone concentration represent the upper 95% range of values obtained in subjects with essential hypertension.

and an anomalous postural decrease in plasma aldosterone concentration.[33] In addition, patients with adenomas are largely unresponsive to changes in sodium balance,[26] and they appear to be exquisitely sensitive to ACTH, unlike patients with hyperplasia, who are more sensitive to angiotensin II infusions.[34] A plasma 18-hydroxycorticosterone value lower than 100 ng/dL or a postural increase in plasma aldosterone, or both, is usually associated with adrenal hyperplasia, but it does not completely rule out the presence of an adenoma.[26]

Localizing Procedures

The adrenal computed tomography (CT) scan should be considered the initial step in localization. It is noninvasive, and all adenomas 1.5 cm in diameter or larger can be located accurately. Only 60% of nodules measuring 1.0 to 1.4 cm in diameter are detected by CT, however, and nodules smaller than 1.0 cm in diameter are very difficult, if not impossible, to detect. The overall sensitivity of localizing adenomas by high-resolution CT scanning exceeds 90%.[35-37] Adrenal venous aldosterone levels should be measured when the results of the adrenal CT scan are ambiguous and biochemical evidence for the presence of a tumor is overwhelming. Bilateral adrenal venous sampling for the measurement of aldosterone concentration is still the most accurate test for localizing aldosterone-producing tumors. When technically successful, and both adrenal veins are entered, the accuracy of comparative adrenal venous aldosterone levels in confirming either a tumor or hyperplasia exceeds 95%.[38] The ratio of ipsilateral to contralateral aldosterone usually is greater than 10:1. Correct placement of the catheter in the adrenal vein is essential and is best evaluated by obtaining simultaneous ACTH-stimulated selective adrenal venous cortisol levels, measured in the same samples as the aldosterone levels. An adrenal vein–to-peripheral vein cortisol ratio of 2:1 indicates that the catheter is in the adrenal vein at the time of sampling. An aldosterone ratio of 10:1 or greater in the presence of symmetrical ACTH-induced cortisol response is diagnostic of an aldosterone-

producing adenoma. Unfortunately, this procedure is invasive and technically demanding, and it requires considerable skill and experience. There is an appreciable incidence of complications, including adrenal and iliac venous thrombosis and extravasation of dye into the gland, which can lead to adrenal insufficiency.

A Simplified Approach to the Diagnosis of Primary Aldosteronism

A simplified approach to the diagnosis of primary aldosteronism is shown in Figure 9-8. In untreated patients who have spontaneous hypokalemia (serum potassium <3 mEq/L), inappropriate kaliuresis (urinary potassium >30 mEq/24 hour), PRA less than 1 ng/mL/hour, plasma aldosterone greater than 22 ng/dL, and an aldosterone excretion rate greater than 14 µg/24 hours when the urinary sodium concentration is 250 mEq/24 hours or higher, the diagnosis is incontrovertible. Under these conditions, additional biochemical studies to differentiate a tumor from hyperplasia can be performed, followed by an adrenal CT scan to determine which adrenal gland could be the site of an adenoma. Patients who are normokalemic but who have a history of becoming significantly hypokalemic during conventional diuretic therapy or who have persistent hypokalemia despite attempts at potassium repletion should have a salt-loading test. This can be accomplished in the outpatient setting (see Table 9-2). An aldosterone excretion rate greater than 14 µg/24 hours when the urinary sodium is at least 250 mEq/24 hours suggests excessive aldosterone production. Additional studies can then be performed to confirm and localize a tumor.

Therapeutic Choices

Medical therapy is indicated in patients with adrenal hyperplasia, in those with adenoma who are poor surgical risks, and in those with bilateral adrenal adenomas that may require bilateral adrenalectomy. Total bilateral adrenalectomy has no

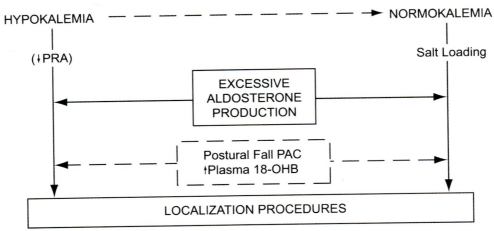

Figure 9–8 Algorithm for the diagnosis of primary aldosteronism. 18-OHB, 18-hydroxycorticosterone; PAC, plasma aldosterone concentration; PRA, plasma renin activity. (From Bravo EL. Primary aldosteronism. *Urol Clin North Am.* 1989:**16**:481-486.)

place in the management of primary aldosteronism, because adrenal insufficiency may be more difficult to treat than hypertension caused by aldosteronism. The hypertension associated with primary aldosteronism is salt and water dependent and is best treated by sustained salt and water depletion (Fig. 9-9).[39-41] The usual doses of diuretics are hydrochlorothiazide, 12.5 to 50 mg/day, or furosemide, 80 to 180 mg/day, in combination with either spironolactone, 100 to 200 mg/day, or amiloride, 10 to 20 mg/day. These combinations usually result in prompt correction of hypokalemia and normalization of BP within 2 to 4 weeks (Fig. 9-10).[40] In some cases, the addition of either a β-adrenergic blocker or a vasodilator may be needed to normalize BP. Spironolactone and amiloride are both capable of controlling BP and normalizing the serum potassium concentration in patients with primary aldosteronism.[42] However, spironolactone may be more efficacious. In 11 of 24 patients who took both amiloride and spironolactone at different times in the course of long-

term (>5 years) medical therapy, BP was 123 ± 4.6 (standard error [SE])/82 ± 1.8 (SE) mm Hg with spironolactone and 134 ± 3.9 (SE)/80 ± 2.5 (SE) mm Hg with amiloride. The serum potassium concentration during spironolactone therapy was 4.6 ± 0.2 (SE) mEq/L, and it was 4.1 ± 0.1 (SE) mEq/L with amiloride. None of the differences was statistically significant, perhaps because of the small number of patients. However, spironolactone was associated with more adverse effects. In 17 patients started on a spironolactone regimen, the most common complaints included breast tenderness in 13, breast engorgement in 8, muscle cramps in 7, and sexual dysfunction in 5. These adverse effects had no relation to dose. The only adverse effect noted with amiloride was muscle cramping, which was usually related to dose. This study also showed that the medical management of primary aldosteronism in reliable patients is an acceptable alternative to surgery if such therapy is warranted by overriding co-morbid conditions or strong preference. During long-term follow-up, no strokes, myocar-

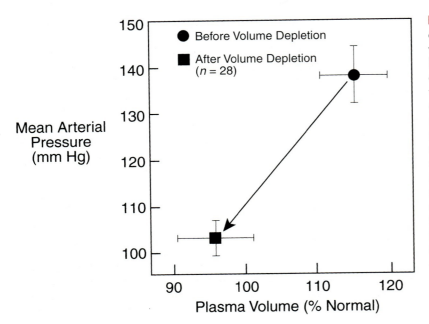

Figure 9–9 The effect of adequate volume depletion on the blood pressure of patients with primary aldosteronism and resistant hypertension. Spironolactone (200 mg/day) and hydrochlorothiazide (50 to 100 mg/day) were added to current therapy. Blood pressure and plasma volume values were those obtained after 8 to 12 weeks of continued therapy. Mean arterial pressure was significantly reduced in all. For the group as a whole, it fell from 138 ± 2 to 103 ± 9 (SEM) mm Hg (*P* < .01). Associated with reductions in mean arterial pressure were decreases in plasma volume (from 114% ± 3% to 97% ± 2% [SEM] normal) (*P* < .01). (From Bravo EL. Primary aldosteronism. Issues in diagnosis and management. *Endocrinol Metab Clin North Am.* 1994;**23**:271-282.)

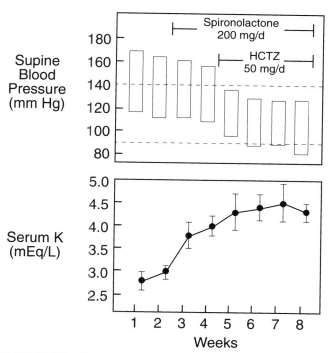

Figure 9–10 Diuretic therapy in primary aldosteronism. The effect of spironolactone combined with hydrochlorothiazide (HCTZ) on blood pressure and serum potassium (K) concentrations in patients with aldosterone-producing tumors. (From Bravo EL, Dustan HP, Tarazi RC. Spironolactone as a nonspecific treatment for primary aldosteronism. *Circulation.* 1973;**48**:491-498.)

dial infarctions, or heart failure episodes occurred in any patient. None of the patients experienced any malignant transformation of their tumors. Only 5 of 24 patients had a noticeable increase (>0.5 cm) in the size of the adrenal tumor, as measured by CT. Eplerenone, a selective aldosterone receptor antagonist, may be used in place of spironolactone. However, no studies to date have compared the efficacy of eplerenone with that of spironolactone in patients with primary hyperaldosteronism. Agents that block transmembrane calcium flux and inhibit in vitro aldosterone production induced by angiotensin II, ACTH, and potassium[43] are potent direct arteriolar vasodilators, and in some studies, they are reported to have natriuretic properties.[44] For these reasons, calcium channel blockers should be ideally suited for treating the hypertension associated with excessive aldosterone production. In a study by Bravo and colleagues,[45] nifedipine (30 to 80 mmg/day) was given to eight hypertensive patients with solitary adenomas for at least 4 weeks, followed by the addition of spironolactone (100 to 200 mg/day) for 4 weeks, after which nifedipine was discontinued, and patients remained on spironolactone alone. The following factors were assessed in the fourth week of each phase of the study: weekly averages of supine home BPs, plasma volume, PRA, plasma aldosterone concentration, and serum electrolyte levels. Nifedipine decreased BP, but not to normal levels, and it did not alter plasma volume, PRA, aldosterone, or serum potassium concentrations. Spironolactone normalized BP and serum potassium concentration, reduced plasma volume, and increased PRA and plasma aldosterone concentration. Nifedipine in combination with spironolactone did not result in a greater antihypertensive effect than spironolactone alone. These results suggest that nifedipine is not as efficacious as spironolactone in the treatment of primary aldosteronism.

In the majority of patients, surgical excision of an aldosterone-producing adenoma leads to normotension, as well as reversal of the biochemical defects. At the very least, surgery renders BP easier to control with medications. Neither the duration and severity of hypertension nor the degree of target organ involvement has any relation to arterial pressure response after surgery.[46] One year postoperatively, about 70% of patients are normotensive. The restoration of normal potassium homeostasis is permanent.

Patients planning to undergo surgery should receive drug treatment for at least 8 to 10 weeks, both to decrease BP and to correct metabolic abnormalities. These patients have a significant potassium deficiency that must be corrected preoperatively because hypokalemia increases the risk of cardiac arrhythmias during anesthesia. Prolonged control of BP (≥3 months before surgery) permits the perioperative use of intravenous fluids without producing hypertension and decreases morbidity. Administration of antihypertensive medications usually is continued until surgery, and glucocorticoid administration is not needed preoperatively. After removal of an aldosterone-producing adenoma, selective hypoaldosteronism usually occurs, even in patients whose PRA had been stimulated with long-term diuretic therapy.[47] Potassium supplementation therefore should be given cautiously, and serum potassium values should be monitored closely. Residual mineralocorticoid activity is often sufficient to prevent excessive renal retention of potassium, provided sodium intake is adequate. If hyperkalemia does occur, furosemide in doses of 80 to 160 mg/day should be started. Treatment with fludrocortisone is not often necessary. If it is needed, 0.1 mg/day may be used as the initial dose, and adequate salt intake should be continued. Abnormalities in aldosterone production can persist for as long as 3 months after tumor removal.

Glucocorticoid-Remediable Aldosteronism

GRA is an inherited autosomal dominant disorder that mimics an aldosterone-producing adenoma.[48] The disorder is caused by a genetic mutation that results in a hybrid or chimeric gene product that fuses nucleotide sequences of the 11β-hydroxylase and aldosterone synthase genes.[49] This chimeric gene arose from unequal crossing between the 11β-hydroxylase and aldosterone synthase genes. These two genes are located in close proximity on human chromosome 8, are 95% homologous in nucleotide sequence, and have an identical intron-exon structure. The structure of the duplicated gene contains 5′ regulatory sequences conferring the ACTH responsiveness of 11β-hydroxylase, fused to more distal coding sequences of the aldosterone synthase gene (Fig. 9-11). This hybrid gene is expected to be regulated by ACTH and to have aldosterone synthase activity. It allows ectopic expression of aldosterone synthase activity in the ACTH-regulated zona fasciculata, which normally produces cortisol.[50] Aldosterone synthase oxidizes the C-18 carbon of a steroid precursor, such as corticosterone or cortisol, thus leading to the production of aldosterone and the hybrid steroids 18-hydroxycortisol and 18-oxycortisol (Fig. 9-12). This abnormal gene duplication

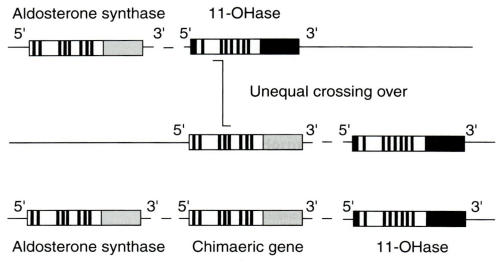

Figure 9–11 The diagram depicts unequal crossing over between aldosterone synthase and 11β-hydroxylase (11-OHase) genes. Each gene is represented by a *wide bar*, with the location of exons indicated by either *black* (11-OHase) or *stippled* (aldosterone synthase) bands. One of the two products of unequal crossing over will have a chimeric gene fusing sequences of the normal aldosterone synthase and 11-OHase genes. In this example, unequal crossing over is depicted as occurring in the intron between exons 3 and 4. (From Lifton RP, Dluhy RG, Powers M, et al. A chimaeric 11β-hydroxylase/aldosterone synthase gene causes glucocorticoid-remediable aldosteronism and human hypertension. *Nature*. 1992;**355**:262-265.)

can direct genetic screening for this disorder with a small blood sample. An important clinical clue is the age of onset of hypertension. Patients with GRA typically are diagnosed with high BP as children; conversely, patients with other mineralocorticoid excess disorders, such as aldosterone-producing adenomas and idiopathic hyperplasia, usually are diagnosed in their 30s to 60s. A strong family history of hypertension, often associated with early death of affected family members from cerebrovascular accidents, is seen in some families with GRA.

No controlled studies of treatment of patients with GRA have been conducted. Theoretically, the suppression of ACTH with exogenous glucocorticoid should correct all GRA abnormalities. However, this therapy may be limited by complications of glucocorticoid administration. Another concern with glucocorticoid treatment is that patients may undergo a brief period of mineralocorticoid insufficiency when therapy is initiated before the renin-angiotensin axis recovers fully. Additional treatment modalities include mineralocorticoid receptor blockade with spironolactone and inhibition of the mineralocorticoid-sensitive distal tubule sodium channel with amiloride.

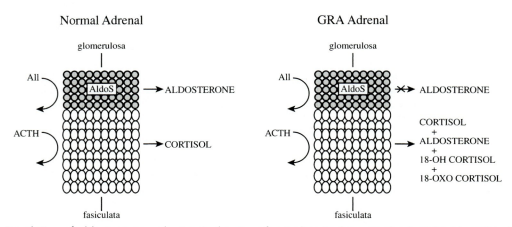

Figure 9–12 Regulation of aldosterone production in the zona fasciculata in the normal adrenal and model of the physiologic abnormalities in the adrenal cortex in glucocorticoid-remediable aldosteronism (GRA). Ectopic expression of aldosterone synthase (AldoS) enzymatic activity in the adrenal fasciculata results in GRA. ACTH, adrenocorticotropic hormone; AII, angiotensin II; 18-OH cortisol, 18-hydroxycortisol; 18-OXO cortisol, 18-oxycortisol. (From Lifton RP, Dluhy RG, Powers M, et al. Hereditary hypertension caused by chimaeric gene duplications and ectopic expression of aldosterone synthase. *Nat Genet*. 1992;**2**:66-74.)

References

1. Liddle GW, Bledsoe T, Coppage WS. A familial renal disorder simulating primary aldosteronism but with negligible aldosterone secretion. *Trans Assoc Am Physicians*. 1963;**76**: 199-213.

2. White PC, Speiser PW. Steroid 11 beta-hydroxylase deficiency and related disorders. *Endocrinol Metab Clin North Am*. 1994;**23**:325-339.

3. Biglieri EG, Herron MA, Brust N. 17-Hydroxylation deficiency in man. *J Clin Invest*. 1966;**45**:1946-1954.

4. Saadi HF, Bravo EL, Aron DC. Feminizing adrenocortical tumor: Steroid hormone response to ketoconazole. *J Clin Endocrinol Metab*. 1990;**70**:540-543.

5. Azziz R, Boots LR, Parker CR Jr, et al. 11 beta-hydroxylase deficiency in hyperandrogenism. *Fertil Steril*. 1991;**55**: 733-741.

6. Biglieri EG, Kater CE, Brust N, et al. The regulation and diseases of deoxycorticosterone. *In*: Mantero F, Takeda R, Scoggins BA, et al. (eds). The Adrenal and Hypertension from Cloning to Clinic. New York: Raven Press, 1989, pp. 355-374.

7. Lamberts SW, Poldermans D, Zweens M, de Jong FH. Familial cortisol resistance: Differential diagnostic and therapeutic aspects. *J Clin Endocrinol Metab*. 1986;**63**:1328-1333.

8. Malchoff CD, Malchoff DM. Glucocorticoid resistance in humans. *Trends Endocrinol Metab*. 1995;**6**:89-95.

9. Edwards CR, Stewart PM, Burt D, et al. Localisation of 11 beta-hydroxysteroid dehydrogenase—tissue specific protector of the mineralocorticoid receptor. *Lancet*. 1988;**2**:986-989.

10. Funder JW, Pearce PT, Smith R, Smith AI. Mineralocorticoid action: Target tissue specificity is enzyme, not receptor, mediated. *Science*. 1988;**242**:583-585.

11. Howlett TA, Drury PL, Perry L, et al. Diagnosis and management of ACTH-dependent Cushing's syndrome: Comparison of the features in ectopic and pituitary ACTH production. *Clin Endocrinol (Oxf)*. 1986;**24**:699-713.

12. Christy NP, Laragh JH. Pathogenesis of hypokalemic alkalosis in Cushing's syndrome. *N Engl J Med*. 1961;**265**:1083.

13. Ritchie CM, Sheridan B, Fraser R, et al. Studies on the pathogenesis of hypertension in Cushing's disease and acromegaly. *Q J Med*. 1990;**76**:855-867.

14. Cost WS. Quantitative estimation of adrenocortical hormones and their alpha-ketotic metabolites in urine. II. Pathological adrenocortical hyperfunction. *Acta Endocrinol (Copenh)*. 1963;**42**:39.

15. Phillipou G. Investigation of urinary steroid profiles as a diagnostic method in Cushing's syndrome. *Clin Endocrinol*. 1982;**16**:433-439.

16. Ulick S, Wang JZ, Blumenfeld JD, Pickering TG. Cortisol inactivation overload: A mechanism of mineralocorticoid hypertension in the ectopic adrenocorticotropin syndrome. *J Clin Endocrinol Metab*. 1992;**74**:963-967.

17. Walker BR, Campbell JC, Fraser R, et al. Mineralocorticoid excess and inhibition of 11 beta-hydroxysteroid dehydrogenase in patients with ectopic ACTH syndrome. *Clin Endocrinol*. 1992;**37**:483-492.

18. Tsigos C, Kamilaris TC, Chrousos GP. Adrenal diseases. *In*: Moore WT, Eastman RC (eds). Diagnostic Endocrinology. Philadelphia: BC Decker, 1996, pp 125-156.

19. Oldfield EH, Chrousos GP, Schulte HM, et al. Preoperative lateralization of ACTH-secreting pituitary microadenomas by bilateral and simultaneous inferior petrosal venous sinus sampling. *N Engl J Med*. 1985;**312**:100-103.

20. Mampalam TJ, Tyrrell JB, Wilson CB. Transsphenoidal microsurgery for Cushing disease: A report of 216 cases. *Ann Intern Med*. 1988;**109**:487-493.

21. Aron DC, Findling JW, Fitzgerald PA, et al. Cushing's syndrome: Problems in management. *Endocr Rev*. 1982;**3**:229-244.

22. Howlett TA, Plowman PN, Wass JA, et al. Megavoltage pituitary irradiation in the management of Cushing's disease and Nelson's syndrome: Long-term follow-up. *Clin Endocrinol (Oxf)*. 1989;**31**:309-323.

23. Lamberts SW, Krenning EP, Reubi JC. The role of somatostatin and its analogs in the diagnosis and treatment of tumors. *Endocr Rev*. 1991;**12**:450-482.

24. Tabarin A, Navarranne A, Guerin J, et al. Use of ketoconazole in the treatment of Cushing's disease and ectopic ACTH syndrome. *Clin Endocrinol*. 1991;**34**:63-69.

25. Luton JP, Mahoudeau JA, Bouchard P, et al. Treatment of Cushing's disease by o,p'-DDD: Survey of 62 cases. *N Engl J Med*. 1979;**300**:459-464.

26. Bravo EL, Tarazi RC, Dustan HP, et al. The changing clinical spectrum of primary aldosteronism. *Am J Med*. 1983;**74**: 641-651.

27. Conn JW. The evolution of primary aldosteronism: 1954-1967. *Harvey Lect*. 1966;**62**:257-291.

28. Ferriss JB, Beevers DG, Brown JJ, et al. Clinical, biochemical and pathological features of low-renin ("primary") hyperaldosteronism. *Am Heart J*. 1978;**95**:375-388.

29. George JM, Wright L, Bell NH, Bartter FC. The syndrome of primary aldosteronism. *Am J Med*. 1970;**48**:343-356.

30. Lins PE, Adamson U. Plasma aldosterone-plasma renin activity ratio: A simple test to identify patients with primary aldosteronism. *Acta Endocrinol (Copenh)*. 1986;**113**:564-569.

31. Biglieri EG, Irony I, Kater CE. Identification and implications of new types of mineralocorticoid hypertension. *J Steroid Biochem*. 1989;**32**:199-204.

32. Biglieri EG, Schambelan M. The significance of elevated levels of plasma 18- hydroxycorticosterone in patients with primary aldosteronism. *J Clin Endocrinol Metab*. 1979;**49**:87-91.

33. Ganguly A, Melada GA, Luetscher JA, Dowdy AJ. Control of plasma aldosterone in primary aldosteronism: Distinction between adenoma and hyperplasia. *J Clin Endocrinol Metab*. 1973;**37**:765-775.

34. Fraser R, Beretta-Piccoli C, Brown JJ, et al. Response of aldosterone and 18-hydroxycorticosterone to angiotensin II in normal subjects and patients with essential hypertension, Conn's syndrome, and nontumorous hyperaldosteronism. *Hypertension*. 1981;**3**:I87-I92.

35. Geisinger MA, Zelch MG, Bravo EL, et al. Primary hyperaldosteronism: Comparison of CT, adrenal venography, and venous sampling. *AJR Am J Roentgenol*. 1983;**141**:299-302.

36. Linde R, Coulam C, Battino R, et al. Localization of aldosterone-producing adenoma by computed tomography. *J Clin Endocrinol Metab*. 1979;**49**:642-645.

37. White EA, Schambelan M, Rost CR, et al. Use of computed tomography in diagnosing the cause of primary aldosteronism. *N Engl J Med*. 1980;**303**:1503-1507.

38. Melby JC, Spark RF, Dale SL, et al. Diagnosis and localization of aldosterone-producing adenomas by adrenal-vein catheterization. *N Engl J Med*. 1967;**277**:1050-1056.

39. Tarazi RC, Ibrahim MM, Bravo EL, Dustan HP. Hemodynamic characteristics of primary aldosteronism. *N Engl J Med*. 1973; **289**:1330-1335.

40. Bravo EL, Dustan HP, Tarazi RC. Spironolactone as a nonspecific treatment for primary aldosteronism. *Circulation*. 1973;**48**:491-498.

41. Bravo EL, Fouad-Tarazi FM, Tarazi RC, et al. Clinical implications of primary aldosteronism with resistant hypertension. *Hypertension*. 1988;**11**:I207-I211.

42. Ghose RP, Hall PM, Bravo EL. Medical management of aldosterone-producing adenomas. *Ann Intern Med*. 1999;**131**:105-108.

43. Schiffrin EL, Lis M, Gutkowska J, et al. Role of Ca^{2+} in response of adrenal glomerulosa cells to angiotensin II, ACTH, K^+ and ouabain. *Am J Physiol*. 1981;**241**:E42-E48.

44. Kiowski W, Bertel O, Erne P, et al. Hemodynamic and reflex responses to acute and chronic antihypertensive therapy with the calcium entry blocker nifedipine. *Hypertension.* 1983;**5 (Suppl I)**:I70-I74.

45. Bravo EL, Fouad FM, Tarazi RC. Calcium channel blockade with nifedipine in primary aldosteronism. *Hypertension.* 1986;**8 (Suppl I)**:I191.

46. Bravo EL. Pheochromocytoma and mineralocorticoid hypertension. *In:* Glassock RJ (ed). Current Therapy in Nephrology and Hypertension. 4th ed. St. Louis: Mosby–Year Book, 1998, pp 330-334.

47. Bravo EL, Dustan HP, Tarazi RC. Selective hypoaldosteronism despite prolonged pre- and postoperative hyperreninemia in primary aldosteronism. *J Clin Endocrinol Metab.* 1975;**41**: 611-617.

48. Ganguly A, Grim CE, Weinberger MH. Anomalous postural aldosterone response in glucocorticoid-suppressible hyperaldosteronism. *N Engl J Med.* 1981;**305**:991-993.

49. Lifton RP, Dluhy RG, Powers M, et al. A chimaeric 11 beta-hydroxylase/aldosterone synthase gene causes glucocorticoid-remediable aldosteronism and human hypertension. *Nature.* 1992;**355**:262-265.

50. Lifton RP, Dluhy RG, Powers M, et al. Hereditary hypertension caused by chimaeric gene duplications and ectopic expression of aldosterone synthase. *Nat Genet.* 1992;**2**:66-74.

Secondary Hypertension: Pheochromocytoma

William F. Young, Jr.

Catecholamine-secreting tumors that arise from chromaffin cells of the adrenal medulla and the sympathetic ganglia are termed *pheochromocytomas* and *extra-adrenal catecholamine-secreting paragangliomas* ("extra-adrenal pheochromocytomas"), respectively. Many clinicians use the term "pheochromocytoma" to refer to both adrenal pheochromocytomas and extra-adrenal catecholamine-secreting paragangliomas because the tumors have similar clinical presentations and are treated with similar approaches.

CLINICAL PRESENTATION

Although catecholamine-secreting tumors are rare (annual incidence of 2 to 8 cases per million people),[1] it is important to suspect, confirm, localize, and resect these tumors because the associated hypertension is curable with surgical removal of the tumor, the risk of a lethal paroxysm exists, and at least 10% of the tumors are malignant. These tumors occur with equal frequency in men and women, primarily in the third, fourth, and fifth decades. Patients harboring catecholamine-secreting tumors may be asymptomatic. However, symptoms usually are present and result from the pharmacologic effects of excess circulating catecholamine concentrations. The resulting hypertension may be sustained or paroxysmal. Episodic symptoms may occur in spells, or paroxysms, that can be extremely variable in presentation but typically include forceful heartbeat, pallor, tremor, and diaphoresis. Spells may be either spontaneous or precipitated by postural change, anxiety, medications (e.g., metoclopramide, anesthetic agents), exercise, or maneuvers that increase intra-abdominal pressure. Although the types of spells experienced across the patient population are highly variable, spells tend to be stereotypical for each patient. However, the clinician must recognize that most patients with spells do not have a pheochromocytoma (Table 10-1).[2]

Additional clinical signs of catecholamine-secreting tumors include hypertension, hypertensive retinopathy, orthostatic hypotension, constipation (megacolon may be the presenting symptom),[3] painless hematuria and paroxysmal attacks induced by micturition (associated with urinary bladder paragangliomas), hyperglycemia and diabetes mellitus, hypercalcemia, and erythrocytosis. Thus, the presentation of patients with catecholamine-secreting tumors may mimic other disorders (Table 10-2). Some of the co-secreted hormones that may dominate the clinical presentation include corticotropin (or adrenocorticotropin, leading to Cushing's syndrome), parathyroid hormone–related peptide (hypercalcemia), vasoactive intestinal polypeptide (watery diarrhea), and growth hormone–releasing hormone (acromegaly).[4-7] The symptomatic presentations of pheochromocytoma that are most commonly missed by clinicians are cardiomyopathy and heart failure.[8-10] Many physical examination findings can be associated with genetic syndromes that predispose to pheochromocytoma; these findings include retinal angiomas, marfanoid body habitus, café au lait spots, axillary freckling, subcutaneous neurofibromas, and mucosal neuromas on the eyelids and tongue.

A "rule of 10" has been quoted for describing the characteristics of catecholamine-secreting tumors: 10% are extra-adrenal, 10% occur in children, 10% are multiple or bilateral, 10% recur after surgical removal, 10% are malignant, 10% are familial, and 10% of benign sporadic adrenal pheochromocytoma occur as adrenal incidentalomas.[11,12] None of these "rules" are precisely 10%. For example, recent studies suggest that up to 20% of catecholamine-secreting tumors are familial.[13]

Pheochromocytomas are localized to the adrenal glands and have an average size of 4.5 cm (Fig. 10-1).[14] Paragangliomas are found where chromaffin tissue exists: along the para-aortic sympathetic chain, within the organ of Zuckerkandl (at the origin of the inferior mesenteric artery), in the wall of the urinary bladder, and in the sympathetic chain in the neck or mediastinum.[15,16] In early postnatal life, the extra-adrenal sympathetic paraganglionic tissues are prominent; these tissues then degenerate, leaving residual foci associated with the vagal nerves, carotid vessels, aortic arch, pulmonary vessels, and mesenteric arteries. Odd locations for paragangliomas include the neck, intra-atrial cardiac septum,[17] spermatic cord, vagina, scrotum, and sacrococcygeal region.

SYNDROMIC PHEOCHROMOCYTOMA AND PARAGANGLIOMA: ROLE FOR GENETIC TESTING

Approximately 10% to 20% of patients with catecholamine-secreting tumors have associated germline mutations (inherited mutations present in all cells of the body) in genes known to cause genetic disease.[13,18,19] The familial neurocrestopathic syndromes associated with adrenal pheochromocytoma include familial pheochromocytoma; multiple endocrine neoplasia type 2A (MEN 2A: pheochromocytoma, medullary thyroid carcinoma [MTC], and hyperparathyroidism) and type 2B (MEN 2B: pheochromocytoma, MTC, mucosal neuromas, thickened corneal nerves, intestinal ganglioneuromatosis, and marfanoid body habitus); neurofibromatosis type 1 (NF1); von Hippel–Lindau disease (VHL: pheochromocytoma, retinal angiomas, cerebellar hemangioblastoma, renal and pancreatic cysts, and renal cell carcinoma); and

Table 10-1 Differential Diagnosis of Pheochromocytoma-type Spells

Endocrine
Pheochromocytoma
"Hyperadrenergic spells"
Thyrotoxicosis
Primary hypogonadism (menopausal syndrome)
Medullary thyroid carcinoma
Pancreatic tumors (e.g,, insulinoma)
Hypoglycemia
Carbohydrate intolerance

Cardiovascular
Labile essential hypertension
Cardiovascular deconditioning
Pulmonary edema
Syncope
Orthostatic hypotension
Paroxysmal cardiac arrhythmia and torsade de pointes
Angina
Renovascular disease

Psychological
Anxiety and panic attacks
Somatization disorder
Hyperventilation
Factitious (e.g., drugs, Valsalva maneuver)

Pharmacologic
Withdrawal of adrenergic inhibitor
Monoamine oxidase inhibitor therapy and decongestant
Sympathomimetic ingestion
Illegal drug ingestion (cocaine, phencyclidine [PCP], lysergic acid diethylamide [LSD])
Chlorpropamide-alcohol flush
Vancomycin ("red man syndrome")

Neurologic
Postural orthostatic tachycardia syndrome (POTS)
Autonomic neuropathy
Migraine headache
Diencephalic epilepsy (autonomic seizures)
Stroke
Cerebrovascular insufficiency

Other
Unexplained flushing spells
Mast cell disease
Carcinoid syndrome
Recurrent idiopathic anaphylaxis

Table 10-2 Conditions That Pheochromocytoma May Mimic or Cause

Resistant essential hypertension
Renovascular hypertension
Myocardial ischemia
Dilated cardiomyopathy
Hypertrophic obstructive cardiomyopathy
Pulmonary edema: cardiogenic and noncardiogenic
Adult respiratory distress syndrome
Syncope
Cardiac arrhythmia
Apical left ventricular hypertrophy
Stroke
Vasculitis
Multiple organ failure with disseminated intravascular coagulopathy
Hemobilia, jaundice, and pancreatic infarction
Hypermetabolism with weight loss and fever (interleukin-6)
Hyperthyroidism
Diabetes mellitus
Orthostatic hypotension (adrenomedullin)
Cushing's syndrome (ectopic corticotropin-releasing hormone/corticotropin)
Primary aldosteronism (possible aldosterone-stimulation factor yet to be identified)
Acromegaly (growth hormone–releasing hormone)
Primary hyperparathyroidism (parathyroid hormone–related peptide)
Watery diarrhea (vasoactive intestinal polypeptide)
Constipation/ostipation (adrenomedullin)
Acute abdomen
Psychiatric disorders (e.g., panic attacks)

Catecholamine-secreting paragangliomas may be associated with familial paraganglioma, NF1, VHL, the Carney triad, and, rarely, MEN 2. From the Mayo Clinic of Rochester, Minnesota, series of 236 patients with paraganglioma, 29 patients (12.3%) had a documented family history of paragangliomas; 19 of these had familial paraganglioma, 5 had VHL, and 1 had MEN 2B.[16] Four patients presented with the Carney triad.[16,26] Genetic testing is available for nearly all these disorders. Families should be offered genetic counseling before genetic tests are performed. To obtain informative genetic testing results, a symptomatic family member should always be tested first.

Multiple Endocrine Neoplasia Type 2

MEN 2A is an autosomal dominant syndrome.[23] The MEN 2A phenotype includes pheochromocytoma (usually bilateral adrenal neoplasms), MTC, and hyperparathyroidism. Almost all patients with MEN 2A have MTC, which is typically detected before the pheochromocytoma is identified.[27] Very rarely, the patient with MEN 2A may have an extra-adrenal catecholamine-secreting paraganglioma. Approximately 15% of patients with MEN 2A develop hyperparathyroidism.[28] The prevalence of MEN 2A is approximately 1 in 35,000 individuals. Numerous mutations throughout the *RET* proto-

familial paraganglioma (Table 10-3).[20-24] Additional neurocutaneous syndromes associated with catecholamine-secreting tumors include ataxia-telangiectasia, tuberous sclerosis, and Sturge-Weber syndrome. Other diagnoses associated with catecholamine-secreting tumors that do not appear to be inherited are the Carney triad (gastric leiomyosarcoma, pulmonary chondroma, and extra-adrenal catecholamine-secreting tumors),[25] cholelithiasis, and renal artery stenosis.

oncogene have been documented in individuals with MEN 2A. The *RET* proto-oncogene, located on chromosome 10q11.2, encodes a receptor tyrosine kinase. Pheochromocytoma is most frequently associated with mutations in codon 634 (located in exon 11) of the *RET* proto-oncogene. Mutations in codon 634 are found in approximately 80% of all patients with MEN 2A. Variants of MEN 2A include MEN 2A with Hirschsprung's disease and MEN 2A with cutaneous lichen amyloidosis.

MEN 2B is also an autosomal dominant syndrome, and it represents approximately 5% of all MEN 2 cases. This genetic condition is also very rarely associated with extra-adrenal catecholamine-secreting paraganglioma. The MEN 2B phenotype includes pheochromocytoma (usually bilateral adrenal neoplasms), MTC, mucosal neuromas, thickened corneal nerves, intestinal ganglioneuromatosis, and marfanoid body habitus.[27,29] The mucosal neuromas are typically located in the lips, buccal mucosa, conjunctiva, eyelids, and on the anterior tongue. Like MEN 2A, MEN 2B is caused by mutations in the *RET* proto-oncogene. MEN 2B is primarily associated with mutations in codon 918 (located in exon 16).

Overall, pheochromocytoma occurs in approximately 50% of patients with MEN 2. More than 95% of patients with MEN 2A and more than 98% of patients with MEN 2B have identifiable mutations in the *RET* proto-oncogene. Mutation analysis is commercially available and should be considered in patients with: bilateral pheochromocytoma, co-phenotype disorders, tumor onset at a young age (e.g., <21 years of age), or a family history of pheochromocytoma.

von Hippel–Lindau Disease

VHL is an autosomal dominant syndrome.[24] The VHL phenotype includes pheochromocytoma (usually bilateral adrenal neoplasms), retinal angiomas, cerebellar hemangioblastoma, epididymal cystadenoma, renal and pancreatic cysts, and renal cell carcinoma. Rarely, these patients may have an extra-adrenal catecholamine-secreting paraganglioma.[16] The prevalence of VHL is approximately 1 in 35,000 individuals. Patients are classified as having VHL type 1 (without pheochromocytoma) or VHL type 2 (with pheochromocytoma).[27] Approximately 20% of patients with VHL have the type 2 phenotype. VHL type 2 is further characterized into three subtypes: (1) patients with *type 2A* lack renal cell carcinoma and have a low frequency of hemangioblastoma and retinal angioma, (2) patients with *type 2B* have renal cell carcinoma and variable expression of hemangioblastoma and retinal angiomas, and (3) patients with *type 2C* have pheochromocytoma only. VHL-associated pheochromocytomas have a noradrenergic phenotype and secrete primarily norepinephrine.[30] The *VHL* tumor suppressor gene is located on chromosome 3p25-26. More than 300 *VHL* mutations have been identified. In up to 97% of VHL cases, pheochromocytoma is associated with missense mutations (rather than truncating or null mutations) in the *VHL* gene. Nearly 100%

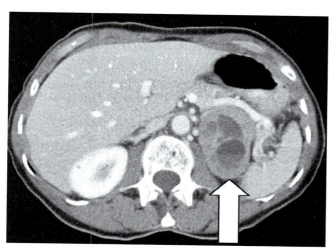

Figure 10–1   A computed tomography (CT) scan of the abdomen with intravenous contrast from a 68-year-old woman with a 5-year history of spells of headache, palpitations, nausea, and dizziness. The 24-hour urine studies were abnormal: metanephrines, 4402 µg (normal, <400 µg); normetanephrines, 4220 µg (normal, <900 µg); norepinephrine, 248 µg (normal, <170 µg); epinephrine, 183 µg (normal, <35 µg); and dopamine, 146 µg (normal, <700 µg). The CT image shows a typical 6.0 × 4.9-cm complex (cystic and solid) left adrenal mass consistent with pheochromocytoma *(arrow)*. Following α- and β-adrenergic blockade, the patient underwent laparoscopic removal of a 95-g pheochromocytoma. Postoperatively, the patient's 24-hour urinary metanephrines and catecholamines normalized.

Table 10-3   Autosomal Dominant Syndromes Associated with Pheochromocytoma and Paraganglioma

Syndrome	Gene*	Typical Tumor Location
MEN 2A and 2B	*RET* proto-oncogene	Adrenal medulla: bilateral
von Hippel–Lindau disease	*VHL*	Adrenal medulla: bilateral
Neurofibromatosis type 1	*NF1*	Adrenal-periadrenal
Familial paraganglioma	*SDHD*	Head and neck, rarely adrenal
Familial paraganglioma	*SDHB*	Abdomen and pelvis, rarely adrenal
Familial paraganglioma	*SDHC*	Head and neck

MEN, multiple endocrine neoplasia; *NF1*, neurofibromatosis type 1 gene; *SDHB*, succinate dehydrogenase B gene; *SDHC*, succinate dehydrogenase C gene; *SDHD*, succinate dehydrogenase D gene; *VHL*, von Hippel–Lindau tumor suppressor gene.

of patients with VHL have identifiable mutations in the *VHL* gene. Mutation analysis is commercially available and should be considered in patients with: bilateral pheochromocytoma, co-phenotype disorders, tumor onset at a young age (e.g., <21 years of age), or a family history of pheochromocytoma.

Neurofibromatosis Type 1

Approximately 2% of patients with NF1 develop a catecholamine-secreting neoplasm (typically an adrenal pheochromocytoma). The prevalence of NF1, an autosomal dominant syndrome, is approximately 1 in 3000 individuals. NF1 is caused by mutations in a tumor-suppressor gene (*NF1*) located on chromosome 17q11.2. Utilizing a multistep testing protocol, more than 95% of mutations within the *NF1* gene can be identified. However, unless a patient with a catecholamine-secreting tumor presents with additional clinical characteristics consistent with a diagnosis of NF1 (e.g., multiple café au lait spots, axillary and inguinal freckling, subcutaneous fibromas, macrocephaly), genetic testing for the *NF1* gene is not recommended.

Familial Paraganglioma

Familial paraganglioma is an autosomal dominant syndrome characterized by paragangliomas that are most often located in the head and neck, but they also occur in the thorax, abdomen, pelvis, and urinary bladder. The occurrence of catecholamine hypersecretion in familial paraganglioma depends on tumor location; approximately 5% of head and neck paragangliomas and 50% of abdominal paragangliomas are hormone producing.[16] The average age at diagnosis is 30 to 35 years, and it can vary greatly within a family (average of 14.3 ± 9.6 years difference; range, 0 to 37 years).[31] Familial paraganglioma is caused by mutations in the succinate dehydrogenase (SDH; succinate:ubiquinone oxidoreductase) subunit genes *SDHB*, *SDHC*, *SDHD*, which compose portions of mitochondrial complex II.[32] Most germline mutations in *SDHD*, located on chromosome 11q23, have been identified in multigenerational families with head and neck paragangliomas.[33] In families with *SDHD* mutations, penetrance depends on the parent of origin: the disease is not manifest when the mutation is inherited from the mother but is highly penetrant when inherited from the father.[32] Mutations in *SDHB*, located on chromosome 1p35-36, and *SDHC*, located on chromosome 1q21, have been associated with families that have abdominal as well as head and neck paraganglioma.[34-36] In families with *SDHB* and *SDHC* mutations, no imprinting effects have been observed in inheritance pattern. The *SDH* gene mutation detection rate in individuals with familial paraganglioma is currently unknown. *SDHB*, *SDHC*, and *SDHD* mutation analysis is commercially available and should be considered in all patients with paraganglioma because of the high prevalence of *SDH* mutations in this population. In addition, *SDHB* mutations have been associated with increased risk of malignant paraganglioma.[36-38] Patients with *SDHB* mutations are also at increased risk of renal cell carcinoma and papillary thyroid cancer.[38] Finally, large germline deletions of *SDHB* and *SDHD* have been identified in families with paraganglioma[39]; these large deletions are not detected by mutation analysis methodologies that molecular diagnostic laboratories currently offer.

Carney Triad or Syndrome

The Carney triad or syndrome is a rare disorder that primarily affects young women, and it is characterized by gastric stromal sarcoma, pulmonary chondroma, paraganglioma, adrenal cortical adenoma, and esophageal leiomyomas.[26] The longest reported interval between detection of the first and second components of the syndrome is 26 years (mean, 8.4 years; median, 6 years).[26] The Carney triad is a chronic, persistent, and indolent disease. Although the disorder may be inherited, the responsible gene has yet to be identified.

DIAGNOSTIC INVESTIGATION

Case Finding

Pheochromocytoma should be suspected in patients with hypertension accompanied by one or more of the following: hyperadrenergic spells (e.g., self-limited episodes of nonexertional palpitations, diaphoresis, headache, tremor, and pallor), resistant hypertension, a familial syndrome that predisposes to catecholamine-secreting tumors (e.g., MEN 2), an incidentally discovered adrenal mass, or a history of gastric stromal tumor or pulmonary chondromas (Carney triad). The diagnosis must be confirmed biochemically by demonstrating the presence of increased urine or plasma concentrations of catecholamines or their metabolites (including metanephrines).

Most laboratories now measure catecholamines and metanephrines by high-performance liquid chromatography with electrochemical detection or with tandem mass spectroscopy.[40] These techniques have overcome the problems with fluorometric analysis (e.g., false-positive results caused by α-methyldopa and other drugs with high native fluorescence).

At Mayo Clinic, the single most reliable test for identifying catecholamine-secreting tumors is measurement of metanephrines in a 24-hour urine collection[12,41]; this conclusion is shared by other groups.[42,43] If clinical suspicion is high, then urinary catecholamines (epinephrine, norepinephrine, and dopamine) are measured in addition to the 24-hour urine metanephrines. Fractionated plasma free metanephrines, which are products of intrapheochromocytoma catecholamine metabolism, are also obtained.[44] Some groups have advocated that fractionated plasma free metanephrines should be a first-line test for pheochromocytoma.[45,46] However, other groups have found that fractionated plasma free metanephrines lack the necessary specificity to be recommended as a first-line test; therefore, this measurement should be reserved for high-suspicion cases. High-suspicion cases include patients who have one or more of the following: resistant hypertension, spells, a family history of pheochromocytoma, a genetic syndrome that predisposes to pheochromocytoma (e.g., MEN 2), a past history of resected pheochromocytoma and now have recurrent hypertension or spells, or an incidentally discovered adrenal mass that has imaging characteristics consistent with pheochromocytoma (e.g., marked enhancement with intravenous contrast medium on computed tomography [CT], high signal intensity on T2-weighted magnetic resonance imaging [MRI], cystic and hemorrhagic changes, larger size [e.g., >4 cm], or bilaterality).[12,41] In addition, measuring fractionated plasma free metanephrines is a good first-line test in pediatric patients, because obtaining a complete 24-hour urine collection is often difficult in children.

A study that compared the diagnostic efficacy of the two main pheochromocytoma testing methods in an outpatient population found that the sensitivity of fractionated plasma free metanephrines was 97%, and the sensitivity of urinary total metanephrines and catecholamines was 90%.[41] The specificity was 85% for fractionated plasma free metanephrines and 98% for urinary total metanephrines and catecholamines. The likelihood ratios for positive tests were 6.3 for fractionated plasma metanephrines and 58.9 for urinary total metanephrines and catecholamines. In this study, an adrenal pheochromocytoma was missed by urinary testing in two patients with familial syndromes and in one asymptomatic patient with an incidentally discovered adrenal mass. A dopamine-secreting extra-adrenal paraganglioma was missed by plasma testing in one patient. Therefore, in the common clinical setting, when sporadic pheochromocytoma is suspected, 24-hour urinary metanephrines and catecholamines provide adequate sensitivity and a lower false-positive rate than fractionated plasma free metanephrines.

A recent review of the literature that examined the diagnostic efficacy of measuring fractionated plasma free metanephrines in the biochemical investigation for pheochromocytoma found that a normal result adequately ruled out pheochromocytoma[47]; however, a positive result only moderately increased the likelihood of disease, especially when sporadic pheochromocytoma is suspected. The plasma normetanephrine fraction is responsible for most false-positive results, and the concentration of plasma normetanephrine increases with age.[41] During screening for sporadic pheochromocytoma, the false-positive rate of fractionated plasma free metanephrines can be significantly reduced by using age-dependant cutoffs for interpretation of the results.[48] Reducing the false-positive rate may save expenditures related to confirmatory imaging.[49] Because fractionated plasma free metanephrines are highly specific, their true value comes from normal results that rule out pheochromocytoma.

For patients with episodic hypertension, the 24-hour urine collection should be started with the onset of a spell. When the 24-hour urine is collected in this manner, patients with pheochromocytoma have one or both the following findings: (1) levels of 24-hour urine catecholamines that are increased more than twofold higher than the upper normal limit (e.g., norepinephrine >170 μg, or epinephrine >35 μg, or dopamine >700 μg) or (2) levels of urinary metanephrines (e.g., >400 μg) or normetanephrine (e.g., >900 μg) that are significantly increased to more than the upper normal limit. In 130 patients with benign sporadic adrenal pheochromocytomas who were surgically treated at Mayo Clinic from 1978 to 1995, the following were noted: (1) 24-hour urinary total metanephrines (metanephrine and normetanephrine) were increased to more than the upper normal limit in 94% of patients, (2) 24-hour urinary norepinephrine or epinephrine was increased more than twofold higher than the upper normal limit in 93% of patients, and (3) diagnostic increases occurred in either 24-hour urine metanephrines or catecholamines in 99% of patients.[12] Over a span of 20 years at Mayo Clinic, histamine and glucagon stimulation testing was performed in 542 patients in whom pheochromocytoma was strongly suspected, despite normal 24-hour urinary cate-

Table 10-4   Medications That May Increase Measured Levels of Catecholamines and Metanephrines

Tricyclic antidepressants
Levodopa
Drugs containing catecholamines (e.g., decongestants)
Amphetamines
Buspirone, and most psychoactive agents
Withdrawal from clonidine and other drugs
Ethanol
Acetaminophen and phenoxybenzamine (may increase measured levels of fractionated plasma metanephrines in some assays)

cholamine or metanephrine excretion. Of these patients, none had positive stimulation test results.[50] Therefore, because of currently available methods, there is no longer a role for provocative histamine and glucagon testing.

Although it is preferred that patients not receive any medication during the diagnostic evaluation, treatment with most medications may be continued, with some exceptions (Table 10-4). Tricyclic antidepressants are the agents that interfere most frequently with the interpretation of 24-hour urine catecholamines and metabolites. To screen for catecholamine-secreting tumors effectively, treatment with tricyclic antidepressants and other psychoactive agents listed in Table 10-4 should be tapered and discontinued at least 2 weeks before any hormonal assessments. In addition, catecholamine secretion may be appropriately increased in situations of physical stress or illness (e.g., stroke, obstructive sleep apnea). Therefore, the clinical circumstances under which measurements of catecholamines and metanephrines are made must be assessed in each case.

Clonidine Suppression Test

The high false-positive rate for plasma catecholamines and metanephrines triggered the development of a confirmatory test—the clonidine suppression test—to distinguish pheochromocytoma from false-positive elevations. Clonidine (0.3 mg) is administered orally; plasma catecholamines or metanephrines are measured before and 3 hours after the dose. In patients with essential hypertension, plasma catecholamine concentrations decrease (norepinephrine and epinephrine <500 pg/mL or a >50% fall in norepinephrine), as do plasma normetanephrine concentrations (into the normal range or a >40% fall). However, these concentrations remain elevated in patients with pheochromocytoma.[51,52]

Clinicians have used many other approaches to screen for and to confirm the presence of catecholamine-secreting tumors. Although plasma catecholamines are convenient to collect, they are not as sensitive as 24-hour urinary measurements, and they add little information to the diagnostic evaluation.[53] Plasma concentrations of catecholamines are affected by diuretic treatment, smoking, and renal insufficiency. The plasma levels of chromogranin A, which is co-stored and co-secreted with catecholamines, are increased in 80% to 90% of patients with catecholamine-secreting tumors.[54,55] Moreover, plasma levels of neuropeptide Y are increased in up to 87% of patients with these tumors.[56]

Renal Failure

Measurements of urinary catecholamines and metabolites may be invalid in patients with advanced renal insufficiency.[57] Serum chromogranin A levels have poor diagnostic specificity in these patients.[58] In hemodialyzed patients who do not have pheochromocytoma, plasma norepinephrine and dopamine concentrations are increased threefold and twofold, respectively, higher than the upper normal limit.[59,60] However, standard normal ranges can be used for interpreting plasma epinephrine concentrations.[61] Therefore, when patients with renal failure have plasma norepinephrine concentrations that are increased more than threefold higher than the upper normal limit or epinephrine that is increased to more than the upper normal limit, pheochromocytoma should be suspected.[57] One study found that plasma concentrations of free metanephrines are increased approximately twofold in patients with renal failure; this finding may be useful in the biochemical evaluation patients with marked renal insufficiency or renal failure.[62] However, an earlier study suggested that concentrations of fractionated plasma free metanephrines could not distinguish between 10 patients with pheochromocytoma and 11 patients with end-stage renal disease who required long-term hemodialysis.[63]

Factitious Pheochromocytoma

As with other factitious disorders, factitious pheochromocytoma can be difficult to confirm.[64] The patient usually has a medical background. The patient may "spike" the 24-hour urine container or self-administer catecholamines.[65,66]

Localization

Localization studies should not be initiated until biochemical studies have confirmed the diagnosis of a catecholamine-

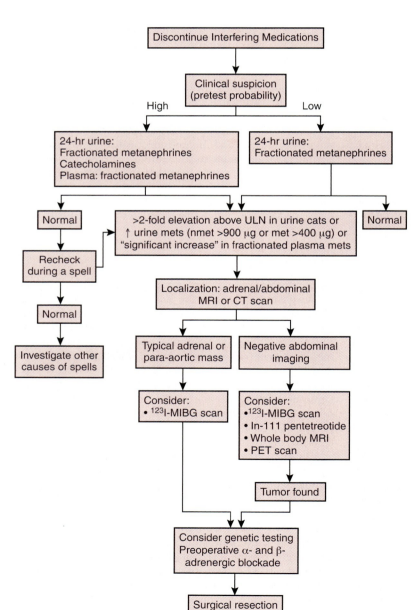

Figure 10–2 Evaluation and treatment of catecholamine-secreting tumors. Clinical suspicion is triggered by the following: paroxysmal symptoms (especially hypertension); hypertension that is intermittent, unusually labile, or resistant to treatment; family history of pheochromocytoma or associated conditions; or incidentally discovered adrenal mass. The details are discussed in the text. cats, catecholamines; CT, computed tomography; ^{123}I-MIBG, ^{123}I-meta-iodobenzylguanidine; In-111, indium-111; met, metanephrine; MRI, magnetic resonance imaging; nmet, normetanephrine; PET, positron emission tomography; ULN, upper limit of normal. (Modified from Young WF Jr. Pheochromocytoma: 1926-1993. *Trends Endocrinol Metab.* 1993;**4**:122.)

secreting tumor (Fig. 10-2). The first localization test should be computer-assisted imaging of the adrenal glands and abdomen (MRI or CT) (sensitivity, >95%; specificity, >65%) (Fig. 10-3).[67] Approximately 90% of these tumors are found in the adrenal glands, and 98% are found in the abdomen.[68] If the results of abdominal imaging are negative, scintigraphic localization with iodine-123–meta-iodobenzylguanidine (^{123}I-MIBG) is indicated (Fig. 10-4). This radiopharmaceutical agent accumulates preferentially in catecholamine-secreting tumors; however, this procedure is not as sensitive as initially hoped (sensitivity, 80%; specificity, 99%).[69] In a study of 282 patients with catecholamine-secreting tumors that were surgically confirmed, the sensitivities of imaging studies were 89% for CT, 98% for MRI, and 81% for ^{131}I-MIBG.[70] Catecholamine-secreting paragangliomas are found where chromaffin tissue is located (e.g., along the para-aortic sympathetic chain, within the organ of Zuckerkandl at the origin of the inferior mesenteric artery, in the wall of the urinary bladder, and in the sympathetic chain in the neck or mediastinum).[15] Tumor size is correlated with the degree of increase in plasma free metanephrine concentration,[71] but not with the degree of increase in catecholamine concentrations.[72] In one study, tumor diameter was strongly correlated with summed plasma concentrations and urinary outputs of metanephrine and normetanephrine ($r = 0.81$ and 0.77; $P < .001$).[71] All the tumors associated with a plasma metanephrine concentration that was greater than 15% of the combined increases of normetanephrine and metanephrine were either located in the adrenal glands or appeared to be recurrences of previously resected adrenal tumors. The density of the image (black is less dense) on CT scans is attributed to x-ray attenuation. The extremes of the CT density spectrum are air (black) and bone (white). The Hounsfield scale is a semiquantitative method of measuring x-ray attenuation.

Typical Hounsfield unit (HU) values are as follows: air, 0 HU; adipose tissue, −20 to −150 HU; kidney, 20 to 50 HU. If an adrenal mass measures less than 0 HU on nonenhanced CT, the likelihood that it is a benign adenoma is close to 100%. A study of patients who underwent helical CT (17 with pheochromocytoma, 11 with adrenocortical carcinoma, 23 with adrenal adenoma, and 16 with metastasis to the adrenal gland) found the following: (1) on nonenhanced CT scans, the mean attenuation of adenomas (8 HU) was significantly lower than the mean attenuation of pheochromocytomas (44 HU), adrenocortical carcinomas (39 HU), and metastases (34 HU) ($P < .001$); (2) on 10-minute delayed contrast-enhanced CT scans, the mean attenuation of adenomas (32 HU) was significantly lower than the mean attenuations of pheochromocytomas (83 HU), carcinomas (72 HU), and metastases (66 HU) ($P < .001$).[73] When adenomas were compared with carcinomas, pheochromocytomas, and metastases at optimal threshold values (50% for absolute percentage of enhancement loss and 40% for relative percentage of enhancement loss at 10 minutes), the diagnostic sensitivity and specificity for adenomas were 100%.[73] In the past, there was concern that administering ionic contrast medium to patients with pheochromocytoma could precipitate a hypertensive crisis.[74] However, with the availability of nonionic contrast medium, although it may be prudent to have the patient receive an α-adrenergic blocker before imaging, it is not mandatory.[75]

If a typical (<10-cm) unilateral adrenal pheochromocytoma is found on CT or MRI, ^{123}I-MIBG scintigraphy is superfluous, and the results may confuse the clinician.[76,77] However, if a paraganglioma is identified on CT or MRI, then ^{123}I-MIBG scintigraphy is indicated, because the patient has an increased risk of having additional paragangliomas and malignant disease. Performing preoperative ^{123}I-MIBG

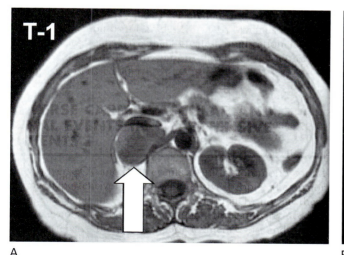
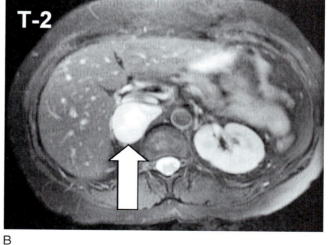

A   B

Figure 10–3   A magnetic resonance imaging (MRI) scan of the abdomen from a 59-year-old woman with an 8-year history of episodic diaphoresis, headache, palpitations, and tremor. Hypertension was diagnosed only recently. The fractionated plasma free metanephrines were abnormal: metanephrines, 4.3 nmol/L (normal, <0.5 nmol/L); and normetanephrines, 1.24 nmol/L (normal, <0.9 nmol/L). The MRI images show a typical 3.2 × 4.0-cm complex (cystic and solid) right adrenal mass consistent with pheochromocytoma (arrow) that has increased signal intensity on T2-weighted images. **A,** T1-weighted image. **B,** T2-weighted image. Following α- and β-adrenergic blockade, the patient underwent laparoscopic removal of a 28-g pheochromocytoma. Postoperatively, the fractionated plasma free metanephrines normalized.

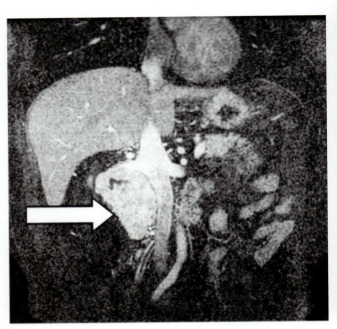

A

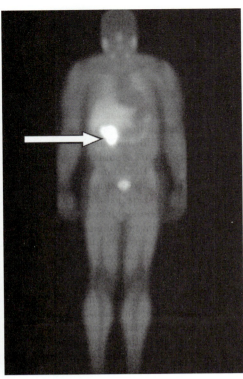

B

Figure 10–4   Magnetic resonance imaging (MRI) and iodine-123 (^{123}I)-meta-iodobenzylguanidine (MIBG) imaging from a 48-year-old man. Pheochromocytoma was suspected in this previously normotensive man after a single dose of metoclopramide was administered; within minutes, he developed chest pressure, shortness of breath, tachycardia, and diaphoresis. His blood pressure rose to 240/130 mm Hg, and he developed pulmonary edema. The echocardiogram showed severe global hypokinesis (ejection fraction was 20% to 25%). Pheochromocytoma was appropriately suspected and was confirmed with a 24-hour urine test for fractionated metanephrines and catecholamines: metanephrines, 120 µg (normal, <400 µg); normetanephrines, 13,901 µg (normal, <900 µg); norepinephrine, 597 µg (normal, <170 µg); epinephrine, 3.8 µg (normal, <35 µg); and dopamine, 222 µg (normal, <700 µg). **A,** Coronal abdominal MRI image shows a 9.6 × 6.2-cm retroperitoneal mass located next to the inferior vena cava and just below the right renal vein *(arrow)*. **B,** ^{123}I-MIBG whole-body scan shows a large intense area of uptake in the right upper quadrant of the abdomen that corresponds to the mass seen on MRI; no other abnormal uptake is seen. Following α- and β-adrenergic blockade, the patient underwent laparoscopic removal of an 11 × 7 × 5-cm paraganglioma that was arising near the right renal hilum. Postoperatively, the 24-hour urinary fractionated metanephrines and catecholamines normalized.

scintigraphy in patients with large (>10-cm) adrenal pheochromocytomas may be indicated to identify metastatic disease; however, finding metastatic disease preoperatively does not usually change the surgical treatment plan.

Localizing procedures that can also be used, but are rarely required, include central venous sampling and computer-assisted imaging of the chest, neck, and head. Results of selective venous sampling for catecholamines are frequently misleading because of periodic secretion; however, some medical centers have had successful results.[78,79] Other localizing studies, such as somatostatin-receptor imaging with indium-111 (^{111}In)-labeled pentetreotide, may also be considered.[80,81] Positron emission tomography scanning[82] with fluorine-18 (^{18}F)-fluorodeoxyglucose (FDG) or carbon-11 (^{11}C)-hydroxyephedrine or 6-^{18}F-fluorodopamine is capable of identifying paragangliomas that may be detected with less expensive techniques,[83] but this procedure should be reserved for identifying sites of metastatic disease in ^{123}I-MIBG–negative patients (Fig. 10-5).[84]

TREATMENT

The treatment of choice for pheochromocytoma is complete surgical resection. Careful preoperative pharmacologic preparation is crucial to successful treatment. Most catecholamine-secreting tumors are benign and can be totally excised. Tumor excision usually cures hypertension.

Preoperative Management

Some form of preoperative pharmacologic preparation is indicated in all patients with catecholamine-secreting neoplasms. However, no randomized, controlled trials that compare the different approaches have been undertaken. Combined α- and β-adrenergic blockade is one approach to control the patient's blood pressure (BP) and to prevent intraoperative hypertensive crises.[85] α-Adrenergic blockade should be started 7 to 10 days preoperatively to normalize BP and to expand the contracted blood volume. Target BPs are less than

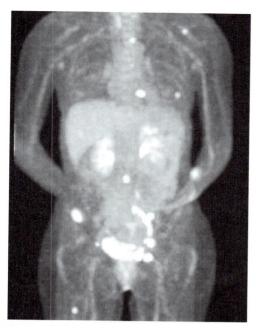

Figure 10–5   Fluoride-18 fluorodeoxyglucose (FDG) positron emission tomography (PET) scan from a 43-year-old woman who had a 2.5-cm urinary bladder paraganglioma resected 7 years previously. The patient developed recurrent signs and symptoms of a catecholamine-secreting tumor. The fractionated plasma free metanephrines were abnormal: metanephrines, 0.25 nmol/L (normal, <0.5 nmol/L); and normetanephrines, 16.0 nmol/L (normal, <0.9 nmol/L). The FDG-PET scan shows bony and nodal metastatic disease involving the third and sixth thoracic vertebral bodies, third lumbar vertebra, right femur, left second costochondral junction, anterior left fifth rib, posterior left ninth rib, left scapula, posterior midsacrum, right anterior iliac crest, posterior left innominate bone, right acetabulum, and left external iliac and inguinal lymph node chains.

120/80 mm Hg (seated), with systolic BP higher than 90 mm Hg (standing); both targets should be modified for patient age and co-morbid disease. On the second or third day of α-adrenergic blockade, patients are encouraged to start a diet high in sodium, because of the catecholamine-induced volume contraction and the orthostasis associated with α-adrenergic blockade. Once adequate α-adrenergic blockade is achieved, β-adrenergic blockade may be initiated, which typically occurs 2 to 3 days preoperatively.

α-Adrenergic Blockade

Phenoxybenzamine is the preferred drug for preoperative preparation to control BP and arrhythmias.[85,86] It is an irreversible, long-acting, nonspecific α-adrenergic blocking agent.[87] The initial dose is 10 mg one or two times daily, and the dose is increased by 10 to 20 mg every 2 to 3 days as needed to control BP and spells. The final target dosage of phenoxybenzamine is 20 to 100 mg daily. The patient should be cautioned regarding the orthostasis that occurs almost universally. The selective α_1-adrenergic blocking agents pra-

zosin, terazosin, and doxazosin are preferable to phenoxybenzamine when long-term pharmacologic treatment is indicated (e.g., for metastatic pheochromocytoma) because they have more favorable side effect profiles. However, these agents are not routinely used in the preoperative situation because they fail to achieve complete α-adrenergic blockade.

β-Adrenergic Blockade

The β-adrenergic antagonist should be administered only after α-adrenergic blockade is effective; β-adrenergic blockade alone may cause more severe hypertension owing to the unopposed α-adrenergic stimulation. Preoperative β-adrenergic blockade is indicated to control the tachycardia associated with both the high circulating catecholamine concentrations and the α-adrenergic blockade. The clinician should exercise caution if the patient is asthmatic or has heart failure. Chronic catecholamine excess can produce myocardiopathy,[88] a finding that may become evident after initiation of β-adrenergic blockade, which can result in acute pulmonary edema. Therefore, when the β-adrenergic blocker is administered, it should be used cautiously and at a low dose. For example, a patient is usually given 10 mg of propranolol every 6 hours to start. On the second day of treatment, the β-adrenergic blockade (assuming the patient is tolerating the β-adrenergic blocker) is converted to a single, long-acting dose. The dose is then increased as necessary to control the tachycardia (goal heart rate is 60 to 80 beats/minute). Labetalol (a combined α- and β-adrenergic blocker) has been shown to be effective in the treatment of hypertension associated with pheochromocytoma. However, some instances of paradoxical hypertensive responses have been reported while patients are taking labetalol. These cases are presumably the result of incomplete α-adrenergic blockade. Therefore, the safe use of labetalol as primary therapy is controversial; the primary role for this agent may be medically managing patients with metastatic disease.

Catecholamine Synthesis Inhibitor

α-Methylparatyrosine (metyrosine) should be used with caution and only when other agents have been ineffective. Although some centers have used this agent preoperatively, most centers reserve it primarily for those patients who cannot be treated with the typical combined α- and β-adrenergic blockade protocol for cardiopulmonary reasons. Metyrosine inhibits catecholamine synthesis by blocking the enzyme tyrosine hydroxylase. Metyrosine's side effects can be disabling and they include sedation, depression, diarrhea, anxiety, nightmares, crystalluria and urolithiasis, galactorrhea, and extrapyramidal manifestations.

Calcium Channel Blockers

Calcium channel blockers (CCBs), which block norepinephrine-mediated calcium transport into vascular smooth muscle, have been used successfully at several medical centers preoperatively to prepare patients with pheochromocytoma.[89-91] Nicardipine is the most commonly used CCB. It is given orally to control BP preoperatively and is then infused intravenously intraoperatively. In a study conducted between 1988 to 1996 in France, 70 patients with pheochromocytoma were operated on and managed with CCBs.[90] Nicardipine was used in 61 patients, and other CCBs were used in the remaining patients. Based on patients' plasma volume and BP control, the duration of preoperative treatment ranged from 24 hours to several weeks. Intraoperatively, nicardipine infusion was started after intubation, adjusted according to systolic BP, and stopped before ligation of the tumor venous drainage. Elevated systolic BP (values >200 mm Hg) occurred in 10 patients and was effectively controlled by nicardipine in all cases. Heart rates faster than 100 beats/minute occurred in 51 patients and were easily controlled by esmolol. Arrhythmias were infrequent, and only one patient required treatment.[90] No surgical deaths occurred in 113 patients with pheochromocytoma who were managed perioperatively with CCBs and who were operated on at the Cleveland Clinic in Cleveland, Ohio.[91] This study showed that preoperative α-adrenergic blockade is not essential in patients with pheochromocytoma. When CCBs are used as the primary mode of antihypertensive therapy, they may be just as effective as α- and β-adrenergic blockade.

Acute Hypertensive Crises

Acute hypertensive crises may occur before or during operation, and they should be treated intravenously with sodium nitroprusside, phentolamine, or nicardipine. Sodium nitroprusside is an ideal vasodilator for intraoperative management of hypertensive episodes because of its rapid onset of action and short duration of effect. This agent is administered as an intravenous infusion, 0.5 to 5.0 µg/kg/minute; the maximum dose should not exceed 800 µg/minute. Phentolamine is available in lyophilized form in 5-mg vials; the initial infused dose should be 1 mg, followed by repeat 5-mg boluses or a continuous infusion. Nicardipine can be started at an infusion rate of 5 mg/hour and titrated for BP control (maximum = 15 mg/hour).

Anesthesia and Surgery

Resecting a catecholamine-secreting tumor is a high-risk surgical procedure, and an experienced surgeon and anesthesiologist team is required. The last oral doses of α- and β-adrenergic blockers can be administered early in the morning on the day of operation. Fentanyl, ketamine, and morphine should be avoided because they can potentially stimulate catecholamine release from a pheochromocytoma.[92] In addition, parasympathetic nervous system blockade with atropine should be avoided because of the associated tachycardia. Induction of anesthesia may be achieved with intravenous injection of propofol, etomidate, or barbiturates, in combination with synthetic opioids.[92] Most anesthetic gases can be used, but halothane and desflurane should be avoided.[92] Cardiovascular and hemodynamic variables must be monitored closely. Continuous measurement of intra-arterial pressure and heart rhythm is required. When patients have heart failure or decreased cardiac reserve, monitoring of pulmonary capillary wedge pressure is indicated. Surgical survival rates are 98% to 100%. Four perioperative deaths occurred in a series of 165 patients operated on in Paris, France from 1975 to 1997.[93] No surgical mortalities resulted in 113 patients with pheochromocytoma operated at the Cleveland Clinic from 1977 to 1994.[91] Adverse perioperative events or complications occurred in 32% of 143 patients

operated at Mayo Clinic from 1983 to 1996.[14] The most common adverse event was sustained hypertension in 36 patients. In this Mayo Clinic series, there were no perioperative deaths, myocardial infarctions, or cerebrovascular events. The preoperative and perioperative treatment approach outlined here is the same for adults and pediatric patients.[94,95]

In the past, an anterior midline abdominal surgical approach was usually used for resecting adrenal pheochromocytoma. However, the procedure of choice for patients with solitary intra-adrenal pheochromocytomas that are smaller than 8 cm in diameter is now the laparoscopic approach.[96] In a series of 39 patients with pheochromocytoma who underwent laparoscopic adrenalectomy, the mean duration of hospitalization was only 1.7 days.[97] If the pheochromocytoma is in the adrenal gland, the entire gland should be removed. Laparoscopic adrenalectomy for pheochromocytoma should be converted to open adrenalectomy for difficult dissection, invasion, adhesions, or surgeon inexperience.[98] If the tumor is malignant, as much of the tumor should be removed as possible. If a bilateral adrenalectomy is planned preoperatively, the patient should receive glucocorticoid stress coverage while awaiting transfer to the operating room. Glucocorticoid coverage should be initiated in the operating room if unexpected bilateral adrenalectomy is necessary. Cortical-sparing bilateral adrenalectomies have been used to treat patients with MEN 2 and VHL.[99,100]

An anterior midline abdominal surgical approach is indicated for abdominal paragangliomas. The midline abdomen should be inspected carefully. Paragangliomas of the neck, chest, and urinary bladder require specialized approaches. "Unresectable" cardiac pheochromocytomas may require cardiac transplantation.[101]

Hypotension may occur after surgical resection of the pheochromocytoma, and it should be treated with fluids and colloids. Postoperative hypotension is less frequent in patients who have had adequate preoperative α-adrenergic blockade. If both adrenal glands were manipulated during surgery, adrenocortical insufficiency should be considered as a potential cause of postoperative hypotension. Because hypoglycemia can occur in the immediate postoperative period, blood glucose levels should be monitored, and the fluid given intravenously should contain 5% dextrose.

BP is usually normal by the time of hospital discharge. Some patients remain hypertensive for up to 4 to 8 weeks postoperatively. Long-standing, persistent hypertension does occur and may be related to accidental ligation of a polar renal artery, resetting of baroreceptors, hemodynamic changes, structural changes of the blood vessels, altered sensitivity of the vessels to pressor substances, functional or structural renal changes, or coincident primary hypertension.

Long-Term Postoperative Follow-up

Approximately 1 to 2 weeks after surgery, catecholamines and metanephrines should be measured by collecting a 24-hour urine. If the levels are normal, the resection of the pheochromocytoma should be considered complete. The survival rate after removal of a benign pheochromocytoma is nearly that of age- and sex-matched physiologically normal controls. Increased levels of catecholamines and metanephrines detected postoperatively are consistent with residual tumor, either a second primary lesion or occult metastases. If bilateral adrenalectomy was performed, lifelong glucocorticoid and mineralocorticoid replacement therapy should be prescribed. Twenty-four-hour urinary excretion of catecholamines and metanephrines or plasma metanephrines should be checked annually for life. The annual biochemical testing assesses for metastatic disease, tumor recurrence in the adrenal bed, or delayed appearance of multiple primary tumors.[102] The highest tumor recurrence rates are found in patients who have one or more of the following: a positive family history, a right-sided adrenal tumor, or a paraganglioma.[103] Follow-up computerized imaging is not needed unless the metanephrine or catecholamine levels become elevated or the original tumor was associated with minimal catecholamine excess.

Consider genetic testing for patients with one or more of the following: a family history of pheochromocytoma, a paraganglioma, or any signs that suggest a genetic origin (e.g., retinal angiomas, axillary freckling, café au lait spots, cerebellar tumor, MTC, hyperparathyroidism). In addition, all first-degree relatives of the patient with a pheochromocytoma or a paraganglioma should have biochemical testing (e.g., 24-hour urine for fractionated metanephrines and catecholamines). When a patient has an identified mutation, genetic testing of first-degree relatives should proceed in a stepwise fashion (i.e., parents first).[104]

MALIGNANT PHEOCHROMOCYTOMA

The distinction between benign and malignant catecholamine-secreting tumors is difficult to make based on clinical, biochemical, or histopathologic characteristics. MIB-1 is a monoclonal antibody that is immunoreactive with Ki-67, a nuclear antigen that is detectable only during the proliferative stages of the cell cycle and is a surrogate measure of the biologic processes that are present in phenotypically aggressive neoplasms. The MIB-1 labeling index is the fraction of tumor cells that are labeled by Ki-67. In one study, the MIB-1 labeling index of more than 3% was 100% specific and 50% sensitive for malignant pheochromocytoma.[105] In another study, logistic regression showed that the proliferative index ($P = .0072$), size ($P = .0022$), and extra-adrenal location ($P = .0012$) of the primary tumor were independently predictive for malignancy.[106] However, malignancy is generally determined by finding direct local invasion or disease metastatic to sites that do not normally have chromaffin tissue, such as lymph nodes, bone, lung, and liver. Malignancy is rare in patients who have adrenal familial syndromes, but it is common in patients with familial paraganglioma caused by mutations in *SDHB*. Patients with *SDHB* mutations are more likely to develop malignant disease and neoplasms other than paraganglioma (e.g., renal cell carcinoma).[36-38] A study of 90 malignant and 60 benign pheochromocytomas found that the risk of malignancy increases as the size of all pheochromocytomas increases; however, tumor size does not reliably predict malignancy in pheochromocytomas with local disease only.[98]

Although the 5-year survival rate for patients with malignant pheochromocytoma is less than 50%, the prognosis is variable. Approximately 50% of patients have an indolent form of the disease, with life expectancy of more than 20 years, and the other 50% of patients have rapidly progressive disease with death occurring within 1 to 3 years. Metastatic sites include local tissue invasion, liver, bone, lung, and lymph nodes. Endobronchial metastases have been reported.[107] Metastatic lesions should be resected if possible. Skeletal metastatic lesions that are painful or threaten structural function can be treated with external radiation therapy or cryoablation therapy. External radiotherapy can also be used to treat unresectable soft tissue lesions.[108] Local tumor irradiation with therapeutic doses of ^{131}I-MIBG has produced partial and temporary responses in approximately one third of patients.[109-113] A review of 116 patients with malignant pheochromocytoma or paraganglioma summarized the experiences with ^{131}I-MIBG therapy at 24 centers in 10 countries from 1983 to 1996. Of the studied patients, the following outcomes were documented: initial symptomatic improvement in 76%, tumor responses in 30%, and hormonal responses in 45%.[114] Five patients (4.3%) had complete tumor and hormonal responses that ranged from 16 to 58 months at the time of reporting. Of the 89 patients for whom follow-up data were available, 45% of responders had relapses, with recurrent or progressive disease after a mean interval of 29.3 ± 31.1 months (median, 19 months). Of patients who initially responded to ^{131}I-MIBG therapy, death following treatment was reported in 33% after a mean of 23.2 months (median, 22 months). Of nonresponding patients, death following treatment was reported in 45% after a mean of 14.3 ± 8.3 months (median, 13 months).[114] Sporadic dramatic responses to ^{131}I-MIBG treatment have been reported,[115] and there may be a role for high-dose ^{131}I-MIBG treatment in patients with high ^{131}I-MIBG uptake and rapidly advancing disease that has been unsuccessfully treated with other approaches.[113] Thrombotic therapy of large, unresectable liver metastases and radiofrequency ablation of small liver metastases are options to be considered. Radiofrequency ablation involves the percutaneous or intraoperative placement of an electrode into the lesion with guidance from ultrasound or CT. The needle tip contains multiple curved electrodes that can be deployed to span a lesion up to 7 cm in diameter. The radiofrequency signal produces ionic agitation in the tissue and results in frictional heating with controllable temperatures of 95° to 100° C. This temperature is maintained for approximately 10 minutes, with the goal of destroying the tumor and a 1-cm margin of surrounding normal tissue. Pacak and colleagues reported radiofrequency ablation to a single rib lesion in a patient with metastatic pheochromocytoma.[116] When catecholamine-containing cells are destroyed, there is concern that a hypertensive crisis could be provoked. Therefore, when radiofrequency ablation or cryoablation is considered, the patient should be prepared with α- and β-adrenergic blockade and tyrosine hydroxylase inhibition. In selected cases, long-acting octreotide is beneficial in controlling BP.[117,118]

Combination chemotherapy may be considered if the tumor is aggressive and the patient's quality of life is affected. In a nonrandomized, single-arm trial, the efficacy of chemotherapy (CVD protocol: cyclophosphamide, 750 mg/m² body surface area on day 1; vincristine, 1.4 mg/m² on day 1; and dacarbazine, 600 mg/m² on days 1 and 2 and every 21 days) was studied in 14 patients with malignant pheochromocytoma.[119] The combination CVD protocol produced a complete and partial tumor response rate of 57% (median duration, 21 months; range, 7 to >34). All responding patients had objective improvement in performance status and BP. Hypertensive episodes may be induced by CVD chemotherapy.[120] Hypertension and spells can be controlled with combined α- and β-adrenergic blockade or inhibition of catecholamine synthesis with metyrosine.

Managing patients with malignant pheochromocytoma can be frustrating because curative options are limited. Clearly, innovative prospective protocols are needed to identify new treatment options for this neoplasm.[121]

PHEOCHROMOCYTOMA IN PREGNANCY

Pheochromocytoma in pregnancy can cause the death of both the fetus and the mother. The treatment of hypertensive crises is the same as for nonpregnant patients, except nitroprusside is contraindicated; the fetus is very susceptible to cyanide toxicity. Although some controversy exists regarding the most appropriate management,[122] pheochromocytomas should be removed promptly if they are diagnosed during the first two trimesters of pregnancy. Preoperative preparation is the same as for nonpregnant patients. If medical therapy is chosen, or if the pregnancy is in the third trimester, one operation is recommended to perform a cesarean section and to remove the pheochromocytoma at the same time. Spontaneous labor and delivery should be avoided.

References

1. Stenstrom G, Svardsudd K. Phaechromocytoma in Sweden, 1958-81: An analysis of the National Cancer Registry Data. *Acta Med Scand.* 1986;**220**:225-232.
2. Young WF Jr, Maddox DE. Spells: In search of a cause. *Mayo Clin Proc.* 1996;**70**:757-765.
3. Sweeney AT, Malabanan AO, Blake MA, et al. Megacolon as the presenting feature in pheochromocytoma. *J Clin Endocrinol Metab.* 2000;**85**:3968-3972.
4. O'Brien TO, Young WF Jr, Davila DG, et al. Cushing's syndrome associated with ectopic production of corticotropin-releasing hormone, corticotropin, and vasopressin by a phaeochromocytoma. *Clin Endocrinol (Oxf).* 1992;**37**:460-467.
5. Mune T, Katakami H, Kato Y, et al. Production and secretion of parathyroid hormone-related protein in pheochromocytoma: Participation of an alpha-adrenergic mechanism. *J Clin Endocrinol Metab.* 1993;**76**:757-762.
6. Smith SL, Slappy AL, Fox TP, et al. Pheochromocytoma producing vasoactive intestinal peptide. *Mayo Clin Proc.* 2002;**77**:97-100.
7. Saito H, Sano T, Yamasaki R, et al. Demonstration of biological activity of growth hormone–releasing hormone–like substance produced by a pheochromocytoma. *Acta Endocrinol (Copenh).* 1993;**129**:246-250.
8. Schifferdecker B, Kodali D, Hausner E, et al. Adrenergic shock: An overlooked clinical entity? *Cardiol Rev.* 2005;**13**:69-72.
9. Gordon RY, Fallon JT, Baran DA: Case report: A 32-year-old woman with familial paragangliomas and acute cardiomyopathy. *Transplant Proc.* 2004;**36**:2819-2822.
10. Kim J, Reutrakul S, Davis DB, et al. Multiple endocrine neoplasia 2A syndrome presenting as peripartum cardiomyopathy due to catecholamine excess. *Eur J Endocrinol.* 2004;**151**:771-777.
11. Manger WM, Gifford RW Jr. Diagnosis. *In:* Manger WM, Gifford RW Jr (eds). Clinical and Experimental Pheochromocytoma, 2nd ed. Cambridge, Mass: Blackwell Science, 1996, pp 205-332.
13. Kudva YC, Sawka AM, Young WF Jr. Clinical review 164: The laboratory diagnosis of adrenal pheochromocytoma. The Mayo Clinic experience. *J Clin Endocrinol Metab.* 2003;**88**:4533-4539.
13. Neumann HP, Bausch B, McWhinney SR, et al. Germ-line mutations in nonsyndromic pheochromocytoma. *N Engl J Med.* 2002;**346**:1459-1466.
14. Kinney MA, Warner ME, van Heerden JA, et al. Perianesthetic risks and outcomes of pheochromocytoma and paraganglioma resection. *Anesth Analg.* 2000;**91**:1118-1123.
15. O'Riordain DS, Young WF Jr, Grant CS, et al. Clinical spectrum and outcome of functional extraadrenal paraganglioma. *World J Surg.* 1996;**20**:916-922.
16. Erickson D, Kudva YC, Ebersold MJ, et al. Benign paragangliomas: Clinical presentation and treatment outcomes in 236 patients. *J Clin Endocrinol Metab.* 2001;**86**:5210-5216.
17. Osranek M, Bursi F, Gura GM, et al. Echocardiographic features of pheochromocytoma of the heart. *Am J Cardiol.* 2003;**91**:640-643.
18. Elder EE, Elder G, Larsson C. Pheochromocytoma and functional paraganglioma syndrome: No longer the 10% tumor. *J Surg Oncol.* 2005;**89**:193-201.
19. Gimm O, Koch CA, Januszewicz A, et al. The genetic basis of pheochromocytoma. *Front Horm Res.* 2004;**31**:45-60.
20. Gross DJ, Avishai N, Meiner V, et al. Familial pheochromocytoma associated with a novel mutation in the von Hippel–Lindau gene. *J Clin Endocrinol Metab.* 1996;**81**:147-149.
21. Atuk NO, McDonald T, Wood T, et al. Familial pheochromocytoma, hypercalcemia, and von Hippel–Lindau disease: A ten year study of a large family. *Medicine (Baltimore).* 1979;**58**:209-218.
22. Brauch H, Kishida T, Glavac D, et al. von Hippel–Lindau (VHL) disease with pheochromocytoma in the Black Forest region of Germany: Evidence for a founder effect. *Hum Genet.* 1995;**95**:551-556.
23. Eng C, Clayton D, Schuffenecker I, et al. The relationship between specific *RET* proto-oncogene mutations and disease phenotype in multiple endocrine neoplasia type 2: International *RET* mutation consortium analysis. *JAMA.* 1996;**276**:1575-1579.
24. Atuk NO, Stolle C, Owen JA Jr, et al. Pheochromocytoma in von Hippel–Lindau disease: Clinical presentation and mutation analysis in a large multigenerational kindred. *J Clin Endocrinol Metab.* 1998;**83**:117-120.
25. Carney JA. The triad of gastric epithelioid leiomyosarcoma, pulmonary chondroma, and functioning extra-adrenal paraganglioma: A five-year review. *Medicine (Baltimore).* 1983;**62**:159-169.
26. Carney JA. Gastric stromal sarcoma, pulmonary chondroma, and extra-adrenal paraganglioma (Carney triad): Natural history, adrenocortical component, and possible familial occurrence. *Mayo Clin Proc.* 1999;**74**:543-552.
27. Maher ER, Eng C. The pressure rises: update on the genetics of phaeochromocytoma. *Hum Mol Genet.* 2002;**11**:2347-2354.
28. Howe JR, Norton JA, Wells SA Jr. Prevalence of pheochromocytoma and hyperparathyroidism in multiple endocrine neoplasia type 2A: Results of long-term follow-up. *Surgery.* 1993;**114**:1070-1077.
29. O'Riodain DS, O'Brien T, Crotty TB, et al. Multiple endocrine neoplasia type 2B: More than an endocrine disorder. *Surgery.* 1995;**118**:936-942.
30. Koch C, Mauro D, McClellan MW, et al. Pheochromocytoma in von Hippel–Lindau disease: Distinct histopathologic phenotype compared to pheochromocytoma in multiple endocrine neoplasia type 2. *Endocr Pathol.* 2002;**13**:17-27.
31. Young AL, Young WF Jr. Benign paragangliomas. *In:* Linos D, van Heerden JA (eds). Adrenal Glands: Diagnostic Aspects and Surgical Therapy. New York: Springer-Verlag, 2005, pp 201-209.
32. Baysal BE, Ferrell RE, Willett-Brozick JE, et al. Mutations in SDHD, a mitochondrial complex II gene, in hereditary paraganglioma. *Science.* 2000;**287**:848-851.

33. Baysal BE, Willett-Brozick JE, Lawrence EC, et al. Prevalence of SDHB, SDHC and SDHD germline mutations in clinic patients with head and neck paragangliomas. *J Med Genet.* 2002;**39**:178-183.

34. Niemann S, Muller U. Mutations in SDHC cause autosomal dominant paraganglioma, type 3. *Nat Genet.* 2000;**26**:268-270.

35. Astuti D, Latif F, Dallol A, et al. Gene mutation in the succinate dehydrogenase subunit SDHB cause susceptibility to familial pheochromocytoma and to familial paraganglioma. *Am J Hum Genet.* 2001;**69**:49-54.

36. Young AL, Baysal BE, Deb A, et al. Familial malignant catecholamine-secreting paraganglioma with prolonged survival associated with mutation in the succinate dehydrogenase B gene. *J Clin Endocrinol Metab.* 2002;**87**:4101-4105.

37. Gimenez-Roqueplo AP, Favier J, et al. Mutations in SDHB gene are associated with extra-adrenal and/or malignant phaeochromocytomas. *Cancer Res.* 2003;**63**:5615-5621.

38. Neumann HP, Pawlu C, Peczkowska M, et al. Distinct clinical features of paraganglioma syndromes associated with SDHB and SDHD gene mutations. *JAMA.* 2004;**292**:943-951.

39. McWhinney SR, Pilarski RT, Forrester SR, et al. Large germline deletions of mitochondrial complex II subunits SDHB and SDHD in hereditary paraganglioma. *J Clin Endocrinol Metab.* 2004;**89**:5694-5699.

40. Taylor RL, Singh RJ. Validation of liquid chromatography–tandem mass spectrometry method for analysis of urinary conjugated metanephrine and normetanephrine for screening of pheochromocytoma. *Clin Chem.* 2002;**48**:533-539.

41. Sawka AM, Jaeschke R, Singh RJ, et al. A comparison of biochemical tests for pheochromocytoma: Measurement of fractionated plasma metanephrines compared with the combination of 24-hour urinary metanephrines and catecholamines. *J Clin Endocrinol Metab.* 2003;**88**:553-558.

42. Hernandez FC, Sanchez M, Alvarez A, et al. A five-year report on experience in the detection of pheochromocytoma. *Clin Biochem.* 2000;**33**:649-655.

43. Witteles RM, Kaplan EL, Roizen MF. Sensitivity of diagnostic and localization tests for pheochromocytoma in clinical practice. *Arch Intern Med.* 2000;**160**:2521-2524.

44. Eisenhofer G, Keiser H, Friberg P, et al. Plasma metanephrines are markers of pheochromocytoma produced by catechol-O-methyltransferase within tumors. *J Clin Endocrinol Metab.* 1998;**83**:2175-2185.

45. Raber W, Raffesberg W, Bischof M, et al. Diagnostic efficacy of unconjugated plasma metanephrines for the detection of pheochromocytoma. *Arch Intern Med.* 2000;**160**:2957-2963.

46. Lenders JW, Pacak K, Walther MM, et al. Biochemical diagnosis of pheochromocytoma: Which test is best? *JAMA.* 2002;**287**:1427-1434.

47. Sawka AM, Prebtani AP, Thabane L, et al. A systematic review of the literature examining the diagnostic efficacy of measurement of fractionated plasma free metanephrines in the biochemical diagnosis of pheochromocytoma. *BMC Endocr Disord.* 2004;**4**:2. http://www.biomedcentral.com/1472-6823/4/2. Accessed on March 27, 2005.

48. Sawka AM, Thabane L, Gafni A, et al. Measurement of fractionated plasma metanephrines for exclusion of pheochromocytoma: can specificity be improved by adjustment for age? *BMC Endocr Disord.* 2005;**5**:1. http://www.biomedcentral.com/1472-6823/5/1. Accessed March 27, 2005.

49. Sawka AM, Gafni A, Thabane L, et al. The economic implications of three biochemical screening algorithms for pheochromocytoma. *J Clin Endocrinol Metab.* 2004;**89**:2859-2866.

50. Young WF Jr. Phaeochromocytoma: How to catch a moonbeam in your hand. *Eur J Endocrinol.* 1997;**136**:28-29.

51. Sjoberg RJ, Simcic KJ, Kidd GS. The clonidine suppression test for pheochromocytoma: Review of its utility and pitfalls. *Arch Intern Med.* 1992;**152**:1193-1197.

52. Eisenhofer G, Goldstein DS, Walther MM, et al. Biochemical diagnosis of pheochromocytoma: How to distinguish true-from false-positive results. *J Clin Endocrinol Metab.* 2003;**88**:2656-2666.

53. Lenders JWM, Keiser HR, Goldstein DS, et al. Plasma metanephrines in the diagnosis of pheochromocytoma. *Ann Intern Med.* 1995;**123**:101-109.

54. Hsiao RJ, Parmer RJ, Takiyyuddin MA, et al. Chromogranin A storage and secretion: sensitivity and specificity for the diagnosis of pheochromocytoma. *Medicine (Baltimore).* 1991;**70**:33-45.

55. Stridsberg M, Husebye ES. Chromogranin A and chromogranin B are sensitive circulating markers for phaeochromocytoma. *Eur J Endocrinol.* 1997;**136**:67-73.

56. Mouri T, Sone M, Takahashi K, et al. Neuropeptide Y as a plasma marker for phaeochromocytoma, ganglioneuroblastoma and neuroblastoma. *Clin Sci (Lond).* 1992;**83**:205-211.

57. Godfrey JA, Rickman OB, Williams AW, et al. Pheochromocytoma in a patient with end-stage renal disease. *Mayo Clin Proc.* 2001;**76**:953-957.

58. Canale MP, Bravo EL. Diagnostic specificity of serum chromogranin-A for pheochromocytoma in patients with renal dysfunction. *J Clin Endocrinol Metab.* 1994;**78**:1139-1144.

59. Chauveau D, Martinez F, Houhou S, et al. Malignant hypertension secondary to pheochromocytoma in a hemodialyzed patient. *Am J Kidney Dis.* 1993;**21**:52-53.

60. Stumvoll M, Radjaipour M, Seif F. Diagnostic considerations in pheochromocytoma and chronic hemodialysis: Case report and review of the literature. *Am J Nephrol.* 1995;**15**:147-151.

61. Morioka M, Yuihama S, Nakajima T, et al. Incidentally discovered pheochromocytoma in long-term hemodialysis patients. *Int J Urol.* 2002;**9**:700-703.

62. Eisenhofer G, Huysmans F, Pacak K, et al. Plasma metanephrines in renal failure. *Kidney Int.* 2005;**67**:668-677.

63. Marini M, Fathi M, Ballotton M. [Determination of serum metanephrines in the diagnosis of pheochromocytoma]. *Ann Endocrinol (Paris).* 1994;**54**:337-342.

64. Stern TA, Cremens CM. Factitious pheochromocytoma: One patient history and literature review. *Psychosomatics.* 1998;**39**:283-287.

65. Spitzer D, Bongartz D, Ittel TH, et al. Simulation of a pheochromocytoma: Munchausen syndrome. *Eur J Med Res.* 1998;**3**:549-553.

66. Sawka AM, Singh RJ, Young WF Jr. False positive biochemical testing for pheochromocytoma caused by surreptitious catecholamine addition to urine. *Endocrinologist.* 2001;**11**:421-423.

67. Jackson JA, Kleerekoper M, Mendlovic D. Endocrine grand rounds: a 51-year-old man with accelerated hypertension, hypercalcemia, and right adrenal and paratracheal masses. *Endocrinologist.* 1993;**3**:5.

68. van Gils APG, Falke THM, van Erkel AR, et al. MR imaging and MIBG scintigraphy of pheochromocytomas and extraadrenal functioning paragangliomas. *Radiographics.* 1991;**11**:37-57.

69. Shapiro B, Gross MD, Fig L, et al. Localization of functioning sympathoadrenal lesions. *In:* Biglieri EG, Melby JC (eds). Endocrine Hypertension. New York: Raven Press, 1990, pp 235-255.

70. Jalil ND, Pattou FN, Combemale F, et al. Effectiveness and limits of preoperative imaging studies for the localisation of pheochromocytomas and paragangliomas: A review of 282 cases. French Association of Surgery (AFC), and the French Association of Endocrine Surgeons (AFCE). *Eur J Surg.* 1998;**164**:23-28.

71. Eisenhofer G, Lenders JW, Goldstein DS, et al. Pheochromocytoma catecholamine phenotypes and prediction of tumor size and location by use of plasma free metanephrines. *Clin Chem.* 2005;**51**:735-744

72. Ito Y, Fujimoto Y, Obara T. The role of epinephrine, norepinephrine, and dopamine in blood pressure disturbances in patients with pheochromocytoma. *World J Surg.* 1992;**16**:759-763.

73. Szolar DH, Korobkin M, Reittner P, et al. Adrenocortical carcinomas and adrenal pheochromocytomas: Mass and enhancement loss evaluation at delayed contrast-enhanced CT. *Radiology.* 2005;**234**:479-485.

74. Konen E, Konen O, Katz M, et al. Are referring clinicians aware of patients at risk from intravenous injection of iodinated contrast media? *Clin Radiol.* 2002;**57**:132-135.

75. Mukherjee JJ, Peppercorn PD, Reznek RH, et al. Pheochromocytoma: effect of nonionic contrast medium in CT on circulating catecholamine levels. *Radiology.* 1997;**202**:227-231.

76. Miskulin J, Shulkin BL, Doherty GM, et al. Is preoperative iodine 123 meta-iodobenzylguanidine scintigraphy routinely necessary before initial adrenalectomy for pheochromocytoma? *Surgery.* 2003;**134**:918-922.

77. Taieb D, Sebag F, Hubbard JG, Mundler O, et al. Does iodine-131 meta-iodobenzylguanidine (MIBG) scintigraphy have an impact on the management of sporadic and familial phaeochromocytoma? *Clin Endocrinol (Oxf).* 2004;**61**:102-108.

78. Newbould EC, Ross GA, Dacie JE, et al. The use of venous catheterization in the diagnosis and localization of bilateral phaeochromocytomas. *Clin Endocrinol (Oxf).* 1991;**35**:55-59.

79. Walker IA. Selective venous catheterization and plasma catecholamine analysis in the diagnosis of phaeochromocytoma. *J R Soc Med.* 1996;**89**:216P-218P.

80. Lamberts SW, Bakker WH, Reubi JC, et al. Somatostatin-receptor imaging in the localization of endocrine tumors. *N Engl J Med.* 1990;**323**:1246-1249.

81. Tenenbaum F, Lumbroso J, Schlumberger M, et al. Comparison of radiolabeled octreotide and meta-iodobenzylguanidine (MIBG) scintigraphy in malignant pheochromocytoma. *J Nucl Med.* 1995;**36**:1-6.

82. Pacak K, Eisenhofer G, Carrasquillo JA, et al. Diagnostic localization of pheochromocytoma: The coming of age of positron emission tomography. *Ann N Y Acad Sci.* 2002;**970**:170-176.

83. Hwang JJ, Uchio EM, Patel SV, et al. Diagnostic localization of malignant bladder pheochromocytoma using 6-^{18}F fluorodopamine positron emission tomography. *J Urol.* 2003;**169**:274-275.

84. Shulkin BL, Wieland DM, Schwaiger M, et al. PET scanning with hydroxyephedrine: An approach to the localization of pheochromocytoma. *J Nucl Med.* 1992;**33**:1125-1131.

85. Young WF Jr. Pheochromocytoma: 1926-1993. *Trends Endocrinol Metab.* 1993;**4**:122-127.

86. Dabrowska B, Pruszczyk P, Dabrowski A, et al. Influence of alpha-adrenergic blockade on ventricular arrhythmias, QTc interval and heart rate variability in phaeochromocytoma. *J Hum Hypertens.* 1995;**9**:925-929.

87. Frishman WH, Kotob F. Alpha-adrenergic blocking drugs in clinical medicine. *J Clin Pharmacol.* 1999;**39**:7-16.

88. Frustaci A, Loperfido F, Gentiloni N, et al. Catecholamine-induced cardiomyopathy in multiple endocrine neoplasia: A histologic, ultrastructural, and biochemical study. *Chest.* 1993;**99**:383-385.

89. Bravo EL. Pheochromocytoma: An approach to antihypertensive management. *Ann N Y Acad Sci.* 2002;**970**:1-10.

90. Combemale F, Carnaille B, Tavernier B, et al. Exclusive use of calcium channel blockers and cardioselective beta-blockers in the pre- and peri-operative management of pheochromocytoma. 70 cases. *Ann Chir.* 1998;**52**:341-345.

91. Ulchaker JC, Goldfarb DA, Bravo EL, et al. Successful outcomes in pheochromocytoma surgery in the modern era. *J Urol.* 1999;**161**:764-767.

92. Memtsoudis SG, Swamidoss C, Psoma M. Anesthesia for adrenal surgery. *In:* Linos D, van Heerden JA (eds). Adrenal Glands: Diagnostic Aspects and Surgical Therapy. New York: Springer-Verlag, 2005, pp 287-297.

93. Plouin PF, Duclos JM, Soppelsa F, et al. Factors associated with perioperative morbidity and mortality in patients with pheochromocytoma: Analysis of 165 operations at a single center. *J Clin Endocrinol Metab.* 2001;**86**:1480-1486.

94. Hack HA. The perioperative management of children with phaeochromocytoma. *Paediatr Anaesth.* 2000;**10**:463-476.

95. Reddy VS, O'Neill JA Jr, Holcomb GW 3rd, et al. Twenty-five-year surgical experience with pheochromocytoma in children. *Am Surg.* 2000;**66**:1085-1091.

96. Assalia A, Gagner M. Laparoscopic adrenalectomy. *Br J Surg.* 2004;**91**:1259-1274.

97. Cheah WK, Clark OH, Horn JK, et al. Laparoscopic adrenalectomy for pheochromocytoma. *World J Surg.* 2002;**26**:1048-1051.

98. Shen WT, Sturgeon C, Clark OH, et al. Should pheochromocytoma size influence surgical approach? A comparison of 90 malignant and 60 benign pheochromocytomas. *Surgery.* 2004;**136**:1129-1137.

99. Lee JE, Curley SA, Gagel RF, et al. Cortical-sparing adrenalectomy for patients with bilateral pheochromocytoma. *Surgery.* 1996;**120**:1064-1071.

100. Walther MM, Keiser HR, Choyke PL, et al. Management of hereditary pheochromocytoma in von Hippel–Lindau kindreds with partial adrenalectomy. *J Urol.* 1999;**161**:395-398.

101. Jeevanandam V, Oz MC, Shapiro B, et al. Surgical management of cardiac pheochromocytoma: Resection versus transplantation. *Ann Surg.* 1995;**221**:415-419.

102. van Heerden JA, Roland JA, Carney JA, et al. Long-term evaluation following resection of apparently benign pheochromocytoma(s)/paraganglioma(s). *World J Surg.* 1990;**14**:325-329.

103. Amar L, Servais A, Gimeniz-Roqueplo AP, et al. Year of diagnosis, features at presentation, and risk of recurrence in patients with pheochromocytoma or secreting paraganglioma. *J Clin Endocrinol Metab.* 2005;**90**:2110-2116.

104. McDonnell CM, Benn DE, Marsh DJ, et al. K40E: A novel succinate dehydrogenase (SDH)B mutation causing familial phaeochromocytoma and paraganglioma. *Clin Endocrinol (Oxf).* 2004;**61**:510-514.

105. Clarke MR, Weyant RJ, Watson CG, et al. Prognostic markers in pheochromocytoma. *Hum Pathol.* 1998;**29**:522-526.

106. van der Harst E, Bruining HA, Jaap Bonjer H, et al. Proliferative index in phaeochromocytomas: Does it predict the occurrence of metastases? *J Pathol.* 2000;**191**:175-180.

107. Sandur S, Dasgupta A, Shapiro JL, et al. Thoracic involvement with pheochromocytoma: A review. *Chest.* 1999;**115**:511-521.

108. Naguib M, Caceres M, Thomas CR Jr, et al. Radiation treatment of recurrent pheochromocytoma of the bladder: Case report and review of the literature. *Am J Clin Oncol.* 2002;**25**:42-44.

109. Krempf M, Lumbroso J, Mornex R, et al. Use of m-[^{131}I]iodobenzylguanidine in the treatment of malignant pheochromocytoma. *J Clin Endocrinol Metab.* 1991;**72**:455-461.

110. Shapiro B, Sisson JC, Wieland DM, et al. Radiopharmaceutical therapy of malignant pheochromocytoma with [131-I]-metaiodobenzylguanidine: Results from ten years of experience. *J Nucl Biol Med.* 1991;**35**:269-276.

111. Sisson JC. Radiopharmaceutical treatment of pheochromocytomas. *Ann NY Acad Sci.* 2002;**970**:54-60.

112. Safford SD, Coleman RE, Gockerman JP, et al. Iodine-131 metaiodobenzylguanidine is an effective treatment for malignant pheochromocytoma and paraganglioma. *Surgery.* 2003;**134**:956-962.

113. Rose B, Matthay KK, Price D, et al. High-dose ^{131}I-metaiodobenzylguanidine therapy for 12 patients with malignant pheochromocytoma. *Cancer.* 2003;**98**:239-248.

114. Loh KC, Fitzgerald PA, Matthay KK, et al. The treatment of malignant pheochromocytoma with iodine-131 metaiodobenzylguanidine (^{131}I-MIBG): A comprehensive review of 116 reported patients. *J Endocrinol Invest.* 1997;**20**:648-658.

115. Pujol P, Bringer J, Faurous P, et al. Metastatic phaeochromocytoma with a long-term response after iodine-131 metaiodobenzylguanidine therapy. *Eur J Nucl Med.* 1995;**22**:382-384.

116. Pacak K, Fojo T, Goldstein DS, et al. Radiofrequency ablation: A novel approach for treatment of metastatic pheochromocytoma. *J Natl Cancer Inst.* 2001;**93**:648-649.

117. Lamarre-Cliché M, Gimenez-Roqueplo AP, Billaud E, et al. Effects of slow-release octreotide on urinary metanephrine excretion and plasma chromogranin A and catecholamine levels in patients with malignant or recurrent phaeochromocytoma. *Clin Endocrinol (Oxf).* 2002;**57**:629-634.

118. Lehnert H, Mundschenk J, Hahn K. Malignant pheochromocytoma. *Front Horm Res.* 2004;**31**:155-162.

119. Averbuch SD, Steakley CS, Young RC, et al. Malignant pheochromocytoma: Effective treatment with a combination of cyclophosphamide, vincristine, and dacarbazine. *Ann Intern Med.* 1988;**109**:267-273.

120. Wu LT, Dicpinigaitis P, Bruckner H, et al. Hypertensive crises induced by treatment of malignant pheochromocytoma with a combination of cyclophosphamide, vincristine, and dacarbazine. *Med Pediatr Oncol.* 1994;**22**:389-392.

121. Eisenhofer G, Bornstein SR, Brouwers FM, et al. Malignant pheochromocytoma: Current status and initiatives for future progress. *Endocr Relat Cancer.* 2004;**11**:423-436.

122. Harper MA, Murnaghan GA, Kennedy L, et al. Phaeochromocytoma in pregnancy: Five cases and a review of the literature. *Br J Obstet Gynaecol.* 1989;**96**:594-606.

Secondary Hypertension: Sleep Apnea

Gianfranco Parati, Grzegorz Bilo, Carolina Lombardi, and Giuseppe Mancia

DEFINITIONS AND DIAGNOSIS

In normal subjects, sleep is characterized by major changes in the physiologic mechanisms responsible for cardiovascular (CV) regulation, including an increase in parasympathetic activity and a reduction in sympathetic drive. These changes lead to marked reductions in blood pressure (BP) and heart rate.[1-3] In parallel, a change in breathing patterns occurs: respiration becomes slower and more regular than in the awake period. These changes in part derive from reduced physical activity at night, but they are also determined by the neural changes related to sleep itself.[3] Therefore, any alteration in the physiology of sleep may result in important changes in the nocturnal modulation of BP and heart rate.

Increasingly frequent problems affecting sleep are alterations in breathing patterns at night that lead to concomitant alterations in the neural and CV effects of sleep. These conditions, known as *sleep-disordered breathing* (SDB) syndromes, include habitual snoring, sleep apnea, Cheyne-Stokes breathing syndrome, and sleep hypoventilation syndrome (Table 11-1).[4,5] The full clinical picture including sleep apnea and its associated symptoms, often also extending to daytime (Table 11-2), is termed *sleep apnea syndrome* (SAS).

SASs are characterized by multiple cessations of respiration during sleep that induce partial arousals and interfere with the physiologic cyclic shift between the various sleep stages. These sleep structure alterations have been associated with daytime somnolence. Airflow arrests and reductions lasting more than 10 seconds are considered significant. Apnea is defined as complete breathing cessation, and hypopnea is a reduction in breathing amplitude of 50% or more. The usual duration of apnea and hypopnea episodes is 20 to 30 seconds, with a possible prolongation up to 1 minute. The occurrence of more or less frequent oxygen desaturations, or of electroencephalographic arousals, is considered an additional diagnostic tool to identify these conditions.[4,5]

Apneas are typically classified as being *central*, predominating in central sleep apnea syndromes (CSAS), *obstructive*, predominating in obstructive sleep apnea syndromes (OSAS), or *mixed*. The criterion differentiating between OSAS and CSAS is the concomitant presence or absence of efforts to breathe, respectively.

Obstructive sleep apnea is the result of upper airway obstruction, which may be the effect of the upper airway collapse, facilitated by anatomic (e.g., obesity, acromegaly, adenotonsillar hypertrophy, myxedema, micrognathia), neuromuscular (myotonic dystrophy or other neuromuscular diseases), or toxic (sedative drugs, alcohol consumption) factors or by a combination of these.[4-6]

Apneas of central origin are caused by a dysfunction of neural centers that regulate respiration, whether idiopathic (primary), of organic causes (e.g., lower brainstem lesions), or induced by conditions external to the central nervous system (chronic obstructive pulmonary disease, heart failure, medications).

In *apneas of mixed origin*, airway collapse typically depends initially upon a central mechanism and subsequently upon an obstructive one.

Currently, the diagnosis of these disorders is based on sleep studies. These studies involve overnight monitoring of numerous parameters (e.g., nasal air flow, snoring sounds, abdominal and thoracic movements, blood oxygen saturation, intraesophageal pressure, electrocardiogram), usually in a controlled hospital setting. An extensive monitoring including at least 12 channels is termed polysomnography and constitutes the gold standard for the diagnosis and classification of SASs.[5]

The diagnosis and evaluation of the severity of SASs are most commonly based on the apnea-hypopnea index (AHI), defined as the average number of apneas and hypopneas per sleep hour. Alternatively, the term *respiratory disturbance index* (RDI) is also used. This index is calculated by adding the number of apnea episodes to the number of hypopneas and to that of respiratory efforts–related arousals (RERA). The American Academy of Sleep Medicine Task Force recommends an AHI greater than 5 and the presence of symptoms as criteria for a diagnosis of OSAS.[5] Other indices of OSAS severity are sometimes used, including the oxygen desaturation index (ODI, i.e., the average number of significant oxygen desaturations per hour of sleep) and the arousal index (the number of electroencephalographic arousals per hour of sleep). A recently proposed index is the cross-power index (CPI, i.e., the integral of the cross-spectrum modulus between concomitant fluctuations in systolic BP and oxygen saturation).[7]

Subjects who have an AHI of less than 5 but who generally snore most of the night are classified as *habitual snorers* and do not meet criteria for the formal diagnosis of OSAS.

Given the cost and limited availability of polysomnography, in practice, screening for OSAS is based on the presence of symptoms, and it may be further aided by questionnaire-based methods (e.g., the Berlin questionnaire).[8]

The main clinical consequences of SASs are related to the CV and metabolic changes they induce, including arterial hypertension (discussed later), and to the relative sleep deprivation and daytime tiredness and/or sleepiness caused by reduced quantity and impaired quality of sleep. The latter, apart from a general reduction in a patient's quality of life, may lead to important complications, such as car and work accidents or episodes of sudden falls.[9]

Table 11-1 Classification of Sleep Disordered Breathing Syndromes

Habitual snoring
Sleep apnea syndromes (SASs)
    Obstructive sleep apnea syndrome (OSAS)
    Central sleep apnea syndrome (CSAS)
    Mixed sleep apnea syndrome
Cheyne-Stokes breathing syndrome
Sleep hypoventilation syndrome

Table 11-2 Clinical Features of Obstructive Sleep Apnea Syndrome

Daytime
Excessive daytime sleepiness
Impaired concentration
Irritability/personality change
Decreased libido

Night-time
Snoring
Unrefreshing sleep
Choking episodes during sleep
Witnessed apneas
Restless sleep
Nicturia

From Management of Obstructive Sleep Apnoea/hypopnoea in Adults: A National Clinical Guideline. Edinburgh, Scotland: Scottish Inercollegiate Guidelines Network, 2003.

EPIDEMIOLOGY OF OBSTRUCTIVE SLEEP APNEA SYNDROME

The prevalence of SDB depends on the definition applied (see earlier) and on the population under study. It is estimated that about 20% of the general population displays obstructive apneas (AHI ≤ 5), whereas a full clinical picture of OSAS is seen in around 1% to 5% of men and in 0.5% to 1% of women.[4,10,11] The prevalence of habitual snoring is even higher, reaching about 25% to 35%.[10,11] The overall prevalence of sleep apneas increases with age, but this increase depends mainly on central apneas, whereas OSAS displays a peak of prevalence in middle-aged subjects,[12] with a decline after the age of 65 years.[10] Men are much more frequently affected by OSAS than women, and although the prevalence tends to increase importantly in postmenopausal women who do not receive hormone replacement therapy, it remains lower in women than in men in the same age stratum.[13]

The major epidemiologic factor associated with the presence of OSAS is increased body mass. The increasing prevalence of OSAS in Western countries parallels the progressive increase in the prevalence of overweight and obesity; OSAS is seen in about 40% of obese men and in a slightly smaller percentage of obese women. Approximately 70% of patients with OSAS are obese.[10,14]

Although OSAS is a condition affecting mainly adults, its presence in children should not be neglected, not only because of its relatively high prevalence (2% in children aged 2 to 8 years, apparently related to adenotonsillar hypertrophy) but also because of its clinical consequences, including hypertension, nocturnal enuresis, growth retardation, and cognitive impairment.[15]

OBSTRUCTIVE SLEEP APNEA SYNDROME AS A CAUSE OF SECONDARY HYPERTENSION: CLINICAL EVIDENCE AND MECHANISMS

Although arterial hypertension is a common finding in patients with OSAS, the complex link between these two phenomena is still far from being fully explained. This is because both conditions frequently appear on a common background of obesity, metabolic syndrome, and increased sympathetic activity. Nevertheless, sufficient evidence is available to support the view that hypertension and OSAS are linked with each other through the following: (1) an association related to common underlying causes, mainly obesity; and (2) a causal relationship, in which OSAS causes an elevation in BP, through acute (transient BP peaks immediately following apnea episodes) and chronic (elevated BP both day and night) mechanisms.

Association between Obstructive Sleep Apnea Syndrome and Hypertension

Population studies on the association between OSAS and hypertension demonstrated that the latter condition may be present in more than 50% of patients with OSAS, a percentage approximately 1.5 to 2 times higher than in OSAS-free subjects.[16,17] A strikingly high prevalence of OSAS was seen in patients with drug-resistant hypertension (96% in men and 65% in women), a finding suggesting that OSAS may be one of the most important causes of refractory hypertension. Indeed, in patients with refractory hypertension, a careful sleep history is mandatory, and a screening procedure (e.g., the Berlin questionnaire[8]) is highly recommended, followed by a sleep study whenever SDB is suspected.[18]

However, because of many epidemiologic, genetic, clinical, hematologic, biochemical, and physiologic similarities between OSAS and arterial hypertension (Table 11-3),[19] it was hypothesized that these two conditions merely coexist within the common framework of underlying obesity and associated metabolic changes. This possibility was considered in numerous cross-sectional and case-control studies. Multivariate analyses of study results, by taking into consideration potential confounders, have indeed consistently demonstrated a significant and independent association between OSAS and hypertension that is clinically relevant. A common finding in these studies was a significantly higher BP in patients with OSAS during the day, but even more so at night, a finding reflected by a reduced nocturnal BP fall or a "nondipping" profile.[20] The difference in BP between persons with and those without OSAS varied among studies, but a clinically and epidemiologically relevant increase of about 10 mm Hg for systolic and 5 mm Hg for diastolic BP was frequently reported.[16,20] When the risk of hypertension was expressed as an odds ratio, after adjusting for confounders, the excess risk

Table 11-3   Similarities between Obstructive Sleep Apnea Syndrome and Essential Hypertension

Similar Epidemiologic Findings
Increased prevalence of obesity and central obesity
More common in middle-aged men than women
More common in older than younger women
More common in black than white individuals
More common with alcohol abuse: alcohol an important cause of hypertension and can also worsen obstructive sleep apnea and snoring

Similar Genetic Characteristics
Similar hereditary pattern present for obstructive sleep apnea and essential hypertension

Similar Clinical Findings
Improvement with weight loss
Increased prevalence of the following:
Snoring
Cardiovascular complications
Renal damage
Cognitive dysfunction
Headaches
Impotence
Nondipping blood pressure during sleep
Increased blood pressure variability
Diabetes and insulin resistance

Similar Hematologic and Biochemical Findings
Increased sympathetic activity
Elevated atrial natriuretic factor
Reduced renin levels during sleep
Elevated hematocrit
Hyperuricemia
Elevated ratio of vasoconstrictor to vasodilator prostaglandins
Reduced testosterone levels in men
Reduced endothelium-dependent relaxation factor (nitric oxide)
Reduced blood fibrinolytic activity
Increased platelet activation and aggregation
Elevated erythropoietin levels
Elevated plasma fibrinogen levels
Elevated endothelin
Increased peripheral resistance
Elevated leptin levels
Elevated von Willebrand factor
Elevated digitalis-like factors
Increased oxidative stress
Abnormal lipid peroxidation
Elevated C-reactive protein

Similar Changes in Physiologic Mechanisms (Mainly Autonomic) Responsible for Cardiovascular and Respiratory Regulation
Increased chemoreceptor reflex sensitivity as seen by exaggerated pressor response and ventilation response to hypoxia
Reduced baroreceptor reflex sensitivity

Modified from Silverberg DS, Oksenberg A. Are sleep-related breathing disorders important contributing factors to the production of essential hypertension? *Curr Hypertens Rep.* 2001;**3**:209-215.

seen in different studies ranged from 1.3-fold to as high as 9.7-fold, depending on the population under study and on the method used to define OSAS.[11,21,22] Some discrepancies have been noted among studies regarding whether BP levels correlate with the severity of OSAS,[11] but at least in two large studies a clear-cut dose-effect relationship was seen.[16,21] In one of these studies, the increase in severity of OSAS by one apneic episode per hour of sleep increased the risk of having hypertension by approximately 1% (Fig. 11-1).[16]

Although these studies have clearly shown the existence of an independent association between OSAS and hypertension, they provide no information on whether the relationship is one of cause and effect. The only clinically significant evidence available to support the view that OSAS actually causes hypertension (even if it is not the sole cause in most patients) and that the risk of developing hypertension in OSAS is dose dependent (i.e., related to OSAS severity) was provided by the longitudinal part of the Wisconsin Sleep Cohort Study. In 709 subjects followed for 4 years, after adjustment for baseline hypertension status, body mass index, neck and waist circumferences, age, sex, alcohol and cigarette use, odds ratios for developing hypertension were 1.42, 2.03, and 2.89 for baseline AHI of 0.1 to 4.9, 5 to 14.9, and greater than 15.0, respectively, when compared with subjects with an AHI of 0.[23]

Information on factors associated with the development of hypertension in the population with SDB is still limited. It appears that an elevated risk of hypertension is mainly seen in young and nonobese subjects with severe OSAS,[17] in contrast to the tendency toward increased hypertension with advancing age observed in the general population. The mechanisms responsible for this association remain poorly understood. It could be hypothesized, however, that the lower CV reactivity and impaired CV control mechanisms that characterize elderly subjects could render them partly resistant to the effects of repeated nocturnal airway obstruction and hypoxia, which increase BP through a hypoxia-related activation of the same mechanisms.

Although OSAS is certainly the most important type of SDB in terms of hypertension development, habitual snoring without clinically relevant apnea also seems to play an independent role in determining increased BP.[24] It also appears relevant in pregnant women. In this population, habitual snoring is prevalent and is independently predictive of maternal hypertension and fetal growth retardation.[25]

Pathophysiologic Mechanisms Linking Obstructive Sleep Apnea Syndrome with Hypertension

Obstructive sleep apneas are known to influence BP and heart rate directly and acutely. This type of apnea is also responsible for increases and fluctuations in BP and heart rate that are initially confined to nighttime and subsequently extend to daytime. These changes are the consequence of (1) the mechanical effects of repeated Müller's maneuvers (i.e., the abrupt fall in intrathoracic pressure caused by an attempt to inspire, despite partly or completely obstructed upper airways), (2) the effect of chemoreceptor stimulation by hypoxemia and hypercapnia, and (3) arousal followed by restart of breathing after apnea. This process leads to a typical hemodynamic pattern consisting of two distinct phases (Fig. 11-2):

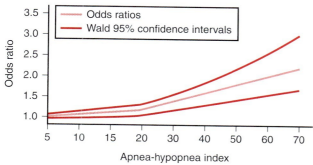

Figure 11–1   Age-, gender-, and body mass index–adjusted odds ratios for hypertension associated with apnea-hypopnea index levels of 5, 15, 30, 40, 50, 60 and 70. (From Lavie P, Herer P, Hoffstein V. Obstructive sleep apnoea syndrome as a risk factor for hypertension: Population study. *BMJ.* 2000;**320**:479-482.)

1. The first phase consists of the hemodynamic changes associated with the respiratory efforts against obstructed airways (Müller's maneuver) combined with the effects of chemoreflex stimulation. The former depend on a complex interaction of factors: increased venous return to the right ventricle, shifting of the interventricular septum to the left, impaired filling of the left ventricle, reduced stroke volume, and pulsus paradoxus (decreased systolic BP during attempted inspiration) related to changes of transmural pressure in the aorta. Initially, the hemodynamic effects of Müller's maneuver prevail, leading to an abrupt fall in sympathetic activity and a reduction of BP; later, a progressive fall in oxygen tension and an increase in carbon dioxide tension activate chemoreceptors and lead to a concomitant increase in sympathetic activity and an initial rise of BP.[6,26]

2. The restarting of breathing usually occurs after arousal (owing to hypoxemia and hypercapnia) and is characterized by hyperventilation and a further withdrawal of parasympathetic activity, accompanied by a reduction in baroreflex sensitivity. The occurrence of these changes on the background of markedly increased sympathetic activity leads to an abrupt increase in BP and heart rate.[6,27]

As a consequence of the foregoing pattern, the average values of BP and heart rate are higher in the sleep periods between successive apneas, characterized by resumption of ventilation, than during apnea. The difference is approximately 25 mm Hg for mean BP and 10 to 15 beats/minute for heart rate (Fig. 11-3).[28]

The involvement of autonomic factors has been confirmed by the observations that apneic episodes are associated with signs of sympathetic excitation independent of the effects of obesity alone.[29] In patients with severe OSAS, the occurrence of repeated and frequent apnea-related surges in sympathetic activity may directly contribute to an increase in average nocturnal BP levels. This may translate into the absence of the physiologic nocturnal BP fall (nondipping) or even into a higher mean BP level at night than during the day (reverse dipping); in fact, both phenomena are frequently observed in patients with OSAS, even if daytime values remain within normal limits. OSAS may be the most important cause of nondipping in the general population (Fig. 11-4).[19,30]

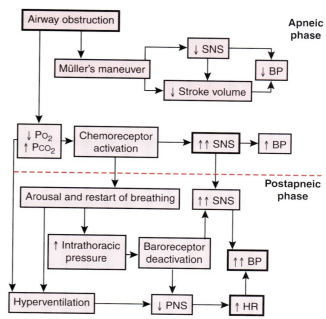

Figure 11–2   Acute physiologic changes during and immediately following an obstructive apneic episode. BP, blood pressure; HR, heart rate; PNS, parasympathetic nervous system activity; SNS, sympathetic nervous system activity.

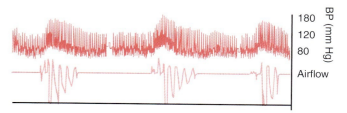

Figure 11–3   Original tracings showing the changes in continuous noninvasive finger blood pressure (BP) at the time of the apnea-hyperventilation cycles characterizing the obstructive sleep apnea syndrome.

Although the acute hemodynamic effects of apnea are easily conceivable, the mechanisms responsible for the development of chronic hypertension and, in particular, for the extension of high BP levels into the daytime are poorly understood. Several possible explanations have been suggested (Fig. 11-5).

Changes in Chemoreflexes, Arterial Baroreflexes, and Sympathetic Activity

Numerous experiments performed in subjects with OSAS provide clear evidence of the persistence of an enhanced efferent sympathetic activity to the muscle region in humans who also suffer from daytime OSAS; these findings are independent of obesity, hypertension, or gender.[31] However, the mechanisms responsible for sustained elevation of sympathetic neural activity are still largely unknown. Alterations in the chemoreflex and baroreflex control of sympathetic CV modulation appear to be of particular importance. Indeed,

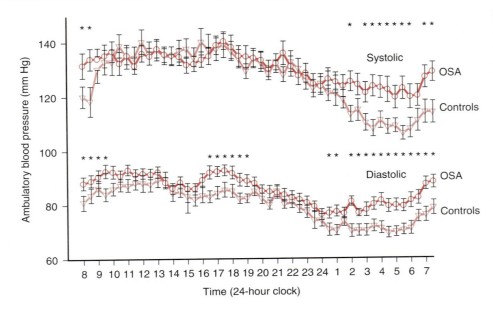

Figure 11–4 The 24-hour systolic and diastolic blood pressure profiles for patients with obstructive sleep apnea and their matched controls. Data are given as mean ± standard error of the mean. Note the clearly reduced nocturnal fall in blood pressure in the patients with obstructive sleep apnea (OSA). *Asterisks* indicate times at which the individual differences are statistically significant. (From Davies CWH, Crosby JH, Mullins RL, et al. Case-control study of 24 hour ambulatory blood pressure in patients with obstructive sleep apnoea and normal matched control subjects. *Thorax.* 2000;**55**:736-740.)

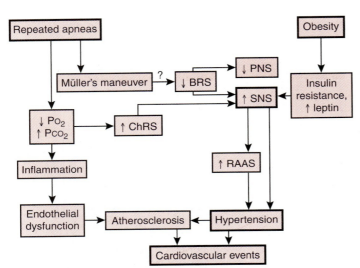

Figure 11–5 Main mechanisms involved in the pathogenesis of cardiovascular disease in obstructive sleep apnea syndromes. The role of obesity was included. BRS, baroreflex sensitivity; ChRS, chemoreflex sensitivity; PNS, parasympathetic nervous system activity; RAAS, renin-angiotensin-aldosterone system activity; SNS, sympathetic nervous system activity.

the sensitivity of chemoreflex-mediated increase in sympathetic activity in response to hypoxia is enhanced in OSAS,[32] whereas arterial baroreflex sensitivity is reduced during both day and night.[27]

Systemic Humoral Changes

The information on possible changes in the renin-angiotensin system in OSAS is limited and frequently conflicting. Higher angiotensin-converting enzyme activity[33] and higher aldosterone excretion[34] in patients with OSAS than in controls, as seen in some studies, suggest that the renin-angiotensin-aldosterone system may be involved in the pathogenesis of

OSAS-related hypertension. However, it is not clear whether this involvement is merely secondary to other changes (e.g., sympathetic activation) or whether the system has an independent role.

Endothelial Function and Inflammation

Studies on the pathogenesis of CV diseases including hypertension have shown an important role played by generalized inflammatory processes, paralleled by impaired endothelial function. Such changes occur also in OSAS, probably as a result of repeated exposure to hypoxia.

Data that support the involvement of endothelial dysfunction in OSAS include elevated levels of circulating endothelin-1, reduction of levels of nitric oxide metabolites, impairment of endothelium-dependent vasodilation, and enhanced sensitivity to vasoconstrictors.[35-38]

An important mechanism in the pathogenesis of hypoxia-induced endothelial dysfunction in OSAS may be increased generation of free radicals, similar to that observed in the oxidative stress provoked by ischemia and reperfusion. Oxidative stress leads to a generalized inflammatory response in other conditions as well as in patients with OSAS; elevated levels of several markers of inflammation, including C-reactive protein, tumor necrosis factor-α, and interleukin-6 have been observed.[39-41] The foregoing changes may lead to a chronic increase in vascular resistance and, as a consequence, to arterial hypertension, in parallel with an acceleration of atherosclerosis.

Metabolic Consequences of Obstructive Sleep Apnea Syndrome

Elevated levels of leptin, a hormone involved in the pathogenesis of obesity and metabolic syndrome, were repeatedly demonstrated in OSAS, even after adjustment for body fat.[41,42] Other metabolic alterations typical of the metabolic syndrome, such as insulin resistance, have also been observed; the degree of these alterations correlated with the severity of OSAS.[41,43] The origin of these changes is uncertain, but both hypoxia and fragmented sleep may be involved. The epidemiologic association and pathophysiologic similarities between OSAS and metabolic syndrome make some authors believe that the former should be considered an additional element of the latter (the so-called Z syndrome).

Impact of Obstructive Sleep Apnea Syndrome on Central Nervous System Mechanisms

Sleep disturbance is an important source of generalized stress. Fragmented sleep, repeated arousals, and oxygen desaturation were shown to be among the most important determinants of an abnormal circadian rhythm of BP.[44] Furthermore, fragmented sleep in habitual snorers is related to an increased risk of hypertension, even in subjects without OSAS.[45]

CLINICAL IMPORTANCE OF HYPERTENSION RELATED TO OBSTRUCTIVE SLEEP APNEA SYNDROME

The investigation of the prognostic importance of OSAS is strongly influenced by the concomitant presence of important risk factors for CV disease, above all abdominal obesity, but also insulin resistance, diabetes, dyslipidemia, increased sympathetic activity, and worsened respiratory function.[46] These factors can hardly be accounted for in studies exploring the prognostic relevance of OSAS, and this makes the interpretation of their results extremely difficult.

In one of the first studies on this issue, He and colleagues not only showed an association between OSAS and CV mortality, but also demonstrated that this association is dose dependent. The risk of death in this study was linearly related to the AHI, with a tendency of the slope of this relationship to increase when the AHI was higher than 20.[47] The most convincing evidence on the prognostic importance of OSAS comes from a 7-year follow-up study of a cohort of middle-aged men without diabetes or hypertension at baseline. The risk of CV morbidity was independently increased by the presence of OSAS (36.7% of subjects with OSAS developed CV disease versus 6.6% of subjects without OSAS) (Fig. 11-6).[48] These results were further supported by the demonstration of an increased CV risk in untreated patients with severe OSAS.[49] When focusing specifically on particular types of CV consequences of OSAS, associations with coronary heart disease, heart failure, cardiac arrhythmias, and cerebrovascular diseases were observed.[50,51] Some data suggest that OSAS may be of particular importance in predicting cerebrovascular complications and less important in predicting coronary events.[52] A particular difficulty that affects cross-sectional studies on the association between OSAS and cerebrovascular events lies in that, in many cases, SDB occurs or worsens after a stroke.[51] According to a recent longitudinal cohort study, OSAS is a significant risk factor for the composite outcome of death and stroke, independent of other risk factors including hypertension and atrial fibrillation.[51a]

The prognostic consequences of OSAS are not equal in all populations. The occurrence of OSAS does not appear to influence morbidity and mortality in elderly patients.[52] Some data are available to indicate that snoring by itself can also be a risk factor, especially in younger persons.[53]

Some studies have dealt with intermediate endpoints, such as left ventricular structure and function or structural and functional changes in large arteries. Although in some of these studies, a relationship between OSAS and left ventricular mass or diastolic dysfunction was seen, it appears that it was exclusively related to hypertension and not to OSAS itself.[54] Conversely, an acceleration of atherosclerotic changes in carotid arteries was seen in patients with OSAS.[55] Taken together, these data may thus corroborate the hypothesis that OSAS is independently associated with adverse consequences in the cerebral (or peripheral) circulation, whereas its cardiac effects seem to be mediated by other changes, such as hypertension. This hypothesis requires further confirmation, however.

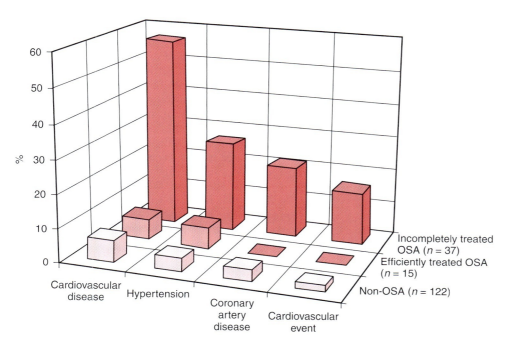

Figure 11-6 Incidence of cardiovascular disease events during 7 years of follow-up in otherwise healthy middle-aged men at baseline. This figure shows the proportion of individuals with an incidence of cardiovascular event, coronary artery disease, hypertension, and overall cardiovascular disease in those with incompletely treated obstructive sleep apnea (OSA), those with efficiently treated OSA, and those without OSA. (From Peker Y, Hedner J, Norum J, et al. Increased incidence of cardiovascular disease in middle-aged men with obstructive sleep apnea: A 7-year follow-up. *Am J Respir Crit Care Med.* 2002;**166**:159-165.)

MANAGEMENT OF HYPERTENSIVE PATIENTS WITH OBSTRUCTIVE SLEEP APNEA SYNDROME

One of the key features defining any type of secondary hypertension is the observation that by treating the underlying condition, BP is improved. Currently, the treatment of choice in OSAS is the nocturnal application of either classic or modified nasal continuous positive airway pressure (CPAP).[4] By increasing pressure in the airways, CPAP prevents the collapse of the upper airways and the occurrence of obstructive apneas. This leads to a major reduction in the frequency of apneas and to a disappearance of apnea-related BP and heart rate peaks.[56] A reduction in the pressor response to apneas was also seen on the first night after CPAP suspension,[7] a finding suggesting that regular CPAP may, at least in part, reverse the adverse changes in CV regulation caused by OSAS.

Numerous clinical studies have assessed the possible association between the application of CPAP in OSAS and prolonged arterial BP reduction. Unfortunately, some of these studies were affected by methodologic problems, the most important being the lack of proper control groups and inadequate BP measurement techniques. Only a few placebo-controlled studies are currently available, but even these do not provide definitive answers.

In contrast to the discouraging results of studies using oral preparations as placebo, in two analyses in which CPAP at subtherapeutic pressures was used as a physical placebo in control groups, significant BP reductions were demonstrated in active treatment groups, particularly when daytime BP was considered.[57,58] The average reductions of BP induced by effective CPAP in one of these studies, characterized by a particularly long treatment time (9 weeks), were 10.0 mm Hg during the day and 10.3 mm Hg at night (Fig. 11-7).[57]

Convincing evidence that treatment of severe OSAS may be beneficial for CV risk reduction was presented in a recent analysis of observational data. When compared with OSAS-free subjects, the subjects with severe OSAS but no CPAP treatment displayed a three times higher risk of CV events, both fatal and nonfatal, even after adjustment for major risk factors. No excess risk was seen in subjects who received CPAP treatment, but this was the case also in a subgroup of subjects with mild and moderate OSAS and no CPAP treatment.[49]

The mechanisms underlying the BP-lowering effect of CPAP were investigated in numerous studies, most of them focusing on changes in autonomic CV control. CPAP reduced sympathetic and increased parasympathetic activity, increased stroke volume and cardiac output, and decreased systemic vascular resistance.[59] These changes can be mediated by an increase in baroreflex sensitivity, but also by changes in some non-neural mechanisms (Fig. 11-8).[60] An improvement in baroreflex sensitivity by long-lasting CPAP treatment was shown by studies making use of spontaneous baroreflex analysis, which allows the sensitivity of arterial baroreflex control of heart rate to be assessed through computer analysis of the interactions between spontaneous systolic BP fluctuations and the subsequent reflex fluctuations in R-R interval of the electrocardiogram.[2,7,27,60] The decrease in BP and risk reduction achieved with CPAP therapy in OSAS patients may be also derived from an improvement in metabolic parameters[43] or endothelial function.[61]

Apart from CPAP, some other strategies for treating OSAS have also been developed, including oral appliances and sur-

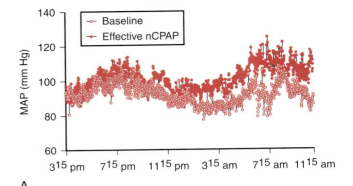

A

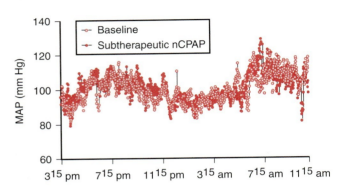

B

Figure 11–7 Time course of mean arterial pressure (MAP) before *(closed circles)* and during *(open circles)* treatment with therapeutic (**A**) and subtherapeutic (**B**) nasal continuous positive airway pressure (nCPAP). (From Becker HF, Jerrentrup A, Ploch T, et al. Effect of nasal continuous positive airway pressure treatment on blood pressure in patients with obstructive sleep apnea. *Circulation.* 2003;**107**:68-73.)

gical procedures (the most popular being uvulopalatoplasty). The efficacy of these methods is questionable, however, and their effects on BP are being studied.

An issue of great importance is the choice of the most suitable antihypertensive drug or drugs to be administered to patients with OSAS and high BP. Because increased sympathetic activity appears to be one of the key mechanisms, a possible benefit from the administration of adrenergic blocking agents was hypothesized. Although some data are available to support this hypothesis,[62] they do not appear sufficient to allow definitive recommendation of this class of drugs in treating OSAS-related hypertension, especially in light of the possible aggravation of the metabolic changes frequently present in patients with OSAS. Other suggestions focus on the use of drugs that interfere with the renin-angiotensin-aldosterone system or long-acting calcium channel blockers belonging to the dihydropyridine subclass.

CONCLUSIONS

The evidence reviewed in this chapter emphasizes the association between SDB, in particular OSAS, and arterial hypertension, and it provides some insight into the mechanisms potentially involved in this association. The clinical implica-

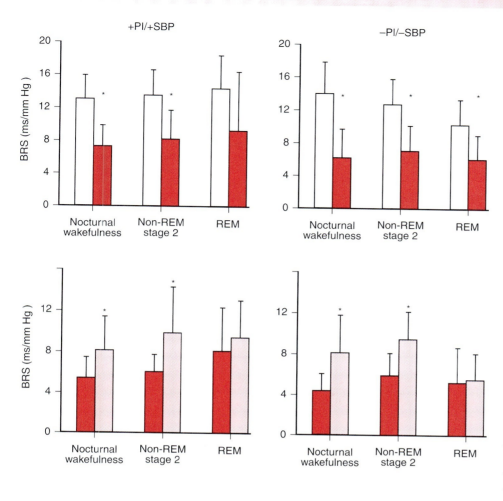

Figure 1–8 **Top,** Spontaneous baroreflex control of heart rate during sleep in normal subjects *(white bars)* and untreated patients with obstructive sleep apnea syndrome (OSAS, *red bars).* Asterisks indicate significant differences between control and OSAS groups (*P* < .0005). **Bottom,** Effect of long-term continuous positive airway pressure (CPAP) on baroreflex control of heart rate during sleep. *Red bars,* untreated OSAS; *orange bars,* first night of CPAP withdrawal after long-term CPAP treatment; *asterisks,* significant differences between pretreatment and post-treatment studies; BRS, baroreflex sensitivity; +PI/+SBP and –PI/–SBP, hypertension/ bradycardia and hypotension/ tachycardia sequences, respectively; REM, rapid eye movement. (Modified from Bonsignore MR, Parati G, Insalaco G, et al. Continuous positive airway pressure treatment improves baroreflex control of heart rate during sleep in severe obstructive sleep apnea syndrome. *Am J Respir Crit Care Med.* 2002;**166**:279-286.)

tions of the demonstrated link between hypertension and OSAS include the need for more systematic search for SDB among hypertensive patients at the time of their diagnostic evaluation, ranging from an accurate sleep history to performance of full polysomnography when appropriate. This demanding diagnostic approach should be considered in obese patients with hypertension and in those hypertensive patients who display a reproducible attenuation or disappearance of the physiologic nocturnal BP reduction (i.e., "nondippers") during 24-hour ambulatory BP monitoring. Given the potential benefits of CPAP in these patients, detection of SDB and its adequate treatment by properly titrated CPAP could represent important steps toward better control of BP in hypertensive patients, in particular in patients with refractory hypertension.

Because of the large scale of the problem in the general population and evidence that even mild OSAS (which is quite common) can induce a significant increase in BP, OSAS has important implications for both clinical medicine and public health. OSAS should be addressed much more extensively by hypertension guidelines. At present, the 2003 seventh report of the Joint National Committee merely mentions OSAS as a potentially identifiable cause of secondary hypertension,[63] without discussing the diagnosis and treatment of OSAS in any detail. Moreover, the 2003 European Society of Hypertension and European Society of Cardiology guidelines for hypertension management fail to address the issue at all.[64]

References

1. Somers VK, Dyken ME, Mark AL, Abboud FM. Sympathetic-nerve activity during sleep in normal subjects. *N Engl J Med.* 1993;**328**:303-307.
2. Parati G, Di Rienzo M, Bertinieri G, et al. Evaluation of the baroreceptor-heart rate reflex by 24-hour intra-arterial blood pressure monitoring in humans. *Hypertension.* 1988;**12**:214-222.
3. Mancia G, Zanchetti A. Cardiovascular regulation during sleep. *In:* Orem J (ed.). Handbook of Physiology during Sleep. New York: Academic Press, 1980, pp 1-55.
4. Management of Obstructive Sleep Apnoea/Hypopnoea in Adults: A National Clinical Guideline. Edinburgh, Scotland: Scottish Intercollegiate Guidelines Network, 2003.
5. American Academy of Sleep Medicine Task Force. Sleep-related breathing disorders in adults: Recommendations for syndrome definition and measurement techniques in clinical research. *Sleep.* 1999;**22**:667-689.
6. Parati G, Ongaro G, Bonsignore MR, et al. Sleep apnoea and hypertension. *Curr Opin Nephrol Hypertens.* 2002;**11**:201-214.
7. Castiglioni P, Bonsignore MR, Insalaco G, et al. Signal processing procedures for the evaluation of the cardiovascular effects in the obstructive sleep apnea syndrome *Comput Cardiol.* 2001;**28**:221-224.
8. Netzer NC, Stoohs RA, Netzer CM, et al. Using the Berlin Questionnaire to identify patients at risk for the sleep apnea syndrome. *Ann Intern Med.* 1999;**131**:485-491.
9. George CF, Smiley A. Sleep apnea and automobile crashes. *Sleep.* 1999;**22**:790-795.

10. Young T, Peppard PE, Gottlieb DJ. Epidemiology of obstructive sleep apnea: A population health perspective. *Am J Respir Crit Care Med.* 2002;**165**:1217-1239.

11. Duran J, Esnaola S, Rubio R, Iztueta A. Obstructive sleep apnea-hypopnea and related clinical features in a population-based sample of subjects aged 30 to 70 years. *Am J Respir Crit Care Med.* 2001;**163**:685-689.

12. Bixler EO, Vgontzas AN, Ten Have T, et al. Effects of age on sleep apnea in men: I. Prevalence and severity. *Am J Respir Crit Care Med.* 1998;**157**:144-148.

13. Bixler EO, Vgontzas AN, Lin H-M, et al. Prevalence of sleep-disordered breathing in women: Effects of gender. *Am J Respir Crit Care Med.* 2001;**163**:608-613.

14. Wolk R, Shamsuzzaman ASM, Somers VK. Obesity, sleep apnea, and hypertension. *Hypertension.* 2003;**42**:1067-1074.

15. Gozal D, O'Brien LM. Snoring and obstructive sleep apnea in children: Why should we treat? *Paediatr Respir Rev.* 2004;**5 (Suppl A)**:S371-S376.

16. Lavie P, Herer P, Hoffstein V. Obstructive sleep apnoea syndrome as a risk factor for hypertension: Population study. *BMJ.* 2000;**320**:479-482.

17. Grote L, Ploch T, Heitmann J, et al. Sleep-related breathing disorder is an independent risk factor for systemic hypertension. *Am J Respir Crit Care Med.* 1999;**160**:1875-1882.

18. Logan AG, Perlikowski SM, Mente A, et al. High prevalence of unrecognized sleep apnea in drug-resistant hypertension. *J Hypertens.* 2000;**19**:2271-2277.

19. Silverberg DS, Oksenberg A. Are sleep-related breathing disorders important contributing factors to the production of essential hypertension? *Curr Hypertens Rep.* 2001;**3**:209-215.

20. Davies CWH, Crosby JH, Mullins RL, et al. Case-control study of 24 hour ambulatory blood pressure in patients with obstructive sleep apnoea and normal matched control subjects. *Thorax.* 2000; **55**:736-740.

21. Nieto FJ, Young TB, Lind BK, et al. Association of sleep-disordered breathing, sleep apnea, and hypertension in a large community-based study. *JAMA.* 2000;**283**:1829-1836.

22. Ohayon MM, Guilleminault C, Priest RG, et al. Is sleep-disordered breathing an independent risk factor for hypertension in the general population (13,057 subjects)? *J Psychosom Res.* 2000;**48**:593-601.

23. Peppard PE, Young T, Palta M, Skatrud J. Prospective study of the association between sleep-disordered breathing and hypertension. *N Engl J Med.* 2000;**342**:1378-1384.

24. Young T, Finn L, Hla M, et al. Snoring as a part of a dose-response relationship between sleep-disordered breathing and blood pressure. *Sleep.* 1996;**19**:S202-S205.

25. Franklin KA, Holmgren PA, Johnsson F, et al. Snoring, pregnancy-induced hypertension, and growth retardation of the fetus. *Chest.* 2000;**117**:137-141.

26. Somers VK, Dyken ME, Skinner JL. Autonomic and hemodynamic responses and interactions during the Müeller maneuver in humans. *Auton Nerv Syst.* 1993;**44**:253-259.

27. Parati G, Di Rienzo M, Bonsignore MR, et al. Autonomic cardiac regulation in obstructive sleep apnea syndrome: Evidence from spontaneous baroreflex analysis during sleep. *J Hypertens.* 1997;**15**:1621-1626.

28. Tun Y, Okabe S, Hida W, et al. Nocturnal blood pressure during apnoeic and ventilatory periods in patients with obstructive sleep apnoea. *Eur Respir J.* 1999;**14**:1271-1277.

29. Narkiewicz K, van de Borne PJ, Cooley RL, et al. Sympathetic activity in obese subjects with and without obstructive sleep apnea. *Circulation.* 1998;**98**:772-776.

30. Stradling JR, Barbour C, Glennon J, et al. Which aspects of breathing during sleep influence the overnight fall of blood pressure in a community population? *Thorax.* 2000;**55**: 393-398.

31. Phillips BG, Somers VK. Neural and humoral mechanism mediating cardiovascular responses to obstructive sleep apnea. *Respir Physiol.* 2000;**119**:181-187.

32. Narkiewicz K, van de Borne PJH, Pesek CA, et al. Selective potentiation of peripheral chemoreflex sensitivity in obstructive sleep apnea. *Circulation.* 1999;**99**:1183-1189.

33. Barcelò A, Elorza MA, Barbè F, et al. Angiotensin converting enzyme in patients with sleep apnoea syndrome: Plasma activity and gene polymorphism. *Eur Respir J.* 2001;**17**:728-732.

34. Calhoun DA, Nishizaka KM, Zaman MA, Harding SM. Aldosterone excretion among subjects with resistant hypertension and symptoms of sleep apnea. *Chest.* 2004;**125**:112-117.

35. Saarelainen S, Seppala E, Laasonen K, Hasan J. Circulating endothelin-1 in obstructive sleep apnea. *Endothelium.* 1997;**5**: 115-118.

36. Schulz R, Schmidt D, Blum A, et al. Decreased plasma levels of nitric oxide derivatives in obstructive sleep apnoea: Response to CPAP therapy. *Thorax.* 2000;**55**:1046-1051.

37. Kato M, Roberts-Thomson P, Phillips BG, et al. Impairment of endothelium-dependent vasodilation of resistance vessels in patients with obstructive sleep apnea. *Circulation.* 2000;**102**: 2607-2610.

38. Kraiczi H, Hedner J, Yüksel P, et al. Increased vasoconstrictor sensitivity in obstructive sleep apnea. *J Appl Physiol.* 2000;**89**: 493-498.

39. Prabhakar NR. Sleep apneas: An oxidative stress? *Am J Respir Crit Care Med.* 2002;**165**:859-860.

40. Yokoe T, Minoguchi K, Matsuo H, et al. Elevated levels of C-reactive protein and interleukin-6 in patients with obstructive sleep apnea syndrome are decreased by nasal continuous positive airway pressure. *Circulation.* 2003;**107**:1129-1134.

41. Vgontzas AN, Papanicolaou DA, Bixler EO, et al. Sleep apnea and daytime sleepiness and fatigue: Relation to visceral obesity, insulin resistance, and hypercytokinemia. *J Clin Endocrinol Metab.* 2000;**85**:1151-1158.

42. Marik PE. Leptin, obesity and obstructive sleep apnea. *Chest.* 2000;**118**:569-570.

43. Punjabi NM, Sorkin JD, Katzel LI, et al. Sleep-disordered breathing and insulin resistance in middle-aged and overweight men. *Am J Respir Crit Care Med.* 2002;**165**:677-682.

44. Noda A, Yasuma F, Okada T, et al. Influence of movement arousal on circadian rhythm of blood pressure in obstructive sleep apnea syndrome. *J Hypertens.* 2000;**18**:539-544.

45. Morrell MJ, Finn L, Kim H, et al. Sleep fragmentation, awake blood pressure, and sleep-disordered breathing in a population-based study. *Am J Respir Crit Care Med.* 2000;**162**:2091-2096.

46. Kiely JL, McNicholas WT. Cardiovascular risk factors in patients with obstructive sleep apnoea syndrome. *Eur Respir J.* 2000;**16**: 128-133.

47. He J, Kryger MH, Zorick FJ, et al. Mortality and apnea index in obstructive sleep apnea: Experience in 385 male patients. *Chest.* 1988;**94**:9-14.

48. Peker Y, Hedner J, Norum J, et al. Increased incidence of cardiovascular disease in middle-aged men with obstructive sleep apnea: A 7-year follow-up. *Am J Respir Crit Care Med.* 2002;**166**:159-165.

49. Marin JM, Carrizo SJ, Vicente E, Agusti AGN. Long-term cardiovascular outcomes in men with obstructive sleep apnoea-hypopnoea with or without treatment with continuous positive airway pressure: An observational study. *Lancet.* 2005;**365**: 1046-1053.

50. Quan SF, Gersh BJ, National Center on Sleep Disorders Research, National Heart, Lung and Blood Institute. Cardiovascular consequences of sleep-disordered breathing: past, present and future: Report of a workshop from the National Center on Sleep Disorders Research and the National Heart, Lung and Blood Institute. *Circulation.* 2004;**109**:951-957.

51. Mohsenin V. Sleep-related breathing disorders and risk of stroke. *Stroke.* 2001;**32**:1271-1278.

51a. Yaggi HK, Concato J, Kernan WN, et al. Obstructive sleep apnea as a risk factor for stroke and death. *N Engl J Med.* 2005;**353**:2034–2041.

52. Mooe T, Franklin KA, Holmström K, et al. Sleep-disordered breathing and coronary artery disease: Long-term prognosis. *Am J Respir Crit Care Med.* 2001;**164**:1910-1913

53. Lindberg E, Janson C, Svärdsudd K, et al. Increased mortality among sleepy snorers: A prospective population based study. *Thorax.* 1998;**53**:631-637.

54. Niroumand M, Kuperstein R, Sasson Z, et al. Impact of obstructive sleep apnea on left ventricular mass and diastolic function. *Am J Crit Care Med.* 2001;**163**:1632-1636.

55. Silvestrini M, Rizzato B, Placidi F, et al. Carotid artery wall thickness in patients with obstructive sleep apnea syndrome. *Stroke.* 2002;**33**:1782-1785.

56. Bonsignore MR, Marrone O, Insalaco G, Bonsignore G. The cardiovascular effects of obstructive sleep apnoeas: Analysis of pathogenetic mechanisms. *Eur Respir J.* 1994;**7**:786-805.

57. Dimsdale JE, Loredo JS, Profant J. Effect of continuous positive airway pressure on blood pressure. *Hypertension.* 2000;**35**:144-147.

58. Becker HF, Jerrentrup A, Ploch T, et al. Effect of nasal continuous positive airway pressure treatment on blood pressure in patients with obstructive sleep apnea. *Circulation.* 2003;**107**:68-73.

59. Nelesen RA, Yu H, Ziegler MG, et al. Continuous positive airway pressure normalizes cardiac autonomic and hemodynamic responses to a laboratory stressor in apneic patients. *Chest.* 2001;**119**:1092-1101.

60. Bonsignore MR, Parati G, Insalaco G, et al. Continuous positive airway pressure treatment improves baroreflex control of heart rate during sleep in severe obstructive sleep apnea syndrome. *Am J Respir Crit Care Med.* 2002;**166**:279-286.

61. Imadojemu VA, Gleeson K, Quraishi SA, et al. Impaired vasodilator responses in obstructive sleep apnea are improved with continuous positive airway pressure therapy. *Am J Respir Crit Care Med.* 2002;**165**:950-953.

62. Kraiczi H, Hedner J, Yüksel P, et al. Comparison of atenolol, amlodipine, enalapril, hydrochlorothiazide, and losartan for antihypertensive treatment in patients with obstructive sleep apnea. *Am J Resp Crit Care Med.* 2000;**161**:1423-1428.

63. Chobanian AV, Bakris GL, Black HR, et al., and the National High Blood Pressure Education Program Coordinating Committee. The Seventh Report of the Joint National Committee on Prevention, Detection, Evaluation, and Treatment of High Blood Pressure: The JNC 7 report. *JAMA.* 2003;**289**:2560-2572.

64. European Society of Hypertension-European Society of Cardiology. 2003 European Society of Hypertension–European Society of Cardiology guidelines for the management of arterial hypertension. *J Hypertens.* 2003;**21**:1011-1053.

Chapter 12

Rare and Unusual Forms of Hypertension

Ehud Grossman and Franz H. Messerli

Most patients with hypertension have essential hypertension or well-known forms of secondary hypertension, such as those associated with renal disease, renal artery stenosis, or common endocrine diseases (hyperaldosteronism or pheochromocytoma). Physicians are less aware of rare and unusual forms of hypertension. These may include overestimation of the true blood pressure (BP) because of technical problems of BP measurement or rare diseases that usually go unrecognized. In this chapter, we discuss some rare and unusual causes of hypertension.

TECHNICAL PROBLEMS OF BLOOD PRESSURE MEASUREMENT

The diagnosis of hypertension is based on BP measurements with a sphygmomanometer. BP levels of 140/90 mm Hg and higher are arbitrarily considered hypertensive, whereas BP levels of 139/89 mm Hg or less are considered normal or prehypertensive.[1] The precise diagnosis of hypertension is based on the assumption that BP measurements are very accurate and can separate 140 from 139 mm Hg. However, many factors may affect the accuracy of office BP measurements, and many patients may therefore be falsely labeled as hypertensive or normotensive. Moreover, some technical problems in BP measurement may give erroneously elevated BP levels and lead to a wrong diagnosis of hypertension. We briefly discuss some common technical problems that may increase BP levels.

Clearly, it is a great challenge to determine BP accurately (see Chapter 5). The accurate measurement of BP is the sine qua non for successful management. The guidelines for BP measurement emphasize the importance of using validated devices that undergo periodic maintenance and calibration.[2,3] For example, a cuff that is too narrow or not centered or a leaky bulb valve may increase the BP reading. Rouse and Marshall assessed the accuracy of sphygmomanometers in general practices.[4] Of 1462 sphygmomanometers, 9.2% gave inaccurate readings by more than 5 mm Hg. These authors concluded that because of this inaccuracy, women who are less than 35 years old may be misclassified as hypertensive and may receive inappropriate treatment. False BP readings may be attributed not only to faulty equipment but also to poor technique. If the patient's arm is much below heart level, or if the patient supports his or her own arm with effort, BP will appear falsely high. A loose cuff or a bladder that balloons outside the cuff also leads to falsely high readings.

Mejia and colleagues evaluated 15 patients with refractory hypertension by simultaneous cuff and intra-arterial BP measurements.[5] The average cuff diastolic reading was 11.4 mm Hg higher than the intra-arterial reading. Seven patients had normal mean intra-arterial BP. Of these patients, three had a cuff diastolic pressure that was more than 15 mm Hg higher than the intra-arterial reading. This phenomenon was called "cuff inflation hypertension" because the marked rise of intra-arterial BP occurred during cuff inflation and rapidly returned to baseline when the cuff was fully deflated. This phenomenon recurred during each cuff inflation and deflation. In one patient the intra-arterial pressure increased from 132/65 mm Hg before cuff inflation to 150/90 mm Hg during inflation.

Certain groups of people merit special consideration for BP measurement. These include the elderly, who often have isolated systolic hypertension, and obese people, in whom the inflatable bladder may be too small for the arm size, thereby leading to "cuff hypertension."[6,7]

In some elderly patients with very rigid, calcified arteries, more pressure in the bladder is needed to compress the brachial artery; this gives rise to falsely high readings, a phenomenon termed *pseudohypertension*.[8] The possibility of pseudohypertension (cuff diastolic BP ≥15 mm Hg higher than simultaneously determined intra-arterial pressure) should be suspected in elderly patients who have little or no target organ damage, despite markedly high BP readings, and who suffer inordinate postural symptoms despite cautious therapy. The Osler maneuver, in which the radial pulse remains palpable after the pressure in the balloon has occluded the brachial artery, has been suggested to identify this entity.[8] However, this maneuver is not diagnostic because of marked intraobserver and interobserver disagreement[9] and because it is frequently present in elderly people with normal BP.[10] An automatic oscillometric recorder or finger BP measurement may help to diagnose this entity,[11] but only direct intra-arterial reading is diagnostic.

Another common phenomenon that may lead to inaccurate BP readings in elderly patients is an *auscultatory gap*—a silent interval that may be present between the systolic and the diastolic pressures. An unrecognized auscultatory gap may lead to serious underestimation of systolic pressure or overestimation of diastolic pressure. Cavallini and associates evaluated 168 patients with hypertension who were otherwise healthy and were not receiving medications.[12] Classic auscultatory gaps were present in 21% of the patients. Female sex, arterial stiffness, and atherosclerotic plaques were independently associated with the presence of auscultatory gaps. To avoid the error caused by an auscultatory gap, it is recommended first to estimate the systolic pressure by palpation, then to inflate the cuff 30 mm Hg above the level of radial pulse disappearance. The systolic pressure is determined when Korotkoff sounds first appear, and the diastolic pressure is measured when the sounds disappear. To avoid overestimation of the diastolic pressure, it is necessary to confirm the disappearance of the sounds by listening as the pressure falls another 10 to 20 mm Hg.

RARE AND UNUSUAL CAUSES OF HYPERTENSION

Iatrogenic Causes

Hypertension related to drugs and other substances represents an important, modifiable, unnoticed source of secondary hypertension.[13] An accurate and detailed medical history should include specific inquiries concerning foods, poisons, and medications, such as vitamins and dietary supplements, that patients often do not consider to be drugs and therefore frequently omit from their history. Identification of such substances is important because their elimination can obviate the need for unnecessary, costly, and potentially dangerous evaluations and treatments. When drug-induced or chemically induced hypertension is identified, discontinuation of the causative agent is recommended.[13]

Steroids

Hypertension occurs in about 20% of patients treated with high doses of synthetic corticosteroids. Oral cortisol increases BP in a dose-dependent fashion. At a dose of 80 to 200 mg/day, the peak increase in systolic pressure is of the order of 15 mm Hg. The increase in BP is apparent within 24 hours. The mechanism of glucocorticoid-induced hypertension remains uncertain and seems to be multi-factorial. Glucocorticoid-induced hypertension is more common in elderly patients and in patients with positive family history of essential hypertension. Certain exogenous compounds such as liquorice, phenylbutazone, carbenoxolone, 9-α-fluoroprednisolone, and 9-α-fluorocortisol have mineralocorticoid activity and, when ingested in excessive quantities, may produce arterial hypertension, characterized by increased exchangeable sodium and blood volume, hypokalemia with metabolic alkalosis, and suppressed plasma renin and aldosterone levels. Prolonged use of high-dose ketoconazole may alter enzymatic degradation of steroids and lead to mineralocorticoid-related hypertension. Skin ointments, antihemorrhoidal preparations, ophthalmic drops, and nasal sprays may contain substances with mineralocorticoid activity (9-α-fluoroprednisolone) or sympathetic amines. Their excessive use may cause severe arterial hypertension. Discontinuation of these substances is recommended to lower BP. However, when steroid treatment is mandatory, a diuretic is the drug of choice because volume overload is the main mechanism by which steroids raise BP; careful monitoring of potassium concentrations is necessary.

Sex Hormones

Oral contraceptives induce hypertension in approximately 5% of users of high-dose pills that contain at least 50 μg of estrogen and 1 to 4 mg of progestin, and small increases in BP have been reported even among users of modern low-dose formulations. Women with a history of high BP during pregnancy, those with a family history of hypertension, cigarette smokers, obese, black, or diabetic women, and those with renal disease may respond with a greater increase in BP. Compared with women who have never used oral contraceptives, users of oral contraceptives have an increased risk of development of hypertension (risk ratio, 1.8; 95% confidence interval, 1.5 to 2.3). However, only in a small percentage of women can hypertension be attributed to oral contraceptive use. The risk of hypertension decreases quickly with cessation of oral contraceptives, and past users appear to have only a slightly increased risk. The increased BP is usually minimal, although severe hypertensive episodes, including malignant hypertension, have been reported. Cessation of the oral contraceptive is recommended when new-onset hypertension occurs.

Postmenopausal estrogen replacement therapy has minimal effect on arterial pressure, and rare cases of estrogen-induced hypertension represent an idiosyncratic reaction to this therapy. The use of estrogen replacement therapy has been associated with increased cardiovascular morbidity and mortality, and therefore it is not routinely recommended.[14-17] Men receiving estrogen for the treatment of prostatic cancer may also exhibit an increase in BP, but this therapy is no longer as common as it once was. Danazol, a semisynthetic androgen used in the treatment of endometriosis and hereditary angioedema, has been reported to induce hypertension as a result of fluid retention.

Anesthetics and Narcotics

Several anesthetic and narcotic agents such as ketamine hydrochloride, desflurane, and sevoflurane may induce hypertension. The simultaneous use of vasoconstrictors (felypressin) with topical cocaine can result in severe hypertension. Hypertensive responses to naloxone (an opiate antagonist), especially during attempted reversal of narcotic-induced anesthesia in hypertensive patients, have also been reported. Naloxone seems to reverse the antihypertensive effects of clonidine acutely and can thereby cause a hypertensive emergency.

Drugs Affecting the Sympathetic Nervous System

Phenylephrine, a sympathomimetic agent with potent vasoconstrictor activity, has been reported to increase BP severely following its administration in an ophthalmic solution. Dipivefrin, an epinephrine prodrug used topically in the management of chronic simple glaucoma, can also increase BP in treated hypertensive patients.

The concomitant use of sympathomimetic agents and β-blockers can severely increase arterial pressure because of unopposed α-adrenergic vasoconstriction. Antiemetic agents such as metoclopramide, alizapride, and prochlorperazine have been reported to increase BP transiently in patients treated with cisplatin.

Yohimbine hydrochloride—an α₂-adrenoceptor antagonist that was approved for treatment of impotence—may significantly increase BP in hypertensive patients. Glucagon may induce severe hypertension in patients with pheochromocytoma. Blocking α-adrenoceptors by either intravenous phentolamine or oral agents such as phenoxybenzamine or doxazosin may prevent catastrophic cardiovascular events.

Cocaine intoxication is characterized by α-adrenergic overactivity associated with increased BP. Cocaine use is associated with acute but not chronic hypertension.

Sibutramine is a novel serotonin and norepinephrine reuptake inhibitor that is used as an antiobesity drug. Sibutramine reduces food intake by enhancing the physiologic response of postingestive satiety and increases energy expenditure. By activating the sympathetic nervous system, the drug increases heart rate and BP in obese normotensive subjects. In obese hypertensive patients, the BP reduction achieved by weight loss negates the potential BP increase related to the drug. Nevertheless, obese patients treated with sibutramine should be monitored periodically for changes in BP.[18]

Clozapine is an antipsychotic agent used for schizophrenic symptoms in patients refractory to classical antipsychotics. This drug may raise BP by sympathetic activation. Several case reports of pseudopheochromocytoma syndrome associated with clozapine have been described. BP and sympathetic overactivity were normalized on discontinuation of treatment.

Immunosuppressive Agents

Cyclosporine A, a potent, orally active immunosuppressive drug, may induce arterial hypertension. The incidence of cyclosporine-associated hypertension (CAH) varies with the patient population under evaluation. The greatest experience to date has been with patients undergoing organ transplantation, and kidney recipients represent the largest single group. CAH is also common in patients with autoimmune disease and dermatologic disorders. The risk of CAH is unrelated to sex or race, but it is dose related, and it increases with age of the patient and with preexisting hypertension or high serum creatinine levels. Although most patients present with mild to moderate asymptomatic BP elevation, others may rapidly develop severe hypertension and encephalopathy. BP usually falls after the withdrawal or substitution of cyclosporine immunosuppression, but hypertension may not remit completely. Furthermore, it is often not possible to discontinue therapy. Calcium antagonists have been used successfully, but some of these agents can increase cyclosporine blood levels. This approach can be an advantage in another way because it decreases the required dose of expensive cyclosporine. Multidrug therapy is usually necessary to control CAH.

Tacrolimus, another immunosuppressive agent that inhibits calcineurin, may also induce hypertension. However, it produces less hypertension than cyclosporine A, and therefore conversion to tacrolimus may be considered in patients with CAH. Rapamycin, a novel immunosuppressive agent that does not inhibit calcineurin, produces little nephrotoxicity or hypertension.

Over-the-Counter Drugs

Most nonprescription anorexic agents contain combinations of an antihistamine and an adrenergic agonist (usually phenylpropanolamine, ephedrine, pseudoephedrine, or caffeine). All act by potentiating presynaptic norepinephrine release and by directly activating adrenergic receptors. α-Adrenergic intoxication induced by nasal decongestant and cough medications containing massive doses of oxymetazoline hydrochloride, phenylephrine hydrochloride, or ephedrine hydrochloride has been reported to result in severe hypertension. Phenylpropanolamine is the active ingredient in most diet aids and in many decongestant agents, and it is also used as a substitute for amphetamine. Little if any increase in BP occurs with standard doses of phenylpropanolamine, but the use of excessive doses may result in severe hypertension.

Caffeine can acutely and transiently increase BP by increasing peripheral resistance. The reaction to caffeine is more pronounced in men than in women and in those with a positive family history than in those with a negative family history. Concomitant medications, such as monoamine oxidase inhibitors, antihypertensive drugs, oral contraceptives, and nonsteroidal anti-inflammatory drugs (NSAIDs) seem to increase the risk of hypertension. A recent meta-analysis by Noordzij and associates showed that regular caffeine intake increases BP. When ingested through coffee, however, the BP-raising effect of caffeine is small.[19]

Antidepressant Agents

Monamine oxidase inhibitors can induce severe hypertension when patients consume foods containing tyramine. Some investigators have reported that monoamine oxidase inhibitors cause a severe hypertensive reaction even without use of concomitant medications. Among the various monoamine oxidase inhibitors, tranylcypromine is the most hazardous, whereas moclobemide and brofaromine are the least likely to induce a hypertensive reaction. These drugs exert their effects by delaying the metabolism of sympathomimetic amines and 5-hydroxytryptophan and by increasing the storage of norepinephrine in postganglionic sympathetic neurons.

Tricyclic antidepressants block the reuptake of the neurotransmitters in synapses in the central nervous system. There are some reports that these agents increase BP, mainly in patients with panic disorders.

Buspirone, a serotonin receptor type 1α agonist, has also been reported to increase BP. It is speculated that buspirone increases BP by its metabolite, 1-2-pyrimidinyl piperazine, which is an α_2-adrenoceptor antagonist, and therefore should not be used concomitantly with a monamine oxidase inhibitor. A small but sustained and dose-dependent increase in BP seems to occur with other serotonin agonists as well. Venlafaxine has a dose-dependent effect on BP that is clinically significant at high doses. Episodes of severe hypertension were described in patients treated with other antidepressant agents such as fluoxetine, fluoxetine and selegiline in combination, and thioridazine.

Antineoplastic Agents

Several alkylating agents can increase BP. In one series, 15 of 18 patients treated with multiple alkylating agents following autologous bone marrow transplantation developed hypertension. Hypertensive reactions associated with paclitaxel treatment have been reported.

Recombinant Human Erythropoietin

Recombinant human erythropoietin (r-HuEPO) has revolutionized the treatment of anemia in patients with renal failure, both in the predialysis phase and the postdialysis phase. Not only does this treatment improve well-being, but also it positively influences cardiac function and permits cardiac hypertrophy to regress. r-HuEPO can lead to an increase in BP that appears to be dose related. Systemic hypertension has been reported to develop, or to worsen, in 20% to 30% of patients treated with r-HuEPO worldwide. The greatest increases in BP affect daytime systolic and nighttime diastolic BP. Hypertension may develop in some patients as early as 2 weeks, and in others as late as 4 months, after the start of r-HuEPO treatment.

Hypertension has not proved to be a serious general problem in patients treated with r-HuEPO; however, a few cases of hypertensive crisis with encephalopathy have been reported. Several risk factors for the development, or worsening, of hypertension after r-HuEPO therapy have been identified. They include the presence of preexisting hypertension, a rapid increase in hematocrit before r-HuEPO administration, a low baseline hematocrit before r-HuEPO administration, high doses and intravenous route of administration, the presence of native kidneys, a genetic predisposition to hypertension, and possibly a younger age. There are several potential mechanisms by which r-HuEPO therapy may increase BP in hemodialysis-treated patients. These mechanisms include increased blood viscosity, the loss of hypoxic vasodilation, the activation of neuro-humoral systems (catecholamines, the renin-angiotensin system), and especially a direct vascular effect. This last mechanism is supported by several sets of data, and many factors may be involved in its pathogenesis (increased cell calcium uptake; imbalance in local vasoactive agents, with increased synthesis of endothelin-1; a mitogenic effect; or a platelet-dependent mechanism). By optimizing dialysis treatment, paying close attention to volume regulation, and administering r-HuEPO subcutaneously and in a fashion to increase hematocrit gradually, the occurrence of BP increases can be minimized.

Hemodynamically, r-HuEPO increases BP by a marked increase in peripheral resistance associated with only a mild decrease in cardiac output. The hypertension associated with r-HuEPO has not generally been too difficult to control. In one study, 42% of patients with r-HuEPO–induced hypertension had their BP controlled with a single agent. Fluid removal with dialysis is also helpful. If these measures are unsuccessful, the dose of r-HuEPO should be lowered, or therapy should be held for several weeks. Phlebotomy of 500 mL of blood may rapidly lower BP in patients with refractory hypertension. In the past several years, patients with mild chronic renal insufficiency and anemia have been receiving r-HuEPO to raise their hemoglobin levels. The drug is often associated with an increase in BP and increases the need for additional antihypertensive therapy. In general, these patients feel better, and the benefit of a higher hematocrit appears to outweigh the additional drugs required to reach their target BP.

Bromocriptine

Bromocriptine mesylate is commonly used for prolactin inhibition and for suppression of puerperal lactation. Although bromocriptine often has a hypotensive effect, severe hypertension with subsequent stroke has been reported in the postpartum period. Patients with pregnancy-induced hypertension are at increased risk to develop hypertension. The use of bromocriptine for suppression of lactation is no longer approved by the Food and Drug Administration.

Disulfiram

Disulfiram is commonly used as a pharmacologic adjunct in the treatment of alcoholism. Administration of 500 mg/day of disulfiram for 2 to 3 weeks has been reported to increase BP slightly. A low dose of 125 mg/day of this agent may also increase BP. It seems that changes in peripheral or central noradrenergic activity are responsible for the increase in arterial pressure.

Alcohol

Excessive alcohol use has clearly been shown to raise BP and can also increase resistance to antihypertensive therapy. The BP effects of alcohol are independent of obesity, salt intake, cigarette smoking, and potassium intake. A dose-response relationship exists for the hypertensive effects of alcohol. Moderation of alcohol intake in those who drink excessively is recommended as part of the initial management for patients with hypertension. A reasonable approach is to limit daily alcohol consumption to no more than approximately 2 oz of alcohol for men and 1 oz for women.

Nonsteroidal Anti-inflammatory Drugs

NSAIDs can induce an increase in BP and can interfere with antihypertensive treatment, often by nullifying its effect. Two meta-analyses demonstrated that, after pooling data drawn from published reports of randomized trials of younger adults, the use of NSAIDs produced a clinically significant increment in mean BP of 5 mm Hg. Elderly patients, those with preexisting hypertension, salt-sensitive patients, patients with renal failure, and patients with renovascular hypertension are at a higher risk to develop severe hypertension when they are treated with NSAIDs. The mechanisms whereby NSAIDs raise BP are not fully understood. Inhibiting the intrarenal synthesis of prostaglandins from arachidonic acid via cyclooxygenase (COX)-1 and COX-2, the two isoforms of COX, is probably the main mechanism of action. Interference with both the control of vascular resistance and the regulation of extracellular volume homeostasis has been incriminated, but several other putative mechanisms such as moderation of adrenergic activity or resetting of the baroreceptor response may also be involved. NSAIDs may interact with some antihypertensive agents such as diuretics, β-blockers, and angiotensin-converting enzyme inhibitors, but they do not interact as strongly with calcium antagonists, α-blockers, and centrally acting drugs. NSAIDs vary considerably in their effect on BP. In a recent meta-analysis, Aw and colleagues showed that selective COX-2 inhibitors increased BP slightly, but not significantly more than the nonselective agents,[20] but significant inhomogeneity exists across the three COX-2 selective agents. Patients receiving celecoxib experience less increase in BP compared with those receiving rofecoxib, whether compared in head-to-head trials, in meta-analyses against placebo, or against nonselective NSAIDs.[19] A recent study by Sowers and associates showed that treatment with rofecoxib, but not celecoxib or naproxen, induced a significant increase in 24-hour systolic BP.[21] It is wise to balance the risk of an increase in BP against the expected benefit of treatment with an NSAID. In patients who take NSAIDs, calcium antagonists would appear to be preferred to other antihypertensive agents.

Heavy Metals

Several studies show that cumulative exposure to lead, even at low levels sustained by the general population, may increase the risk of hypertension. Some studies suggest that arsenic exposure also may induce hypertension in humans. Several studies suggest that cadmium exposure may increase BP. However, in a recent study, environmental exposure to cadmium was not associated with higher conventional BP or

24-hour ambulatory BP measurements or with an increased risk for hypertension.

Scorpion and Black Widow Spider Venom

The venom of scorpions (especially South American species) and of black widow spiders commonly produces a clinical picture of profuse perspiration, lacrimation, vomiting, convulsion, and cardiovascular collapse. However, hypertension and bradycardia occur occasionally. Hypertension is mediated by a massive discharge of catecholamines into the circulation produced by the venom, and β- or α-blockade is therefore effective in this condition.

Amphotericin B

Amphotericin B remains the mainstay of therapy for serious fungal infections. A few cases of severe hypertension associated with the use of amphotericin B deoxycholate have been reported in the literature, and recently one case report of hypertension associated with a lipid-containing preparation of the medication has been described.

Antiviral Treatment in Human Immunodeficiency Virus Infection

One case report of severe hypertension and renal atrophy associated with the protease inhibitor indinavir has been described. Hypertensive crisis secondary to phenylpropanolamine interacting with triple-drug therapy for human immunodeficiency virus prophylaxis has also been reported. In addition, potential drug interactions exist between antiretroviral medications, particularly the protease inhibitors, and antihypertensive medications.[22]

Coarctation of the Aorta

Coarctation of the aorta is a constriction of the lumen of aorta located most commonly near the ligamentum arteriosum and the origins of the left subclavian artery. This lesion makes up approximately 7% of all cases of congenital heart disease.[23] Hypertension with weak or absent femoral pulses in a young person is the most common presentation. Other common signs include the presence of a systolic murmur over the anterior chest, bruits over the back, and visible notching of the posterior ribs on a chest radiograph. Symptoms may not be present until late in life. Coarctation may be associated with other congenital heart diseases. Atypical aortic coarctation in adults most likely represents Takayasu's arteritis, or pulseless disease, which usually affects the aortic arch and may also involve the descending aorta.[24] Two-dimensional echocardiography with Doppler interrogation is usually used to confirm the diagnosis. Computed tomography or magnetic resonance angiography can also be used to confirm the diagnosis. Before the advent of effective surgery, the mean age of death was 34 years,[25] and the usual cause of death was heart failure, aortic dissection or rupture, endocarditis, endarteritis, or intracranial hemorrhage. Surgical correction or percutaneous balloon dilatation angioplasty is currently used to repair the coarctation. BP may paradoxically increase immediately after surgical correction, but this rise is usually transient.[26] The long-term outcome of patients after coarctation repair is certainly better than it is for those who do not undergo repair, but survival after surgery is less than in the general population.[27] Late complications include hypertension in as many as 70% of patients 30 years after surgery, recoarctation, aortic aneurysm formation and rupture, sudden death, ischemic heart disease, heart failure, and cerebrovascular accidents. Because of the late complications, careful follow-up is required.

Hormonal Disturbances

Cushing's Syndrome

Cushing's syndrome is chronic glucocorticoid excess, with various causes, that typically produces hypertension. The pathogenetic mechanisms of Cushing's syndrome can be divided into those dependent and those not dependent on corticotropin (formerly adrenocorticotropin or adrenocorticotropic hormone). The most common form, which is termed *Cushing's disease* and accounts for 60% to 80% of cases in most series, is generally the result of overproduction of corticotropin from a pituitary adenoma, in most cases a microadenoma (<1 cm in diameter).[28] Hyperplasia of pituitary corticotrophs has been described in a minority of patients in whom no tumor could be found.[28,29] Stressful life events have been shown to have a pathogenic role in hypothalamic-pituitary forms of Cushing's syndrome.[30]

Ectopic production of corticotropin may derive from several types of tumors.[31-33] Most patients with ectopic corticotropin syndrome have small cell lung carcinoma. Plasma corticotropin concentrations in these patients are extremely high, and therefore hyperpigmentation, hypertension, edema, hypokalemia, weakness, and glucose intolerance are generally present. However, the typical Cushing's habitus is not present in many cases, whereas anorexia, weight loss, and other signs of malignant disease are common. Other cases of ectopic production of corticotropin result from more indolent tumors, such as bronchial, thymic, and pancreatic carcinoids. Patients with this form of Cushing's syndrome have characteristics typical of Cushing's disease.[34] Most ectopic tumors are benign, and some are so small that they are difficult to locate even with sophisticated morphologic procedures. Forms of autonomous adrenal hyperfunction include adrenocortical adenomas or carcinomas and the rarer primary nodular adrenal hyperplasia. Adrenal masses discovered by imaging studies for unrelated reasons (incidentalomas) are almost always nonhyperfunctioning adrenocortical adenomas. Their natural history is still under investigation; however, a few such lesions evolve toward overt Cushing's syndrome.[35] Finally, iatrogenic or factitious Cushing's syndrome may be rarely associated with exogenous administration of corticotropin. Long-term treatment with glucocorticoids (e.g., dexamethasone or prednisone) or, in rare cases, with megestrol acetate may produce clinical features of hypercortisolism.

Hypertension is present in approximately 80% of patients with Cushing's syndrome and is the result of one of several mechanisms. These include a sodium-retaining action of cortisol, through binding to either mineralocorticoid receptors[36] or nonreceptor mechanisms, increased production of mineralocorticoids (usually noted in patients with adrenal tumors), reduced activity of various vasodepressor mechanisms, in particular endothelial nitric oxide,[37] increased levels of renin substrate, and an increased responsiveness to various pressors. Some other mechanisms may also be involved, including an increase in erythropoietin.[38]

Certain features, such as weakness associated with proximal muscle wasting, skin atrophy, easy bruising after minor trauma, extensive ecchymoses, purple striae produced by the rapid enlargement of the trunk and abdomen, hypertension, and psychological changes, strongly suggest hypercortisolism. Some patients present with only isolated symptoms, and even the most common findings, such as truncal obesity and hypertension, may be absent in some cases.[39,40]

Biochemical abnormalities associated with hypercortisolism include neutrophilic leukocytosis, hyperglycemia, hypokalemia, hypercholesterolemia, and a hypercoagulable state.[41] For screening of hypercortisolism, a urinary free cortisol assay and an overnight 1-mg dexamethasone suppression test are suggested. The sensitivity of urinary free cortisol is 95% to 100%, and the specificity is 94% to 98%. Because of the variability of cortisol secretion from day to day, three 24-hour urine collections are required. Urinary free cortisol measurements may be less accurate in diagnosing patients with renal failure and low glomerular filtration rate (<30 mL/minute). The dexamethasone suppression test that uses a single 1-mg dose at midnight, after which the plasma cortisol concentration is measured at 8 AM the next day, has a sensitivity of 98%.[40] A level of less than 5 μg/dL essentially excludes Cushing's syndrome. False-positive results are seen in approximately 10% of patients who do not have Cushing's syndrome, especially obese patients or patients with endogenous depression, alcoholism, psychological stress, high concentrations of corticosteroid-binding globulin, glucocorticoid resistance, decreased absorption of dexamethasone; those taking drugs that stimulate enzyme activity in the liver; those presenting with abnormal cortisol metabolism; and those unable to follow directions. False-negative tests can occur in chronic renal failure and in hypothyroidism. When the screening test is positive, further evaluation should be done, first to confirm the diagnosis of Cushing's syndrome and second to identify the cause of the syndrome. To confirm the diagnosis, a low dose of 0.5 mg dexamethasone every 6 hours for 2 days should be given, and plasma cortisol should be measured 6 hours after the last of the eight doses. If plasma cortisol is higher than 5 μg/dL or urinary cortisol is higher than 10 μg/day, the diagnosis of Cushing's disease is nearly always confirmed. In hospitalized patients, a single blood cortisol measurement taken from an indwelling catheter during sleep at midnight indicates the presence of Cushing's syndrome when values are greater than 5 μg/dL with a sensitivity of 100%.[42] An increase in plasma cortisol and corticotropin in response to intravenous administration of the vasopressin analogue, desmopressin, suggests the diagnosis of pituitary-dependent Cushing's disease.

Once Cushing's syndrome has been diagnosed, the anatomic cause needs to be determined accurately to guide therapy. To distinguish corticotropin-dependent from corticotropin-independent hypercortisolism, corticotropin can be measured. Concentrations lower than the limit of detection indicate autonomous adrenal hyperfunction. In pituitary and ectopic sources of the hormone, the plasma corticotropin levels are usually high. The levels are extremely high in patients with an ectopic source, especially in small cell lung carcinoma. The high-dose dexamethasone suppression test, together with the corticotropin-releasing hormone stimulation test, is the most useful in distinguishing pituitary from ectopic corticotropin-dependent Cushing's syndrome. Most pituitary but not ectopic corticotropin-secreting tumors have corticotropin-releasing hormone receptors and show exaggerated corticotropin and cortisol responses to corticotropin-releasing hormone administration. For localization of pituitary or ectopic corticotropin-producing tumors and adrenal masses, computed tomography and magnetic resonance imaging scans of the pituitary and the adrenal are helpful. The finding of an incidental adrenal mass does not necessarily means adrenal hyperfunction; conversely, a normal pituitary gland on scanning does not exclude Cushing's disease because 40% to 50% of the pituitary tumors are so small that they are not recognized.

The choice of therapy depends on the cause of the syndrome. For pituitary tumors, transsphenoidal microsurgical removal of pituitary tumors has become the treatment of choice. If the syndrome recurs and the patient is not a suitable candidate for reoperation, pituitary irradiation is appropriate. For adrenal tumors, or ectopic tumors that cannot be resected, removal of the adrenal gland or glands may be helpful. Various drugs that act at the hypothalamic-pituitary level or on adrenocortical steroid synthesis or at the receptor level may be used in certain cases.[40]

Until definitive therapy is provided, the hypertension should be treated with antihypertensive agents. Because excess fluid volume is the main mechanism, a thiazide diuretic in combination with an aldosterone antagonist is an appropriate initial choice.

Hypothyroidism

Hypothyroidism may be associated with diastolic hypertension. Streeten and colleagues found diastolic hypertension in 16 of 40 (40%) patients who became hypothyroid after radioiodine treatment for hyperthyroidism.[43] The same authors also diagnosed hypothyroidism in 3.6% of 688 patients with newly diagnosed hypertension. Hypertension was resolved by thyroid hormone replacement therapy in one third of the patients. In contrast, Bergus and associates found no association between hypothyroidism and diastolic hypertension.[44] The mechanism by which hypothyroidism may increase diastolic BP is not clear. Biondi and associates showed that patients with hypothyroidism tend to have impaired cardiac diastolic relaxation and decreased contractility, thereby leading to low cardiac output.[45] To maintain tissue perfusion in the setting of low cardiac output, peripheral resistance increases by a combination of increased responsiveness of α-adrenergic receptors and increased levels of sympathetic nervous system activity.[46] This compensatory increase in peripheral resistance tends to raise diastolic more than systolic BP, as usually seen in hypothyroidism.[47]

Hyperthyroidism

Patients with hyperthyroidism tend to have elevated systolic and low diastolic BP as a result of high cardiac output and reduced peripheral resistance.[48] The isolated systolic hypertension and tachycardia in hyperthyroidism generally respond well to β-blockers[47] while one waits for the definitive treatment of the disease to be effective.

Hyperparathyroidism

Hypertension is common in patients with primary hyperparathyroidism.[49] Patients have increased arterial stiffness and impaired endothelium-mediated vasodilatation that may cause elevated BP.[50,51] The relationship between hyperparathyroidism and hypertension is not so clear, however, because hypertension usually does not recede after surgical treatment.[52] Moreover, no correlation was found between BP and either serum calcium or parathyroid hormone levels in 194 patients with primary hyperparathyroidism.[53] Therefore, hypertension is not an indication for surgery for otherwise asymptomatic hyperparathyroidism. Thiazide diuretics should be avoided in these patients because these drugs may cause or exacerbate hypercalcemia. If a diuretic is required, furosemide can be used safely, because it causes hypocalcemia and hypercalciuria.

Acromegaly

Acromegaly is a clinical condition caused by chronic growth hormone (GH) hypersecretion. In the majority of cases, excess GH is produced by a pituitary adenoma. Secondary pituitary hyperplasia induced by excess GH-releasing hormone secreted from the hypothalamus or an ectopic source can also be responsible for excess GH production, but this is a very rare cause of acromegaly.[54] Acromegaly is rare, with an annual incidence of about 3 per million and a prevalence of about 40 per million.[55,56] The diagnosis of acromegaly should be based on elevated serum levels of a specific immunoreactive peptide, insulin growth factor-I (IGF-I), and on the lack of GH suppression during an oral glucose tolerance test. Excess GH secretion before puberty leads to increased height and gigantism. After cessation of bone growth, the characteristic clinical features include enlargement of the distal parts of the skeleton such as the ears, nose, jaw, fingers, and toes, together with soft tissue overgrowth. In the largest series of patients with acromegaly, 98% had acral growth and coarsened facial features, and 90% had soft tissue swelling. The excess GH also stimulates excessive growth of other tissues, thus causing organomegaly and multiple symptoms, including excessive respiration, headache, visual field impairment, peripheral neuropathy, paresthesias, osteoarthritis, and impotence.[57]

Hypertension is an important complication of acromegaly that contributes to the increased morbidity and mortality seen in this condition. The prevalence of hypertension in acromegalic patients ranges from 18% to 60% in different clinical series,[58] with a mean prevalence of approximately 35%. This wide range may result from the different criteria used to define hypertension and the different techniques used for measuring BP (conventional sphygmomanometer versus 24-hour ambulatory BP monitoring). In one series, hypertension was more common in acromegalic patients than in controls, and BP fell significantly in female patients after successful surgical treatment.[59] In a Japanese series, 37.5% of patients with acromegaly were hypertensive, a much higher prevalence than the general population in Japan.[60] In the largest series (500 patients), half of patients were hypertensive or were taking antihypertensive drugs.[57] The prevalence of hypertension is lower in all studies reported so far when the definition is based on 24-hour ambulatory BP monitoring, rather than office BP readings: 17% versus 42%[61] or 40%

versus 56%.[62] Patients with acromegaly exhibit an impaired nocturnal BP fall and are more likely to be nondippers than controls.[61-62] The cause of hypertension in acromegaly remains unclear, and several mechanisms may be involved; sodium retention and volume expansion are common. Clinical and experimental studies suggest either an indirect, systemic mechanism underlying the GH-induced and IGF-I–induced tubular sodium and water absorption or a direct effect of GH or IGF-I on renal tubular handling of sodium. However, the mechanisms underlying the antinatriuretic action of GH excess are not fully understood. A direct activation of distal tubular sodium channels by IGF-I has been suggested. Some data indicate that the renin-angiotensin-aldosterone system (RAAS) is stimulated by GH and IGF-I in rats, in physiologically normal humans, and in acromegalic patients, but others show little change in RAAS activity during GH administration.[63-65] It seems that plasma renin activity is less suppressed than would be expected, given the sodium retention in this disease. Some of this may result from increased prolactin levels, which could stimulate the secretion of aldosterone.[66] Karlberg and Ottosson found low renin concentrations, with an inappropriately elevated aldosterone levels, in 16 of 24 acromegalic patients.[67] These observations suggest that aldosterone secretion is not suppressed and is not related to concomitantly obtained plasma renin levels.[67,68] Reduction in atrial natriuretic peptide by GH and IGF-I may also contribute to the reduced natriuresis seen in patients with acromegaly.[69] Acromegaly is often associated with metabolic disorders, such as diabetes mellitus, impaired glucose tolerance, insulin resistance, and hyperinsulinemia. Hyperinsulinemia causes sodium and water retention, activation of the sympathetic nervous system, activation of the RAAS, and vascular hypertrophy, thereby leading to hypertension. The evidence for overactivity of the sympathetic nervous system is equivocal, but the normal nocturnal fall in norepinephrine levels and BP is blunted in acromegalic patients. Normalization of circadian sympathetic activity and BP profile was achieved in patients whose acromegaly was completely cured.[70] Sleep apnea may contribute to the absence of a nocturnal BP fall in acromegaly, as it does in persons without acromegaly. Because sleep apnea occurs in 60% to 75% of acromegalic patients, it may constitute an important risk factor for hypertension and cardiovascular morbidity in this disease.[71] Hemodynamically, cardiac output is increased in patients with acromegaly, compared with age-and sex-matched controls.[72] The increased output reflects increases in both heart rate and stroke volume. Augmented peripheral blood flow causing increased cardiac output may also be a factor in the development of hypertension in acromegaly.[72] Hypertension may accelerate cardiomyopathy in patients with acromegaly and therefore should be identified and treated appropriately.

References

1. Chobanian AV, Bakris GL, Black HR, et al., and the National High Blood Pressure Education Program Coordinating Committee. The Seventh Report of the Joint National Committee on Prevention, Detection, Evaluation, and Treatment of High Blood Pressure: The JNC 7 report. *JAMA.* 2003;**289**:2560-2572.
2. O'Brien E, Asmar R, Beilin L, et al. European Society of Hypertension recommendations for conventional, ambulatory

and home blood pressure measurement. *J Hypertens.* 2003;**21**:821-848.

3. O'Brien E, Asmar R, Beilin L, et al. Practice guidelines of the European Society of Hypertension for clinic, ambulatory and self blood pressure measurement. *J Hypertens.* 2005;**23**:697-701.

4. Rouse A, Marshall T. The extent and implications of sphygmomanometer calibration error in primary care. *J Hum Hypertens.* 2001;**15**:587-591.

5. Mejia AD, Egan BM, Schork NJ, Zweifler AJ. Artefacts in measurement of blood pressure and lack of target organ involvement in the assessment of patients with treatment-resistant hypertension. *Ann Intern Med.* 1990;**112**:270-277.

6. Baker RH, Ende J. Confounders of auscultatory blood pressure measurement. *J Gen Intern Med.* 1995;**10**:223-231.

7. Campbell NR, Hogan DB, McKay DW. Pitfalls to avoid in the measurement of blood pressure in the elderly. *Can J Public Health.* 1994;**85 (Suppl 2)**:S26-S28.

8. Messerli FH, Ventura HO, Amodeo C. Osler's maneuver and pseudohypertension. *N Engl J Med.* 1985;**312**:1548-1551.

9. Oliner CM, Elliott WJ, Gretler DD, Murphy MB. Low predictive value of positive Osler manoeuvre for diagnosing pseudohypertension. *J Hum Hypertens.* 1993;**7**:65-70.

10. Wright JC, Looney SW. Prevalence of positive Osler's manoeuver in 3387 persons screened for the Systolic Hypertension in the Elderly Program (SHEP). *J Hum Hypertens.* 1997;**11**:285-289.

11. Zweifler AJ, Shahab ST. Pseudohypertension: A new assessment. *J Hypertens.* 1993;**11**:1-6.

12. Cavallini MC, Roman MJ, Blank SG, et al. Association of the auscultatory gap with vascular disease in hypertensive patients. *Ann Intern Med.* 1996;**124**:877-883.

13. Grossman E, Messerli FH. High blood pressure: A side effect of drugs, poisons, and food. *Arch Intern Med.* 1995;**155**:450-460.

14. Cushman M, Kuller LH, Prentice R, et al. Estrogen plus progestin and risk of venous thrombosis. *JAMA.* 2004;**292**:1573-1580.

15. Rossouw JE, Anderson GL, Prentice RL, et al. Risks and benefits of estrogen plus progestin in healthy postmenopausal women: Principal results From the Women's Health Initiative randomized controlled trial. *JAMA.* 2002;**288**:321-333.

16. Wassertheil-Smoller S, Hendrix SL, Limacher M, et al. Effect of estrogen plus progestin on stroke in postmenopausal women. The Women's Health Initiative: A randomized trial. *JAMA.* 2003;**289**:2673-2684.

17. Waters DD, Alderman EL, Hsia J, et al. Effects of hormone replacement therapy and antioxidant vitamin supplements on coronary atherosclerosis in postmenopausal women: A randomized controlled trial. *JAMA.* 2002;**288**:2432-2440.

18. Arterburn DE, Crane PK, Veenstra DL. The efficacy and safety of sibutramine for weight loss: A systematic review. *Arch Intern Med.* 2004;**164**:994-1003.

19. Noordzij M, Uiterwaal CS, Arends LR, et al. Blood pressure response to chronic intake of coffee and caffeine: A meta-analysis of randomized controlled trials. *J Hypertens.* 2005;**23**:921-928.

20. Aw TJ, Haas SJ, Liew D, Krum H. Meta-analysis of cyclooxygenase-2 inhibitors and their effects on blood pressure. *Arch Intern Med.* 2005;**165**:490-496.

21. Sowers JR, White WB, Pitt B, et al. The effects of cyclooxygenase-2 inhibitors and nonsteroidal anti-inflammatory therapy on 24-hour blood pressure in patients with hypertension, osteoarthritis, and type 2 diabetes mellitus. *Arch Intern Med.* 2005;**165**:161-168.

22. Chow DC, Souza SA, Chen R, et al. Elevated blood pressure in HIV-infected individuals receiving highly active antiretroviral therapy. *HIV Clin Trials.* 2003;**4**:411-416.

23. Prisant LM, Mawulawde K, Kapoor D, Joe C. Coarctation of the aorta: A secondary cause of hypertension. *J Clin Hypertens (Greenwich).* 2004;**6**:347-350, 352.

24. Numano F, Okawara M, Inomata H, Kobayashi Y. Takayasu's arteritis. *Lancet.* 2000;**356**:1023-1025.

25. Campbell M. Natural history of coarctation of the aorta. *Br Heart J.* 1970;**32**:633-640.

26. Choy M, Rocchini AP, Beekman RH, et al. Paradoxical hypertension after repair of coarctation of the aorta in children: Balloon angioplasty versus surgical repair. *Circulation.* 1987;**75**:1186-1191.

27. Bobby JJ, Emami JM, Farmer RD, Newman CG. Operative survival and 40 year follow up of surgical repair of aortic coarctation. *Br Heart J.* 1991;**65**:271-276.

28. Mampalam TJ, Tyrrell JB, Wilson CB. Transsphenoidal microsurgery for Cushing disease: A report of 216 cases. *Ann Intern Med.* 1988;**109**:487-493.

29. Kruse A, Klinken L, Holck S, Lindholm J. Pituitary histology in Cushing's disease. *Clin Endocrinol (Oxf).* 1992;**37**:254-259.

30. Sonino N, Fava GA, Boscaro M. A role for life events in the pathogenesis of Cushing's disease. *Clin Endocrinol (Oxf).* 1993;**38**:261-264.

31. Becker M, Aron DC. Ectopic ACTH syndrome and CRH-mediated Cushing's syndrome. *Endocrinol Metab Clin North Am.* 1994;**23**:585-606.

32. Wigg SJ, Ehrlich AR, Fuller PJ. Cushing's syndrome secondary to ectopic ACTH secretion from metastatic breast carcinoma. *Clin Endocrinol (Oxf).* 1999;**50**:675-678.

33. Arnaldi G, Angeli A, Atkinson AB, et al. Diagnosis and complications of Cushing's syndrome: A consensus statement. *J Clin Endocrinol Metab.* 2003;**88**:5593-5602.

34. Perry LA, Grossman AB. The role of the laboratory in the diagnosis of Cushing's syndrome. *Ann Clin Biochem.* 1997;**34**:345-359.

35. Barzon L, Scaroni C, Sonino N, et al. Risk factors and long-term follow-up of adrenal incidentalomas. *J Clin Endocrinol Metab.* 1999;**84**:520-526.

36. Ulick S. Cortisol as mineralocorticoid. *J Clin Endocrinol Metab.* 1996;**81**:1307-1308.

37. Mangos GJ, Walker BR, Kelly JJ, et al. Cortisol inhibits cholinergic vasodilation in the human forearm. *Am J Hypertens.* 2000;**13**:1155-1160.

38. Whitworth JA, Mangos GJ, Kelly JJ. Cushing, cortisol, and cardiovascular disease. *Hypertension.* 2000;**36**:912-916.

39. Ross EJ, Linch DC. Cushing's syndrome—killing disease: Discriminatory value of signs and symptoms aiding early diagnosis. *Lancet.* 1982;**2**:646-649.

40. Boscaro M, Barzon L, Fallo F, Sonino N. Cushing's syndrome. *Lancet.* 2001;**357**:783-791.

41. Casonato A, Pontara E, Boscaro M, et al. Abnormalities of von Willebrand factor are also part of the prothrombotic state of Cushing's syndrome. *Blood Coagul Fibrinolysis.* 1999;**10**:145-151.

42. Newell-Price J, Trainer P, Besser M, Grossman A. The diagnosis and differential diagnosis of Cushing's syndrome and pseudo-Cushing's states. *Endocr Rev.* 1998;**19**:647-672.

43. Streeten DH, Anderson GH Jr, Howland T, et al. Effects of thyroid function on blood pressure: Recognition of hypothyroid hypertension. *Hypertension.* 1988;**11**:78-83.

44. Bergus GR, Mold JW, Barton ED, Randall CS. The lack of association between hypertension and hypothyroidism in a primary care setting. *J Hum Hypertens.* 1999;**13**:231-235.

45. Biondi B, Fazio S, Palmieri EA, et al. Left ventricular diastolic dysfunction in patients with subclinical hypothyroidism. *J Clin Endocrinol Metab.* 1999;**84**:2064-2067.

46. Fletcher AK, Weetman AP. Hypertension and hypothyroidism. *J Hum Hypertens.* 1998;**12**:79-82.

47. Saito I, Saruta T. Hypertension in thyroid disorders. *Endocrinol Metab Clin North Am.* 1994;**23**:379-386.

48. Fraser R, Davies DL, Connell JM. Hormones and hypertension. *Clin Endocrinol (Oxf).* 1989;**31**:701-746.

49. Toft AD. Surgery for primary hyperparathyroidism—sooner rather than later. *Lancet*. 2000;**355**:1478-1479.

50. Smith JC, Page MD, John R, et al. Augmentation of central arterial pressure in mild primary hyperparathyroidism. *J Clin Endocrinol Metab*. 2000;**85**:3515-3519.

51. Nilsson IL, Aberg J, Rastad J, Lind L. Endothelial vasodilatory dysfunction in primary hyperparathyroidism is reversed after parathyroidectomy. *Surgery*. 1999;**126**:1049-1055.

52. Silverberg SJ. Editorial: Cardiovascular disease in primary hyperparathyroidism. *J Clin Endocrinol Metab*. 2000;**85**:3513-3514.

53. Lumachi F, Ermani M, Luisetto G, et al. Relationship between serum parathyroid hormone, serum calcium and arterial blood pressure in patients with primary hyperparathyroidism: Results of a multivariate analysis. *Eur J Endocrinol*. 2002;**146**:643-647.

54. Ezzat S, Asa SL, Stefaneanu L, et al. Somatotroph hyperplasia without pituitary adenoma associated with a long standing growth hormone–releasing hormone–producing bronchial carcinoid. *J Clin Endocrinol Metab*. 1994;**78**:555-560.

55. Alexander L, Appleton D, Hall R, Ross WM, Wilkinson R. Epidemiology of acromegaly in the Newcastle region. *Clin Endocrinol (Oxf)*. 1980;**12**:71-79.

56. Etxabe J, Gaztambide S, Latorre P, Vazquez JA. Acromegaly: An epidemiological study. *J Endocrinol Invest*. 1993;**16**:181-187.

57. Ezzat S, Forster MJ, Berchtold P, et al. Acromegaly: Clinical and biochemical features in 500 patients. *Medicine (Baltimore)*. 1994;**73**:233-240.

58. Bondanelli M, Ambrosio MR, degli Uberti EC. Pathogenesis and prevalence of hypertension in acromegaly. *Pituitary*. 2001;**4**:239-249.

59. Kraatz C, Benker G, Weber F, et al. Acromegaly and hypertension: Prevalence and relationship to the renin-angiotensin-aldosterone system. *Klin Wochenschr*. 1990;**68**:583-587.

60. Ohtsuka H, Komiya I, Aizawa T, Yamada T. Hypertension in acromegaly: Hereditary hypertensive factor produces hypertension by enhancing IGF-I production. *Endocr J*. 1995;**42**:781-787.

61. Minniti G, Moroni C, Jaffrain-Rea ML, et al. Prevalence of hypertension in acromegalic patients: Clinical measurement versus 24-hour ambulatory blood pressure monitoring. *Clin Endocrinol (Oxf)*. 1998;**48**:149-152.

62. Pietrobelli DJ, Akopian M, Olivieri AO, et al. Altered circadian blood pressure profile in patients with active acromegaly: Relationship with left ventricular mass and hormonal values. *J Hum Hypertens*. 2001;**15**:601-605.

63. Ho KY, Weissberger AJ. The antinatriuretic action of biosynthetic human growth hormone in man involves activation of the renin-angiotensin system. *Metabolism*. 1990;**39**:133-137.

64. Moller J, Frandsen E, Fisker S, et al. Decreased plasma and extracellular volume in growth hormone deficient adults and the acute and prolonged effects of GH administration: A controlled experimental study. *Clin Endocrinol (Oxf)*.1996;**44**:533-539.

65. Wyse B, Waters M, Sernia C. Stimulation of the renin-angiotensin system by growth hormone in Lewis dwarf rats. *Am J Physiol*. 1993;**265**:E332-E339.

66. Marks P, Vincent R, Wilson B, Delassale A. Aldosterone in acromegaly. *Am J Med Sci*. 1984;**287**:16-19.

67. Karlberg BE, Ottosson AM. Acromegaly and hypertension: Role of the renin-angiotensin-aldosterone system. *Acta Endocrinol (Copenh)*. 1982;**100**:581-587.

68. Mantero F, Opocher G, Armanini D, et al. Plasma renin activity and urinary aldosterone in acromegaly. *J Endocrinol Invest*. 1979;**2**:13-18.

69. Moller J, Jorgensen JO, Moller N, et al. Expansion of extracellular volume and suppression of atrial natriuretic peptide after growth hormone administration in normal man. *J Clin Endocrinol Metab*. 1991;**72**:768-772.

70. Bondanelli M, Ambrosio MR, Franceschetti P, et al. Diurnal rhythm of plasma catecholamines in acromegaly. *J Clin Endocrinol Metab*. 1999;**84**:2458-2467.

71. Grunstein RR, Ho KY, Sullivan CE. Sleep apnea in acromegaly. *Ann Intern Med*. 1991;**115**:527-532.

72. Thuesen L, Christensen SE, Weeke J, et al. A hyperkinetic heart in uncomplicated active acromegaly: Explanation of hypertension in acromegalic patients? *Acta Med Scand*. 1988;**223**:337-343.

Risk Stratification

The Natural History of Untreated Hypertension

William J. Elliott

One of the great triumphs of preventive medicine since the 1880s has been the recognition of elevated blood pressure (BP) as a "strong, graded, and independent risk factor" for adverse cardiovascular (CV) outcomes (including coronary heart disease [CHD], stroke, renal failure, and CV death), which was followed by development of effective and well-tolerated drug therapies for this condition that significantly reduce these risks.[1] The purpose of this chapter is to review the important, albeit generally older, information from epidemiologic studies and clinical trials that led to the clear and inescapable conclusion that elevated BP is associated with adverse CV and, perhaps to a lesser degree, renal outcomes. The framework of the discussion is shown in Figure 13-1, which broadly characterizes the progression of prehypertension to hypertension to target organ damage to adverse clinical events and finally to death. These issues are covered in reverse order of their usual chronology in human patients.

CAUSES OF MORTALITY IN HYPERTENSIVE PATIENTS

Elevated BP was recognized as an important risk factor for all-cause mortality even before it could be accurately and objectively measured. It took less than 20 years from the development of the Korotkoff method of indirect BP measurement to publications linking elevated BP measurements to excess mortality.[2] Early analyses by the life insurance industry showed a clear-cut relationship between BP and the risk of a payout related to death.[3] Even today, age and BP are the two most important determinants of the premiums that will be paid by a person seeking a life insurance policy.[4] The medical profession, however, was far behind the business community in recognizing the importance of lowering elevated BP. Despite reports from several centers that the administration of antihypertensive drugs to individuals with diastolic BPs higher than 130 mm Hg reduced morbidity and even mortality,[5,6] the widely held view into the late 1960s was that lowering the BP did not affect the unknown underlying reasons for the vascular complications that followed it and therefore could not be recommended.[7] Only in 1971 were sufficient outcomes data available from the Pooling Project of the Council on Epidemiology of the American Heart Association that showed a significant risk for mortality and morbidity for persons with diastolic BPs between 90 and 114 mm Hg.[8] Controversies surrounding the rationale and early development of antihypertensive therapy, from the perspective of a person who was prominent in this battle, are nicely summarized in a book by Marvin Moser, MD.[9]

Ultimately, mortality is the final event in the natural history of all diseases, so it is perhaps simplest to consider the various causes of death in large populations and to compare the life span and reasons for mortality among hypertensive and nonhypertensive persons. Unfortunately, this is difficult, both because of the very long duration of follow-up required for any large cohort and because hypertension is a major risk factor for other clinical events and diseases that are more commonly recognized as an immediate and/or direct cause of death. It is seldom simple to estimate the proportion of deaths, for example, from heart disease or stroke that can be directly attributed to preexisting hypertension. As a result, vital statistics data typically very much underestimate the true risk for death that is attributable to hypertension. Projections from the World Health Organization suggest that hypertension will increase in importance worldwide during the first half of the 21st century, even though it is currently the number 1 cause of preventable death.[10] In the year 2025, an estimated 1.56 billion hypertensive people are expected to inhabit the Earth (giving a prevalence of hypertension of ~29.2%), a 60% increase from the year 2000, when the global prevalence was only 26.4%.[11] Most persons who will become hypertensive over the next 20 years are expected to be residents of economically developing countries, not the developed countries where hypertension is already so prevalent.

Unfortunately, few population-based reports indicate causes of death among only hypertensive people. Even if these did exist, however, their interpretation would be challenging. It is much more likely that death may be significantly *postponed* when and if BP is lowered than that the ultimate cause of death would be changed. Thus, recent vital statistics data indicating that heart disease has remained the number 1 killer of U.S. citizens since 1918,[12] despite dramatic improvements in population-based estimates of BP awareness, treatment, and control, are consistent with this hypothesis.[13] So, too, is the finding that *age-adjusted* stroke and CHD mortality rates have decreased by about 60% and 50%, respectively, since the National High Blood Pressure Education Program began in the United States in 1972.[13] The second, and perhaps most important, challenge to the interpretation of vital statistics information derived from death certificates is that hypertension is seldom listed as a "significant contributing cause of death," even when the immediate cause is clearly related to hypertension (e.g., stroke). Thus, data derived from death certificates are seldom a reliable measure of the attributable risk associated with risk factors such as hypertension.

It is nonetheless interesting to examine the existing data, despite these caveats. In the Prospective Studies Collaboration, mortality data from 958,074 people without a history of prior

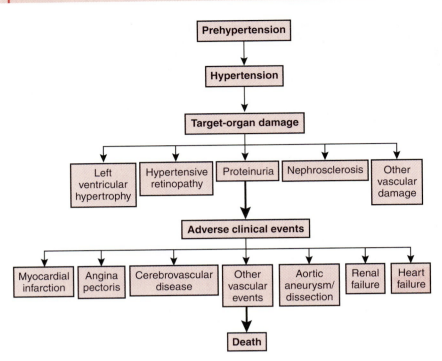

Figure 13–1 Schematic model of the natural history of (untreated) hypertension, showing the progression from prehypertension to hypertension, to target organ damage, to clinical events, and eventually to death.

CV disease enrolled in 61 observational studies were broken down by age and BP, appropriately corrected for regression-dilution bias.[14] During a variable duration of follow-up (average, 13.3 years), 122,716 deaths were reported. Because many of these studies were started when the threshold value for diagnosis of hypertension was higher than it is today (e.g., 160/95 mm Hg), it was not possible to do analyses restricted to a prior diagnosis of hypertension. Nonetheless, there was approximately a twofold higher risk of death, either from stroke or from ischemic heart disease, for every 20/10 mm Hg increase in usual BP. Systolic BP was a better predictor than diastolic BP for death from either heart disease (93% versus 73%, respectively) or stroke (89% versus 83%, respectively), whereas pulse pressure was not predictive (43% for heart disease, 37% for stroke). The total number of deaths from stroke was 11,960 (or ~10% of the total). Ischemic heart disease accounted for 34,283 deaths (~28% of the total), and a further 10,092 deaths were attributed to other vascular causes (or ~8% of the total). About 50% of the deaths were attributed to non-CV causes, and the remaining 4% of the deaths had unknown causes. These data, which are surprisingly similar to recent U.S. vital statistics data,[12] suggest that ischemic heart disease kills about three times more people (with and without hypertension) than stroke and about four times more people than other vascular diseases. However, some of the data in the Prospective Collaborative Studies compilation were derived from populations and eras in which antihypertensive drug therapy was available. This is likely to have had a disproportionate effect on these endpoints, with a larger reduction in stroke deaths than other causes. These data therefore hint that, in a large collection of data from around the world, hypertensive patients die more commonly of heart disease than of stroke or other vascular diseases. The number of individuals from minority populations in these studies is small, however; vital statistics and other data from blacks (including African Americans and

Australian Aboriginals) indicate that this rank ordering of events may be different in specific populations.

In several very early cohort studies conducted before antihypertensive drug therapy was available, this conclusion can also be corroborated. One of the first reports of mortality associated with BP was that of Theodore Caldwell Janeway, who became Sir William Osler's successor as Chair of Medicine at Johns Hopkins in Baltimore.[2] Janeway and his father practiced medicine and cardiology in New York City for nearly 30 years. From 1903 to 1912, he measured BP objectively using a mercury column and a cuff around the arm in 9208 new patients in his private consulting rooms. Using painstaking cataloging methods that were unusual for the day, Janeway determined that 212 "hypertensive" patients died during the 9 years: 33% from heart disease, 14% from stroke, 23% from renal failure, and 30% from non-CV causes. Despite the relatively small number of deaths and the lack of modern statistical tools, he concluded that systolic BP was a strong predictor of cardiac and CV death. Very similar results were reported by Henry A. Christian at Harvard University in Cambridge, Massachusetts, and others in 1926.[15] A 50-year follow-up of 293 elderly hypertensive patients showed a somewhat higher proportion dying of heart disease (45%),[16] but this figure was quite similar to that found in a series of 144 hypertensive Australians (41%).[17] Putting these and other observations together suggests that, in the era before antihypertensive therapy, heart disease accounted for about 39% ± 6% (weighted average ± standard deviation) of deaths in hypertensive people, stroke was responsible for 21% ± 9%, renal failure for 14% ± 8%, and other diseases for 25% ± 8%.

Two investigators followed the clinical course of a large number of hypertensive patients for 20 to 50 years, before the advent of antihypertensive therapy; these may be the least confounded studies of the natural history of hypertension, even if they are very old. In a series of 500 consecutive hypertensive patients in the United States (150 from before the onset of hypertension, and 350 from an early stage of hypertension, without target organ damage), Perera reported that most of these patients developed cardiac complications.[18] Although their mean age at diagnosis was only 32 years, over 20 years of average follow-up, 59% to 74% developed left ventricular hypertrophy (LVH), as assessed by electrocardiogram or chest radiograph, respectively, after which they lived only 6 or 8 more years on average. Fully 50% of these patients developed heart failure, which was followed by death after only 4 years. Only 16% developed angina pectoris, but its onset was followed by a mean survival time of only 5 years. These relatively young patients with hypertension had a very abbreviated life span; they typically died of complications of hypertension in their early 50s. During 50 years of follow-up of 271 men and 629 women with an initial BP of 160/100 mm Hg or higher, Bechgaard noted excessive mortality (mostly resulting from cardiac complications, particularly among the men) during the first 10 years, after which survival was similar to that expected for their age.[16] Even in individuals whose BPs were not quite so high at presentation, the prognosis was generally poor, with premature stroke and heart disease killing most of these patients in their late 40s or early 50s.[19]

Even before effective antihypertensive therapy became available, the causes of death among hypertensive people differed according to the severity of the hypertension, as well as the degree of target organ damage present at diagnosis. Perhaps the most striking example of the early work in this area came from the Mayo Clinic, where the Keith-Wagener-Barker classification of hypertensive retinopathy had previously been developed.[20] In 1950, of 100 patients seen there with grade IV Keith-Wagener-Barker fundi, 59% died of renal failure (as opposed to 22% with heart disease), whereas there was a graded increase in deaths from heart disease (from 28% to 46% to 52%) from grade I to grade III.[21] Of greater importance than how they died, however, were the differences in how quickly death occurred: those with grade IV fundi had a median survival time of about 6 months, with each lower grade having progressively longer median survival (16 versus 64 versus >90 months for grades III versus II versus I, respectively).[22] These data have their greatest implication for the prognosis associated with various levels of target organ damage, as discussed later.

ADVERSE CARDIOVASCULAR AND RENAL EVENTS IN HYPERTENSIVE PATIENTS

Many adverse CV and renal events are more commonly found among hypertensive than normotensive people; the major events are listed in Figure 13-1. Unfortunately, not all these adverse events have been shown to be significantly reduced by antihypertensive therapy (e.g., aortic aneurysm), and not all have been linked to hypertension in studies of the general population (e.g., epistaxis). Consideration in this chapter is given to the four with the greatest public health implications: ischemic heart disease, stroke, heart failure, and renal failure.

Ischemic Heart Disease

Even after the advent of effective antihypertensive drug therapy, ischemic heart disease ranks as the most common

major consequence of hypertension in the general population. There is little doubt from many epidemiologic studies done all over the world that elevated BP is strongly related to eventual development of ischemic heart disease, but the absolute risk of developing it depends on geography,[23] as well as age, and on the absence or presence (and severity) of other CV risk factors (see Chapter 16). Contrary to popular belief, only about 5% to 20% of individuals who present with incident CHD were completely free of CV risk factors in the past.[24,25] Of all the risk factors, hypertension has the greatest population-wide prevalence, even in countries where it is not the risk factor with the greatest attributable risk for CHD.[11,26] Attribution of risk for CHD across traditional risk factors is difficult because hypertension, dyslipidemia, diabetes, obesity, and physical inactivity "cluster," that is, they are found more commonly together in individual people than would be expected by chance. This confounds statistical methods that seek to quantify the effect of "independent" risk factors when they are, in fact, interrelated.[26]

The most comprehensive correlation of BP and risk of fatal or nonfatal CHD was a now-classic meta-analysis of nine prospective observational studies involving 418,343 people, 4260 CHD deaths, and 596 nonfatal myocardial infarctions (MIs).[27] Although the number of subjects and studies is far smaller than in the subsequent publication,[14] this analysis included all three epidemiologic studies of incident *nonfatal* CHD events (Puerto Rico, Honolulu, and Framingham, Massachusetts). In each of these, there were 50% to 300% more nonfatal than fatal events; other data suggest that the composite endpoint of fatal or nonfatal CHD has about a 50% to 100% higher incidence than fatal CHD, depending on the population studied. In each of these analyses, every study showed an identical trend for the direct relationship between the usual BP level and CHD risk, whether the study used only fatal cases or both fatal and nonfatal events. Despite using data from only 4 of more than 40 years of follow-up from the Framingham Heart Study, the overall data show a "highly significant, positive, continuous, and apparently independent" association of the risk of CHD events with diastolic BP (Fig. 13-2). Further analyses of these data indicated that, for each 7.5 mm Hg reduction in usual diastolic BP, a 29% ± 1% reduction in CHD risk was observed. Overall, a difference in usual diastolic BP across the five categories (~30 mm Hg) resulted in a five- to sixfold increase in CHD risk. No significant differences in these estimates were noted for the different studies, for men versus women, or for studies that reported only fatal versus fatal or nonfatal CHD events.

Since 1917, ischemic heart disease has ranked as the number 1 cause of death in the United States. Population-wide data from the National Health and Nutrition Examination Survey of 1999 to 2000 and other sources indicate that about 13 million persons in the United States had CHD in 2002.[28] About 7.1 million of these persons had a previous MI, and in 2002, 494,382 deaths resulted from CHD (179,514 from acute MI), with about 865,000 people having a first or recurrent MI and a total burden of disease of about 1.2 million fatal or nonfatal MIs that year.[28] Although it is difficult to estimate, for the entire population, the proportion of these events that can be attributed to hypertension, about half of the people who suffer a first MI have BP higher than 160/95 mm Hg (the old definition of hypertension).[28]

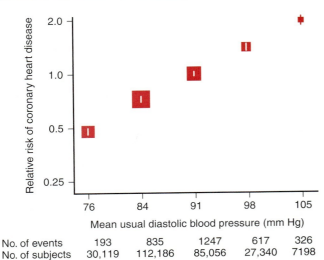

| No. of events | 193 | 835 | 1247 | 617 | 326 |
| No. of subjects | 30,119 | 112,186 | 85,056 | 27,340 | 7198 |

Figure 13–2 The "highly significant, positive, continuous, and apparently independent" relation of usual diastolic blood pressure to the relative risk of fatal or nonfatal coronary heart disease, in 418,343 people involved in nine prospective observational studies. The *squares* are proportional to the number of events at each level of diastolic blood pressure; the *vertical bars* are the 95% confidence limits for the relative risk estimates. Serial blood pressure measurements were obtained in the clinic setting, and statistical adjustments were performed to account for repeated measurements that typically regress toward a mean value over time. (Modified from MacMahon S, Peto R, Cutler J, et al. Blood pressure, stroke, and coronary heart disease: I. Prolonged differences in blood pressure: Prospective observational studies corrected for the regression dilution bias. *Lancet.* 1990;**335**:765-774.)

Fatal or nonfatal CHD is the endpoint for which risk calculators were developed by the Framingham Heart Study investigators (see Chapter 16). The simplest of these was adopted by the Third Adult Treatment Panel of the National Cholesterol Education Program.[29] At the extremes, these equations indicated that untreated systolic BP greater than 160 mm Hg does not increase the 10-year risk of CHD in a very young and low-risk man or woman, but it does increase the risk by 16% in an older woman with other risk factors. In high-risk people, untreated systolic BP between 140 and 159 mm Hg increases the 10-year risk of CHD by more than 6% (in a man) or more than 13% (in a woman). This methodology, of course, ignores the much higher risk associated with higher levels of BP, but it does provide an estimate of the incremental risk of CHD with untreated hypertension. In the 36-year follow-up of the original Framingham cohort, hypertension was associated with a increase in risk for CHD of 2.0-fold in men (age-adjusted rates: 45.4 versus 22.7 per 1000, hypertensive versus normotensive, respectively) and 2.2-fold in women (21.3 versus 9.5).[30] In the Framingham Heart Study, CHD included MI, angina pectoris, sudden death, other coronary deaths, and coronary insufficiency syndrome (which could be categorized today as acute coronary syndrome).

Individuals who were screened for participation in the Multiple Risk Factor Intervention Trial (MRFIT) form a large data set that has been examined for the relative importance of various CV risk factors (including BP) and the subsequent risk for fatal CHD. After an average of 12 years of follow-up, 6327 deaths from CHD occurred among the 316,099 nondiabetic white men who had no prior history of CHD.[31] Even though some of the men received antihypertensive drug therapy after screening, there were strong, independent associations for both systolic and diastolic BP at baseline with subsequent CHD mortality, although systolic BP was a stronger predictor than diastolic BP.

The epidemiologic evidence summarized earlier provides strong support for the view that CHD is part of the natural history of elevated (but untreated) BP, but these data are confounded by temporal trends (especially after antihypertensive drug therapy became available) and by the concern that these associations, albeit strong, direct, and highly significant, may not be causal. The best "experimental evidence" that CHD events can be prevented by lowering BP comes from clinical trials, which have the added advantages that follow-up is generally assiduous and that outcomes are commonly adjudicated by a blinded panel of experts. It is therefore useful to address the natural history of (untreated) hypertension by examining the incidence of CHD events during clinical trials in which one group is given either placebo or no treatment. The major disadvantages of this approach are that the trials are generally somewhat remote to contemporary practice (because it is no longer ethical to give only placebo or no treatment to hypertensive people) and that the event rates are confounded by "crossovers" (people originally assigned to placebo or no treatment whose BP rises to such a dangerous level that they are given open-label drug therapy or those who stop active treatment).

Investigators have conducted 23 clinical trials with a placebo/no treatment arm, in which each randomized arm included at least 25 subjects who experienced a CHD event (CHD death or nonfatal MI). The absolute risk of a CHD event varied greatly in these studies, probably because they enrolled widely different individuals. Figure 13-3 shows, on the x-axis, the wide range of absolute risk for CHD (calculated as CHD events/1000 patient-years of follow-up) across these 23 trials and the corresponding absolute benefit of treatment (seen in the arm that received active antihypertensive drug therapy). The number of CHD events prevented (per 1000 patient-years of treatment) is significantly correlated ($r = 0.72$, $P < .001$) with the absolute risk of CHD events in the untreated group (i.e., those with an unaltered natural history of untreated hypertension). This relationship has important economic implications because those at highest absolute risk derive the most benefit from therapy. The correlation improves slightly when the 12 trials that used no antihypertensive drug therapy in the placebo group are analyzed separately ($r = 0.83$, $P < .001$).

A few trials that are not included in Figure 13-3 deserve additional comment. In the first Veterans Affairs (VA) trial, the only trial that enrolled individuals with no other medical problems except a baseline diastolic BP between 115 and 129 mm Hg (and no severe target organ damage) after 6 days in hospital on a low-sodium diet, 70 men were given placebo and were followed for an average of 16 months. Two men suffered a first MI, and another had sudden cardiac death; no such events occurred in the 73 men in the drug-treated group.[32] In the second VA trial, 186 men with diastolic BP

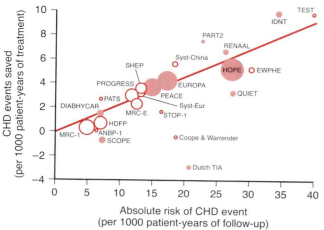

Figure 13–3 Correlation (*r* = 0.73, *P* < .001, unweighted, or *r* = 0.80, *P* < .001, weighted for number of events) between the absolute risk of a coronary heart disease (CHD) event (calculated per 1000 patient-years of follow-up) in 23 clinical trials involving placebo or no treatment only (*open circles, n* = 12) or placebo or no treatment atop other antihypertensive drugs (*closed circles*), and the number of CHD events prevented per 1000 patient-years of treatment. The values on the x-axis denote the wide variability of the natural history of (untreated) hypertension in control groups in clinical trials. The *circles* are drawn encompassing an area proportional to the number of CHD events in the trial. The acronyms of the trials are as follows: ANBP-1, Australian National Blood Pressure trial no. 1; Coope & Warrender, Coope and Warrender study; DIABHYCAR, Diabetes and Hypertension Cardiovascular Events with Ramipril; Dutch TIA, Dutch Transient Ischemic Attack trial; EUROPA, European Trial on Reduction of Cardiac Events with Perindopril in Stable Coronary Artery Disease; EWPHE, European Working Party on Hypertension in the Elderly; HDFP, Hypertension Detection and Follow-up Program; HOPE, Heart Outcomes Prevention Evaluation; IDNT, Irbesartan Diabetes Nephropathy Trial; MRC-E, Medical Research Council Trial in the Elderly; MRC-1, Medical Research Council Trial (in mild hypertension); PART2, Prevention of Atherosclerosis with Ramipril Trial no. 2; PATS, Post-stroke Antihypertensive Treatment Study; PEACE, Prevention of Events with Angiotensin-Converting Enzyme Inhibition; PROGRESS, Perindopril Protection against Recurrent Stroke Study; QUIET, Quinapril Ischemic Events Trial; RENAAL, Reduction of Endpoints in Non–Insulin Dependent Diabetes Mellitus with the Angiotensin II Antagonist Losartan trial; SCOPE, Study on Cognition and Prognosis in the Elderly; SHEP, Systolic Hypertension in the Elderly Program; STOP-1, Swedish Trial in Old Patients with Hypertension no. 1; Syst-China, Systolic Hypertension in China trial; Syst-Eur, Systolic Hypertension in Europe trial; TEST, Tenormin after Stroke and TIA.

between 90 and 114 mm Hg after the same 6 days of hospitalized bed rest and a low-sodium diet were given placebo and were followed for an average of 3.3 years.[33] In this group, 13 fatal or nonfatal CHD events occurred in the placebo group, as opposed to 11 in the treated group. The authors believed that one reason for the absence of a substantive drop in CHD

events in this trial was the failure to change other risk factors, such as cigarette smoking and dyslipidemia. These investigators also showed that among those patients with diastolic BPs between 105 and 114 mm Hg, 75% fewer morbid events occurred in the treatment group, compared with the placebo-treated group; for those with diastolic BPs between 90 and 104 mm Hg, however, the difference was only 35% (and the odds ratio, which can be calculated today, is not significant). Because of the high prevalence of "mild" hypertension (diastolic BP between 90 and 114 mm Hg), the United States Public Health Service funded a randomized, placebo-controlled, prospective trial in six clinics that enrolled 389 men and women younger than 55 years of age, 196 of whom were randomized to placebo.[34] Surprisingly, this trial finished its planned 7 years of follow-up (and even followed the participants for another 3 years), because no significant differences were seen in outcomes between the randomized groups. However, individuals with stroke or whose BPs exceeded threshold values were removed from blinded therapy and were given drug treatment. If only the events that occurred during blinded therapy are considered, six fatal or nonfatal MIs occurred in the actively treated group, as compared with seven in the placebo group; for the entire duration of follow-up, these numbers grow (15 versus 20), but they still do not achieve statistical significance.

The trials at the extremes of absolute risk for CHD events (in Fig. 13-3) are also worthy of comment. Having a very elevated BP (e.g., as in the first VA trial, discussed earlier, with 32 CHD events/1000 patient-years of observation, but not shown in Figure 13-3 because only 3 CHD events were recorded) is only one way to have a very high absolute risk of CHD. Individuals enrolled in several secondary prevention trials (e.g., Heart Outcomes Prevention Evaluation, Tenormin after Stroke and TIA) also have an absolute risk that is greater than 20 events/1000 patient-years. Similarly, subjects in those trials that enrolled much older patients (e.g., European Working Party on Hypertension in the Elderly) have a higher absolute risk simply because of their advanced age. On the contrary, the three studies with the lowest absolute risk (<7 events/1000 patient-years: first Medical Research Council Trial, Hypertension Detection and Follow-up Program, Australian National Blood Pressure trial no. 1) each prevented less than one CHD event for every 1000 patient-year of treatment.

Stroke

An elevated risk of stroke has been recognized as part of the natural history of untreated hypertension for centuries, even before it was possible to measure BP objectively. Stroke typically occurs sooner in the natural history of untreated hypertension than CHD, with the larger risk associated with the highest levels of BP. Before the advent of effective drug therapy, stroke and hypertensive encephalopathy were the two major causes of death in patients with "malignant hypertension." In fact, in a recent meta-analysis involving 32 studies and 10,892 patients, elevated diastolic BP was a major predictor of death (odds ratio, 1.71; 95% confidence interval [CI], 1.33 to 2.48) and death or dependency after stroke,[35] even though, according to current guidelines, BP should seldom be lowered in the setting of an acute stroke.[36] In nearly every epidemiologic study and clinical trial, the relative risk for stroke attributable to BP is greater than that for CHD. Although about 80% of strokes in the developed nations are the result of ischemic stroke, the less common hemorrhagic stroke is even more closely associated with elevations in BP, because the acute rupture of an intracerebral (Charcot-Bouchard) aneurysm can be pathophysiologically linked to increased BP in an intracerebral artery. The probability of stroke-related death, as assessed by the Prospective Studies Collaborative, is clearly and significantly related to the usual BP.[14] This analysis, however, does not address the problem of nonfatal stroke, which ranks first or second in the most common causes of permanent disability in most of the world.

The now-classic 1990 meta-analysis of 7 large epidemiologic cohort studies that originally included 599 fatal and 244 nonfatal strokes[27] has been updated and now includes 45 prospective cohort studies involving 448,415 people followed for an average of 16 years.[37] Strokes were reported in 13,397 people; 9824 of these were from the 23 studies that recorded only fatal strokes. Because the stroke subtype was not available for all studies, the authors were unable to perform separate analyses for ischemic versus hemorrhagic stroke. Nonetheless, their conclusions were quite similar, whether examining only fatal strokes or the composite of fatal and nonfatal strokes: For each 10 mm Hg increase in usual diastolic BP, the risk of stroke increased by 84%. The effect was particularly pronounced in younger people, although a significant trend exists also up to age 80 years. No significant differences were noted between men and women, although in some ethnicities (e.g., African Americans), the trend was even stronger. Figure 13-4 summarizes the findings of these data regarding the relationship of fatal or nonfatal stroke with BP and age. Unlike the situation in CHD, the 1990 meta-analysis of the effects of antihypertensive drug therapy showed nearly all the expected reduction in stroke (−46% ± 2%), as compared with the expected improvement based on epidemiologic studies (−42% ± 6%).[38]

Stroke has remained the number 3 cause of death in the United States since 1958, when it was displaced from the second position by cancer. Current estimates are that about 700,000 people experience a new or recurrent stroke in the United States each year, and about 500,000 have a first stroke.[28] In the United States, nearly 90% of the strokes are ischemic, approximately 9% are hemorrhagic, and a further 3% are subarachnoid hemorrhages. Approximately 2.6% of the population (or 5.4 million people) have experienced a stroke, and in 2003, 157,803 people died of a stroke. Major risk factors for stroke in U.S. populations include hypertension (two- to threefold increase in 29% of the population), atrial fibrillation (fivefold increase in 1% of the population), smoking (60% increase in 24% of the population), and diabetes (twofold increase in 10% of the population).

The Framingham Heart Study has excellent data about the contribution of hypertension to stroke risk. These have not been put together into a risk calculator in the same way that 10-year CHD risk has been estimated, but several investigators suggest that the calculations for CHD risk can be increased by about 33%, which gives a reasonable estimate of the risk of CV events, of which the major contributor (aside from CHD) is stroke. In the 36-year follow-up of the original Framingham cohort, hypertension (defined then as BP ≥160/95 mm Hg) was associated with a highly significant 3.8-fold age-adjusted biennial risk of stroke for men (12.4 versus 3.3 events per 100) and a 2.6-fold increase for women (6.2 versus 2.4 events per

100).[30] In Framingham, the absolute risk for stroke was about 3.5-fold lower in hypertensive men and women than for CHD; the increment for CHD over stroke in nonhypertensive men was approximately 6.8-fold, and in women it was approximately fourfold.

Perhaps because early clinical trials of antihypertensive drugs showed a relatively uniform and very impressive reduction in the incidence of stroke, relatively little has been written from the large U.S. epidemiologic databases (e.g., VA Hypertension Clinics) regarding the risk of stroke in hypertensive people. However, the 230 stroke deaths observed in MRFIT screenees that were included in the 1990 meta-analysis by MacMahon and colleagues show the graded increase in risk across the usual diastolic BP at baseline.[27] These data on the risk of fatal stroke with increasing levels of diastolic BP were later published in detail.[39] There were 765 deaths from stroke in their original cohort of 353,340 men over 12 years of follow-up. Subarachnoid hemorrhage accounted for 139, intracranial hemorrhage accounted for 227, and 399 were nonhemorrhagic (or ischemic) stroke. For all subtypes of stroke, systolic BP was a stronger predictor for stroke death than was diastolic BP, but both showed a significant increase in risk as the baseline BP increased, as did the number of cigarettes smoked per day.

Beginning with the first VA trial, nearly all early studies that randomized some participants to placebo or no treatment showed an impressive effect on stroke. In fact, the first terminating event in the first VA trial was a stroke in the placebo group, which occurred 4 months after randomization. When the study was terminated, four strokes and one transient

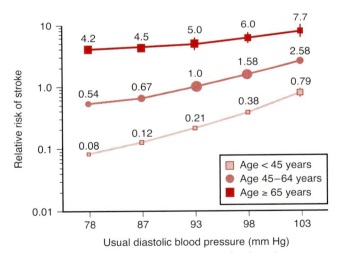

Figure 13–4 Relative risk of fatal or nonfatal stroke in 448,415 persons followed for an average of 13 years, during which time 13,397 fatal or nonfatal strokes were observed. The normalized relative risk of 1.0 was assigned to the middle-aged (45 to 64 years old) individuals with usual diastolic BP of 91 mm Hg, as in Figure 13-1. Note the exponential scale on the y-axis. Symbols encompass area in proportion to the number of strokes for each group, standard deviations are shown when they extend beyond the symbol. (Data recalculated from Figure 6 and data in Prospective Studies Collaboration. Cholesterol, diastolic blood pressure, and stroke: 13,000 strokes in 450,000 people in 45 prospective cohorts. *Lancet.* 1995;**346**:1647-1653.)

ischemic attack occurred among the 70 men assigned to placebo, and only one nondebilitating stroke occurred in the actively treated group.[32] Although this was not analyzed separately at the time, in today's world, the impressive 81% relative risk reduction for stroke or transient ischemic attack outweighs the fact that it is not statistically significant (95% CI, −60% to 2%). The second VA trial enrolled 380 patients with diastolic BPs between 90 and 114 mm Hg and noted a significant reduction in stroke (20 versus 5; relative risk reduction, 74%; 95% CI, 32% to 90%).[33] The 389 "mildly" hypertensive people enrolled in the U.S. Public Health Service Cooperative study also had a reduction in stroke risk (6 versus 1, *P* = .13), but the results of this study may have been confounded by crossovers related to uncontrolled hypertension.[34]

Figure 13-5 shows the large variability in stroke risk (along the x-axis) for individuals enrolled in 12 trials comparing effective antihypertensive drug therapy with only placebo or no treatment in the "control group." Trials that experienced very little BP difference between the two randomized groups (e.g., trials in which either other antihypertensive drugs were allowed or β-blockers were given to normotensive people) were excluded from this analysis. The highest-risk patients were those with a previous history of neurologic events (e.g., Perindopril Protection against Recurrent Stroke Study, Post-stroke Antihypertensive Treatment Study, Hypertension-Stroke Cooperative Study Group) or those of advanced age (e.g., the first Swedish Trial in Old Patients with Hypertension). In these high-risk people, antihypertensive

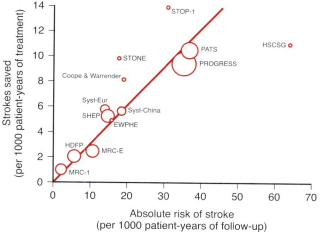

Figure 13–5 Correlation (*r* = 0.77, *P* < .001, unweighted, or *r* = 0.84, *P* < .001, weighted for number of strokes) between the absolute risk of stroke (calculated per 1000 patient-years of follow-up) in 12 clinical trials involving effective antihypertensive therapy versus placebo or no treatment and the number of strokes prevented per 1000 patient-years of treatment. The values on the x-axis denote the wide, 28-fold variability of the natural history of (untreated) hypertension progressing to stroke in control groups in clinical trials. The *circles* are drawn encompassing an area proportional to the number of strokes in the trial. The acronyms of the trials are identical to those in Figure 13-3, with the addition of the following: HSCSG, Hypertension-Stroke Cooperative Study Group; STONE, Shanghai Trial of Nifedipine in the Elderly.

drug therapy is quite effective and even cost-effective in preventing a stroke, as shown by the corresponding values on the y-axis (strokes prevented per 1000 patient-years of treatment). On the contrary, very low-risk people, such as those in the first Medical Research Council trial on mild hypertension, had only one stroke prevented for every 850 patients treated for a year, a finding that dampened enthusiasm for lowering BP for some years in Great Britain.

Cardiovascular Death

As is clear from the earlier discussion regarding the relationship of BP with death from either ischemic heart disease or stroke in the data gathered by the Prospective Studies Collaborative, an impressive association exists between usual systolic or diastolic BP and CV death, which does include a few causes of death besides that related to ischemic heart disease and stroke. In fact, the Prospective Studies Collaborative collected 10,092 "other vascular" deaths, among their total of more than 56,000 CV deaths. The "other vascular" deaths were analyzed separately, however, and no composite of CV deaths was examined. It is nonetheless clear that the same "strong, graded, and independent" effect of BP on other vascular death was seen as for both stroke and CHD mortality.[14]

In the United States during 2003, CV death was experienced by 34% of those who died: 684,462 deaths from heart disease (28%) and a further 157,803 deaths (6.45%) attributed to stroke.[12] In 2002, CV disease was listed as a primary or contributing cause of death on about 1.4 million death certificates (or ~60% of the total). In the United States, CV death accounts for more deaths than the next five leading causes of death combined (cancer, chronic lung disease, accidents, diabetes, influenza/pneumonia).[12] In 2001, premature death (i.e., at age <65 years) from cardiac causes was most common among Native Americans/Alaskan Natives (at 36%), followed by Hispanics (23.5%), blacks (31.5%), and whites (14.7%). Men also had higher rates of premature cardiac death (24%), as compared with women (10%).[40]

Investigators from the MRFIT published an analysis of 25,721 CV disease–related deaths after an average of 22 years of average follow-up among their 342,815 men without diabetes or history of MI who were originally screened for their study.[41] Although the focus of the article was ostensibly pulse pressure, it included an extensive analysis of the effects of both systolic and diastolic BPs on the risk of CV mortality. The major conclusion was that both systolic and diastolic BPs were better predictors than systolic BP, diastolic BP, or pulse pressure alone. After adjustment for baseline age, race, cholesterol, and daily number of cigarettes consumed, a significant, graded increase was noted across the baseline levels of systolic, diastolic, and pulse pressure for the risk of CV death. This increase was seen even in those who were only 35 to 44 years old at the time of screening. As would be expected, the older men (45 to 57 years old at screening) had a slightly higher predictive value of pulse pressure than the younger men.

As had been the case previously with "malignant hypertension," the very early clinical trials in hypertension also showed impressive reductions in CV death with treatment, compared with those given placebo. In the first VA trial, five CV deaths occurred in 70 patients in the placebo-treated group, whereas none of the 73 died in the drug-treated group. Although this would not be considered statistically significant today, two deaths were caused by dissecting aortic aneurysms, and one each resulted from a ruptured aortic aneurysm and presumed MI (sudden cardiac death).[32] In the second VA trial, 19 of 186 patients in the placebo-treated group had a CV death, as opposed to only 8 of 194 in the drug-treated group.[33] This corresponds today to a significant relative risk reduction of 60% (95% CI, 10% to 82%).

The experience with CV death in control groups from clinical trials that gave some enrollees placebo or no treatment may be the best way to summarize the time dependence and variability of CV death as perhaps the ultimate expression of the natural history of (untreated) hypertension. As with CHD and stroke, there was wide (16-fold) variability in the risk of CV death in the 17 trials that reported a total of more than 75 CV deaths (the x-axis of Fig. 13-6). The correlation between the number of CV deaths prevented and the absolute risk of a CV event is again highly significant, and it improves (to $r = 0.77$, $P < .001$) if one limits the data to trials that did not begin with antihypertensive drug therapy for subjects in their control groups (i.e., excluding Heart Outcomes Prevention Evaluation, European Trial on Reduction of Cardiac Events with Perindopril in Stable Coronary Artery Disease, Prevention of Events with Angiotensin-Converting Enzyme Inhibition, Irbesartan Diabetes Nephropathy Trial).

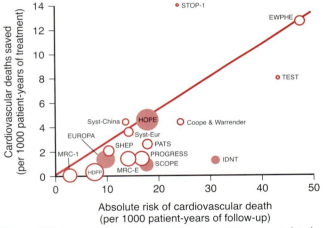

Figure 13–6   Correlation ($r = 0.70$, $P < .002$, unweighted, or $r = 0.79$, $P < .001$, weighted for number of cardiovascular deaths) between the absolute risk of cardiovascular death (calculated per 1000 patient-years of follow-up) in 17 clinical trials with more than 75 cardiovascular deaths in both groups and the number of cardiovascular deaths prevented per 1000 patient-years of treatment. The values on the x-axis denote the wide, 16-fold variability of the natural history of (untreated) hypertension progressing to cardiovascular death in control groups in clinical trials. *Open circles* denote trials in which the "control" group did not receive antihypertensive drugs; *closed circles* denote trials in which antihypertensive drugs were given to the control group. The *circles* are drawn encompassing an area proportional to the number of cardiovascular deaths in the trial. The acronyms of the trials are identical to those in Figure 13-3.

Heart Failure

Before the advent of effective antihypertensive therapy, heart failure was fairly uncommon in the general population. The initial feature was typically acute pulmonary edema, resulting from acute left ventricular dysfunction and a hypertensive emergency in young people with very elevated BPs. This was a common cause of death in case series of "accelerated/ malignant" hypertension, but chronic heart failure, as seen today most commonly in older people, was rare. Most younger patients with moderate to severe hypertension in the era before antihypertensive treatment died before they were old enough to manifest chronic heart failure. Thus, part of the reason for the recent increase in the incidence and prevalence of chronic heart failure is thought to be the effective treatment and better BP control in young but severely hypertensive individuals, treatment that prevents episodes of acute pulmonary edema. Instead, today, chronic left ventricular dysfunction typically manifests in older people who have had too many years of either poorly controlled hypertension (e.g., heart failure with preserved ventricular function, often seen as a consequence of LVH) or major cardiac damage from MI or viral infection.[42]

Perhaps because of its low incidence and prevalence before the advent of antihypertensive drug therapy, heart failure was not commonly categorized in many of these early epidemiologic studies. A recent survey of the literature found only 10 population-based studies of the prevalence of heart failure in the entire literature in which left ventricular systolic performance was evaluated by echocardiography; the overall prevalence, which increased with age, ranged between 2.1% and 8.8%.[43]

In contrast to these data, in 2002, about 4.9 million persons in the United States had diagnosed heart failure, and about 500,000 were new diagnoses that year. The age-dependent increase in prevalence is striking after age 55 years, and the prevalence is nearly 10% in those more than 75 years old. In 2001, 52,828 U.S. residents died of heart failure, and this discharge diagnosis has ranked number 1 for Medicare beneficiaries at acute care hospitals since the late 1990s. Recent data suggest that hypertension and diabetes are the two major risk factors for heart failure, especially in women, in whom body mass index and chronic kidney disease are also important. In most patients, heart failure is associated with systolic or diastolic dysfunction, both of which have hypertension as a major risk factor.[44] Conversely, once heart failure has been diagnosed, the probability of finding the usual contributory risk factors in that population are reversed: hypotension is a much bigger risk factor for death than is hypertension.[45]

Heart failure has been most clearly linked to antecedent hypertension in the Framingham Heart Study. In the 24-year follow-up, 75% of the people who developed heart failure had a previous history of hypertension, and a further 5% to 8% had elevated BP when heart failure was first diagnosed (typically as acute pulmonary edema).[42] An analysis of the Framingham data concluded that systolic BP and pulse pressure were strong predictors of future heart failure (which developed in 11% of the original Framingham Heart Study participants, 55% of which was subsequent to a MI).[46] The 36-year follow-up of the original Framingham cohort (who were largely untreated for hypertension for at least 15 years) indicates a fourfold increase in the risk of heart failure for men and a threefold increase in women for hypertension versus BP lower than 140/90 mm Hg, with biennial age-adjusted rates of 13.9 and 6.3 for hypertensive men and women, versus 3.5 and 2.1 for normotensive men and women, respectively.[30] The lifetime risk for heart failure in the Framingham Offspring Study was 21% for men and 20.3% for women at 40 years of age, but it is doubled if the baseline BP (in 1971) was 160/90 mm Hg or higher, as opposed to less than 140/90 mm Hg.[47] These data may have been confounded by antihypertensive treatment (which was widely available in Framingham beginning in the mid-1960s), so the natural history of untreated hypertension may result in a different lifetime risk.

Even very early clinical trials in hypertension showed impressive reductions in heart failure with treatment, compared with patients given placebo, a finding suggesting that the natural history of untreated hypertension includes heart failure early in its course. Despite an average age of only 51 years of participants in the first VA trial, two episodes of heart failure occurred in 70 patients in the placebo-treated group, compared with none of the 73 in the drug-treated group.[32] In the second VA trial, which had an average age of 52 years, 11 episodes of heart failure occurred in the 194 patients originally given placebo, and heart failure did not occur at all in the drug-treated group.[33] This finding corresponds today to a significant relative risk reduction of 95% (95% CI, 20% to 99%). Only four clinical trials that compared active antihypertensive drugs versus placebo/no treatment have observed more than 11 cases of heart failure in both arms of the trials. The largest numbers of patients with newly diagnosed heart failure (150) were seen in the Systolic Hypertension in the Elderly Program, in which 102 of 2371 patients originally given placebo developed heart failure over an average of 4.5 years of follow-up (or roughly 24 events/1000 patient-years of follow-up). In comparison, the group given chlorthalidone and atenolol, if needed, enjoyed a relative risk reduction of 52%.[48] In the Systolic Hypertension in Europe trial, 43 of the 2297 patients with isolated systolic hypertension who were treated with placebo developed heart failure (~7.6 events/1000 patient-years); this was reduced by 36% in the group given antihypertensive drugs.[49] In the Swedish Trial in Old Patients with Hypertension, 39 of the 815 patients given placebo developed heart failure (~23 events/1000 patient-years) over 2.1 years, but the rate was reduced by half in those given antihypertensive drugs.[50] In the Systolic Hypertension in China trial, heart failure was diagnosed in only 12 of the 2394 patients, but twice as many of the patients who were originally given placebo were affected as those given antihypertensive drug therapy.[51] A summary of all early treatment trials identified that heart failure occurred in 240 of 6923 subjects given placebo or no treatment, as opposed to 112 of 6914 individuals given drug therapy, a more than 50% reduction.[52]

The natural history of heart failure thus has changed from a reasonably common event with a high case-fatality rate in severely hypertensive young patients in the 1920s to 1960s to a more chronic condition found mostly among the elderly now. Effective antihypertensive therapy is doubtless part of the reason for this change.

Renal Failure

Ever since Richard Bright made the connection between elevated BP and renal disease, hypertension has been continu-ously reaffirmed as one of the most important factors contributing to the natural history of renal failure. The most impressive recent data about the importance of BP as a contributor to renal failure come from a meta-analysis of clinical trial data in nondiabetic patients in which an angiotensin-converting enzyme inhibitor was compared with another type of antihypertensive drug; these data no doubt underestimate the rate of progression of untreated hypertension to renal failure because the BPs were controlled, at least to some degree, in the patients who did not receive the angiotensin-converting enzyme inhibitor.[53] Over a 4-year period of follow-up, about 20% of the 919 patients with chronic kidney disease developed end-stage renal disease (ESRD), and about 45% doubled their baseline serum creatinine or developed ESRD. Both these endpoints were reduced by about 36% in those patients who were randomized to angiotensin-converting enzyme inhibitor therapy. More importantly, the optimal systolic BP for avoiding doubling of serum creatinine or ESRD was 110 to 129 mm Hg, and this was particularly true for individuals who began with more than 1 g/day of proteinuria (Fig. 13-7).

In the United States, ESRD has doubled in prevalence since the mid-1990s, with more than 100,000 new cases joining the 324,000 people already receiving dialysis (or having a kidney transplant) in 2002. Hypertension is typically underrecognized as a contributor to the epidemic of ESRD. Although diabetes mellitus has been ranked first as the cause

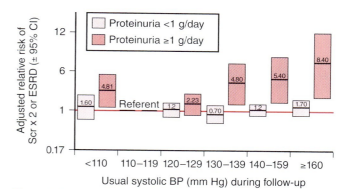

Figure 13–7 Relationship of in-trial blood pressure and risk of doubling serum creatinine (Scr × 2) or developing end-stage renal disease (ESRD) in nine randomized, placebo-controlled trials of angiotensin-converting enzyme inhibitors in patients with nondiabetic chronic kidney disease. Other antihypertensive medications were used in the "placebo-groups" of these trials, so the natural history of blood pressure (BP) to deteriorating renal function is likely underestimated by these data. Nonetheless, the data show that a systolic BP of 110 to 129 mm Hg is the best for avoiding progressive renal disease, particularly in those individuals who begin with proteinuria greater than 1 g/day *(red bars)*. Each *vertical bar* represents the upper and lower limits of the 95% confidence intervals (CI) for each blood pressure; the *line in the middle* is the point estimate for each group. Note the exponential scale used on the y-axis. (Data from Jafar TH, Stark PC, Schmid CH, et al. Progression of chronic kidney disease: The role of blood pressure control, proteinuria, and angiotensin-converting enzyme inhibition. A patient-level meta-analysis. *Ann Intern Med.* 2003;**139**:244-

of ESRD for more than 10 years, the 2003 estimates suggest that hypertension and diabetes coexist in about 39% of newly dialyzed patients, with "pure" hypertension being more common than "pure" diabetes (33% versus 15%). Hypertension is thus at least a contributing cause of more than 50% of cases of incident ESRD.

Unfortunately, no prospective data on ESRD are available from the Framingham Heart Study, primarily because in the original cohort of 5209, fewer than two cases would be expected, given the U.S. population incidence for the time frame from 1948 to 1998. Much larger databases are necessary to detect enough cases of ESRD to assess the role of BP in the natural history of ESRD. The two biggest sources of data are the screenees for the MRFIT and the Hypertension Clinics in the U.S. Department of Veterans Affairs Medical System. Both data sets show an impressive correlation of both systolic and diastolic BP with the future risk of ESRD.[54,55] In the MRFIT screenees, 814 of the 332,544 men who were originally 35 to 47 years of age developed ESRD or died of it during 16 years of follow-up. A strong, graded, and significant relationship existed between the risk of ESRD and either systolic or diastolic BP, even after adjustment for eight other risk factors (including demographics and diseases such as diabetes, heart disease, and dyslipidemia).[54] The adjusted risk of ESRD for those with BP of 210/120 mm Hg or higher was 22.1 times the risk for those with BP lower than 120/80 mm Hg. Even after adjustment for serum creatinine and urinary protein excretion rate at baseline, the significant relationship of BP and ESRD persisted. In the 32 VA Hypertension Screening and Treatment Program Clinics, 11,912 men seen from 1974 to 1976 were followed for about 15 years through the VA system and the U.S. Renal Data System.[55] In a proportional hazards model, the 245 patients who developed ESRD had a significantly higher risk of elevated pretreatment systolic BP (2.8-fold increased risk for systolic BP between 165 and 180 mm Hg, and 7.6-fold increased risk for systolic BP >180 mm Hg).

Although most people today think that renal failure is a relatively late occurrence in the natural history of hypertension, in the early experience with "malignant hypertension" and even in the initial trials of antihypertensive therapy, renal failure was occasionally noted in those who did not receive antihypertensive treatment. In the first VA trial, progressive renal disease was seen in two patients in the placebo-treated group during 18 months of follow-up, but not in patients who received antihypertensive drugs. In the second VA trial, three patients sustained irreversible renal damage in the placebo-treated arm, as opposed to none in the drug-treated arm. Although these differences are not statistically significant, the finding that renal failure was completely prevented by antihypertensive treatment in both studies but was seen in the placebo-treated arms of these trials should serve as a vivid reminder that renal complications are seen even in the short term in some hypertensive patients. Although no renal failure was noted in the patients with "mild hypertension" enrolled in the U.S. Public Health Services Cooperative Study, 200 cases of "renal insufficiency" (serum creatinine ≥2.0 mg/dL and a 25% increment over the baseline value) were seen over 8.3 years of average follow-up among the 10,940 patients in the Hypertension Detection and Follow-up Program, 99 in the "Stepped Care" group and 101 in the "Referred Care" group. In the Australian National Blood Pressure Trial, only three patients developed "renal insufficiency" (serum creatinine ≥2.0 mg/dL), two of whom were originally assigned to placebo. In most of the rest of the clinical trials that had a placebo or no-treatment group, renal failure and "renal insufficiency" were uncommon, perhaps because nearly all studies employed an "opt-out" threshold, in which all patients whose BP exceeded a very high level (typically 200/120 mm Hg) were removed from their originally assigned treatment arm and were given open-label effective antihypertensive drugs.

Other Cardiovascular Endpoints

The three other CV endpoints that were commonly seen in hypertensive patients before the advent of effective antihypertensive drugs were aortic dissection, peripheral vascular disease (typically presenting as intermittent claudication, but sometimes with arterial occlusion requiring amputation), and vascular dementia. The first two were much more common among individuals with very high BPs and were seldom noted in trials of "mild hypertension." For example, in the first VA trial, two deaths resulted from dissecting aortic aneurysm and another from a ruptured abdominal aortic aneurysm; no such events were seen in the drug-treated group. One case of peripheral arterial insufficiency developed in the placebo group of the U.S. Public Health Service trial, but other early clinical trials did not commonly report this endpoint. The association of elevated BP and vascular dementia has been a topic of renewed interest since the finding in the Systolic Hypertension in Europe trial that antihypertensive drug therapy significantly reduced the incidence of dementia by 50% over placebo, but the incidence was small in both groups: 21 cases of 2297 in the placebo group, and 11 cases of 2885 in the drug-treated group. Subsequent analyses indicated that the reduction was primarily in Alzheimer's dementia (15 versus 8), which is generally attributed to a degenerative, inflammatory process, rather than to neuronal dropout related to vascular injury (as in Binswanger's dementia). Several other clinical trials, including the Systolic Hypertension in the Elderly Program, the Medical Research Council Trial in the Elderly, and the Study on Cognition and Prognosis in the Elderly, did not show much improvement with effective antihypertensive drugs over placebo in prevention of vascular dementia. Prevention of dementia was noted in the Perindopril Protection against Recurrent Stroke Study only in those patients who suffered a recurrent stroke. Unfortunately, little attention was paid to early dementia in the era before effective drug therapy, perhaps because the devastating effects of premature stroke, MI, heart failure, and renal disease typically occurred much earlier in the natural history of hypertension than vascular dementia.

SUBCLINICAL TARGET ORGAN DAMAGE

Left Ventricular Hypertrophy

LVH has been a recognized complication of untreated or undertreated hypertension for many years, even before the electrocardiogram was developed. Perhaps because the left ventricle hypertrophies, like any other muscle during training, in response to an elevated afterload, it can be thought of as the "hemoglobin A_{1c} of BP," because it can reflect both the severity and duration of elevation of the BP. A more detailed discussion of the role of LVH in the current evaluation and treatment of hypertension can be found in Chapter 15. In early series of hypertensive patients (before the advent of drug therapy), LVH was very commonly found at diagnosis (usually ~40% to 60% were affected), and a much higher prevalence was found during follow-up. In a summary of early treatment trials, LVH was found in 216 of 6098 subjects given placebo or no treatment for 3 to 5 years, compared with only 140 of 6150 given active antihypertensive drug therapy.[52] Data from the Framingham Heart Study indicate that LVH was much less common once antihypertensive agents became available, even when all other risk factors were similar.[56] The most recent direct evidence that antihypertensive drug therapy reduces LVH and prevents CV events comes from the Losartan Intervention for Endpoint Reduction in Hypertension Study.[57]

Retinopathy

Although not widely appreciated by physicians today, hypertensive retinopathy played a very important role in the assessment of target organ damage in the era before antihypertensive drugs were available. Papilledema, the hallmark of "malignant hypertension," and the lower grades of Keith-Wagener-Barker retinopathy encompassed one early classification scheme for hypertension that had important prognostic implications. The natural history of hypertension complicated by grade IV funduscopic changes was so poor that the condition was named malignant hypertension because few cancers were associated with a worse short-term mortality rate. Hypertensive retinopathy seldom led to blindness, but the high risk of CV events justified its inclusion in early systems to predict outcomes, including death. The natural history of high-grade hypertensive retinopathy has not been carefully elucidated, but papilledema generally resolves within a few days after effective antihypertensive therapy is begun. Several population-based studies have shown the prevalence of hypertensive retinopathy to range between 5% and 15%, depending on the site, age of patients, and how many diabetic patients are in the sample.[58] The incidence of hypertensive retinopathy and progression of this disease through its usual stages have both been much reduced since the advent of antihypertensive therapy.[58]

Microalbuminuria

Proteinuria (>300 mg/day) is a clear sign of major renal damage, and it has long been associated with an increased risk of both CV and renal adverse outcomes. In addition, in several but not all studies, urinary protein excretion between 30 and 300 mg/day was also a predictor of these problems. Whether this results only from glomerular damage (e.g., from diabetes or persistently high BP) or is independent of these is controversial (see Chapter 29 for one side of this debate). The link between microalbuminuria and the natural history of deterioration of renal function is now widely accepted. Perhaps because 24-hour urine collections were not commonly carried out in the days before antihypertensive therapy became available, few unconfounded data about the natural history of microalbuminuria exist. Nonetheless, the presence of microalbuminuria is now considered evidence of target organ damage

(see Chapter 15), and many sets of guidelines recommend screening for microalbuminuria during the initial evaluation of a person with either hypertension or diabetes.

Carotid Intima-Media Thickness

Several clinical trials of antihypertensive agents have studied the progression of carotid arterial stenoses (see Chapter 22 for details). Nearly all these trials show progressive stenosis in the placebo-treated group. Nonetheless, it is difficult to interpret these data in light of the higher risk of cerebrovascular disease and stroke when antihypertensive drugs did not confound the natural history of (untreated) hypertension. It is nonetheless likely that progressive carotid arterial stenosis contributed to the higher rate of embolic stroke, and hypertension, diabetes, and dyslipidemia are probably the biggest risk factors for both problems.

Binswanger's Lesions

Magnetic resonance imaging has prompted a resurgence of interest in typically asymptomatic lacunar infarcts in periventricular and other white matter areas within the brain that had previously been diagnosed only at autopsy. Several studies have since shown that these lesions are associated with progressive dementia and, at least in epidemiologic studies, are more commonly linked to hypertension. Thus, the natural history of (untreated) hypertension is likely to include subclinical white matter lacunar infarcts, which correlate in number and size with prior BP levels (see Chapters 15 and 33 for more details). Some data indicate that these lesions may also be the result of nocturnal hypotension in older individuals, because they may be more likely to occur in the "watershed areas" of the brain that are hypoperfused during the night (when patients should not note any symptoms) in those persons whose BPs drop more than 20% compared with their daytime BP averages or in whom the morning surge in BP is greater than normal.[59,60]

Progression to Higher Stages of Hypertension

One aspect of hypertension that has received very little attention since the advent of effective antihypertensive therapy is the natural history of elevated BP to ascend to higher levels. Accelerated/malignant hypertension is seldom a term we use today, but decades ago, it was a common reason for admission to hospital. This was perhaps the most easily recognized form of hypertension that had progressed to dangerous levels, and many of the early clinical trials in hypertension documented a substantive (and nearly complete) reduction in the incidence of accelerated/malignant hypertension. A summary of nearly all the placebo-controlled early outcomes trials in hypertension indicated that 1493 of 13,342 subjects in the placebo or no-treatment groups progressed in stages of hypertension, as compared with only 95 of 13,389 in the drug-treated groups.[52]

PREHYPERTENSION

Although no specific cohorts so far recruited have primarily been studied for the natural history of progression of prehypertension (defined by the Seventh Report of the Joint National Committee on Prevention, Detection, Evaluation, and Treatment of High Blood Pressure[13] as BP ranging from 120 to 139/80 to 89 mm Hg) to hypertension (BP ≥140/90 mm Hg), and thereafter to clinical events, several important studies have shed light on this issue. Both meta-analyses by the Prospective Studies Collaborative have stressed that stroke morbidity and mortality, as well as ischemic heart disease mortality, are increased, in a graded fashion, for individuals with BPs higher than the lowest studied (typically 115/75 mm Hg).[14,37] Although age is clearly very important, the risk of CV events in these prospective cohort studies does show a significant, age-dependent increase, even for cohorts that start with a BP lower than 140/90 mm Hg. The average over all age groups is a doubling of CV mortality for every 20/10 mm Hg increase in BP.[14]

Perhaps the most specific information about the elevated long-term risk for either morbid or mortal CV events associated with prehypertension (compared with those with BP <120/80 mm Hg) comes from the Framingham Heart Study.[61] During an average of 11.1 years of follow-up of 6859 initially normotensive participants (2880 with BP <120/80 mm Hg, 2185 with BP 120 to 129/80 to 85 mm Hg, and 1794 with BP 130 to 139/85 to 89 mm Hg), a significant gradient for CV event risk was seen across each of the three groups, in both genders. Even after statistical adjustment for other time-dependent CV risk factors (e.g., diabetes, body mass index, cholesterol, and smoking), the risk for CV events for men was 1.1 for BP 120 to 129/80 to 85 mm Hg, 1.8 for BP 130 to 139/85 to 89 mm Hg, and 2.9 for BP of 140/90 mm Hg or higher, as compared with 1.3, 1.6, and 2.0 for women. Perhaps more importantly, these data showed that all men and nearly all women more than 65 years of age with BPs of 130 to 139/85 to 89 mm Hg have a 10-year absolute risk of CV events that exceeds 20%, which is recommended by several worldwide guidelines as the threshold for antihypertensive therapy.

Some of the excess risk in prehypertension can be attributed to a higher risk of subsequently developing hypertension. Like weight and many other physical characteristics, BP tends to "track" over time, with individuals originally in the upper tertile staying in the highest third of the population, even as it increases as one ages. A total of 14,407 normotensive participants in the first National Health and Nutrition Examination Survey had BPs measured (once, as in the original study) after 9.5 years.[62] Despite using the now-outdated 160/95 mm Hg threshold, an incidence of approximately 5% (over 10 years) per decade of age was observed among both men and women, from 25 to 64 years of age. The incidence of hypertension was not much different for those in the 65- to 74-year age group, compared with the 55 to 64 year olds, perhaps because it was already present in most of them at the first examination. As with the original study, more hypertension developed among African Americans than among whites.

The rates of progression of prehypertension to hypertension were also specifically examined in the Framingham Heart Study. Prehypertensive individuals were two to three times more likely to develop hypertension than normotensive persons over a 26-year follow-up period.[63] More recently, the relatively short-term (3-year) incidence of hypertension was examined.[64] In multivariable logistic regression analyses, the largest predictors among 9845 participants in either the original cohort or Framingham Offspring Study were higher

baseline BPs (multivariable odds ratio for men and women, 11.6 and 5.5, respectively, for BP 130 to 139/85 to 89 mm Hg), age (1.6 and 1.2), weight gain (1.3 and 1.2), and baseline body mass index (1.1 and 1.0). Even over as short a term as 3 years, a significant trend was noted in the incidence of hypertension across baseline BPs: 29.6%, 13.5%, and 4.0% for those aged 35 to 64 years (BPs 130 to 139/85 to 89, 120 to 129/80 to 85, and <120/80 mm Hg, respectively). Similar results were seen in 65 to 94 year olds (40.1%, 19.8%, and 12.2%). In fact, in Framingham, the lifetime risk (over 25 years of follow-up) for developing hypertension was about 90% for both men and women, whether starting observations at 55 or 65 years of age.[65] In the same group, the lifetime risk for receiving drug therapy for hypertension was about 70%. Framingham participants with prehypertension were also significantly more likely to develop any form of hypertension: isolated diastolic hypertension (about threefold greater than those with BP <120/80 mm Hg), systolic/diastolic hypertension (about three- to eightfold greater), or isolated systolic hypertension (three- to fivefold greater). Isolated diastolic hypertension appeared more commonly in younger, overweight men, whereas risk factors for isolated systolic hypertension included older age, female gender, and increased body mass index during follow-up.[66] These data suggest that, if one avoids dying of a competing cause, some type of hypertension is nearly certain to be observed by age 90 years. Because of this natural history of prehypertension, preventive measures (e.g., achieving and attaining ideal body weight, sodium restriction, and exercise) can be recommended for essentially everyone.

SUMMARY

Even though elevated BP is a strong, graded, and continuous risk factor for major adverse CV and renal events (including death), the natural history of untreated hypertension is quite variable. Hypertension is but one of several major CV risk factors that affect the probability of an adverse event. Treatment of hypertension reduces (but does not eradicate) the risk of most CV events, in proportion to the individual's absolute risk before treatment. This is the major reason for advocating treatment of all risk factors and for focusing attention on individuals with prehypertension, who may well benefit from preventing or postponing a transition to frank hypertension.

References

1. Chobanian AV, Bakris GL, Black HR, et al., and the National High Blood Pressure Education Program Coordinating Committee. The Seventh Report of the Joint National Committee on Prevention, Detection, Evaluation, and Treatment of High Blood Pressure: The JNC 7 Report. *JAMA*. 2003;**289**:2560-2572.
2. Janeway TC. Nephritic hypertension: Clinical and experimental studies. *Am J Med Sci*. 1913;**145**:625-635.
3. Society of Actuaries. Blood Pressure: Report of the Joint Committee on Mortality of the Association of Life Insurance Medical Directors and the Actuarial Society of America. New York: Society of Actuaries, 1925.
4. Gubner RS. Systolic hypertension: A pathogenetic entity. Significance and therapeutic considerations. *Am J Cardiol*. 1962;**9**:773-776.

5. Sokolow M, Perloff D. Five-year survival of consecutive patients with malignant hypertension treated with antihypertensive agents. *Am J Cardiol.* 1960;**6**:858-863.

6. Mohler ER, Fries ED. Five-year survival of patients with malignant hypertension treated with antihypertensive agents. *Am Heart J.* 1960;**60**:329-335.

7. Goldring W, Chasis H. Antihypertensive drug therapy: An appraisal. *Arch Intern Med.* 1965;**115**:523-525.

8. Paul O. Risks of mild hypertension: A ten-year report. *Br Heart J.* 1971;**33 (Suppl)**:116-121.

9. Moser M. The Treatment of Hypertension: A Story of Myths, Misconceptions, Controversies and Heroics, 2nd ed. Darien, CT: Le Jacq Communications, 2002, pp 1-94.

10. Ezzati M, Lopez AD, Rodgers A, et al., and the Comparative Risk Assessment Collaborating Group. Selected major risk factors and global and regional burden of disease. *Lancet.* 2002;**360**:1347-1360.

11. Kearney PM, Whelton M, Reynolds K, et al. Global burden of hypertension: Analysis of worldwide data. *Lancet.* 2005;**365**:217-223.

12. Hoyert DL, Kung H-C, Smith BL. Deaths: Preliminary data for 2003. *Natl Vital Stat Rep.* 2005;**53**:1-98.

13. Chobanian A, Bakris G, Black H, et al. JNC 7-complete version: Seventh Report of the Joint National Committee on Prevention, Detection, Evaluation, and Treatment of High Blood Pressure. *Hypertension.* 2004;**42**:1206-1252.

14. Prospective Studies Collaborative. Age-specific relevance of usual blood pressure to vascular mortality: A meta-analysis of individual data for one million adults in 61 prospective studies. *Lancet.* 2002;**360**:1903-1913.

15. Nichols JB, Christian HA, Shropshire W, et al. Abstract of discussion on papers of Drs. Paullin and Andrews. *JAMA.* 1926;**87**:930-932.

16. Bechgaard P. The natural history of arterial hypertension in the elderly: A fifty year follow-up study. *Acta Med Scand Suppl.* 1983;**696**:9-14.

17. Bauer GE. Modifications in the mortality pattern of hypertensive disease (a ten-year prospective study). *Aust NZ J Med.* 1972;**2**:21-27.

18. Perera GA. Hypertensive vascular disease: Description and natural history. *J Chronic Dis.* 1955;**1**:33-42.

19. Bechgaard P. Arterial hypertension: Follow-up study of 1000 hypertensives. *Acta Med Scand Suppl.* 1946;**172**:1-78.

20. Keith NM, Wagener HP, Kernohan JW. The syndrome of malignant hypertension. *Arch Intern Med.* 1928;**41**:141-153.

21. Smith DE, Odel HM, Kerohan JW. Causes of death in hypertension. *Am J Med.* 1950;**9**:516-527.

22. Keith NM, Wagener HP, Barker NW. Some different types of essential hypertension: Their course and prognosis. *Am J Med Sci.* 1939;**197**:332-339.

23. van den Hoogen PC, Feskens EJ, Nagelkerke NJ, et al. The relation between blood pressure and mortality due to coronary heart disease among men in different parts of the world: Seven Countries Study Research Group. *N Engl J Med.* 2000;**342**:1-8.

24. Greenland P, Knoll MD, Stamler J, et al. Major risk factors as antecedents of fatal and nonfatal coronary heart disease events. *JAMA.* 2003;**290**:891-897.

25. Khot UN, Khot MB, Bajzer CT, et al. Prevalence of conventional risk factors in patients with coronary heart disease. *JAMA.* 2003;**290**:898-904.

26. Yusuf S, Hawken S, Ounpuu S, et al. Effect of potentially modifiable risk factors associated with myocardial infarction in 52 countries (the INTERHEART study): Case-control study. The INTERHEART Study Investigators. *Lancet.* 2004;**364**:937-952.

27. MacMahon S, Peto R, Cutler J, et al. Blood pressure, stroke, and coronary heart disease: I. Prolonged differences in blood pressure: Prospective observational studies corrected for the regression dilution bias. *Lancet.* 1990;**335**:765-774.

28. American Heart Association. Heart Disease and Stroke Statistics—2005. Dallas, Tex: American Heart Association, 2004.

29. Executive Summary of the Third Report of the National Cholesterol Education Program (NCEP) Expert Panel on Detection, Evaluation, and Treatment of High Blood Cholesterol in Adults (Adult Treatment Panel III). *JAMA.* 2001;**285**:2486-2497.

30. Kannel WB. Blood pressure as a cardiovascular risk factor: Prevention and treatment. *JAMA.* 1996;**275**:1571-1576.

31. Neaton JD, Wentworth D. Serum cholesterol, blood pressure, cigarette smoking, and death from coronary heart disease: Overall findings and differences by age for 316,099 white men. Multiple Risk Factor Intervention Trial Research Group. *Arch Intern Med.* 1992;**152**:56-64.

32. Veterans Administration Cooperative Study Group on Antihypertensive Agents. Effects of treatment on morbidity in hypertension: Results in patients with diastolic blood pressure averaging 115 through 129 mm Hg. *JAMA.* 1967;**202**:1028-1034.

33. Veterans Administration Cooperative Study Group on Antihypertensive Agents. Effects of treatment on morbidity in hypertension: II. Results in patients with diastolic blood pressure averaging 90 through 114 mm Hg. *JAMA.* 1970;**213**:1143-1152.

34. Smith WM. U.S. Public Health Service Hospitals Cooperative Study Group: Treatment of mild hypertension. Results of a ten-year intervention trial. *Circ Res.* 1977;**40 (Suppl. 1)**:98-105.

35. Willmot M, Leonardi-Bee J, Bath PM. High blood pressure in acute stroke and subsequent outcome: A systematic review. *Hypertension.* 2004;**43**:18-24.

36. Messerli FH, Hanley DF Jr, Gorelick PB. Blood pressure control in stroke patients: What should the consulting neurologist advise? *Neurology.* 2002;**59**:23-25.

37. Prospective Studies Collaboration. Cholesterol, diastolic blood pressure, and stroke: 13,000 strokes in 450,000 people in 45 prospective cohorts. *Lancet.* 1995;**346**:1647-1653.

38. Collins R, Peto R, MacMahon S, et al. Blood pressure, stroke, and coronary heart disease: 2. Short-term reductions in blood pressure: Overview of randomised drug trials in their epidemiological context. *Lancet.* 1990;**335**:827-838.

39. Neaton JD, Wentworth DN, Cutler J, et al. Risk factors for death for different types of stroke: Multiple Risk Factor Intervention Trial Research Group. *Ann Epidemiol.* 1993;**3**:493-499.

40. Centers for Disease Control and Prevention (CDC). Disparities in premature deaths from heart disease—50 States and the District of Columbia, 2001. *MMWR—Morb Mortal Wkly Rep.* 2004;**53**:121-125.

41. Domanski M, Matchell G, Pfeffer M, et al. Pulse pressure and cardiovascular disease–related mortality: Follow-up Study of the Multiple Risk Factor Intervention Trial (MRFIT). MRFIT Research Group. *JAMA.* 2002;**287**:2677-2683.

42. Vasan RS, Levy D. The role of hypertension in the pathogenesis of heart failure: A clinical mechanistic overview. *Arch Intern Med.* 1996;**156**:1789-1796.

43. Hogg K, Swedberg K, McMurray J. Heart failure with preserved left ventricular systolic function: Epidemiology, clinical characteristics, and prognosis. *J Am Coll Cardiol.* 2004;**43**:317-327.

44. Kenchaiah S, Narula J, Vasan RS. Risk factors for heart failure. *Med Clin North Am.* 2004;**88**:1145-1172.

45. Kalantar-Zadeh K, Block G, Horwitch T, Fonarow GC. Reverse epidemiology of conventional cardiovascular risk factors in patients with chronic heart failure. *J Am Coll Cardiol.* 2004;**43**:1439-1444.

46. Haider AW, Larson MG, Franklin SS, Levy D. Systolic blood pressure, diastolic blood pressure, and pulse pressure as predictors of risk for congestive heart failure in the Framingham Heart Study. *Ann Intern Med.* 2003;**138**:10-16.

47. Lloyd-Jones DM, Larson MG, Leip EP, et al. Lifetime risk for developing congestive heart failure: The Framingham Heart Study. *Circulation.* 2002;**106**:3068-3072.

48. Kostis JB, Davis BR, Cutler J, et al. Prevention of heart failure by antihypertensive drug treatment in older persons with isolated systolic hypertension: SHEP Cooperative Research Group. *JAMA.* 1997;**278**:212-216.

49. Staessen JA, Fagard R, Thijs L, et al., for the Systolic Hypertension-Europe (Syst-EUR) trial investigators. Morbidity and mortality in the placebo-controlled European Trial on Isolated Systolic Hypertension in the Elderly. *Lancet.* 1997;**350**:757-764.

50. Dahlöf B, Lindholm LH, Hansson L, et al. Morbidity and mortality in the Swedish Trial in Old Patients with Hypertension (STOP-Hypertension). *Lancet.* 1991;**338**: 1281-1285.

51. Liu L, Wang J, Gong L, et al., for the Systolic Hypertension in China (Syst-China) collaborative group. Comparison of active treatment and placebo in older Chinese patients with isolated systolic hypertension. *J Hypertens.* 1998;**16**:1823-1829.

52. Moser M, Hebert PR. Prevention of disease progression, left ventricular hypertrophy and congestive heart failure in hypertension treatment trials. *J Am Coll Cardiol.* 1996;**27**: 1214-1218.

53. Jafar TH, Stark PC, Schmid CH, et al. Progression of chronic kidney disease: The role of blood pressure control, proteinuria, and angiotensin-converting enzyme inhibition. A patient-level meta-analysis. *Ann Intern Med.* 2003;**139**:244-252.

54. Klag MJ, Whelton PK, Randall BL, et al. Blood pressure and end-stage renal disease in men. *N Engl J Med.* 1996;**334**:13-18.

55. Perry HM Jr, Miller P, Fornoff JR, et al. Early predictors of 15-year end-stage renal disease in hypertensive patients. *Hypertension.* 1995;**25**:587-594.

56. Mosterd DA, D'Agostino RB, Silbershatz H, et al. Trends in the prevalence of hypertension, antihypertensive therapy, and left ventricular hypertrophy from 1950 to 1989. *N Engl J Med.* 1999;**340**:1221-1227.

57. Dahlöf B, Devereux RB, Kjeldsen SE, et al. Cardiovascular morbidity and mortality in the Losartan Intervention for Endpoint Reduction in Hypertension Study (LIFE): A randomised trial against atenolol. The LIFE Study Group. *Lancet.* 2002;**359**:995-1003.

58. Wong TY, Klein R, Klein BEK, et al. Retinal microvascular abnormalities and their relationship with hypertension cardiovascular disease, and mortality. *Surv Ophthalmol.* 2001;**46**:59-80.

59. Kario K, Pickering TG, Matsuo T, et al. Stroke prognosis and abnormal nocturnal blood pressure falls in older hypertensives. *Hypertension.* 2001;**38**:852-857.

60. Kario K, Pickering TG, Umeda Y, et al. Morning surge in blood pressure as a predictor of silent and clinical cerebrovascular disease in elderly hypertensives: A prospective study. *Circulation.* 2003;**107**:1401-1406.

61. Vasan RS, Larson MG, Leip EP, et al. Impact of high-normal blood pressure on the risk of cardiovascular disease. *N Engl J Med.* 2001;**345**:1291-1297.

62. Cornoni-Huntley J, LaCroix AZ, Havlik RJ. Race and sex differentials in the impact of hypertension in the United States: The National Health and Nutrition Examination Survey I Epidemiologic Follow-up Study. *Arch Intern Med.* 1989;**149**:780-788.

63. Leitshuh M, Cupples LA, Kannel W, et al. High-normal blood pressure progression to hypertension in the Framingham Heart Study. *Hypertension.* 1991;**17**:22-27.

64. Vasan RS, Larson MG, Leip EP, et al. Assessment of frequency of progression to hypertension in non-hypertensive participants in the Framingham Heart Study: A cohort study. *Lancet.* 2001;**358**:1682-1686.

65. Vasan RS, Beiser A, Seshadri S, et al. Residual lifetime risk for developing hypertension in middle-aged women and men: The Framingham Heart Study. *JAMA.* 2002;**287**:1003-1010.

66. Franklin SS, Pio JR, Wong ND, et al. Predictors of new-onset diastolic and systolic hypertension: The Framingham Heart Study. *Circulation.* 2005;**111**:1121-1127.

The Special Problem of Isolated Systolic Hypertension

Stanley S. Franklin

With the aging of our population and the advent of effective antihypertensive therapy, there has been a shift toward a more slowly evolving form of hypertension that is predominately systolic and affects middle-aged and older persons. An age-associated rise in systolic blood pressure (SBP), occurring as a consequence of increased arterial stiffness, was once considered an inconsequential part of the aging process. The dictum of that previous era stated that a person's proper SBP was 100 plus his or her age (in years). Indeed, hypertension was largely defined using only the criterion of elevated diastolic blood pressure (DBP) until the Fifth Report of the Joint National Committee on Detection, Evaluation, and Treatment of High Blood Pressure in 1993 (JNC V).[1] This slowly rising SBP with aging, out of proportion with the rise in DBP, is referred to as *isolated systolic hypertension* (ISH). Previously, ISH was defined as an SBP of 160 mm Hg or higher and a DBP of less than 95 or 90 mm Hg. With the recognition of its true cardiovascular risk, ISH was redefined as an SBP of 140 or higher and a DBP less than 90 mm Hg in the 1993 JNC V classification.[1] This form of hypertension is frequently complicated by a history of co-morbid atherosclerotic events, such as coronary heart disease (CHD), thrombotic or hemorrhagic stroke, and slowly progressive heart and renal failure. It has become the most common and the most difficult form of hypertension to treat successfully and hence a public health problem of major proportion. The purpose of this chapter is to provide a better understanding of ISH and how to treat it effectively.

EPIDEMIOLOGY

Both cross-sectional and longitudinal population studies,[2,3] including the Framingham Heart Study,[4] demonstrate that SBP rises from adolescence through most of adulthood. In contrast, DBP initially increases with age, levels off at age 50 to 55 years, and then actually decreases after age 60 to 65 years. Thus, pulse pressure (PP), defined by the difference between peak SBP and end DBP, increases after age 50 to 55 years, a change that is accelerated from the age of 60 to 65 years and beyond. The rise in SBP and DBP up to age 50 to 55 years results in isolated diastolic hypertension (SBP <140 mm Hg and DBP ≥90 mm Hg) and systolic-diastolic hypertension (SBP ≥140 mm Hg and DBP ≥90 mm Hg).[5] Diastolic hypertension can best be explained by the dominance of peripheral vascular resistance (Fig. 14-1). In contrast, after the sixth decade of life, increasing PP and decreasing DBP are surrogate measurements for central (elastic) artery stiffening (see Fig. 14-1). Indeed, the fall in DBP with increasing aortic stiffness is explained by a diminished hydraulic buffering system that leads to greater peripheral runoff of stroke volume during

systole. Thus, with less blood remaining in the aorta at the beginning of diastole, and with diminished elastic recoil, DBP decreases with increased steepness of diastolic decay.

Although increased peripheral vascular resistance may initiate essential hypertension, acceleration of large artery stiffness is the driving force leading to the steeper rise of SBP after age 50 years and the fall in DBP after age 60 years, which results in the development of ISH. Liao and associates, utilizing high-resolution B-mode ultrasound examination of the common carotid artery, showed that arterial stiffness was associated with a risk of future ISH, independent of established risk factors and the level of BP.[6] In addition, the Framingham Heart Study showed that persons with untreated hypertension (Fig. 14-2, groups 3 and 4) have accelerated stiffening of elastic arteries, as suggested by the earlier decrease in DBP and increase in PP as compared with normotensive groups (see Fig. 14-2, groups 1 and 2).[4] This process, in turn, may set up a vicious cycle of worsening hypertension and further increases in elastic artery stiffness. These findings were confirmed by Benetos and colleagues, who found that annual rates of progression in pulse wave velocity were higher in hypertensive patients than in normotensive persons, a finding suggesting accelerated progression of arterial stiffness among hypertensive patients.[7] Moreover, in the presence of diseases that accelerate arterial stiffness, ISH can develop at an earlier age. In a type 1 diabetic population free of kidney disease, investigators noted a 15- to 20-year earlier decrease in DBP, increase in PP, and development of ISH compared with aged-matched nondiabetic persons, a finding suggesting accelerated vascular aging.[8] In summary, the relation between arterial stiffness and ISH may be bidirectional, and it reflects not only normal aging but also various disease conditions.

The Third National Health and Nutrition Examination Survey demonstrated that three out of four adults with hypertension are 50 years of age or older.[5] Moreover, 80% of those with untreated or inadequately treated hypertension in this age group have ISH, which by definition consists of elevated PP. In addition to ISH's being the predominant form of geriatric hypertension, evidence indicates that widened PP may complement SBP as a predictor of cardiovascular risk.

PULSE PRESSURE AND CARDIOVASCULAR RISK

Using almost the same Framingham cohort as the previous study, 1924 men and women between 50 and 79 years of age at baseline, with no clinical evidence of CHD and free from antihypertensive drug therapy, were followed for up to 20 years.[9] In this population, CHD risk was inversely correlated with DBP at any level of SBP higher than 120 mm Hg, a finding suggesting that PP is an important component of risk. A far greater increase in CHD risk was noted with increments in PP for a given SBP than with increments in SBP with a constant PP. The Framingham Heart Study supports the findings of earlier studies[10-12] that PP may be useful as an adjunct to SBP in predicting risk and that CHD events are more closely related to the pulsatile stress of elastic artery stiffness during systole (as reflected in a rise in PP) than to the steady-state stress of resistance during diastole (as reflected in a parallel rise in SBP and DBP). A meta-analysis of eight trials by Staessen and colleagues (Fig. 14-3),[13] and three additional studies,[14-16] showed the same relation for predicting CHD risk. Furthermore, the value of PP in predicting risk in elderly persons has been confirmed by 24-hour conventional,[17] and intra-arterial,[18] ambulatory blood pressure (BP) monitoring.

Although PP is a well-established surrogate risk marker for cardiovascular risk, few studies have examined the prognostic effect of PP on cardiac and cerebrovascular events separately. In middle-aged populations, where there is predominately diastolic hypertension, mean arterial pressure (MAP) is a superior predictor of stroke events than PP, whereas the reverse is true for CHD events.[12-14,17] Conversely, in older populations with predominantly ISH, PP either independent of or complementary to MAP is a predictor of stroke events.[19] This finding is not surprising, in that the MAP equation tends to underestimate peripheral resistance in an elderly population with predominant ISH.[4] Additional evidence indicates that pulsatile stress may play an important role in cerebral function. One study demonstrated that 24-hour ambulatory PP, independent of MAP, is a predictor of prognosis following stroke.[20] Another study suggests that PP is a better predictor of Alzheimer's dementia than is MAP.[21]

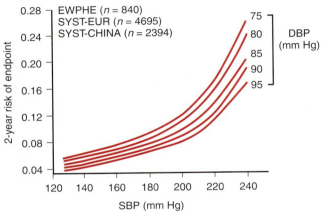

Figure 14-3 Risk of death associated in control patients with systolic blood pressure (SBP) at baseline at fixed levels of diastolic blood pressure (DBP). The 2-year probability of death was standardized to female sex, mean age (70 years), no previous cardiovascular complications, and nonsmoking. EWPHE, European Working Party on Hypertension in the Elderly; SYST-CHINA, Systolic Hypertension in China trial; SYST-EUR, Systolic Hypertension in Europe trial. (Modified from Staessen JA, Gasowski, Wang JG, et al. Risks of untreated and treated isolated systolic hypertension in the elderly meta-analysis of outcome trials. *Lancet.* 2000;**104**: 865-872.)

Age (Years)	DBP (mm Hg)	SBP (mm Hg)	MAP (mm Hg)	PP (mm Hg)	Hemodynamics
30–49	↑	↑	↑	→ or ↑	R>S
50–59	→	↑	→	↑↑	R=S
≥60	↓	↑	→ or ↓	↑↑↑↑	S>R

R = small-vessel resistance
S = large-vessel stiffness

Figure 14-1 Hemodynamic patterns of age-related changes in blood pressure. ↑, increase; ↓, decrease; →, no change; DBP, diastolic blood pressure; MAP, mean arterial pressure; PP, pulse pressure; SBP, systolic blood pressure. (Modified from Franklin SS, Gustin W, Wong ND, et al. Hemodynamic patterns of age-related changes in blood pressure: The Framingham Heart Study. *Circulation.* 1997;**96**:308-315.)

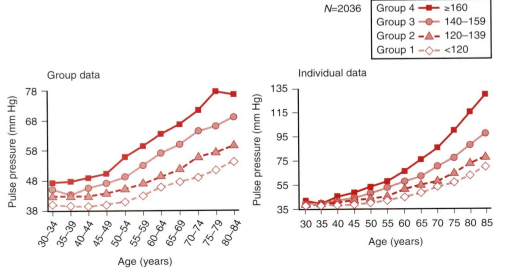

Figure 14-2 Pulse pressure by age. Group averaged data *(left)* and averaged individual regression analysis *(right)* for all subjects and with deaths, myocardial infarction, and congestive heart failure excluded. Curves are plotted based on blood pressure predicted values at 5-year age intervals by systolic blood pressure groupings. (Modified from Franklin SS, Gustin W, Wong ND, et al. Hemodynamic patterns of age-related changes in blood pressure: The Framingham Heart Study. *Circulation.* 1997;**96**: 308-315.)

BLOOD PRESSURE IN THE ASSESSMENT OF CORONARY HEART DISEASE RISK?

The Framingham Heart Study also examined the relationship between BP and CHD risk as a function of age.[22] From the age of 20 to 79 years, investigators noted a continuous, graded shift from DBP to SBP and eventually to PP as predictors of CHD risk (Fig. 14-4). From age 60 years onward, when considered with SBP, DBP was negatively related to CHD risk, so PP emerged as the best predictor.[22] In contrast to the findings in elderly persons, all three BP indices in the Framingham study were equally predictive of CHD risk in the transitional ages of 50 to 59 years.[22] In the younger group (<50 years of age), DBP was a more powerful predictor of CHD risk than SBP, and PP itself was not predictive.

Not only do SBP elevations predominate as hypertensive patients age, but also the SBP appears to be a more accurate staging criterion on which to base and evaluate treatment. The JNC 7 and the World Health Organization–International Society of Hypertension guidelines classify stage 1 hypertension as an SBP of 140 to 159 mm Hg or a DBP of 90 to 99 mm Hg.[23,24] Stage 2 or greater classifications begin at an SBP or a DBP that exceeds these levels.[23,24] Lloyd-Jones and colleagues analyzed data from patients who were not receiving antihypertensive therapy in the Framingham Heart Study and found a disparity between the SBP and the DBP in slightly more than 35% of the 3656 untreated patients.[25] In these discordant patients, 31.6% were classified into a higher stage based on an elevated SBP, versus 3.8% on the basis of the DBP alone. When added to the proportion of patents with congruent stages of SBP and DBP (64.6%), SBP as the sole criterion provided the correct classification in approximately 96% of cases.

As suggested by their age-dependent divergent patterns of onset, diastolic hypertension and ISH may be two distinct disorders with significant overlap. The conversion from diastolic hypertension to ISH in the older age group has been attributed to burned-out diastolic hypertension.[26] Although some people who have had untreated or poorly treated diastolic hypertension at a younger age develop ISH as they become older, data from the Framingham Study suggest that only about 40% of patients acquire ISH in this manner.[27] The majority of people who developed ISH did so without going through a stage of elevated DBP (Fig. 14-5).[27] The bias toward DBP over SBP by earlier generations of physicians may be, in part, a result of the emphasis on hypertension as a young person's condition. However, with the aging of the population since the 1950s, hypertension has become largely a condition affecting older persons, that is, those with the ISH subtype.[5]

HEMODYNAMICS OF ISOLATED SYSTOLIC HYPERTENSION

PP is determined by arterial stiffness, by stroke volume, and, to a lesser extent, by the ejection rate of the left ventricle. In contrast, MAP is determined by cardiac output and total peripheral resistance. By definition, ISH is characterized by an increase in PP, but not necessarily by an increase in MAP. Thus, in older subjects, brachial PP is regarded as a surrogate measure of arterial stiffness.[28,29]

ETIOLOGY OF ARTERIAL STIFFNESS

By middle age, long-standing cyclic stress in the media of elastic-bearing arteries produces fatigue and eventual fracturing of elastin, along with structural changes of the extracellular matrix that include proliferation of collagen and deposition of calcium.[30] This degenerative process, termed arteriosclerosis, is the pathologic process that results in

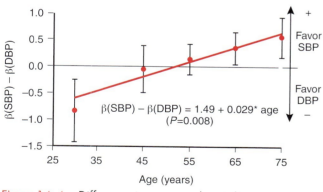

Figure 14–4 Difference in coronary heart disease prediction between systolic blood pressure (SBP) and diastolic blood pressure (DBP) as function of age. Difference in ß coefficients (from Cox proportional hazards regression) between SBP and DBP is plotted as a function of age, obtaining this regression line: $\beta(SBP) - \beta(DBP) = -1.49848 + 0.0290 \times age$ ($P = .008$). (Modified from Franklin SS, Larson MG, Khan SA, et al. Does the relation of blood pressure to coronary heart disease risk change with aging? The Framingham Heart Study. *Circulation*. 2001;**103**: 1245-1249.)

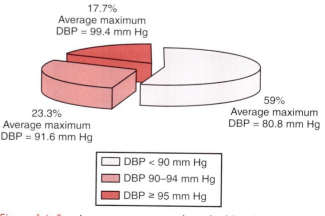

Figure 14–5 Average maximum diastolic blood pressure (DBP) reached before the development of isolated systolic blood pressure for those who reached a diastolic blood pressure of less than 90 mm Hg, from 90 to 94 mm Hg, and 95 mm Hg or higher, respectively. (Modified from Franklin SS, Pio JR, Wong ND, et al. Predictors of new-onset diastolic and systolic hypertension: The Framingham Heart Study. *Circulation*. 2005;**111**:1121-1127.)

increased central elastic arterial stiffness with widening of PP. Other disease processes, such as type 1 and type 2 diabetes,[31,32] obesity,[33] hypercholesterolemia,[34] generalized atherosclerosis,[35] smoking,[36] and chronic renal failure,[37] can accelerate aging of central elastic arteries with earlier development of arterial stiffness. Arterial stiffness is also accompanied by the phenomenon of early wave reflection.

WAVE REFLECTION AND RISK

The central pressure waveform is produced by two major components, a forward traveling wave, generated by ventricular ejection, and a reflected wave arriving back from the periphery.[30] In young subjects, the reflected pressure waves return to the ascending aorta in diastole and serve to elevate mean DBP, thus boosting coronary artery perfusion.[30] The summation of the incident pressure wave with the reflected wave in young adults produces a normal phenomenon of pressure amplification of PP and SBP from the aorta to the brachial artery.[30] Between the ages of 20 and 70 years, as arteries stiffen, the pulse wave velocity doubles. In older individuals, the reflected pressure wave returns to the ascending aorta earlier during late systole and increases or "augments" the central SBP and PP, thus decreasing pressure amplification and simultaneously contributing to increase cardiac afterload.[30]

Paradoxically, the heart "sees" SBP only in the ascending aorta, and pressure wave amplification distorts the relationship between central and peripheral SBP, as measured at the brachial artery by the sphygmomanometer. Therefore, central and not peripheral SBP, regardless of age, determines cardiac afterload and hence cardiac risk. The changing pattern of age-related brachial artery BP components that predict CHD risk results from altered peripheral resistance, aortic stiffness, and early wave reflection, all acting in concert to raise SBP, decrease DBP, and abolish pressure amplification. This leads to an age-related shift from sphygmomanometrically determined DBP to SBP and ultimately to ISH with wide PP as the predictors of cardiac risk.[22] These findings represent a significant paradigm shift in our understanding of how we use brachial artery cuff BP components to predict cardiovascular risk.

CAVEATS IN DIAGNOSING HYPERTENSIVE CARDIOVASCULAR RISK

BP variability represents an important barrier to the assessment of cardiovascular risk. Only when office or clinic BP mercury sphygmomanometry is performed in a rigorous and standardized manner can one minimize inherent BP variability (see Chapter 5). The calculation of PP is less precise and accurate than individual BP components because of the summation of measurement errors for SBP and DBP. Furthermore, intra-arterial DBP measurements are higher than simultaneously recorded brachial cuff measurements, especially in older individuals.[38] Thus, the true prevalence of ISH in elderly persons may be underestimated. Despite this imprecision and inaccuracy of brachial cuff BP measurement, many observational studies in elderly persons, as previously noted, have shown a stronger relation of brachial cuff PP as

compared with SBP or MAP in predicting cardiovascular events. In the few studies of elderly persons that failed to show superiority of PP over SBP or MAP in predicting cardiovascular events, systematic errors may have occurred. One possible source of error is the clinic or office alerting reaction, often called white-coat tendency.[39] The alerting reaction tends to inflate PP falsely as a result of a greater rise in SBP than DBP. Indeed, studies show that cardiovascular events are better predicted by 24-hour ambulatory PP than by office PP.[39]

In middle-aged, healthy populations with both systolic and diastolic hypertension, SBP and MAP may be equal or superior to PP as predictors of cardiovascular risk.[40-42] In these populations, such high colinearity exists between SBP and PP that it becomes impossible to show an advantage of one index over another in predicting risk. Only when SBP increases and DBP decreases does the superiority of PP over SBP as a predictor of cardiovascular risk become apparent in uncomplicated hypertension. With advanced age and after adjustment for cardinal risk factors, PP becomes an independent predictor of CHD risk. Therefore, despite the high colinearity between SBP with PP, the latter predominates as the single best predictor of CHD risk because of the contribution of pulsatile stress in a minority of subjects with discordantly low DBP values. The MAP equation grossly underestimates vascular resistance after age 50 to 60 years as DBP plateaus and then falls.[4] Hence, beyond middle age, PP becomes a better predictor and MAP a poorer predictor of cardiovascular risk. Paradoxically, the value of MAP has been highlighted with the publication of meta-analyses by the Prospective Studies Collaboration and the Asia Pacific Cohort Studies Collaboration, using 61 and 37 observational cohort studies, respectively.[43,44] These investigators concluded that MAP, in both the young and old, was a far superior predictor of CHD risk than PP. Their conclusions are in disagreement with the proven importance of arterial stiffness and early wave reflection as important risk factors in middle-aged and elderly individuals with ISH and the superiority of DBP as a predictor of cardiovascular risk in the young.[22] The Prospective Studies Collaboration and Asia Pacific Cohort Studies Collaboration studies included persons with single BP measurements and persons receiving antihypertensive medication. The majority of the population cohorts in these meta-analyses did not consider PP and MAP as independent variables. A meta-analysis of a smaller number of well-done observational studies, rather than the multiple diverse studies included in the Prospective Studies Collaboration and Asia Pacific Cohort Studies Collaboration, may have provided a different picture of the importance of DBP in the young and SBP and PP in the old as predictors of cardiovascular risk.

The preponderance of evidence supports PP as a surrogate risk marker for arterial stiffness in elderly persons, although at times an imperfect one. Clearly, these findings call into question the prevailing belief that elevation of SBP and DBP contribute equally to cardiovascular risk. However, evidence supporting the reduction of PP instead of SBP as a therapeutic goal remains scant. In addition, we have little information on the utility of using PP and SBP together, rather than SBP alone, to classify hypertensive risk. Because most people with systolic hypertension are more than 50 years of age and have ISH, the focus should be on high-risk systolic hypertension. From a practical viewpoint, effective antihypertensive therapy most often lowers both SBP and PP simultaneously. Furthermore, a public health recommendation that focuses on PP may detract from the importance of SBP in the diagnosis and treatment of hypertension. On the basis of prevailing data, it would be premature to modify current treatment guidelines that focus primarily on lowering SBP in middle-aged and elderly persons for the prevention of cardiovascular events.

PATHOPHYSIOLOGY OF ISOLATED SYSTOLIC HYPERTENSION

Increased PP may be a surrogate marker for several possible pathologic mechanisms, all originating from the underlying increased central arterial stiffness and early wave reflection. Increased aortic pulsatile afterload is a major factor in the development of left ventricular hypertrophy with increased coronary blood flow requirements. In addition, increased turbulent flow leads to endothelial dysfunction, with a greater propensity for coronary atherosclerosis and for rupture of unstable atherosclerotic plaques.

Whereas reflected waves normally return during early diastole and thereby enhance coronary perfusion, this increased boost is absent in elderly persons with ISH; the decline in DBP, however, rarely falls to the critical level (~60 mm Hg) required to disturb coronary flow autoregulation.[45] Thus, it is unlikely that the reduction in DBP that occurs in most patients with ISH compromises coronary perfusion. Nonetheless, a potential imbalance exists between systolic demand and coronary supply. Furthermore, cardiac ejection into the stiff arterial system results in more coronary perfusion during the systolic period, thus making the heart more vulnerable to changes in systolic pressure and systolic heart function. In addition to arterial stiffening, the left ventricle itself develops systolic stiffness, perhaps an adaptive change to facilitate cardiac ejection and to maintain matched coupling of heart to arteries. This is particularly notable in hearts that develop ventricular hypertrophy, a common occurrence in elderly patients and particularly those with ISH. A stiffer left ventricle coupled to a stiffer arterial system can contribute to increased cardiovascular risk in several ways, as shown by the studies of Kass and associates.[46-49] First, late-systolic wall stress is increased, as are the cardiac energy costs imposed on the heart to deliver cardiac output to the systemic circulation. Second, the imposition of high late-systolic load that often rises markedly during stress demand slows cardiac relaxation rates, potentially leading to incomplete diastolic relaxation, elevated diastolic pressures, and compromised cardiac reserve. This mechanism is important in patients with heart failure symptoms who have apparent preservation of left ventricular function. Finally, loss of arterial distensibility appears to alter vascular mechanosignaling, so the normal augmentations of nitric oxide release and vasoprotective mechanisms are compromised. Many of these disturbances in cardiovascular function characterize the elderly person with long-standing ISH and markedly elevated PP. In summary, diastolic dysfunction and heart failure result from the combination of elevated cardiac afterload presented to a compromised left ventricle, which is unable to handle the load. Thus, cardiovascular risk is defined by both (1) increased SBP, which is a marker of cardiac afterload, and (2) concordant decreased DBP, resulting in further increased PP, which is a marker of vascular-cardiac stiffness and a predictor of diastolic dysfunction.

THERAPEUTIC BENEFITS

During the past few decades, the treatment approach for elderly hypertensive patients has steadily evolved. In the early 1970s, prevailing wisdom questioned the benefit of administering antihypertensive agents to patients more than 65 years old.[50] Beginning in the early 1990s, the publication of three major placebo-controlled studies that specifically addressed the treatment of ISH in older patients changed the perception of the significance of SBP control. In 1991, the landmark Systolic Hypertension in the Elderly Program first established that ISH increased the risk of adverse cardiovascular events and that older patients benefited from treatment.[51] The Systolic Hypertension in Europe and the Systolic Hypertension in China trials corroborated these findings.[52,53] Staessen and colleagues conducted a meta-analysis of 11,825 patients who participated in these major trials, as well as an additional 3868 subjects with ISH 60 years old or older who participated in five other trials.[13] This analysis found that antihypertensive treatment significantly reduced fatal and nonfatal coronary events by 23% ($P = .001$), fatal and nonfatal strokes by 30% ($P < .0001$), cardiovascular events by 26% ($P < .0001$), cardiovascular mortality by 18% ($P = .01$), and total mortality by 13% ($P = .02$).[13] Additionally, a highly significant 49% reduction in fatal and nonfatal heart failure was reported using data from the Systolic Hypertension in the Elderly Program ($P < .001$).[51] These results clearly demonstrate that antihypertensive treatment in ISH patients who are more than 60 years old reduces morbidity and mortality. Furthermore, these studies negate prior assumptions that age-related changes in BP are safe and reinforce the emerging paradigm that treatment will benefit patients with elevated SBP, even when these patients have normal diastolic pressure.

Based on a 2001 estimate, life expectancy in the United States is 77 years,[54] thus raising the question of the benefit of antihypertensive agents in patients who are older than that. A meta-analysis of several trials that included 1670 patients 80 years old or older suggests even very old patients may benefit from antihypertensive treatment.[55] In these patients, active treatment produced a 34% reduction in stroke ($P = .014$), a 39% reduction in heart failure ($P = .01$), and a 22% reduction in major cardiovascular events ($P = .01$). The reduction in coronary events was not statistically significant, and a nonsignificant 6% increase in mortality was observed.[55] These results imply that although antihypertensive treatment may not extend the lives of octogenarians, treatment may enhance the quality of their remaining years through prevention of strokes, heart failure, and major cardiovascular complications.

THERAPEUTIC TARGET GOALS

The JNC 7 and the World Health Organization/International Society of Hypertension provide guidelines for the optimal reduction of BP to achieve maximum benefit from antihypertensive therapy.[23,56] These guidelines, based on observational as well as on outcome data, suggest that low-risk patients be treated to a target goal of SBP lower than 140 mm Hg. For high-risk subjects, the therapeutic target is SBP less than 130 mm Hg. In addition to reaching target BP, the paramount goal of therapy in patients with ISH is to achieve the maximum reduction in overall cardiovascular risk through simultaneous treatment of all reversible risk factors.

SELECTION OF ANTIHYPERTENSIVE DRUG THERAPY

Treatment approaches with the capability of minimizing arterial stiffness include a variety of approved agents; however, most conventional antihypertensive drugs fall short of optimally reducing age-related increases in PP.[57] Optimal treatment of ISH should reduce not only peripheral resistance but also, more importantly, large artery stiffness and the early wave reflection generated by that stiffness. The question of which drug class is best suited to start first in patients with ISH remains controversial, although diuretics and calcium channel blockers were shown to be effective in reducing cardiovascular events in the major intervention studies.[51-53] Furthermore, in the ISH substudy of the Losartan Intervention for Endpoint Reduction in Hypertension study, which was a trial of patients with hypertension and left ventricular hypertrophy, losartan, an angiotensin II receptor blocker, was superior to atenolol, a β-blocker, in preventing fatal and nonfatal strokes.[58] Importantly, a diuretic was an add-on drug in more than 70% of both therapeutic arms of the trial, a finding suggesting that the combination of a diuretic and an angiotensin II receptor blocker is effective in stroke prevention in patients with ISH. In practice, a combination of two or more drug classes will be necessary for BP control in the majority of patients with ISH, especially when SBP is higher than 160 mm Hg.[23]

Therapeutic benefit of antihypertensive drugs in ISH may result from at least five different mechanisms. First, reduction of peripheral resistance downstream will decrease large artery stiffness upstream by diminishing intramural pressure and decreasing the stretch on elastic arteries; antihypertensive agents that dilate blood vessels work in this manner.[59] Second, vasodilation of small arteries will shorten the artery reflection sites, decrease early wave reflection, decrease aortic late SBP peaking, and hence decrease cardiac afterload.[28] Nitrates, in doses that do not affect peripheral vascular resistance, can decrease early wave reflection and can change the significant central PP component to lower the left ventricular load on the heart, even without a significant change in arterial stiffness.[60] Third, long-term reduction in cardiac afterload will eventually result in regression of left ventricular hypertrophy, regression of vascular smooth muscle hypertrophy, and remodeling of small blood vessels toward a normal wall-to-lumen ratio.[61] Indeed, the ability of angiotensin-converting enzyme inhibitors and angiotensin receptor blockers to promote regression of left ventricular hypertrophy and arterial remodeling may have important long-term benefits in reducing arterial stiffness.[28] Fourth, therapy that blocks excessive aldosterone at the tissue level may over time result in regression of fibrosis in the heart, renal mesangium, and large blood vessels; spironolactone may prove to be of value in this area.[28] Fifth, some antihypertensive agents appear to possess properties that specifically influence arterial stiffness. In animal models, and more recently in humans, advanced glycation end product crosslinking breakers have been shown to prevent arterial stiffening.[62] In the future, these agents may be extremely important treatment options for patients who do not reach SBP targets. Although poorly understood, reduced-sodium diets to achieve negative salt balance, with or without the use of diuretics, can influence arterial stiffness.[28,29]

The optimal strategy in treating ISH is to maximize SBP reduction while minimizing the reduction in DBP. As demonstrated in patients receiving antihypertensive therapy from Koch-Weser in 1973,[63] the higher the PP (in part, age related), the greater the fall in SBP as compared with the fall in DBP. Antihypertensive therapy that decreases vascular resistance will result in a parallel reduction in SBP and DBP.[30] In contrast, drug-induced reduction in large artery stiffness will result in a fall in SBP and a rise in DBP.[30] Therefore, antihypertensive therapy maximizes the decrease in PP and minimizes the further reduction in DBP, in direct proportion to the age of the patient and the extent of large artery stiffness.

ACHIEVING THERAPEUTIC GOALS

The realization that antihypertensive treatment of patients who are more than 60 years old correlates with improved outcomes makes awareness of hypertension and access to treatment important factors in achieving therapeutic goals. Since the 1970s, awareness of hypertension has steadily increased; however, in the most recent National Health and Nutrition Examination Survey (1999 to 2000), awareness was approximately 69%, the same as in the previous survey conducted more than 5 years earlier. Thus, a substantial proportion (31%) of hypertensive persons in the United States continue to be unaware of having hypertension, with nearly one half of these persons more than 65 years old.[64]

Furthermore, of the patients treated, many remain at higher than recommended BP goals. Nearly 60% of hypertensive patients receive antihypertensive therapy, but only about 25% achieve the recommended SBP of 140 mm Hg.[64] Not unexpectedly, most treatment failures occur in patients older than 50 years. Only 14% of reported failures occurred in patients younger than this age cutoff, whereas 86% of treatment failures occurred in older individuals, most of whom had ISH, access to health care, and relatively frequent contact with physicians.[5,65] Analyzing treatment failures by age reveals the age-related discrepancy in the successful control of both facets of BP. Approximately 50% of younger patients in whom treatment failed had both SBP and DBP that were not at target goals, a finding representing a concordant failure in this younger population. In stark contrast, older patients who failed to achieve treatment goals had discordant failure. Only 17% of patients age 50 years or older had DBP higher than their goal, but fully 82% had SBP higher than their goal.[5]

The tendency toward discordant failure amplifies with increasing age. Using data from the Framingham study, Lloyd-Jones and colleagues demonstrated age-related changes in the ability to reach the target DBP and SBP goals.[66] More patients older than 75 years than less than 60 years old achieved their DBP goal (92% versus 85%, respectively). In contrast, the SBP target progressively became more difficult to achieve: in patients less than age 60 years, 69% reached their SBP target goal; in those ages 61 to 75 years, 48% of patients reached goal; and in those more than 75 years old, only 34% reached goal.[66]

That the target SBP apparently becomes more difficult to achieve with aging may be explained by a failure in the treatment approach. In the past, treatment guidelines focused on the DBP and relegated the control of SBP to minimal importance. Some clinicians feared reaching an excessively low DBP and therefore were reluctant to lower the SBP even at SBPs higher than 150 or 140 mm Hg as long as the DBP remained at or lower than its target. Failure to use optimal polypharmacy and, in particular, failure to incorporate diuretics as part of polypharmacy may have hampered the ability to control ISH. In addition, not treating to the lower target goals in high-risk patients with diabetes and with kidney disease likely further contributed to the disappointingly high incidence of treatment failures. Although several aspects involving treatment approaches may explain the failure to optimally control ISH overall, one must conclude that substantial numbers of patients with systolic hypertension are truly resistant to currently available medications, even when these agents are used properly. This category of patients includes the following: patients with stage 2 ISH in whom the SBP is much higher than 160 mm Hg; those with left ventricular hypertrophy and diastolic dysfunction; those with complicated hypertension in terms of diabetes, CHD, renal disease, or peripheral vascular disease; and those who are truly resistant to an appropriate three-drug regimen. Indeed, many elderly patients with ISH fall into this category.

SUMMARY

Once considered an inconsequential part of the aging process, the development of ISH represents a late manifestation of increased arterial stiffness in the middle-aged and elderly population. Its inherent increased risk for vascular events highlights the importance of its control. Furthermore, overwhelming evidence indicates that pharmacologic treatment of ISH reduces cardiovascular events in elderly persons. Paradoxically, ISH remains more difficult to control than diastolic hypertension, and most middle-aged and elderly hypertensive patients fail to achieve recommended targets. In part, the lack of strict control of ISH in the aged population lies in the hemodynamic differences between diastolic and systolic hypertension. Younger patients tend toward isolated diastolic hypertension or combined systolic-diastolic hypertension, primarily driven by increased peripheral resistance and more easily and effectively treated by antihypertensive medications. In contrast, older patients develop ISH in association with increased arterial stiffness that is less amenable to current therapies. This barrier to control of ISH can be overcome largely by an aggressive polypharmacologic approach to therapy.

References

1. Fifth Joint National Committee on Prevention, Detection, Evaluation, and Treatment of High Blood Pressure (JNC V). *Arch Intern Med.* 1993;**153**:154-183.
2. Whelton PK, He J, Klag MJ. Blood pressure in Westernized populations. *In:* Swales JD (ed.). Textbook of Hypertension. Oxford: Blackwell Scientific Publications, 1994.
3. Burt VL, Whelton P, Roccella EJ, et al. Prevalence of hypertension in the US adult population: Results from the Third National Health and Nutrition Examination Survey, 1988-1991. *Hypertension.* 1995;**25**:305-313.
4. Franklin SS, Gustin W, Wong ND, et al. Hemodynamic patterns of age-related changes in blood pressure: The Framingham Heart Study. *Circulation.* 1997;**96**:308-315.
5. Franklin SS, Jacobs MJ, Wong ND, et al. Predominance of isolated systolic hypertension among middle-aged and elderly US hypertensives. *Hypertension.* 2001;**37**:869-874.
6. Liao D, Arnett DK, Tyroler HA, et al. Arterial stiffness and the development of hypertension: The ARIC study. *Hypertension.* 1999;**34**:201-206.
7. Benetos A, Adamopoulos C, Bureau J-M, et al. Determinants of accelerated progression of arterial stiffness in normotensive subjects and in treated hypertensive subjects over a 6-year period. *Circulation.* 2002;**105**:1202-1207.
8. Ronnback M, Fagerudd J, Forsblom C, et al. Altered age-related blood pressure pattern in type 1 diabetes. *Circulation.* 2004;**110**:1076-1082.
9. Franklin SS, Khan SA, Wong ND, et al. Is pulse pressure useful in predicting risk for coronary heart disease? The Framingham Heart Study. *Circulation.* 1999;**100**:354-360.
10. Darne B, Girerd X, Safar M, et al. Pulsatile versus steady component of blood pressure: A cross-sectional analysis and a prospective analysis on cardiovascular mortality. *Hypertension.* 1989;**13**:392-400.
11. Fang J, Madhavan S, Cohen H, et al. Measures of blood pressure and myocardial infarction in treated hypertensive patients. *J Hypertens.* 1995;**13**:413-419.
12. Benetos A, Safar M, Rudnichi A, et al. Pulse pressure: A predictor of long-term cardiovascular mortality in a French male population. *Hypertension.* 1997;**30**:1410-1415.
13. Staessen JA, Gasowski, Wang JG, et al. Risks of untreated and treated isolated systolic hypertension in the elderly meta-analysis of outcome trials. *Lancet.* 2000;**104**:865-872.
14. Millar JA, Lever AF, Burke V. Pulse pressure as a risk factor for cardiovascular events in the MRC mild hypertension trial. *J Hypertens.* 1999;**17**:1065-1072.
15. Sesso HD, Stampfer MJ, Rosner B, et al. Systolic and diastolic blood pressure, pulse pressure, and mean arterial pressure as predictors of cardiovascular disease risk in men. *Hypertension.* 2000;**36**:801-807.
16. Vaccarino V, Holford TR, Krumholz HM. Pulse pressure and risk for myocardial infarction and heart failure in the elderly. *J Am Coll Cardiol.* 2000;**36**:130-138.
17. Verdecchia P, Schillaci G, Borgione C, et al. Ambulatory pulse pressure: A potent predictor of total cardiovascular risk in hypertension. *Hypertension.* 1998;**32**:983-988.
18. Khattar RS, Swales JD, Dore C, et al. Effect of aging on the prognostic significance of ambulatory systolic, diastolic, and pulse pressure in essential hypertension. *Circulation.* 2001;**104**:783-789.
19. Domanski MJ, Davis BR, Pfeffer MA, et al. Isolated systolic hypertension: Prognostic information provided by pulse pressure. *Hypertension.* 1999;**34**:375-380.
20. Aslanyan S, Weir CJ, Lees KR. Elevated pulse pressure during the acute period of ischemic stroke is associated with poor stroke outcome. *Stroke.* 2004;**35**:e153-e155.
21. Qiu C, Winblad B, Viitanen M, et al. Pulse pressure and risk of Alzheimer disease in persons aged 75 years and older: A community-based longitudinal study. *Stroke.* 2003;**34**: 594-599.
22. Franklin SS, Larson MG, Khan SA, et al. Does the relation of blood pressure to coronary heart disease risk change with aging? The Framingham Heart Study. *Circulation.* 2001;**103**:1245-1249.
23. Chobanian AV, Bakris GL, Black HR, et al., and the National High Blood Pressure Education Program Coordinating Committee. The Seventh Report of the Joint National

Committee on Prevention, Detection, Evaluation, and Treatment of High Blood Pressure: The JNC 7 report. *JAMA*. 2003;**289**:2560-2572.

24. World Health Organization. 2003 World Health Organization–International Society of Hypertension statement on the management of hypertension. *J Hypertens*. 2003;**21**:1983-1992.

25. Lloyd-Jones DM, Evans JC, Larson GM, et al. Differential control of systolic and diastolic blood pressure: Factors associated with lack of blood pressure control in the community. *Hypertension*. 2000;**36**:594-599.

26. Bulpitt CJ, Palmer AJ, Fletcher AE, et al. Proportion of patients with isolated systolic hypertension who have burned-out diastolic hypertension. *J Hum Hypertens*. 1995;**9**:675-679.

27. Franklin SS, Pio JR, Wong ND, et al. Predictors of new-onset diastolic and systolic hypertension: The Framingham Heart Study. *Circulation*. 2005;**111**:1121-1127.

28. Van Bortel LMAB, Struijker-Boudier HAJ, Safar ME. Pulse pressure, arterial stiffness, and drug treatment of hypertension. *Hypertension*. 2001;**38**:914-921.

29. Safar ME, Levy BL, Struijker-Boudier HAJ. Current perspectives on arterial stiffness and pulse pressure in hypertension and cardiovascular diseases. *Circulation*. 2003;**107**:2864-2869.

30. Nichols WW, O'Rourke MF. McDonald's Blood Flow in Arteries: Theoretical, Experimental and Clinical Principles, 4th ed. London: Arnold, 1998, pp 349-376.

31. Wilkinson IB, MacCallum H, Rooijmans DF, et al. Increased augmentation index and systolic stress in type 1 diabetes mellitus. *Q J Med*. 2000;**93**:441-448.

32. Brooks B, Molyneaux L, Yue DK. Augmentation of central arterial pressure in type 1 diabetes. *Diabetes Care*. 1999;**22**:1722-1727.

33. Westerbacka J, Vehkavaar S, Bergholm R, et al. Marked resistance of the ability of insulin to decrease wave reflection in the aorta characterizes human obesity. *Diabetes*. 1999;**48**:821-827.

34. Wilkinson IB, Prasad K, Hall IR, et al. Increased central pulse pressure and augmentation index in subjects with hypercholesterolemia. *J Am Coll Cardiol*. 2002;**39**:1005-1011.

35. Weber T, Auer J, O'Rourke MF, et al. Arterial stiffness, wave reflections, and the risk of coronary artery disease. *Circulation*. 2004;**109**:184-189.

36. Mahmud A, Feely J. Effect of smoking on arterial stiffness and pulse pressure amplification. *Hypertension*. 2003;**41**:183-187.

37. Safar ME, Blacher J. Pannier B, et al. Central pulse pressure and mortality in end-stage renal failure. *Hypertension*. 2003;**39**:735-738.

38. Zweifer AJ, Shahab ST. Pseudohypertension: A new assessment. *J Hypertens*. 1993;**11**:1-6.

39. Verdecchia P, Schillaci G, Reboldi G, et al. Different prognostic impact of 24-hour mean blood pressure and pulse pressure on stroke and coronary artery disease in essential hypertension. *Circulation*. 2001;**103**:2579-2584.

40. Antikainen RL, Jousiliahti P, Vanhanen H, Tuomilehto J. Excess mortality associated with increased pulse pressure among middle-aged men and women is explained by high systolic blood pressure. *J Hypertens*. 2000;**18**:417-423.

41. Miura K, Daviglus ML, Dyer AR, et al. Relationship of blood pressure to 25-year mortality due to coronary heart disease, cardiovascular diseases, and all causes in young adult men: The Chicago Heart Association Detection Project in industry. *Arch Intern Med*. 2001;**161**:1501-1508.

42. Domanski M, Mitchell G, Pfeffer M, et al. Pulse pressure and cardiovascular disease-related mortality. *JAMA*. 2002;**287**:2677-2683.

43. Prospective Studies Collaboration. Age-specific relevance of usual blood pressure to vascular mortality: A meta-analysis of individual data for one million adults in 61 prospective studies. *Lancet*. 2002;**360**:1903-1913.

44. Asia Pacific Cohort Studies Collaboration. Blood pressure indices and cardiovascular disease in the Asia Pacific Region: A pooled analysis. *Hypertension*. 2003;**42**:69-75.

45. Somes GW, Pahor M, Shorr RI, et al. The role of diastolic blood pressure when treating isolated systolic hypertension. *Arch Intern Med*. 1991;**265**:3255-3264.

46. Kass DA, Bronzwaer JGF, Paulus WJ. What mechanisms underlie diastolic dysfunction in heart failure? *Circ Res*. 2004;**94**:1533-1542.

47. Chen CH, Nakayama M, Nevo E, et al. Coupled systolic-ventricular and vascular stiffening with age: Implications for pressure regulation and cardiac reserve in the elderly. *J Am Coll Cardiol*. 1998;**32**:1221-1227.

48. Kawaguchi M, Hay I, Fetics B, et al. Combined ventricular systolic and arterial stiffening in patients with heart failure and preserved ejection fraction: Implications for systolic and diastolic reserve limitations. *Circulation*. 2003;**107**:714-720.

49. Peng X, Haldar S, Deshpande S, et al. Wall stiffness suppresses Akt/eNOS and cytoprotection in pulse-perfused endothelium. *Hypertension*. 2003;**41**:378-381.

50. Fry J. Natural history of hypertension: A case for selective non-treatment. *Lancet*. 1974;**2**:431-433.

51. SHEP Cooperative Research Group. Prevention of stroke by antihypertensive drug treatment in older persons with isolate systolic hypertension: Final results of the Systolic Hypertension in the Elderly Program (SHEP). *JAMA*. 1991;**265**:3255-3264.

52. Staessen JA, Fagard R, Thijs L, et al. Randomized double-blind comparison of placebo and active treatment for older patients with isolated systolic hypertension. *Lancet*. 1997;**350**:757-764.

53. Wang J-G, Staessen JA, Gong L, et al. Chinese trial on isolated systolic hypertension in the elderly. *Arch Intern Med*. 2000;**160**:211-220.

54. Arias E. United States life tables, 2001. *Natl Vital Stat Rep*. 2004;**52**:1-38.

55. Gueyffier F, Bulpitt C, Boissel J-P, et al. Antihypertensive drugs in very old people: A subgroup meta-analysis of randomized controlled trials. *Lancet*. 1999;**353**:793-796.

56. World Health Organization–International Society of Hypertension Guidelines Subcommittee. World Health Organization–International Society of Hypertension guidelines for the management of hypertension, 1999. *J Hypertens*. 1999;**17**:151-183.

57. Mourad J-J, Blacher J, Blin P, et al. Conventional antihypertensive drug therapy does not prevent the increase of pulse pressure with age. *Hypertension*. 2001;**38**:958-962.

58. Kjeldsen SE, Dahlof B, Devereux RB, et al. Effects of losartan on cardiovascular morbidity and mortality in patients with isolated systolic hypertension and left ventricular hypertrophy: A Losartan Intervention for Endpoint Reduction (LIFE) substudy. *JAMA*. 2002;**288**:1491-1498.

59. Smulyan H, Safar ME. Systolic blood pressure revisited. *J Am Coll Cardiol*. 1997;**29**:1407-1413.

60. Stokes GS, Barin ES, Gilfillan KL. Effects of isosorbide mononitrate and AII inhibition on pulse wave reflection in hypertension. *Hypertension*. 2003;**41**:297-301.

61. Schiffrin El, Deng LY, Larochelle P. Progressive improvement in the structure of resistance arteries of hypertensive patients after 2 years of treatment with an angiotensin I-converting enzyme inhibitor: Comparison with effects of a β-blocker. *Am J Hypertens*. 1995;**8**:229-236.

62. Kass D, Shapiro EP, Kawaguchi M, et al. Improved arterial compliance by a novel advanced glycation end product crosslink breaker. Circulation. 2001;**104**:1464-1470.

63. Koch-Weser J. Correlation of pathophysiology and pharmacotherapy in primary hypertension. *Am J Cardiol.* 1973,**32**:499-510.

64. Hajjar I, Kotchen TA. Trends in prevalence, awareness, treatment, and control of hypertension in the United States, 1988-2000. *JAMA.* 2003;**290**:199-206.

65. Hyman DJ, Pavlik VN. Characteristics of patients with uncontrolled hypertension in the USA. *N Engl J Med.* 2001; **345**:479-486.

66. Lloyd-Jones DM, Evans JC, Larson GM, et al. Differential control of systolic and diastolic blood pressure: Factors associated with lack of blood pressure control in the community. *Hypertension.* 2000;**36**:594-599.

Chapter 15

Assessment of Hypertensive Target Organ Damage

Joseph L. Izzo, Jr., Philip R. Liebson, Philip B. Gorelick, James J. Reidy, and Albert Mimran

Many different pathologic changes accompany the syndrome of hypertension. Broadly speaking, chronic hypertension eventually damages the heart and blood vessels, with secondary effects on the function of the brain, eyes, and kidneys. In general, the degree of hypertensive target organ damage (TOD) is proportional to the duration and severity of hypertension, sometimes called the total blood pressure (BP) burden over a lifetime. The presence of any given form of TOD signals the likelihood that other major target organs have also been damaged and clearly identifies a condition of increased risk for overall morbidity and mortality. Patterns of TOD also affect treatment strategies; according to the Seventh Report of the Joint National Committee on the Prevention, Detection, Evaluation, and Treatment of High Blood Pressure (JNC 7), both the appropriate BP target and the specific medications recommended for treatment of hypertension depend on the pattern of TOD present.[1] Thus, careful assessment of TOD is a vital part of the management of any patient with hypertension. This chapter is organized by organ system, with pathophysiology and assessment techniques included for each form of hypertensive TOD, along with a clinical overview.

GENERAL APPROACH

Whether or not clinically significant hypertensive TOD is present should be established in any hypertensive patient, but all possible diagnostic tests cannot and should not be performed in all patients. Thus, appropriate testing requires reasonable clinical suspicion that a particular form of TOD is likely. A few tests are recommended in all patients, including a careful history and physical examination, with particular attention paid to the assessment of the heart, peripheral vasculature, eyes, and central nervous system. Each patient should also have a routine blood sample for electrolytes and serum creatinine, fasting glucose and lipid profile (high-density lipoprotein and low-density lipoprotein cholesterol and triglycerides), a urinalysis, and a resting electrocardiogram (ECG). Additional tests to assess particular forms of hypertensive TOD depend on the clinical circumstances and require clinical judgment.

HYPERTENSIVE HEART DISEASE

The spectrum of hypertensive heart disease (Table 15-1) includes left ventricular hypertrophy (LVH) and left ventricular (LV) systolic or diastolic dysfunction that may lead to heart failure (HF). Hypertension also exacerbates ischemic heart disease (IHD). In clinical practice, often no clear-cut separation exists among these intermediate categories, but early signs of hypertensive heart disease are associated with an adverse prognosis, even if symptoms are not yet present. Many of the specific diagnostic and therapeutic interventions in hypertension, coronary heart disease, and HF (discussed in Chapters 17 to 24, 27, and 28) are not reviewed here.

Left Ventricular Hypertrophy

Demographic Associations

Important factors predisposing to LVH include age, BP, and obesity.[2,3] LVH is more prevalent in women and blacks than in men and whites.[4-6] Over the age range of 30 to 70 years, the prevalence of echocardiographically detectable LVH increases from less than 10% to more than 30% in men and to more than 50% in women.[2] Although LVH is exacerbated by obesity,[7] patients usually have no accompanying impairment in LV systolic performance with increasing weight. BP is the most important determinant of LVH, whether hypertension is established by office, home, or ambulatory BP monitoring.[8] In a population with stage 1 hypertension but without overt IHD, the prevalence of LVH varies between 15% and 32%, depending on LV mass indexing criteria and body habitus.[9] Patterns of LVH also vary with the type of hypertension. In combined systolic-diastolic hypertension, eccentric hypertrophy is more common than concentric hypertrophy,[9,10] whereas in isolated systolic hypertension, concentric LVH is the predominant abnormality, even at lower levels of mean arterial pressure.[2] The prevalence of LVH may be declining in the United States as a result of increased use of antihypertensive agents.[11]

Pathogenesis

Left Ventricular Geometry and Remodeling

Increased LV mass is commonly classified as *eccentric* or *concentric* hypertrophy to describe the type of adaptation of cardiac myofibrils. In eccentric hypertrophy (e.g., the athletic heart), myofibrillar units are added in sequence, leading to an elongated ventricular chamber with increased end-diastolic volume, normal end-diastolic pressures, and enhanced contractile efficiency. In concentric hypertrophy, myofibrillar units are added in parallel to offset the effects of increased afterload; the result is a uniform thickening of the heart muscle. Early in the course of concentric LVH, subtle evidence of ventricular dysfunction is seen such as decreased fractional shortening of cardiac myofibrils,[12] impaired diastolic relax-

Table 15-1 Cardiac Target Organ Damage: Noninvasive Evaluation

1. LVH

Electrocardiography

Sokolow-Lyon criteria (S_{V1} + $R_{V5 or 6}$) > 3.5 mV
Cornell voltage criteria (S_{V3} + R_{aVL}) > 2.8 mV
Cornell product (S_{V3} + R_{aVL}) × QRS duration > 244 V.s
LV strain (downsloping ST depression V_4 to V_6)

Echocardiography

M-mode cube formula
   LV mass = 1.05 [(LVDD + IVS + PW)^3 − LVDD^3]
   LVH = indexed LV mass >97.5th percentile of normal
      population

Types

Concentric hypertrophy: LVH + Th/R > 0.43
Eccentric hypertrophy: LVH + Th/R ≤ 0.43

2. Ischemic Heart Disease

Angina/prior myocardial infarction

Electrocardiography
   Significant Q waves in appropriate leads.
Echocardiography
   Segmental wall motion abnormalities
Stress echocardiography
   Segmental wall motion abnormalities
   Perfusion abnormalities (power Doppler-contrast)

Prior coronary revascularization

History/record documentation

3. Heart Failure (LV Dysfunction)

Clinical

Left ventricular S_3 gallop
Pulmonary rales
Decreased maximum oxygen consumption

Chest radiograph

Enlarged heart
Pulmonary venous redistribution
Pulmonary infiltrates

Echocardiography

Systolic: LVEF <50%, fractional shortening <0.29,
   dilated LV
Diastolic: Reversed mitral Doppler E/A ratio (abnormal
   relaxation)
   Markedly increased E/A ratio (restriction)
   Abnormal pulmonary vein S/D ratio
   Abnormal mitral annulus Doppler ratio: E'/A'

E/A ratio, ratio of E wave to A wave; IVS, end-diastolic intraventricular septal thickness; LV, left ventricular; LVH, left ventricular hypertrophy; LVDD, left ventricular end-diastolic dimension; LVEF, left ventricular ejection fraction; PW, end-diastolic posterior wall thickness; S/D ratio, systolic-to-diastolic ratio; Th/R, ratio of end-diastolic (IVS + PW)/LVDD (or 2 PW/LVDD).

ation, and reduced coronary blood flow reserve. Later in life, concentric LVH leads to more advanced LV diastolic dysfunction and eventually predisposes patients to systolic HF, dysrhythmias, and sudden cardiac death. Because increased LV mass can be physiologic or pathologic, cardiac function and dimensions must be considered. The simplest indicator that differentiates concentric from eccentric LVH is the ratio of ventricular wall thickness to chamber radius (Th/R). In concentric hypertrophy, Th/R is increased, whereas in eccentric hypertrophy, Th/R is normal.

Central Systolic Blood Pressure and Cardiac Load

Chronic increases in central systolic BP and cardiac afterload promote concentric LVH. Cardiac load and oxygen consumption are the product of heart rate and the integral of the systolic interval of the central pressure waveform. The contribution of the arterial tree to cardiac load includes a series of ventricular-vascular interactions that can be separated into three major components: (1) residual systemic (diastolic) pressure, (2) *early-systolic* interactions involving early ventricular contraction and aortic elasticity, and (3) *late-systolic* interactions involving reflected pressure waves and central systolic pressure augmentation. The pattern of LV remodeling in hypertensive heart disease is related to parallel changes in arterial structure and function. In general, patients with stiff central arteries (wide pulse pressure [PP], high ratio of PP to stroke volume, or high pulse wave velocity [PWV]) tend to have concentric remodeling or hypertrophy and more adverse outcomes than do patients with eccentric hypertrophy or concentric remodeling without LVH.[13,14]

Other Associations

LVH is also a risk factor for other forms of hypertensive TOD, including stroke, chronic kidney disease (CKD), and IHD.[15] LVH is also associated with endothelial dysfunction and reduced coronary reserve independent of systemic BP.[16,17] No association has been found between myocardial blood flow and LV mass, although a heterogeneous pattern of regional defects has been reported with increased LV mass.[18] Both genetics and environment appear to play roles in the development of LVH, but LVH is predominantly an acquired characteristic. In young patients with mild hypertension who have never been treated,[19] the presence of the angiotensinogen 825T allele or an aldosterone synthase polymorphism is weakly associated with increased LV mass index.[20,21] LV mass is greater in persons with the T-1370G endothelin allele, but only in those of low socioeconomic status.[22]

Assessment

Electrocardiography

The Cornell product (see Table 15-1) is generally preferred, in part because it is more reliable in obese patients,[23] yet its sensitivity is only 50% to 60% that of echocardiography or necropsy.[24] The Cornell product and echocardiography have been reported to predict cardiovascular mortality independently.[25] The classic strain pattern (ST-T abnormalities in the lateral precordial leads) on the ECG correlates reasonably with echocardiographic signs of LVH and is the strongest ECG marker of increased morbidity and mortality.[26] In people with hypertension and LVH shown on the ECG, relative wall thickness (Th/R) is independently correlated with higher systolic pressure, lower stroke volume,[27] and increased risk for coronary events.[28,29]

Echocardiography

The findings on echocardiography evolve as hypertension progresses, and adjustment for calculated LV end-systolic stress is necessary to account for differences in LV inotropy. An early sign is reduced LV midwall fractional shortening, which can occur with normal LV ejection fraction.[29] Midwall fractional shortening is lower than the fifth percentile in 16% of hypertensive patients, despite only a corresponding 2% reduction in endocardial fractional shortening.[30] Midwall fractional shortening abnormalities also predict LV dysfunction during exercise in asymptomatic hypertensive individuals.[31] Widespread application of echocardiographic screening for LVH has been limited by cost-to-benefit considerations; as a result, a limited echocardiographic study has been proposed.[32] Technical differences, including the use of varying criteria for Th/R ratio, make interstudy comparisons difficult.[3] Echocardiography has been validated against a necropsy-based cube formula for LV end-diastolic intraventricular septal and posterior wall thicknesses and chamber dimensions (see Table 15-1).[33] Echocardiographic visualization may be suboptimal in up to 20% of studies, especially in obese patients, in whom two-dimensional and even three-dimensional approaches may be needed.

Other Imaging Techniques

LV mass can be accurately quantitated using newer computer-assisted imaging techniques such as magnetic resonance imaging (MRI) and computed tomography (CT), which are more sensitive and accurate than echocardiography. As the cost of these techniques is reduced and more clinical experience is gained, they are expected to become increasingly useful in the quantitation of LV mass and the accompanying assessment of functional and structural alterations in hypertension and related diseases.

Ambulatory Blood Pressure Monitoring

Ambulatory BP monitoring over 24 hours provides a close correlation with hypertensive TOD, including LV mass and albuminuria.[34] Better correlations with LV mass are also found with self-measured average home BPs than with clinic BPs.[35] Thus, white-coat hypertension, which may be present in as many as 20% of hypertensive patients,[36] has been associated with increased LV mass in some,[37] but not all, studies.[36,38] Overall, 24-hour BP load (the proportion of BPs higher than normal during ambulatory BP monitoring) is a reasonable surrogate for hypertensive TOD, including LV midwall fractional shortening abnormalities.[39] Echocardiographically detectable LVH is very common in patients with refractory hypertension (persistent increase in ambulatory 24-hour BP despite the use of at least three antihypertensive agents for at least 3 months) compared with those with adequate BP control (40% to 55% versus 16% to 22% depending on method of indexing LV mass).[40]

Assessment Overview

The presence of LVH is clear proof that the BP burden is increased, cardiovascular risk is increased, and antihypertensive drug therapy is warranted. The Cornell voltage-duration product is recommended for initial screening of all patients with hypertension using an ECG. Echocardiography, which is more sensitive than the ECG, should be considered in any individual with exercise-induced fatigue or dyspnea. Echocardiography is also fully indicated in any patient with a suspicion of IHD, in valvular disease, and in patients with chronic edema. Th/R and systolic and diastolic wall motion abnormalities should be quantitated. Newer imaging studies, such as MRI, are attractive alternatives to echocardiography. Ambulatory BP correlates strongly with concentric LVH. Regression of echocardiographically detectable LVH has been demonstrated with effective antihypertensive therapy, but it is not necessary to follow patients with serial echocardiographic studies documenting LVH regression.

Ischemic Heart Disease

IHD, a common problem in patients with hypertension, is exacerbated by the increased cardiac work needed to sustain the increased central systolic pressure and is further worsened by LVH. Hypertension also tends to accelerate the process of atherogenesis, by enhancing the pathogenesis of IHD through increased shear forces and mechanical strain on large and small blood vessels. Progression of atherosclerosis also heavily depends on non–BP-dependent changes in arterial walls, especially increased cholesterol oxidation and local inflammation. A more complete discussion of IHD and hypertension is provided in Chapter 27.

Assessment Overview

Because hypertension is an independent risk factor for IHD, the presence of subclinical myocardial ischemia must be considered in all middle-aged and elderly patients. Cardiovascular risk factors should be assessed (e.g., Framingham Heart Study risk score) for all patients with hypertension because a high-risk profile such as diabetes plus one or more additional IHD risk factors affects prognosis and treatment. Typical clinical presentations of active myocardial ischemia and a history of a prior infarction or revascularization afford an easy diagnosis of IHD, but atypical presentations of IHD must be considered, especially in patients with diabetes, in whom IHD may be silent. A resting ECG (Q waves, ST-segment–T-wave abnormalities) or ambulatory monitoring with an ECG may yield adequate evidence of ischemia, but physical or pharmacologic stress tests are more sensitive. Echocardiographic or nuclear studies may reveal segmental LV wall motion abnormalities. CT can identify the presence of coronary calcification, but it gives no direct information about blood flow or myocardial disease. Intra-arterial ultrasonography remains limited in its usage. Newer noninvasive forms of angiography using MRI (MRA) or CT are promising. Invasive coronary angiography remains the gold standard for the diagnosis of coronary artery disease, but positron emission technology can differentiate viable from nonviable myocardium.

Left Ventricular Dysfunction and Heart Failure

Overt HF is a natural consequence of the interplay between LVH and IHD. Regardless of the cause of cardiac dysfunction, a combination of systolic and diastolic dysfunction ultimately leads to symptomatic heart disease that can be categorized by disease state (using the American College of Cardiology–American Heart Association recommendations) and functional performance (New York Heart Association functional scores).

Demographics

Increased risk for HF occurs in individuals with LVH,[41,42] obesity,[43] female gender, or African-American ethnicity.[44] LV function is highly correlated with 24-hour systolic BP and either LV mass index or LV filling rate ($r = 0.69$ and -0.60, respectively).[45] PP and systolic pressure confer a greater risk than diastolic pressure for the development of HF: for each 20 mm Hg increase in systolic BP or 16 mm Hg increase in PP, the risk of HF roughly doubles.[46]

Pathogenesis

Systolic versus Diastolic Dysfunction

It is now standard practice to define HF functionally (systolic versus diastolic dysfunction, also known as HF with preserved systolic function). The most common cause of LV systolic dysfunction is IHD, with post–myocardial infarction segmental dyskinesia leading to ventricular enlargement and reduced LV ejection fraction. Patients with LV systolic dysfunction almost always have a degree of diastolic dysfunction, but the reverse is not always true. Isolated diastolic dysfunction is common in patients with LVH, many of whom have normal or supranormal contractility. In some normotensive nonobese young men, especially those with sleep apnea syndrome, diastolic dysfunction may precede LVH.[47] The classic presentation of diastolic dysfunction is "flash pulmonary edema," in which resting LV ejection fraction is normal.[48]

Ventricular Failure

The development of symptomatic systolic dysfunction ultimately depends on progressive loss of myocytes as a result of infarction, apoptosis, or other degenerative mechanisms that accelerate the age-related decline in LV function.[49] The spectrum of LV dysfunction in hypertension includes progressive changes in systolic and diastolic performance, especially impaired midwall fractional shortening and relaxation, with or without overt symptoms. Systemic hypertension plays an important role in the process through direct increases in afterload and oxygen consumption. In subjects with systolic hypertension associated with increased aortic stiffness, increased reflection of pressure waves adds to the late-systolic pressure load (systolic pressure augmentation), thus increasing LV afterload and mass. In many hypertensive patients, especially those with kidney disease, increased preload further exacerbates the problem by adding a volume overload component. LV dilatation tends to increase LV wall stress and thus further compromises oxygen consumption and stimulates maladaptive increases in LV wall thickness that cannot fully compensate for the increased cardiac afterload. Compensatory increases in circulating neurohormones such as catecholamines, angiotensin II, and aldosterone secondarily increase preload or afterload in a variety of ways, including increased vasoconstriction and fluid retention.[50] These progressive functional abnormalities are further exacerbated by limitation of coronary flow reserve and abnormal myocardial collagen deposition, which increases ventricular stiffness.

Assessment of Heart Failure: Overview

HF remains first and foremost a clinical diagnosis, based on a thorough history and physical examination. New York Heart Association functional status (grades I to IV) should be assessed in all patients, and each case should be staged according to accepted guidelines (e.g., American College of Cardiology–American Heart Association stages A to D). Grading and staging are not exact, owing to the nonspecific nature of the usual clinical symptoms (e.g., dyspnea, fatigue) and signs (e.g., peripheral edema, jugular venous distention, S_3 gallop, basilar rales, lateralized apex beat). A chest radiograph is almost always indicated if one suspects HF, but findings can be vague (e.g., increase in heart size, pulmonary parenchymal haziness, pulmonary venous redistribution). The assessment of systolic and diastolic ventricular function is usually made by echocardiography. Assessment of LV systolic performance should include measured chamber sizes, indices of fractional shortening or midwall function, description of segmental wall motion abnormalities, and calculation of LV ejection fraction. Assessment of diastolic function should include measurements of ventricular wall thickness and mass as well as indices of diastolic relaxation. Echocardiographic Doppler mitral flow studies (E/A wave ratio) should be considered to estimate atrial pressures. Nuclear techniques are alternatives to echocardiography to assess segmental perfusion defects and diastolic relaxation parameters and are particularly accurate in determining LV ejection fraction and mass.

HYPERTENSIVE ARTERIOPATHY

Arteriosclerosis and Atherogenesis

Functional and structural alterations in the arterial tree are causally related to the development of chronic hypertension, which, in turn directly damages large and small arteries (see Chapter 32). Two independent degenerative processes affecting large arteries often interact: *arteriosclerosis* (stiffening of arteries resulting from diffuse noninflammatory changes in the composition of the tunica media of large arteries that lead to systolic hypertension) and *atherogenesis* (patchy occlusive inflammatory vascular disease leading to IHD and peripheral arterial disease [PAD]). Small vessel constriction and vascular smooth muscle hypertrophy lead to increased systemic vascular resistance and mean arterial pressure. Isolated systolic hypertension and wide PP result from increased central arterial stiffness superimposed on increased systemic vascular resistance.[51] Atherosclerosis commonly affects the aorta and the carotid, coronary, renal, and ileofemoral, but not brachial, arteries. PAD is a designation usually reserved for atherosclerotic occlusive disease in the lower body, with claudication and impotence as common symptoms. The presence of PAD confers roughly the same overall risk as known IHD.

Arterial Compartments

The arterial tree can be divided functionally into three major compartments: large central arteries, muscular conduit arteries, and small arteries and arterioles.[52] A critical principle is that these different vascular compartments react differently to aging and disease. Second, each compartment operates independently and interdependently with the other compartments. Thus, no single artery or regional circulation can serve as a surrogate for the other compartments. The structural and functional properties of arteries depend on the vessel size and on wall thickness and composition (proportions of collagen, elastin, and vascular smooth muscle).

Central arteries (aorta, innominate, proximal carotids) have relatively thin walls and are relatively elastic, serving as a circulatory "damper" to convert cardiac pulsation into a more continuous flow pattern. Stiffness of the central arterial compartment, most reliably represented by characteristic aortic impedance (Zc), is the principal determinant of the width of the PP. Zc is higher in individuals with smaller aortic diameters (usually women) or with aging (via increased wall thickness and collagen content). Large central arteries are also subject to atherosclerotic degeneration, which is usually patchy and thus has a limited effect on arterial stiffness. Fusiform aneurysms also occur, particularly in the abdominal aorta.

Muscular conduit arteries (second- and third-order arteries) have smaller internal diameters than the central vessels and a greater proportional wall thickness (wall-to-lumen ratio), and they are intrinsically stiffer than central arteries. Decreasing diameters of conduit arteries leads to a progressive increase in input impedance, a property that leads to widening of PP (PP amplification). This phenomenon is important because brachial cuff BP is not necessarily a good surrogate for central arterial or microcirculatory pressures,[51,53] a finding suggesting that cuff BPs may need to be replaced by newer techniques to provide a clearer picture of hypertensive TOD. Some muscular conduits (e.g., coronary arteries) are also subject to atherosclerosis, at least in the first few centimeters of major vessels that directly branch off the aorta.

Small arteries and arterioles (<0.5 mm in diameter) generate systemic vascular resistance by their intrinsic myogenic tone, by neurogenic and humorally mediated constriction, and as a result of hypertrophy of arteriolar smooth muscle, which encroaches on the vascular lumen. In arterioles, the relationship between the endothelium and the underlying vascular smooth muscle is quite intimate, and endothelially derived vasodilators can buffer constrictor responses to acute changes in flow or pressure. Arteriolar constriction also promotes pulse wave reflection.[54]

Arterial Assessment Techniques

Large Arterial Stiffness

PWV varies directly with wall stiffness and is related to wall thickness and elasticity and inversely to arterial radius.[52] PWV represents the average stiffness of the arterial tree between the measurement sites, but it has many drawbacks, most notably that PWV is a "lumped parameter" that measures properties of arterial segments with intrinsically different radii and wall composition. Carotid-femoral PWV, the most common index, is blind to changes in the proximal aorta, where most of the systolic damping function occurs. Changes in carotid-femoral PWV thus represent adaptations of more distal vessels that most likely represent late consequences of hypertension. As a result, although PWV is an independent predictor of cardiovascular disease risk,[55] it is marginally superior to PP in that regard.[56]

Characteristic aortic impedance, a much more sensitive indicator of aortic function than PWV, is also proportional to wall thickness and elastance, but it is 2.5 times more sensitive to changes in aortic diameter.[52] Application of characteristic impedance to medical practice is technically difficult because simultaneous pressure and flow tracings are required, usually by carotid tonometry and LV outflow tract Doppler velocity. Changes in characteristic aortic impedance occur early in the syndrome of systolic hypertension and can differentiate benefits of different antihypertensive drug classes.[57]

Augmentation Index

Antegrade and retrograde (reflected) pressure waves that travel within the arterial tree sum to determine the morphology of the pressure wave at any point. Reflected waves are affected by three major properties: the magnitude of the reflection coefficient, the distance of the principal reflecting site from the aortic root, and PWV. The most commonly used wave reflection parameter is central augmentation index,[58] the proportion of central PP resulting from the primary reflected wave. The augmentation index can be estimated noninvasively by applying a generalized transfer function to the tonometric measurement of a peripheral arterial systolic waveform.[59] In general, the augmentation index is most directly related to the degree of distal vasoconstriction, although much of the literature propagates the incorrect interpretation that the augmentation index is a reliable indicator of arterial stiffness.[52,54]

Other Indicators of Large Vessel Stiffness

The Windkessel model (diastolic pulse contour analysis) has been said to yield information about central and peripheral arterial properties, but this approach has multiple theoretical and practical flaws and unclear utility.[60] Newer imaging techniques such as gated MRI may offer new insights and clinical approaches that allow more accurate arterial diameters to be calculated for the study of compliance or distensibility.

Ankle-Brachial Index

When an artery's diameter is reduced by 70% or more, flow and pressure distal to the stenosis are reduced. Accordingly, clinically significant PAD in the lower extremity can be diagnosed using the ankle-brachial index (ABI, the ratio of Doppler flow in the posterior tibial or dorsalis pedis artery to that of the brachial artery). An ABI lower than 0.9 is highly suspicious of clinically significant PAD and is considered to be an IHD risk equivalent. Patients are also at increased risk of IHD when ABI is high (~>1.4), a finding suggesting that abnormal PP amplification may be harmful.

Arteriosclerosis and increased central arterial stiffness widen PP and contribute heavily to the pathogenesis of systolic hypertension. A sensitive stiffness index would be a potentially relevant clinical indicator, but current techniques are best characterized as research tools. Arteries of different sizes do not change uniformly with aging or hypertension and do not display uniform changes in arterial stiffness. Thus, studies of peripheral arterial stiffness have uncertain relevance. The augmentation index gives information about wave reflection, which depends on the function and structure of distal arteries and arterioles. Intermittent claudication is the cardinal sign of atherosclerotic PAD, but buttock pain and impotence may also occur. Late symptoms include marked reductions in tissue temperature, ulceration, and gangrene. Reduced ABI occurs during the middle phases of PAD and is the only arterial assessment technique that has been widely applied to clinical practice. ABI is somewhat insensitive, however.

HYPERTENSIVE CEREBROVASCULAR DISEASE

Stroke Syndromes

Demographics

A diagnosis of hypertension, whether based on systolic BP, diastolic BP, PP, or isolated systolic hypertension, is a strong risk factor for acute brain infarction, but the risk of ischemic stroke, the most common form, is most closely related to systolic BP.[61] Starting at 115 mm Hg, for each 20 mm Hg increase in systolic BP, the relative risk of stroke increases by about two- to threefold in subjects aged 60 to 79 years, across gender, geographic regions, and stroke subtypes and for fatal and nonfatal stroke. A weaker association of hypertension with single lacunar infarcts is seen,[62] but multiple lacunar infarcts are associated more closely with hypertension and diabetes mellitus.[62] Additional factors such as cigarette smoking, IHD, and other vascular factors may contribute.

Pathogenesis

The brain and cardiovascular system are adversely affected by hypertension and atherosclerosis,[63-65] but whereas the heart often recovers from temporary ischemia, the brain is frequently irreversibly damaged by similar degrees of oxygen deprivation. Brain damage can occur by several mechanisms, most notably acute ischemic stroke, cardiac embolic stroke, lacunar stroke, and hemorrhagic stroke.

Large Artery (Atherothrombotic) Infarction

Large artery infarction is caused by atherosclerosis of the extracranial cerebral arteries, often as a result of plaque rupture in a proximal artery with downstream embolization of atherosclerotic debris. Occlusion or high-grade stenosis of the extracranial internal carotid artery can also cause ischemia or downstream brain infarction.[66] The size of the infarct depends, at least in part, on the size of the artery where the embolism lodges. Large artery occlusions (e.g., main stem of the middle cerebral artery or the internal carotid artery) typically result in large infarcts. Watershed infarcts may also occur with atherothrombotic occlusion of a large cerebral artery. Distal artery occlusion usually results in smaller infarcts unless a shower of emboli occurs. The availability of collateral circulation may be another important determinant of size of the infarct.

Cardiac Embolic Infarction

Cardiac embolic infarction is often associated with atrial fibrillation, thrombus formation after myocardial infarction, cardiomyopathy, mechanical prosthetic valves, and other conditions.[67] The presence of hypertension in persons with atrial fibrillation heightens the risk of subsequent stroke. Strokes resulting from cardioembolic disease are often large and abrupt in onset, but the mode of onset and vascular territory are neither specific nor sensitive clues. The presence of multiple infarctions in different vascular territories and the finding of systemic embolism heighten the likelihood of a cardiac source.[67] Common sites where emboli of cardiac origin lodge are the middle and posterior cerebral arteries.

Lacunar Infarction

Lacunes (little lakes, as the term suggests) are small, deep brain infarcts resulting from occlusion of penetrating branches of larger cerebral arteries. Lacunar infarcts range in size from a few cubic millimeters to approximately 15 mm^3. The underlying pathologic process is believed to be lipohyalinosis, which is a degenerative, occlusive disease of smaller penetrating arteries; this disease of uncertain origin is related to hypertension and atherosclerosis, but it can also result from microatheromata, arteriopathies, or microemboli.[68] Lacunar infarcts follow penetrating vessel territories (basal ganglia, thalamus, pons, internal capsule, and cerebral white matter). Based on the presenting features and location of lacunar infarctions, four common clinical lacunar syndromes have been described. *Pure motor hemiparesis* occurs when the disease affects the posterior limb of internal capsule, lower pons, or midportion of the cerebral peduncle. *Pure sensory stroke* occurs with disease of the sensory relay nuclei of posteroventral thalamus. *Dysarthria–clumsy hand syndrome* occurs with lesions at the basis pontis at the junction of the upper and middle two thirds or the genu of the internal capsule. *Ataxic-hemiparesis* is the result of lesions of the basis pontis at the junction of the upper and middle thirds or the posterior limb of the internal capsule.

Acute Brain Hemorrhage

Hypertension is the most important preventable and modifiable risk factor for parenchymatous brain hemorrhage, which tends to occur in the distribution of small penetrating arteries (e.g., lenticulostriate arteries, thalamic perforating arteries) that constitute a resistance system for the basal ganglia, thalamus, and pons. These small penetrating arteries are affected by chronic hypertension and lipohyalinosis, the same pathologic change associated with lacunar infarction. In parenchymatous brain hemorrhage, the small penetrating arteries exhibit frayed and thinned walls or small Charcot-Bouchard aneurysms that may rupture.[69]

Assessment Overview

Physical Findings

Typical acute neurologic symptoms or signs of cerebral infarction may include monocular visual loss (e.g., amaurosis fugax), hemiparesis, cortical sensory loss, or higher cortical dysfunction (e.g., aphasia, constructional or dressing apraxia). The degree of cortical dysfunction depends predominantly on whether the dominant or nondominant cerebral hemisphere is ischemic.

Imaging Studies

Noninvasive studies such as extracranial and intracranial MRA or carotid ultrasound duplex imaging are employed to define the location and extent of occlusive cerebrovascular arterial lesions. Brain CT and MRI can determine the site and extent of ischemic brain injury. Cranial CT has advanced our knowledge of subcortical infarction.[70] However, CT is not sensitive for the acute diagnosis of lacunar infarction. The diagnosis of primary lacunar infarction is made after exclusion of large artery atherothrombotic occlusive disease, cardiac source embolism, and nonatherosclerotic causes of stroke, by diagnostic studies such as intracranial and extracranial MRA, carotid ultrasound, transthoracic or transesophageal echocardiography, and conventional cerebral angiography. Studies of hypercoagulable states are occasionally appropriate. MRI pulse sequences, especially diffusion-weighted imaging sequences, are an exciting new development to identify subcortical and acute lacunar lesions. CT is a sensitive diagnostic tool for detecting parenchymatous brain hemorrhage, and more recently, brain MRI has been recognized as a valuable means for detecting this condition. The diagnosis of cardiac embolic disease depends on adequate sensitivity of the cardiac imaging modality. Transthoracic echocardiography is often insufficiently sensitive to rule out a cardiac embolic source. Transesophageal echocardiography is more sensitive than transthoracic echocardiography,[67] particularly for identifying left atrial sources, atrial septal defects, and aortic atheroma. A routine ECG and an ambulatory ECG are helpful to identify cardiac rhythm disturbances such as atrial fibrillation.

Dementia

Vascular cognitive impairment (VCI) is a major hypertension-related public health problem. VCI (dementia) is commonly present in individuals said to have Alzheimer's disease, and it is likely that most dementia is actually "mixed dementia." VCI includes a spectrum of problems associated with stroke and small vessel disease, ranging from mild to moderate to severe cognitive deficits. It is estimated that up to approximately 25% to 33% of patients have significant VCI at 3 months after a stroke. The population-attributable risk of hypertension in VCI is approximately 66%.[71] Hypertension may be linked to VCI via the occurrence of hypertension-related cortical or subcortical infarcts and white matter disease that may be exacerbated by diabetes mellitus or dyslipidemia.[71] It is not yet clear whether BP lowering or use of different classes of antihypertensive agents prevents VCI. Some secondary analyses suggest that treatment with dihydropyridine calcium antagonists or angiotensin-converting enzyme inhibitors is associated with a lower risk of dementia or less cognitive decline in recurrent stroke. It also remains to be determined whether substantial BP lowering is beneficial from a cognitive standpoint in persons who already have VCI.[63] A variety of assessment tools is available for the evaluation of cognitive function.[61,64]

Hypertensive Encephalopathy

Hypertensive encephalopathy is now uncommon, probably because of a greater awareness of hypertension, the more widespread use of antihypertensive agents, and more effective BP control.[72] Encephalopathy results from a sudden increase in BP to very high levels (e.g., mean arterial pressure >150 mm Hg in adults). As mean pressure increases, the early increase in cerebrovascular resistance (part of normal cerebral autoregulation) gives way to vascular collapse, with increased vascular permeability, acute fibrinoid change of the vessel walls, brain edema, thrombosis, and microinfarcts. Eclampsia is considered a special case of hypertensive encephalopathy. Treatment of hypertensive encephalopathy may result in complete neurologic recovery, and subsequent control of BP prevents recurrence.

Assessment of hypertensive encephalopathy includes a careful history that may reveal headache, nausea, vomiting, confusion, depressed level of consciousness, focal neurologic symptoms, or convulsions. Visual symptoms suggest parieto-occipital brain involvement. The cardinal physical finding is papilledema. Brain swelling and other focal perfusion defects can be detected by brain CT or MRI.

HYPERTENSIVE RETINOPATHY

Low-vision states are known complications of hypertensive retinopathy,[73] but the association often escapes clinical awareness. Various clinical classification systems based on the physical appearance of the retinal arterial system have been proposed, but older classification systems are considered obsolete as a result of a better understanding of the pathophysiology of hypertensive retinopathy.[74-77] A review of the world's recent literature suggests that standard funduscopy is neither sensitive nor specific for reliably detecting changes caused by hypertension.[78] Current standards suggest that pathophysiologic changes in each of the three main divisions of the ocular circulation (retinal, choroidal, and optic nerve) should be described separately because of their different features and implications (Table 15-2). Retinal capillaries are composed of nonfenestrated vascular endothelium, which forms the blood-retinal barrier. In contrast, the choriocapillaris is fenestrated and serves no barrier function. There is an efficient autoregulatory system of retinal blood flow, whereas the choroidal system has no such autoregulation. Unlike the choroidal vasculature, the retinal vasculature lacks sympathetic innervation.

Optic Fundus in Hypertension

In *early hypertension*, a relatively common finding is inner retinal ischemic spots (or "cotton-wool spots") that represent focal ischemia of the inner retina (Fig. 15-1). These lesions are white, range from 0.5 to 1 mm, have irregular shapes with feathery margins, and are located along the peripapillary arteriolar arcades. The lesions are present at the level of the retinal nerve fiber layer and gradually fade over 3 to 6 weeks. Inner retinal ischemic spots can be seen in a wide variety of other conditions, such as human immunodeficiency viral disease and systemic lupus erythematosus. Microaneurysms, small intraretinal hemorrhages, and retinal edema in the macular region (punctate, pale white lesions beneath the retina at the level of the choroid) may occur along with focal serous retinal detachment.

In *late hypertension*, retinal arterial changes include increased tortuosity of the retinal arterioles with focal or generalized arteriosclerosis (copper wiring). One may also see cystoid macular edema as a result of failed retinal autoregulation. Lipid exudates in the retina typically located within the major arterial arcades may persist for months. Eventually, patients have retinal nerve fiber loss in areas previously

Table 15-2   Hypertensive Retinal Changes

Retinal Vascular Changes	Choroidal Vascular Changes	Optic Nerve Changes
Focal intraretinal periarteriolar transudates (FIPTs)	Focal infarction of the RPE and outer retina	Optic nerve edema
Inner retinal ischemic (cotton-wool) spots (IRIS)	Elschnig's spots	Optic nerve pallor
Retinal capillary changes	Polymorphic RPE atrophy	
Microaneurysms	Serous retinal detachment	
Arteriovenous shunt vessels		
Retinal venous changes		
Arteriovenous nicking		
Venous dilation and tortuosity		
Retinal arteriolar changes		
Arteriolar narrowing		
Copper wire appearance		
Silver wire appearance		
Increased permeability of the retinal vascular bed		
Retinal and macular edema		
Retinal lipid exudates		
Focal retinal nerve fiber loss		

RPE, retinal pigment epithelium.

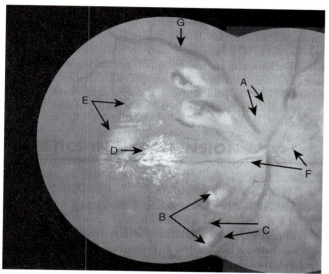

Figure 15–1   A photograph of the optic fundus from a 34-year-old white man with malignant hypertension (blood pressure 240/135 mm Hg). Optic nerve edema is present (blurred disk margin, A), as well as inner retinal ischemic spots (B), nerve fiber layer hemorrhages along the vascular arcades (C), lipid exudates in the macular region (D), focal serous retinal detachment (E), diffuse arteriolar narrowing (F), and venous engorgement (G).

affected by inner retinal ischemic spots. Other changes in the retinal venous circulation include narrowing of retinal venules as they cross retinal arterioles (arteriovenous nicking), dilation, and tortuosity.

In *malignant hypertension,* edema of the optic nerve occurs secondary to vasoconstriction of the peripapillary circulation. It is believed that this process results from diffusion of angiotensin II and other endogenous vasoconstrictors from the peripapillary choroidal circulation into the prelaminar region of the optic nerve. Focal intraretinal periarteriolar transudates are the consequence of leakage of dilated pre-

capillary retinal arterioles located in the deeper layers of the retina during the early phases of malignant hypertension. Focal intraretinal periarteriolar transudates are typically located along the major arterioles, are dull white, round to oval, range in size from pinpoint to 0.5 mm, and are typically multiple. These opacities usually fade away 2 to 3 weeks after the onset of the hypertensive episode.

CHRONIC KIDNEY DISEASE

CKD is a highly morbid, extremely costly condition that affects increasing numbers of people worldwide (see Chapter 29). In 2003, nearly half a million persons in the United States had end-stage renal disease (and required dialysis or renal transplantation), and this number is expected to grow inexorably over the next 20 years.

Pathophysiology

Age, Reduced Glomerular Filtration Rate, and Coronary Heart Disease Risk

Glomerular filtration rate (GFR) declines with age, and the slope of the age-related rate of decline in GFR is markedly affected by the presence of other diseases and risk factors such as hypertension and diabetes.[79,80] In healthy people, beginning in the fourth decade of life, GFR declines at a rate of about 1 mL/minute/year. The presence of hypertension or diabetes accelerates the age-related decline in kidney function by as much as 10-fold, thus leading to premature CKD, dialysis, or transplantation. Stage 3 CKD as a cardiovascular risk factor is at least as powerful as diabetes or prior myocardial infarction.[79,80]

Pathologic Features

The presence of early but significant glomerulopathy is signaled by the appearance of microalbuminuria, which is often an indicator of glomerular hyperfiltration, glomerular capillary hypertension, and increased basement membrane permeability. Vascular disease in general and glomerular capillary hypertension in particular are essential elements that predispose to focal glomerulosclerosis, a progressive condition common to virtually all forms of progressive renal disease and perhaps to the age-related decline in renal function. Mononuclear cell infiltration and increasing degrees of albuminuria also occur, further accelerating the rate of decline in GFR. When hypertension is left untreated, patients have accelerated progression to ongoing glomerulosclerosis and tubular dropout. In hypertensive kidney disease, progressive thickening of the afferent arterioles (nephrosclerosis) seems to be an attempt of the glomerulus to reduce glomerular capillary hypertension. In the end, however, it exacerbates nephron ischemia.

Assessment of Kidney Function

Definition of Chronic Kidney Disease

The diagnosis of CKD is based on abnormal findings in *either* of two major categories: impaired excretory function (reduced GFR; Table 15-3) or the presence of albuminuria, which is considered an important marker of glomerular damage and generalized microcirculatory disease.[79] A GFR of less than 60 mL/minute (stage 3 CKD) or the presence of overt albuminuria (>300 mg/day) defines the nominal boundary of clinically significant CKD.[79-81]

Albuminuria

Detection of microalbuminuria requires a specific assay, because standard urine dipsticks become positive only when levels are higher than approximately 150 mg/L on spot urine, whereas specific microalbumin test strips can detect less than 10 mg albumin/L. Quantitation of albuminuria no longer depends on the collection of a 24-hour urine, which is often unreliable. Current recommendations are to perform repeated spot urine tests for albumin-to-creatinine ratio, which replaces 24-hour determinations in most cases. The excretion of more than 30 mg of albumin/g creatinine defines the presence of stage 1 CKD. When patients have more than 300 mg of albumin/g creatinine, stage 3 CKD is generally present. The approximate threshold for albuminuria in the nephrotic syndrome begins at about 1500 to 2000 mg albumin/g creatinine on spot urine or 1500 to 2000 mg/day of albumin excretion.

Serum Creatinine and Estimated Glomerular Filtration Rate

Because of errors in timed urine collections, serum creatinine is often more reliable than creatinine clearance. Yet early recognition of CKD is impaired by reliance on serum creatinine measurements because small changes in serum creatinine, representing marked reductions in GFR, are often overlooked on casual inspection (e.g., a persistent increase in serum creatinine from 0.8 to 1.2 mg/dL represents a 33% reduction in GFR). Another confounder of serum creatinine is its dependence on muscle mass. In an effort to remedy these diagnostic issues and to improve the diagnosis, the Modification of Diet in Renal Disease study formula for estimation of GFR (*e*GFR) is now reported along with serum creatinine by most large clinical laboratories. The *e*GFR includes an adjustment for age, gender, race, and can include further adjustment for albumin, and urea nitrogen (see Table 15-3).[79,81]

Urinalysis and Other Markers of Renal Damage

Simple urinalysis is often omitted from the assessment of kidney function, but it carries major importance for assessing the presence of macroproteinuria, red or white blood cells, and hyaline or granular casts, any or all of which may signal glomerular or tubular disease. Renal blood flow and GFR can be estimated from standard nuclear medicine techniques, and the filtration fraction (FF = GFR/renal plasma flow) can be calculated. Increased FF resulting from reduced renal blood flow can be seen with nephrosclerosis, but increased FF also occurs as a consequence of dehydration, thus making FF much less specific for assessment of progressive renal damage. β_2-Microglobulin is the marker of tubular damage most often used in research studies. Newer markers of glomerular filtration include cystatin C, a cysteine protease inhibitor that is produced by nearly all human cells, is fully filtered by the glomerulus, and metabolized in the proximal tubule. Cystatin C concentration may be a better surrogate for GFR than serum creatinine because it is not affected by age, sex, or muscle mass.[81,82]

Assessment Overview

Albuminuria, elevated serum creatinine, or reduced GFR should be staged according to recent guidelines.[79] Any abnormality in renal function is a major risk factor for end-stage

Table 15-3 Progression and Staging of Chronic Kidney Disease

CKD Stage	eGFR (mL/min)	Albuminuria	Comment
1	90–120	Microalbuminuria (>30 mg/g creatinine)	Earliest sign of renal damage
2	60–90	Increasing microalbuminuria common	Progressive disease or aging effect
3	30–60	If macroalbuminuria (albumin excretion >300 mg/g creatinine) present, stage 3 CKD established irrespective of *e*GFR	
4	15–30	Macroalbuminuria usually present	
5	<15	End-stage renal disease	Dialysis or transplantation indicated

CKD, chronic kidney disease; *e*GFR, estimated glomerular filtration rate.

kidney disease and for IHD.[78,79] Renal function varies physiologically, so modest changes in renal indicators are more likely to represent modest hemodynamic changes than to signify kidney damage. To establish the presence of significant renal disease, repeat testing is necessary, and it is wise to establish a graphic trend for renal function indicators to highlight the temporal relationship between the onset of renal dysfunction and the occurrence of a clinical predisposing condition (e.g., hypotension) or the start of a particular therapy. Serum creatinine is a highly imperfect indicator that may be replaced in the future with a better indicator of GFR such as cystatin C.

SUMMARY

Hypertensive TOD reflects the severity and duration of hypertension and should be the focus of the physical examination and laboratory survey done for every hypertensive patient at diagnosis. The major types of TOD include several aspects of cardiac structure and function (typically best evaluated with an echocardiogram), hypertensive arteriopathy (for which ABI testing is most commonly performed), hypertensive cerebrovascular disease (for which CT or MRI of the brain is typically considered), hypertensive retinopathy (with description of specific changes), and CKD (for which serum creatinine, eGFR, and spot urine for the albumin-to-creatinine ratio are typically recommended). None of the foregoing tests are perfectly sensitive or specific for each type of TOD, and therefore they may not be necessary in all cases. Nonetheless, when hypertensive TOD is detected, the patient can be classified as having a greater stage of hypertension, using the most recent classification system.[83] TOD is a strong indication for antihypertensive therapy, with the objective of reversing or at least retarding the progression of target organ dysfunction from elevated BP.

References

1. Chobanian AV, Bakris GL, Black HR, et al. Seventh Report of the Joint National Committee on Prevention, Detection, Evaluation, and Treatment of High Blood Pressure. *Hypertension.* 2003;**42**:1206-1252.
2. Levy D, Anderson KM, Savage DD, et al. Echocardiographically detected left ventricular hypertrophy: Prevalence and risk factors. The Framingham Heart Study. *Ann Intern Med.* 1988;**108**:7-13.
3. de Simone G, Daniels SR, Kimball TR, et al. Evaluation of concentric left ventricular hypertrophy in humans: Evidence for age-related systematic underestimation. *Hypertension.* 2005;**45**:64-68.
4. Post WS, Hill MN, Dennison CR, et al. High prevalence of target organ damage in young, African American inner-city men with hypertension. *J Clin Hypertens (Greenwich).* 2003;**5**:24-30.
5. Arnett DK, Hong Y, Bella JN, et al. Sibling correlation of left ventricular mass and geometry in hypertensive African Americans and whites: The HyperGEN Study. *Am J Hypertens.* 2001;**14**:1226-1230.
6. East MA, Jollis JG, Nelson CL, et al. The influence of left ventricular hypertrophy on survival in patients with coronary artery disease: Do race and gender matter? *J Am Coll Cardiol.* 2003;**41**:949-954.
7. Schmieder RE, Messerli FH. Does obesity influence early target organ damage in hypertensive patients? *Circulation.* 1993;**87**:1482-1488.

8. Mancia G, Carugo S, Grassi G, et al. Prevalence of left ventricular hypertrophy in hypertensive patients with and without blood pressure control: Data from the PAMELA population. Pressioni Arteriose Monitorate e Loro Associazioni. *Hypertension.* 2002;**39**:744-749.
9. Liebson PR, Grandits GA, Dianzumba S, et al. Comparison of five antihypertensive monotherapies and placebo for change in left ventricular mass in patients receiving nutritional-hygienic therapy in the Treatment of Mild Hypertension Study (TOMHS). *Circulation.* 1995;**91**:698-706.
10. Ganau A, Devereux RB, Roman MJ, et al. Patterns of left ventricular hypertrophy and geometric remodeling in essential hypertension. *J Am Coll Cardiol.* 1992;**19**:1552-1558.
11. Mostero A, D'Agostino RB, Silbershatz H, et al. Trends in the prevalence of hypertension, antihypertensive therapy, and left ventricular hypertrophy from 1950 to 1989. *N Engl J Med.* 1999;**340**:1221-1227.
12. Saba PS, Ganau A, Devereux RB, et al. Impact of arterial elastance as a measure of vascular load on left ventricular geometry in hypertension. *J Hypertens.* 1999;**17**:1007-1015.
13. Roman MJ, Pickering TG, Schwartz JE, et al. Relation of arterial structure and function to left ventricular geometric patterns in hypertensive patients. *J Am Coll Cardiol.* 1996;**28**:751-756.
14. Cuspidi C, Macca G, Michev I, et al. Left ventricular concentric remodelling and extracardiac target organ damage in essential hypertension. *J Hum Hypertens.* 2002;**16**:385-390.
15. Struijker Boudier HA, Cohuet GM, Baumann M, Safar ME. The heart, macrocirculation and microcirculation in hypertension: A unifying hypothesis. *J Hypertens.* 2003;**21** (**Suppl 3**):S19-S23.
16. Zeiher AM, Drexler H, Saurbier B, Just H. Endothelium-mediated coronary blood flow modulation in humans: Effects of age, atherosclerosis, hypercholesterolemia and hypertension. *J Clin Invest.* 1993;**92**:652-662.
17. Hamasaki S, Al Suwaidi J, Higano ST, et al. Attenuated coronary flow reserve and vascular remodeling in patients with hypertension and left ventricular hypertrophy. *J Am Coll Cardiol.* 2000;**35**:1654-1660.
18. Gimelli A, Schneider-Eicke J, Neglia D, et al. Homogeneously reduced versus regionally impaired myocardial blood flow in hypertensive patients: Two different patterns of myocardial perfusion associated with the degree of hypertrophy. *J Am Coll Cardiol.* 1998;**31**:366-373.
19. Lajemi M, Gautier, S, Poirier O, et al. Endothelial gene variants and aortic and cardiac structure in never treated hypertensives. *Am J Hypertens.* 2001;**14**:755-760.
20. Semplicini A, Siffert W, Sartori M, et al. G protein β_3 subunit gene 825T allele is associated with increased left ventricular mass in young subjects with mild hypertension. *Am J Hypertens.* 2001;**14**:1191-1195.
21. Stella P, Bigatti G, Tizzoni L, et al. Association between aldosterone synthase (CYP11B2) polymorphism and left ventricular mass in human essential hypertension. *J Am Coll Cardiol.* 2004;**43**:265-270.
22. Dong Y, Wang X, Zhu H, et al. Endothelin-1 gene and progression of blood pressure and left ventricular mass: Longitudinal findings in youth. *Hypertension.* 2004;**44**:884-890.
23. Okin PM, Jern S, Devereux RB, et al. Effect of obesity on electrocardiographic left ventricular hypertrophy in hypertensive patients: The Losartan Intervention for Endpoint (LIFE) Reduction in Hypertension Study. *Hypertension.* 2000;**35**:13-18.
24. Casale PN, Devereux RB, Alonso DR, et al. Improved sex-specific criteria of left ventricular hypertrophy for clinical and computer interpretation of electrocardiograms: Validation with autopsy findings. *Circulation.* 1987;**75**:565-572.
25. Sundström J, Lind L, Ärnlöv J, et al. Echocardiographic and electrocardiographic diagnoses of left ventricular hypertrophy predict mortality independently of each other in a population of elderly men. *Circulation.* 2001;**103**:2346-2351.

26. Okin PM, Devereux RB, Fabsitz RR, et al. Quantitative assessment of electrocardiographic strain predicts increased left ventricular mass: The Strong Heart Study. *J Am Coll Cardiol.* 2002;**40**:1395-1400.

27. Bella JN, Wachtell K, Palmieri V, et al. Relation of left ventricular geometry and function to systemic hemodynamics in hypertension: The LIFE study. Losartan Intervention for Endpoint Reduction in Hypertension Study. *J Hypertens.* 2001;**19**:127-134.

28. Kannel WB, Gordon T, Castelli WP, Margolis JR. Electrocardiographic left ventricular hypertrophy and risk of coronary heart disease: The Framingham Study. *Ann Intern Med.* 1970;**72**: 813-822.

29. de Simone G, Devereux RB, Koren MJ, et al. Midwall left ventricular mechanics: An independent predictor of cardiovascular risk in arterial hypertension. *Circulation.* 1996;**93**:259-265.

30. de Simone G, Devereux RB, Roman MJ, et al. Assessment of left ventricular function by the midwall functional shortening/end-systolic stress relation in human hypertension. *J Am Coll Cardiol.* 1994;**23**:1444-1451.

31. Schussheim AE, Devereux RB, de Simone G, et al. Usefulness of subnormal midwall fractional shortening in predicting left ventricular exercise dysfunction in asymptomatic patients with systemic hypertension. *Am J Cardiol.* 1997;**79**:1070-1074.

32. Black HR, Weltin G, Jaffe CC. The limited echocardiogram: a modification of standard echocardiograph for use in routine evaluation of patients with systemic hypertension. *Am J Cardiol.* 1991;**67**:1027-1030.

33. Devereux RB, Alonso DR, Lutas EM, et al. Echocardiographic assessment of left ventricular hypertrophy: Comparison with necropsy finding. *Am J Cardiol.* 1986;**57**:450-458.

34. Mancia G, Zanchetti A, Agabiti-Rosei E, et al. Ambulatory blood pressure is superior to clinic blood pressure in predicting treatment-induced regression of left ventricular hypertrophy: SAMPLE Study Group. Study on Ambulatory Monitoring of Blood Pressure and Lisinopril Evaluation. *Circulation.* 1997;**95**: 1464-1470.

35. Tsunoda S, Kawano Y, Horio T, et al. Relationship between home blood pressure and longitudinal changes in target organ damage in treated hypertensive patients. *Hypertens Res.* 2002;**25**:167-173.

36. Cavallini MC, Roman MJ, Pickering TG, et al. Is white coat hypertension associated with arterial disease or left ventricular hypertrophy? *Hypertension.* 1995;**26**:413-419.

37. Liu JE, Roman MJ, Pini R, et al. Cardiac and arterial target organ damage in adults with elevated ambulatory and normal office blood pressure. *Ann Intern Med.* 1999;**131**:564-572.

38. Palatini P, Mormino P, Santonastaso M, et al. Target-organ damage in stage I hypertensive subjects with white coat and sustained hypertension: Results from the HARVEST study. *Hypertension.* 1998;**31**:57-63.

39. Mule G, Nardi E, Andronico G, et al. Relationships between 24-h blood pressure load and target organ damage in patients with mild-to-moderate essential hypertension. *Blood Press Monit.* 2001;**6**:115-123.

40. Cuspidi C, Macca G, Sampieri L, et al. High prevalence of cardiac and extracardiac target organ damage in refractory hypertension. *J Hypertens.* 2001;**19**:2063-2070.

41. Casale PN, Devereux RB, Milner M, et al. Value of echocardiographic measurement of left ventricular mass in predicting cardiovascular morbid events in hypertensive men. *Ann Intern Med.* 1986;**105**:173-178.

42. Levy D, Larson MG, Vasan RS, et al. The progression from hypertension to heart failure. *JAMA.* 1996;**275**:1557-1562.

43. Messerli FH. Cardiomyopathy of obesity: A not-so-Victorian disease. *N Engl J Med.* 1986;**314**:378-380.

44. Dunlap SH, Sueta CA, Tomasko L, Adams KF Jr. Association of body mass, gender and race with heart failure primarily due to hypertension. *J Am Coll Cardiol.* 1999;**34**:1602-1608.

45. White WB. Blood pressure load and target organ effects in patients with essential hypertension. *J Hypertens.* 1991; **9 (Suppl)**:S39-S42.

46. Haider AW, Larson MG, Franklin SS, Levy D. Systolic blood pressure, diastolic blood pressure, and pulse pressure as predictors of risk for congestive heart failure in the Framingham Heart Study. *Ann Intern Med.* 2003;**138**:10-16.

47. Aeschbacher BC, Hutton D, Fuhrer J, et al. Diastolic dysfunction precedes myocardial hypertrophy in the development of hypertension. *Am J Hypertens.* 2001;**14**: 106-113.

48. Gandhi SK, Powers JC, Nomeir AM, et al. The pathogenesis of acute pulmonary edema associated with hypertension. *N Engl J Med.* 2001;**344**:17-22.

49. Williams RS. Apoptosis and heart failure. *N Engl J Med.* 1999;**341**:759-760.

50. Izzo JL Jr, Gradman AH. Mechanisms and management of hypertensive heart disease: From left ventricular hypertrophy to heart failure. *Med Clin North Am.* 2004;**88**:1257-1271.

51. Izzo JL Jr. Arterial stiffness and the systolic hypertension syndrome. *Curr Opin Cardiol.* 2004;**19**:341-352.

52. Mitchell GF, Izzo JL Jr. Evaluation of arterial stiffness. In: Izzo JL Jr, Black HR (eds.). Hypertension Primer, 3rd ed. Dallas, Tex: American Heart Association, 2003, pp 351-355.

53. Wilkinson IB, Franklin SS, Hall IR, et al. Pressure amplification explains why pulse pressure is unrelated to risk in young subjects. *Hypertension.* 2001;**38**:1461-1466.

54. Wilkinson IB, MacCallum H, Hupperetz PC, et al. Changes in the derived central pressure waveform and pulse pressure in response to angiotensin II and noradrenaline in man. *J Physiol (Lond).* 2001;**530**:541-550.

55. Boutouyrie P, Tropeano AI, Asmar R, et al. Aortic stiffness is an independent predictor of primary coronary events in hypertensive patients: A longitudinal study. *Hypertension.* 2002;**39**:10-15.

56. Domanski MJ, Davis BR, Pfeffer MA, et al. Isolated systolic hypertension: Prognostic information provided by pulse pressure. *Hypertension.* 1999;**34**:375-380.

57. Mitchell GF, Izzo JL Jr, Lacourciere Y, et al. Omapatrilat reduces pulse pressure and proximal aortic stiffness in patients with systolic hypertension: Results of the Conduit Hemodynamics of Omapatrilat International Research (CHOIR) study. *Circulation.* 2002;**105**:2955-2961.

58. O'Rourke MF, Kelly RP. Wave reflection in the systemic circulation and its implications in ventricular function. *J. Hypertens.* 1993;**11**:327-337.

59. Karamanoglu M, O'Rourke MF, Avolio AP, Kelly RP. An analysis of the relationship between central aortic and peripheral upper limb pressure waves in man. *Eur Heart J.* 1993;**14**:160-167.

60. Manning TS, Shykoff BE, Izzo JL Jr. Validity and reliability of diastolic pulse contour analysis (Windkessel model) in humans. *Hypertension.* 2002;**39**:963-968.

61. Gorelick PB. New horizons for stroke prevention: PROGRESS and HOPE. *Lancet Neurol.* 2002;**1**:149-156.

62. Davis SM, Parsons MW. MRI and other neuroimaging modalities for subcortical stroke. In: Donnan G, Norrving B, Bamford J, Bogousslavsky J (eds.). Subcortical Stroke, 2nd ed. New York: Oxford University Press, 2002, pp 124-136.

63. Gorelick PB. Risk factors for vascular dementia and Alzheimer disease. *Stroke.* 2004;**35 (Suppl I)**:2620-2622.

64. Gorelick PB. William M. Feinberg lecture: Cognitive vitality and the role of stroke and cardiovascular disease risk factors. *Stroke.* 2005;**36**:875-879.

65. Pedelty L, Gorelick PB. Chronic management of blood pressure after stroke. *Hypertension.* 2004;**44**:1-5.

66. Albers GW, Amarenco P, Easton JD, et al. Antithrombotic and thrombolytic therapy for ischemic stroke. *Chest.* 2001;**119**: 300S-320S.

67. Sacco RL, Adams R, Albers G, et al. Guidelines for prevention of stroke in patients with ischemic stroke or transient ischemic attack: A statement for healthcare professionals from the American Heart Association/American Stroke Association Council on Stroke: Co-sponsored by the Council on Cardiovascular Radiology and Intervention: *The American Academy of Neurology affirms the value of this guideline. Stroke.* 2006;**37**:577-617.

68. Boiten J, Lodder J. Risk factors for lacunar infarction. *In:* Donnan G, Norrving B, Bamford J, Bogousslavsky J (eds.). Subcortical Stroke, 2nd ed. New York: Oxford University Press, 2002, pp 87-97.

69. Kase C, Mohr JP, Caplan LR. Intracerebral hemorrhage. *In:* Barnett HJM, Mohr JP, Stein BM, Yatsu FM (eds.). Stroke: Pathophysiology, Diagnosis and Management, 3rd ed. New York: Churchill Livingstone, 1998, pp 649-700.

70. Gorelick PB. Stroke prevention therapy beyond antithrombotics: Unifying mechanisms in ischemic stroke pathogenesis and implications for therapy. An invited review. *Stroke.* 2002;**33**:862-875.

72. Gorelick PB. Prevention. *In:* Bowler JV, Hachinski V (eds.). Vascular Cognitive Impairment: Preventable Dementia. New York: Oxford University Press, 2003, pp. 308-320.

73. Dinsdale HB, Mohr JP. Hypertensive encephalopathy. *In:* Barnett HJM, Mohr JP, Stein BM, Yatsu FM (eds.). Stroke: Pathophysiology, Diagnosis and Management, 3rd ed. New York, NY: Churchill Livingstone, 1998, pp. 869-872.

73. Liebreich R. Ophthalmoskopischer Befund bei Morbus Brightii. *Albrecht von Graefes Arch Ophthalmol.* 1859;**5**:265-268.

74. Keith NM, Wagener HP, Barker NW. Some different types of essential hypertension: their course and prognosis. *Am J Med Sci.* 1939;**197**:332-343.

75. Hayreh SS. Classification of hypertensive fundus and their order of appearance. *Ophthalmologica.* 1989;**198**:247-260.

76. Hayreh SS. Hypertensive fundus changes. *In:* Guyer DR, Yanuzzi LA, Chang S, et al. (eds.). Retina-Vitreous-Macula. Philadelphia: WB Saunders, 1999, vol I, pp 345-371.

77. Wong TY, Mitchell P. Hypertensive retinopathy. *N Engl J Med.* 2004;**351**:2510-2517.

78. van den Born BJ, Hulsman CA, Hoekstra JB, et al. Value of routine funduscopy in patients with hypertension: Systematic review. *BMJ.* 2005;**331**:73-76.

79. K/DOQI clinical practice guidelines on hypertension and antihypertensive agents in chronic kidney disease. *Am J Kidney Dis.* 2004;**43 (5 Suppl 2)**:1-290.

80. Sarnak MJ, Levey AS, Schoolwerth AC, et al. Kidney disease as a risk factor for development of cardiovascular disease: A statement from the American Heart Association Councils on Kidney in Cardiovascular Disease, High Blood Pressure Research, Clinical Cardiology, and Epidemiology and Prevention. *Hypertension.* 2003;**42**:1050-1065.

81. Stevens LA, Levey AS. Measurement of kidney function. *Med Clin North Am.* 2005;**89**:457-473.

80. Newman DJ, Thakkar H, Edwards RG, et al. Serum cystatin C measured by automated immunoassay: A more sensitive marker of changes in GFR than serum creatinine. *Kidney Int.* 1995;**47**:312-318.

82. Fliser D, Ritz E. Serum cystatin C concentration as a marker of renal dysfunction in the elderly. *Am J Kidney Dis.* 2001;**37**: 79-83.

83. Giles T, Berk B, Black HR, et al. Position paper: Expanding the definition and classification of hypertension. *J Clin Hypertens (Greenwich).* 2005;**7**:505-512.

Chapter 16

Prediction of Global Cardiovascular Risk in Hypertension

Peter W. F. Wilson

TRADITIONAL RISK FACTORS

Origins

Coronary heart disease (CHD) is typically the clinical consequence of arteriosclerosis, a process that becomes evident in adolescence and early adulthood. Manifest disease is often not apparent until after the age of 40 years, and CHD has been reported more commonly in men than in women before the age of 75 years.[1]

Risk factors for CHD were first noted in the late 1950s and early 1960s. Analyses described higher levels of cholesterol, blood pressure (BP), and cigarette smoking that acted in concert to increase the chances of developing CHD over a follow-up interval, because single factors were generally not responsible for the development of clinical vascular events (Fig. 16-1). Since that time, a variety of advances led to the development of key factors that are easy to assess and are consistently related to greater risk of initial CHD events, including age, gender, BP, lipids, smoking, and diabetes mellitus.

Age and Gender

The first events in clinical CHD vary according to age and sex. Angina pectoris has historically been the most common first vascular disease event in women, followed by myocardial infarction (MI) and CHD death. In men, an MI is typically the most common first CHD event, followed by angina pectoris and CHD death.

CHD in women tends to occur after menopause, and rates are significantly higher than for other common diseases of aging, including fractures, cerebrovascular disease, breast cancer, and uterine cancer. Decreased estrogen production after menopause has been thought to be an important determinant of increased risk for CHD in older women. Observational studies undertaken in the 1970s and 1980s consistently demonstrated lower CHD rates in women who were using postmenopausal estrogens.[2-4] Meta-analyses of observational studies estimated a 50% reduction in risk of a first heart attack with postmenopausal estrogens,[5] but randomized clinical trials from the Heart and Estrogen/Progestin Replacement Study and the Women's Health Initiative prevention trial have not confirmed the observational study reports, although lipids may be changed in a favorable direction by hormonal replacement therapy. It is now recommended that women not take estrogens to prevent CHD.[6]

Lipids

Higher cholesterol levels typically raise the risk for CHD. Among more than 350,000 middle-aged men who were screened for the Multiple Risk Factor Intervention Trial, higher cholesterol levels led to increased risk of cardiovascular disease (CVD) death.[7] Using a cholesterol level of 200 mg/dL as the comparison, a level of 250 mg/dL led to a twofold risk, and a level of 300 mg/dL led to a threefold risk of CVD death.

Subfractions of blood cholesterol also help to determine vascular disease risk. For instance, lower levels of high-density lipoprotein cholesterol (HDL-C) augment the risk for CHD, MI, and CHD death, even when the total cholesterol levels are relatively low. In an early report, the 12-year incidence of MI was positively related to cholesterol level and inversely to HDL-C level in women in the Framingham Heart Study (Fig. 16-2).[8] At a total cholesterol level lower than 211 mg/dL, the HDL-C levels were inversely related to the risk of developing MI in women. Similar results were obtained for men and in other studies, findings that helped to provide the rationale for total cholesterol, as well as HDL-C, screening to assess CVD risk. Similar results were obtained for men in the Framingham Heart Study and in other studies in which similar analyses were undertaken, such as the Copenhagen Male Study.[9]

Lipid-lowering therapies to prevent CHD have improved greatly since the 1980s and have shown that lowering of total cholesterol and low-density lipoprotein cholesterol (LDL-C), along with raising of HDL-C levels, leads to a reduced risk of initial and recurrent CHD events.[10] In general, more cholesterol lowering has led to a greater reduction in the risk of initial and recurrent CHD in these studies.[11] The effectiveness of therapy in these trials has largely been based on intention to treat, not on the ability to reach predefined target levels of cholesterol or LDL-C.

Blood Pressure

The age-adjusted prevalence of high BP decreased from the late 1970s to 1990s for several ethnic groups in the United States, but higher BP in the frankly elevated range or in borderline categories persists as a very important antecedent of CHD. In U.S. national data from the 1990s, it was reported that approximately 5% of persons with high BP were treated, and only 27% to 29% had their hypertension under control. A sizable fraction, ranging from 27% to 41% of persons with high BP, were unaware that they were affected.[12] In the U.S. national survey of 1999 to 2000, the rate of awareness was 70%, treatment was being received in 59%, and control (≤140/90 mm Hg) was achieved in 31%.

Although medical education has stressed the importance of elevations in diastolic BP, on a population basis the systolic BP levels appear to be more highly related to the development of clinical CHD. Taken simply, systolic and diastolic hypertension each confer a relative risk of 1.6 for CVD. Combined systolic and diastolic hypertension imparts a relative risk of 2.0.[13] Wider pulse pressure is also related to CVD outcomes, especially in older persons, because diastolic BPs typically are lower in elderly persons than those observed in middle age.[14]

BP levels that do not meet the criteria for definite hypertension increase the risk for a first major vascular event. Long-term comparisons have shown that the risk of CVD is increased in persons with what was formerly called "high-normal BP" (systolic BP 130 to 139 mm Hg or diastolic BP 85 to 89 mm Hg). Because high-normal BP is a common condition, this level of BP accounts for a sizable fraction of CVD

events and, on a population basis, is nearly as important as hypertension itself.[15]

Summary analyses of antihypertensive drug treatment trials show convincing results that lower BP levels generally reduce the risk of CHD and cerebrovascular events. Newer efforts are also directed at the investigation of simultaneously lowering BP and lipids, such as in the Antihypertensive and Lipid-Lowering Treatment to Prevent Heart Attack Trial, a study with more than 40,000 U.S. participants, and the Anglo-Scandinavian Cardiac Outcomes Trial, which used BP medications and a different statin.[16,17]

Smoking

Current smoking of cigarettes generally doubles the risk of vascular outcomes. Both regular and filter cigarettes have similar adverse effects on CHD risk. Low-tar and low-nicotine cigarettes do not appear to reduce risk for cardiovascular events, although they not increase the risk for pulmonary diseases or lung cancer as greatly as the higher-tar and nicotine products.[18]

Passive smoking can lead to an increased risk for CHD that is approximately 30% greater than the risk for nonsmokers.[19] Persons exposed to environmental smoke have increased intima-media thickness of their carotid arteries, an indication of subclinical arteriosclerosis, in comparison with nonsmokers.[20]

Diabetes Mellitus

The risk of CHD is generally increased twofold among younger men and threefold among younger women with type 2 diabetes mellitus.[21] Finnish data suggested that the risk for a heart attack in a person with diabetes is very similar to the risk for a nondiabetic person who has had a heart attack. This result led to the concept of type 2 diabetes mellitus as a "CHD risk equivalent," and it emphasizes the need for aggressive treatment of risk factors in persons with type 2 diabetes mellitus to prevent CVD events.[22]

Recommendations to reduce the risk of CVD in persons with type 2 diabetes mellitus are generally more aggressive than for persons without diabetes mellitus. For example, an LDL-C lower than 100 mg/dL is the target for all persons

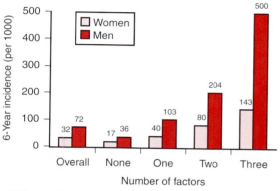

Figure 16–1 Risk of coronary heart disease over 6 years of follow-up according to presence of elevated blood pressure (>160/95 mm Hg), elevated cholesterol (>260 mg/dL), and left ventricular hypertrophy in the original Framingham Heart Study cohort. (From Kannel WB, Dawber TR, Kagan A, et al. Factors of risk in the development of coronary heart disease—six year follow-up experience: The Framingham Study. *Ann Intern Med.* 1961;**55**:33-50.)

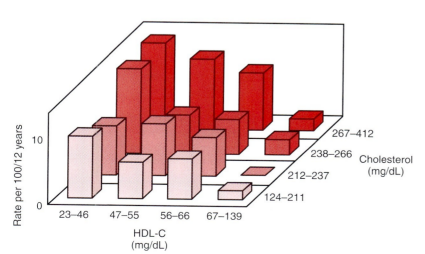

Figure 16–2 Risk of a myocardial infarction over 12 years of follow-up in women in the Framingham Heart Study according to quintile of cholesterol and quartile of high-density lipoprotein cholesterol (HDL-C). (From Abbott RD, Wilson PW, Kannel WB, et al. High density lipoprotein cholesterol, total cholesterol screening, and myocardial infarction. the Framingham Study. *Arteriosclerosis.* 1988;**8**:207-211.)

with diabetes mellitus. Similarly, the recommended BP target for persons with type 2 diabetes mellitus is less than 130/80 mm Hg, lower than for persons without diabetes or chronic kidney disease. The basis for these aggressive approaches came from subgroup analyses of treatment effects for BP and lipid lowering in type 2 diabetic patients in randomized clinical trials, and the American Diabetes Association has taken a very proactive stance over the past several years, including annual updates on guidelines in many instances.[23] Evidence for an aggressive attitude toward controlling risk factors in persons with type 2 diabetes mellitus has been published in a Danish trial with a combination of therapies for hyperglycemia, hypertension, dyslipidemia, and microalbuminuria.[24]

Observational studies have supported concerted glucose control as a CVD prevention strategy. Moreover, clinical trials have shown impressive prevention of small vessel disease in the eye and kidney with glucose and glycosylated hemoglobin reduction, with a smaller degree of added benefit for atherosclerotic events with more aggressive glucose control.[25]

MULTIVARIABLE CORONARY HEART DISEASE RISK ESTIMATION

Risk for CVD events can be estimated with prediction equations that use several variables, largely including the factors mentioned in this chapter. A score sheet, pocket calculator, and a computer have been used to estimate risk for CHD over a prescribed follow-up interval that typically ranges from a few years to a decade or more. The variables of age, systolic BP, smoking, cholesterol, HDL-C, and diabetes mellitus are commonly used to estimate risk for initial CHD events; separate equations are used for men and women, and the risk varies according to the combinations of risk factors (Fig. 16-3).[26] This approach has been validated in the United States across several observational studies. Various population

research techniques are used in this setting, including testing the ability of the variables to discriminate new cases from noncases and calibrating equations for use in other locales, by comparing the experience with population studies in the United States and elsewhere.

Estimation of CHD risk is generally valid for middle-class, white populations in North America and Europe, where risk factors and heart disease rates approximate the experience of studies such as the Framingham Heart Study that provided the estimates. It is useful for clinicians to estimate a patient's risk from the available data and then compare those 10-year CHD estimates with other estimates (Fig. 16-4). In this way, persons can be compared with others with "low" or "lowest" risk who are the same age and sex. The distributions of 10-year "hard CHD risks" (i.e., death from CHD or nonfatal MI) for Framingham men and women were recently published, and it can be seen that age and sex are extremely important determinants of risk (Figs. 16-5 and 16-6).[27] Overestimates of CHD risk may be obtained in other locales, especially where CHD risk in the general population is low, such as in Hawaii,[28,29] and caution should be taken when using CHD risk estimating equations in those or similar areas. In the case of using Framingham-based estimates for CHD risk in areas of the world where CHD risk is generally low, these estimates typically overestimate the risk of CHD in the other locale unless statistical adjustments are made.[30]

Using a slightly different set of variables, equations that estimate CHD risk have been developed in Germany to predict initial CHD events in men.[31] European investigators from several countries have also developed algorithms to estimate risk of CHD disease mortality.[32] For persons with type 2 diabetes mellitus, British investigators have developed a CHD risk estimating equation, and this approach includes factoring in levels of glycosylated hemoglobin and duration of diabetes mellitus.[33]

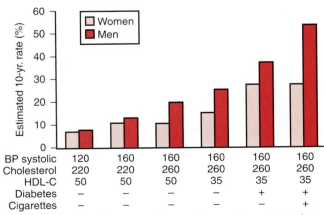

Figure 16-3   Total coronary heart disease risk estimated according to combinations of risk factors for 55-year-old men or women from the Framingham Heart Study. BP, blood pressure; HDL-C, high-density lipoprotein cholesterol. (Estimated from equations developed by Wilson. Data from Wilson PW, D'Agostino RB, Levy D, et al. Prediction of coronary heart disease using risk factor categories. *Circulation.* 1998;**97**:1837-1847.)

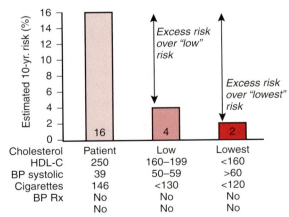

Figure 16-4   Estimated 10-year risk of "hard" coronary heart disease events (myocardial infarction or coronary death) in a 55-year-old man according to levels of various risk factors. (Developed from equations used in The Third Report of the Adult Treatment Panel of the National Cholesterol Education Panel. Executive Summary of The Third Report of The National Cholesterol Education Program [NCEP] Expert Panel on Detection, Evaluation, and Treatment of High Blood Cholesterol in Adults [Adult Treatment Panel III]. *JAMA.* 2001;**285**:2486-2497.)

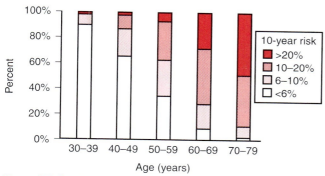

Figure 16-5 Estimated 10-year "hard" coronary heart disease risk in men in the Framingham Heart Study according to age group at baseline. (From Pasternak RC, Abrams J, Greenland P, et al. 34th Bethesda Conference: Task force #1. Identification of coronary heart disease risk: Is there a detection gap? *J Am Coll Cardiol.* 2003;**41**:1863-1874.)

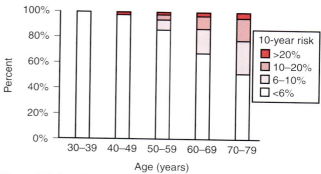

Figure 16-6 Estimated 10-year "hard" coronary heart disease risk in women in the Framingham Heart Study according to age group at baseline. (From Pasternak RC, Abrams J, Greenland P, et al. 34th Bethesda Conference: Task force #1. Identification of coronary heart disease risk: Is there a detection gap? *J Am Coll Cardiol.* 2003;**41**:1863-1874.)

Estimating CHD risk can help clinicians to match the estimated risk of CHD with the intensity of risk factor management. Using a multivariable equation approach is a dynamic process, and new information is constantly being evaluated because it may change the approach. It is important to assess whether new information improves the overall prediction of CHD within a population. Accuracy and precision of the new measurement, standardization of the technique, low correlation with existing predictive variables, validation in other observational studies, and biologic relevance are examples of features that need to be considered before the inclusion of newer variables into risk estimating approaches.[34,35]

EUROPEAN APPROACH

By the late 1990s, concern had arisen among European scientists regarding how well Framingham algorithms predicted CHD risk in their region. A large-scale, multinational European effort was undertaken to address this issue. This consortium included data from 12 European countries; most participants were white, and the study was called the Systematic Coronary Risk Evaluation (SCORE) Project. The investigators analyzed data sets from several observational studies; more than 200,000 men and women were represented, and the experience included 2.7 million person-years of follow-up. The large number of countries, the different collection methods, and the difficulty in ensuring accuracy in CHD events across the different regions led to limitations. Fatal CVD was the vascular disease outcome that was estimated, because data were insufficient to assess CHD morbidity.[32]

The SCORE Project undertook validation efforts within the participating groups, and the investigators reported that the risk of CVD death could be estimated with good discrimination. The area under the receiver-operator characteristic curve ranged from 0.71 to 0.84 for the participating countries. The SCORE scientists also reported that HDL-C information did not markedly improve the capability of CHD risk estimation in their data, a result that differed from the North American experience. These investigators showed that CHD

mortality risk varied considerably across Europe, and population samples from higher latitudes typically experienced greater risk than those closer to the Equator. Because of these differences, these investigators provided two CVD death risk estimation algorithms and recommended that the high-risk algorithm be used for persons from countries with a high risk of CVD (Russia, Scotland, Sweden, and the United Kingdom) and that a different CVD risk algorithm be used for regions where CVD risk was lower (France and southern Germany).

The SCORE investigators noted limitations in vascular disease risk estimation, including the error related to use of measurements from a single clinic visit, the potential effects of a regression-dilution bias, the use of principal risk factors only, and absence of information such as family history of premature vascular CHD. Because the SCORE system unfortunately used only CVD mortality and had little representation of minority groups, its utility may be limited outside Europe.

LIFESTYLE AND CORONARY HEART DISEASE RISK

Nutrition, physical activity, and obesity are key lifestyle and environmental features that generally underlie the development of risk factors. Prevention programs often emphasize the importance of these features. For example, greater dietary intake of cholesterol and saturated fat has been related to higher cholesterol levels in several populations.[36,37] There is great interest in popular diets, but long-term vascular disease outcome data are generally not available, and observational data continue to be the mainstay of nutritional guidelines for overall consumption of calories, fat, and carbohydrates. Dietary cholesterol guidelines promulgated by expert committees now recommend consumption of a variety of foods, including fruits, vegetables, and grains; a healthy body weight, desirable cholesterol level in the blood, and desirable BP levels are all important.[38]

Alcohol intake in the range of more than two drinks a day in men and more than one drink a day in women has consistently been related to a slightly increased risk for hypertension but a reduced risk for CHD.[39] Favorable effects on HDL-C levels are thought to be important in exerting this effect, as well as anti-inflammatory and antiplatelet effects. Greater alcohol intake is not without hazards, and a greater risk of gastrointestinal bleeding, hemorrhagic stroke, accidents, suicide, and cirrhosis may occur with increased intake.

Obesity

Excess adiposity has been defined by the World Health Organization. Two general measures are used: the body mass index, which is calculated by dividing the body weight in kilograms by the height in meters squared; and abdominal girth, which is the greatest circumference of the abdomen when a subject is standing.[40] Overweight is considered present when the body mass index is 25 to 29.9 kg/m^2, and obesity is present when the body mass index is greater than 30 kg/m^2. Increased abdominal adiposity is defined as more than 90 cm for women and more than 100 cm for men.

The prevalence of obesity has increased dramatically since the 1970s in the United States.[41] Data from U.S. surveys from 1960 to 2000 have shown that the prevalence of obesity has more than doubled from 10% to 27% in men and from 16% to 34% in women. Correspondingly, the prevalence of overweight has also increased, and it is now estimated that more than 50% of adults in the United States are either overweight or obese.[1,40] A similarly worrisome pattern is occurring in adolescents.

Obesity contributes to the development of several CHD risk factors, especially hypertension, diabetes mellitus, low HDL-C, elevated triglycerides, and elevated levels of inflammatory markers. Weight gain, even relatively modest increases, during adult years is highly related to developing a greater risk factor burden.[42] Obesity augments the effects of traditional risk factors and accounts for approximately 23% of CHD in men and 15% in women in long-term analyses of Framingham data.[43] When obesity is considered as an additional risk factor for the development of CHD over and above the traditional risk factors, there is no added benefit of knowing the level of obesity. The absence of an effect potentially has many sources, because adiposity is highly related to BP, low HDL-C, diabetes mellitus, age, and inflammatory markers.

NEWER ISSUES FOR MULTIVARIABLE CORONARY HEART DISEASE RISK ASSESSMENT

Lifetime Risk

The lifetime risk of CHD is highly related to sex and age. At age 40 years, the Framingham men experienced a 49% risk of developing CHD (angina pectoris, MI, or CHD death) before death. The lifetime incidence was lower for older persons who had never experienced CHD, and at age 70 years, the lifetime risk for CHD in men was only 35% (Fig. 16-7). The lifetime risks for CHD in women were lower at each age in comparison with men. Overall, the lifetime risk for CHD was approximately 40% in men and 30% in women.[44] In contrast, the lifetime risk for developing breast cancer in women is approx-

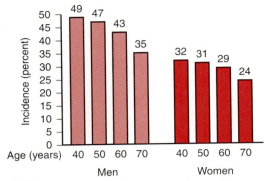

Figure 16–7 Lifetime risk for coronary heart disease according to age group at baseline for participants in the Framingham Heart Study. (From Lloyd-Jones DM, Larson MG, Beiser A, et al. Lifetime risk of developing coronary heart disease. *Lancet.* 1999;**353**:89-92.)

imately 10%, a rate that is much lower than a woman's lifetime risk for CHD. Lifetime risk estimates bridge the traditional 5- to 10-year CHD risk estimates to a distant horizon, but this approach has not been incorporated into CHD risk estimating strategies in common use in the United States and Europe.

Inflammation

Various factors related to hematologic, endothelial, and inflammatory processes have been studied for their relation to CHD. A European investigation assessed the relations between recurrent CHD and levels of fibrinogen, von Willebrand factor antigen, tissue plasminogen activator (t-PA) antigen, and C-reactive protein in persons with angina pectoris. Each of these markers was highly related to greater risk of subsequent CHD in categoric analyses that used quintiles of each factor.[45] Subsequent research in a large number of studies has shown that inflammatory markers, especially C-reactive protein, are highly related to an increased risk of atherosclerotic events,[46] including initial and recurrent CVD, as well as stroke.[47-50] Measurement of inflammatory markers, specifically high-sensitivity C-reactive protein (hs-CRP), is now considered a reasonable adjunct to the major risk factors for further assessment of the absolute risk for CHD primary prevention.

Blood levels of the amino acid homocysteine have been studied for its relation to CVD risk. Investigations in the early 1990s showed that lower intake of B vitamins (folate, vitamin B$_6$, vitamin B$_{12}$) was related to greater concentrations of homocysteine.[51] Persons with higher homocysteine levels experienced greater risk for CVD, and the results were stronger in the earlier reports than in more recent investigations.[52,53] Folate fortification of cereals and grains was undertaken in the United States during the late 1990s to reduce the risk of neural tube defects during pregnancy, and it appears to have reduced the frequency of elevated homocysteine levels in the free-living population. Additional folate intake from supplementary vitamins and multivitamins may be contributing to a reduced importance for homocysteine as a CVD risk factor. Homocysteine may still be an important contributor to greater CHD risk in specific situations, such persons with impaired kidney function.[54,55]

Newer Lipid Biomarkers

Many different lipoprotein particles have been identified, and several techniques are available to assess their density, diameter, electrophoretic characteristics, and nuclear magnetic resonance properties. Initially, the LDL particles received the most attention, because apolipoprotein B is present in the LDL fraction. Research interest has spread to investigate the role of all particle groups because newer methods have allowed rapid assessment of the numbers and concentrations of lipoprotein particles.[56-58] The smaller, denser LDL particles may be associated with greater risk, but the added usefulness of these measurements for the assessment of CVD risk in prospective studies is not assured at this time.[59]

Lipoprotein (a) [Lp(a)] is an accepted determinant of CVD risk, and this particle includes an LDL moiety linked to a protein chain that bears homology to plasminogen. The length of the apolipoprotein (a) varies and is heritable. Various methods have been undertaken to assay Lp(a),[60] but standardization has been difficult because the particle varies in composition from person to person.[61] Levels of Lp(a) are higher in Africans and in African Americans than in whites.[62] In African populations, the particle concentrations follow a normal statistical distribution, but Lp(a) levels are lower, and the distribution is skewed in whites. Lp(a) has generally been shown to be a CVD risk factor, especially at the higher concentrations (>30 mg/dL) in whites, and routine screening for Lp(a) levels has been recommended for persons with premature CVD that is not explained by conventional risk factor levels.[63]

Metabolic Syndrome and Insulin Resistance

Several CVD risk factors occur at a frequency greater than expected, and insulin resistance is thought to account for clustering of these traits, especially higher BP, impaired fasting glucose, increased triglycerides, decreased HDL-C, and greater abdominal adiposity. The presence of three or more of these five abnormalities has been named the metabolic syndrome, and some of the criteria are sex specific. The metabolic syndrome is present in approximately 24% of adults in the United States according to survey data from the early 1990s, and the prevalence is highly related to age, ranging from 7% in persons at 20 to 29 years to 43% in persons 60 to 69 years old.[64] The presence of the metabolic syndrome in adults confers an increased risk of diabetes mellitus, CHD, and CVD-related death.[65]

Subclinical Cardiovascular Disease

Modern techniques can provide assessment of subclinical vascular disease in smaller arteries. The carotid arteries have been studied with B-mode ultrasound and more recently with magnetic resonance imaging. Greater carotid stenosis in older persons has correlated with the burden of smoking, BP, and cholesterol across the adult years,[66] and increased intima-media thickening of the carotid arteries in elderly persons has been shown to be predictive of the subsequent development of CVD.[67] The usefulness of this testing is limited by the need for accurate measurements and trained sonographers.

Over the past few years, scanning of the coronary arteries for the presence of calcification has been proposed as a useful strategy to identify persons at high risk for the development of clinical CVD.[68] Data from groups without possible self-referral bias are limited at present, but large investigations such as the Multi-Ethnic Study of Atherosclerosis should provide a critical assessment of the added usefulness of these newer screening modalities in nonselected population cohorts.[69]

Kidney Disease

Proteinuria was noted in the 1980s to be related to an increased risk of CHD. More recent research has focused on microalbuminuria (>30 mg of albumin/g urinary creatinine) as a marker of renal impairment in persons with hypertension or diabetes mellitus. Modest decrements in estimated glomerular filtration rate and the presence of microalbuminuria are important predictors of decline in renal function and the development of CVD.[70] Assessment of albumin excretion is now recommended at regular intervals for persons with diabetes mellitus or hypertension.

Long-term treatment of hypertension and type 2 diabetes mellitus has led to extension of life, but chronic kidney failure may occur. These two diseases are now the most common diagnoses for persons who need to start long-term dialysis. Once renal failure has developed, the prognosis is quite poor. Atherosclerosis appears to enter an accelerated phase, and death from CVD or from cardiac failure is quite common.

CORONARY HEART DISEASE RISK ESTIMATION IN THE AFRICAN-AMERICAN POPULATION

Various issues relating to CHD risk estimation are important for estimating CHD in high-risk population groups such as African-Americans. The usual CHD risk variables exhibit differences in effects, prevalence, or treatment in African Americans, and these differences can affect the accuracy of prediction.

In comparisons of relative risks for CHD in the Atherosclerosis Risk in Communities participants, the relative risk for CHD in persons with diabetes was significantly increased in men (2.19 whites, 1.60 African Americans) and women (2.95 whites, 1.86 African Americans).[71] Different results were evident for the effects of BP on CHD risk in white versus African-American participants. The relative risk for CHD associated with a 20 mm Hg difference for systolic pressure was 1.31 in white men, a relative risk that was significantly greater than 1.00. Conversely, the relative risk for a 20 mm Hg difference in African-American men was only 1.05 and was not statistically significant. The lower relative risk in African-American men could lead a reader to conclude that systolic BP exerts a less important effect in African-American men. However, the relative risk of CHD related to hypertension therapy was 2.00 in African-American men and only 1.13 in white men, a finding indicating that hypertension treatment in African-American men was associated with the much greater risk than anticipated. A reasonable interpretation of these results is that hypertensive African-American men were treated inadequately and may have received therapy later in the course of their hypertension. However, recent clinical trials have convincingly demonstrated the beneficial effects of hypertension therapy on CHD risk in both white and African-American populations. These results also suggest that caution should be exercised when implementing CHD risk algorithms, especially when effects in observational studies are not congruent with the experience of controlled clinical trials.

BP elevation is an important CHD risk predictor, and levels are typically higher in the African-American populations. These differences may be particularly important at higher BP categories. For example, BPs higher than 180/110 mm Hg were uncommon in the all-white Framingham Heart Study experience, but they are more frequently seen in African-American population groups. A second BP consideration is the role of treatment. In years past, there was a greater degree of no treatment, undertreatment, and late treatment of hypertension along African Americans compared with whites in the United States.

A third element related to BP is the myocardium itself, considering left ventricular mass and left ventricular hypertrophy on the electrocardiogram (ECG-LVH). In the 1991 formulation of CHD risk published by the Framingham investigators, ECG-LVH was included as a risk factor. Framingham data obtained during the 1990s showed that the prevalence of ECG-LVH was low, only a few percent, and U.S. national expert committees have not recommended ECG determinations or echocardiographic evaluations at the time of screening for CHD risk. This recommendation may hold for white population groups, but the greater prevalence of ECG-LVH in African Americans, even at the same BP levels, suggests that biologic differences may be operative, and more pronounced adverse effects on CHD risk are possible. Data from observational studies have consistently shown that ECG-LVH leads to a fivefold or greater risk for CHD. Overall, the data suggest that ECG-LVH is a CHD risk equivalent and should be assessed in population groups where it is reasonably common, so aggressive therapy can be instituted and maintained.

Blood cholesterol levels in whites and in African Americans are roughly similar, but a tendency toward higher HDL-C levels has typically been reported for African Americans.[72] This difference may not be obtained among African Americans with higher socioeconomic status or when obesity or type 2 diabetes mellitus is present. Additionally, as mentioned earlier, levels of Lp(a) are typically greater in persons of African ancestry.[73]

Finally, obesity and type 2 diabetes mellitus are more common among African-Americans, but their contribution to CHD risk has not been well characterized for this group. In the African-American Atherosclerosis Risk in Communities participants from Jackson, Mississippi, most of the CHD risk factors appeared to operate along the lines observed for whites in the United States. It has been reported, however, that greater duration of diabetes and microalbuminuria can augment risk of initial CHD events in persons with diabetes.[74] These issues may be particularly important to African Americans with type 2 diabetes mellitus and have not been well studied.

SUMMARY

Summation of risk factors, using modern research methods, provides a quantitative estimate of an individual's odds of manifesting CHD in the future.[75] Even more important, these factors provide a rationale and target for therapies and lifestyle modifications to reduce substantially, but probably not eliminate, the absolute risk for future atherosclerotic events in Westernized societies. Vascular disease risk estimation is possible for persons with hypertension, but consideration of end-organ damage and subclinical disease may prove to be especially important in those individuals.

References

1. American Heart Association. Heart Disease and Stroke Statistics: 2005 Update. Dallas, Tex: American Heart Association, 2004.
2. Chambless LE, Toole JF, Nieto FJ, et al. Association between symptoms reported in a population questionnaire and future ischemic stroke: The ARIC study. *Neuroepidemiology*. 2004;**23**:33-37.
3. Stampfer MJ, Willett WC, Colditz GA, et al. A prospective study of postmenopausal estrogen therapy and coronary heart disease. *N Engl J Med*. 1985;**313**:1044-1049.
4. Bush TL, Cowan LD, Barrett-Connor EL, et al. Estrogen use and all-cause mortality. *JAMA*. 1983;**249**:903-906.
5. Grady D, Rubin SM, Petitti DB, et al. Hormone therapy to prevent disease and prolong life in postmenopausal women. *Ann Intern Med*. 1992;**117**:1016-1037.
6. Hulley S, Grady D, Bush T, et al. Randomized trial of estrogen plus progestin for secondary prevention of coronary heart disease in postmenopausal women: Heart and Estrogen/Progestin Replacement Study (HERS) Research Group. *JAMA*. 1998;**280**:605-613.
7. Neaton JD, Wentworth D. Serum cholesterol, blood pressure, cigarette smoking, and death from coronary heart disease: Overall findings and differences by age for 316,099 white men. Multiple Risk Factor Intervention Trial Research Group. *Arch Intern Med*. 1992;**152**:56-64.
8. Abbott RD, Wilson PW, Kannel WB, et al. High density lipoprotein cholesterol, total cholesterol screening, and myocardial infarction: The Framingham Study. *Arteriosclerosis*. 1988;**8**:207-211.
9. Jeppesen J, Hein HO, Suadicani P, et al. Relation of high TG-low HDL cholesterol and LDL cholesterol to the incidence of ischemic heart disease: An 8-year follow-up in the Copenhagen Male Study. *Arterioscler Thromb Vasc Biol*. 1997;**17**:1114-1120.
10. Gordon DJ, Rifkind BM. High-density lipoprotein: The clinical implications of recent studies. *N Engl J Med*. 1989;**321**: 1311-1316.
11. Durrington P. Dyslipidaemia. *Lancet*. 2003;**362**:717-731.
12. Hyman DJ, Pavlik VN. Characteristics of patients with uncontrolled hypertension in the United States. *N Engl J Med*. 2001;**345**:479-486.
13. Basile JN. The importance of systolic blood pressure control and cardiovascular disease prevention. *Curr Treat Options Cardiovasc Med*. 2003;**5**:271-277.
14. Franklin SS, Larson MG, Khan SA, et al. Does the relation of blood pressure to coronary heart disease risk change with aging? The Framingham Heart Study. *Circulation*. 2001;**103**:1245-1249.
15. Vasan RS, Larson MG, Leip EP, et al. Impact of high-normal blood pressure on the risk of cardiovascular disease. *N Engl J Med*. 2001;**345**:1291-1297.
16. Major outcomes in moderately hypercholesterolemic, hypertensive patients randomized to pravastatin vs. usual care: The Antihypertensive and Lipid-Lowering Treatment to Prevent Heart Attack Trial (ALLHAT-LLT). *JAMA*. 2002;**288**: 2998-3007.

17. Sever PS, Dahlof B, Poulter NR, et al. Prevention of coronary and stroke events with atorvastatin in hypertensive patients who have average or lower-than-average cholesterol concentrations, in the Anglo-Scandinavian Cardiac Outcomes Trial—Lipid Lowering Arm (ASCOT-LLA): A multicentre randomised controlled trial. *Lancet.* 2003;**361**:1149-1158.

18. Palmer JR, Rosenberg L, Shapiro S. "Low yield" cigarettes and the risk of nonfatal myocardial infarction in women. *N Engl J Med.* 1989;**320**:1569-1573.

19. Steenland K. Passive smoking and the risk of heart disease. *JAMA.* 1992;**267**:94-99.

20. Howard G, Burke GL, Szklo M, et al. Active and passive smoking are associated with increased carotid wall thickness: The Atherosclerosis Risk in Communities Study. *Arch Intern Med.* 1994;**154**:1277-1282.

21. Wilson PW. Diabetes mellitus and coronary heart disease. *Am J Kidney Dis.* 1998;**32**:S89-100.

22. Haffner SM, Lehto S, Ronnemaa T, et al. Mortality from coronary heart disease in subjects with type 2 diabetes and in nondiabetic subjects with and without prior myocardial infarction. *N Engl J Med.* 1998;**339**:229-234.

23. American Diabetes Association. Clinical practice recommendations 2005. *Diabetes Care.* 2005;**28 (Suppl 1)**:S1-79.

24. Gaede P, Vedel P, Larsen N, et al. Multifactorial intervention and cardiovascular disease in patients with type 2 diabetes. *N Engl J Med.* 2003;**348**:383-393.

25. Diabetes Control and Complications Trial Research Group. The effect of intensive treatment of diabetes on the development and progression of long-term complications in insulin-dependent diabetes mellitus: The Diabetes Control and Complications Trial Research Group. *N Engl J Med.* 1993;**329**:977-986.

26. Wilson PW, D'Agostino RB, Levy D, et al. Prediction of coronary heart disease using risk factor categories. *Circulation.* 1998;**97**:1837-1847.

27. Pasternak RC, Abrams J, Greenland P, et al. 34th Bethesda Conference: Task force #1. Identification of coronary heart disease risk: Is there a detection gap? *J Am Coll Cardiol.* 2003;**41**:1863-1874.

28. D'Agostino RB Sr, Grundy S, Sullivan LM, et al. Validation of the Framingham coronary heart disease prediction scores: Results of a multiple ethnic groups investigation. *JAMA.* 2001;**286**:180-187.

29. Marrugat J, Solanas P, D'Agostino R, et al. Coronary risk estimation in Spain using a calibrated Framingham function. *Rev Esp Cardiol.* 2003;**56**:253-261.

30. Liu J, Hong Y, D'Agostino RB Sr, et al. Predictive value for the Chinese population of the Framingham CHD risk assessment tool compared with the Chinese Multi-Provincial Cohort Study. *JAMA.* 2004;**291**:2591-2599.

31. Assmann G, Cullen P, Schulte H. Simple scoring scheme for calculating the risk of acute coronary events based on the 10-year follow-up of the prospective cardiovascular Munster (PROCAM) study. *Circulation.* 2002;**105**:310-315.

32. Conroy RM, Pyorala K, Fitzgerald AP, et al. Estimation of ten-year risk of fatal cardiovascular disease in Europe: The SCORE project. *Eur Heart J.* 2003;**24**:987-1003.

33. Stevens RJ, Kothari V, Adler AI, et al. The UKPDS risk engine: A model for the risk of coronary heart disease in type II diabetes (UKPDS 56). *Clin Sci (Lond).* 2001;**101**:671-679.

34. Wilson PW. Metabolic risk factors for coronary heart disease: Current and future prospects. *Curr Opin Cardiol.* 1999;**14**:176-185.

35. Mosca L. C-reactive protein—to screen or not to screen? *N Engl J Med.* 2002;**347**:1615-1617.

36. Keys A, Karvonen JM, Punsar S. HDL serum cholesterol and 24-year mortality of men in Finland. *Int J Epidemiol.* 1984;**13**:428-435.

37. Verschuren WM, Jacobs DR, Bloemberg BP, et al. Serum total cholesterol and long-term coronary heart disease mortality in different cultures: Twenty-five-year follow-up of the seven countries study. *JAMA.* 1995;**274**:131-136.

38. Krauss RM, Eckel RH, Howard B, et al. AHA dietary guidelines: Revision 2000: A statement for healthcare professionals from the Nutrition Committee of the American Heart Association. *Circulation.* 2000;**102**:2284-2299.

39. Kannel WB, Ellison RC. Alcohol and coronary heart disease: The evidence for a protective effect. *Clin Chim Acta.* 1996;**246**:59-76.

40. Expert Panel. Clinical Guidelines on the Identification, Evaluation, and Treatment of Overweight and Obesity in Adults. Bethesda, MD: Public Health Service, National Institutes of Health, National Heart, Lung, and Blood Institute, 1998.

41. Mokdad AH, Serdula MK, Dietz WH, et al. The spread of the obesity epidemic in the United States, 1991-1998. *JAMA.* 1999;**282**:1519-1522.

42. Wilson PW, Kannel WB, Silbershatz H, et al. Clustering of metabolic factors and coronary heart disease. *Arch Intern Med.* 1999;**159**:1104-1109.

43. Wilson PW, D'Agostino RB, Sullivan L, et al. Overweight and obesity as determinants of cardiovascular risk: The Framingham experience. *Arch Intern Med.* 2002;**162**:1867-1872.

44. Lloyd-Jones DM, Larson MG, Beiser A, et al. Lifetime risk of developing coronary heart disease. *Lancet.* 1999;**353**:89-92.

45. Thompson SG, Kienast J, Pyke SD, et al. Hemostatic factors and the risk of myocardial infarction or sudden death in patients with angina pectoris: European Concerted Action on Thrombosis and Disabilities Angina Pectoris Study Group. *N Engl J Med.* 1995;**332**:635-641.

46. Ridker PM, Hennekens CH, Buring JE, et al. C-reactive protein and other markers of inflammation in the prediction of cardiovascular disease in women. *N Engl J Med.* 2000;**342**:836-843.

47. Ridker PM, Cushman M, Stampfer MJ, et al. Plasma concentration of C-reactive protein and risk of developing peripheral vascular disease. *Circulation.* 1998;**97**:425-428.

48. Ridker PM, Glynn RJ, Hennekens CH. C-reactive protein adds to the predictive value of total and HDL cholesterol in determining risk of first myocardial infarction. *Circulation.* 1998;**97**:2007-2011.

49. Ridker PM, Rifai N, Rose L, et al. Comparison of C-reactive protein and low-density lipoprotein cholesterol levels in the prediction of first cardiovascular events. *N Engl J Med.* 2002;**347**:1557-1565.

50. Rost NS, Wolf PA, Kase CS, et al. Plasma concentration of C-reactive protein and risk of ischemic stroke and transient ischemic attack: The Framingham Study. *Stroke.* 2001;**32**:2575-2579.

51. Nathan DM, Singer DE, Hurxthal K, et al. The clinical information value of the glycosylated hemoglobin assay. *N Engl J Med.* 1984;**310**:341-346.

52. Christen WG, Ajani UA, Glynn RJ, et al. Blood levels of homocysteine and increased risks of cardiovascular disease: Causal or casual? *Arch Intern Med.* 2000;**160**:422-434.

53. Homocysteine and risk of ischemic heart disease and stroke: A meta-analysis. *JAMA.* 2002;**288**:2015-2022.

54. Bostom AG, Gohh RY, Liaugaudas G, et al. Prevalence of mild fasting hyperhomocysteinemia in renal transplant versus coronary artery disease patients after fortification of cereal grain flour with folic acid. *Atherosclerosis.* 1999;**145**:221-224.

55. Bostom AG, Selhub J, Jacques PF, et al. Power shortage: Clinical trials testing the "homocysteine hypothesis" against a background of folic acid–fortified cereal grain flour. *Ann Intern Med.* 2001;**135**:133-137.

56. Austin MA, King MC, Vranizan KM, et al. Atherogenic lipoprotein phenotype: A proposed genetic marker for coronary heart disease risk. *Circulation*. 1990;**82**:495-506.

57. Otvos JD, Jeyarajah EJ, Bennett DW, et al. Development of a proton nuclear magnetic resonance spectroscopic method for determining plasma lipoprotein concentrations and subspecies distributions from a single, rapid measurement. *Clin Chem*. 1992;**38**:1632-1638.

58. Reaven GM, Abbasi F, Bernhart S, et al. Insulin resistance, dietary cholesterol, and cholesterol concentration in postmenopausal women. *Metabolism*. 2001;**50**:594-597.

59. Lamarche B, St Pierre AC, Ruel IL, et al. A prospective, population-based study of low density lipoprotein particle size as a risk factor for ischemic heart disease in men. *Can J Cardiol*. 2001;**17**:859-865.

60. Marcovina SM, Albers JJ, Scanu AM, et al. Use of a reference material proposed by the International Federation of Clinical Chemistry and Laboratory Medicine to evaluate analytical methods for the determination of plasma lipoprotein(a). *Clin Chem*. 2000;**46**:1956-1967.

61. Marcovina SM, Hegele RA, Koschinsky ML. Lipoprotein(a) and coronary heart disease risk. *Curr Cardiol Rep*. 1999;**1**:105-111.

62. Gidding SS, Liu K, Bild DE, et al. Prevalence and identification of abnormal lipoprotein levels in a biracial population aged 23 to 35 years (the CARDIA Study): The Coronary Artery Risk Development in Young Adults Study. *Am J Cardiol*. 1996;**78**:304-308.

63. Scanu AM. Lp(a) lipoprotein: Coping with heterogeneity. *N Engl J Med*. 2003;**349**:2089-2090.

64. Ford ES, Giles WH, Dietz WH. Prevalence of the metabolic syndrome among US adults: Findings from the third National Health and Nutrition Examination Survey. *JAMA*. 2002;**287**:356-359.

65. Sattar N, Gaw A, Scherbakova O, et al. Metabolic syndrome with and without C-reactive protein as a predictor of coronary heart disease and diabetes in the West of Scotland Coronary Prevention Study. *Circulation*. 2003;**108**:414-419.

66. Wilson PWF, Hoeg JM, D'Agostino RB, et al. Cumulative effects of high cholesterol levels, high blood pressure, and cigarette smoking on carotid stenosis. *N Engl J Med*. 1997;**337**:516-522.

67. O'Leary DH, Polak JF, Kronmal RA, et al. Carotid-artery intima and media thickness as a risk factor for myocardial infarction and stroke in older adults: Cardiovascular Health Study Collaborative Research Group. *N Engl J Med*. 1999;**340**:14-22.

68. Raggi P, Callister TQ, Cooil B, et al. Identification of patients at increased risk of first unheralded acute myocardial infarction by electron-beam computed tomography. *Circulation*. 2000;**101**:850-855.

69. Bild DE, Bluemke DA, Burke GL, et al. Multi-Ethnic Study of Atherosclerosis: Objectives and design. *Am J Epidemiol*. 2002;**156**:871-881.

70. Culleton BF, Larson MG, Wilson PW, et al. Cardiovascular disease and mortality in a community-based cohort with mild renal insufficiency. *Kidney Int*. 1999;**56**:2214-2219.

71. Chambless LE, Folsom AR, Sharrett R, et al. Coronary heart disease risk prediction in the Atherosclerosis Risk in Communities (ARIC) Study. *J Clin Epidemiol*. 2003;**56**:880-890.

72. Watkins LO, Neaton JD, Kuller LH, et al. High density lipoprotein cholesterol and coronary heart disease incidence in black and white MRFIT usual care men. *Circulation*. 1985;**71**:417a.

73. Mooser V, Seabra MC, Abedin M, et al. Apolipoprotein(a) kringle 4-containing fragments in human urine: Relationship to plasma levels of lipoprotein(a). *J Clin Invest*. 1996;**97**:858-864.

74. Stevens RJ, Coleman RL, Adler AI, et al. Risk factors for myocardial infarction: Case fatality and stroke case fatality in type 2 diabetes. UKPDS 66. *Diabetes Care*. 2004;**27**:201-207.

75. Executive Summary of the Third Report of the National Cholesterol Education Program (NCEP) Expert Panel on Detection, Evaluation, and Treatment of High Blood Cholesterol in Adults (Adult Treatment Panel III). *JAMA*. 2001;**285**:2486-2497.

SECTION 4

Treatment

SECTION CONTENTS

Chapter 17

Diet and Blood Pressure

Lawrence J. Appel

Elevated blood pressure (BP) remains an extraordinarily common and important risk factor for cardiovascular disease (CVD) and chronic renal disease throughout the world.[1] In the United States, according to the National Health and Nutrition Examination Survey conducted in 1999 to 2000, 27% of adults have hypertension (systolic BP ≥140 mm Hg, diastolic BP ≥90 mm Hg or are using antihypertensive medication), and another 31% have prehypertension (systolic BP of 120 to 139 mm Hg or diastolic BP of 80 to 89 mm Hg and not taking medication).[2] Regrettably, the prevalence of hypertension appears to be increasing,[3] and control rates remain low.[4] Systolic BP progressively rises with age, such that hypertension becomes almost ubiquitous among elderly persons. Elevated BP afflicts both men and women. African Americans, on average, have higher BPs than non–African Americans,[3] as well as an increased risk of BP-related diseases, particularly stroke[5,6] and kidney disease.[7]

BP is a strong, consistent, continuous, independent, and etiologically relevant risk factor for CVD and renal disease.[8] Importantly, no evidence exists of a BP threshold, and the risk of CVD increases progressively throughout the full range of BPs, including the prehypertensive range.[9] Investigators have estimated that almost one third of BP-related deaths from coronary heart disease occur in individuals with BP in the nonhypertensive range.[10] Accordingly, prehypertensive individuals not only have a high probability of developing hypertension (~90%[11]), but also carry an excess risk of CVD compared with those with a normal BP (systolic BP <120 mm Hg and diastolic BP <80 mm Hg).

Elevated BP results from environmental factors (including dietary factors), genetic factors, and interactions among these factors. Of the environmental factors that affect BP (diet, physical inactivity, toxins such as lead, and psychosocial factors), dietary factors likely have a predominant role in BP homeostasis. Well-established dietary modifications that lower BP are reduced salt intake, weight loss, and moderation of alcohol consumption (among those who drink). Since the mid-1990s, increased potassium intake and consumption of an overall healthy dietary pattern, termed the *Dietary Approaches to Stop Hypertension (DASH) diet*, have emerged as effective strategies that also lower BP. An extensive review on the role of diet as a means to prevent and treat hypertension has been published recently.[12]

In nonhypertensive individuals, dietary changes that lower BP have the potential to prevent hypertension and reduce the risk of BP-related CV events. Indeed, even an apparently small BP reduction, if applied broadly to an entire population, could have an enormous beneficial impact. For example, it has been estimated that a 3 mm Hg reduction in systolic BP could lead to an 8% reduction in stroke mortality and a 5% reduction in mortality from coronary heart disease (Fig. 17-1).[13] In uncomplicated stage 1 hypertension (systolic BP 140 to 159 mm Hg or diastolic BP 90 to 99 mm Hg), dietary changes can serve as first-line therapy. Among hypertensive patients who are already taking medication, dietary changes, particularly reduced salt intake, can further lower BP and can facilitate medication step-down. In general, the magnitude of BP reduction from dietary changes is greater in hypertensive than in nonhypertensive individuals.

Although dietary changes have been shown to lower BP, considerably less information is available on whether dietary changes blunt the age-related rise in BP. On average, systolic BP rises imperceptibly by approximately 0.6 mm Hg/year. Efforts to prevent this age-associated rise in BP hold the greatest promise as a means to prevent elevated BP and curb the epidemic of BP-related disease. Unfortunately, even the longest diet-BP intervention trials have lasted less than 5 years. Whether the BP reductions observed in these trials have merely shifted the age-associated rise in BP curve downward, without a change in slope (Fig. 17-2A), or have actually reduced its slope (see Fig. 17-2B) cannot be determined. Still, evidence from migration studies[14] and cross-sectional observational studies[15] suggests that dietary factors should reduce the rise in BP with age. Furthermore, a compelling body of research documents the effects of diet on absolute BP levels. The following sections highlight this research.

DIETARY FACTORS THAT REDUCE BLOOD PRESSURE

Weight Loss

Weight is directly associated with BP (see Chapter 31). The importance of this relationship is reinforced by the high and increasing prevalence of obesity throughout the world. In the United States, approximately 65% of adults have a body mass index greater than or equal to 25 kg/m² and therefore are classified as either overweight or obese; more than 30% of adults are obese (body mass index ≥30 kg/m²).[16] In children and adolescents in the United States, the prevalence of overweight is increasing, as is the average BP.[17]

With rare exception, trials have documented that weight loss lowers BP. Reductions in BP occur before, and even without, attainment of a desirable body weight. In a recent meta-analysis that aggregated data across 25 trials, an average weight loss of 5.1 kg reduced systolic BP by a mean of 4.4 mm Hg and diastolic BP by a mean of 3.6 mm Hg.[18] In subgroup analyses, BP reductions were greater in those who lost more weight. Within trials, dose-response analyses[19,20] and observational studies[21] also provide evidence that greater weight loss leads to greater BP reductions.

Other research has documented that modest weight loss, with or without sodium reduction, can prevent hypertension by approximately 20% among overweight, nonhypertensive individuals,[22] and it can facilitate efforts to reduce and even

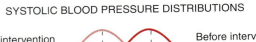

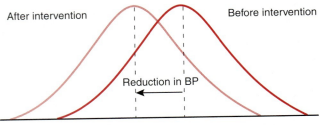

Reduction in BP	% Reduction in mortality		
mm Hg	Stroke	CHD	Total
2	−6	−4	−3
3	−8	−5	−4
5	−14	−9	−7

Figure 17–1 Estimated effects of population-wide shifts in systolic blood pressure (BP) on mortality. CHD, coronary heart disease. (Modified from Stamler R. Implications of the INTERSALT study. *Hypertension.* 1991;**17**:116-I20.)

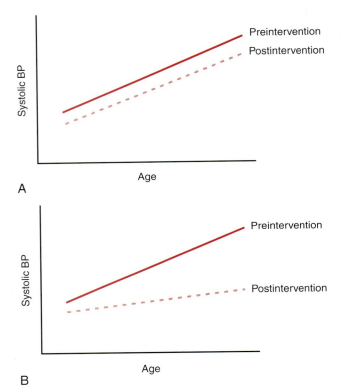

Figure 17–2 **A,** Model in which a dietary intervention shifts the age–blood pressure (BP) curve downward without affecting the slope. **B,** Model in which a dietary intervention shifts the age-BP curve downward and reduces its slope.

withdraw antihypertensive medications.[23,24] Behavioral intervention trials have uniformly achieved short-term weight loss, primarily through a reduction in energy intake. In several instances, substantial weight loss has also been maintained over 3 or more years.[24,25] Regular physical activity is well recognized as a critical factor in sustaining weight loss. Whether weight loss can blunt the age-related rise in BP is uncertain. In one of the longest weight loss trials, individuals

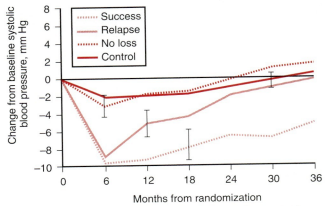

Figure 17–3 Mean systolic blood pressure change in the Trials of Hypertension Prevention (TOHP2) in four groups of participants: those assigned to a weight loss group who successfully maintained weight loss, those assigned to a weight loss group who lost weight but experienced relapse, those assigned to a weight loss group who never lost weight, and the control group. (From Stevens VJ, Obarzanek E, Cook NR, et al. Long-term weight loss and changes in blood pressure: Results of the Trials of Hypertension Prevention, phase II. *Ann Intern Med.* 2001;**134**:1-11.)

who sustained a more than 10-lb weight loss achieved a lower BP that nonetheless still rose over time (Fig. 17-3).[20] In aggregate, available evidence strongly supports weight reduction as an effective approach to prevent and treat hypertension.

Reduced Salt (Sodium Chloride) Intake

On average, as dietary salt intake rises, so does BP. Available types of evidence include animal studies, epidemiologic studies, clinical trials, and meta-analyses of trials. To date, more than 50 randomized trials have been performed. In one of the most recent meta-analyses,[26] a median reduction in urinary sodium of approximately 1.8 g/day (78 mmol/day) lowered systolic and diastolic BP by 2.0 and 1.0 mm Hg in nonhypertensive individuals and by 5.0 and 2.7 mm Hg in hypertensive persons.

The most persuasive evidence on the effects of salt on BP comes from rigorously controlled dose-response studies.[27-29] Each of these trials tested at least three sodium intake levels, and each documented statistically significant, direct, progressive, dose-response relationships. The largest of these trials, the DASH-Sodium trial,[29] tested the effects of three different sodium intakes separately in two diets: the DASH diet (see later) and a control diet more typical of what is usually eaten in the United States. As estimated from 24-hour urine collections, the three sodium intake levels (termed lower, intermediate, and higher) provided 65, 107, and 142 mmol of sodium/day, respectively (corresponding to 1.5, 2.5, and 3.3 g/day).

The main results of this trial are displayed in Figure 17-4. The BP response to sodium reduction, albeit direct and progressive, was nonlinear, that is, the slope of BP change per change in sodium intake was steeper at less than 100 mmol/day than the corresponding slope at values higher than this level. In subgroup analyses of this trial,[30,31] a reduced sodium intake

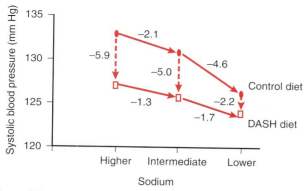

Figure 17–4 Mean systolic blood pressure changes in the DASH-Sodium trial. The sample size was 412, 59% were prehypertensive, and 57% were African American. Solid lines display the effects of sodium reduction in the two diets; *hatched lines* display the effects of the Dietary Approaches to Stop Hypertension (DASH) diet at each sodium level. (Modified from Sacks FM, Svetkey LP, Vollmer WM, et al. Effects on blood pressure of reduced dietary sodium and the Dietary Approaches to Stop Hypertension [DASH] diet. DASH-Sodium Collaborative Research Group. *N Engl J Med.* 2001;**344**:3-10.)

significantly lowered BP in each of the major subgroups studied (i.e., African American, non–African American, men, women). Importantly, sodium reduction significantly lowered BP in nonhypertensive individuals on both diets.

In addition to lowering BP, trials have documented that reduced sodium intake can prevent hypertension (relative risk reduction of approximately 20% with or without concomitant weight loss),[22] can lower BP even in the setting of BP-lowering medications,[32,33] and can improve hypertension control.[23,24] In observational studies, reduced sodium intake is associated with a blunted age-related rise in systolic BP.[15] In observational studies, reduced salt intake is associated with a reduced risk of CVD,[34,35] including heart failure.[36]

Similar to other interventions, the BP response to changes in dietary sodium intake is heterogeneous.[37] Despite attempts to classify individuals in research studies as salt sensitive and salt resistant, the change in BP in response to a change in salt intake is not binary.[38] Rather, the change in BP from reduced sodium intake has a continuous distribution, that is, individuals have greater or lesser degrees of BP reduction. In general, the extent of BP reduction as a result of reduced sodium intake is greater in blacks, in middle-aged and older persons, and in patients with hypertension, diabetes, or kidney disease. These groups tend to have a less responsive renin-angiotensin-aldosterone system.[39] Investigators have hypothesized that salt sensitivity is a phenotype that reflects subclinical kidney dysfunction.[40] As discussed later, genetic and dietary factors also influence the response to sodium. With respect to diet, the rise in BP for a given increase in sodium is blunted in the setting of either the DASH diet[29] or high dietary potassium intake.[41,42]

No trial has tested the effects of reduced sodium intake on clinical CV events. As for most other nutrients, the absence of such a trial does not preclude dietary recommendations. Available evidence indicates that reduced sodium intake

lowers BP and that lower levels of BP should reduce the risk of CVD. Apart from reductions in BP, sodium reduction may also have other favorable effects. In cross-sectional studies, left ventricular mass is directly related to sodium intake[43]; one small trial documented that sodium reduction can reduce left ventricular mass.[44] Importantly, no convincing or consistent evidence indicates harm from reduced sodium intake. Although extreme sodium reduction to less than 20 mmol/day may adversely affect blood lipids and insulin resistance, moderate sodium reduction has no such effects.[26,45] A potential adverse effect of reduced sodium intake is an increase in plasma renin activity, perhaps indicative of stimulation the renin-angiotensin-aldosterone system. However, in contrast to the well-accepted benefits of BP reduction, the clinical relevance of modest rises in plasma renin activity as a result of sodium reduction and other antihypertensive therapies is uncertain. In fact, thiazide diuretics, an antihypertensive drug therapy that also raises plasma renin activity, have been shown to reduce CVD.[46]

Some salt intake is essential. An Institute of Medicine Committee set 1.5 g sodium/day (65 mmol/day) as an adequate intake level to ensure nutrient adequacy.[47] Although lower sodium intake is associated with lower BP,[48] little information exists about the nutrient content of diets at such low levels of sodium intake. Because the relationship between sodium intake and BP is direct and progressive without an apparent threshold, it is difficult to set an upper level of sodium intake, which could also be 1.5 g (65 mmol) sodium/day. Practical considerations related to the current food supply prevent attainment of this level, which is less than the upper limit of 2.3 g/day (100 mmol/day) that has been previously recommended.[8,49]

In summary, available data strongly support current, population-wide recommendations to lower salt intake. Consumers should choose foods low in salt and should limit the amount of salt added to food. However, because more than 75% of consumed salt comes from processed foods,[50] any meaningful strategy to reduce salt intake must involve the efforts of food manufacturers and restaurants. Recent guidelines have recommended that these groups should progressively reduce the salt added to foods by 50% over the next 10 years.[8,51]

Increased Potassium Intake

High potassium intake is associated with lower BP. Available evidence includes animal studies, observational studies, clinical trials, and meta-analyses of these trials. Although data from individual trials have typically been inconsistent, three meta-analyses each documented a significant inverse relationship between potassium intake and BP in nonhypertensive and hypertensive individuals.[52-54] In one meta-analysis,[53] a net increase in urinary potassium excretion of 2 g/day (50 mmol/day) was associated with average systolic and diastolic BP reductions of 4.4 and 2.5 mm Hg in hypertensive patients and of 1.8 and 1.0 mm Hg in nonhypertensive persons. Increased potassium has beneficial effects on BP in the setting of low potassium intake (e.g., 1.3 to 1.4 g/day, or 35 to 40 mmol/day)[55] or much higher intake (e.g., 3.3 g/day, or 84 mmol/day).[56] Importantly, increased potassium intake reduces BP to a greater extent in blacks compared with whites,[53] and therefore it may be a valuable tool in efforts to reduce health disparities related to the prevalence of elevated BP and its complications.

Because high intake of potassium can be achieved through diet and because potassium contained in foods is also accompanied by a variety of other nutrients, the preferred strategy to increase potassium intake is to consume potassium-rich foods, such as fruits and vegetables. In the DASH trial, the two groups that increased fruit and vegetable consumption both lowered BP.[29,57] The DASH diet provides approximately 4.7 g/day (120 mmol/day) of potassium.[58] Another trial documented that increased fruit and vegetable intake lowers BP, but it did not specify the amount of potassium that was provided.[59]

Potassium and sodium interact, such that the effects of potassium on BP depend on the concurrent intake of salt and vice versa. Specifically, increased intake of potassium has greater BP-lowering effects in the setting of higher salt intake, and it has lesser BP effects when salt intake is already low. Conversely, the BP reduction from lower salt intake is greatest when potassium intake is also low. In one trial, high potassium intake (120 mmol/day) blunted the pressor response to increased salt intake in 24 nonhypertensive black men and to a lesser extent in 14 nonblacks (Fig. 17-5).[42] In a 2 by 2 factorial trial that tested the effects of reduced salt intake and increased potassium intake, alone or together, on BP in 212 hypertensive patients,[60] reduced sodium intake lowered BP to the same extent as increased potassium intake; however, the combination did not further lower BP. Overall, these data are consistent with subadditive effects of reduced salt intake and increased potassium intake on BP.

The dearth of dose-response studies precludes a firm recommendation for a specific level of potassium intake as a means to lower BP. However, an Institute of Medicine Committee set the recommended potassium intake level at 4.7 g/day (120 mmol/day).[47] This level is similar to the average total potassium intake in clinical trials,[53] the highest dose in the one available dose-response trial,[42] and the potassium content of the DASH diet.[57]

In the generally healthy population with normal kidney function, potassium intake from foods that is greater than 4.7 g/day (120 mmol/day) poses no risk because excess potassium is readily excreted. However, in individuals whose urinary potassium excretion is impaired, potassium intake less than 4.7 g/day (120 mmol/day) is appropriate because of adverse cardiac effects (arrhythmias) from hyperkalemia. Common drugs that impair potassium excretion are angiotensin-converting enzyme inhibitors, angiotensin receptor blockers, nonsteroidal anti-inflammatory drugs, and potassium-sparing diuretics. Medical conditions associated with impaired renal excretion of potassium include diabetes, chronic kidney disease, end-stage renal disease, severe heart failure, and adrenal insufficiency. Elderly individuals are also at increased risk of hyperkalemia. Available evidence is insufficient to identify the level of kidney function at which patients with chronic kidney disease are at risk for hyperkalemia from high dietary intake of potassium. However, an expert panel recommended that persons with stage 3 or 4 chronic kidney disease, that is, an estimated glomerular filtration rate of less than 60 mL/min/1.73 m², restrict their intake of potassium.[61]

Moderation of Alcohol Consumption

Observational and experimental studies have documented a direct, dose-response relationship between alcohol intake and BP, particularly as the intake of alcohol increases to more than two drinks/day.[62,63] This relationship has been shown to be independent of potential confounders such as age, obesity, and salt intake.[64] Although some studies have shown that the alcohol-BP relationship also extends into the light drinking range, that is, at or less than two drinks/day, this is the range in which alcohol may reduce the risk of coronary heart disease.

A meta-analysis of 15 randomized trials reported that decreased alcohol consumption (median reduction in self-reported alcohol intake of 76%; range, 16% to 100%) lowered systolic and diastolic BP by 3.3 and 2.0 mm Hg, respectively.[63] BP reductions were similar in nonhypertensive and hypertensive persons, and the relationship appeared dose dependent.

In aggregate, available evidence supports moderation of alcohol intake (among those who drink) as an effective strategy to lower BP. The prevailing consensus is that alcohol consumption should be limited to no more than two alcoholic drinks/day in men and to no more than one alcoholic drink/day in women and in lighter-weight persons. One drink is defined as 12 oz of regular beer, 5 oz of wine (12% alcohol), and 1.5 oz of 80 proof distilled spirits.

Dietary Patterns

Vegetarian Diets

Certain dietary patterns, particularly vegetarian diets, have been associated with low BP. In industrialized countries, where elevated BP is extremely commonplace, individuals who consume a vegetarian diet have markedly lower BP than nonvegetarians.[65,66] Some of the lowest BPs observed in industrialized countries have been documented in strict vegetarians

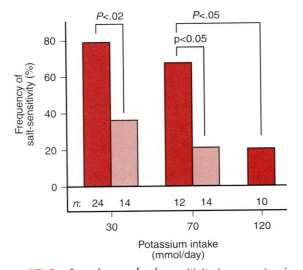

Figure 17–5 Prevalence of salt sensitivity in normotensive individuals (blacks, *red bars*; whites, *orange bars*) at three levels of potassium intake. Salt sensitivity is defined by a salt-induced increase in mean arterial pressure of at least 3 mm Hg. (From Morris RC Jr, Sebastian A, Forman A, et al. Normotensive salt sensitivity: Effects of race and dietary potassium. *Hypertension.* 1999;**33**:18-23.)

living in Massachusetts.[67] Vegetarians may also experience a lower age-related rise in BP.

Several aspects of a vegetarian lifestyle may affect BP. These lifestyle factors include nondietary lifestyle factors (e.g., physical activity), established dietary risk factors (e.g., salt, potassium, weight, alcohol), and other aspects of a vegetarian diet (e.g., high fiber, no meat). To a limited extent, observational studies have controlled for the well-established dietary determinants of BP. For instance, in a study of Seventh-Day Adventists, analyses were adjusted for weight but not for dietary salt or potassium intake.[66] In two clinical trials, one in nonhypertensive persons[68] and another in hypertensive patients,[69] lacto-ovovegetarian diets reduced systolic BP by approximately 5 mm Hg, but they had equivocal effects on diastolic BP.

DASH-Type Dietary Patterns

The DASH trial was a randomized feeding study that tested the effects of three diets on BP.[57] The most effective diet, now termed the DASH diet, emphasized fruits, vegetables, and low-fat dairy products; it included whole grains, poultry, fish, and nuts, and it was reduced in fats, red meat, sweets, and sugar-containing beverages. In terms of nutrients, it was rich in potassium, magnesium, calcium, and fiber, and it was reduced in total fat, saturated fat, and cholesterol; it was also slightly increased in protein.[58] Among all participants, the DASH diet significantly lowered systolic BP by a mean of 5.5 mm Hg and diastolic BP by 3.0 mm Hg, each net of control. The BP-lowering effects of the diets were rapid, occurring within only 2 weeks (Fig. 17-6).

In subgroup analyses, the DASH diet significantly lowered BP in all major subgroups (men, women, African Americans, non–African Americans, hypertensive patients, and non-

hypertensive persons).[70] However, the effects of the DASH diet in the African American participants were striking (systolic and diastolic BP reductions of 6.9 and 3.7 mm Hg, respectively) and were significantly greater than corresponding reductions in white participants (3.3 and 2.4 mm Hg). The effects in hypertensive individuals (systolic and diastolic BP reductions of 11.6 and 5.3 mm Hg, respectively) have obvious clinical significance. The corresponding effects in nonhypertensive individuals (3.5 and 2.2 mm Hg) have major public health importance (see Fig. 17-1). In a subsequent trial that enrolled a similar population,[29] the DASH diet significantly lowered BP at each of three sodium levels (see Fig. 17-4), and the combination of the DASH diet with sodium reduction resulted in the lowest level of BP. Most recently, in the OmniHeart trial, two DASH-style diets that partially replaced some carbohydrate with protein or monounsaturated fat further lowered BP.[58]

Speculation about the effective components of the DASH diet has been considerable. The diet that emphasized fruits and vegetables alone resulted in BP reductions that were approximately half of the total effect of the DASH diet (see Fig. 17-6). Fruits and vegetables are rich in potassium, magnesium, fiber, and many other nutrients. Of these nutrients, potassium is best established as a means to lower BP, particularly in hypertensive patients and in African Americans. In view of the additional BP reduction from the DASH diet beyond that of the fruits and vegetables diet, some other aspect of the DASH diet further lowered BP. Compared with the fruits and vegetables diet, the DASH diet had more vegetables, low-fat dairy products, and fish, and it was lower in red meat, sugar, and refined carbohydrates.

The DASH diet is safe and is broadly applicable to the general population. However, because of its relatively high potassium, phosphorus, and protein content, this diet is not recommended in persons with stage 3 or 4 chronic kidney disease (estimated glomerular filtration rate <60 mL/minute/1.73 m^2).[61]

DIETARY FACTORS WITH LIMITED OR UNCERTAIN EFFECTS

Fish Oil Supplementation

Several predominantly small trials and meta-analyses of these trials have documented that high-dose ω-3 polyunsaturated fatty acid (commonly termed *fish oil*) supplements can reduce BP in hypertensive individuals.[71-73] In nonhypertensive individuals, BP reductions tend to be small or nonsignificant. The effects appears to be dose dependent, with BP reductions occurring at relatively high doses of fish oil, namely, 3 g/day or more. In hypertensive individuals, average systolic and diastolic BP reductions were 4.0 and 2.5 mm Hg, respectively.[73] Side effects, including a fishy taste or smell and belching, are commonplace. In view of these side effects and the high dose required to lower BP, fish oil supplements cannot be routinely recommended as a therapy to lower BP.

Fiber

Fiber consists of the indigestible components of food from plants. Evidence from observational studies and several trials suggests that increased fiber intake may reduce BP.[74] More

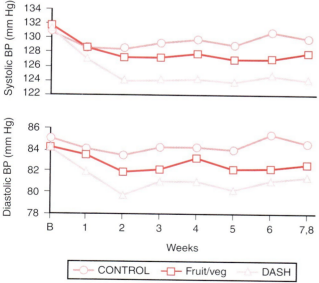

Figure 17–6 Blood pressure by week during the Dietary Approaches to Stop Hypertension (DASH) feeding study in three diets (control diet, fruits and vegetables diet, and the DASH diet. (Modified from Appel LJ, Moore TJ, Obarzanek E, et al. A clinical trial of the effects of dietary patterns on blood pressure: DASH Collaborative Research Group. *N Engl J Med.* 1997;**336**:1117-1124.)

than 40 trials of fiber supplementation have been conducted. Still, most did not have BP as their primary outcome, and many had a multicomponent intervention. In addition, differences in definition and classification of fiber have complicated interpretation of trial findings. A meta-analysis of available trials,[75] restricted to the 20 trials that increased just fiber intake, documented that supplemental fiber (average increase of 14 g/day) was associated with a net systolic BP reduction of 1.6 mm Hg and a diastolic BP reduction of 2.0 mm Hg. Subsequently, in a large randomized trial,[76] supplemental fiber did not significantly reduce BP. Overall, data are insufficient to recommend supplemental fiber or an increased intake of dietary fiber as a means to lower BP.

Calcium and Magnesium

Evidence that increased dietary calcium intake may lower BP comes from a variety of sources including animal studies, observational studies, trials, and meta-analyses. In a meta-analysis of 23 observational studies, Cappuccio and associates noted an inverse association between dietary calcium intake and BP.[77] However, the effect size was relatively small, and evidence indicated publication bias and heterogeneity across studies. Subsequently, meta-analyses of randomized trials documented modest reductions in systolic BP of 0.9 to 1.4 mm Hg and in diastolic BP of 0.2 to 0.8 mm Hg from calcium supplementation (400 to 2000 mg/day).[78-80] Some evidence indicates that the level of dietary calcium intake may affect the pressor response to salt. In three small trials, calcium supplementation mitigated the effects of a high sodium intake on BP.[81-83]

Evidence implicating magnesium as a major determinant of BP is inconsistent. In observational studies, often cross-sectional, a common finding is an inverse association between dietary magnesium and BP, a relationship shown in a pooled analysis of 29 observational studies.[84] However, in a meta-analysis of 20 randomized clinical trials, increased magnesium intake had no clear effect on BP.[85] Overall, evidence is insufficient to recommend either supplemental calcium or magnesium as a means to lower BP.

Intake of Fats Other than ω-3 Polyunsaturated Fatty Acids

Total fat includes saturated fat, ω-3 polyunsaturated fat, ω-6 polyunsaturated fat, and monounsaturated fat. Early studies focused on the effects of total fat intake on BP. However, there is a plausible biologic basis to hypothesize that certain types of fat could raise BP (e.g., saturated fat) and that other types of fat (e.g., ω-3 polyunsaturated fat) could lower it.

Saturated Fat

Several observational studies and a few trials have assessed the effects of saturated fat on BP. In most studies, including two prospective observational studies, the Nurses Health Study and the Health Professionals Follow-up Study, saturated fat intake was not associated with incident hypertension.[86,87] In the few available clinical trials, diet interventions that focused solely on reducing saturated fat had no effect on BP.[88] Because most trials tested diets that were simultaneously reduced in saturated fat and increased in polyunsaturated fat, the absence of a BP effect also suggests no benefit from polyunsaturated fat.

ω-6 Polyunsaturated Fat Intake

Dietary intake of ω-6 polyunsaturated fat (mainly linoleic acid in Western diets) has little or no effect on BP. In an overview of cross-sectional studies that correlated BP with tissue or blood levels of ω-6 polyunsaturated fat, no apparent relationship was noted.[88] Prospective observational studies and clinical trials have likewise been unsupportive.[86-88]

Monounsaturated Fat Intake

Few studies have assessed the effects of monounsaturated fatty acid intake on BP. Most (five of seven) cross-sectional studies did not detect a relationship,[88] and neither of two prospective studies conducted in the United States documented an effect of monounsaturated fat intake on incident hypertension.[86,87] Likewise, evidence from the earliest trials did not support a relationship between monounsaturated fat and BP.[88] However, subsequent trials have documented an inverse association between monounsaturated fat and BP,[89,90] as has one major observational study. In the OmniHeart trial, substitution of carbohydrate with monounsaturated fat lowered BP.[58] Overall, although increased monounsaturated fat may lower BP, this relationship is often confounded by a reduction in carbohydrate intake. Hence, the effects of monounsaturated fat intake are uncertain.

Cholesterol

Few studies have examined the BP effects of dietary cholesterol. In the observational analyses of the Multiple Risk Factor Intervention Trial, significant direct relationships were noted between cholesterol intake (mg/day) and both systolic and diastolic BP.[91] The Keys score was also associated with diastolic BP but not systolic BP. In longitudinal analyses from the Chicago Western Electric Study, investigators found significant positive relationships of change in systolic BP over 8 years with dietary cholesterol as well as the Keys score.[92] Still, despite these two reports, the paucity of evidence precludes any firm conclusion about a relationship between dietary cholesterol and BP.

Protein Intake

An extensive, and generally consistent, body of evidence from observational studies has documented inverse associations between BP and protein intake,[75,93] particularly protein from plants. Two major observational studies, the International Study on Macronutrients and Blood Pressure and the Chicago Western Electric Study, documented significant inverse relationships between protein intake and BP.[92,94] In these studies, protein from plant sources was associated with lower BP, whereas protein from animal sources had no significant effect.

In contrast to the large volume of evidence from observational studies, few trials have examined the effects of increased protein intake on BP. Two trials documented that increased protein intake from soy supplements, in comparison with carbohydrate supplements, can reduce BP. In one trial, supplemental soy protein (total of 25% kcal protein, 12.5% from soy) lowered average 24-hour systolic BP by 5.9 mm Hg and diastolic BP by 2.6 mm Hg in hypertensive individuals.[95] In a large trial conducted in the People's Republic of China, supplemental soy protein, which increased total protein intake from 12% to 16% kcal, lowered average systolic BP by 4.3 mm Hg and diastolic BP by 2.7 mm Hg, net of a control group that received supplemental carbohydrate.[96] In the OmniHeart trial,[58] partial substitution of carbohydrate with protein (about half from plant sources) lowered BP. In aggregate, data from clinical trials, in conjunction with evidence from observational studies, support the hypothesis that increased intake of protein from plants can lower BP.

Vitamin C

Laboratory studies, depletion-repletion studies, and observational studies suggest that increased vitamin C intake and higher vitamin C levels are associated with lower BP. In a systematic review by Ness and colleagues,[97] most cross-sectional studies reported an inverse association between plasma vitamin C levels and BP, and three of four trials reported an inverse association with vitamin C intake. The two non-randomized and four randomized trials were all small, and results were inconsistent; systolic BP reductions ranged from 0 to more than 10 mm Hg. In a subsequent trial, 500 mg/day of vitamin C had no effect on BP over the course of 5 years.[98] In summary, it remains unclear whether an increased intake of vitamin C affects BP.

GENE-DIET INTERACTIONS

A substantial and increasing body of evidence has documented that genetic factors affect BP levels and the BP response to dietary changes. Most of the available research has focused on genetic factors that influence the BP response to dietary salt intake. Several genotypes that affect BP have been identified, and most influence the renin-angiotensin-aldosterone axis or renal salt handling. In a line of research that has focused on mendelian diseases associated with either high or low BP, six genes associated with higher BP and eight genes associated with lower BP have been identified.[99] Of considerable importance is that each of these genes regulates renal salt-handling. Mutations that increase net sodium chloride reabsorption raise BP, whereas mutations that lower sodium chloride reabsorption reduce BP.

A few trials have examined the interactive effects of specific genotypes and the BP response to dietary changes. In three trials, genetic variation of the angiotensinogen gene modified the BP response to changes in salt intake in whites,[27,100,101] as well as the BP responses to weight change[100] and the DASH diet.[102] Polymorphism of the α-adducin gene also appears to affect the BP response to sodium chloride.[103] Finally, angiotensin-converting enzyme insertion-deletion polymorphism may also affect the BP response to weight change.[104]

EFFECTS OF MULTIPLE DIETARY CHANGES

Despite the potential for large BP reductions from simultaneously implementing multiple dietary changes, few trials

have examined the combined effects of multicomponent interventions. In general, multicomponent intervention trials have documented subadditivity, that is, the BP effect of interventions with two or more components is less than the sum of BP reductions from interventions that implement each component alone.[22,60] Despite subadditivity, the BP effects of multicomponent interventions are often large and clinically relevant. One small, but well-controlled, trial tested the effects of a comprehensive program of supervised exercise with provision of prepared meals to accomplish weight loss, sodium reduction, and the DASH diet; participants were medication-treated hypertensive adults. The program substantially lowered daytime ambulatory systolic and diastolic BP by 12.1 and 6.6 mm Hg, respectively, net of control.[105] Subsequently, a behavioral intervention trial, PREMIER, tested the effects of the major lifestyle recommendations (weight loss, sodium reduction, increased physical activity, and the DASH diet).[106] In nonhypertensive persons, mean systolic and diastolic BP reductions were 9.2 and 5.8 mm Hg, respectively (3.1 and 2.0 mm Hg, net of control). In hypertensive individuals, none of whom were taking medication, corresponding BP reductions were 14.2 and 7.4 mm Hg (6.3 and 3.6 mm Hg, net of control).

BEHAVIORAL INTERVENTIONS TO ACCOMPLISH LIFESTYLE MODIFICATIONS

Numerous behavioral intervention trials have tested the BP effects of dietary change. Several theories and models have informed the design of these trials, including social cognitive theory,[107] self-applied behavior modification techniques termed *behavioral self-management*,[108] the relapse prevention model,[109] and the transtheoretical, or stages-of-change model.[110] Application of these theories and models typically leads to a common intervention approach that emphasizes behavioral skills training, self-monitoring, self-regulation, and motivational interviewing.[111] Often, these studies enrolled motivated individuals, selected in part because their self-reported readiness to change. Further, these studies relied on skilled therapists, often health educators or dietitians. At least for weight loss trials, characteristic findings regarding successful behavior change over the short term, usually 6 months or less, with subsequent recidivism. The limited long-term success of these intensive intervention programs highlights the importance of environmental and policy changes that facilitate adoption of desirable lifestyle changes broadly across whole populations.

SPECIAL POPULATIONS

Children

The problem of elevated BP begins early in life, perhaps in utero.[112] Numerous observational studies have documented that BP tracks from childhood into adulthood.[113-115] Hence, efforts to reduce BP in children and to prevent the age-related rise in BP seem prudent, even if direct evidence from clinical trials is sparse. The importance of efforts to reduce BP in children is highlighted by evidence that BP levels and the prevalence of obesity in children and adolescents have both increased between the National Health and Nutrition Examination Survey conducted in 1988 to 1994 and that conducted in 1999 to 2000.[17]

The effects of dietary factors on BP in children were reviewed by Simons-Morton and Obarzanek.[116] Unfortunately, most studies had methodologic limitations, including small sample size, suboptimal BP measurements, and limited dietary contrast. At present, direct evidence from rigorous, well-controlled clinical trials in children and adolescents is sparse. Accordingly, the BP effects of diet in children and adolescents are extrapolated from studies conducted in adults. Such extrapolations are reasonable, because elevated BP is a chronic condition resulting from the insidious rise in BP throughout childhood and adulthood.

Older Persons

Dietary strategies should be especially beneficial as adults age. The age-related rise in BP is particularly prominent in middle-aged and older persons, and the incidence of BP-related CVD is especially high in older persons. Although most diet-BP trials were conducted in middle-aged persons, several were conducted in older individuals.[24,117,118] Other trials have presented results stratified by age. Several important findings emerge. First, evidence is remarkably consistent that older persons are able to make and sustain dietary changes, specifically dietary sodium reduction and weight loss.[24,25] Second, BP reduction from dietary interventions is greater in older persons in comparison with middle-aged individuals.[30,31] Third, because of high attributable risk associated with elevated BP in elderly persons, the beneficial effects of dietary changes on BP should substantial reduce CVD risk substantially.[119]

African Americans

In comparison with whites, African Americans have higher BP,[3] and they are at greater risk of BP-related complications, especially stroke and kidney disease.[5-7] As documented previously, in well-controlled efficacy trials, African Americans achieve greater BP reduction than whites from several non-pharmacologic therapies, specifically sodium reduction, increased potassium intake, and the DASH diet. The potential benefits of modifying these dietary factors is amplified because survey data indicate that African Americans tend to consume high levels of sodium, whereas their potassium intake is less than that of whites.[47] In this setting, the potential benefits of dietary change are substantial and should provide a means to reduce racial disparities in BP and the CV-renal complications of hypertension.[120]

HEALTH CARE PROVIDERS

The clinician's office can be a powerful setting to advocate and accomplish lifestyle change.[121] Through advice and by example, physicians can have a powerful influence on their patients' willingness to make lifestyle changes. Although behavioral counseling is usually beyond the scope of many office practices, simple assessments and provision of advice are typically feasible (e.g., measurement of body mass index).

The success of physician-directed, office-based attempts to achieve lifestyle changes depends on several factors including the skills of the physician and staff, available resources, organizational structure of the office, and the availability of algorithms that incorporate locally available resources.

Individualized, physician-directed efforts should be guided, in large part, by the patient's willingness to adopt lifestyle changes. Motivated patients should be referred to a skilled dietitian, health educator, or behavioral change program, because success will typically require frequent visits and contacts. Still, even without the assistance of ancillary personnel and programs, health care providers should routinely and unambiguously encourage lifestyle modification.

CONCLUSION

A compelling body of evidence supports the concept that multiple dietary factors affect BP. Dietary changes that effectively lower BP are weight loss, reduced salt intake, increased potassium intake, moderation of alcohol intake (among those who drink), and consumption of an overall healthy diet, termed the DASH diet. Other dietary factors may also affect BP, but the effects are small or the evidence is uncertain. For a summary of evidence, see Table 17-1.

In view of the increasing levels of BP in children and adults and the continuing epidemic of BP-related CVD and renal disease, efforts to reduce BP in both nonhypertensive and

Table 17-1 A Summary of the Evidence on the Effects of Dietary Factors and Dietary Patterns on Blood Pressure

	Hypothesized Effect	Evidence
Weight	Direct	++
Sodium chloride (salt)	Direct	++
Potassium	Inverse	++
Magnesium	Inverse	+/−
Calcium	Inverse	+/−
Alcohol	Direct	++
Fat		
Saturated fat	Direct	+/−
ω-3 Polyunsaturated fat	Inverse	++
ω-6 Polyunsaturated fat	Inverse	+/−
Monounsaturated fat	Inverse	+
Protein		
Total protein	Uncertain	+
Vegetable protein	Inverse	+
Animal protein	Uncertain	+/−
Carbohydrate	Uncertain	+
Fiber	Inverse	+
Cholesterol	Direct	+/−
Dietary patterns		
Vegetarian diets	Inverse	++
DASH-type dietary patterns	Inverse	++

+/−, limited or equivocal evidence; +, suggestive evidence, typically from observational studies and some clinical trials; ++, persuasive evidence, typically from clinical trials; DASH, Dietary Approaches to Stop Hypertension.
Modified from reference 12.

hypertensive individuals are warranted. Such efforts will require individuals to change behavior and society to make environmental changes that encourage such changes. The challenges to health care providers, researchers, government officials, and the general public are to develop and to implement effective clinical and public health strategies that lead to sustained dietary changes among individuals and more broadly among populations.

References

1. Kearney PM, Whelton M, Reynolds K, et al. Global burden of hypertension: Analysis of worldwide data. *Lancet*. 2005;**365**: 217-223.
2. Wang Y, Wang QJ. The prevalence of prehypertension and hypertension among US adults according to the new joint national committee guidelines: New challenges of the old problem. *Arch Intern Med*. 2004;**164**:2126-2134.
3. Fields LE, Burt VL, Cutler JA, et al. The burden of adult hypertension in the United States 1999 to 2000: A rising tide. *Hypertension*. 2004;**44**:398-404.
4. Hajjar I, Kotchen TA. Trends in prevalence, awareness, treatment, and control of hypertension in the United States, 1988-2000. *JAMA*. 2003;**290**:199-206.
5. Giles WH, Kittner SJ, Hebel JR, et al. Determinants of black-white differences in the risk of cerebral infarction. The National Health and Nutrition Examination Survey Epidemiologic Follow-up Study. *Arch Intern Med*. 1995;**155**:1319-1324.
6. Ayala C, Greenlund KJ, Croft JB, et al. Racial/ethnic disparities in mortality by stroke subtype in the United States, 1995-1998. *Am J Epidemiol*. 2001;**154**:1057-1063.
7. Klag MJ, Whelton PK, Randall BL, et al. Blood pressure and end-stage renal disease in men. *N Engl J Med*. 1996;**334**:13-18.
8. Chobanian AV, Bakris GL, Black HR, et al. Seventh report of the Joint National Committee on Prevention, Detection, Evaluation, and Treatment of High Blood Pressure. *Hypertension*. 2003;**42**:1206-1252.
9. Lewington S, Clarke R, Qizilbash N, et al., for the Prospective Studies Collaboration. Age-specific relevance of usual blood pressure to vascular mortality: A meta-analysis of individual data for one million adults in 61 prospective studies. *Lancet*. 2002;**360**:1903-1913.
10. Stamler J, Stamler R, Neaton JD. Blood pressure, systolic and diastolic, and cardiovascular risks: US population data. *Arch Intern Med*. 1993;**153**:598-615.
11. Vasan RS, Beiser A, Seshadri S, et al. Residual lifetime risk for developing hypertension in middle-aged women and men: The Framingham Heart Study. *JAMA*. 2002;**287**:1003-1010.
12. Appel LJ, Brands MW, Daniels SR, et al. Dietary approaches to prevent and treat hypertension. *Hypertension*. 2006;**47**:296-308.
13. Stamler R. Implications of the INTERSALT study. *Hypertension*. 1991;**17**:I16-20.
14. He J, Klag MJ, Whelton PK, et al. Migration, blood pressure pattern, and hypertension: The Yi Migrant Study. *Am J Epidemiol*. 1991;**134**:1085-1101.
15. INTERSALT Cooperative Research Group. INTERSALT: An international study of electrolyte excretion and blood pressure. Results for 24 hour urinary sodium and potassium excretion. *BMJ*. 1988;**297**:319-328.
16. Flegal KM, Carroll MD, Ogden CL, Johnson CL. Prevalence and trends in obesity among US adults, 1999-2000. *JAMA*. 2002;**288**:1723-1727.
17. Muntner P, He J, Cutler JA, et al. Trends in blood pressure among children and adolescents. *JAMA*. 2004;**291**:2107-2113.
18. Neter JE, Stam BE, Kok FJ, et al. Influence of weight reduction on blood pressure: A meta-analysis of randomized controlled trials. *Hypertension*. 2003;**42**:878-884.
19. Stevens VJ, Corrigan SA, Obarzanek E, et al. Weight loss intervention in phase 1 of the Trials of Hypertension Prevention: The TOHP Collaborative Research Group. *Arch Intern Med*. 1993;**153**:849-858.
20. Stevens VJ, Obarzanek E, Cook NR, et al. Long-term weight loss and changes in blood pressure: Results of the Trials of Hypertension Prevention, phase II. *Ann Intern Med*. 2001;**134**:1-11.
21. Huang Z, Willett WC, Manson JE, et al. Body weight, weight change, and risk for hypertension in women. *Ann Intern Med*. 1998;**128**:81-88.
22. Trials of Hypertension Prevention Collaborative Research Group. Effects of weight loss and sodium reduction intervention on blood pressure and hypertension incidence in overweight people with high-normal blood pressure: The Trials of Hypertension Prevention, phase II. *Arch Intern Med*. 1997;**157**:657-667.
23. Langford HG, Blaufox MD, Oberman A, et al. Dietary therapy slows the return of hypertension after stopping prolonged medication. *JAMA*. 1985;**253**:657-664.
24. Whelton PK, Appel LJ, Espeland MA, et al. Sodium reduction and weight loss in the treatment of hypertension in older persons: A randomized controlled trial of nonpharmacologic interventions in the elderly (TONE). TONE Collaborative Research Group. *JAMA*. 1998;**279**:839-846.
25. Knowler WC, Barrett-Connor E, Fowler SE, et al. Reduction in the incidence of type 2 diabetes with lifestyle intervention or metformin. *N Engl J Med*. 2002;**346**:393-403.
26. He FJ, MacGregor GA. Effect of modest salt reduction on blood pressure: A meta-analysis of randomized trials. Implications for public health. *J Hum Hypertens*. 2002;**16**: 761-770.
27. Johnson AG, Nguyen TV, Davis D. Blood pressure is linked to salt intake and modulated by the angiotensinogen gene in normotensive and hypertensive elderly subjects. *J Hypertens*. 2001;**19**:1053-1060.
28. MacGregor GA, Markandu ND, Sagnella GA, et al. Double-blind study of three sodium intakes and long-term effects of sodium restriction in essential hypertension. *Lancet*. 1989;**2**: 1244-1247.
29. Sacks FM, Svetkey LP, Vollmer WM, et al. Effects on blood pressure of reduced dietary sodium and the Dietary Approaches to Stop Hypertension (DASH) diet. DASH-sodium Collaborative Research Group. *N Engl J Med*. 2001;**344**:3-10.
30. Vollmer WM, Sacks FM, Ard J, et al. Effects of diet and sodium intake on blood pressure: Subgroup analysis of the DASH-sodium trial. *Ann Intern Med*. 2001;**135**:1019-1028.
31. Bray GA, Vollmer WM, Sacks FM, et al. A further subgroup analysis of the effects of the DASH diet and three dietary sodium levels on blood pressure: Results of the DASH-sodium trial. *Am J Cardiol*. 2004;**94**:222-227.
32. Weir MR, Hall PS, Behrens MT, Flack JM. Salt and blood pressure responses to calcium antagonism in hypertensive patients. *Hypertension*. 1997;**30**:422-427.
33. Appel LJ, Espeland MA, Easter L, et al. Effects of reduced sodium intake on hypertension control in older individuals: Results from the Trial of Nonpharmacologic Interventions in the Elderly (TONE). *Arch Intern Med*. 2001;**161**:685-693.
34. He J, Ogden LG, Vupputuri S, et al. Dietary sodium intake and subsequent risk of cardiovascular disease in overweight adults. *JAMA*. 1999;**282**:2027-2034.
35. Tuomilehto J, Jousilahti P, Rastenyte D, et al. Urinary sodium excretion and cardiovascular mortality in Finland: A prospective study. *Lancet*. 2001;**357**:848-851.
36. He J, Ogden LG, Bazzano LA, et al. Dietary sodium intake and incidence of congestive heart failure in overweight US men and women: First National Health and Nutrition Examination

Survey Epidemiologic Follow-up Study. *Arch Intern Med.* 2002;**162**:1619-1624.

37. Weinberger MH, Miller JZ, Luft FC, et al. Definitions and characteristics of sodium sensitivity and blood pressure resistance. *Hypertension.* 1986;**8**:II127-34.

38. Obarzanek E, Proschan MA, Vollmer WM, et al. Individual blood pressure responses to changes in salt intake: Results from the DASH-sodium trial. *Hypertension.* 2003;**42**:459-467.

39. He FJ, Markandu ND, MacGregor GA. Importance of the renin system for determining blood pressure fall with acute salt restriction in hypertensive and normotensive whites. *Hypertension.* 2001;**38**:321-325.

40. Johnson RJ, Herrera-Acosta J, Schreiner GF, Rodriguez-Iturbe B. Subtle acquired renal injury as a mechanism of salt-sensitive hypertension. *N Engl J Med.* 2002;**346**:913-923.

41. Luft FC, Rankin LI, Bloch R, et al. Cardiovascular and humoral responses to extremes of sodium intake in normal black and white men. *Circulation.* 1979;**60**:697-706.

42. Morris RC Jr, Sebastian A, Forman A, et al. Normotensive salt sensitivity: Effects of race and dietary potassium. *Hypertension.* 1999;**33**:18-23.

43. Schmieder RE, Messerli FH, Garavaglia GE, Nunez BD. Dietary salt intake: A determinant of cardiac involvement in essential hypertension. *Circulation.* 1988;**78**:951-956.

44. Jula AM, Karanko HM. Effects on left ventricular hypertrophy of long-term nonpharmacological treatment with sodium restriction in mild-to-moderate essential hypertension. *Circulation.* 1994;**89**:1023-1031.

45. Harsha DW, Sacks FM, Obarzanek E, et al. Effect of dietary sodium intake on blood lipids: Results from the DASH-sodium trial. *Hypertension.* 2004;**43**:393-398.

46. Psaty BM, Lumley T, Furberg CD, et al. Health outcomes associated with various antihypertensive therapies used as first-line agents: A network meta-analysis. *JAMA.* 2003;**289**:2534-2544.

47. Institute of Medicine. Dietary Reference Intakes: Water, Potassium, Sodium Chloride, and Sulfate. Washington, DC: National Academy Press, 2004.

48. Mancilha-Carvalho Jde J, Souza e Silva NA. The Yanomami Indians in the INTERSALT study. *Arq Bras Cardiol.* 2003;**80**:289-300.

49. Whelton PK, He J, Appel LJ, et al. Primary prevention of hypertension: Clinical and public health advisory from the National High Blood Pressure Education Program. *JAMA.* 2002;**288**:1882-1888.

50. Mattes RD, Donnelly D. Relative contributions of dietary sodium sources. *J Am Coll Nutr.* 1991;**10**:383-393.

51. Havas S, Roccella EJ, Lenfant C. Reducing the public health burden from elevated blood pressure levels in the United States by lowering intake of dietary sodium. *Am J Public Health.* 2004;**94**:19-22.

52. Cappuccio FP, MacGregor GA. Does potassium supplementation lower blood pressure? A meta-analysis of published trials. *J Hypertens.* 1991;**9**:465-473.

53. Whelton PK, He J, Cutler JA, et al. Effects of oral potassium on blood pressure: Meta-analysis of randomized controlled clinical trials. *JAMA.* 1997;**277**:1624-1632.

54. Geleijnse JM, Kok FJ, Grobbee DE. Blood pressure response to changes in sodium and potassium intake: A meta-regression analysis of randomised trials. *J Hum Hypertens.* 2003;**17**:471-480.

55. Brancati FL, Appel LJ, Seidler AJ, Whelton PK. Effect of potassium supplementation on blood pressure in African Americans on a low-potassium diet: A randomized, double-blind, placebo-controlled trial. *Arch Intern Med.* 1996;**156**:61-67.

56. Naismith DJ, Braschi A. The effect of low-dose potassium supplementation on blood pressure in apparently healthy volunteers. *Br J Nutr.* 2003;**90**:53-60.

57. Appel LJ, Moore TJ, Obarzanek E, et al. A clinical trial of the effects of dietary patterns on blood pressure: DASH Collaborative Research Group. *N Engl J Med.* 1997;**336**:1117-1124.

58. Appel LJ, Sacks FM, Carey VJ, et al. Effects of protein, monounsaturated fat, and carbohydrate intake on blood pressure and serum lipids. *JAMA.* 2005;**294**:2455-2464.

59. John JH, Ziebland S, Yudkin P, et al., Oxford Fruit and Vegetable Study Group. Effects of fruit and vegetable consumption on plasma antioxidant concentrations and blood pressure: A randomised controlled trial. *Lancet.* 2002;**359**:1969-1974.

60. Chalmers J, Morgan T, Doyle A, et al. Australian National Health and Medical Research Council dietary salt study in mild hypertension. *J Hypertens Suppl.* 1986;**4**:S629-S637.

61. National Kidney Foundation. K/DOQI clinical practice guidelines on hypertension and antihypertensive agents in chronic kidney disease. *Am J Kidney Dis.* 2004;**43 (Suppl 1)**:S1-S290.

62. Klatsky AL, Friedman GD, Siegelaub AB, Gerard MJ. Alcohol consumption and blood pressure: Kaiser-Permanente Multiphasic Health Examination data. *N Engl J Med.* 1977;**296**:1194-1200.

63. Xin X, He J, Frontini MG, et al. Effects of alcohol reduction on blood pressure: A meta-analysis of randomized controlled trials. *Hypertension.* 2001;**38**:1112-1117.

64. Okubo Y, Miyamoto T, Suwazono Y, et al. Alcohol consumption and blood pressure in Japanese men. *Alcohol.* 2001;**23**:149-156.

65. Sacks FM, Rosner B, Kass EH. Blood pressure in vegetarians. *Am J Epidemiol.* 1974;**100**:390-398.

66. Armstrong B, van Merwyk AJ, Coates H. Blood pressure in Seventh-Day Adventist vegetarians. *Am J Epidemiol.* 1977;**105**:444-449.

67. Sacks FM, Kass EH. Low blood pressure in vegetarians: Effects of specific foods and nutrients. *Am J Clin Nutr.* 1988;**48**:795-800.

68. Rouse IL, Beilin LJ, Armstrong BK, Vandongen R. Blood-pressure-lowering effect of a vegetarian diet: Controlled trial in normotensive subjects. *Lancet.* 1983;**1**:5-10.

69. Margetts BM, Beilin LJ, Vandongen R, Armstrong BK. Vegetarian diet in mild hypertension: A randomised controlled trial. *BMJ (Clin Res).* 1986;**293**:1468-1471.

70. Svetkey LP, Simons-Morton D, Vollmer WM, et al. Effects of dietary patterns on blood pressure: Subgroup analysis of the Dietary Approaches to Stop Hypertension (DASH) randomized clinical trial. *Arch Intern Med.* 1999;**159**:285-293.

71. Appel LJ, Miller ER 3rd, Seidler AJ, Whelton PK. Does supplementation of diet with 'fish oil' reduce blood pressure? A meta-analysis of controlled clinical trials. *Arch Intern Med.* 1993;**153**:1429-1438.

72. Morris MC, Sacks F, Rosner B. Does fish oil lower blood pressure? A meta-analysis of controlled trials. *Circulation.* 1993;**88**:523-533.

73. Geleijnse JM, Giltay EJ, Grobbee DE, et al. Blood pressure response to fish oil supplementation: Meta-regression analysis of randomized trials. *J Hypertens.* 2002;**20**:1493-1499.

74. Whelton SP, Hyre AD, Pedersen B, et al. Effect of dietary fiber intake on blood pressure: A meta-analysis of randomized, controlled clinical trials. *J Hypertens.* 2005;**23**:475-481.

75. He J, Whelton PK. Effect of dietary fiber and protein intake on blood pressure: A review of epidemiologic evidence. *Clin Exp Hypertens.* 1999;**21**:785-796.

76. He J, Streiffer RH, Muntner P, et al. Effect of dietary fiber intake on blood pressure: A randomized, double-blind, placebo-controlled trial. *J Hypertens.* 2004;**22**:73-80.

77. Cappuccio FP, Elliott P, Allender PS, et al. Epidemiologic association between dietary calcium intake and blood pressure: A meta-analysis of published data. *Am J Epidemiol.* 1995;**142**:935-945.

78. Allender PS, Cutler JA, Follmann D, et al. Dietary calcium and blood pressure: A meta-analysis of randomized clinical trials. *Ann Intern Med.* 1996;**124**:825-831.

79. Bucher HC, Cook RJ, Guyatt GH, et al. Effects of dietary calcium supplementation on blood pressure. A meta-analysis of randomized controlled trials. *JAMA.* 1996;**275**:1016-1022.

80. Griffith LE, Guyatt GH, Cook RJ, et al. The influence of dietary and nondietary calcium supplementation on blood pressure: An updated meta-analysis of randomized controlled trials. *Am J Hypertens.* 1999;**12**:84-92.

81. Zemel MB, Gualdoni SM, Sowers JR. Sodium excretion and plasma rennin activity in normotensive and hypertensive black adults as affected by dietary calcium and sodium. *J Hypertens.* 1986;**4**:343S-345S.

82. Saito K, Sano H, Furuta Y, Fukuzaki H. Effect of oral calcium on blood pressure response in salt-loaded borderline hypertensive patients. *Hypertension.* 1989;**13**:219-226.

83. Rich GM, McCullough M, Olmedo A, et al. Blood pressure and renal blood flow responses to dietary calcium and sodium intake in humans. *Am J Hypertens.* 1991;**4**:642S-645S.

84. Mizushima S, Cappuccio FP, Nichols R, Elliott P. Dietary magnesium intake and blood pressure: A qualitative overview of the observational studies. *J Hum Hypertens.* 1998;**12**:447-453.

85. Jee SH, Miller ER 3rd, Guallar E, et al. The effect of magnesium supplementation on blood pressure: A meta-analysis of randomized clinical trials. *Am J Hypertens.* 2002;**15**:691-696.

86. Ascherio A, Rimm EB, Giovannucci EL, et al. A prospective study of nutritional factors and hypertension among US men. *Circulation.* 1992;**86**:1475-1484.

87. Ascherio A, Hennekens C, Willett WC, et al. Prospective study of nutritional factors, blood pressure, and hypertension among US women. *Hypertension.* 1996;**27**:1065-1072.

88. Morris MC. Dietary fats and blood pressure. *J Cardiovasc Risk.* 1994;**1**:21-30.

89. Rasmussen OW, Thomsen C, Hansen KW, et al. Effects on blood pressure, glucose, and lipid levels of a high-monounsaturated fat diet compared with a high-carbohydrate diet in NIDDM subjects. *Diabetes Care.* 1993;**16**:1565-1571.

90. Ferrara LA, Raimondi AS, d'Episcopo L, et al. Olive oil and reduced need for antihypertensive medications. *Arch Intern Med.* 2000;**160**:837-842.

91. Stamler J, Caggiula A, Grandits GA, et al. Relationship to blood pressure of combinations of dietary macronutrients: Findings of the Multiple Risk Factor Intervention Trial (MRFIT). *Circulation.* 1996;**94**:2417-2423.

92. Stamler J, Liu K, Ruth KJ, et al. Eight-year blood pressure change in middle-aged men: Relationship to multiple nutrients. *Hypertension.* 2002;**39**:1000-1006.

93. Obarzanek E, Velletri PA, Cutler JA. Dietary protein and blood pressure. *JAMA.* 1996;**275**:1598-1603.

94. Elliott P, Stamler J, Dyer AR, et al. Association between protein intake and blood pressure: The INTERMAP study. *Arch Intern Med.* 2006;**166**:79-87.

95. Burke V, Hodgson JM, Beilin LJ, et al. Dietary protein and soluble fiber reduce ambulatory blood pressure in treated hypertensives. *Hypertension.* 2001;**38**:821-826.

96. He J, Gu D, Wu X, et al. Effect of soybean protein on blood pressure: A randomized, controlled trial. *Ann Intern Med.* 2005;**143**:1-9.

97. Ness AR, Chee D, Elliott P. Vitamin C and blood pressure: An overview. *J Hum Hypertens.* 1997;**11**:343-350.

98. Kim MK, Sasaki S, Sasazuki S, et al. Lack of long-term effect of vitamin C supplementation on blood pressure. *Hypertension.* 2002;**40**:797-803.

99. Lifton RP, Wilson FH, Choate KA, Geller DS. Salt and blood pressure: New insight from human genetic studies. *Cold Spring Harb Symp Quant Biol.* 2002;**67**:445-450.

100. Hunt SC, Cook NR, Oberman A, et al. Angiotensinogen genotype, sodium reduction, weight loss, and prevention of hypertension: Trials of Hypertension Prevention, phase II. *Hypertension.* 1998;**32**:393-401.

101. Hunt SC, Geleijnse JM, Wu LL, et al. Enhanced blood pressure response to mild sodium reduction in subjects with the 235T variant of the angiotensinogen gene. *Am J Hypertens.* 1999;**12**:460-466.

102. Svetkey LP, Moore TJ, Simons-Morton DG, et al. Angiotensinogen genotype and blood pressure response in the Dietary Approaches to Stop Hypertension (DASH) study. *J Hypertens.* 2001;**19**:1949-1956.

103. Grant FD, Romero JR, Jeunemaitre X, et al. Low-renin hypertension, altered sodium homeostasis, and an alpha-adducin polymorphism. *Hypertension.* 2002;**39**:191-196.

104. Kostis JB, Wilson AC, Hooper WC, et al. Association of angiotensin-converting enzyme DD genotype with blood pressure sensitivity to weight loss. *Am Heart J.* 2002;**144**:625-629.

105. Miller ER 3rd, Erlinger TP, Young DR, et al. Results of the Diet, Exercise, and Weight loss Intervention Trial (DEW-IT). *Hypertension.* 2002;**40**:612-618.

106. Appel LJ, Champagne CM, Harsha DW, et al. Effects of comprehensive lifestyle modification on blood pressure control: Main results of the PREMIER clinical trial. *JAMA.* 2003;**289**:2083-2093.

107. Bandura A. Social Foundations of Thought and Action: A Social Cognitive Theory. Englewood Cliffs, NJ: Prentice-Hall, 1986.

108. Watson DL, Tharp RG. Self-Directed Behavior: Self-Modification for Personal Adjustment, 5th ed. Pacific Grove, Calif: Brooks/Cole, 1989.

109. Marlatt GA, Gordon JR. Relapse Prevention: Maintenance Strategies in the Treatment of Addictive Behaviors. New York: Guilford Press, 1985.

110. Prochaska JO, DiClemente CC. Stages and processes of self-change of smoking: Toward an integrative model of change. *J Consult Clin Psychol.* 1983;**51**:390-395.

111. Miller WR, Rollnick S. Motivational Interviewing: Preparing People to Change Addictive Behavior. New York: Guilford Press, 1991.

112. Barker DJ, Osmond C, Golding J, et al. Growth in utero, blood pressure in childhood and adult life, and mortality from cardiovascular disease. *BMJ.* 1989;**298**:564-567.

113. Gillman MW, Cook NR, Rosner B, et al. Identifying children at high risk for the development of essential hypertension. *J Pediatr.* 1993;**122**:837-846.

114. Bao W, Threefoot SA, Srinivasan SR, Berenson GS. Essential hypertension predicted by tracking of elevated blood pressure from childhood to adulthood: The Bogalusa Heart Study. *Am J Hypertens.* 1995;**8**:657-665.

115. Dekkers JC, Snieder H, Van Den Oord EJ, Treiber FA. Moderators of blood pressure development from childhood to adulthood: A 10-year longitudinal study. *J Pediatr.* 2002;**141**:770-779.

116. Simons-Morton DG, Obarzanek E. Diet and blood pressure in children and adolescents. *Pediatr Nephrol.* 1997;**11**:244-249.

117. Applegate WB, Miller ST, Elam JT, et al. Nonpharmacologic intervention to reduce blood pressure in older patients with mild hypertension. *Arch Intern Med.* 1992;**152**:1162-1166.

118. Cappuccio FP, Markandu ND, Carney C, et al. Double-blind randomised trial of modest salt restriction in older people. *Lancet*. 1997;**350**:850-854.

119. Klag MJ, Whelton PK, Appel LJ. Effect of age on the efficacy of blood pressure treatment strategies. *Hypertension*. 1990;**16**:700-705.

120. Erlinger TP, Vollmer WM, Svetkey LP, Appel LJ. The potential impact of nonpharmacologic population-wide blood pressure reduction on coronary heart disease events: Pronounced benefits in African Americans and hypertensives. *Prev Med*. 2003;**37**:327-333.

121. Miller ER Jr, Erlinger TP, Young DR, et al. Lifestyle changes that reduce blood pressure: Implementation in clinical practice. *J Clin Hypertens (Greenwich)*. 1999;**1**:191-198.

Chapter 18

Diuretic Therapy in Cardiovascular Disease
Domenic A. Sica and Marvin Moser

Modern diuretic therapy evolved from two seemingly unrelated events in the 1930s: the development of sulfanilamide, the first truly effective antibacterial agent, and the characterization of the enzyme carbonic anhydrase. Sulfanilamide was observed to increase sodium (Na^+)/potassium (K^+), and water excretion by inhibiting carbonic anhydrase activity. Recognition of this action proved the impetus for synthesis of compounds, such as acetazolamide, that could inhibit carbonic anhydrase with greater specificity. However, acetazolamide was a short-acting compound, and diuretics with greater potency or duration of action were quickly sought. Chlorothiazide (CTZ) was the first of these new-generation diuretics, and its introduction in 1958 began the modern era of diuretic therapy.

Diuretics are tools of considerable therapeutic importance. First, they effectively reduce blood pressure (BP) while at the same time decreasing the morbidity and mortality from hypertension. Diuretics are currently recommended by the Joint National Committee on Prevention, Detection, Evaluation, and Treatment of Hypertension (JNC 7) as first-line therapy for the treatment of hypertension.[1] In addition, they remain an important component of heart failure (HF) therapy, in that they improve the symptoms of congestion, which typify the more advanced stages of HF. This chapter reviews the mode of action of the various diuretic classes and the physiologic adaptations that follow and sets up the basis for their use in the treatment of hypertension and volume-retaining states. In addition, side effects that are normally encountered during diuretic use are reviewed.

INDIVIDUAL CLASSES OF DIURETICS

The predominant sites of action in the nephron of various diuretic classes are depicted in Figure 18-1. Interclass and intraclass differences exist for all diuretic classes. The diuretic classes of note include carbonic anhydrase inhibitors, loop and distal tubular diuretics, and K^+-sparing agents (Table 18-1).[2]

Carbonic Anhydrase Inhibitors

Acetazolamide is the only carbonic anhydrase inhibitor with relevant diuretic effects. This agent is readily absorbed and undergoes renal elimination by tubular secretion. Its administration is ordinarily accompanied by a brisk alkaline diuresis. Although carbonic anhydrase inhibitors are proximal tubular diuretics (in which the bulk of Na^+ reabsorption occurs), their net diuretic effect is modest, because Na^+ reabsorption in more distal nephron segments offsets proximal Na^+ losses. Acetazolamide use is constrained by both its transient action and the development of metabolic acidosis during prolonged administration. Alternatively, acetazolamide (250 to 500 mg/day) can remedy the metabolic alkalosis that occasionally occurs with thiazide or loop diuretic therapy.

Loop Diuretics

Loop diuretics act predominantly at the apical membrane in the thick ascending limb of the loop of Henle, where they compete with chloride (Cl^-) for binding to the $Na^+/K^+/2Cl^-$ cotransporter, thereby inhibiting Na^+ and Cl^- reabsorption.[3] Loop diuretics also have effects on Na^+ reabsorption within other nephron segments that appear to be qualitatively minor compared with their action at the thick ascending limb. Other clinically important effects of loop diuretics include a decrease in both free water excretion and absorption during water loading and dehydration, respectively, about a 30% increase in fractional calcium (Ca^{2+}) excretion, a significant increase in magnesium (Mg^{2+}) excretion, and a transient increase followed by an ultimate decrease in uric acid excretion.

Loop diuretics can also enhance renal prostaglandin synthesis, particularly the vasodilatory prostaglandin E_2. Angiotensin II, generated following the administration of intravenous loop diuretics, coupled with an increased synthesis of prostaglandin E_2, is the probable reason for the finding that loop diuretics reallocate renal blood flow from the inner to the outer cortex of the kidney. Despite this redeployment of renal blood flow, both total renal blood flow and glomerular filtration rate (GFR) are maintained after loop diuretic administration to physiologically normal subjects.[4]

The available loop diuretics include bumetanide, ethacrynic acid, furosemide, and torsemide. These compounds are heavily protein bound (to albumin). Therefore, to gain access to the tubular lumen (site of action), they must undergo secretion (the same applies to thiazide-type diuretics), which in their case is by way of probenecid-sensitive organic anion transporters localized to the proximal tubule. Tubular secretion of loop diuretics may be slowed in the presence of elevated levels of endogenous organic acids, such as occurs in chronic kidney disease (CKD), and by drugs that share the same transporter, such as salicylates and nonsteroidal anti-inflammatory drugs (NSAIDs). Loop diuretic protein binding can also be decreased by uremic toxins and fatty acids, a change that presumably alters diuretic action but has been incompletely characterized.[5]

Diuretic excretion rates approximate drug delivery to the medullary thick ascending limb and correspond to the observed natriuretic response.[2,5] The relationship between urinary loop diuretic excretion rate and natriuretic effect is that of a sigmoidal curve (Fig. 18-2).[3,5] A normal dose-response relationship (as is typically seen in persons with untreated hypertension) can be adversely distorted (shifted downward and to the right) by a number of clinical conditions ranging from volume depletion (braking phenomenon)

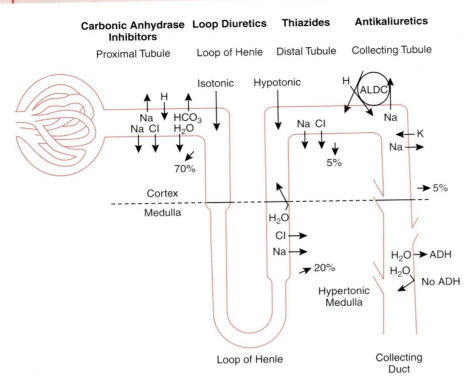

Figure 18–1 Schematic of the nephron illustrating the handling of water and electrolytes by the different segments and the major nephron sites of diuretic action. *Short arrows* represent the approximate percentage of sodium reabsorbed by the various nephron segments. ADH, antidiuretic hormone; ALDO, aldosterone; Cl, chloride; H, hydrogen; K, potassium; Na, sodium.

Table 18-1 Pharmacokinetics of Diuretics

Diuretic	Bioavailability (%)	Half-Life		
		Normal Subjects (hr)	Renal Failure (hr)	Heart Failure (hr)
Loop				
Furosemide	10-100	1.5-2	2.8	2.7
Bumetanide	80-100	1	1.6	1.3
Torsemide	80-100	3-4	4-5	6
Thiazide-type				
Bendroflumethiazide	ND	2-5	ND	ND
Chlorthalidone	64	24-55	ND	ND
Chlorothiazide	30-50	1.5	ND	ND
Hydrochlorothiazide	65-75	2.5	Increased	ND
Indapamide	93	15-25	ND	ND
Polythiazide	ND	26	ND	ND
Trichlormethiazide	ND	1-4	5-10	ND
Distal/Collecting Duct				
Amiloride	?	17-26	100	ND
Triamterene	>80	2-5	Prolonged	ND
Spironolactone	?	1.5	No change	ND
Eplerenone	?	4-6	No change	ND

ND, not determined.

to HF or nephrotic syndrome (disease-state alterations) to various drug therapies.[3,5,6] As an example of the last category, NSAIDs rework this relationship through inhibition of prostaglandin synthesis, with consequent blunting of the diuretic effect. Finally, although the diuretic dose-response relationship can deteriorate in the setting of nephrotic-range proteinuria, the binding of loop diuretics to urinary protein appears not to be involved.[7]

Furosemide is the most widely used diuretic in this class; however, its use is complicated by erratic absorption, with a bioavailability range of 12% to 112%.[8] The coefficient of variation for absorption varies from 25% to 43% for different furosemide products; thus, exchanging one furosemide formulation for another will not standardize the patient's absorption of (and thus response to) oral furosemide.[9] Bumetanide and especially torsemide are more predictably

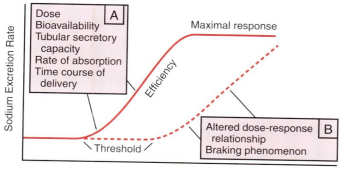

Figure 18–2   Pharmacokinetic (A) and pharmacodynamic (B) determinants of loop diuretic response. The broken line represents an altered dose-response relationship, as is observed in a typical diuretic resistant state. Diuretic delivery necessary to achieve a threshold response can vary substantially in the presence of diuretic resistance.

absorbed than furosemide. The consistency of torsemide's absorption and its longer duration of action are pharmacologic features to consider when loop diuretic therapy is called for in the patient with HF.[9,10] In the setting of long-term therapy of HF, torsemide-treated patients do not have as much fatigue and are less apt to be readmitted for decompensated HF than are patients who are treated with furosemide.[10]

The loop diuretics furosemide, bumetanide, and torsemide are commonly used in patients with CKD. The pharmacokinetic properties of loop diuretics are altered in CKD: renal clearance of these drugs is reduced in parallel with the level of change in renal function. In general, furosemide's pharmacokinetic properties are more significantly changed in CKD than are those of the other loop diuretics, because furosemide is a renally metabolized compound; therefore, both its intact renal clearance and renal metabolism are decreased in CKD.[11] Alternatively, bumetanide and torsemide undergo significant hepatic metabolism, and thus their pharmacokinetic profiles in CKD change only as a function of decreased renal clearance of the intact molecules (see Table 18-1).[11,12]

Thiazide Diuretics

The main site of action for thiazide-type diuretics is the early distal convoluted tubule, where the coupled reabsorption of Na^+ and Cl^- is inhibited (see Fig. 18-1). Besides effects on Na^+ excretion, thiazide diuretics also impair urinary diluting capacity (while preserving urinary concentrating mechanisms), reduce Ca^{2+} and uric acid excretion, and increase Mg^{2+} excretion. This last effect is particularly prominent with long-acting thiazide-type diuretics such as chlorthalidone.[13]

Hydrochlorothiazide (HCTZ) is the most widely used thiazide-type diuretic in the United States. Its absorption is dose proportional, with a bioavailability ranging from 60% to 80%. Its absorption can be reduced (rapidity and extent of absorption) in HF or CKD. The onset of diuresis with HCTZ is rapid (within 2 hours), peaking at 3 to 6 hours and sometimes continuing for as long as 12 hours with only a small fraction of the total natriuretic response occurring beyond 6 hours after administration. The diuretic effect of HCTZ can be extended by administering higher doses (50 to 200 mg)

than those currently used (12.5 to 25.0 mg). Alternatively, if a lengthier period of natriuresis is desired, one can consider a longer-acting thiazide-type diuretic, such as chlorthalidone or metolazone.[14]

The half-life of HCTZ (and other thiazide diuretics) is prolonged in patients with decompensated HF or CKD.[14] Large doses of HCTZ (100 to 200 mg/day) can induce diuresis in patients with CKD, a finding contrary to the belief that these drugs are ineffective in advanced stages of CKD.[15,16] However, the magnitude of the diuretic response in CKD has a specific ceiling controlled by two factors: first, the lowered GFR in CKD reduces the filtered load of Na^+; and second, the distal tubular site of thiazide diuretic action is one in which, even under the best of circumstances, only a modest natriuretic response occurs with a thiazide-type diuretic.[14-16]

Metolazone is a quinazoline diuretic with a chief site of action in the distal tubule and a minor inhibitory effect on proximal Na^+ reabsorption through a carbonic anhydrase–independent mechanism.[17] Metolazone is lipid soluble and has a wide volume of distribution, which plays a role in its prolonged duration of action. The pharmacokinetic features of metolazone are a factor in its effectiveness in the setting of either renal insufficiency or diuretic-resistant situations when it is combined with a loop diuretic.[5,18] Oral metolazone is absorbed slowly and fairly erratically, and this can confound the diagnosis of diuretic resistance in a volume-overloaded patient. *Diuretic resistance*, which is the failure to respond to a diuretic regimen, is usually taken to signify a worsening of the primary volume-retaining state, but with metolazone, it can simply be a consequence of failure to absorb the drug adequately.[5,18]

Distal Potassium-Sparing Diuretics

The two classes of K^+-sparing diuretics are competitive antagonists of aldosterone, such as spironolactone, and compounds that act independent of aldosterone, such as amiloride and triamterene. Drugs in this class inhibit active Na^+ absorption in the late distal tubule and the collecting duct. In so doing, basolateral Na^+,K^+-adenosine triphosphatase (ATPase) activity declines and intracellular K^+ concentration is reduced. The resultant decrease in the electrochemical gradient for both K^+ and hydrogen reduces secretion of these cations. K^+-sparing diuretics also reduce Ca^{2+} and Mg^{2+} excretion.[13] Because K^+-sparing diuretics are capable of only modest natriuresis, their clinical utility resides more in their K^+-sparing properties, especially when more proximally acting diuretics increase distal Na^+ delivery, or in states of hyperaldosteronism.

Spironolactone is highly protein bound and is a well-absorbed, lipid-soluble K^+-sparing diuretic with a 20-hour half-life. The onset of action for spironolactone is characteristically slow, with a peak response at times 48 hours or more after the first dose. 7α-Thiomethylspirolactone and canrenone are two metabolites of spironolactone that are responsible for much of its antimineralocorticoid activity.[19] Spironolactone remains active in states of reduced renal function because it gains access to its site of action independent of glomerular filtration; however, its propensity to cause hyperkalemia precludes its use in many patients with HF or CKD.[20]

Eplerenone is an aldosterone receptor antagonist with a molecular structure that affords selectivity for the aldosterone receptor; accordingly, its lesser affinity for androgen and progesterone receptors results in less gynecomastia than seen with spironolactone.[21] Typically, eplerenone is a very mild diuretic; thus, its antihypertensive effects originate from nondiuretic aspects of its action. Such actions result in a level of BP reduction comparable to that seen with drug classes such as angiotensin-converting enzyme (ACE) inhibitors and Ca^{2+} channel blockers (CCBs).[22,23] The use of eplerenone also results in regression of left ventricular hypertrophy (LVH) (either when it is given alone or when it is administered with an ACE inhibitor),[24] and it has a prominent antiproteinuric effect.[23] In patients with a recent history of acute myocardial infarction and left ventricular (LV) dysfunction or HF, eplerenone reduces morbidity and mortality when it is added to standard of care medical therapy.[21]

Amiloride is a K^+-sparing diuretic that is actively secreted by cationic transporters found in the proximal tubule. Amiloride blocks epithelial Na^+ channels in the luminal membrane of the collecting duct; only a modest natriuretic response can be expected with its use. Amiloride is extensively renally cleared and accumulates (with repetitive doses) in the setting of reduced renal function. If amiloride therapy is needed in patients with CKD (GFR <50 mL/minute), it is prudent either to reduce the dose or to decrease the dosing frequency to reduce the risk of hyperkalemia.

Triamterene, another K^+-sparing diuretic, works independently of a direct antagonism of aldosterone's effects. Triamterene is metabolized to an active phase II sulfate-conjugated metabolite. Both triamterene and its sulfated metabolite are cations and gain access to their intraluminal site of action by proximal tubular secretion. Triamterene and its metabolite accumulate after repetitive administration in CKD. In those unusual circumstances in which its use is considered necessary in CKD, empiric dosage adjustment is advisable because of the potential for hyperkalemia. Because of its weak BP-lowering properties, triamterene is seldom employed as monotherapy for hypertension. It is usually used in combination with a thiazide-type diuretic with the premise behind such a two-diuretic combination being that triamterene reduces the K^+ and Mg^{2+} losses that may accompany thiazide therapy.[25] Triamterene, given together with an NSAID, has been reported to cause acute renal failure, which may last for several days.[26] The mechanism behind this effect is unclear, but it may relate to triamterene's increasing renal vascular resistance (and as much as a 30% decrease in renal blood flow); correspondingly, there is an increase in the urinary excretion of the vasodilator prostaglandins E_2 and $F_{2\alpha}$.[25] The decrease in prostaglandin production that follows NSAID therapy would allow for an exaggerated renal vasoconstrictor effect from triamterene.

ADAPTATION TO DIURETIC THERAPY

Diuretic-induced inhibition of Na^+ reabsorption in one nephron segment elicits important adaptations in other nephron segments. This process not only limits diuretics' antihypertensive and fluid-depleting actions but also contributes to side effects. Although a portion of this resistance to diuretic effect is an expected consequence of the use of these agents, profound diuretic resistance from such adaptations can be encountered in patients with clinical disorders such as HF, cirrhosis, and proteinuric CKD. An understanding of how adaptation to diuretic therapy occurs is essential if the negative features of this process are to be minimized.

The initial dose of a diuretic ordinarily produces brisk diuresis and in most cases ends with a net negative Na^+ balance. The new equilibrium state established is one in which body weight decreases and stabilizes, because adaptive processes intervene and preclude a continued volume loss. In nonedematous patients who are given either a thiazide or a loop diuretic, this adaptation or *braking phenomenon* occurs within a matter of days and limits weight loss to 1 to 2 kg[6]; this finding has been convincingly demonstrated in physiologically normal subjects given the loop diuretics furosemide or bumetanide.[26,27] Furosemide administered to subjects ingesting a high-Na^+ diet (270 mmol/24 hours) produces brisk natriuresis, which results in a negative Na^+ balance for the following 6 hours. This is followed by an 18-hour period in which Na^+ excretion is reduced to a level considerably lower than that of intake. This postdiuresis Na^+ retention corrects for initial Na^+ losses, and the result is no net weight loss. In fact, this same pattern of Na^+ loss and compensatory retention persists for as long as a month after furosemide administration.[4] Na^+ intake, before and after diuretic administration, influences the end effect of the braking phenomenon. For example, if Na^+ intake is kept low, Na^+ balance will remain negative in the hours after the initial natriuresis, with a fall in net body weight.

The pathophysiology of the braking phenomenon is complex. In part, the relationship between natriuresis and the rate of loop diuretic excretion depends on the level of Na^+ intake. In subjects on a low-Na^+ diet, the diuretic response curve is typically shifted to the right, which is indicative of a blunting of the tubular responsiveness to the diuretic (see Fig. 18-2).[26,27] A reduction in extracellular fluid (ECF) volume is an important factor in the genesis of postdiuretic Na^+ retention. Using lithium (Li^+) clearance as a marker of proximal Na^+ handling in the postdiuretic period, overall Na^+ retention can be ascribed to an increase in both proximal and distal tubular Na^+ absorption. It has been suggested that this heightened Na^+ reabsorption may be on the basis of α-stimulation and activation of the renin-angiotensin-aldosterone system (RAAS); however, administration of α-adrenergic antagonists and blockers of the RAAS do not seem to modify the *braking phenomenon* meaningfully.[26-28] A volume-independent component to the process has also been suggested; this may be structural.[4,29,30] Structural hypertrophy in the distal nephron has been demonstrated in rats receiving prolonged infusions of loop diuretics. These structural changes are associated with enhanced rates of distal nephron Na^+ and Cl^- absorption and increased secretion of K^+, a sequence that is independent of aldosterone. These nephron adaptations may contribute to postdiuretic Na^+ retention and to diuretic tolerance in humans and may possibly explain the Na^+ retention occurring up to 2 weeks after discontinuation of diuretic therapy.[4,31]

NEUROHUMORAL RESPONSE TO DIURETICS

Neurohumoral activation by diuretics remains an important consideration in the sustained effectiveness of diuretic therapy in hypertension and HF. The neurohumoral response to a diuretic depends on both its route of administration and the level of drug exposure. Intravenous loop diuretics have an immediate (within minutes) stimulatory effect on the RAAS at the macula densa that is independent of volume depletion or sympathetic nervous system (SNS) activation. This first wave of neurohumoral effects with an intravenous loop diuretic is short-lived but can be of sufficient magnitude to increase afterload and decrease renal blood flow in a dose-dependent fashion. This may diminish the effectiveness of a diuretic for a short time. This sequence of events may provide an explanation for the observation that certain diuretic-treated patients fail to respond to bolus diuretic therapy yet have quite effective diuresis after a loop diuretic infusion.[32] A second-phase response is initiated within 15 minutes of intravenous loop diuretic administration, and it results from an increase in the renal production of prostaglandins. This second response offers a probable explanation for the reduction in preload and ventricular filling pressures that takes place shortly after intravenous loop diuretic administration.[33] The next stage of neurohumoral activation occurs with excess volume removal, and it can occur with either intravenous or oral diuretics. Volume removal can chronically activate the RAAS and increase circulating concentrations of both angiotensin II and aldosterone, which, in turn, can promote Na^+ absorption in proximal and distal tubular locations, respectively. The role of aldosterone excess in electrolyte depletion or persistent hypertension in a diuretic-treated patient is widely underappreciated. In this regard, low-dose spironolactone provides significant additive BP reduction in diuretic-treated patients with resistant hypertension.[34]

DIURETICS IN HYPERTENSION

Hypertension (BP ≥140/90 mm Hg) and the newly defined prehypertension state (BP 120 to 139/80 to 89 mm Hg) are widely prevalent in the United States.[1,35] Worldwide prevalence estimates for hypertension may be as great as 1 billion individuals. Approximately 7.1 million deaths per year may be attributable to hypertension. Cardiac and cerebrovascular events, renal failure progression, and all-cause mortality each increase in a continuous fashion with rising diastolic or systolic BP. The beneficial effects of BP-lowering treatments on the risks of major cardiovascular disease (CVD) and renal events are indisputable. What has been questioned is the comparative effects of regimens based on different initial drug classes or regimens targeting different BP goals. In an analysis undertaken by the Blood Pressure Lowering Treatment Trialists' Collaboration, no significant differences were noted in total major CVD events when regimens based on an initial ACE inhibitor, a CCB, or a diuretic or β-blocker were compared.[36]

The results of such analyses tend to shift the argument from which is the preferred first-line drug in the treatment of hypertension to which compound (or combination of drugs) is most cost-effective. In this regard, diuretic therapy as first-step treatment (or as a component of multidrug therapy) has an established and widely accepted position. All the earlier JNC documents (dating to 1977) and the most recent JNC 7 guidelines have advanced a position favoring the early use of diuretic therapy in the management of hypertension in a stepped-care approach to BP reduction.[1]

Mechanism of Action

Thiazide-type diuretics have been employed in the treatment of hypertension since the 1950s. Despite the enormous experience with these compounds, some questions remain concerning their use. Of the uncertainties concerning thiazide-type diuretics, three are particularly relevant. To what degree is a persistent reduction in ECF volume a prerequisite for continuous BP reduction with these compounds? Do thiazide-type diuretics provide better BP reduction than loop diuretics? Are all thiazide-type diuretics the same in their BP-reducing effect (i.e., is there a class effect)?

Some evidence indicates that a thiazide diuretic is more effective over the long term in lowering BP than a short-acting loop diuretic.[37] However, the exact means by which a thiazide-type diuretic lowers BP is unclear.[38] The effect of a thiazide diuretic on BP may be divided into three sequential phases: acute, subacute, and chronic, which correspond to periods of about 1 to 2 weeks, several weeks, and several months, respectively (Fig. 18-3).[39] In the acute-response phase, the BP-lowering effect of a diuretic is coupled to a reduction in ECF volume and a corresponding fall in cardiac output. The early response (first 2 to 4 days of treatment) to a thiazide-type diuretic, in the setting of a no-salt-added diet (100 to 150 mmol/day), results in a net Na^+ loss of 100 to 300 mmol, which translates into a 1 to 2 L decrease in ECF volume. Plasma Na^+ concentrations are unchanged in the process.

Direct measurements of ECF volume in the *acute*-response phase in hypertensive patients who are treated with thiazide diuretics show an approximate 12% decrease. A similar reduction is noted in plasma volume, a finding suggesting that this acute volume loss arises proportionally from both the plasma and interstitial compartments. This decrease in plasma volume reduces venous return and diminishes cardiac output, the basis for the initial BP decrease with a thiazide diuretic. This change in plasma volume can stimulate both the SNS and the RAAS.[39]

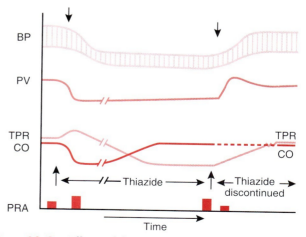

Figure 18–3 Effects of thiazide administration in an "idealized" patient. BP, blood pressure; CO, cardiac output; PRA, plasma renin activity; PV, plasma volume; TPR, total peripheral resistance.

In due course, the thiazide diuretic's effects on volume and cardiac output lessen in importance, although BP remains lowered. During the *subacute* phase of a treatment response (first few weeks), plasma volume returns to slightly less than pretreatment levels, despite the continued administration of a diuretic. The subacute-response phase with thiazide-type diuretics is a transitional period during which both volume and resistance factors contribute to the BP reduction.[40]

Blood Pressure Reduction: Chronic Phase of Therapy

In the *chronic*-response phase of therapy, the vasodepressor influence of a diuretic develops into a process mechanistically driven by a reduction in total peripheral resistance (TPR). No simple explanation exists for the drop in TPR that accompanies long-term diuretic use. The decrease in TPR during prolonged therapy has been attributed to several factors including changes in the ionic content of vascular smooth muscle cells, altered ion gradients across smooth muscle cells or K^+ channel activation, and changes in membrane-bound ATPase activity.[38] The ability of thiazide-type diuretics to reduce BP seems to be linked to the presence of functioning renal tissue; thus, these drugs do not reduce BP in patients undergoing maintenance hemodialysis.[41]

A mechanistic understanding of both the diuretic action and the countervailing forces triggered by diuresis provides a well-reasoned approach to the treatment of hypertension. The early action of diuretics to reduce ECF volume is optimized if dietary Na^+ is restricted at the start of therapy. This limits the repercussions of the braking phenomenon, which is an inevitable occurrence with uninterrupted diuretic use.[5] Some limitation in dietary Na^+ intake may also be germane to how diuretics reduce TPR on a long-term basis. It is believed that intracellular Na^+/Ca^{2+} in vascular smooth muscle cells are favorably adjusted, with the acute volume contraction observed during the first several days of thiazide diuretic therapy. How the development of volume contraction specifically translates into a reduction in TPR remains uncertain.[38,39] Whatever the mechanism, it can be quite long-lived, because a residual BP reduction can be seen several weeks after the withdrawal of thiazide diuretics (even without interposing nonpharmacologic treatments for maintenance of BP control).[42] This residual BP-reducing effect with cessation of thiazide-type diuretics has not been carefully compared with that observed with nondiuretic antihypertensive drug classes.

Another consideration in chronic BP reduction with a diuretic relates to the duration of a natriuretic response. For example, when long-term responses to HCTZ and furosemide are compared in hypertensive patients, diastolic and especially systolic BP decreases more consistently with HCTZ.[43] This difference in effect has been ascribed to vascular adaptations associated with the more gradual and relatively more prolonged thiazide-related diuresis. In the end, during the acute phase of response, a thiazide diuretic may be able to maintain a nominal state of volume contraction more effectively than a loop diuretic.[5] It is thought that this pattern of volume removal lends itself to a greater downward shift in TPR with a thiazide-type diuretic. A direct vasodilator effect of HCTZ had been postulated, but when tested the effect was quite small and occurred only at high local concentrations experimentally obtained by infusion into the human forearm.[44]

Diuretic Class Effect

The concept of class effect has been applied to both loop diuretics and thiazide-type diuretics in respect to the management of hypertension. The loop diuretic effect on BP is a function of at least two processes: first, the manner in which volume removal is effected, and second, the capacity of these compounds to decrease TPR independently. Small doses of the long-acting loop diuretic, torsemide, may cause significant BP reduction in patients with essential hypertension, a process independent of diuresis and not demonstrable with subdiuretic doses of furosemide. Intra-arterially infused furosemide does not directly dilate human forearm arterial vessels even at supratherapeutic concentrations.[45] In bioequivalent doses, however, furosemide is just as effective as torsemide in reducing 24-hour ambulatory BP in patients with stage II to III CKD.[46] Until comparison studies of loop diuretics are conducted in diverse populations, it is premature to presume that these compounds are distinguishable (independent of volume removal) in their BP-reducing ability.

The idea of *class effect* for thiazide-type diuretics is still promulgated by some investigators, but it has minimal experimental support.[2] Much of the recent debate on thiazide-type diuretic class effect has centered on the similarities and differences between chlorthalidone and HCTZ.[47] The concept of class effect with thiazide-type diuretics should be considered in two ways: effect on BP fall and event-rate reduction. These two compounds are fundamentally different diuretics, in that chlorthalidone has a considerably longer duration of diuretic action than HCTZ. This does not mean, however, that chlorthalidone is a superior antihypertensive compound. It is likely that the longer duration of diuretic action with chlorthalidone makes it a stronger antihypertensive compound, milligram to milligram, than HCTZ. The exact dose equivalence between these two compounds is a matter of some debate and one that is not easily resolved. Regarding outcomes, chlorthalidone has been used in several of the major clinical trials in the United States and has had a more consistent pattern of favorable outcomes than is the case with HCTZ.[47-49] Although it is tempting to assume that chlorthalidone is a better outcomes drug, at present this can only be viewed as an assumption.

Diuretics in Clinical Trials

By the mid 1990s, evidence of the effects of BP-lowering regimens—mainly based on diuretics and β-blockers—was available from a series of randomized placebo-controlled clinical trials involving more than 47,000 hypertensive patients.[50-52] Systematic overviews and meta-analyses of these trials reported that reductions in BP of about 10 to 12 mm Hg systolic and 5 to 6 mm Hg diastolic provided relative risk reductions for stroke and coronary heart disease (CHD) of 38% and 16%, respectively, within just a few years of beginning therapy.[50-52] The size of these effects was similar in major subgroups of patients. The few studies that directly compared diuretics and β-blockers detected no overall obvious differences in the risk of either stroke or CHD; however, differences between these two therapies were detected in specific patient groups. For example, in the Medical Research Council trial in the elderly (MRC-2) and in an overview of treatment outcomes in elderly patients, first-line diuretic therapy was superior to β-blockade in preventing cerebrovascular events, fatal stroke, CHD, CVD mortality, and all-cause mortality. In contrast, β-blocker therapy reduced only the risk for cerebrovascular events and was ineffective in preventing CHD, CVD and all-cause mortality.[53]

After 1993, numerous comparative studies of BP-lowering drugs were undertaken. Most of these trials were designed to detect large disparities in relative risk and had insufficient power to identify small to moderate differences among the studied regimens. To maximize the information acquired by these and future trials, a collaborative program of prospectively designed overviews was developed. The first of these overviews became available in 2000, and the second was published in 2003.[36] This important article and other more recent overviews of trials in hypertensive patients comparing ACE inhibitor–based regimens with diuretic or β-blocker–based regimens reported that the endpoint benefits of ACE inhibitors were not significantly better than those provided by diuretics or β-blockers (Fig. 18-4).[36] The overview of trials comparing CCB therapy with diuretic- or β-blocker–based regimens suggests some difference in the effects of the two regimens on cause-specific outcomes, with the risk for stroke slightly less with CCBs than with diuretics (Fig. 18-5). The risk of HF, however, is very significantly higher with a CCB-based regimen.[36] No significant difference was noted between treatment effects of CCB regimens when dihydropyridine or nondihydropyridine CCBs were compared with diuretic/β-blocker regimens.

The largest single trial that provides information about diuretic therapy and outcomes is the Antihypertensive and Lipid-Lowering Treatment to Prevent Heart Attack Trial (ALLHAT).[49,54] A total of 42,448 participants aged 55 years or older (35% African Americans) with hypertension and at least one other CHD risk factor were enrolled in ALLHAT. ALLHAT originally was designed to study ACE inhibition (lisinopril), CCB treatment (amlodipine), and peripheral α-antagonism (doxazosin) compared with therapy with the diuretic (chlorthalidone), with a composite primary outcome of fatal CHD or nonfatal myocardial infarction. The doxazosin arm of the trial was terminated early because of an increased risk of combined CVD (of which HF was a major component) when compared with chlorthalidone.[54]

In ALLHAT, no significant difference was observed between chlorthalidone and either amlodipine or lisinopril in the primary outcome; however, other outcomes showed a greater reduction in total major CVD events with the diuretic. Both stroke and HF were more frequent with lisinopril and HF events were more common with the CCB than with chlorthalidone.[49,54] This difference in event rates in the ACE inhibitor/diuretic comparison was in large measure attributable to outcomes in the African-American subgroup, perhaps related to the smaller BP reduction in that subgroup with the ACE inhibitor–based regimen. This difference in BP control (between primary drug classes) was not unexpected based on study design considerations.

Responsive Patient Populations

When used alone in the nonedematous patient, thiazide diuretics are as effective as most other antihypertensive drug classes, independent of body mass index.[55] Although it is erroneous to offer universal recommendations about anti-hypertensive care on the basis of race, age, or gender, this is still done routinely. In general, African American, elderly, and female hypertensive patients typically respond better to diuretics than do other patients.[56] The same can be said for other salt-sensitive forms of hypertension, such as the hypertension seen with diabetes. However, the basis for the interindividual variability in response to a thiazide diuretic continues to go unexplained, despite the predictability of responses in the foregoing patient groups (black race, old age, and female gender).[56]

Elderly Patients

Certain studies utilizing diuretic-based regimens have been specifically conducted in elderly hypertensive patients (age >60 years): the Systolic Hypertension in the Elderly Program (SHEP), the Swedish Trial in Old Patients (STOP), MRC-2, the European Working Party on High Blood Pressure in the Elderly, and the trial of Coope and Warrender.[57] Significant reductions in stroke similar to those observed in younger patients and greater benefits in terms of protection from myocardial infarction have been demonstrated in these older patients.[58]

Four clinical trials, with a total of almost 35,000 patients, compared diuretics with β-blockers: the International Prospective Primary Prevention Study in Hypertension, the Heart Attack Primary Prevention in Hypertension Research Group, MRC, and MRC-2. In most of these comparative trials, β-blocker therapy was comparable to, but not better than, diuretic therapy with regard to the incidence of stroke, although this observation has been disputed.[58] Findings were mixed with regard to myocardial infarction; two studies favored either a diuretic or a β-blocker over the other. Differences between these classes were quite small, however.

The SHEP, STOP, and MRC-2 trials each found significant reductions in cardiac and cerebrovascular morbidity and mortality associated with diuretic and β-blocker therapy, although the MRC elderly trial reported a significantly better reduction in CHD events with a diuretic compared with a β-blocker. To highlight one of these trials, the SHEP trial was a double-blind, placebo-controlled trial involving 4736 men and women with isolated systolic hypertension who were older than 60 years of age. Patients were randomized to receive a low dose of the diuretic chlorthalidone (12.5 to 25 mg/day) as initial therapy; a β-blocker (atenolol, 25 to 50 mg/day) or reserpine (0.05 to 0.10 mg/day) was then added as needed to reach goal BP (systolic BP <160 or a ≥20 mm Hg decrease in systolic BP).

At the end of the 5-year follow-up period, 46% of the subjects had adequate BP control using only a low dose of chlorthalidone, and BP was equally well controlled irrespective of the serum creatinine level (range, 35 to 212 μmol/L) (Fig. 18-6).[59] Another 23% of patients had their hypertension controlled with the addition of a β-blocker. Outcomes included a statistically significant 36% reduction in stroke and a 27% reduction in CHD, as well as a trend for reduction in all-cause mortality (13%). These benefits were less pronounced in patients with hypokalemia (serum K+ <3.5 mEq/L) in the chlorthalidone-treated group, but they were still better than in the placebo-treated group.[60]

Results of these trials clearly establish the benefit of low-dose diuretics or β-blockers for the treatment of isolated

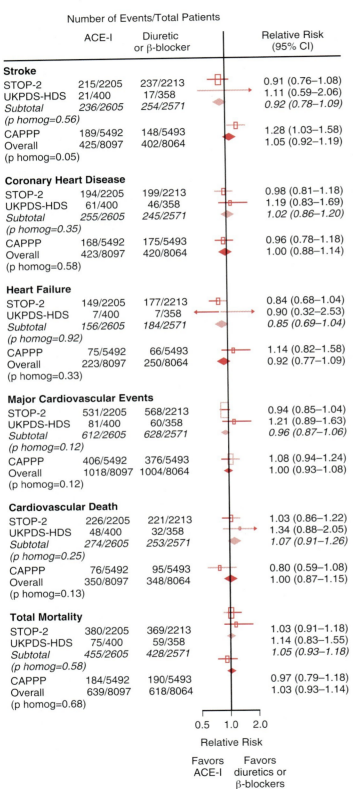

Number of Events/Total Patients

Figure 18–4 Comparisons of angiotensin-converting enzyme inhibitor–based therapy with diuretic-based or β-blocker–based therapy. ACE I, ACE inhibitor; CAPPP, Captopril Prevention Project; CI, confidence interval; p homog, P value from a χ² test for homogeneity; STOP-2, second Swedish Trial in Old Patients; UKPDS-HDS, United Kingdom Prospective Diabetes Study–Hypertension and Diabetes Study. (From Neal B, MacMahon S, Chapman N, Blood Pressure Lowering Treatment Trialists' Collaboration. Effects of ACE inhibitors, calcium antagonists, and other blood-pressure-lowering drugs: Results of prospectively designed overviews of randomised trials. Blood Pressure Lowering Treatment Trialists' Collaboration. *Lancet.* 2000;**356**:1955-1964.)

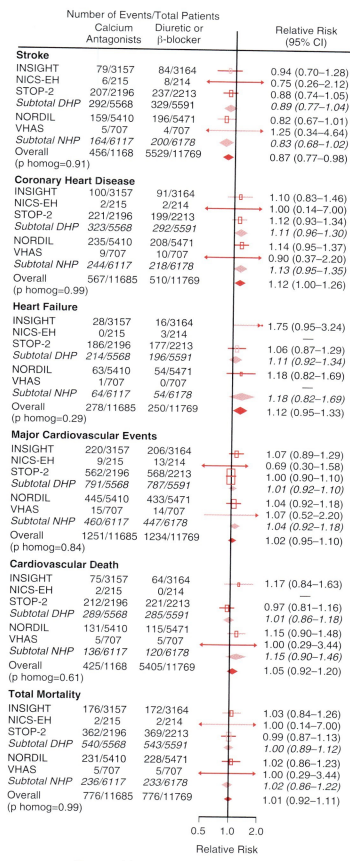

	Number of Events/Total Patients		Relative Risk (95% CI)
	Calcium Antagonists	Diuretic or β-blocker	
Stroke			
INSIGHT	79/3157	84/3164	0.94 (0.70–1.28)
NICS-EH	6/215	8/214	0.75 (0.26–2.12)
STOP-2	207/2196	237/2213	0.88 (0.74–1.05)
Subtotal DHP	*292/5568*	*329/5591*	*0.89 (0.77–1.04)*
NORDIL	159/5410	196/5471	0.82 (0.67–1.01)
VHAS	5/707	4/707	1.25 (0.34–4.64)
Subtotal NHP	*164/6117*	*200/6178*	*0.83 (0.68–1.02)*
Overall (p homog=0.91)	456/1168	5529/11769	0.87 (0.77–0.98)
Coronary Heart Disease			
INSIGHT	100/3157	91/3164	1.10 (0.83–1.46)
NICS-EH	2/215	2/214	1.00 (0.14–7.00)
STOP-2	221/2196	199/2213	1.12 (0.93–1.34)
Subtotal DHP	*323/5568*	*292/5591*	*1.11 (0.96–1.30)*
NORDIL	235/5410	208/5471	1.14 (0.95–1.37)
VHAS	9/707	10/707	0.90 (0.37–2.20)
Subtotal NHP	*244/6117*	*218/6178*	*1.13 (0.95–1.35)*
Overall (p homog=0.99)	567/11685	510/11769	1.12 (1.00–1.26)
Heart Failure			
INSIGHT	28/3157	16/3164	1.75 (0.95–3.24)
NICS-EH	0/215	3/214	—
STOP-2	186/2196	177/2213	1.06 (0.87–1.29)
Subtotal DHP	*214/5568*	*196/5591*	*1.11 (0.92–1.34)*
NORDIL	63/5410	54/5471	1.18 (0.82–1.69)
VHAS	1/707	0/707	—
Subtotal NHP	*64/6117*	*54/6178*	*1.18 (0.82–1.69)*
Overall (p homog=0.29)	278/11685	250/11769	1.12 (0.95–1.33)
Major Cardiovascular Events			
INSIGHT	220/3157	206/3164	1.07 (0.89–1.29)
NICS-EH	9/215	13/214	0.69 (0.30–1.58)
STOP-2	562/2196	568/2213	1.00 (0.90–1.10)
Subtotal DHP	*791/5568*	*787/5591*	*1.01 (0.92–1.10)*
NORDIL	445/5410	433/5471	1.04 (0.92–1.18)
VHAS	15/707	14/707	1.07 (0.52–2.20)
Subtotal NHP	*460/6117*	*447/6178*	*1.04 (0.92–1.18)*
Overall (p homog=0.84)	1251/11685	1234/11769	1.02 (0.95–1.10)
Cardiovascular Death			
INSIGHT	75/3157	64/3164	1.17 (0.84–1.63)
NICS-EH	2/215	0/214	—
STOP-2	212/2196	221/2213	0.97 (0.81–1.16)
Subtotal DHP	*289/5568*	*285/5591*	*1.01 (0.86–1.18)*
NORDIL	131/5410	115/5471	1.15 (0.90–1.48)
VHAS	5/707	5/707	1.00 (0.29–3.44)
Subtotal NHP	*136/6117*	*120/6178*	*1.15 (0.90–1.46)*
Overall (p homog=0.61)	425/1168	5405/11769	1.05 (0.92–1.20)
Total Mortality			
INSIGHT	176/3157	172/3164	1.03 (0.84–1.26)
NICS-EH	2/215	2/214	1.00 (0.14–7.00)
STOP-2	362/2196	369/2213	0.99 (0.87–1.13)
Subtotal DHP	*540/5568*	*543/5591*	*1.00 (0.89–1.12)*
NORDIL	231/5410	228/5471	1.02 (0.86–1.23)
VHAS	5/707	5/707	1.00 (0.29–3.44)
Subtotal NHP	*236/6117*	*233/6178*	*1.02 (0.86–1.22)*
Overall (p homog=0.99)	776/11685	776/11769	1.01 (0.92–1.11)

0.5   1.0   2.0

Relative Risk

Favors calcium antagonists   Favors diuretics or β-blockers

Figure 18–5   Comparisons of calcium antagonist–based therapy with diuretic-based or β-blocker–based therapy. CI, confidence interval; DHP, dihydropyridine; INSIGHT, International Nifedipine GITS Study: Intervention as a Goal in Hypertension Treatment; NHP, nondihydropyridine; NICS-EH, National Intervention Cooperative Study in Elderly Hypertensives Study Group; NORDIL, Nordic Diltiazem; p homog, *P* value from a χ^2 test for homogeneity; STOP-2, second Swedish Trial in Old Patients; VHAS, Verapamil in Hypertension and Atherosclerosis Study. (From Neal B, MacMahon S, Chapman N, Blood Pressure Lowering Treatment Trialists' Collaboration. Effects of ACE inhibitors, calcium antagonists, and other blood-pressure-lowering drugs: Results of prospectively designed overviews of randomised trials. Blood Pressure Lowering Treatment Trialists' Collaboration. *Lancet.* 2000;**356**:1955-1964.)

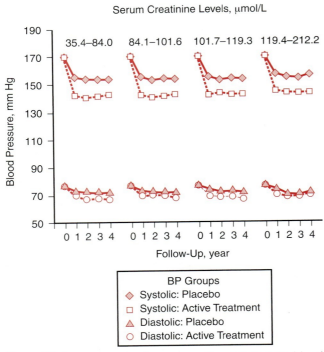

Serum Creatinine Levels, µmol/L

Figure 18–6 Variations of mean systolic and diastolic blood pressure (BP) during follow-up according to treatment and baseline serum creatinine levels in the Systolic Hypertension in the Elderly Program. The graph has been truncated after 4 years. (From Pahor M, Shorr RI, Somes GW, et al. Diuretic-based treatment and cardiovascular events in patients with mild renal dysfunction enrolled in the Systolic Hypertension in the Elderly Program. *Arch Intern Med.* 1998;**158**:1340-1345.)

systolic hypertension in elderly patients and have been the basis for current treatment recommendations advocating diuretic therapy in uncomplicated forms of hypertension. This positioning of diuretics in the management of uncomplicated forms of hypertension has been reinforced by the ALLHAT findings.[49,54]

Black Patients

In black patients, hypertension is more prevalent at a younger age, may be more severe, and is associated with a greater incidence of cardiac, central nervous system, and renal complications than occur in white patients.[61] Although the pathogenesis of hypertension has not been clearly defined, most blacks fall into the low-renin category. This low-renin status cannot be explained by volume expansion alone; no consistent relationship between these two factors has been detected in this population. In addition, the INTERSALT study (International Study of Sodium, Potassium, and Blood Pressure), a multicenter, cross-sectional study that evaluated the relationship between electrolytes and BP, was unable to show a relationship between excessive Na^+ intake and the development of hypertension in blacks.[62] Although not fully resolved, there appears to be a relationship between low K^+ intake and elevated BP in normotensive and hypertensive blacks.[63]

Nonetheless, black patients respond well to diuretic therapy: between 40% and 67% of young patients and between 58% and 80% of elderly patients respond to diuretic monotherapy. Although the absolute BP reduction (−12/−8 mm Hg) in black patients given diuretic therapy is more predictable than with other drug classes given as monotherapy, such as ACE inhibitors, β-blockers, or angiotensin receptor blockers (ARBs), it is often insufficient to reduce BP to goal.[64] In black patients, diuretics often need to be added to nondiuretic drug classes if goal BP is to be reached. This practice of administering multiple antihypertensive agents (including a diuretic) to black patients can occur by beginning therapy with a diuretic or with a diuretic as add-on therapy to other drug classes, such as ACE inhibitors, ARBs, or β-blockers.[65]

Diuretic therapy has been associated with reductions in morbidity and mortality in blacks.[54] Black patients made up approximately half of the study participants in the Veterans Administration Cooperative Study on Antihypertensive Agents and the Hypertension Detection and Follow-up Program (HDFP), both of which were diuretic-based studies. In the Veterans Administration study, HCTZ treatment compared with placebo was associated with a drop in morbid events from 26% to 10% in black patients. In the HDFP study, the reduction in mortality was 18.5% for black men and 27.8% for black women. In ALLHAT, diuretic therapy reduced the primary outcome of fatal CHD and nonfatal myocardial infarction to a similar degree as lisinopril or amlodipine.[54] However, the ability of diuretics to delay or prevent renal dysfunction in hypertensive black patients was called into question by the Multiple Risk Factor Intervention Trial (MRFIT), which did not show a benefit.[66] This study however, included a comparator group of patients who were also treated, and it was not a blinded or placebo-controlled trial, thus making it more difficult to demonstrate a difference in outcomes. More recently, in ALLHAT, initial diuretic therapy did not lead to greater development of end-stage renal disease than did other therapies, although there was limited power for this endpoint in this trial.[54] Investigators have speculated that diuretic therapy may negatively influence renal function if the RAAS becomes overly activated; however, because an ACE inhibitor or an ARB is generally coadministered with a diuretic in most patients with CKD, this is less of an issue.

Regression of Left Ventricular Hypertrophy with Diuretic Therapy

An increase in LV mass has been recognized as a powerful independent risk factor for CVD. With the exception of direct vasodilators used alone, antihypertensive therapy effectively regresses LVH.[67] In 1991, Moser and Setaro compiled an overview of all studies evaluating LVH regression in diuretic-treated hypertensive patients; the findings supported the effectiveness of diuretics in regressing LV mass.[68] Several meta-analyses have also specifically examined LVH regression with different classes of antihypertensive agents.[67,69,70] Using echocardiography, Dahlöf and colleagues analyzed 109 studies comprising 2357 patients and found diuretics to be associated with an 11.3% reduction in LV mass; this finding, however, was in large measure the result of a reduction in LV volume.[69] Alternatively, the reduction of LV mass associated with ACE inhibitor therapy was 15%, with β-blockade it was 8%, and with CCB treatment it was 8.5%, with structural changes largely reflected by a decrease in posterior and intraventricular septal thickness. In another meta-analysis of 39 qualifying trials of ACE inhibitors, CCBs, β-blockers, and diuretics, the decreases in both LV mass index and wall thickness were correlated with the treatment-induced decline in BP, especially systolic BP. Reductions in LV mass of 13%, 9%, 6%, and 7% occurred with ACE inhibitors, CCBs, β-blockers, and diuretics, respectively.[70] In the blinded Treatment of Mild Hypertension Study, diuretics were just as effective as, or even more effective than, other medications in regressing LVH; thus, diuretics are similar to most other drug classes in their ability to regress LVH and are perhaps more effective than β-blockers.[67,69,70]

General Considerations

Diuretics are likely to find their major use in the future as initial therapy or "priming" agents. Their primary mode of sensitization derives from initial volume depletion–related neurohumoral or SNS activation. Even subtle degrees of volume contraction (or RAAS activation), as produced by low-dose thiazide-type diuretic therapy, establish a basis for an enhanced effect of nondiuretic antihypertensive compounds.[65] This additive effect has revived interest in the use of a low-dose diuretic as a part of fixed combination antihypertensive therapy in the primary management of essential hypertension.[65] The concept of using two drugs at low doses for BP control is not recent. It has gathered new support, however, because it is increasingly evident that most patients who receive antihypertensive therapy will achieve their target BP only if multiple drugs are given.[71]

The dose-response relationship for the antihypertensive effect of diuretics has been more completely characterized since the mid-1980s. In the process, many of the alleged negative aspects of diuretic use have not been documented with the currently used lower doses. In the early days of diuretic use, doses were unnecessarily high, driven by the belief that "if a little is good, more is better." It was soon recognized, however, that the dose-BP response for a thiazide-type diuretic (e.g., HCTZ) was relatively flat beyond a daily dose of 25 mg and that much of the negative metabolic experience with diuretics occurred at very high doses (100 to 200 mg/day).[65,72] At lower doses (12.5 to 25 mg of HCTZ), the metabolic changes seen with high-dose thiazide-type diuretic therapy do not appear to be of clinical significance.[72] Recent observations are confusing regarding new-onset diabetes as a consequence of diuretic therapy. For example, the recent 13-year SHEP follow-up trial reported that new-onset diabetes with diuretic therapy does not carry the same risk as preexisting diabetes,[73] whereas a 2004 report, by Verdecchia and colleagues, concluded otherwise.[74]

Strong outcomes data on diuretic therapy are available, and based on these data and the recently completed ALLHAT trial, JNC 7 recommended as initial therapy "thiazide-type diuretics" for most but not all hypertensive patients.[1] In stage 2 hypertension (BP >160/100 mm Hg) and for patients with compelling indications (e.g., an ACE inhibitor for HF), diuretics should be used as part of combination therapy.[75]

ADVERSE EFFECTS OF DIURETICS

Hyponatremia

Hyponatremia an uncommon but possibly serious complication of diuretic therapy.[76,77] Thiazide diuretics are more likely to cause hyponatremia than are loop diuretics. Loop diuretics inhibit Na^+ transport in the renal medulla and preclude the generation of a maximal osmotic gradient. Thus, urinary concentrating ability is impaired with loop diuretics. Alternatively, thiazide-type diuretics increase Na^+ excretion and prevent maximal urine dilution while preserving the kidney's innate concentrating capacity. When diuretic-related hyponatremia occurs, it is usually seen shortly after therapy begins (≤2 weeks) and is most commonly seen in elderly women.[78] Multiple factors contribute to the predisposition of elderly women to diuretic-related hyponatremia, including an exaggerated natriuretic response to a thiazide diuretic, a diminished capacity to excrete free water, and low solute intake (Fig. 18-7).

Controversy surrounds several aspects of the therapy of hyponatremia that also apply to diuretic-related hyponatremia. Mild asymptomatic diuretic-related hyponatremia (typically between 125 and 135 mEq/L) can be treated in a number of ways (which are not necessarily mutually exclusive), including restricting free water intake, restoring K^+ losses if present, withholding diuretics, and converting thiazide to loop diuretic therapy.[79] Symptomatic hyponatremia (generally <125 mEq/L), complicated by seizures or other neurologic sequelae, represents a true medical emergency. A decrease in serum Na^+ to a value less than 125 mEq/L calls for intensive therapy; however, symptomatic hyponatremia should not be rapidly corrected because of an increased risk of osmotic demyelinating syndrome. The risks of ongoing hyponatremia must be weighed against those of too rapid a correction. Current recommendations are for plasma Na^+ not to be corrected by more than 0.5 mEq/L/hour during the first 24 hours of treatment.[80] Initial treatment efforts should be slowed and possibly even stopped once a mildly hyponatremic serum Na^+ (≈125 to 130 mEq/L) has been attained. The duration of hyponatremia (<48 hours) also influences the rate at which hyponatremia should be corrected.

Hypokalemia and Hyperkalemia

A serum K^+ value of less than 3.5 mEq/L, which is the most common criterion for a diagnosis of hypokalemia, may occur in patients treated with loop or thiazide diuretics.[80] During the first several days of thiazide diuretic therapy, plasma K^+ decreases by an average of 0.6 mEq/L (in a dose-dependent manner) in patients not taking K^+ supplements, as compared with an approximately 0.3 mEq/L decrease in patients taking furosemide.[80] It is unusual, however, for serum K^+ values to remain lower than 3.0 mEq/L in diuretic-treated outpatients unless they have high dietary Na^+ intake or are taking a long-acting diuretic, such as chlorthalidone. Mechanisms that contribute to the onset of hypokalemia during diuretic use include increased flow-dependent distal nephron K^+ secretion (more commonly observed with a high Na^+ intake), a fall in distal tubule luminal Cl^- concentration, metabolic alkalosis, and significant secondary hyperaldosteronism (see Fig. 18-7).

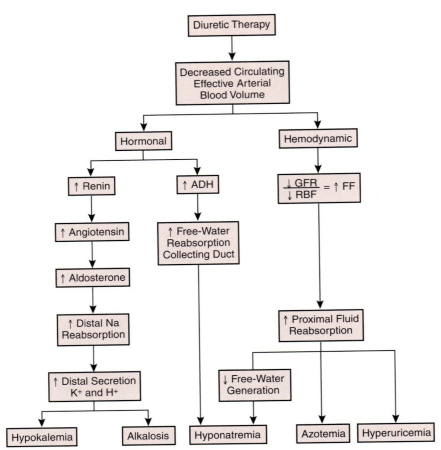

Figure 18–7 Adaptive changes to conserve salt and water in states of extracellular volume depletion resulting in side effects related to diuretic use. ADH, antidiuretic hormone; FF, filtration fraction; GFR, glomerular filtration rate; H, hydrogen; K, potassium; Na, sodium; RBF, renal blood flow.

The cardiac implications of diuretic-induced hypokalemia remain controversial. It would seem logical to infer that arrhythmia-related event rates are coupled to the degree of hypokalemia, but this is in no way an unambiguous relationship (at least in the outpatient setting). This theme is confused by several factors, including the inconstant relationship between serum K^+ concentrations and total body K^+ deficits in the presence of diuretic therapy. Most of the clinical trials evaluating arrhythmia risk (and sudden cardiac death) did not measure serum K^+ values frequently enough or under sufficiently standardized conditions to allow for anything more than an educated guess about the "average" K^+ value at the time of an event. The range of serum K^+ values most commonly associated with increased ventricular ectopy is very small, typically between 3.0 and 3.5 mEq/L. The issue whether hypokalemia produced by transcellular shifts of K^+ carries the same risk as reduced serum K^+ on the basis of body losses has not been settled.

Investigators have observed that even mild degrees of diuretic-induced hypokalemia can be associated with ventricular ectopy.[81] For example, the MRFIT trial found a significant inverse relationship between the serum K^+ concentration and the incidence of premature ventricular contractions.[81] However, this relationship has not been detected in all studies, perhaps because of the short duration of some of these trials.[82]

The hazards central to diuretic-related hypokalemia are most apparent in patients with LVH, HF, or myocardial ischemia, particularly when they become acutely ill and require hospitalization.[83,84] Conversely, several carefully con-trolled studies over a 4-week period in patients with or without LVH who took high-dose HCTZ (100 mg/day) before and after exercise and who had serum K^+ levels lower than 3.5 mmol/L did not report an increase in premature ventricular contractions, couplets, or ventricular tachycardia.[85] As mentioned previously, diuretic-related hypokalemia in outpatients is infrequently severe enough to command urgent attention; however, lowered serum K^+ values create a basis for more significant degrees of hypokalemia when transcellular shifts of K^+ are interposed by, for example, an acute myocardial infarction.[84]

Despite a sometimes increased level of concern about CVD risk (rather than benefit) with diuretic therapy, many clinical trials, including SHEP, STOP, and MRC, showed that low-dose diuretic therapy reduces CVD event rates by 20% to 25%.[48] Perhaps the use of lower doses of thiazides, or their combination with a K^+-sparing diuretic, explains some of these favorable results. However, as noted in the SHEP trial, patients with hypokalemia (serum K^+ <3.5 mEq/L) had a lower benefit from treatment than in similarly treated, but normokalemic, patients.[60]

Two additional treatment issues exist for diuretic-related hypokalemia. First is a hemodynamic benefit of normalizing serum K^+. Supplementation with K^+ (average increase in serum K^+ of 0.56 mEq/L) in hypokalemic (serum K^+ values <3.5 mEq/L) diuretic-treated patients has been associated with a 5.5 mm Hg average decrease in mean arterial pressure.[86] Second, the risk of cardiac arrest among patients receiving combined thiazide and K^+-sparing diuretic therapy

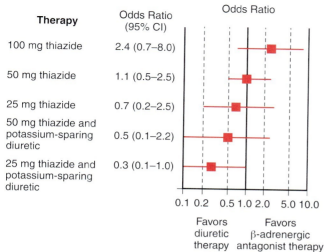

Therapy	Odds Ratio (95% CI)
100 mg thiazide	2.4 (0.7–8.0)
50 mg thiazide	1.1 (0.5–2.5)
25 mg thiazide	0.7 (0.2–2.5)
50 mg thiazide and potassium-sparing diuretic	0.5 (0.1–2.2)
25 mg thiazide and potassium-sparing diuretic	0.3 (0.1–1.0)

Figure 18–8 Risk of primary cardiac arrest associated with thiazide therapy with and without potassium-sparing diuretic therapy, as compared with β-adrenergic antagonist therapy, among patients treated with single antihypertensive drugs. Odds ratios are adjusted for age, gender, pretreatment systolic blood pressure and heart rate, duration of hypertension, current smoking, and diabetes mellitus. CI, confidence interval. (From Siscovick DS, Raghunathan TE, Psaty BM, et al. Diuretic therapy and the risk of primary cardiac arrest. *N Engl J Med.* 1994;**330**:1852-1857.)

was lower than in patients treated with a thiazide alone, with odds ratios for an event increasing significantly as the dose of HCTZ increased from 25 to 100 mg/day. This low-dose combination resulted in a better outcome than with a diuretic and β-blockade (Fig. 18-8).[87]

K^+-sparing diuretics (e.g., triamterene and amiloride) and aldosterone receptor antagonists (e.g., spironolactone and eplerenone) may cause significant hyperkalemia. Hyperkalemia is more likely to develop in patients taking K^+-sparing diuretics in the setting of a reduced GFR (especially elderly patients), in those also receiving KCl supplements or salt substitutes, in patients taking an ACE inhibitor/ARB or an NSAID, and in other situations that predispose patients to hyperkalemia such as metabolic acidosis, hyporeninemic hypoaldosteronism, or heparin therapy (including subcutaneous heparin regimens).[88]

Acid-Base Changes

Mild metabolic alkalosis is a not uncommon feature of thiazide-type diuretic therapy. Severe metabolic alkalosis is much less frequent, and when it occurs, it does so in association with loop diuretic use. The generation of metabolic alkalosis with diuretic therapy is primarily the result of contraction of the ECF space, caused by urinary losses of relatively bicarbonate-free fluid. Diuretic-induced metabolic alkalosis is best managed by the administration of K^+ or NaCl, although NaCl administration may be problematic in patients who are volume expanded (i.e., those with HF). In such patients, a K^+-sparing diuretic or a carbonic anhydrase inhibitor, such as acetazolamide, may be considered. Metabolic alkalosis

also impairs the natriuretic response to loop diuretics and may contribute to diuretic resistance in the patient with HF. All K^+-sparing diuretics can cause hyperkalemic metabolic acidosis, which can represent a serious complication in elderly patients or in those with renal impairment or HF.

Hypomagnesemia

Both thiazide diuretics and loop diuretics increase urine Mg^{2+} excretion. All K^+-sparing diuretics diminish the magnesuria that follows thiazide or loop diuretic use. Prolonged therapy with thiazide or loop diuretics decreases plasma Mg^{2+} concentration on average by 5% to 10%, although some patients develop more severe hypomagnesemia. Cellular Mg^{2+} depletion occurs in up to 50% of patients during thiazide therapy, and it can be present regardless of normal serum Mg^{2+} concentrations. Hypomagnesemia occurs more often in elderly patients and in those receiving continuous high-dose diuretic therapy (e.g., patients with HF). Hypomagnesemia often coexists with hyponatremia and hypokalemia; one study found that 42% of patients with hypokalemia also had low serum Mg^{2+} concentrations.[89] Hypokalemia or hypocalcemia occurring in the presence of hypomagnesemia typically cannot be wholly reversed until the underlying Mg^{2+} deficit is corrected.

The measurement of serum Mg^{2+} continues to be the everyday test for detection of hypomagnesemia.[90] The presence of hypomagnesemia can also be suspected from characteristic electrocardiographic, neurologic, and neuromuscular findings. On an electrocardiogram, hypomagnesemia can present as prolongation of the Q-T and P-R intervals, widening of the QRS complex, ST segment depression, and low T waves, in addition to supraventricular and ventricular tachyarrhythmias. The neurologic changes with hypomagnesemia are nonspecific and are usually marked by mental status changes and neuromuscular irritability. Tetany, one of the most conspicuous and better known manifestations of Mg^{2+} deficiency, is only rarely seen; instead, less specific signs such as tremor, muscle twitching, peculiar movements, focal seizures, generalized convulsions, delirium, and coma are more common findings.

Although a low serum Mg^{2+} level is helpful in making the diagnosis, and is in general indicative of low intracellular stores, normal serum Mg^{2+} values can still be observed in the presence of a significant body deficiency of Mg^{2+}. Thus, serum Mg^{2+} determinations are an unreliable measure of total body Mg^{2+} balance.[91] Intracellular Mg^{2+} measurements and other sophisticated technologies are available to assess Mg^{2+} balance, but they remain clinically impractical. A more useful measure of Mg^{2+} balance is the Mg^{2+} loading test, which is both therapeutic and diagnostic. This test consists of the parenteral administration of Mg sulfate ($MgSO_4$) and a timewise assessment of urinary Mg^{2+} retention, which can be accomplished on an outpatient basis in 1 hour or less. Individuals in a state of normal Mg^{2+} balance eliminate at least 75% of an administered load.[91]

Several theoretical reasons exist to treat diuretic-related hypomagnesemia (beyond simple empiric correction to normalize a laboratory value) including improvement in BP control, decrease in arrhythmias, and resolution of coexisting electrolyte or neuromuscular symptoms. Although there appears to be little additional reduction in BP when Mg^{2+}

deficiency is corrected, some measure of BP reduction seems to be evident when Mg^{2+} supplementation occurs in a nondeficient state. The inconclusive nature of the available studies on Mg^{2+} supplementation as a therapy for hypertension precludes a specific therapeutic recommendation.

It is recommended that Mg^{2+} deficiency be identified when clinically indicated, but particularly in patients with ischemic heart disease or recognized cardiac arrhythmias. In mild deficiency states, Mg^{2+} balance can often be reestablished by simply controlling the contributing factors (limiting diuretic use and Na^+ intake) and allowing dietary Mg^{2+} to correct the deficit.

Parenteral Mg^{2+}, however, is the most efficient way to correct hypomagnesemia and should always be the mode of administration when the need for replacement is urgent. Total body Mg^{2+} deficits are typically in the order of 1 to 2 mEq/kg body weight in the depleted patient. One commonly employed treatment regimen in the Mg^{2+}-depleted patient gives 2 g of $MgSO_4$ (16.3 mEq) intravenously over 30 minutes, followed by a constant infusion providing between 32 and 64 mEq/day until the estimated deficit is corrected.

Various Mg^{2+} salts are available for oral use. Mg^{2+} oxide is a commonly employed Mg^{2+} salt, but it is not very water soluble and has a major cathartic effect; thus, its use can unpredictably influence Mg^{2+} concentrations. Mg^{2+} gluconate is the preferred therapy for oral use; this salt form is very soluble and causes minimal diarrhea. Mg^{2+} carbonate is also not very water soluble and is not as effective as the gluconate salt in correcting hypomagnesemia. Oral Mg^{2+} is not recommended as a means of therapy during urgent situations of Mg^{2+} deficiency, because the high doses needed almost always bring about significant diarrhea. The intramuscular route for Mg^{2+} administration is occasionally used, but it is painful and should be used only if intravenous access is difficult.[90]

Hyperuricemia

Higher-dose thiazide diuretic therapy increases serum urate concentrations by as much as 35%, an effect related to decreased renal clearance of urate. This effect is most evident in people with the highest urate clearance before therapy. Decreased urate clearance may reflect increased reabsorption secondary to diuretic-related ECF volume depletion or competition for tubular secretion, because both thiazide diuretics and urate undergo tubular secretion by the same organic anion transporter pathway.[92] Diuretic-related hyperuricemia is dose dependent and does not typically precipitate a gouty attack unless the patient has an underlying tendency or serum urate concentrations exceed 12 mg/dL.[92] In the blinded MRC trial, patients receiving thiazide diuretics had significantly more withdrawals for gout than did placebo-treated patients (4.4 versus 0.1/1000 patient-years). In the HDFP trial, fewer than 3% of patients experienced a gouty attack, despite the use of high-dose thiazides.

If a gouty attack occurs in a diuretic-treated patient, the diuretic should be discontinued. If this is not feasible, then the lowest effective dose should be given, with careful attention to maintaining euvolemia. An additional alternative in the gouty patient requiring diuretic therapy is the use of the xanthine oxidase inhibitor, allopurinol. Allopurinol should be used cautiously (dose adjusted according to level of renal function)

in patients receiving a thiazide-type diuretic, because allopurinol hypersensitivity reactions are more frequent with this combination than with allopurinol alone. Allopurinol should not be routinely started, as is often the case, in patients with asymptomatic diuretic-related hyperuricemia.[93]

METABOLIC ABNORMALITIES

Hyperglycemia

Prolonged thiazide diuretic therapy impairs glucose tolerance and may occasionally precipitate diabetes mellitus.[54,74,94,95] Short-term metabolic studies, epidemiologic studies, and a variety of clinical trials causally linked the use of thiazide diuretics and the development of type 2 diabetes. However, these studies often involved small numbers of patients and had limited follow-up periods, varying definitions of new-onset diabetes, inadequate comparison groups, and selection criteria that limited the generalizability of the findings.[95] In placebo-controlled trials, diuretic use increased the incidence of new-onset diabetes in fewer than 1% of patients.

Hyperglycemia and carbohydrate intolerance have been associated with diuretic-induced hypokalemia, a condition that inhibits β-cell secretion of insulin. Diuretic-induced changes in glucose metabolism are not conclusively related to hypokalemia, however. Impaired glucose tolerance occurs even when thiazide-type diuretics in relatively low doses are given together with K^+-sparing agents. The glucose intolerance seen with diuretic therapy can be worsened when SNS activity increases, because peripheral glucose utilization decreases in the process. Diuretic-associated glucose intolerance appears to be dose related, less common with loop diuretics, not present with spironolactone, and reversible (to a degree) on withdrawal of the offending agent.[95]

The conclusions of a large, prospective cohort study of 12,550 adults (45 to 64 years old) who did not have diabetes were (after appropriate adjustment for confounders) that hypertensive patients taking thiazide diuretics were not at greater risk for incident diabetes than were patients who did not receive antihypertensive therapy. The diuretic doses were not reported in this cohort study. Because of the perceived variability of this effect, blood glucose should be monitored during thiazide therapy, particularly in patients with either existing diabetes or the metabolic syndrome.[96] Opinion differs regarding the CVD risk with new-onset diabetes compared with that observed in patients with existing diabetes. In ALLHAT, the presence or absence of diabetes or new-onset diabetes did not appear to decrease the beneficial effects of diuretic therapy.[54]

Hyperlipidemia

Short-term thiazide diuretic therapy can cause a dose-dependent elevation in serum total cholesterol levels, a modest increase in low-density lipoprotein cholesterol levels, and raised triglyceride levels with little change in high-density lipoprotein cholesterol.[97-99] These lipid effects have been reported more often in blacks than in whites, in men than in women, and in diabetic patients.[98] All diuretics, including loop diuretics, cause these lipid changes, with the possible exception of indapamide, although data with this agent are not definitive.[99] The mechanisms behind diuretic-induced dyslipidemia remain uncertain, but they may be related to decreased insulin sensitivity or reflex activation of the RAAS and SNS brought about by volume contraction. In support of this latter observation, a diuretic dose low enough to not induce reflex sympathetic activation generally does not cause lipid alterations. The lipid changes with thiazide-type diuretic therapy are short-lived, with unchanged cholesterol levels reported after 1 year of diuretic therapy.[97,99] Moreover, data from HDFP indicate that hypertensive subjects with baseline cholesterol values higher than 250 mg/dL who were treated with diuretics experienced a decline in cholesterol levels from the second to the fifth years of treatment.

Other Adverse Effects

Impotence

Adverse effects of thiazide and thiazide-like diuretics on male sexual function, including decreased libido, erectile dysfunction, and difficulty in ejaculating, have been reported in several studies, with an incidence that varies from 3% to 32%. As an example, in the MRC trial, in which 15,000 hypertensive subjects received placebo, a thiazide diuretic (bendrofluazide), or the β-blocker propranolol for 5 years, impotence was 22-fold and 4-fold higher in those receiving a thiazide compared with placebo or a β-blocker, respectively. In this trial, impotence was the most frequent principal reason for withdrawal from antihypertensive therapy. Another smaller trial reported by Chang and associates confirmed a higher frequency of decreased libido, difficulty in gaining and sustaining an erection, and trouble in ejaculating in patients receiving a thiazide diuretic. Multivariate analysis suggested that the findings were not associated with reduction in serum K[+] levels or BP.[100]

In the Treatment of Mild Hypertension Study, problems with sexual interest, erection, and orgasm were greater among men receiving chlorthalidone compared with those given placebo or atenolol. In this trial, weight loss improved the problem of chlorthalidone-induced sexual dysfunction.[101] In this study, the increase in sexual dysfunction at 1 year with chlorthalidone (compared with other drugs) was not present at 4 years.[102] The mechanism by which thiazides affect erectile function or libido is unclear, but it has been suggested that these drugs wield a direct effect on vascular smooth muscle cells or decrease the response to catecholamines. However, patients with diuretic-related impotence can respond favorably to sildenafil without an associated additional increase in BP.[103]

Impotence and decreased libido are the more frequent sexual side effects of spironolactone. Gynecomastia, another fairly frequent complication of spironolactone therapy, may be associated with mastodynia and is typically bilateral. The sexual side effects of spironolactone have been attributed to endocrine dysfunction: spironolactone is structurally similar to the sex hormones and inhibits the binding of dihydrotestosterone to androgen receptors, thus leading to an increased clearance of testosterone. Eplerenone is another aldosterone receptor antagonist that is more selective than spironolactone, and it apparently does not produce the sexual side effects seen with spironolactone.[104]

Drug Allergy

Photosensitivity dermatitis occurs rarely during thiazide or furosemide therapy. HCTZ more commonly causes photosensitivity than other thiazides. Diuretics may occasionally cause more serious generalized dermatitis and, at times, even necrotizing vasculitis. Cross-sensitivity with sulfonamide drugs may occur with all diuretics, with the exception of ethacrynic acid, which is not structurally related to sulfonamides. Severe necrotizing pancreatitis is an additional serious, rare, life-threatening complication of thiazide therapy, as is acute allergic interstitial nephritis characterized by fever, rash, and eosinophilia. This latter condition may result in permanent renal failure if drug exposure is prolonged.[105] Ethacrynic acid is chemically dissimilar from the other loop diuretics and can be safely substituted in diuretic-treated patients who experience any one of several of these allergic complications.

Carcinogenesis

Twelve clinical studies, three cohort (1,226,229 patients with 802 cases of renal cell carcinoma) and nine case-control studies (4185 cases of renal cell carcinoma and 6010 controls), have evaluated the association between the use of diuretics and renal cell carcinoma. In the case-control studies, the odds were greater for diuretic-treated patients to develop renal cell carcinoma (average odds ratio, 1.55). In several studies, the risk of renal cell carcinoma was related to the duration of diuretic treatment and not to the average daily diuretic dose. Unlike the association between diuretics and renal cell carcinoma, no connection has been found between diuretic use and breast cancer. Finally, no evidence for this risk has been found in any of the prospective long-term controlled clinical trials; thus, the issue of renal cell carcinoma occurring with diuretic therapy remains incompletely resolved.[106]

Adverse Drug Interactions

Loop diuretics can potentiate aminoglycoside nephrotoxicity. By causing hypokalemia, diuretics increase the risk of digitalis toxicity. Plasma Li[+] concentrations can rise during thiazide therapy, with significant volume contraction as a result of the associated increase in Li[+] resorption. However, some diuretics, such as CTZ and furosemide, with significant carbonic anhydrase inhibitory activity, can increase Li[+] clearance, thus leading to a decrease in blood levels. Whole blood Li[+] should be closely monitored in patients who take both Li[+] and diuretics. NSAIDs can both antagonize the effects of diuretics and predispose diuretic-treated patients to a generally reversible form of renal failure. The combination of indomethacin and triamterene may be particularly dangerous in that respect.[107]

CONCLUSIONS

Diuretics should remain an important component of any management plan for hypertension. Of the several available classes of diuretics, the thiazide-type diuretic is the one most commonly used in the treatment of hypertension. The safe and effective use of diuretics in the treatment of hypertension and edema requires an understanding of the pharmacokinetics of these drugs. Thiazide diuretics are generally well tolerated and can be used effectively as either monotherapy or in combination with other antihypertensive agents with the expectation that BP will be lowered and CVD events will be reduced.

References

1. Chobanian AV, Bakris GL, Black HR, et al. Seventh Report of the Joint National Committee on Prevention, Detection, Evaluation, and Treatment of High Blood Pressure. *Hypertension*. 2003;**42**:1206-1252.
2. Brater DC. Diuretic therapy. *N Engl J Med*. 1998;**339**:387-395.
3. Shankar SS, Brater DC. Loop diuretics: From the Na-K-2Cl transporter to clinical use. *Am J Physiol*. 2003;**284**:F11-F21.
4. Loon NR, Wilcox CS, Unwin RJ. Mechanism of impaired natriuretic response to furosemide during prolonged therapy. *Kidney Int*. 1989;**36**:682-689.
5. Sica DA, Gehr TWB. Diuretic combinations in refractory edema states: pharmacokinetic-pharmacodynamic relationships. *Clin Pharmacokinet*. 1996;**30**:229-249.
6. Wilcox CS, Mitch WE, Kelly RA, et al. Response of the kidney to furosemide. I. Effects of salt intake and renal compensation. *J Lab Clin Med*. 1983;**102**:450-458.
7. Agarwal R, Gorski JC, Sundblad K, Brater DC. Urinary protein binding does not affect response to furosemide in patients with nephrotic syndrome. *J Am Soc Nephrol*. 2000;**11**:1100-1105.
8. Murray MD, Haag KM, Black PK, et al. Variable furosemide absorption and poor predictability of response in elderly patients. *Pharmacotherapy*. 1997;**17**:98-106.
9. Vargo DL, Kramer WG, Black PK, et al. Bioavailability, pharmacokinetics, and pharmacodynamics of torsemide and furosemide in patients with congestive heart failure. *Clin Pharmacol Ther*. 1995;**57**:601-609.
10. Murray MD, Deer MM, Ferguson JA, et al. Open-label randomized trial of torsemide compared with furosemide therapy for patients with heart failure. *Am J Med*. 2001;**111**:513-520.
11. Voelker JR, Cartwright-Brown D, Anderson S, et al. Comparison of furosemide to bumetanide in chronic renal insufficiency. *Kidney Int*. 1987;**32**:572-578.
12. Rudy DW, Gehr TW, Matzke GR, et al. The pharmacodynamics of intravenous and oral torsemide in patients with chronic renal insufficiency. *Clin Pharmacol Ther*. 1994;**56**:39-47.
13. Leary WP, Reyes AJ. Diuretic-induced magnesium losses. *Drugs*. 1984;**28 (Suppl 1)**:182-187.
14. Welling PG. Pharmacokinetics of the thiazide diuretics. *Biopharm Drug Dispos*. 1986;**7**:501-535.
15. Knauf H, Mutschler E. Diuretic effectiveness of hydrochlorothiazide and furosemide alone and in combination in chronic renal failure. *J Cardiovasc Pharmacol*. 1995;**26**:394-400.
16. Sica DA, Gehr TWB. Diuretic use in stage 5 chronic kidney disease (CKD) and end-stage renal disease. *Curr Opin Nephrol Hypertens*. 2003;**12**:483-490.
17. Suki WN, Dawoud F, Eknoyan G, et al. Effects of metolazone on renal function in normal man. *J Pharmacol Exp Ther*. 1972;**180**:6-12.
18. Sica DA. Metolazone and its role in edema management. *Congest Heart Fail*. 2003;**9**:100-105.
19. Gardiner P, Schrode K, Quinlan D, et al. Spironolactone metabolism: Steady-state serum levels of the sulfur-containing metabolites. *J Clin Pharmacol*. 1989;**29**:342-347.
20. McLaughlin N, Gehr TWB, Sica DA. Aldosterone receptor antagonism in end-stage renal disease. *Curr Hypertens Rep*. 2004;**6**:327-330.
21. Pitt B, Remme W, Zannad F, et al. Eplerenone, a selective aldosterone blocker, in patients with left ventricular dysfunction after myocardial infarction. *N Engl J Med*. 2003;**348**:1309-1321.
22. Williams GH, Burgess E, Kolloch RE, et al. Efficacy of eplerenone versus enalapril as monotherapy in systemic hypertension. *Am J Cardiol*. 2004;**93**:990-996.
23. White WB, Duprez D, St Hillaire R, et al. Effects of the selective aldosterone blocker eplerenone versus the calcium antagonist amlodipine in systolic hypertension. *Hypertension*. 2003;**41**:1021-1026.
24. Pitt B, Reichek N, Willenbrock R, et al. Effects of eplerenone, enalapril, and eplerenone/enalapril in patients with essential hypertension and left ventricular hypertrophy: The 4E-left ventricular hypertrophy study. *Circulation*. 2003;**108**:1831-1838.
25. Sica DA, Gehr TW. Triamterene and the kidney. *Nephron*. 1989;**51**:454-461.
26. Favre L, Glasson P, Vallotton MB. Reversible acute renal failure from combined triamterene and indomethacin: A study in healthy subjects. *Ann Intern Med*. 1982;**96**:317-320.
27. Kelly RA, Wilcox CS, Mitch WE, et al. Response of the kidney to furosemide. II. Effect of captopril on sodium balance. *Kidney Int*. 1983;**24**:233-239.
28. Wilcox CS, Guzman NJ, Mitch WE, et al. Na$^+$ and BP homeostasis in man during furosemide: Effects of prazosin and captopril. *Kidney Int*. 1987;**31**:135-141.
29. Almeshari K, Ahlstom NG, Capraro FE, et al. A volume-independent component to post-diuretic sodium retention in man. *J Am Soc Nephrol*. 1993;**3**:1878-1883.
30. Ellison DH, Velazquez H, Wright FS. Adaptation of the distal convoluted tubule of the rat: Structural and functional effects of dietary salt intake and chronic diuretic infusion. *J Clin Invest*. 1989;**83**:113-126.
31. Idiopathic edema: Role of diuretic abuse. *Kidney Int*. 1981;**19**:881-891.
32. Pivac N, Rumboldt Z, Sardelic S, et al. Diuretic effects of furosemide infusion versus bolus injection in congestive heart failure. *Int J Clin Pharmacol Res*. 1998;**18**:121-128.
33. Dikshit K, Vyden JK, Forrester JS, et al. Renal and extrarenal hemodynamic effects of furosemide in congestive heart failure after acute myocardial infarction. *N Engl J Med*. 1973;**288**:1087-1090.
34. Nishizaka MK, Zaman MA, Calhoun DA. Efficacy of low-dose spironolactone in subjects with resistant hypertension. *Am J Hypertens*. 2003;**16**:925-930.
35. Hajjar I, Kotchen TA. Trends in prevalence, awareness, treatment, and control of hypertension in the United States, 1988-2000. *JAMA*. 2003;**290**:199-206.
36. Neal B, MacMahon S, Chapman N, Blood Pressure Lowering Treatment Trialists' Collaboration. Effects of ACE inhibitors, calcium antagonists, and other blood-pressure-lowering drugs: Results of prospectively designed overviews of randomised trials. Blood Pressure Lowering Treatment Trialists' Collaboration. *Lancet*. 2000;**356**:1955-1964.
37. Finnerty FA, Maxwell MH, Lunn J, Moser M. Long-term effects of furosemide and hydrochlorothiazide in patients with essential hypertension: A two-year comparison of efficacy and safety. *Angiology*. 1977;**28**:125-133.
38. Hughes AD. How do thiazide and thiazide-like diuretics lower blood pressure? *J Ren Angio Aldo Sys*. 2004;**5**:155-160.
39. Roos JC, Boer P, Koomans HA, et al. Haemodynamic and hormonal changes during acute and chronic diuretic treatment in essential hypertension. *Eur J Clin Pharmacol*. 1981;**19**:107-112.
40. Shah S, Khatri I, Freis ED. Mechanism of antihypertensive effect of thiazide diuretics. *Am Heart J*. 1978;**95**:611-618.
41. Bennett WM, McDonald WJ, Kuehnel E, et al. Do diuretics have antihypertensive properties independent of natriuresis? *Clin Pharmacol Ther*. 1977;**22**:499-504.

42. Nelson MR, Reid CM, Krum H, et al. Short-term predictors of maintenance of normotension after withdrawal of antihypertensive drugs in the second Australian National Blood Pressure Study (ANBP2). *Am J Hypertens*. 2003;**16**:39-45.

43. Holland OB, Gomez-Sanchez CE, Kuhnert LV, et al. Antihypertensive comparison of furosemide with hydrochlorothiazide for black patients. *Arch Intern Med*. 1979;**139**:1015-1021.

44. Pickkers P, Hughes AD, Russel FG, et al. Thiazide-induced vasodilation in humans is mediated by potassium channel activation. *Hypertension*. 1998;**32**:1071-1076.

45. Pickkers P, Dormans TP, Russel FG, et al. Direct vascular effects of furosemide in humans. *Circulation*. 1997;**96**:1847-1852.

46. Carter BL, Ernst ME, Cohen JD. Hydrochlorothiazide versus chlorthalidone: Evidence supporting their interchangeability. *Hypertension*. 2004;**43**:4-9.

47. Mortality after 10 1/2 years for hypertensive participants in the Multiple Risk Factor Intervention Trial. *Circulation*. 1990;**82**:1616-1628.

48. SHEP Cooperative Research Group. Prevention of stroke by antihypertensive drug treatment in older persons with isolated systolic hypertension: Final results of the Systolic Hypertension in the Elderly Program (SHEP). *JAMA*. 1991;**265**:3255-3264.

49. Major outcomes in high-risk hypertensive patients randomized to angiotensin-converting enzyme inhibitor or calcium channel blocker vs diuretic: The Antihypertensive and Lipid-Lowering Treatment to Prevent Heart Attack Trial (ALLHAT). *JAMA*. 2002;**288**:2981-2997.

50. Collins R, Peto R, MacMahon S, et al. Blood pressure, stroke, and coronary heart disease: Part 2. Short-term reductions in blood pressure: Overview of randomised drug trials in their epidemiological context. *Lancet*. 1990;**335**:827-838.

51. Herbert PR, Moser M, Mayer J, Hennekens C. Recent evidence on drug therapy of mild to moderate hypertension and decreased risk of coronary heart disease. *Arch Intern Med*. 1991;**151**:1277-1279.

52. Psaty B, Smith N, Siscovick D, et al. Health outcomes associated with antihypertensive therapies used as first-line agents: A systematic review and meta-analysis. *JAMA*. 1997;**277**:739-745.

53. Messerli FH, Grossman E, Goldbourt U. Are β blockers efficacious as first-line therapy for hypertension in the elderly? A systematic review. *JAMA*. 1998;**279**:1903-1907.

54. Antihypertensive and Lipid-Lowering Treatment to Prevent Heart Attack Trial Collaborative Research Group. Diuretic versus alpha-blocker as first-step antihypertensive therapy: Final results from the Antihypertensive and Lipid-Lowering Treatment to Prevent Heart Attack Trial (ALLHAT). *Hypertension*. 2003;**42**:239-246.

55. Materson BJ, Williams DW, Reda DJ, et al. Response to six classes of antihypertensive medications by body mass index in a randomized controlled trial. *J Clin Hypertens. (Greenwich)* 2003;**5**:197-201.

56. Chapman AB, Schwartz GL, Boerwinkle E, Turner ST. Predictors of antihypertensive response to a standard dose of hydrochlorothiazide for essential hypertension. *Kidney Int*. 2002;**61**:1047-1055.

57. Coope J, Warrender TS. Randomized trial of treatment of hypertension in elderly patients in primary care. *BMJ*. 1986;**293**:1145-1151.

58. Messerli F, Grossman E, Lever AF. Do thiazide diuretics confer protection against stroke? *Arch Intern Med*. 2003;**163**:2557-2560.

59. Pahor M, Shorr RI, Somes GW, et al. Diuretic-based treatment and cardiovascular events in patients with mild renal dysfunction enrolled in the Systolic Hypertension in the Elderly Program. *Arch Intern Med*. 1998;**158**:1340-1345.

60. Franse LV, Pahor M, Di Bari M, et al. Hypokalemia associated with diuretic use and cardiovascular events in the Systolic Hypertension in the Elderly Program. *Hypertension*. 2000;**35**:1025-1030.

61. Douglas JG, Bakris GL, Epstein M, et al. Management of high blood pressure in African Americans: Consensus statement of the Hypertension in African Americans Working Group of the International Society on Hypertension in Blacks. *Arch Intern Med*. 2003;**163**:525-541.

62. INTERSALT Cooperative Research Group. INTERSALT: An international study of electrolyte excretion and blood pressure. Results of 24 h urinary sodium and potassium excretion. *BMJ*. 1988;**297**:319-328.

63. Whelton PK, He J, Cutler JA, et al. Effects of oral potassium on blood pressure: Meta-analysis of randomized controlled clinical trials. *JAMA*. 1997;**277**:1624-1632.

64. Sareli P, Radevski IV, Valtchanova ZP, et al. Efficacy of different drug classes used to initiate antihypertensive treatment in black subjects: Results of a randomized trial in Johannesburg, South Africa. *Arch Intern Med*. 2001;**161**:965-971.

65. Sica DA. Rationale for fixed-dose combinations in the treatment of hypertension: The cycle repeats. *Drugs*. 2002;**62**:443-462.

66. Walker WG, Neaton JD, Cutler JA, et al. Renal function change in hypertensive members of the Multiple Risk Factor Intervention Trial: Racial and treatment effects. *JAMA*. 1992;**268**:3085-3091.

67. Klingbeil AU, Schneider M, Martus P, et al. A meta-analysis of the effects of treatment on left ventricular mass in essential hypertension. *Am J Med*. 2003;**115**:41-46.

68. Moser M, Setaro JF. Antihypertensive drug therapy and regression of left ventricular hypertrophy: A review with a focus on diuretics. *Eur Heart J*. 1991;**12**:1034-1039.

69. Dahlöf B, Pennert K, Hansson L. Reversal of left ventricular hypertrophy in hypertensive patients: A meta-analysis of 109 treatment studies. *Am J Hypertens*. 1992;**5**:95-110.

70. Schmieder RE, Martus P, Klingbeil A. Reversal of left ventricular hypertrophy in essential hypertension. *JAMA*. 1996;**275**:1507-1513.

71. Hansson L, Zanchetti A, Carruthers SG, et al. Effect of intensive blood-pressure lowering and low-dose aspirin in patients with hypertension: Principal results of the Hypertension Optimal Treatment (HOT) randomised trial. *Lancet*. 1998;**351**:1755-1762.

72. Moser M. Why are physicians not prescribing diuretics more frequently in the management of hypertension? *JAMA*. 1998;**270**:1813-1816.

73. Kostis JB, Wilson AC, Freudenberger RS, et al. Long-term effect of diuretic-based therapy on fatal outcomes in subjects with isolated systolic hypertension with and without diabetes. *Am J Cardiol*. 2005;**95**:29-35.

74. Verdecchia P, Reboldi G, Angeli F, et al. Adverse prognostic significance of new diabetes in treated hypertensive subjects. *Hypertension*. 2004;**43**:963-969.

75. Moser M, Setaro J. Continued importance of diuretics and β-adrenergic blockers in the management of hypertension. *Med Clin North Am*. 2004;**88**:167-187.

76. Chow KM, Szeto CC, Wong TY, Leung CB, et al. Risk factors for thiazide-induced hyponatraemia. *Q J Med*. 2003;**96**:911-917.

77. Ashraf N, Locksley R, Arieff AI. Thiazide-induced hyponatremia associated with death or neurologic damage in outpatients. *Am J Med*. 1981;**70**:1163-1168.

78. Sonnenblick M, Friedlander Y, Rosin AJ. Diuretic-induced severe hyponatremia: Review and analysis of 129 reported patients. *Chest*. 1993;**103**:601-606.

79. Decaux G, Soupart A. Treatment of symptomatic hyponatremia. *Am J Med Sci*. 2004;**326**:25-30.

80. Morgan DB, Davidson C. Hypokalemia and diuretics: An analysis of publications. *BMJ*. 1980;**280**:905-908.

81. MacMahon S, Collins G, Rautaharju P, et al. Electrocardiographic left ventricular hypertrophy and effects of antihypertensive drug therapy in hypertensive patients in the Multiple Risk Factor Intervention Trial. *Am J Cardiol.* 1989;**63**:202-210.

82. Medical Research Council, Working Party on Mild to Moderate Hypertension. Ventricular extrasystoles during thiazide treatment: Substudy of MRC Mild Hypertension Trial. *BMJ.* 1983;**287**:1249-1253.

83. Macdonald JE, Struthers AD. What is the optimal serum potassium level in cardiovascular patients? *J Am Coll Cardiol.* 2004;**43**:155-161.

84. Sica DA, Struthers AD, Cushman WC, et al. Importance of potassium in cardiovascular disease. *J Clin Hypertens.* 2003;**4**;198-206.

85. Papademetriou V, Burris JF, Notargiacomo A, et al. Thiazide therapy is not a cause of arrhythmia in patients with systemic hypertension. *Arch Intern Med.* 1988;**148**:1272-1276.

86. Kaplan NM, Carnegie A, Raskin P, et al. Potassium supplementation in hypertensive patients with diuretic-induced hypokalemia. *N Engl J Med.* 1985;**312**:746-749.

87. Siscovick DS, Raghunathan TE, Psaty BM, et al. Diuretic therapy and the risk of primary cardiac arrest. *N Engl J Med.* 1994;**330**:1852-1857.

88. Sica DA, Hess M. Aldosterone receptor antagonism: Interface with hyperkalemia in heart failure. *Congest Heart Fail.* 2004;**10**:259-264.

89. Whang R, Oei TO, Aikawa JK, et al. Predictors of clinical hypomagnesemia: Hypokalemia, hypophosphatemia, hyponatremia, and hypocalcemia. *Arch Intern Med.* 1984;**144**:1794-1796.

90. Sica DA, Frishman WH, Cavusoglu E. Magnesium, potassium, and calcium as potential cardiovascular disease therapies. *In:* Frishman W, Sonnenblick E, Sica DA (eds.). Cardiovascular Pharmacotherapeutics, 2nd ed. New York: McGraw-Hill, 2003, pp 177-190.

91. Rob PM, Dick K, Bley N, et al. Can one really measure magnesium deficiency using the short-term magnesium loading test? *J Intern Med.* 1999;**246**:373-378.

92. Sica DA, Schoolwerth A. Renal handing of organic anions and cations and renal excretion of uric acid. *In:* Brenner B, Rector F (eds.). *The Kidney,* 7th ed. Philadelphia: WB Saunders, 2004, pp 637-662.

93. Gurwitz JH, Kalish SC, Bohn RL, et al. Thiazide diuretics and the initiation of anti-gout therapy. *J Clin Epidemiol.* 1997;**50**:953-959.

94. Furman BL. Impairment of glucose intolerance produced by diuretics and other drugs. *Pharmacol Ther.* 1981;**12**:613-649.

95. Sowers JR, Bakris GL. Antihypertensive therapy and the risk of type 2 diabetes mellitus. *N Engl J Med.* 2000;**342**:969-970.

96. Gress TW, Nieto FJ, Shahar E, et al. Hypertension and antihypertensive therapy as risk factors for type 2 diabetes mellitus. *N Engl J Med.* 2000;**342**:905-912.

97. Mantel-Teeuwisse AK, Kloosterman JM, Maitland-van der Zee AH, et al. Drug-induced lipid changes: A review of the unintended effects of some commonly used drugs on serum lipid levels. *Drug Saf.* 2001;**24**:443-456.

98. Kasiske BL, Ma JZ, Kalil RSN, Louis TA. Effects of antihypertensive therapy on serum lipids. *Ann Intern Med.* 1995;**122**:133-141.

99. Lakshman MR, Reda DJ, Materson BJ, et al. Diuretics and beta-blockers do not have adverse effects at 1 year on plasma lipid and lipoprotein profiles in men with hypertension. *Arch Intern Med.* 1999;**159**:551-558.

100. Chang SW, Fine R, Siegel D, et al. The impact of diuretic therapy on reported sexual function. *Arch Intern Med.* 1991;**151**:2402-2408.

101. Wassertheil-Smoller S, Blaufox MD, Oberman A, et al. Effect of antihypertensives on sexual function and quality of life: The TAIM study. *Arch Intern Med.* 1991;**114**:613-620.

102. Grimm RH Jr, Grandits GA, Prineas RJ, et al. Long-term effects on sexual function of five antihypertensive Drugs and Nutritional Hygienic Treatment in hypertensive Men and Women. Treatment of Mild Hypertension Study (TOMHS). *Hypertension.* 1997;**29**:8-14.

103. Pickering TG, Shepherd AM, Puddey I, et al. Sildenafil citrate for erectile dysfunction in men receiving multiple antihypertensive agents: A randomized controlled trial. *Am J Hypertens.* 2004;**17**:1135-1142.

104. Williams GH, Burgess E, Kolloch RE, et al. Efficacy of eplerenone versus enalapril as monotherapy in systemic hypertension. *Am J Cardiol.* 2004;**93**:990-996.

105. Schwarz A, Krause PH, Kunzendorf U, et al. The outcome of acute interstitial nephritis: Risk factors for the transition from acute to chronic interstitial nephritis. *Clin Nephrol.* 2000;**54**:179-190.

106. Grossman E, Messerli FH, Goldbourt U. Does diuretic therapy increase the risk of renal cell carcinoma? *Am J Cardiol.* 1999;**83**:1090-1093.

107. Favre L, Glasson P, Vallotton MB. Reversible acute renal failure from combined triamterene and indomethacin: A study in healthy subjects. *Ann Intern Med.* 1982;**96**:317-320.

β-Blockers in Hypertension

William H. Frishman

The Seventh Report of the Joint National Committee on Detection, Evaluation, and Treatment of High Blood Pressure (JNC 7) from the National High Blood Pressure Education Program of the National Heart Lung and Blood Institute reiterated the recommendation of JNC III through VI that β-adrenergic blockers are appropriate alternatives as first-line treatment for hypertension.[1] These recommendations are based on the reduction of morbidity and mortality when these drugs were used in large clinical trials. Although no consensus exists regarding the mechanisms by which β-blocking drugs lower blood pressure, it is probable that some or all of the modes of action referred to in Table 19-1 are involved.[2]

Thirteen orally active β-adrenergic blockers are approved in the United States for the treatment of hypertension (Table 19-2). In addition, intravenous labetalol is approved for the management of hypertensive emergencies. Oral bisoprolol, in combination with a very low dose of diuretic, is available as a first-line antihypertensive treatment, the first such β-blocker combination so approved for the treatment of hypertension.[3] The various β-blocking agents differ in terms of the presence or absence of intrinsic sympathomimetic activity, membrane stabilizing activity, β_1 selectivity, α-adrenergic blocking activity, and relative potencies and duration of action. Nevertheless, all β-blockers studied to date appear to have favorable blood pressure–lowering effects when they are used in appropriate doses.[4,5]

PHARMACODYNAMIC PROPERTIES

Membrane Stabilizing Activity

At concentrations much higher than therapeutic levels, certain β-blockers have a quinidine-like or local anesthetic membrane stabilizing effect on the cardiac action potential. No evidence indicates that membrane stabilizing activity is responsible for any direct negative inotropic effect of the β-blockers, because drugs with and without this property can depress left ventricular function. However, membrane stabilizing activity can manifest clinically with massive β-blocker intoxications.[2,4]

β_1 Selectivity

When used in low doses, β_1-selective blocking agents such as acebutolol, betaxolol, bisoprolol, esmolol, atenolol, and metoprolol inhibit cardiac β_1-receptors but have less influence on bronchial and vascular β-adrenergic receptors (β_2). In higher doses, however, β_1-selective blocking agents also block β_2-receptors. Accordingly, β_1-selective agents may be safer than nonselective agents in patients with obstructive pulmonary disease, because β_2-receptors remain available to mediate

adrenergic bronchodilatation. However, even selective β-blockers may aggravate bronchospasm in certain patients, so these drugs should be used with caution in patients with bronchospastic disease.[2,4]

A second theoretical advantage is that, unlike nonselective β-blockers, β_1-selective blockers in low doses may not block the β_2-receptors that mediate dilatation of arterioles. It is possible that leaving the β_2-receptors unblocked and responsive to epinephrine may be functionally important in some patients with asthma, hypoglycemia, hypertension, or peripheral vascular disease who are treated with β-adrenergic blocking drugs.[2,4]

Intrinsic Sympathomimetic Activity or Partial Agonist Activity

Certain β-adrenergic receptor blockers possess partial agonist activity at β_1-adrenergic receptor sites, β_2-adrenergic receptor sites, or both. In a β-blocker, this property is identified as a slight cardiac stimulation that can be blocked by propranolol. The β-blockers with this property slightly activate the β-receptor in addition to preventing the access of natural or synthetic catecholamines to the receptor. In the treatment of patients with arrhythmias, angina pectoris, and hypertension, drugs with mild to moderate partial agonist activity appear to be as efficacious as β-blockers lacking this property. It is still debated whether the presence of partial agonist activity in a β-blocker constitutes an overall advantage or disadvantage in cardiac therapy. Drugs with partial agonist activity cause less slowing of the heart rate at rest than do propranolol and metoprolol, although the increments in heart rate with exercise are similarly blunted. β-Blocking agents with nonselective partial agonist activity reduce peripheral vascular resistance and may also cause less depression or atrioventricular conduction compared with drugs lacking this property.[2-6] However, drugs with partial agonist activity appear to be less protective against recurrent events in survivors of myocardial infarction than β-blockers without this property.

α-Adrenergic Activity

Carvedilol and labetalol are β-blockers with antagonistic properties at both α- and β-adrenergic receptors, with direct vasodilator activity. Like other β-blockers, they are useful in the treatment of hypertension and angina pectoris. However, unlike most β-blocking drugs, the additional α-adrenergic blocking actions of carvedilol and labetalol lead to a reduction in peripheral vascular resistance that may maintain cardiac output. Evidence indicates that carvedilol can provide a more favorable effect on the metabolic profile in patients with diabetes mellitus and hypertension than β-blockers without concomitant α-blocking activity.[7,8] In a recent study, carvedilol was shown not to affect glycemic control, although it improved some components of the metabolic syndrome relative to metoprolol in diabetic patients with hypertension.[8]

Nitric Oxide Potentiating Activity

A new generation of β-blockers is being evaluated (nebivolol, nipradilol) that have vasodilating activity related to an α-β-blocker enhancement of nitric oxide activity.[9] Whether this additional property will confer greater benefit in the treatment of cardiovascular disease has yet to be determined.

Table 19-1 Proposed Mechanisms to Explain the Antihypertensive Actions of β-Blockers

1. Reduction in cardiac output
2. Central nervous system effect
3. Inhibition of renin secretion (and possibly other steps in the renin-angiotensin-aldosterone cascade)
4. Reduction in plasma volume
5. Reduction in vasomotor tone
6. Reduction in peripheral vascular resistance
7. Improvement in vascular compliance
8. Resetting of baroreceptor levels
9. Effects on prejunctional β-receptors: reduction in norepinephrine release
10. Attenuation of pressor response to catecholamines with exercise and stress

Modified from Frishman WH, Silverman R. Physiologic and metabolic effects. *In:* Frishman WH (ed.). Clinical Pharmacology of the β-Adrenoceptor Blocking Drugs, 2nd ed. Norwalk, Conn: Appleton-Century-Crofts, 1984, pp 27-49.

PHARMACOKINETIC PROPERTIES

Although the β-adrenergic blocking drugs as a group have similar therapeutic effects, their pharmacokinetic properties are markedly different (Tables 19-3 and 19-4). Their varied aromatic ring structures lead to differences in completeness of gastrointestinal absorption, amount of first-pass hepatic metabolism, lipid solubility, protein binding, extent of distribution in the body, penetration into the brain, concentration in the heart, rate of hepatic biotransformation, pharmacologic activity of metabolites, and renal clearance of a drug and its metabolites that may influence the clinical usefulness of these drugs in some patients (Fig. 19-1).[2,4,7,10]

The β-blockers can be divided by their pharmacokinetic properties into two broad categories: those eliminated by hepatic metabolism, which tend to have relatively short plasma half-lives; and those eliminated unchanged by the kidney, which tend to have longer half-lives. Propranolol and metoprolol are both lipid soluble, are almost completely absorbed by the small intestine, and are largely metabolized by the liver. They tend to have highly variable bioavailability and relatively short plasma half-lives. Their plasma half-lives can also be influenced by gene polymorphisms of the cytochrome P-450A system in the liver.[11-13] A lack of correlation between the duration of clinical pharmacologic effect and plasma half-life may allow these drugs to be administered once or twice daily.[2,4]

In contrast, agents such as atenolol and nadolol are more water soluble, are incompletely absorbed through the gut, and are eliminated unchanged by the kidney. They tend to have less variable bioavailability in patients with normal renal function, in addition to longer half-lives, which allow once-daily dosing. The longer half-lives may be useful in patients who find adherence to frequent β-blocker administration a problem.[2,4]

Table 19-2 Pharmacodynamic Properties of β-Adrenergic Blocking Drugs Used for Hypertension in the United States

Drug	β_1-Blockade Potency Ratio (Propranolol = 1.0)	Relative β_1-Selectivity	Intrinsic Sympathomimetic Activity	Membrane Stabilizing Activity
Acebutolol	0.3	+	+	+
Atenolol	1.0	++	0	0
Betaxolol	1.0	++	0	+
Bisoprolol*	10.0	++	0	0
Carteolol	10.0	0	+	0
Carvedilol†	10.0	0	0	++
Labetalol‡	0.3	0	+?	0
Metoprolol	1.0	++	0	0
Nadolol	1.0	0	0	0
Penbutolol	1.0	0	+	0
Pindolol	6.0	0	++	+
Propranolol	1.0	0	0	++
Timolol	6.0	0	0	0

*Bisoprolol is also approved as a first-line antihypertensive therapy in combination with a very low dose diuretic.
†Carvedilol has additional α_1-adrenergic blocking activity without peripheral β_2-agonism.
‡Labetalol has additional α_1-adrenergic blocking activity and direct vasodilatory activity (β_2-agonism); it is available for use in intravenous form for hypertensive emergencies.
Modified from Frishman WH. Alpha and beta-adrenergic blocking drugs. *In:* Frishman WH, Sonnenblick EH, Sica DA (eds.). Cardiovascular Pharmacotherapeutics, 2nd ed. New York: McGraw Hill, 2003, pp 67-97.

Table 19-3   Pharmacokinetic Properties of β-Adrenoceptor Blocking Drugs Used in Hypertension

Drug	Extent of Absorption (% of Dose)	Extent of Bioavailability (% of Dose)	Dose-Dependent Bioavailability (Major First-Pass Hepatic Metabolism)	Interpatient Variations in Plasma Levels	β-Blocking Plasma Concentrations	Protein Binding (%)	Lipid Solubility*
Acebutolol	≈90	≈40	Yes	7-fold	0.2–2.0 µg/mL	25	Low
Atenolol	≈50	≈40	No	4-fold	0.2–5.0 µg/mL	<5	Low
Betaxolol	>90	≈80	No	2-fold	0.005–0.05 µg/mL	50	Low
Bisoprolol	>90	≈88	No		0.005–0.02 µg/mL	≈30	Low
Carteolol	≈90	≈90	No	2-fold	40–160 ng/mL	20–30	Low
Carvedilol	>90	≈30	Yes	5–10- fold	10–100 ng/mL	98	Moderate
Celiprolol	≈30	≈30	No	3-fold		22–24	Low
Esmolol†	NA	NA	NA	5-fold	0.15–1.0 µg/mL	55	Low
Labetalol	>90	≈33	Yes	10-fold	0.7–3.0 µg/mL	≈50	Moderate
Metoprolol	>90	≈50	Yes	10-fold	50–100 ng/mL	12	Moderate
Metoprolol LA‡	>90	65–70	Yes	10-fold	35-323 ng/mL	12	Moderate
Nadolol	≈30	≈30	No	7-fold	50–100 ng/mL	≈30	Low
Nebivolol	>90	12–96	Yes	7-fold	1.5 ng/mL	98	High
Oxprenolol	≈90	19–74	Yes	5-fold	80–100 ng/mL	80	Moderate
Penbutolol	>90	≈100	No	4-fold	5–15 ng/mL	80-98	High
Pindolol	>90	≈90	No	4-fold	50–100 ng/mL	57	Moderate
Propranolol	>90	30–70	Yes	20-fold	50–100 ng/mL	93	High
Propranolol LA‡ Propranolol CR§	>90	30–40	Yes	20–30-fold	20–100 ng/mL	93	High
Sotalol	≈70	≈90	No	4-fold	1–3.2 µg/mL	0	Low
Timolol	>90	≈75	Yes	7-fold	5–10 ng/mL	≈10	Low-Moderate

*Determined by the distribution ratio between octanol and water.
†Ultra short-acting β-blocker available only in intravenous form.
‡Propranolol and metoprolol succinate are available in an extended-release (LA) formulation.
§Propanolol is also available in a delayed-release/extended-release (CR) formulation designed to be taken orally at bedtime.
Modified from Frishman WH. Alpha- and beta-adrenergic blocking drugs. *In:* Frishman WH, Sonnenblick EH, Sica DA (eds.). Cardiovascular Pharmacotherapeutics, 2nd ed. New York: McGraw Hill, 2003, pp 67-97.

Extended-release formulations of metoprolol and propranolol are available that allow once-daily dosing of these drugs. Both long-acting propranolol and metoprolol provide much smoother curves of daily plasma levels than do comparable divided doses of conventional propranolol and metoprolol. In addition, a delayed-release/extended-release chronotherapeutic formulation of propranolol is available that is taken at night to address circadian variations in blood pressure, in an attempt to blunt early morning elevations while providing 24-hour blood pressure control.[14,15] Although early morning blood pressure peaks have been associated with increased cardiovascular and cerebrovascular events, the clinical significance of early morning pressure blunting with delayed-release drugs has not yet been shown.[16] Sublingual and nasal spray formulations that can provide immediate β-blockade have been tested in clinical trials.[2,4]

Ultra–short-acting β-blockers are available and may be useful when a short duration of action is desired (e.g., in patients with questionable heart failure). One of these compounds, esmolol, a β₁-selective drug, has been shown to be useful in the treatment of perioperative hypertension and supraventricular tachycardias. Blood and hepatic esterases metabolize this drug rapidly, independently of disease status, and this accounts for its short half-life (~7 to 15 minutes).[17]

EFFECTS ON BLOOD PRESSURE

β-Adrenergic blockers, alone and in combination with other antihypertensive agents, reduce blood pressure at rest and during exercise in patients with combined systolic and diastolic hypertension and in those with isolated systolic hypertension.[18-21] β-Blockers are also available in combination formulations with diuretics in very low and conventional diuretic doses and (in Europe) in a formulation combining long-acting metoprolol with felodipine.[22] The effects of β-blockers in hypertensive patients may relate to the presence of specific genetic polymorphisms of both the β₁- and β₂-adrenergic receptors.[23-28] Some of these polymorphisms may also provide a genetic basis for hypertension.[23-27] Uncommonly, a paradoxical elevation of systolic pressure occurs during β-blockade in persons with severe aortic stenosis, presumably as a result of the increased stroke volume caused by rate slowing in the setting of increased impedance. Escalating doses of β-blockers

Table 19-4 Elimination Characteristics of β-Adrenoceptor Blocking Drugs Used in Hypertension

Drug	Elimination Half-Life (hr)	Total Body Clearance (mL/min)	Urinary Recovery of Unchanged Drug (% of Dose)	Total Urinary Recovery (% of Dose)	Predominant Route of Elimination	Active Metabolites	Drug Accumulation in Renal Disease
Acebutolol	3–4*	480	≈40	>90	RE (≈40% unchanged and HM)	Yes	Yes
Atenolol	6–9	130	≈40	>95	RE	No	Yes
Betaxolol	15	350	15	>90	HM	No	Yes
Bisoprolol	9–12	260	50	>98	RE + HM	No	Yes
Carteolol	5–6	497	40–68	90	RE	Yes	Yes
Carvedilol	7–10	600†	<2	16	HM	Yes	No
Celiprolol	5	500	≈90	≈30	RE (≈50% unchanged and HM)	Yes	No
Esmolol	≈9 min	19,950	1–2	71–88	Red blood cells	No	Yes
Labetalol	3–4	2,700	<1	>90	HM	No	No
Metoprolol	3–4	1,100	≈3	>95	HM	No	No
Metoprolol LA	3–4	1,100	≈3	>95	HM	No	No
Nebivolol‡	8–27	—	<1	—	HM	No	Yes
Oxprenolol‡	2	—	<3	—	HM	—	No
Penbutolol	27	350	50–70	>90	RE	No	No
Pindolol	3–4	400	≈40	>90	RE (≈40% unchanged and HM)	No	No
Propranolol	3–4	1,000	<1	>90	HM	Yes	No
Propranolol LA§ Propranolol CR	10	1,000	<1	>90	HM	Yes	No
Timolol	4–5	660	≈20	65	RE (≈20% unchanged and HM)	No	No

*Acebutolol has an active metabolite with an elimination half-life of 8 to 13 hours.
†Plasma clearance.
‡Nebivolol, a β-blocking drug with nitric oxide–enhancing effect, and oxprenolol, a nonselective β-blocker with partial agonism, are not available in the United States.
§Includes the extended-release (LA) and delayed-release/extended-release (CR) formulations.
HM, hepatic metabolism; RE, renal excretion.
Modified from Frishman WH, Silverman R. Physiologic and metabolic effects. In: Frishman WH (ed.). Clinical Pharmacology of the β-Adrenoceptor Blocking Drugs, 2nd ed. Norwalk, Conn: Appleton-Century-Crofts, 1984, pp 27-49.

and combined α-β-blockers can induce salt and water retention, thus making diuretics a not uncommon adjunctive therapy.[29] The β-blocking drugs are considered to be an alternative first-line treatment for hypertension and are also indicated for patients having concomitant angina pectoris, arrhythmias, hypertrophic cardiomyopathy, congestive cardiomyopathy, hyperdynamic circulations, essential tremor, or migraine headaches.[2,6,29-35] Some β-adrenergic blockers reduce the risk of mortality in survivors of acute myocardial infarction, with and without heart failure.[36,37] Some drugs can be used with caution in pregnancy, and they appear to be especially useful in treating and preventing perioperative hypertension.[38,39] Evidence also indicates that β-blockers can reduce levels of C-reactive protein, an inflammatory marker of cardiovascular risk.[40]

Most antihypertensive drugs, including β-blockers, may reduce left ventricular mass and wall thickness.[41,42] However, in a study of patients with stage 2 hypertension and electrocardiographic evidence of left ventricular hypertrophy, losartan had a greater effect on left ventricular hypertrophy regression than did atenolol, despite similar blood pressure control.[43,44] In this study, losartan was also more effective in preventing the primary composite endpoint of myocardial infarction, stroke, or cardiovascular death.[45] A recent meta-analysis concluded that atenolol may have less protective effect on cardiovascular endpoints than other antihypertensive treatments, including other β-blockers.[46]

Some β-adrenergic blockers (those not having partial agonist activity) may not be as effective as other antihypertensive treatments in black patients. Similar observations have been

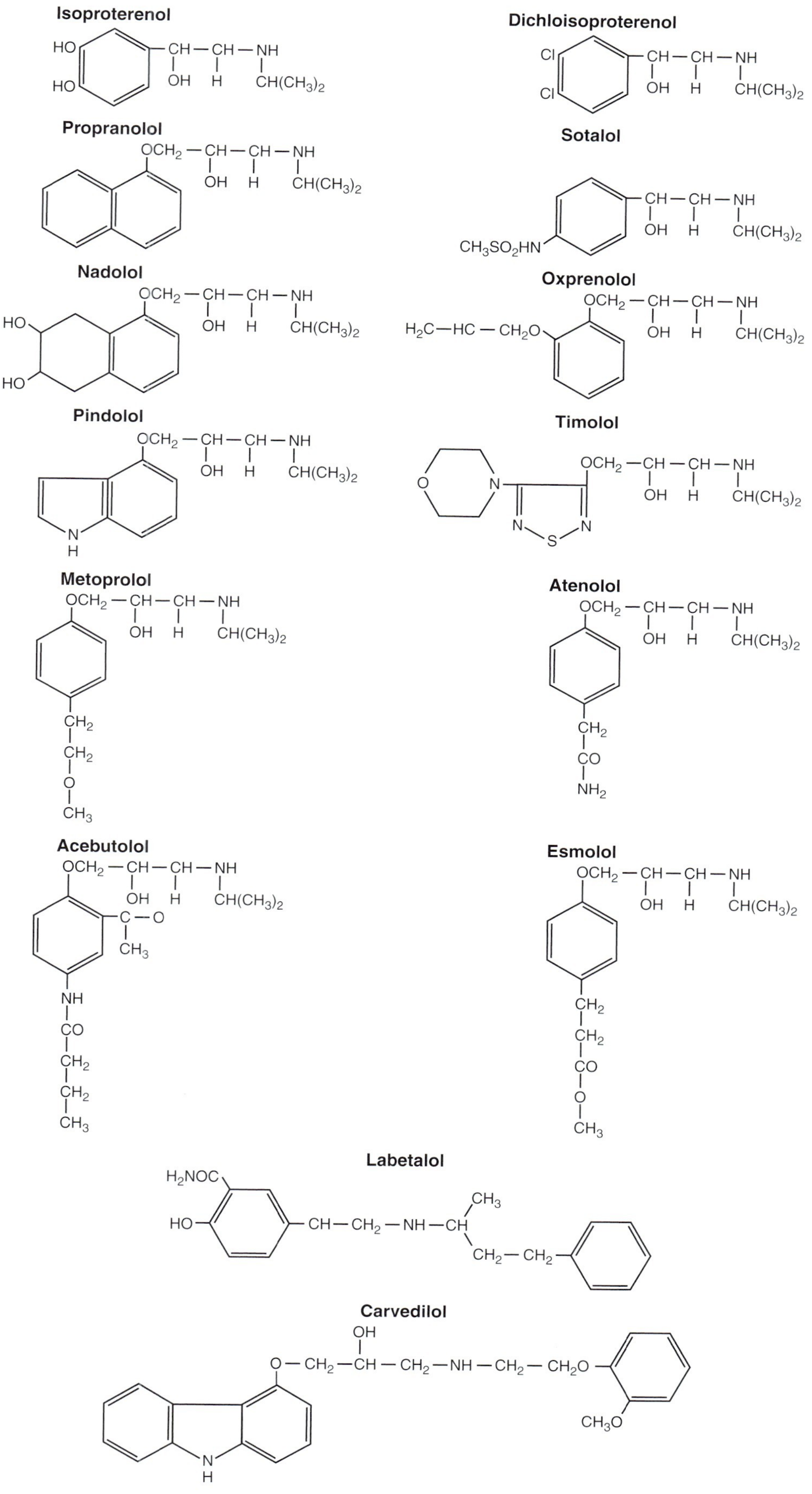

Figure 19–1 Molecular structure of the β-adrenergic agonist isoproterenol and some β-adrenergic blocking drugs.

made in older patients.[47,48] However, when combined with a diuretic, β-blockers appear to be as effective as other combination treatment regimens in both black and elderly patients.[2,4]

The α-β-blocker labetalol is the only β-blocker indicated for parenteral management of hypertensive emergencies and for treatment of intraoperative and postoperative hypertension. It can also be used in oral form to treat patients with hypertensive urgencies.[2,4]

ADVERSE EFFECTS AND CONTRAINDICATIONS

β-Adrenergic blockers should not be used in patients with moderate to severe asthma, unstable heart failure resulting from systolic dysfunction, heart block (greater than first degree), or the sick sinus syndrome (without a pacemaker).[2-6] The β_1-selective blockers and the α-β-blockers appear to be safe to use in patients with chronic obstructive pulmonary disease and mild reactive airways disease.[49,50] The α-β-blocker, carvedilol, reduced morbidity and mortality in patients with stable New York Heart Association class II to IV heart failure who were receiving diuretics, angiotensin-converting enzyme inhibitors, or digoxin.[30,51,52] The β_1-selective agents bisoprolol and the extended-release formulation of metoprolol also reduced morbidity and mortality in patients with stable New York Heart Association class II to III heart failure.[53,54]

β-Blockers should be used with caution in patients with insulin-dependent diabetes because these agents may worsen glucose intolerance and may mask the symptoms of and prolong recovery from hypoglycemia. There is probably a shorter recovery period from hypoglycemia with β_1-selective adrenergic blockers.[2,4] β-Blockers should not be discontinued abruptly in patients with known ischemic heart disease.[2-6] In a prospective cohort study, investigators found that antihypertensive therapy with β-blockers was associated with a greater incidence of type 2 diabetes than was therapy with angiotensin-converting enzyme inhibitors, diuretics, or calcium blockers.[55] However, this increased risk of new-onset diabetes must be weighed against the proven benefit of β-blockers in reducing the risk of cardiovascular events, especially in secondary prevention.[56-58]

β-Blockers may increase levels of plasma triglycerides and reduce those of high-density lipoprotein cholesterol.[59] Despite this effect, β-blockers without intrinsic sympathomimetic activity are the only agents conclusively shown to decrease the rate of sudden death, overall mortality, and recurrent myocardial infarction in survivors of acute myocardial infarction.[36] β-Blockers with intrinsic sympathomimetic activity or α-blocking activity have little or no adverse effects on plasma lipids.[7,59]

Dreams, hallucinations, insomnia, and depression can occur during therapy with β-blockers.[5,60] These symptoms provide evidence of drug entry into the central nervous system and may be more common with the highly lipid-soluble β-blockers (propranolol, metoprolol), which presumably penetrate the central nervous system better. Investigators have claimed that β-blockers with less lipid solubility (atenolol, nadolol) cause fewer central nervous system side effects.[61,62] This claim is intriguing, but its validity has not been corroborated by clinical trials[63] or other extensive clinical experiences.[64,65]

There are special considerations when β-blockers are combined with other drugs.[11,66,67] Combinations of diltiazem or verapamil with β-blockers may have additional sinoatrial and atrioventricular node depressant effects and may also promote negative inotropy.[66] Combinations of β-blockers and reserpine may cause marked bradycardia and syncope. Combination with phenylpropanolamine, pseudoephedrine, ephedrine, and epinephrine can cause elevations in blood pressure because of unopposed α-receptor–induced vasoconstriction.

SUMMARY

β-Adrenergic blockers remain important drug treatments for the management of systemic hypertension and are useful in patients with hypertension who also have concomitant angina pectoris, heart failure, or arrhythmias. β-Adrenergic blockers have also been shown conclusively to reduce the risk of mortality and nonfatal reinfarction in survivors of acute myocardial infarction. β-Adrenergic blockers can be differentiated from one another by the presence or absence of intrinsic sympathomimetic activity, membrane stabilizing activity, β_1-receptor selectivity, α_1-adrenergic blocking activity, solubilities, and routes of elimination.

References

1. Chobanian AV, Bakris GL, Black HR, et al., and the National High Blood Pressure Education Program Coordinating Committee. The Seventh Report of the Joint National Committee on Prevention, Detection, Evaluation and Treatment of High Blood Pressure: The JNC 7 Report. *JAMA*. 2003;**289**:2560-2572.
2. Frishman WH, Sonnenblick EH. β-Adrenergic blocking drugs and calcium channel blockers. *In:* Alexander RW, Schlant RC, Fuster V (eds.). Hurst's The Heart, 9th ed. New York: McGraw-Hill, 1998, pp 1583-1618.
3. Frishman WH, Bryzinski BS, Coulson LR, et al. A multifactorial trial design to assess combination therapy in hypertension: Treatment with bisoprolol and hydrochlorothiazide. *Arch Intern Med*. 1994;**154**:1461-1468.
4. Frishman WH. Alpha and beta-adrenergic blocking drugs. *In:* Frishman WH, Sonnenblick EH, Sica DA (eds.). Cardiovascular Pharmacotherapeutics, 2nd ed. New York: McGraw-Hill, 2003, pp 67-97.
5. Frishman WH. Alpha and beta-adrenergic blocking drugs. *In:* Frishman WH, Sonnenblick EH, Sica DA (eds.). Cardiovascular Pharmacotherapeutics Manual, 2nd ed. New York: McGraw-Hill, 2004, pp 19-57.
6. Frishman WH, Silverman R. Physiologic and metabolic effects. *In:* Frishman WH (ed.). Clinical Pharmacology of the β-Adrenoceptor Blocking Drugs, 2nd ed. Norwalk, Conn: Appleton-Century-Crofts, l984, pp 27-49.
7. Reiter MJ. Cardiovascular drug class specificity: β-Blockers. *Prog Cardiovasc Dis* 2004;**47**:11-33.
8. Bakris GL, Fonseca V, Katholi RE, et al. Metabolic effects of carvedilol vs. metoprolol in patients with type 2 diabetes mellitus and hypertension: A randomized controlled trial. *JAMA*. 2004;**292**:2227-2236.
9. Sule SS, Frishman WH. Nebivolol. New therapy update. *Cardiol Rev*. 2006;**14**:259-264.
10. Frishman WH, Alwarshetty M. Beta-adrenergic blockers in systemic hypertension: Pharmacokinetic considerations related to the JNC-VI and WHO-ISH guidelines. *Clin Pharmacokinet*. 2002;**41**:505-516.

11. Frishman WH, Opie LH, Sica DA. Adverse cardiovascular drug interactions and complications. *In:* Fuster V, Alexander RW, O'Rourke RA, et al. (eds.). Hurst's The Heart, 11th ed. New York: McGraw-Hill, 2004, pp 2169-2188.

12. Kirchheiner J, Heesch C, Bauer F, et al. Impact of ultrarapid metabolizer genotype of cytochrome P450 2D6 on metoprolol pharmacokinetics and pharmacodynamics. *Clin Pharm Ther.* 2004;**76**:302-312.

13. Cheng JWM. Cytochrome P450-mediated cardiovascular drug interactions. *Heart Dis.* 2000;**2**:254-258.

14. Sica D, Frishman WH, Manowitz N. Pharmacokinetics of propranolol after single and multiple dosing with sustained release propranolol or propranolol CR (Innopran XL™), a new chronotherapeutic formulation. *Heart Dis.* 2003;**5**:176-181.

15. Sica DA, Neutel JM, Weber MA, Manowitz N. The antihypertensive efficacy and safety of a chronotherapeutic formulation of propranolol in patients with hypertension. *J Clin Hypertens (Greenwich).* 2004;**6**:231-241.

16. Black HR, Elliott WJ, Grandits G, et al. Principal results of the Controlled Onset Verapamil Investigation of Cardiovascular End Points (CONVINCE) trial. *JAMA.* 2003;**289**:2073-2082.

17. Frishman WH, Murthy VS, Strom JA, Hershman D. Ultrashort-acting β-adrenoreceptor blocking drug: Esmolol. *In:* Messerli FH (ed.). Cardiovascular Drug Therapy, 2nd ed. Philadelphia: WB Saunders, 1996, pp 507-516.

18. Systolic Hypertension in the Elderly Program Cooperative Research Group. Implications of the Systolic Hypertension in the Elderly Program. *Hypertension.* 1993;**21**:335-343.

19. Materson BJ, Reda DJ, Cushman WC, et al., for the Department of Veterans Affairs Cooperative Study Group on Antihypertensive Agents. Single-drug therapy for hypertension in men: A comparison of six antihypertensive agents with placebo. *N Engl J Med.* 1993;**328**:914-921.

20. Psaty BM, Smith NL, Siscovick DS, et al. Health outcomes associated with antihypertensive therapies used as first-line agents: A systematic review and meta-analysis. *JAMA.* 1997;**277**:739-745.

21. Kokkinos P, Chrysohoon C, Panagiotakos D, et al. Beta-blockade mitigates exercise blood pressure in hypertensive male patients. *J Am Coll Cardiol.* 2006;**47**:794-798.

22. Frishman WH, Hainer JW, Sugg J, M-FACT Study Group. A factorial study of combination hypertension treatment with metoprolol succinate extended release and felodipine extended release results of the Metoprolol Succinate-Felodipine Antihypertension Combination Trial (M-FACT). *Am J Hypertens.* 2006;**19**:388-395.

23. Bengtsson K, Melander O, Orho-Melander M, et al. Polymorphism in the β_1-adrenergic receptor gene and hypertension. *Circulation.* 2001;**104**:187-190.

24. Sofowora GG, Dishy V, Muszkat M, et al. A common β_1-adrenergic receptor polymorphism (Arg389Gly) affects blood pressure response to β-blockade. *Clin Pharmacol Ther.* 2003;**73**:366-371.

25. Liu J, Liu Z-Q, Tan Z-R, et al. Gly389Arg polymorphism of β_1-adrenergic receptor is associated with the cardiovascular response to metoprolol. *Clin Pharmacol Ther.* 2003;**74**:372-379.

26. Dishy V, Sofowora GG, Xie H-G, et al. The effect of common polymorphisms of the β_2-adrenergic receptor on agonist-mediated vascular desensitization. *N Engl J Med.* 2001;**345**:1030-1035.

27. Kato N, Sugiyama T, Morita H, et al. Association analysis of β_2-adrenergic receptor polymorphisms with hypertension in Japanese. *Hypertension.* 2001;**37**:286-292.

28. Masuo K, Katsuya T, Fu Y, et al. β2- and β3-adrenergic receptor polymorphisms are related to the onset of weight gain and blood pressure elevation over 5 years. *Circulation.* 2005;**111**:3429-3434.

29. Frishman WH, Sica DA. β-Adrenergic blockers. *In:* Izzo JL Jr, Black HR (eds.). Hypertension Primer, 3rd ed. Dallas, Tex: American Heart Association, 2005, pp 417-421.

30. Frishman WH. Carvedilol. *N Engl J Med.* 1998;**339**:1759-1765.

31. Abrams J, Frishman WH, Bates SM, et al. Pharmacologic options for treatment of ischemic disease. *In:* Antman ED (ed.). Cardiovascular Therapeutics: A Companion to Braunwald's Heart Disease, 2nd ed. Philadelphia: WB Saunders, 2002, pp 97-153.

32. Fihn SD, Williams SV, Daley J, Gibbons RJ. Guidelines for the management of patients with chronic stable angina: Treatment. *Ann Intern Med.* 2001;**135**:616-632.

33. Heidenreich PA, McDonald KM, Hastie T, et al. Meta-analysis of trials comparing β-blockers, calcium antagonists and nitrates for stable angina. *JAMA.* 1999;**281**:1927-1936.

34. LeJemtel TH, Sonnenblick EH, Frishman WH. Diagnosis and management of heart failure. *In:* Fuster V, Alexander RW, O'Rourke RA, et al. (eds.). Hurst's The Heart, 11th ed. New York: McGraw-Hill, 2004, pp 723-762.

35. Frishman WH, Cavusoglu E. β-Adrenergic blockers and their role in the therapy of arrhythmias. *In:* Podrid PJ, Kowey PR (eds.). Cardiac Arrhythmias: Mechanisms, Diagnosis and Management. Baltimore: Williams & Wilkins 1995, pp 421-433.

36. Frishman WH. Role of β-adrenergic blockade. *In:* Fuster V, Topol EJ, Nabel EG (eds.). Atherothrombosis and Coronary Artery Disease, 2nd ed. Philadelphia: Lippincott Williams & Wilkins, 2005, pp 1239-1247.

37. CAPRICORN Investigators. Effect of carvedilol on outcome after myocardial infarction in patients with left ventricular dysfunction: The CAPRICORN randomized trial. *Lancet.* 2001;**357**:1385-1390.

38. Qasqas SA, McPherson C, Frishman WH, Elkayam U. Cardiovascular pharmacotherapeutic considerations during pregnancy and lactation. *Cardiol Rev.* 2004;**12**:201-221, 240-261.

39. Auerbach AD, Goldman L. β-Blockers and reduction of cardiac events in noncardiac surgery: Clinical applications. *JAMA.* 2002;**287**:1445-1447.

40. Jenkins NP, Keevil BG, Hutchinson IV, Brooks NH. Beta blockers are associated with lower C-reactive protein concentrations in patients with coronary artery disease. *Am J Med.* 2002;**112**:269-274.

41. Devereux RB. Left ventricular hypertrophy and angiotensin II antagonists. *Am J Hypertens.* 2001;**14**:174-182.

42. Hachamovitch R, Strom JA, Sonnenblick EH, Frishman WH. Left ventricular hypertrophy in hypertension and the effects of antihypertensive drug therapy. *Curr Probl Cardiol.* 1988;**13**:371-421.

43. Okin PM, Devereux RB, Jerns S, et al. Regression of electrocardiographic left ventricular hypertrophy by losartan versus atenolol: The Losartan Intervention for Endpoint Reduction in Hypertension (LIFE) study. *Circulation.* 2003;**108**:684-690.

44. Devereux RB, Dahlof B, Gerdts E, et al. Regression of hypertensive left ventricular hypertrophy by losartan compared with atenolol: The Losartan Intervention for Endpoint Reduction in Hypertension (LIFE) trial. *Circulation.* 2004;**110**:1456-1462.

45. Dahlof B, Devereux RB, Kjeldsen SE, et al. Cardiovascular morbidity and mortality in the Losartan Intervention for Endpoint Reduction in Hypertension study (LIFE): A randomized trial against atenolol. *Lancet.* 2002;**359**:995-1003.

46. Carlberg B, Samuelsson O, Lindholm LH. Atenolol in hypertension: Is it a wise choice? *Lancet.* 2004;**364**:1684-1689.

47. Messerli FH, Frossman E, Goldbourt U. Are β-blockers efficacious as first-line therapy for hypertension in the elderly? *JAMA.* 1998;**279**:1903-1907.

48. Messerli FH, Beevers DG, Franklin SS, Pickering TG. β-Blockers in hypertension—the emperor has no clothes: An open letter to present and prospective drafters of new guidelines for the treatment of hypertension. *Am J Hypertens.* 2003;**16**:870-873.

49. Salpeter SR, Ormiston TM, Salpeter EE. Cardioselective β-blockers in patients with reactive airway disease: A meta-analysis. *Ann Intern Med.* 2002;**137**:715-725.

50. Sirak TE, Jelic S, LeJemtel TH. Therapeutic update: Non-selective beta- and alpha-adrenergic blockade in patients with coexistent chronic obstructive pulmonary disease and chronic heart failure. *J Am Coll Cardiol.* 2004;**44**:497-502.

51. Packer M, Fowler MB, Roecker EB et al., for the COPERNICUS Study Group. Effect of carvedilol on morbidity of patients with severe chronic heart failure: Results of the Carvedilol Prospective Randomized Cumulative Survival (COPERNICUS) Study. *Circulation.* 2002;**106**:2194-2199.

52. Poole-Wilson PA, Swedberg K, Cleland JGF, et al. for the COMET Investigators. Comparison of carvedilol and metoprolol on clinical outcomes in patients with chronic heart failure in the Carvedilol or Metoprolol European Trial (COMET): Randomized controlled trial. *Lancet.* 2003;**362**:7-13.

53. CIBIS II. The Cardiac Insufficiency Bisoprolol Study II: A randomized trial. *Lancet.* 1999;**353**:9-13.

54. Hjalmarson A, Goldstein S, Fagerberg B et al., for the MERIT-HF Study Group. Effect of controlled-release metoprolol on total mortality, hospitalizations and well-being in patients with heart failure: The Metoprolol CR/XL Randomized Intervention Trial in Congestive Heart Failure (MERIT-HF). *JAMA.* 2000;**283**:1295-1302.

55. Gress TW, Nieto J, Shahar E, et al., for the Atherosclerosis Risk in Communities Study. Hypertension and antihypertensive therapy as risk factors for type 2 diabetes mellitus. *N Engl J Med.* 2000;**342**:905-912.

56. Sowers JR, Bakris GL. Antihypertensive therapy and the risk of type 2 diabetes mellitus [editorial]. *N Engl J Med.* 2000;**342**:969-970.

57. Dunne F, Kendall MJ, Martin U. β-Blockers in the management of hypertension in patients with type 2 diabetes mellitus. *Drugs.* 2001;**61**:429-435.

58. Kostis JB, Wilson AC, Freudenberger RS, et al. Long-term effect of diuretic-based therapy on fatal outcomes in subjects with isolated systolic hypertension with and without diabetes. *Am J Cardiol.* 2005;**95**:29-35.

59. Shachter NS, Zimetbaum P, Frishman WH. Lipid-lowering drugs. *In:* Frishman WH, Sonnenblick EH, Sica DA (eds.). Cardiovascular Pharmacotherapeutics, 2nd ed. New York: McGraw-Hill 2003, pp 317-353.

60. Frishman WH, Razin A, Swencionis C, Sonnenblick EH. Beta-adrenoceptor blockade in anxiety states: A new approach to therapy. Update. *Cardiovasc Rev Rev.* 1992;**13**:8-13.

61. Frishman WH. Atenolol and timolol: Two new systemic adrenoceptor antagonists. *N Engl J Med.* 1982;**306**:1456-1462.

62. Frishman WH. Nadolol: A new β-adrenoceptor antagonist. *N Engl J Med.* 1981;**305**:678-684.

63. Ko DT, Hebert PR, Coffey CS, et al. Beta-blocker therapy and symptoms of depression, fatigue, and sexual dysfunction. *JAMA.* 2002;**288**:351-357.

64. Wurzelman J, Frishman MW, Aronson M, et al. Neuropsychiatric effects of antihypertensive drugs in the old old. *Cardiol Clin.* 1987;**5**:689-699.

65. Perez-Stable EJ, Halliday R, Gardiner PS, et al. The effects of propranolol on cognitive function and quality of life: A randomized trial among patients with diastolic hypertension. *Am J Med.* 2000;**108**:359-365.

66. Frishman WH, Sica DA. Calcium channel blockers. *In:* Frishman WH, Sonnenblick EH, Sica DA (eds.). Cardiovascular Pharmacotherapeutics, 2nd ed. New York: McGraw-Hill, 2003, pp 105-130.

67. Opie LH. Cardiovascular drug interactions. *In:* Frishman WH, Sonnenblick EH, Sica DA (eds.). Cardiovascular Pharmacotherapeutics, 2nd ed. New York: McGraw-Hill, 2003, pp 875-891.

Angiotensin-Converting Enzyme Inhibitors

Domenic A. Sica

Angiotensin-converting enzyme (ACE) inhibitors were originally developed as antihypertensive agents, but their efficacy in treating or preventing progressive renal, cardiac, and vascular disease was soon recognized.[1,2] In the United States, 10 ACE inhibitors are available, and additional agents are marketed in other countries. Individual agents are now approved for heart failure (HF), post–myocardial infarction (post-MI) status, diabetic nephropathy, and primary prevention of cardiovascular events in high-risk patients without left ventricular dysfunction (Tables 20-1 and 20-2).[2]

PHARMACOLOGY

In 1981, captopril, the first orally active ACE inhibitor, was introduced. Shortly thereafter, the longer-acting compounds enalapril maleate and lisinopril became available. Enalapril is a prodrug requiring in vivo esterolysis (in the liver and intestinal wall) to yield enalaprilat, the active acid, which can be given intravenously. Except for captopril and lisinopril, all ACE inhibitors are given orally as ethyl esters, because the parent acids are poorly absorbed and have limited and erratic biovailability.[2] In the presence of hepatic impairment (e.g., in advanced HF), the conversion of an ACE inhibitor's ester to the active acid metabolite takes place efficiently in the intestinal wall, with little adverse therapeutic consequence.

ACE inhibitors can be divided into three structurally heterogeneous groups, based on the ligand that binds to ACE: sulfhydryl-, phosphinyl-, and carboxyl-containing compounds. The sulfhydryl moiety in captopril has been implicated in the maculopapular skin rash and dysgeusia seen more commonly with this ACE inhibitor compared with other agents. Otherwise, these distinguishing chemical features of various ACE inhibitors have not played a prominent role in their pharmacology. Allegations of free-radical scavenging by a sulfhydryl group (in captopril) and improved penetration of a phosphinyl group (in fosinopril) into diseased myocardium remain largely unproven in humans.

Rate and extent of absorption, plasma protein binding, systemic half-life, and mode of clearance can further differentiate ACE inhibitors. With the possible exceptions of route of elimination and tissue binding, however, these differences do not have an impact on the ACE inhibitors' blood pressure (BP)-lowering effects, if comparable doses are given and adequate frequency of administration is maintained (see Table 20-2).[2]

Route of Elimination

In the presence of chronic kidney disease (CKD), the prodrugs ramipril, enalapril, fosinopril, trandolapril, and benazepril do not accumulate in plasma despite repetitive administration, a finding suggesting that these compounds either undergo some biliary clearance or their conversion to the pharmacologically active acids is independent of renal function. Each of these five prodrugs is marginally active, so their failure to accumulate in CKD matters little. ACE inhibitor accumulation in CKD is really important only if there is a buildup of the active acidic metabolites. Fosinoprilat and trandolaprilat, the active acidic metabolites of fosinopril and trandolapril, are the only metabolites that undergo both renal and hepatic elimination. Other ACE inhibitors are cleared renally, by filtration and tubular secretion, and they do accumulate, even in early CKD. This appears not to be associated with a meaningful increase in the frequency of cough or angioneurotic edema, but when ACE inhibitor concentrations rise, BP can be significantly reduced, and end-organ underperfusion can occur.

Tissue Binding

The second potentially differentiating pharmacologic feature of ACE inhibitors is tissue binding. ACE inhibitors can be arbitrarily classified according to their binding affinity for tissue ACE, which depends on binding affinity, potency, lipophilicity, and depot effect.[3] The degree to which tissue ACE is blocked by an ACE inhibitor corresponds both to the drug's natural binding affinity and the free inhibitor concentration within that tissue compartment. The tissue-based free inhibitor concentration is in a constant state of flux and is calculated by summing the amount of ACE inhibitor conveyed to tissues and the residual ACE inhibitor released from tissue depot sites. The quantity of ACE inhibitor transferred to tissues is determined by several pharmacologic variables, including dose frequency and amount, absolute bioavailability, plasma half-life, and the potential for tissue penetration. When blood levels of an ACE inhibitor are high, generally in the first half of the dosing interval, tissue retention of an ACE inhibitor is not needed for a durable level of ACE inhibition. However, during the second half of the dosing interval, as ACE inhibitor blood levels decrease, two factors—inhibitor binding affinity and tissue retention—assume added importance if effective ACE inhibition is to continue.[3]

Varying degrees of tissue ACE inhibition across ACE inhibitors appear to have little impact on their ability to reduce BP similarly. Most of the studies that claim a difference in BP lowering, based on differential tissue-binding of tested ACE inhibitors, did not use equivalent doses.

Some investigators have claimed that ACE inhibitors with a high tissue affinity provide BP-independent end-organ protection, as with the ACE inhibitor, ramipril, in the Heart Outcomes Prevention Evaluation (HOPE).[4] In several studies, endothelial function more regularly improves with higher-affinity tissue ACE compounds, such as quinapril and ramipril. If improvement in endothelial dysfunction is accepted as a

Table 20-1   United States Food and Drug Administration–Approved Indications for Angiotensin-Converting Enzyme Inhibitors

Drug	Hypertension	Heart Failure	Diabetic Nephropathy	High-Risk Patients without Left Ventricular Dysfunction
Benazepril	•			
Captopril	•	• (Post-MI)*	• ‡	
Enalapril	•	• †		
Fosinopril	•	•		
Lisinopril	•	• (Post-MI)*		
Moexipril	•			
Perindopril	•			•
Quinapril	•	•		
Ramipril	•	• (Post-MI)		•
Trandolapril	•	• (Post-MI)		

*Captopril and lisinopril are indicated for heart failure both after myocardial infarction and as adjunctive therapy in general.
†Enalapril is indicated for asymptomatic left ventricular dysfunction.
‡Captopril is indicated in the treatment of type 1 diabetic nephropathy only.
MI, myocardial infarction.

Table 20-2   Angiotensin-Converting Enzyme Inhibitors: Dosage Strengths and Treatment Guidelines

Drug	Trade Name (in United States)	Usual Total Dose and/or Range (in mg): Hypertension (Frequency/day)	Usual Total Dose and/or Range (in mg): Heart Failure (Frequency/day)	Fixed-Dose Combination*
Benazepril	Lotensin	20–40 (1)	Not FDA approved for heart failure	Lotensin HCT, Lotrel
Captopril	Capoten	12.5–100 (2–3)	18.75–150 (3)	Capozide†
Enalapril	Vasotec	5–40 (1–2)	5–40 (2)	Vaseretic, Lexxel
Fosinopril	Monopril	10–40 (1)	10–40 (1)	Monopril-HCT
Lisinopril	Prinivil, Zestril	2.5–40 (1)	5–20 (1)	Prinzide, Zestoretic
Moexipril	Univasc	7.5–30 (1)	Not FDA approved for heart failure	Uniretic
Perindopril	Aceon	2–16 (1)	Not FDA approved for heart failure	
Quinapril	Accupril	5–80 (1)	10–40 (1–2)	Accuretic
Ramipril	Altace	2.5–20 (1)	10 (2)	
Trandolapril	Mavik	1–8 (1)	1–4 (1)	Tarka

*These fixed-dose combinations typically contain a thiazide-like diuretic other than for Tarka, which contains the calcium channel blocker verapamil; Lotrel, which contains the calcium channel blocker amlodipine; or Lexxel, which contains the calcium channel blocker felodipine extended release.
†Capozide is indicated for first-step treatment of hypertension.
FDA, U.S. Food and Drug Administration.

surrogate for protection from clinical events, then relevant differences may exist among ACE inhibitors. However, head-to-head comparisons of different ACE inhibitors do not convincingly support the claim of overall superiority for lipophilic ACE inhibitors.[5]

Application of Pharmacologic Differences

Because little truly separates one long-acting ACE inhibitor from another in the treatment of hypertension, the cost of an ACE inhibitor has assumed added importance.[6] *Class effect* is a commonly used phrase to justify use of a less costly ACE inhibitor when a higher-priced agent in the class has been the one specifically shown to have benefits in complex disease states, such as HF, diabetic nephropathy, or prevention of cardiovascular events in high-risk patients.[4,7,8] The concept of class effect, already vague in its definition, becomes even more

hazy when "true" dose equivalence for a non-BP endpoint, such as rate of progression to end-stage renal disease or survival in HF or after MI, is considered for the various ACE inhibitors.[9-11] Determining ACE inhibitor dose equivalence from outcomes trials is befuddled by differing dose frequency, titration requirements, and level of renal function in enrolled patients.[12,13] The last factor is particular relevant to elderly patients, because senescence-related changes in renal function extend the functional half-life of a renally cleared ACE inhibitor and make it difficult to establish true dose equivalence among various ACE inhibitors.

Evidence-based medicine attributes the benefits in outcomes trials to the compound tested, for the outcome studied, at the per protocol dose. This and the occurrence of unanticipated problems with specific agents may be the best arguments against class effect, when not all agents of the class have demonstrated similar benefits. It is risky for clinicians to estimate equivalent doses among the various ACE inhibitors *if* an ACE inhibitor substitution policy is mandated, because there are few outcomes data on which one can base such an estimate.

MECHANISM OF ACTION AND HEMODYNAMIC EFFECTS

The site of ACE inhibitor activity (within the renin-angiotensin-aldosterone [RAA] axis) can be localized to ACE, a pluripotent enzyme, which catalyzes the conversion of angiotensin I to angiotensin II and facilitates the degradation of bradykinin to a range of vasoactive peptides. However, ACE inhibition fails to suppress production of angiotensin II by alternative enzymatic pathways, such as chymase and other tissue-based proteases.[14] These alternative pathways are the predominant means of angiotensin II generation in certain tissues, including the myocardium and the vasculature.[14] With long-term ACE inhibitor administration, these alternative pathways up-regulate, and this process returns angiotensin II concentrations to pretherapy levels *(angiotensin II escape)*. Substrate for these alternative pathways is obtained from the increase in angiotensin I levels arising from a disinhibition of renin secretion by ACE inhibition.

Because ACE inhibitors reduce angiotensin II levels for only a short time (typically weeks), other mechanisms for their persistent BP-lowering effects must be present.[14] One possibility is an increase in the concentrations of the vasodilator, bradykinin, which enhances the release of nitric oxide, stimulates the production of endothelium-derived hyperpolarizing factor, and stimulates prostacyclin production.[15] Moreover, ACE is also responsible for the degradation

of angiotensin (1-7), an angiotensin peptide (of an autocrine/paracrine nature) that offsets some of the pleotropic (renal and vascular) effects of angiotensin II. Angiotensin (1-7) concentrations increase in response to low sodium intake, which may, in part, explain the additional BP reduction seen with ACE inhibition in the setting of dietary sodium restriction.[16] The contribution of angiotensin "fragments" (many of which are physiologically active) and of prostaglandins and nitric oxide to the antihypertensive effect of ACE inhibitors is being actively studied.

Alternatively, nonsteroidal anti-inflammatory drugs and selective cyclooxygenase-2 inhibitors, such as celecoxib, attenuate the BP-lowering effect of numerous antihypertensive agents, including ACE inhibitors.[17] This occurs more commonly in salt-sensitive hypertensive patients, including many elderly and African-American patients.[17,18]

The possible interaction of aspirin and the antihypertensive and cardioprotective effects of an ACE inhibitor may depend on the dose of aspirin.[19,20] Low-dose aspirin (100 mg/day or less) appears to not attenuate the BP-lowering effects of ACE inhibitors. For example, in the Hypertension Optimal Treatment (HOT) study, long-term aspirin use (at 75 mg/day) did not interfere with the BP-lowering (and possibly the cardioprotective) effect of antihypertensive drug combinations, which often included an ACE inhibitor.[19] However, higher doses (generally >236 mg/day) can blunt the antihypertensive response to an ACE inhibitor and can possibly offset the clinical benefits of ACE inhibitors in HF.[20]

A reduction in central and peripheral sympathetic nervous system activity accounts for some of the antihypertensive effect of an ACE inhibitor (Table 20-3). ACE inhibitors do not interfere with circulatory reflexes or baroreceptor function; thus, they do not cause reflex tachycardia when BP is reduced.

Table 20-3   Predominant Hemodynamic Effects of Angiotensin-Converting Enzyme Inhibitors

Hemodynamic Parameter	Effect	Clinical Significance
Cardiovascular		
Total peripheral resistance	Decreased	These parameters contribute to a general decrease in systemic blood pressure
Mean arterial pressure	Variably decreased	
Cardiac output	Increased or no change	
Stroke volume	Increased or no change	
Preload and afterload	Decreased	
Pulmonary artery pressure	Decreased	
Right atrial pressure	Decreased	
Renal		
Renal blood flow	Usually increased	Contributes to the renoprotective effect of these agents
Glomerular filtration rate	Variable, usually unchanged but may decrease in renal or heart failure	
Efferent arteriolar resistance	Decreased	
Filtration fraction	Decreased	
Sympathetic Nervous System		
Biosynthesis of norepinephrine	Decreased	Enhances blood pressure–lowering effect and resets baroreceptor function
Reuptake of epinephrine	Inhibited	
Circulating catecholamines	Decreased	

This property accounts for the low incidence of postural hypotension and provides an important safety benefit in elderly patients, who are at higher risk for orthostatic hypotension.[21] ACE inhibitors also improve endothelial function, facilitate vascular remodeling, and favorably modify the viscoelastic properties of structurally abnormal blood vessels in patients with hypertension.[22] These vascular effects are a likely explanation for the incremental and persistent reduction in BP that attends long-term ACE inhibitor administration.

BLOOD PRESSURE–LOWERING EFFECT

All ACE inhibitors available in the United States are approved for the treatment of hypertension (see Table 20-1). All current hypertension guidelines worldwide now endorse ACE inhibitors as an option for first-line therapy in patients with essential hypertension, especially in those with a high coronary artery disease (CAD) risk profile, diabetes with renal disease and proteinuria, and HF, as well as those patients who have had an MI.[1,23,24]

Apart from these "compelling indications," ACE inhibitors are a suitable option in the treatment of hypertension in a wide variety of patients.[25,26] Enthusiasm for the use of ACE inhibitors extends beyond the issue of effectiveness in BP lowering, because these agents are at best comparably efficacious to most other drug classes, including diuretics, β-blockers, and calcium channel blockers (CCBs). Response rates with ACE inhibitors range from 40% to 70% in stage 1 or 2 hypertension, with level of sodium intake and ethnicity the major confounders. When interpreting the results of clinical trials with ACE inhibitors, a distinction should be made between the mean reduction in BP (which is typically significant) and the percentage of individuals who are poor, average, and excellent responders (which may vary considerably across different studies).

No reliable predictors of the vasodepressor response to ACE inhibition exist. Although ACE gene polymorphism and specific genotypes have been suggested to predict the antihypertensive response to an ACE inhibitor, such findings have not been sufficiently consistent to justify routine genotyping.[27] There has also been an inconsistent relationship between the pretreatment or post-treatment plasma renin activity and the fall in BP with an ACE inhibitor. However, when hypertension is accompanied by significant RAA axis activation, such as in renal artery stenosis, the acute BP response to an ACE inhibitor can be profound.

Certain patient groups are more responsive to ACE inhibitor monotherapy (high-renin and young hypertensive patients age 6 to 16 years) than others, including low-renin, salt-sensitive, and volume-expanded individuals such as diabetic and African-American hypertensive patients.[2,28] However, the BP response to an ACE inhibitor can be highly variable in African-American and diabetic patients, and some patients in these groups experience significant falls in BP.[29,30] The low-renin state, characteristic of elderly hypertensive patients, differs from other low-renin forms of hypertension in that it represents senescence-related changes in the RAA axis. Elderly patients generally respond well to ACE inhibitors at usual doses, although senescence-related renal impairment, which reduces the elimination of most ACE inhibitors, confounds analysis of dose-specific treatments.

Results from numerous head-to-head trials support the comparable antihypertensive efficacy (and tolerability) of the various ACE inhibitors, *if* comparable doses have been given (see Table 20-2). However, the ACE inhibitors differ with regard to the time to onset and the duration of effect, which may relate to the absorption and tissue distribution characteristics of a specific compound. Whereas many ACE inhibitors are available for oral administration, enalaprilat is the lone ACE inhibitor for intravenous use.[2] ACE inhibitors labeled as "once-daily" vary in their ability to reduce BP for a full 24 hours, as defined by a trough-to-peak ratio greater than 50%, so many patients require a second dose each day to maintain the desired BP. The dosing frequency for ACE inhibitors may be highly individualized, for example, in patients with age-related renal impairment. These patients may have 24-hour BP control with a single daily dose (perhaps at a higher dose than usual).[31,32]

When an ACE inhibitor falls short in reducing BP, the observed initial BP response offers a useful clue to subsequent management. If the initial BP-reducing effect is minimal, switching to an alternative drug class is justified unless a "compelling indication" for the ACE inhibitor exists. However, ACE inhibitor nonresponders fairly regularly "respond" after a diuretic or CCB is added to the regimen. This observation suggests that very few patients should have an ACE inhibitor discontinued simply on the basis of an initial failure to respond.

If the initial BP response is modest, one can increase the dose (by doubling a once-daily dose or shifting to twice-daily drug administration), with the understanding that the dose-response curve for ACE inhibitors, like that of many antihypertensive agents, is relatively steep at the traditional initial doses. Increasing the dose of an ACE inhibitor typically does not increase the peak effect; rather, it prolongs the duration of response. In fact, several of the shorter-acting ACE inhibitors, such as enalapril, can function as true once-a-day medications if high enough doses are given. ACE inhibitors can take several weeks to reach their maximal BP-lowering effect, owing to vascular remodeling or improvement in endothelial function.[22]

COMBINATIONS WITH OTHER AGENTS

The BP-lowering ability of an ACE inhibitor is improved by the concurrent administration of a diuretic, particularly in salt-sensitive patients.[33] The underlying principle for the marketed fixed-dose combinations of an ACE inhibitor and a low-dose thiazide-type diuretic is one of diuretic-induced sodium depletion, thus activating the RAA axis and shifting BP to an angiotensin II–dependent mode. Even minimally natriuretic doses (12.5 mg/day) of thiazide-type diuretics reduce BP when given with an ACE inhibitor. This phenomenon points to a volume-independent component to this pattern of BP response.[33]

A β-blocker can be given with an ACE inhibitor, although the incremental benefit for BP lowering is typically minor. A presumed physiologic basis for this combination is that β-blockade blunts the reactive rise in plasma renin activity that characterizes ACE inhibitor therapy.[33] In reality, when a significant drop in BP accompanies the addition of a β-blocker to an ACE inhibitor, it often occurs in tandem with a meaningful reduction in pulse rate. Alternatively, this combination can be considered for use in the setting of CAD, in which any BP decrease is a secondary consideration to the prevention of recurrent MIs or death.

In the Antihypertensive and Lipid-lowering Treatment to Prevent Heart Attack Trial (ALLHAT), the β-blocker atenolol was the most commonly added second-step medication.[26] Although the average BP was reduced when atenolol was added to lisinopril in ALLHAT, the additional BP reduction in African Americans was marginal. Moreover, it can be further inferred that BP was less effectively reduced overall with the combination of lisinopril and atenolol, because hydralazine was required as step 3 therapy more often in the lisinopril-treated group than in either the diuretic or the CCB treatment arms of ALLHAT.

Adding a peripheral α-antagonist, such as doxazosin, to an ACE inhibitor can further reduce BP, albeit without a clear mechanistic basis.[34] The BP-lowering effect of an ACE inhibitor is also improved by the addition of either a dihydropyridine or a nondihydropyridine CCB. Several fixed-dose combination products with these drug classes are currently available.[1] Combined ACE inhibitor and CCB treatment (benazepril and amlodipine) is more effective than high doses of either individual agent (despite similarly reduced BP levels) in improving arterial compliance and regressing left ventricular mass.[35] In addition, a verapamil-trandolapril–based treatment was as effective in reducing cardiovascular endpoints as an atenolol-hydrochlorothiazide combination in hypertensive patients with CAD.[36] The addition of an ACE inhibitor to a CCB is also of benefit in lessening CCB-related peripheral edema. Preliminary findings suggest that CCB therapy may attenuate the drop in glomerular filtration rate (GFR) that can accompany ACE inhibitor therapy.[37] This finding has some bearing on ACE inhibitor use in elderly patients, because one reason for underuse of these agents in older subjects is fear of a further decline in already impaired renal function.

The efficacy of both ACE inhibitors and angiotensin receptor blockers (ARBs) as individual antihypertensive classes is well established. The observation that angiotensin II escape occurs with prolonged ACE inhibitor therapy has encouraged the belief that the addition of an ARB to an ACE inhibitor regimen may incrementally reduce BP by blocking the effect of that angiotensin II generated during the "escape" process. Despite some encouraging data in heart failure and proteinuria, evidence is insufficient to support a broad recommendation for the regular combination of these two drug classes in BP management.[38]

Finally, ACE inhibitors regress left ventricular hypertrophy induced by the potent vasodilator, minoxidil, which is often needed in complex medical regimens. In addition, if an acute reduction in BP is needed, oral or sublingual captopril (onset of action <15 minutes) can be administered. An additional option for the management of hypertensive emergencies is intravenous enalaprilat, with a dose of 0.625 mg representing a maximum acute dose (higher doses may only extend the duration of action). ACE inhibitors should be administered with care in patients with obvious (or suspected) activation of the RAA axis (e.g., renal artery stenosis, prior effective treatment with diuretics, or in the borderline hypotensive state immediately after MI). In such patients, sudden and occasionally extreme drops in BP sometimes follow the first dose of an ACE inhibitor.

HYPERTENSION ASSOCIATED WITH OTHER CONDITIONS

Cardiac Disorders

ACE inhibitors regress left ventricular hypertrophy and alter ventricular geometry. This is important because left ventricular hypertrophy portends a significant future risk of sudden death or MI. ACE inhibitors can be safely utilized in patients with CAD, because these drugs do not increase myocardial sympathetic tone in a reflex fashion.[4,39-41] Moreover, they are indicated for secondary prevention after an acute MI.[2] Although ACE inhibitors are not coronary vasodilators, they improve cardiac hemodynamics such that myocardial oxygen consumption and ischemia decrease (see Table 20-3). However, quinapril, at 80 mg/day, did not improve transient ischemia in a normotensive CAD cohort free of left ventricular dysfunction.[39]

Two of three studies of in patients with stable CAD (or other vascular disease) have shown impressive benefits of ACE inhibitors, when these drugs were used with all other appropriate therapies. Whereas ramipril (in HOPE) and perindopril (in the European Trial on Reduction of Cardiac Events with Perindopril in Stable Coronary Artery Disease [EUROPA]) were successful,[4,40] the more recent Prevention of Events with Angiotensin-Converting Enzyme Inhibition (PEACE) trial, conducted with trandolapril in patients with stable CAD and preserved left ventricular function, noted no significant reduction in the incidence of cardiovascular death, MI, or coronary revascularization.[41] One possible explanation for the significant differences among these studies' results is that patients in PEACE were very extensively treated with other effective therapies (e.g., aspirin, statins), so very few events could have been prevented by the ACE inhibitor.

ACE inhibitors can also be cautiously used in two other patient types: pediatric cancer survivors previously exposed to anthracyclines[42] and symptomatic patients with aortic stenosis (particularly if there is a component of aortic insufficiency). However, patients with aortic stenosis, left ventricular dysfunction, and low BP are prone to symptomatic hypotension.[43] Although ACE inhibitors slow calcium accumulation in aortic valves, they do not delay the hemodynamic progression of aortic stenosis.[44]

Systolic Hypertension and Peripheral Arterial Disease

ACE inhibitors are effective in reducing BP in either isolated systolic hypertension or systolic-predominant forms of hypertension, perhaps because of improved vessel compliance and reduced central aortic pressures.[22,45,46] In patients with cerebrovascular disease, ACE inhibitors maintain cerebral autoregulation in the setting of lowered BP, a property of particular importance to elderly hypertensive patients.[47]

ACE inhibitors dilate both large- and small-caliber arteries and can be used safely in patients with peripheral arterial disease.[48] In HOPE, 3099 of the patients had peripheral arterial disease—defined by an ankle-brachial index of less than 0.90. Ramipril reduced the risk of fatal and nonfatal ischemic events in patients with peripheral arterial disease who had symptomatic or subclinical disease.[48]

Diabetes

ACE inhibitors are preferred agents in hypertensive diabetic patients because they reduce BP and protect target organs (especially kidneys); this feature is likely to be independent of BP lowering.[49] In diabetic patients, it is often necessary to coadminister a diuretic, because ACE inhibitor monotherapy only modestly reduces BP in the typical low-renin, volume-expanded hypertensive diabetic patient.[33]

In addition, ACE inhibitors protect diabetic retinae. In the EURODIAB Controlled Trial of Lisinopril in Insulin-Dependent Diabetes Mellitus (EUCLID) study, lisinopril reduced retinopathy progression by approximately 50%, and it significantly lessened the risk of progression to proliferative retinopathy.[50] Although these findings support the importance of the RAA system in the eye, and ACE inhibitors can prevent major ophthalmic complications, tight BP control (independent of drug class) remains the most important consideration in retinopathy-prone diabetic patients.[51] A concluding consideration in the hypertensive diabetic patient is the effect of ACE inhibition on lipids and insulin sensitivity, especially in obese hypertensive patients. ACE inhibitors have not yet demonstrated a consistent effect on serum lipids. In addition to being effective in lowering BP in obese patients, in the Captopril Prevention Project (CAPPP),[52] the HOPE study,[4] ALLHAT,[26] and PEACE,[41] the ACE inhibitors captopril, ramipril, lisinopril, and trandolapril (respectively) decreased

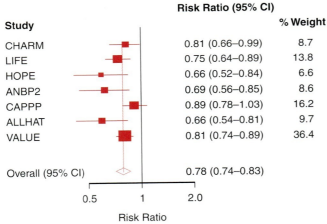

Figure 20–1 Meta-analysis of new-onset diabetes in selected comparative outcomes trials involving the use of renin-angiotensin system blockade versus non–renin angiotensin system blockade. Relative weights were assigned according to the contribution of each study based on the size of the treatment groups and the number of events observed. ALLHAT, Antihypertensive and Lipid-lowering Treatment to Prevent Heart Attack Trial; ANBP2, second Australian National Blood Pressure study; CAPPP, Captopril Prevention Project; CHARM, Candesartan in Heart Failure Assessment of Reduction in Mortality and Morbidity; HOPE, Heart Outcomes Prevention Evaluation; LIFE, Losartan Intervention for Endpoint reduction; VALUE, Valsartan Antihypertensive Long-Term Use Evaluation. (From Jandeleit-Dahm KA, Tikellis C, Reid CM, et al. Why blockade of the renin-angiotensin system reduces the incidence of new-onset diabetes. *J Hypertens.* 2005;**23**:463-473.)

the incidence of type 2 diabetes mellitus. Because a similar reduction in incident diabetes was observed with ARBs in Losartan Intervention for Endpoint Reduction (LIFE),[53] Valsartan Antihypertensive Long-Term Use Evaluation (VALUE),[54] Study on Cognition and Prognosis in the Elderly (SCOPE),[55] and Candesartan in Heart Failure Assessment of Reduction in Mortality and Morbidity (CHARM)[56] (Fig. 20-1),[57] angiotensin II probably affects insulin sensitivity, but the exact mechanism remains uncertain.[57]

END-ORGAN EFFECTS AND RECENT CLINICAL TRIALS

Renal Effects

The seventh report of the Joint National Committee on Prevention, Detection, Evaluation, and Treatment of High Blood Pressure (JNC 7) endorses the use of ACE inhibitors in hypertensive patients with CKD both to slow its rate of progression and to reduce BP.[1] However, the renoprotective features of ACE inhibitors are not substitutes for tight BP control or general health care measures such as smoking cessation, which restores the positive effects of BP control and ACE inhibitor therapy in diabetic patients with CKD.[58]

JNC 7 recommends a goal BP of less than 130/80 mm Hg in CKD.[1] In hypertensive patients with CKD, ACE inhibitor monotherapy (without concomitant diuretic administration) rarely produces a significant lowering of BP, because of the volume dependency of CKD-related hypertension. For example, in the African American Study of Kidney Disease and Hypertension (AASK), patients treated with ramipril and randomized to a mean arterial BP of 102 to 107 mm Hg required, on average, three additional medications (nearly always including a diuretic) to reach this goal BP.[59]

Both macroproteinuria and microalbuminuria are strong indicators of the rate of CKD progression. Because microalbuminuria may herald the progression to overt diabetic nephropathy, several guideline committees now recommend screening all diabetic patients for it. The diagnostic criterion for the stages of proteinuria (macroproteinuria or microalbuminuria) has been arbitrarily established (by various authoritative bodies) at a cutpoint higher or lower than 300 to 500 mg/day. These partition values for urine albumin excretion should not be taken to mean that the incremental risk with proteinuria exists solely by progressing from microalbuminuria to macroproteinuria, because there appears not to be a specific threshold value for the risk associated with microalbuminuria.[60]

Proteinuria is also an independent risk factor for fatal and nonfatal cardiovascular events (see also Chapter 29).[61] Proteinuria is now a recommended therapeutic target for both diabetic and nondiabetic renal disease. ACE inhibitors and ARBs, given separately or together, effectively reduce protein excretion and thereby emerge as important tools in the treatment of patients with microalbuminuria or macroalbuminuria (with or without hypertension). With combination ACE inhibitor and ARB therapy, the antiproteinuric effect may result from favorable renal hemodynamic effects, in addition to improvements in glomerular permselectivity.

ACE inhibitors have renoprotective effects in various settings, including established type 1 insulin-dependent diabetic nephropathy,[8] early type 2 diabetic nephropathy,[4] normotensive type 1 diabetes with microalbuminuria,[62] and an assortment of nondiabetic renal diseases.[63-67] Head-to-head comparisons of an ACE inhibitor and an ARB in nephropathy are rare.[68] In one such study, the ARB telmisartan (80 mg/day) and the ACE inhibitor enalapril (20 mg/day) comparably slowed the rate of renal functional deterioration in patients with type 2 diabetes and early nephropathy, a finding suggesting that little difference exists between these two drug classes.[69] Combination ACE inhibitor and ARB therapy is a treatment option in proteinuric renal diseases; the best long-term data come from nondiabetic glomerular disease, in which the combination of trandolapril and losartan was more renoprotective than either drug alone.[70]

Whether the agent (ACE inhibitor or an ARB) or the achieved BP is more important for renoprotection is debatable. Intensive BP control (<130/80 mm Hg) in elderly patients with type 2 diabetes and preserved renal function stabilized renal function, regardless of whether the initial therapy was an ACE inhibitor or a CCB.[71] Experimental data suggest that much of the renoprotective effect of ACE inhibition is BP dependent and is underappreciated unless the effect on 24-hour BP load is determined.[72]

The benefits of ACE inhibitor therapy in nondiabetic renal disease have become clear. In AASK, ramipril was more effective than amlodipine at slowing the rate of decline in GFR in patients with hypertensive nephrosclerosis and a urinary protein-to-creatinine ratio greater than 0.22 (urinary protein excretion >300 mg/24 hours).[66] A meta-analysis concluded that ACE inhibitors conferred renal benefit in nondiabetic patients with more than 0.5 g/day of proteinuria.[63,65] In many studies in this meta-analysis, the target BP was less than 140/90 mm Hg, which leaves open the issue of whether the renoprotective effects of ACE inhibitors (compared with other antihypertensive agents) could be less prominent with a lower achieved BP.

ACE inhibitor therapy does not always result in positive renal outcomes in every nephropathic state. In the Ramipril Efficacy in Nephropathy (REIN) study, patients with chronic proteinuric nephropathies were randomly assigned to treatment with either ramipril or placebo (in addition to conventional antihypertensive therapy). The ACE inhibitor significantly reduced the rate of proteinuria, decline in GFR, and risk of end-stage renal disease in patients with more than 3 g/day of proteinuria; conversely, during the study period, patients with proteinuria less than 2 g/24 hours, type 2 diabetes, or polycystic kidney disease did not appreciably benefit.[73]

ACE inhibitor regimens proven to slow the rate of CKD progression include the following: benazepril, 10 mg/day; captopril, 25 mg three times daily; enalapril, 5 to 10 mg/day; and ramipril, 2.5 to 5 mg/day.[2] Each of these ACE inhibitors is renally cleared; thus, reduced drug clearance in the presence of CKD is likely to have prolonged their respective pharmacologic effects, as well as augmented the effects of what otherwise would be considered small doses. Whereas the positive effects of ACE inhibition are greatest when baseline urinary protein excretion is high (>3 g/24 hours), the ACE inhibitor dose offering optimal renoprotection is debatable. For example, low-dose ramipril (1.25 mg/day) in addition to conventional antihypertensive therapy had little effect on the cardiovascular and renal outcomes of patients with type 2

diabetes and albuminuria, despite a slight decrease in BP and urinary albumin excretion.[74] Conversely in HOPE, high-dose ramipril (10 mg/day) prevented or delayed progression of microalbuminuria.[75]

Dose titration of an ACE inhibitor should be based on the individual's therapeutic endpoint, because reductions in protein excretion, lipid parameters, and BP differ in their response to upward titration of an ACE inhibitor. Although the antiproteinuric effect of trandolapril plateaued in the Combination Treatment of Angiotensin II Receptor Blocker and Angiotensin-Converting Enzyme Inhibitor in Nondiabetic Renal Disease (COOPERATE) trial at 3 mg/day,[70] in chronic proteinuric nondiabetic nephropathies, up-titration of the ACE inhibitor lisinopril to maximum tolerated doses improved hypertriglyceridemia by a direct, dose-dependent effect and improved hypercholesterolemia indirectly (through increases in serum albumin and thereby oncotic pressure).[76] These lipid benefits were more obvious at high doses of lisinopril, at which the BP-lowering and antiproteinuric effects had already plateaued (Fig. 20-2).[76]

Therapies directed at reducing the production or the effects of angiotensin II offer a mixture of benefits involving hemodynamic, cellular, and lipid-related pathways. ACE inhibitors reduce GFR in tandem with glomerular capillary pressures.[77] Such falls in GFR (typically a 10% to 15% decline) are usually reversible and, in fact, are predictive of renal protection in the long term. Such reductions in GFR can be misconstrued to represent a "nephrotoxic" process and serve as an incorrect excuse to discontinue an ACE inhibitor. Elderly patients are more liable to GFR reductions with ACE inhibitors because of their typically more advanced microvascular and macrovascular renal disease (see the later section on side effects). The differential diagnosis of a severely elevated

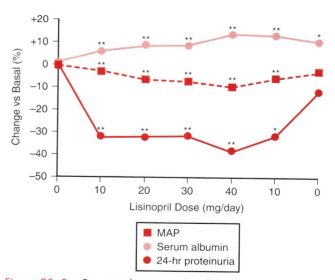

Figure 20–2 Percent changes versus baseline in mean arterial pressure (MAP), 24-hour urinary protein excretion rate, and serum albumin at different lisinopril doses in 22 patients with nondiabetic proteinuric nephropathies. *P < .05; **P < .01 versus baseline. (Modified from Ruggenenti P, Mise N, Pisoni R, et al. Diverse effects of increasing lisinopril doses on lipid abnormalities in chronic nephropathies. *Circulation.* 2003;**107**:586-592.)

serum creatinine level immediately after instituting an ACE inhibitor includes overdiuresis, renal artery disease, and unrecognized left ventricular dysfunction. These seldom require investigation unless the serum creatinine level increases by more than 20%.[77] There is no specific level of renal function at which an ACE inhibitor should not be started, unless clinically important hyperkalemia is expected to develop.

Many factors are involved in the antiproteinuric effect of ACE inhibition (Table 20-4),[78] in addition to other renal effects. First, low sodium intake and diuretic therapy improve both the antiproteinuric and antihypertensive response to ACE inhibition.[79] Second, short-term dietary protein restriction enhances the ACE inhibitor–mediated reductions in protein excretion in nephrotic patients, a finding suggesting that the combination of dietary protein restriction and ACE inhibition could prove more effective than ACE inhibition alone in slowing the progression of CKD. Third, timing of drug administration may be important, because the antiproteinuric effect of ACE inhibition wanes during the nocturnal hours despite persistent 24-hour BP lowering.

Finally, ACE activity varies according to inherited variations in the structure of the gene coding for ACE. Two common forms of the ACE gene, I (insertion) and D (deletion), give rise to three potential genotypes: II, ID, and DD. The DD genotype is associated with higher circulating ACE levels and a heightened pressor response to infused angiotensin I, as compared with the II genotype, with the ID genotype exhibiting intermediate characteristics.

The observation that DD genotype patients were at increased risk for MI and ischemic cardiomyopathy offered an early clue that an inherited variation in ACE activity could be clinical significant. Soon thereafter, it was noted that renal function declined more rapidly in patients with CKD who had the DD genotype. Moreover, when DD genotype patients are given ACE inhibitors, the anticipated reduction in urine protein excretion and decrease in the rate of CKD progression are less than in patients with the II genotype. High-dose ACE

Table 20-4 Mechanisms Explaining the Antiproteinuric Effect of Renin-Angiotensin System Blockade

Decrease in systemic blood pressure
Decrease in intraglomerular pressure
Direct effect of angiotensin-converting enzyme inhibition on decreasing growth factors
    Vascular endothelial growth factor
    Transforming growth factor-β
    Connective tissue growth factor
Effect on podocyte-specific proteins involved in glomerular permeability
    Increase in nephrin expression
Decrease in advanced glycation products
Decrease in activity of intracellular signaling pathways
    Protein kinase C
    Nuclear factor-κB
Improvement in tubular processing of albumin

Modified from Lassila M, Cooper ME, Jandeleit-Dahm K. Antiproteinuric effect of RAS blockade: New mechanisms. *Curr Hypertens Rep.* 2004;**6**:383-392.

inhibitor therapy diminishes the impact of the ACE D allele, and the benefits of such a dosage regimen are most evident in DD genotype patients.[80] Although ACE genotyping offers some promise in selecting patients with HF or CKD who are likely to be more responsive to ACE inhibition, studies thus far are not definitive enough to warrant more widespread use of genotyping.[80]

Cardiac Effects

ACE inhibitor therapy produces positive outcomes in several cardiac conditions including HF[7] and post-MI status,[81] as well as in the hypertensive patient with established vascular disease[4,40,41] or at high cardiovascular risk.[4,25, 82] These drugs also reduce the risk of new-onset or recurrent atrial fibrillation,[83] and they have been suggested as important therapies for patients during and after coronary artery bypass surgery.[84] ACE inhibitors have benefits both in normotensive and hypertensive individuals,[4,25] in diabetic patients,[85] and in patients with varying risk profiles including those with renal disease.[4,25,40,41,86] These beneficial effects have been observed with several ACE inhibitors, a finding suggesting a class effect for the favorable cardiac outcomes benefits with these compounds.

Heart Failure

As demonstrated in both placebo-controlled and open-label trials, ACE inhibitors improve HF-related functional capacity and cognitive function and, most importantly, lower the risk of death and hospitalization from HF.[7,81,85] Outcome-based clinical trials have established ACE inhibitors as first-line therapy for HF.[85,87] ACE inhibitors decrease angiotensin II production (at least in the short-term),[14] thereby readjusting the neurohumoral imbalances of HF and, in addition, affect bradykinin, which is not part of ARBs' effects.[88]

Low doses of ACE inhibitors improve exercise tolerance and HF symptoms,[13,85] and they stem the weight loss seen in progressive HF. However, improvement in HF mortality requires high-dose ACE inhibitor therapy.[85] Optimal frequency of ACE inhibitor dosing in HF is unresolved, because few comparative studies have addressed the question. When formally studied (at least for surrogate markers of HF), twice-daily regimens appeared superior to once-daily treatment schemes.[89] Twice-daily regimens were also used in nearly all registration trials of "long-acting ACE inhibitors" for the HF indication.[82,87] Until evidence to the contrary emerges, the treatment of HF should involve sequential dose titration to doses proven to reduce mortality in randomized clinical trials. The ability to reach these doses in the patient with HF can prove challenging, because treatment-limiting side effects (e.g., systemic hypotension or a significant decline in GFR) can accompany high-dose ACE inhibitor therapy. Reaching goal ACE inhibitor doses requires a clear understanding of the relationship of volume status, BP, and the desired ACE inhibitor dose.[90]

Several ACE inhibitors—including captopril, fosinopril, lisinopril, quinapril, ramipril, and trandolapril—have demonstrated improvements in HF outcomes.[81,85] Despite these convincing data, prescription practices for ACE inhibitor use in HF are suboptimal. Only a modest fraction (50% to 75%) of patients with HF who are eligible for ACE inhibitor therapy actually receive it; nonprescribing is more common when renal impairment coexists with HF.[86] Moreover, ACE inhibitor doses used in "real-world practice" are typically less than one half the dose proven effective in randomized, controlled mortality trials.[85] In one series, only 274 of 767 hospitalized patients who were discharged alive (with the diagnosis of acute MI) received an ACE inhibitor. The average daily doses of the four ACE inhibitors used in the study were as follows: captopril, 69.8 ± 36.9 mg; enalapril, 13.6 ± 8.1 mg; lisinopril, 11.0 ± 7.2 mg; and ramipril, 8.4 ± 4.5 mg. These doses remained unchanged after 6 months, except for captopril, which saw its mean daily dose rise to 84.4 ± 36.7 mg.[91]

Factors predicting optimal dosing of ACE inhibitors include the treatment setting (prior hospitalization or specialty clinic follow-up), the prescribing physician (cardiology specialty versus family practitioner or general internist), patient status (increased severity of symptoms, male sex, younger age), and the drug (lower frequency of administration). Underdosing of ACE inhibitors negatively affects the economics of HF, because it is associated with more frequent HF-related hospitalizations.[92] Finally, some question has emerged regarding whether African Americans with HF respond less well to ACE inhibitors than do whites. Because African Americans with HF have improved outcomes with ACE inhibitors compared with placebo, worries about whether the increment is as large as one could hope should not be a reason to deny African-American patients these therapies.[93]

Post–Myocardial Infarction Status

Enalapril, captopril, lisinopril, and trandolapril have each been shown to reduce morbidity and mortality significantly in the post-MI patient (with a wide range of ventricular dysfunction).[81] In a hemodynamically stable patient (systolic BP >100 mm Hg) following an MI, oral ACE inhibitor therapy should be initiated (generally within the first 24-hours of the event), particularly if the MI resulted in reduced left ventricular function. The hemodynamic effects and overall benefits of ACE inhibition are secured early after an MI; 30-day survival increases by 40% in the first day, 45% in days 2 to 7, and approximately 15% thereafter. These benefits may be attributed to an early effect on infarct expansion, a reduction in neurohumoral activity, or an increase in collateral coronary flow. Recent trends show a promising increase in ACE inhibitor prescriptions in patients discharged followed an acute MI.

Currently, captopril, lisinopril, ramipril, and trandolapril are approved specifically for post-MI left ventricular dysfunction, and enalapril is indicated in asymptomatic left ventricular dysfunction (see Table 20-1).[2] The consistency of these survival findings across various individual drugs implies, but does not prove, a class effect for this aspect of ACE inhibitor therapy. Too few data are available to conclude that clinically significant differences exist across these ACE inhibitors in the post-MI setting, especially given the lack of head-to-head trials and the differing trial designs and patient enrollment.[10,11]

Coronary Artery Disease

Several trials have been completed that assess the utility of ACE inhibitors in modifying cardiac endpoints.[4,25,26,40,41] These trials have compared ACE inhibitor therapy either with placebo[4,40,41] or with an active comparator such as a thiazide diuretic.[25,26] Some of these trials have served as the basis for the belief that ACE inhibitors favorably influence cardiac outcomes; however, in meta-analyses, there appear to be nonsignificant differences in total major cardiovascular events among regimens based on ACE inhibitors, CCBs, diuretics, or β-blockers.[94] This is particularly true given the unequal BP reduction favoring therapies other than ACE inhibitor regimens.[94] ALLHAT showed a slightly smaller reduction in total major cardiovascular events—as was the case for both stroke and HF—with the ACE inhibitor lisinopril than with the diuretic chlorthalidone, a finding largely attributable to lesser reductions in BP in the African-American cohort.[26]

Stroke

Given the considerable public health impact of stroke and the recognition of important nonmodifiable (age, gender, race/ethnicity) and modifiable (BP, diabetes, lipid profile, and lifestyle) risk factors, early prevention strategies are worthy of implementation. After a patient has experienced a stroke, the focus of care becomes the prevention of a second event by a combination of antiplatelet, lipid-lowering, and antihypertensive therapies. Despite the clear risk reduction with these treatment strategies, new approaches are always being sought. One "new" approach is to use an agent, such as an ACE inhibitor or an ARB, that may offer protection from stroke in excess of what could have been expected from BP reduction and favorable changes in the hemodynamic profile.[95]

Data supporting ACE inhibitors in reducing stroke rates (beyond the decline anticipated with BP reduction) have been mixed. For example, in ALLHAT, the stroke rate was 15% greater with the ACE inhibitor lisinopril than with the thiazide-type diuretic chlorthalidone.[26] However, this increase in stroke rate with an ACE inhibitor was found only in the African-American cohort in this study, a group that responded rather poorly to the BP-lowering effects of the lisinopril regimen. Similar negative data for secondary stroke protection with ACE inhibitors are found with perindopril in the Perindopril Protection Against Recurrent Stroke Study (PROGRESS).[96] In PROGRESS, 6105 hypertensive and non-hypertensive patients who had sustained a stroke or a transient ischemic attack (without major disability) within the past 5 years were randomized to perindopril (4 mg/day) with or without indapamide (2.5 mg/day). Diuretic therapy was given at the discretion of the treating physician.

In PROGRESS, active treatment reduced BP by an average of 9/4 mm Hg, and reduced recurrent stroke risk by 28% compared with placebo. This risk reduction extended to all forms of stroke (major disabling, hemorrhagic, ischemic, or unknown), to diabetic and nondiabetic patients, and to patients with and without hypertension (similar BP reductions in both hypertensive and normotensive patients). However, the greatest benefit was seen in the group given both perindopril and indapamide, in which BP decreased 12/5 mm Hg, compared with two placebos. Surprisingly, patients who received perindopril monotherapy had only a 5% reduction in recurrent stroke and a 4% reduction in cardiovascular events, despite a 5/3 mm Hg fall in BP, whereas patients who received both antihypertensive drugs enjoyed highly significant 43% and 40% reductions in those endpoints, respectively.[96]

In contrast, HOPE showed that ACE inhibitor therapy with ramipril lowered stroke risk in both hypertensive and normotensive individuals.[4] Compared with placebo, ramipril reduced the risk of any stroke by 32% and that of fatal stroke by 61%. Benefits were consistent across baseline BPs, drugs used, and subgroups defined by the presence of absence of previous stroke, peripheral arterial disease, diabetes, or hypertension.[97] Based on HOPE, the recent American Heart Association guidelines for the primary prevention of stroke recommend ramipril to prevent stroke in high-risk patients and in patients with diabetes and hypertension.[98]

In choosing an antihypertensive regimen in the poststroke patient, factors beyond a putative cerebroprotective effect of ACE inhibition deserve consideration. First, the ability of this drug class to preserve (if not improve) cerebral autoregulatory ability and vasomotor reactivity in the presence of BP reduction offers the possibility that these drugs may be better tolerated, particularly in elderly patients.[99] Second, the neurotransmitter substance P plays a major role in the sensory pathways for both cough and swallowing. ACE inhibitors impede the breakdown of substance P, and they may be useful in patients (particularly Asians) prone to aspiration pneumonia, as may occur in the poststroke patient.[100] In further support of this theory, a significantly lower rate of pneumonia has been observed in elderly ACE inhibitor-treated hypertensive patients (compared with treatment with an ARB).[101] Finally, ACE inhibitors with or without diuretics decrease cognitive decline (as in PROGRESS and HOPE), stroke-related dementia (in PROGRESS), and perhaps in mild to moderate Alzheimer's disease (Fig. 20-3).[102] The mechanism for these effects of ACE inhibitor therapy is still unresolved.[97,103]

SIDE EFFECTS

Shortly after their release, ACE inhibitors were associated with a syndrome of "functional renal insufficiency." This was first reported in patients with critical renal artery stenosis and a solitary kidney. Other conditions predisposing to a similar process include dehydration, use of nonsteroidal anti-inflammatory drugs, HF, and microvascular renal disease.[90] A fall in glomerular afferent arteriolar flow is thought to be the initiating event. When this occurs, glomerular filtration transiently declines in a vulnerable kidney. In response to this reduction in glomerular filtration, angiotensin II production increases within the kidney, and postglomerular (i.e., efferent) arteriolar constriction occurs. This reestablishes hydrostatic (and thereby filtering) pressures within the more proximal glomerular capillary bed.

The abrupt decrease in angiotensin II activity, either by reduced production with an ACE inhibitor or by blocked receptors with an ARB, will give rise to abrupt dilation of the efferent arteriole. In combination with a reduction in systemic BP, this hemodynamic adjustment reduces hydrostatic pressures, and the GFR plunges. This type of "functional renal insufficiency" is best treated by discontinuation of the offending agent, prompt (yet careful) volume expansion (if intravascular volume contraction is a contributing factor), and, if warranted on clinical grounds, evaluation for renal artery stenosis (Fig. 20-4).[90]

A situation analogous to that of functional renal insufficiency is exposure to ACE inhibitors during the second or third trimester of pregnancy. This situation has resulted in a "Black Box Warning" for all ACE inhibitors and all ARBs.

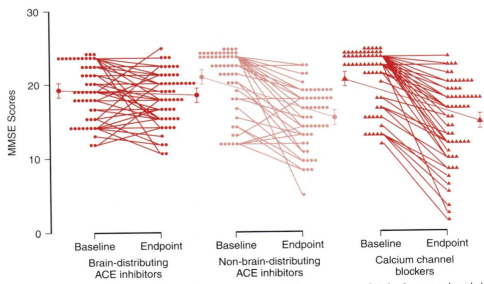

Figure 20–3 Baseline and final Mini-Mental Status Examination (MMSE) scores in individuals treated with brain distributing angiotensin-converting enzyme (ACE) inhibitor group (perindopril or captopril; *red circles*), non–brain-distributing ACE inhibitor group (enalapril or imidapril; *orange circles*), or calcium channel blocker group (nifedipine or nilvadipine; *triangles*). There were no significant differences in the baseline MMSE scores among the three groups. The mean 1-year decline in MMSE scores in the participants of brain-distributing ACE inhibitors was significantly lower compared with those of the non–brain-distributing ACE inhibitor or calcium channel blocker treatment groups. (From Ohrui T, Tomita N, Sato-Nakagawa, et al. Effects of brain-penetrating ACE inhibitors on Alzheimer disease progression. *Neurology.* 2004;**63**: 1324-1325.)

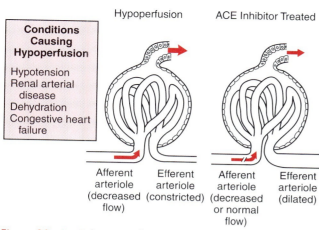

Hypoperfusion   ACE Inhibitor Treated

Conditions Causing Hypoperfusion

Hypotension
Renal arterial disease
Dehydration
Congestive heart failure

Afferent arteriole (decreased flow)   Efferent arteriole (constricted)   Afferent arteriole (decreased or normal flow)   Efferent arteriole (dilated)

Figure 20–4   Schematic illustration of settings in which angiotensin-converting enzyme (ACE) inhibitor therapy may worsen renal function. Conditions causing renal hypoperfusion include systemic hypotension, high-grade renal artery stenosis, extracellular fluid volume contraction (simplified here "dehydration"), and administration of vasoconstrictor agents (nonsteroidal anti-inflammatory drugs or cyclosporine, not shown), and congestive heart failure. These conditions typically increase renin secretion and angiotensin II production. Angiotensin II constricts the efferent arteriole to a greater extent than the afferent arteriole, such that glomerular hydrostatic pressure and the glomerular filtration rate (GFR) can be maintained despite hypoperfusion. When these conditions occur in ACE inhibitor–treated patients, both the formation and effect of angiotensin II are diminished, and GFR may decrease. (Modified from Schoolwerth AC, Sica DA, Ballermann BJ, Wilcox CS. Renal considerations in angiotensin converting enzyme inhibitor therapy: A statement for healthcare professionals from the Council on the Kidney in Cardiovascular Disease and the Council for High Blood Pressure Research of the American Heart Association.

With such exposure, BP and renal perfusion drop in tandem, with resultant in utero acute renal failure. Oligohydramnios develops thereafter, along with specific abnormalities thought to be secondary to reduced amniotic fluid volume (limb deformities, cranial ossification defects, lung hypoplasia, and tubular dysgenesis).[104] Given the lack of documented teratogenicity, inadvertent use of an ACE inhibitor in the first trimester of pregnancy is not a justifiable reason for abortion.[104]

Hypotension is not a specific side effect of ACE inhibitors; rather, it represents a physiologic extension of the drug's desired effect and is more common when a patient becomes dehydrated (e.g., postexercise or with an intercurrent febrile or gastrointestinal illness). Hyperkalemia can develop with ACE inhibitor therapy. However, this is an uncommon finding unless a specific predisposition to hyperkalemia exists, such as in diabetes and HF with renal insufficiency (in patients receiving potassium-sparing diuretics or potassium supplements).[105] Conversely, ACE inhibitors curb the potassium loss that accompanies diuretic therapy.

A dry, irritating, nonproductive cough is a common complication of ACE inhibitor use, with an incidence between 0% and 44%, but about 8% to 10% in the largest and best-conducted studies. Cough is a class phenomenon with ACE inhibitors and has been attributed to an increase in bradykinin and other vasoactive peptides, such as substance P, which may play a second messenger role in setting off the cough reflex. ACE inhibitor–related cough has been variably described as a risk factor for the likelihood of developing angioedema.[106,107] No therapy to suppress or eliminate ACE inhibitor–associated cough has been successful. The sensible clinical approach for suspected ACE inhibitor–related cough is to stop the drug and to reassess the patient several weeks later. Disappearance of the cough can then be taken as evidence for an ACE inhibitor–related problem; rechallenge is typically not needed, but it is probably safer than in a patient with ACE inhibitor–associated angioedema.

Nonspecific side effects of ACE inhibitors are infrequent, with the exception of leukopenia, skin rash, and dysgeusia, which are more common with captopril. ACE inhibitors (as a class) may induce or exacerbate psoriasis, a phenomenon attributed to an increase in skin kinin levels with ACE inhibition. Unlike certain other antihypertensive drugs, ACE inhibitors do not cause headaches and in fact can be used for migraine prophylaxis.[108] In addition, ACE inhibitors reduce the likelihood of nitrate- and dialysis-related headaches.[109,110]

Angioneurotic edema is a potentially life-threatening complication of ACE inhibitors that about three times more common in black patients. In the largest study ever to have this complication as the primary endpoint, 86 of 12,634 patients (or 0.68%) developed angioedema with enalapril, 1.62% in blacks and 0.55% in whites.[111] The incidence is greatest within the first 2 to 4 weeks of starting ACE inhibitor therapy, but it can be delayed many months. Continuing use of ACE inhibitors in spite of angioedema results in a markedly increased rate of angioedema recurrence with serious morbidity.[112] When patients with a history of angioedema with an ACE inhibitor are given an ARB, angioedema can occasionally recur, but it is generally milder and rarely life-threatening.[113] ACE inhibitor angioedema may respond poorly to standard therapy for angioedema (antihistamines, steroids, and supportive care). In refractory cases, the use of fresh frozen plasma (possibly by providing ACE to break down accumulated bradykinin) was associated with resolution of the angioedema.[114]

Angioedema of the intestine, which is more common in women, can also occur with ACE inhibitor therapy. A typical clinical presentation is one of abdominal pain and diarrhea with or without facial or oropharyngeal swelling (Fig. 20-5).[115] This process can be intermittent, developing even several years after ACE inhibitor therapy has been initiated.[116]

ACE inhibitors have also been associated with anemia. These drugs suppress the production of erythropoietin in a dose-dependent manner, and this presents a particular problem when ACE inhibitors are administered in the presence of HF or CKD.[117] Patients with HF and ACE inhibitor–related anemia have an increased mortality risk compared with those patients with HF who never develop anemia.[117] ACE inhibitor–associated anemia is, in part, related to N-acetyl-seryl-aspartyl-lysyl-proline accumulation in plasma. This substance is degraded mainly by ACE and is a potent natural inhibitor of hematopoietic stem cell proliferation. ACE inhibitors may be preferred in patients who need suppression of red cell production (e.g., post-transplant erythrocytosis[118] or high-altitude

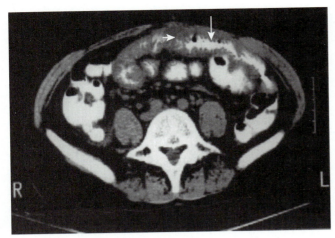

Figure 20–5 Abdominal computed tomography was performed in a 58-year-old woman with acute abdominal pain, nausea, vomiting, and abdominal distention. The patient had had recurrent swelling of the tongue and pharynx during therapy with lisinopril, but the medication had been continued. On the scan, the mucosa of a loop of small intestine is markedly thickened, and the irregularities within the wall are most consistent with the presence of edema (*short arrow*). The valvulae conniventes are prominent and widened (*long arrow*), resulting in a severely narrowed lumen. All the patient's symptoms resolved within 24 hours after the discontinuation of lisinopril. (Modified from Gregory KW, Davis RC. Images in clinical medicine: Angioedema of the intestine. *N Engl J Med.* 1996;**334**:1641.)

polycythemia); a 4 to 5 g/dL fall in hemoglobin has been reported after ACE inhibitor therapy.[119]

CONCLUSIONS

ACE inhibitors are commonly used drugs in clinical medicine. These compounds not only reduce BP but also have cardioprotective and renoprotective effects. ACE inhibitors can be expected to provide the greatest end-organ protection in patients with HF and proteinuric renal disease, as well as in the post-MI setting. Dosing guidelines exist for each of these settings, although these are not commonly followed in clinical practice. ACE inhibitor–related side effects can be physiologic, such as with hypotension or functional renal insufficiency, or nonphysiologic, such as with cough or angioneurotic edema.

References

1. Chobanian AV, Bakris GL, Black HR, et al. Joint National Committee on Prevention, Detection, Evaluation, and Treatment of High Blood Pressure: Seventh Report of the Joint National Committee on Prevention, Detection, Evaluation, and Treatment of High Blood Pressure. *Hypertension.* 2003;**42**:1206-1252.
2. Sica DA, Gehr TWB, Frishman WH. The renin-angiotensin axis: Angiotensin converting enzyme inhibitors and angiotensin-receptor blockers. *In:* Frishman W, Sonnenblick S, Sica DA (eds.), Cardiovascular Pharmacotherapeutics, 2nd ed. New York: McGraw-Hill, 2003, pp 131-156.
3. Dzau VJ, Bernstein K, Celermajer D, et al. The relevance of tissue angiotensin-converting enzyme: Manifestations in mechanistic and endpoint data. *Am J Cardiol.* 2001;**88** (**Suppl 9**):1L-20L.
4. Yusuf S, Sleight P, Pogue J, et al. Effects of an angiotensin-converting enzyme inhibitor, ramipril, on cardiovascular events in high-risk patients: The Heart Outcomes Prevention Evaluation Study Investigators. *N Engl J Med.* 2000;**342**: 145-153.
5. Zeitz CJ, Campbell DJ, Horowitz JD. Myocardial uptake and biochemical and hemodynamic effects of ACE inhibitors in humans. *Hypertension.* 2003;**41**:482-487.
6. Huskamp HA, Deverka PA, Epstein AM, et al. The effect of incentive-based formularies on prescription-drug utilization and spending. *N Engl J Med.* 2003;**349**:2224-2232.
7. SOLVD investigators. Effect of enalapril on survival in patients with reduced left ventricular ejection fractions and congestive heart failure. *N Engl J Med.* 1991;**325**:293-302.
8. Lewis EJ, Hunsicker LG, Bain RP, Rohde RD. The effect of angiotensin converting enzyme inhibition on diabetic nephropathy: The Collaborative Study Group. *N Engl J Med.* 1993;**329**:1456-1462.
9. Sica DA. The HOPE Study: ACE inhibitors—are their benefits a class effect or do individual agents differ? *Curr Opin Nephrol Hypertens.* 2001;**10**:597-601.
10. Sauer WH, Baer JT, Berlin JA, Kimmel SE. Class effect of angiotensin-converting enzyme inhibitors on prevention of myocardial infarction. *Am J Cardiol.* 2004;**94**:1171-1173.
11. Pilote L, Abrahamowicz M, Rodrigues E, et al. Mortality rates in elderly patients who take different angiotensin-converting enzyme inhibitors after acute myocardial infarction : A class effect? *Ann Intern Med.* 2004;**141**:102-112.
12. Segura J, Christiansen H, Campo C, Ruilope LM. How to titrate ACE inhibitors and angiotensin receptor blockers in renal patients: According to blood pressure or proteinuria? *Curr Hypertens Rep.* 2003;**5**:426-429.
13. Tang WH, Vagelos RH, Yee YG, et al. Neurohormonal and clinical responses to high- versus low-dose enalapril therapy in chronic heart failure. *J Am Coll Cardiol.* 2002;**39**:70-78
14. Petrie MC, Padmanabhan N, McDonald JE, et al. Angiotensin converting enzyme and non-ACE dependent angiotensin II generation in resistance arteries from patients with heart failure and coronary heart disease. *J Am Coll Cardiol.* 2001;**37**:1056-1061.
15. Tom B, Dendorfer A, Danser AH. Bradykinin, angiotensin (1-7), and ACE inhibitors: How do they interact? *Int J Biochem Cell Biol.* 2003;**35**:792-801.
16. Kocks MJ, Lely AT, Boomsma F, et al. Sodium status and angiotensin-converting enzyme inhibition: Effects on plasma angiotensin (1-7) in healthy men. *J Hypertens.* 2005;**23**: 597-602
17. Morgan T, Anderson A. The effect of nonsteroidal anti-inflammatory drugs on blood pressure in patients treated with different antihypertensive drugs. *J Clin Hypertens.* 2003; **5**:53-57, 2003.
18. Izhar M, Alausa T, Folker A, et al. Effects of COX inhibition on blood pressure and kidney function in ACE inhibitor–treated blacks and Hispanics. *Hypertension.* 2004;**43**:573-577.
19. Zanchetti A, Hansson L, Leonetti G, et al. Low-dose aspirin does not interfere with the blood pressure-lowering effects of antihypertensive therapy. *J Hypertens.* 2002;**20**:1015-1022.
20. Cleland JG, John J, Houghton T. Does aspirin attenuate the effect of angiotensin-converting enzyme inhibitors in hypertension or heart failure? *Curr Opin Nephrol Hypertens.* 2001;**10**:625-631.
21. Hajjar I. Postural blood pressure changes and orthostatic hypotension in the elderly patient: Impact of antihypertensive medications. *Drugs Aging.* 2005;**22**:55-68.

22. Schiffrin EL. Effects of antihypertensive drugs on vascular remodeling: Do they predict outcome in response to antihypertensive therapy? *Curr Opin Nephrol Hypertens.* 2001;**10**:617-624.

23. Guidelines Committee. 2003 European Society of Hypertension–European Society of Cardiology guidelines for the management of arterial hypertension. *J Hypertens.* 2003;**21**:1011-1053.

24. Khan NA, McAlister FA, Campbell NR, et al. The 2004 Canadian recommendations for the management of hypertension: Part II. Therapy. *Can J Cardiol.* 2004;**20**:41-54.

25. Wing LM, Reid CM, Ryan P, et al. A comparison of outcomes with angiotensin-converting enzyme inhibitors and diuretics for hypertension in the elderly. *N Engl J Med.* 2002;348:583-592.

26. ALLHAT Officers and Coordinators for the ALLHAT Collaborative Group. Major outcomes in high-risk hypertensive patients randomized to angiotensin converting enzyme inhibitor or calcium channel blocker vs diuretic: The Antihypertensive and Lipid-Lowering Treatment to Prevent Heart Attack Trial (ALLHAT). *JAMA.* 2002;**288**:1981-1997.

27. Li X, Du Y, Du Y, Huang X. Correlation of angiotensin-converting enzyme gene polymorphism with effect of antihypertensive therapy by angiotensin-converting enzyme inhibitor. *J Cardiovasc Pharmacol Ther.* 2003;**8**:25-30.

28. Soffer B, Zhang Z, Miller K, et al. A double-blind, placebo-controlled, dose-response study of the effectiveness and safety of lisinopril for children with hypertension. *Am J Hypertens.* 2003;**16**:795-800.

29. Mokwe E, Ohmit SE, Nasser SA, et al. Determinants of blood pressure response to quinapril in black and white hypertensive patients. *Hypertension.* 2004;**43**:1-6.

30. Sehgal AR. Overlap between whites and blacks in response to antihypertensive drugs. *Hypertension.* 2004;**43**:566-572.

31. Pescatello LS, Franklin BA, Fagard R, et al. American College of Sports Medicine position stand: Exercise and hypertension. *Med Sci Sports Exerc.* 2004;**36**:533-553.

32. Elung-Jensen T, Heisterberg J, Kamper AL, et al. Blood pressure response to conventional and low-dose enalapril in chronic renal failure. *Br J Clin Pharmacol.* 2003;**55**:139-146.

33. Sica DA. Rationale for fixed-dose combinations in the treatment of hypertension: The cycle repeats. *Drugs.* 2002;**62**:443-462.

34. Black HR, Sollins JS, Garofalo JL. The addition of doxazosin to the therapeutic regimen of hypertensive patients inadequately controlled with other antihypertensive medications: A randomized, placebo-controlled study. *Am J Hypertens.* 2000;**13**:468-474.

35. Neutel JM, Smith DH, Weber MA. Effect of antihypertensive monotherapy and combination therapy on arterial distensibility and left ventricular mass. *Am J Hypertens.* 2004;**17**:37-42.

36. Pepine CJ, Handberg EM, Cooper-DeHoff RM, et al. A calcium antagonist vs a non-calcium antagonist hypertension treatment strategy for patients with coronary artery disease. *JAMA.* 2003;**290**:2805-2816.

37. Zuccala G, Onder G, Pedone C, et al. Use of calcium antagonists and worsening renal function in patients receiving angiotensin-converting-enzyme inhibitors. *Eur J Clin Pharmacol.* 2003;**58**:695-699.

38. Sica DA. Combination angiotensin-converting enzyme inhibitor and angiotensin receptor blocker therapy: Its role in clinical practice. Practical aspects of combination therapy with angiotensin-receptor blockers and angiotensin-converting enzyme inhibitors. *J Clin Hypertens.* 2003;**5**:414-420.

39. Pepine CJ, Rouleau JL, Annis K, et al. Effects of angiotensin-converting enzyme inhibition on transient ischemia: The Quinapril Anti-Ischemia and Symptoms of Angina Reduction (QUASAR) trial. *J Am Coll Cardiol.* 2003;**42**:2049-2059

40. Fox KM. European Trial on Reduction of Cardiac Events with Perindopril in Stable Coronary Artery Disease investigators: Efficacy of perindopril in reduction of cardiovascular events among patients with stable coronary artery disease. Randomised, double-blind, placebo-controlled, multicentre trial (the EUROPA study). *Lancet.* 2003;**362**:782-788.

41. Braunwald E, Domanski MJ, Fowler SE, et al. Angiotensin-converting-enzyme inhibition in stable coronary artery disease: The PEACE Trial Investigators. *N Engl J Med.* 2004;**351**:2058-2068.

42. Silber JH, Cnaan A, Clark BJ, et al. Enalapril to prevent cardiac function decline in long-term survivors of pediatric cancer exposed to anthracyclines. *J Clin Oncol.* 2004;**22**:820-828.

43. Chockalingam A, Venkatesan S, Subramaniam T, et al. Safety and efficacy of angiotensin-converting enzyme inhibitors in symptomatic severe aortic stenosis: Symptomatic Cardiac Obstruction-Pilot Study of Enalapril in Aortic Stenosis (SCOPE-AS). *Am Heart J.* 2004;**147**:E19.

44. Rosenhek R, Rader F, Loho N, et al. Statins but not angiotensin-converting enzyme inhibitors delay progression of aortic stenosis. *Circulation.* 2004;**110**:1291-1295.

45. Morgan T, Anderson AI, MacInnis RJ. ACE inhibitors, beta-blockers, calcium blockers, and diuretics for the control of systolic hypertension. *Am J Hypertens.* 2001;**14**:241-247.

46. Morgan T, Lauri J, Bertram D, Anderson A. Effect of different antihypertensive drug classes on central aortic pressure. *Am J Hypertens.* 2004;**17**:118-123

47. Walters MR, Bolster A, Dyker AG, Lees KR. Effect of perindopril on cerebral and renal perfusion in stroke patients with carotid disease. *Stroke.* 2001;**32**:473-478.

48. Ostergren J, Sleight P, Dagenais G, et al. Impact of ramipril in patients with evidence of clinical or subclinical peripheral arterial disease. *Eur Heart J.* 2004;**25**:17-24.

49. American Diabetes Association. Position Statement: Hypertension management in adults with diabetes. *Diabetes Care.* 2004;**27**:S65-S67.

50. Sjolie AK, Chaturvedi N. The retinal renin-angiotensin system: Implications for therapy in diabetic retinopathy. *J Hum Hypertens.* 2002;**16** (**Suppl 3**):S42-S46.

51. UKPDS 69. Risks of progression of retinopathy and vision loss related to tight blood pressure control in type 2 diabetes mellitus. *Arch Ophthalmol.* 2004;**122**:1631-1640.

52. Hansson L, Lindholm L, Niskanen L, et al. Effect of angiotensin-converting-enzyme inhibition compared with conventional therapy on cardiovascular morbidity and mortality in hypertension: The Captopril Prevention Project (CAPPP) randomised trial. *Lancet.* 1999;**353**:611-616.

53. Lindholm LH, Ibsen H, Borch-Johnsen K, et al. Risk of new-onset diabetes in the Losartan Intervention for Endpoint Reduction in Hypertension study. *J Hypertens.* 2002;**20**:1879-1886.

54. Julius S, Kjeldsen SE, Weber M, et al. Outcomes in hypertensive patients at high cardiovascular risk treated with regimens based on valsartan or amlodipine: The VALUE randomised trial. *Lancet.* 2004;**363**:2022-2031.

55. Lithell H, Hansson L, Skoog I, et al. The Study on Cognition and Prognosis in the Elderly (SCOPE): Principal results of a randomized double-blind intervention trial. *J Hypertens.* 2003;**21**:875-886.

56. Pfeffer MA, Swedberg K, Granger CB, et al. Effects of candesartan on mortality and morbidity in patients with chronic heart failure: The CHARM overall programme. *Lancet.* 2003;**362**:759-768.

57. Jandeleit-Dahm KA, Tikellis C, Reid CM, et al. Why blockade of the renin-angiotensin system reduces the incidence of new-onset diabetes. *J Hypertens.* 2005;**23**:463-473.

58. Chuahirun T, Simoni J, Hudson C, et al. Cigarette smoking exacerbates and its cessation ameliorates renal injury in type 2 diabetes. *Am J Med Sci.* 2004;**327**:57-67.

59. Wright JT Jr, Agodoa L, Contreras G, et al. Successful blood pressure control in the African American Study of Kidney Disease and Hypertension. *Arch Intern Med.* 2002;**162**:1636-1643.

60. Wachtell K, Ibsen H, Olsen MH, et al. Albuminuria and cardiovascular risk in hypertensive patients with left ventricular hypertrophy: The LIFE study. *Ann Intern Med.* 2003;**139**:901-906.

61. Donnelly R, Yeung JM, Manning G. Microalbuminuria: A common, independent cardiovascular risk factor, especially but not exclusively in type 2 diabetes. *J Hypertens.* 2003;**21 (Suppl 1)**:S7-S12.

62. Viberti G, Mogensen CE, Groop LC, Pauls JF. Effect of captopril on progression to clinical proteinuria in patients with insulin-dependent diabetes mellitus and microalbuminuria: European Microalbuminuria Captopril Study Group. *JAMA.* 1994;**271**:275-279.

63. Jafar TH, Stark PC, Schmid CH, et al. Progression of chronic kidney disease: The role of blood pressure control, proteinuria, and angiotensin-converting enzyme inhibition. A patient-level meta-analysis. *Ann Intern Med.* 2003;**139**:244-252.

64. Giatras I, Lau J, Levey A, et al, for the Angiotensin-Converting Enzyme Inhibition and Progressive Renal Disease Study Group. Effect of angiotensin-converting enzyme inhibitors on the progression of nondiabetic renal disease: A meta-analysis of randomized trials. *Ann Intern Med.* 1997;**127**:337-347.

65. Jafar T, Schmid C, Landa M, et al. The effect of angiotensin-converting-enzyme inhibitors on the progression of non-diabetic renal disease: A pooled analysis of individual patient data from 11 randomized controlled trials. *Ann Intern Med.* 2001;**135**:73-87.

66. Agodoa LY, Appel L, Bakris GL, et al. Effect of ramipril vs. amlodipine on renal outcomes in hypertensive nephrosclerosis: A randomized controlled trial. *JAMA.* 2001;**285**:2719-2728.

67. Kanno Y, Okada H, Yamaji Y, et al. Angiotensin-converting enzyme inhibitors slow renal decline in IgA nephropathy, independent of tubulointerstitial fibrosis at presentation. *Q J Med.* 2005;**98**:199-203.

68. Strippoli GF, Craig M, Decks JJ, et al. Effects of angiotensin converting enzyme inhibitors and angiotensin II receptor antagonists on mortality and renal outcomes in diabetic nephropathy: Systematic review. *BMJ.* 2004;**329**:828-839.

69. Barnett AH, Bain SC, Bouter P, et al. Angiotensin-receptor blockade versus converting enzyme inhibition in type 2 diabetes and nephropathy. *N Engl J Med.* 2004;**351**:1952-1961.

70. Nakao N, Yoshimura A, Morita H, et al. Combination Treatment of Angiotensin II Receptor Blocker and Angiotensin-Converting Enzyme Inhibitor in Nondiabetic Renal Disease (COOPERATE): A randomised controlled trial. *Lancet.* 2003;**361**:117-124.

71. Estacio RO, Esler A, Mehler P. Effects of aggressive blood pressure control in normotensive type 2 diabetic patients on albuminuria, retinopathy and strokes. *Kidney Int.* 2002;**61**:1086-1097.

72. Griffin KA, Abu-Amarah I, Picken M, Bidani AK. Renoprotection by ACE inhibition or aldosterone blockade is blood pressure–dependent. *Hypertension.* 2003;**41**:201-206.

73. Ruggenenti P, Perna A, Gherardi G, et al. Chronic proteinuric nephropathies: Outcomes and response to treatment in a prospective cohort of 352 patients with different patterns of renal injury. *Am J Kidney Dis.* 2000;**35**:1155-1165.

74. Marre M, Lievre M, Chatellier G, et al. Effects of low dose ramipril on cardiovascular and renal outcomes in patients with type 2 diabetes and raised excretion of urinary albumin: Randomised, double blind, placebo controlled trial (the DIABHYCAR study). *BMJ.* 2004;**328**:495.

75. Mann JF, Gerstein HC, Yi QL, et al. Development of renal disease in people at high cardiovascular risk: Results of the HOPE randomized study. *J Am Soc Nephrol.* 2003;**14**:641-647.

76. Ruggenenti P, Mise N, Pisoni R, et al. Diverse effects of increasing lisinopril doses on lipid abnormalities in chronic nephropathies. *Circulation.* 2003;**107**:586-592.

77. Bakris GL, Weir MR. Angiotensin-converting enzyme inhibitor-associated elevations in serum creatinine: Is this a cause for concern? *Arch Intern Med.* 2000;**160**:685-693.

78. Lassila M, Cooper ME, Jandeleit-Dahm K. Antiproteinuric effect of RAS blockade: New mechanisms. *Curr Hypertens Rep.* 2004;**6**:383-392.

79. Esnault V, Ekhlas A, Delcroix C, et al. Diuretic and enhanced sodium restriction results in improved antiproteinuric response to RAS blocking agents. *J Am Soc Nephrol.* 2005;**16**:474-481.

80. Rudnicki M, Mayer G. Pharmacogenomics of angiotensin converting enzyme inhibitors in renal disease: Pathophysiological considerations. *Pharmacogenomics.* 2003;**4**:153-162.

81. Flather MD, Yusuf S, Kober L, et al. Long-term ACE inhibitor therapy in patients with heart failure or left-ventricular dysfunction: A systematic overview of data from individual patients. ACE-Inhibitor Myocardial Infarction Collaborative Group. *Lancet.* 2000;**355**:1575-1581.

82. Lopez-Sendon J, Swedberg K, McMurray J, et al. Expert consensus document on angiotensin converting enzyme inhibitors in cardiovascular disease: The Task Force on ACE inhibitors of the European Society of Cardiology. *Eur Heart J.* 2004;**25**:1454-1470.

83. L'Allier PL, Ducharme A, Keller PF, et al. Angiotensin converting enzyme inhibition in hypertensive patients is associated with a reduction in the occurrence of atrial fibrillation. *J Am Coll Cardiol.* 2004;**44**:159-164.

84. Lazar HL. Role of angiotensin-converting enzyme inhibitors in the coronary artery bypass patient. *Ann Thorac Surg.* 2005;**79**:1081-1090.

85. Shekelle PG, Rich MW, Morton SC, et al. Efficacy of ACE inhibitors and beta-blockers in the management of left ventricular systolic dysfunction according to race, gender, and diabetic status: A meta-analysis of major clinical trials. *J Am Coll Cardiol.* 2003;**41**:1529-1538.

86. Ezekowitz J, McAlister FA, Humphries KH, et al. The association among renal insufficiency, pharmacotherapy, and outcomes in 6,427 patients with heart failure and coronary artery disease. *J Am Coll Cardiol.* 2004;**44**:1587-1592.

87. American College of Cardiology/American Heart Association Task Force on Practice Guidelines. ACC/AHA Guidelines for the Evaluation and Management of Chronic Heart Failure in the Adult: Executive Summary. A Report of the American College of Cardiology/American Heart Association Task Force on Practice Guidelines. *Circulation.* 2001;**104**:2996-3007.

88. Cruden NL, Witherow FN, Webb DJ, et al. Bradykinin contributes to the systemic hemodynamic effects of chronic angiotensin-converting enzyme inhibition in patients with heart failure. *Arterioscler Thromb Vasc Biol.* 2004;**24**:1043-1048.

89. Hirooka K, Koretsune Y, Yoshimoto S, et al. Twice-daily administration of a long-acting angiotensin-converting enzyme inhibitor has greater effects on neurohumoral factors than a once-daily regimen in patients with chronic congestive heart failure. *J Cardiovasc Pharmacol.* 2004;**43**:56-60.

90. Schoolwerth AC, Sica DA, Ballermann BJ, Wilcox CS. Renal considerations in angiotensin converting enzyme inhibitor therapy: A statement for healthcare professionals from the Council on the Kidney in Cardiovascular Disease and the Council for High Blood Pressure Research of the American Heart Association. *Circulation.* 2001;**104**:1985-1991.

91. Chen YT, Wang Y, Radford MJ, Krumholz HM. Angiotensin-converting enzyme inhibitor dosages in elderly patients with heart failure. *Am Heart J*. 2001;**141**:410-417.

92. Schwartz JS, Wang YR, Cleland JG, et al. High- versus low-dose angiotensin converting enzyme inhibitor therapy in the treatment of heart failure: An economic analysis of the Assessment of Treatment with Lisinopril and Survival (ATLAS) trial. *Am J Manag Care*. 2003;**9**:417-424.

93. Dries DJ, Yancy CW, Strong MA, Drazner MH. Racial response to angiotensin-converting enzyme therapy in systolic heart failure. *Congest Heart Fail*. 2004;**10**:30-33.

94. Turnbull F, for the Blood Pressure Lowering Treatment Trialists' Collaboration. Effects of different blood-pressure-lowering regimens on major cardiovascular events: Results of prospectively designed overviews of randomised trials. *Lancet*. 2003;**362**:1527-1535.

95. Davis SM, Donnan GA. Blood pressure reduction and ACE inhibition in secondary stroke prevention: Mechanism uncertain. *Stroke*. 2003;**34**:1335-1336.

96. PROGRESS Collaborative Group. Randomised trial of a perindopril-based blood-pressure–lowering regimen among 6105 individuals with previous stroke or transient ischaemic attack. *Lancet*. 2001;**358**:1033-1041.

97. Bosch J, Yusuf S, Pogue J, et al. Use of ramipril in preventing stroke: Double blind randomised trial. *BMJ*. 2002;**324**:699-702.

98. Goldstein LB, Adams R, Becker K, et al. Primary prevention of ischemic stroke: A statement for healthcare professionals from the Stroke Council of the American Heart Association. *Stroke*. 2001;**32**:280-299.

99. Walters M, Muir S, Shah O, Lees K. Effect of perindopril on cerebral vasomotor reactivity in patients with lacunar infarction. *Stroke*. 2004;**35**:1899-1902.

100. Ohkubo T, Chapman N, Neal B, et al. Effects of an angiotensin-converting enzyme inhibitor-based regimen on pneumonia risk. *Am J Respir Crit Care Med*. 2004;**169**:1041-1045.

101. Arai, T, Yasuda, Y, Takaya, T, et al Angiotensin-converting enzyme inhibitors, angiotensin-II receptor antagonists, and pneumonia in elderly hypertensive patients with stroke. *Chest*. 2001;**119**,660-661.

102. Ohrui T, Tomita N, Sato-Nakagawa, et al. Effects of brain-penetrating ACE inhibitors on Alzheimer disease progression. *Neurology*. 2004;**63**:1324-1325.

103. Tzourio C, Anderson C, Chapman N, et al. Effects of blood pressure lowering with perindopril and indapamide therapy on dementia and cognitive decline in patients with cerebrovascular disease. *Arch Intern Med*. 2003;**163**:1069-1075.

104. Jacqz-Aigrain F, Koren G. Effects of drugs on the fetus. *Semin Fetal Neonatal Med*. 2005;**10**:139-147.

105. Palmer B. Managing hyperkalemia caused by inhibitors of the renin-angiotensin-aldosterone system. *N Engl J Med*. 2004;**351**:585-592.

106. Dykewicz MS. Cough and angioedema from angiotensin-converting enzyme inhibitors: New insights into mechanisms and management. *Curr Opin Allergy Clin Immunol*. 2004;**4**:267-270.

107. Morimoto T, Gandhi TK, Fiskio JM, et al. An evaluation of risk factors for adverse drug events associated with angiotensin-converting enzyme inhibitors. *J Eval Clin Pract*. 2004;**10**:499-509.

108. Rahimtoola H, Buurma H, Tijssen CC, et al. Reduction in the therapeutic intensity of abortive migraine drug use during ACE inhibition therapy: A pilot study. *Pharmacoepidemiol Drug Saf*. 2004;**13**:41-47.

109. Onder G, Pahor M, Gambassi G, et al. Association between ACE inhibitors use and headache caused by nitrates among hypertensive patients: Results from the Italian group of pharmacoepidemiology in the elderly. *Cephalalgia*. 2003;**23**:901-906.

110. Leinisch-Dahlke E, Schmidt-Wilcke T, Kramer BK, May A. Improvement of dialysis headache after treatment with ACE inhibitors but not angiotensin II receptor blockers: A case report with pathophysiological considerations. *Cephalalgia*. 2005;**25**:71-74.

111. Kostis JB, Packer M, Black HR, et al. Omapatrilat and enalapril in patients with hypertension: The Omapatrilat Cardiovascular Treatment vs. Enalapril (OCTAVE) trial. *Am J Hypertens*. 2003;**17**:103-111.

112. Cicardi M, Zingale LC, Bergamaschini L, Agostoni A. Angioedema associated with angiotensin-converting enzyme inhibitor use: Outcome after switching to a different treatment. *Arch Intern Med*. 2004;**164**:910-913.

113. Granger CB, McMurray JJ, Yusuf S, et al. Effects of candesartan in patients with chronic heart failure and reduced left ventricular systolic function intolerant to angiotensin-converting enzyme inhibitors: The CHARM-Alternative trial. *Lancet*. 2003;**362**:772-776.

114. Warrier MR, Copilevitz CA, Dykewicz MS, Slavin RG. Fresh frozen plasma in the treatment of resistant angiotensin-converting enzyme inhibitor angioedema *Ann Allergy Asthma Immunol*. 2004;**92**:573-575.

115. Gregory KW, Davis RC. Images in clinical medicine: Angioedema of the intestine. *N Engl J Med*. 1996;**334**:1641.

116. Orr KK, Myers JR. Intermittent visceral edema induced by long-term enalapril administration. *Ann Pharmacother*. 2004;**38**:825-827.

117. Ishani A, Weinhandl E, Zhao Z, et al. Angiotensin-converting enzyme inhibitor as a risk factor for the development of anemia, and the impact of incident anemia on mortality in patient with left ventricular dysfunction. *J Am Coll Cardiol*. 2005;**45**:391-399.

118. Yildiz A, Cine N, Akkaya V, et al. Comparison of the effects of enalapril and losartan on post-transplantation erythrocytosis in renal transplant recipients: Prospective randomized study. *Transplantation*. 2001;**72**:542-545.

119. Plata R, Cornejo A, Arratia C, et al. Angiotensin-converting-enzyme inhibition therapy in altitude polycythaemia: A prospective randomised trial. *Lancet*. 2002;**359**:663-666.

Chapter 21

Angiotensin Receptor Blockers

William J. Elliott and Henry R. Black

The renin-angiotensin-aldosterone cascade plays an important role in many cardiovascular and renal diseases, including hypertension, heart failure, renal artery stenosis, and diabetic and nondiabetic nephropathies. Angiotensin II, one of the most powerful endogenous vasoconstrictors, is produced by limited and very specific proteolysis of its precursor protein, angiotensin I. The most notable of the hydrolytic enzymes that catalyze this conversion is angiotensin-converting enzyme (ACE), although several others can play a role. Probably even more important than cathepsin G is a chymostatin-sensitive serine protease, human cardiac chymase, which is found in much higher levels in the ventricles of damaged hearts (from heart failure, myocardial infarction [MI], or after angioplasty). Angiotensin II can also be formed by direct and proteolysis of angiotensinogen by several somewhat "promiscuous" enzymes, including tissue plasminogen activator, cathepsin G, and tonin.

Angiotensin II has many diverse effects once it reaches its receptors. In addition to constricting vascular smooth muscle cells directly and thereby producing hypertension when those cells are in small arterioles, angiotensin II increases myocardial contractility, stimulates aldosterone release by the adrenal gland (leading to salt and water retention and exacerbating hypertension), and stimulates catecholamine release from sympathetic nerve endings, which serves to raise blood pressure (BP) even further. Angiotensin II is also involved in cell growth and proliferation, with its greatest impact in human biology and disease in the heart, kidney, and cerebral vessels.

The first clinically useful method of inhibiting the formation of angiotensin II involved ACE inhibitors. On a short-term basis, these agents effectively block the conversion of angiotensin I to angiotensin II through ACE, but they raise several other concerns. First, many biologically active small peptides, including bradykinin, substance P, and other tachykinins are usually metabolized by ACE (under its other name, kininase II) into biologically inactive protein fragments. Inhibition of kininase II by ACE inhibitors is thought to be one of the reasons for the increased rates of cough and angioedema seen with these drugs, although this connection has not been definitively proven. Second, in hypertension and especially in heart failure, chronic inhibition of ACE often results in a compensatory increase in renin and angiotensin I, which can then be metabolized by ACE that is not inhibited or by non-ACE pathways into still more angiotensin II. In many disease states, formation of angiotensin II by chymase, cathepsin G, and other pathways provides a "bypass" around the inhibited ACE and results in continued angiotensin II production, even in the presence of an ACE inhibitor.

The angiotensin II receptor blockers (ARBs) were initially developed at DuPont Laboratories in Wilmington, Delaware, by Timmermans and colleagues in an effort to overcome these problems with ACE inhibitors.[1] In addition to providing an entire new class of antihypertensive drugs with many other potential applications, these investigations led to a whole new arena in molecular pharmacology and a much greater understanding of angiotensin II and its many receptors, most of which would be unknown without specific pharmacologic probes and modern molecular biologic techniques.[2]

PHARMACOLOGY

Currently, seven ARBs are available for use in the United States, and several more are marketed in other countries or are awaiting regulatory approval by the U.S. Food and Drug Administration (FDA) (Table 21-1). Although all these agents specifically inhibit the angiotensin II subtype 1 (AT_1) receptor at very low drug concentrations, some clear differences, as well as subtle nuances, exist among these drugs.

All the ARBs were specifically developed to have a high affinity for the AT_1 receptor.[3] These receptors are widespread in humans and are found in particularly high concentrations in smooth muscle cells, heart, liver, kidneys, liver, aorta, lung, and testes. Within the normal heart, AT_1 receptors are found in large numbers on myocytes, on vascular smooth muscle cells, on fibroblasts, and even in the conduction system. AT_1-receptor activation by angiotensin II stimulates growth and proliferation of both myocytes and vascular smooth muscle cells. The effects of angiotensin II in normal human adults result from activation of the AT_1 receptor, although in fetal development, or in disease, the AT_2 receptor also plays a role. An entire family of antagonists of the AT_2 receptor was synthesized by the Parke-Davis Company and helped to elucidate the role of this receptor, but these antagonists have not developed into a useful therapeutic modality. Several other subtypes of angiotensin II receptors have been identified, and some have been cloned, but only the AT_1 receptors are blocked by the -sartan family of drugs. AT_3 receptors were first isolated from amphibians and later from human neuroblastoma cells. AT_4 receptors specifically bind the hexapeptide, angiotensin IV, or LVV-hemorphin 7; their role in health and disease is still being investigated.[4] Both AT_1 and AT_2 receptors are single polypeptides that belong to the superfamily of G-protein–coupled receptors that traverse the membrane of the cell wall seven times.[3] They share about 35% of their amino acid sequences and are highly conserved across species.

The role of the AT_2 receptor is somewhat less clear than that of the AT_1 receptor. The AT_2 receptor is found in great numbers in fetal tissue, as well as in small numbers in the adrenal, brain, heart (myocytes and fibroblasts), and uterus (especially myometrium). In injured tissues, and in diseased animals, it up-regulates, and its numbers increase. Because blockade of the AT_1 receptor with an ARB allows unopposed

Table 21-1 Pharmacologic Properties of Angiotensin II Receptor Blockers Available in the United States

Parameter	Losartan Potassium	Valsartan	Irbesartan	Candesartan Cilexetil	Telmisartan	Eprosartan	Olmesartan Medoxomil
U.S. trade name Manufacturer/marketer	Cozaar Merck & Co., Inc.	Diovan Novartis Pharmaceuticals Corporation	Avapro Bristol-Myers Squibb/sanofi~aventis Partnership	Atacand AstraZeneca, L.P.	Micardis Boehringer-Ingleheim/Abbott Laboratories	Teveten Kos	Benicar Sankyo Pharma, Inc./Forest Laboratories
Doses available (mg)	50, 100	40, 80, 160, 320	75, 150, 300	4, 8, 16, 32	40, 80	400, 600	5, 20, 40
Usual initial dose (mg/day)	50	80	150	8	40	600	20
Dosing frequency	1-2	1	1	1-2	1	1-2	1
Oral bioavailability	33%	23%	60%-80%	15%	42%-58%	13%	26%
Prodrug?	Yes	No	No	Yes	No	No	Yes
Active metabolite?	EXP3174	No	No	Candesartan	No	No	Olmesartan
Plasma elimination half-life (hr)	1.5-2 or (6-9, for EXP3174)	6	11-15	5-9	24	5-9	12-15
Renal/hepatic elimination (%)	10/90 or (50/50 for EXP3174)	30/70	1/99	60/40	1/99 3	0/70	10/90 (Age-dependent)
Trough-to-peak ratio (at dose, in mg)	58-78 (50-100)	69-76 (80-160)	>60 (≥150)	80 (8-16)	≥97 (20-80)	67 (600)	57-70 (5-80)
Dose adjustment for: Creatinine clearance <30 mL/min?	No	Caution	Caution	Caution	No	No	No
Hepatic impairment?	Yes, decrease by 50%	Caution	No	No	Caution	No	No
Dialyzable?	No	No	No	No	No	No	Uncertain
FDA-approved for hypertension	Yes	Yes	Yes	Yes	Yes	Yes	Yes
Severe hypertension	Yes	No	No	No	No	No	No
Prevention of ESRD in type 2 diabetic nephropathy	Yes	No	No	No	No	No	No
Prevention of progression of type 2 diabetic nephropathy	Yes	No	Yes	No	No	No	No
Heart failure	No	Yes*	No	Yes	No	No	No
Prevention of stroke in hypertensive patients with left ventricular hypertrophy	Yes	No	No	No	No	No	No

* Also indicated for left ventricular dysfunction after myocardial infarction.
ACE, angiotensin-converting enzyme; ESRD, end-stage renal disease; FDA, Food and Drug Administration.

stimulation of the AT_2 receptor, much work in animal models has revealed that stimulation of the AT_2 receptor often results in inhibition of cell growth, cell differentiation, and apoptosis. These effects are typically opposite those seen with activation of the AT_1 receptor and are blocked specifically by one or more of the Parke-Davis compounds. It has been difficult, however, to demonstrate these or other effects of stimulation of the AT_2 receptor in healthy humans.

Binding Characteristics

As with all receptor antagonists, various pharmacokinetic and physical chemical characteristics can be developed to describe the interactions of the drugs and their binding sites. Attempts have been made to link these attributes of a specific agent with its BP-lowering effects, but these efforts have not been very successful. Molecular pharmacology can distinguish between competitive and noncompetitive, surmountable and insurmountable, and reversible and irreversible binding of the agent and its receptor. Typically irreversible binding occurs with a covalent bond formed between the two; this does not occur with the AT_1 receptor and any -sartan drug. *Surmountable binding* is best described as displacement by a ligand of a drug that was preincubated with the receptor; some ARBs display this behavior after a low concentration of angiotensin II is added to the preincubated receptor and ARB complex. *Competitive binding* refers instead to the experimental situation in which both the drug and the natural ligand are added to the receptor without preincubation. All AT_1-receptor antagonists used in clinical medicine bind competitively to the AT_1 receptor, but with a slow dissociation. This accounts, in large measure, for the finding that drugs with a relatively short plasma elimination half-life are effective in lowering BP for many hours longer than would be predicted from their pharmacokinetic parameters.

Differences in Elimination

The available ARBs differ somewhat in their plasma elimination half-lives and routes of elimination or metabolism (see Table 21-1). The extremes for the former are losartan and telmisartan. Losartan has a very short intrinsic elimination half-life of about 2 hours, but it is metabolized to EXP3174, which both lowers BP and has its own elimination half-life of 6 to 8 hours. Unfortunately, it has a very low oral bioavailability, so it was not developed further. In contrast, telmisartan has an intrinsic plasma elimination half-life of at least 24 hours, which has been used to advantage in "skipped-dose" studies to demonstrate that BP control is sustained 48 hours after its last administration, compared with losartan (the drug with the shortest elimination half-life).[5,6] Strictly speaking, both candesartan cilexetil and olmesartan medoxomil are prodrugs, but these are both hydrolyzed early in the gastrointestinal tract to their active compounds. This "extra step" was necessary because both active compounds are erratically and poorly absorbed when they are given orally.

Some differences also exist in the ratio of hepatic to renal elimination of the ARBs (see Table 21-1). Both irbesartan and telmisartan are largely excreted by the liver. However, little modification of the dose is needed for individuals with hepatic impairment. Only a few patients have been discovered who lack the hepatic enzyme system responsible for metabo-

lism of losartan to EXP3174; generally, no reduction in losartan dose is required for hepatic impairment, either. The only ARB that occasionally requires dose reduction in renally impaired patients is losartan.

Metabolic Effects

Generally, the ARBs have few metabolic effects. Like ACE inhibitors, they improve insulin sensitivity, and in several clinical trials, they reduced the incidence of diabetes (see later). The ARBs have little effect on cholesterol or other lipid metabolism, but they all raise serum potassium in a dose-dependent manner, consistent with their negative feedback on aldosterone.

Among the ARBs, losartan has the unique ability to lower serum urate and increase urinary uric acid concentrations. This ability has been attributed to a specific effect of losartan (and not EXP3174) on renal tubular handling of urate in the proximal tubule that is independent of blockade of the AT_1 receptor. Despite the withdrawal of several other uricosuric drugs, this property of losartan stimulated a great deal of epidemiologic research on the role of serum urate as a possible independent cardiovascular risk factor.[7] Some investigators attributed the improvement in cardiovascular outcomes in the Losartan Intervention for Endpoint Reduction in Hypertension (LIFE) trial to a highly significant losartan-induced reduction in serum uric acid levels, because the BP differences across groups were quite small. This interpretation has not been widely accepted, especially because most of the volunteers in the LIFE trial who were originally given losartan took hydrochlorothiazide (HCTZ) or another diuretic as their second-line drug, which would tend to raise serum uric acid levels.

Important Drug Interactions

The ARBs were all developed at a time when avoidance of drug-drug interactions was considered very important and desirable for a marketed product to be successful. As a result, few candidates were accepted for clinical testing if the extensive preclinical studies indicated that the drug shared hepatic enzyme systems with other commonly used drugs. The only two surprises that have been noted are telmisartan and digoxin or warfarin. Despite good assays that suggested there should be little interaction of telmisartan with either of these drugs, the human clinical trials did show a significant, but variable (person-to-person), increase in serum digoxin levels, as well as a somewhat unpredictable increase in activity of warfarin when the two drugs were given to the same person. The molecular mechanisms of these two drug-drug interactions are still unknown. As a result, when telmisartan is given to a person who is already taking either digoxin or warfarin, a reduction in dose of either drug, followed by more frequent blood testing, is recommended.

Clinical Importance of Pharmacologic Differences

These pharmacologic differences across the seven agents in the ARB class are less impressive than those seen for essentially any other commonly used class of antihypertensive drugs. As a result, many formulary committees and other authorities have seen little reason to differentiate one from another, despite some differences in antihypertensive efficacy and use in outcomes-based clinical trials (discussed later).

MECHANISMS OF ACTION AND HEMODYNAMIC AND OTHER EFFECTS

Blood Pressure–Lowering Effect

Because AT_1-receptor blockers interact relatively specifically at this receptor alone, they antagonize many effects of angiotensin II on BP. In nearly all studies, ARBs block, in a dose-dependent manner, the pressor response to intravenously infused angiotensin II. It has been impossible, however, to determine which of the various responses is primarily involved in the BP-lowering effect: vascular smooth muscle contraction, synthesis, and effects of aldosterone in the kidney or involvement of other systems and mediators (e.g., AT_2 receptors). Suffice it that, in the case of every ARB, a dose-dependent decrease in BP has been seen in large numbers of patients, whether studied with office measurements or with 24-hour ambulatory BP monitoring.

Differences among Agents

Early studies of ARBs were directed to establishing their dose-dependent BP-lowering effects as significantly better than placebo and to exploring the upper and lower ends of the dose-response curves. As a result, few of the early studies showed much difference across the ARBs in terms of BP reduction. In fact, a meta-analysis of 142 studies showed little or no difference across the drugs available in 2000.[8] This conclusion was challenged nearly immediately.[9] Many other head-to-head studies succeeded in demonstrating significant differences across the usual starting doses or even higher doses of several of these drugs.[10-12] In most of these studies, losartan, the first ARB to market, was used as the comparator. Because its dose-response curve is rather flat between 50 and 100 mg/day and its duration of effect was rather short, a common study design was to test the BP-lowering efficacy of the usual starting dose,[11] and a second- or third-step dose, against 50 to 100 mg/day of losartan.[10,12] Most such studies did show a significant difference, with the comparator drug having more BP-lowering efficacy than losartan. Candesartan succeeded in having this comparative BP-lowering information added to its FDA-approved product information in 2002. Most authors have now accepted that significant differences exist in BP-lowering across the ARBs,[13] although it has been easiest to demonstrate these differences in studies that limit the doses to the initially recommended level[14] or use trough BPs in the assessment.[5,15]

Headache and Migraine

The ARBs are the first class of antihypertensive drug without a pathognomonic side effect. In fact, in several placebo-controlled studies, there were fewer adverse effects with the ARB than with placebo. This finding challenges the long-standing view that hypertension is an asymptomatic condition. When seven trials involving 2673 hypertensive patients with a baseline diastolic BP of less than 110 mm Hg were combined, headache frequency was significantly reduced in patients who received irbesartan (versus placebo), with more reduction in those patients who achieved lower diastolic BPs.[16] A prospective crossover trial randomized 60 Norwegian patients with a history of migraine headaches (two to six attacks/month) to either placebo or candesartan, 16 mg/day, for 12 weeks, after 4 weeks of open-label placebo treatment. The primary endpoint was the number of days with headache, which was significantly reduced (by 26%, $P < .001$) in the candesartan-treated group. Similarly, the secondary endpoints, hours with headache, days with migraine, hours with migraine, headache severity (by visual analog scale), disability score, and the number of work days lost were all significantly reduced in the candesartan-treated group.[17] The mechanism of the effect is uncertain, but it may involve local vasoconstriction mediated by angiotensin II, because similar properties of lisinopril in migraine prophylaxis have recently been demonstrated.

Prevention of Atrial Fibrillation

Animal experiments, and case-control studies in humans, have suggested that an ACE inhibitor or an ARB is associated with fewer episodes of atrial fibrillation. In the first randomized, prospective trial, patients with at least a week of atrial fibrillation who were scheduled for electrical cardioversion were given amiodarone and then were additionally randomized to placebo or irbesartan. The primary endpoint was the time to recurrent atrial fibrillation. Although some withdrawals and exclusions occurred, individuals who were given irbesartan had a significantly greater (42%) relative probability of remaining free of atrial fibrillation during the 60 to 710 days of follow-up.[18] Although this result was striking and controversial, a second, similar study compared 0, 150, and 300 mg/day of irbesartan in 300 patients undergoing cardioversion and amiodarone therapy (400 mg/day). The higher dose was associated with the least recurrence (23%), followed by the 150 mg/day dose (35%), followed by amiodarone alone (48%).[19] In the LIFE study, only 150 patients randomized to losartan developed atrial fibrillation, compared with 221 in the atenolol-treated group (33% relative risk reduction, $P < .001$). In addition, significantly fewer cardiovascular events (the primary endpoint of LIFE) occurred in patients who developed atrial fibrillation who were randomized to losartan.[20] These data suggest that blockade of the renin-angiotensin system may be beneficial in preventing atrial fibrillation, but more trials with this as the primary outcome measure will be needed to be certain. It is also possible that the ability of losartan to reduce left ventricular hypertrophy (LVH) may extend to reducing the size of the cardiac atria.

Antiproteinuric Effects

Early studies showed that, as with ACE inhibitors, proteinuria is reduced by ARBs, independently of BP control. The most comprehensive and elegant of these studies was the second Irbesartan Microalbuminuria for Type 2 Diabetes Mellitus in Hypertensive Patients (IRMA-2) trial, in which 610 European hypertensive diabetic patients with microalbuminuria were randomized to placebo (plus other antihypertensive drugs, not including ARBs or ACE inhibitors, as needed) or irbesartan (150 or 300 mg/day). The primary endpoint occurred after two urine collections showed protein excretion of more than about 288 mg/day and an increase by 15% compared with baseline.[21] BP was reduced to about the same degree in all three groups, but only those patients who received 300 mg/day had significant prevention of proteinuria during the 2 years of follow-up. The BP independence of the effects of ARBs on proteinuria was more closely studied in the Microalbuminuria Reduction with Valsartan (MARVAL) trial, in which 332 patients with type 2 diabetes were randomized to either valsartan (80 to 160 mg/day) or amlodipine (5 to 10 mg/day), followed by bendrofluazide and doxazosin as needed. At 24 weeks, the albumin excretion rate was significantly reduced (by 44%) in the valsartan-treated group, but not in the amlodipine-treated group (only 8%), despite similar BP reductions (−11.2/−6.6 versus −11.6/−6.5 mm Hg, respectively).[22]

Three other studies contrasted the antiproteinuric effects of ARBs and ACE inhibitors, and two studied the combination. In the Candesartan and Lisinopril Microalbuminuria (CALM) study, 199 hypertensive European patients with type 2 diabetes, aged 30 to 75 years, were enrolled in 37 centers in four countries. These patients were first randomized to half-maximal doses of either candesartan or lisinopril (for 12 weeks) and were then randomized again to either continued monotherapy or the combination (for a further 12 weeks). Although BP was significantly lower with the combination than with either monotherapy alone, the combination also reduced urinary protein excretion more than the ARB alone (by 34%), but not significantly more than the ACE inhibitor alone (by 18%).[23] The interpretation of this study was confounded by the half-maximal doses and the differential BP response to the combination. In a separate study in Japanese hypertensive patients with nephrotic range proteinuria (discussed later), full-dose ARB in combination with full-dose ACE inhibitor resulted in a further reduction in proteinuria than did either monotherapy alone, with no differences in BP over 3 years.[24] In the only head-to-head trial of an ARB (telmisartan) versus an ACE inhibitor (enalapril), in 250 patients with type 2 diabetes and early nephropathy (18% with proteinuria at baseline), no significant changes were reported in the protein excretion rates (a secondary endpoint) in either group over 5 years of follow-up.[25]

COMBINATIONS WITH OTHER ANTIHYPERTENSIVE AGENTS

The combination of an ARB and a diuretic has a good theoretical and practical basis, in that angiotensin II levels typically rise after diuretic administration, and this effect then improves the BP-lowering efficacy of the ARB. Thus, even in patients who do not respond adequately to ARB monotherapy, the addition of a low-dose diuretic typically results in a significant BP reduction. All seven ARBs available in the United States are marketed in a combination product with HCTZ. In each case, the ARB also attenuates some of the hypokalemic (and probably diabetogenic) potential of the diuretic.

Few properly controlled, blinded, randomized studies have investigated the use of an ARB in combination with a β-blocker or an α-blocker. Community-based, open-label experience suggests that either combination may be effective

in lowering BP,[26] but there seems little rationale for these combinations, because they would not be expected to have synergistic actions and perhaps only additive effects on BP.[27]

Experience with the combination of an ARB and an ACE inhibitor is growing, especially in heart failure and proteinuric renal diseases (discussed later). It appears, however, that the combination has little effect on BP, and it may not be synergistic, especially if either drug is given at full dose.[24] Appropriate surveillance and concern about hyperkalemia are recommended, because both classes of drugs can precipitate this problem.

The combination of an ARB and a calcium channel blocker (CCB) is enigmatic and intriguing, especially because the combination of an ACE inhibitor and a dihydropyridine CCB clearly has a beneficial effect on pedal edema, compared with a higher dose of CCB alone.[28] Few properly done, randomized controlled trials have studied the effects of an ARB on CCB-associated pedal edema. The literature about ACE inhibitor–associated reductions in pedal edema is voluminous, but it became so only after fixed-dose combination products were being prepared for market. There is little doubt that CCBs and ARBs lower BP very well together; in the Reduction in Endpoints in Non–Insulin-Dependent Diabetes Mellitus with the Angiotensin II Antagonist Losartan (RENAAL) trial, CCBs were used in more than 80% of the patients in an effort to control BP (see later).

OUTCOMES-BASED CLINICAL TRIALS IN HYPERTENSION

So far, seven randomized clinical trials involving an ARB have reported the numbers of patients who have suffered one or more cardiovascular endpoints (including death) during follow-up. These include Irbesartan Diabetic Nephropathy Trial (IDNT),[29,30] RENAAL,[31,32] LIFE,[33] the Study on Cognition and Prognosis in the Elderly (SCOPE),[34] Acute Candesartan Cilexetil Evaluation in Stroke Survivors (ACCESS),[35] Valsartan Antihypertensive Long-Term Use Evaluation (VALUE),[36] and Morbidity and Mortality after Stroke—Eprosartan vs. Nitrendipine for Secondary Prevention (MOSES) trial.[37] In addition, seven other trials have been done with ARBs in patients with heart failure: Evaluation of Losartan in the Elderly (ELITE),[38] Evaluation of Losartan in the Elderly II (ELITE II),[39] Randomized Evaluation of Strategies for Left Ventricular Dysfunction (RESOLVD),[40] Valsartan Heart Failure Trial (Val-HeFT),[41] Optimal Trial in Myocardial Infarction with the Angiotensin II Antagonist Losartan (OPTIMAAL),[42] Valsartan in Acute Myocardial Infarction (VALIANT),[43] and Candesartan in Heart Failure: Assessment of Reduction in Mortality and Morbidity (CHARM, see later). Because ARBs became available only after other drugs had been proven effective in reducing endpoints in hypertension or heart failure, it was unethical to compare ARBs with placebo or no treatment. As a result, other frequently used drugs with expected efficacy in preventing cardiovascular events (compared with placebo or no treatment) were used in these studies as "active controls." Despite this disadvantage, ARBs did show efficacy comparable to that of other drugs in preventing cardiovascular events (Fig. 21-1), and they were better than other drugs in preventing diabetes mellitus in the studies that reported this endpoint (Fig. 21-2).

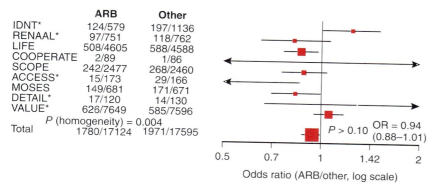

Figure 21–1 Meta-analysis of cardiovascular events in randomized clinical trials involving angiotensin II receptor blockers. For acronyms of trials, see text.

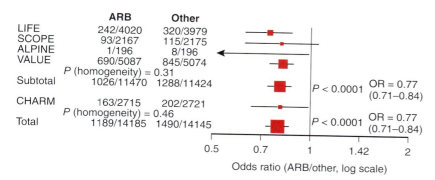

Figure 21–2 Meta-analysis of the incidence of diabetes in randomized clinical trials involving angiotensin II receptor blockers. For acronyms of trials, see text.

Two large clinical trials were conducted in high-risk hypertensive patients with no other major inclusion criterion: SCOPE and VALUE. The patients in these two trials were at high risk for cardiovascular events, based solely on their age (SCOPE) or on a combination of traditional cardiac risk factors that included age (VALUE). In SCOPE, 4937 patients between 70 and 89 years old (with Mini-Mental Status Examination scores ≥ 24 points) were first given HCTZ at 12.5 mg/day, and they had uncontrolled BPs (160 to 179/90 to 99 mm Hg) with this agent.[34] These patients were then randomized to either candesartan or any other active antihypertensive drug therapy that did not include either an ARB or an ACE inhibitor. After about 3.7 years of follow-up, BP was slightly better in the group randomized to the ARB (drop of 22/11 versus 18/9 mm Hg), but the primary endpoint (new major adverse cardiovascular events) was not quite significantly lower (242 versus 268 patients) in the group given candesartan. Analysis of individual endpoints showed fewer strokes (89 versus 115, and a 28% reduction in nonfatal stroke, P = .04), but slightly more MIs (70 versus 63), and no significant decrease in cardiovascular death (145 versus 152) in the candesartan-treated group. The prespecified secondary endpoint, cognitive function, was not significantly different across randomized groups, but two of three measures of quality of life favored the group given candesartan. So far, this is the only clinical trial that has compared other antihypertensive drugs with ARBs as second-line therapy, a position congruent with the recommendations of the Seventh Report of the Joint National Committee on Prevention, Detection, Evaluation, and Treatment of High Blood Pressure (JNC 7).[44,45]

The largest reported study using ARBs in hypertension is VALUE, which randomized 15,313 hypertensive patients at 942 clinical sites in 31 countries to either valsartan (80 to 160 mg/day) or amlodipine (5 to 10 mg/day).[36] If needed, HCTZ and then other antihypertensive drugs (again not including an ACE inhibitor, an ARB, or a CCB) could be added to achieve a BP lower than 140/90 mm Hg. Because stroke was considered to be primarily a BP-related endpoint, and not particularly benefited by effects of AT_1 blockade (i.e., "beyond BP control"), the designers of VALUE chose a composite endpoint of cardiac events as their primary endpoint. Furthermore, their initial hypothesis was that patients receiving the ARB-based regimen would have fewer cardiac events than those receiving the CCB-based regimen, *for the same level of BP control.* Unfortunately, in the first 2 months after randomization, there was a significant difference in BP reductions across the two regimens, of about 4.5/2.5 mm Hg, favoring the amlodipine-treated group. This difference decreased somewhat in magnitude, but it remained more than 2.2/2 mm Hg during the entire 4.2 years of (average) follow-up, which stopped when a prespecified number of primary events had occurred. Overall, valsartan-treated patients had a hazard ratio for a first primary endpoint of 1.03 (95% confidence interval [CI], 0.94 to 1.14; P = .49), but the ratio was much higher during the first few months of follow-up, when BP was not as well-controlled. Stroke followed a similar pattern, but fatal or nonfatal MI was significantly more common (by 19%, P = .02) in the valsartan-treated group. The heart failure rate slightly favored valsartan, but new-onset diabetes was 23% less common in the valsartan-treated group. Several types of supplemental analyses were undertaken to attempt to control for the BP differences across randomized groups; one showed that patients who achieved BP control during the first 6 months of follow-up had a significant reduction in the primary endpoint, as well as in death, stroke, and heart failure hospitalizations, irrespective of the initial drug to which they were randomized.[46] Similar analyses based on BP response at 1 month after randomization showed somewhat less impressive results, but the trends were in the same direction. Attempts to match patients from each randomized group based on the median BP response at 6 months discarded about one third of the patients, but the hazard ratios for nearly all endpoints did not significantly favor the group originally given valsartan. Perhaps not surprisingly, given the tolerability profile of the ARBs, edema and hypokalemia were both more common with amlodipine, but many other side effects (including dizziness, headache, diarrhea, angina, and syncope) were significantly more common in patients given valsartan initially. Some of these problems may have resulted from the additional medications required to achieve BP control. The main message of VALUE was that early BP control is important for reducing cardiovascular events, whether the initial therapy is an ARB or a CCB.

Patients with Specific Problems

Kidney Disorders

In addition to the clinical trials discussed previously that used urinary protein excretion as a primary endpoint, three very important studies randomized patients with chronic kidney disease to an ARB and observed the composite renal endpoint of doubling of serum creatinine, end-stage renal disease, or (in two very similar studies) all-cause mortality. The first two trials were done in patients with type 2 diabetic nephropathy and major proteinuria and resulted in a specific indication for both these drugs in this condition in the United States.

In IDNT, 1715 hypertensive patients with type 2 diabetes (average BP during placebo run-in, 160/87 mm Hg) and abnormal serum creatinine levels (average, 1.67 mg/dL, but not ≥ 3.0 mg/dL) and proteinuria greater than 900 mg/day (average, 2.9 g/day) were randomized to initial therapy with amlodipine, placebo, or irbesartan. Doses were escalated thereafter (to an average of 9.1, 0, or 269 mg/day, respectively), and other drugs were added (on average, 3.0, 4.0, and 3.0, respectively), to achieve the target BP of less than 140/90 mm Hg (the existing standard for diabetic patients and patients with renal disease when the study started). At study end, the BPs were 141/77, 144/80, and 140/77 mm Hg, respectively. During an average of 2.6 years of follow-up, there was a significant reduction in the primary endpoint only among those randomized to the ARB (23% versus amlodipine and 20% versus placebo); these data led to an FDA-approved indication for irbesartan to prevent the progression of nephropathy in patients with hypertension and type 2 diabetes. Protein excretion rates were also more greatly reduced in the group receiving the ARB (−6%, −10%, −33%, respectively, compared with baseline). Because IDNT carried a "positive control" that had BPs during follow-up that were very similar to those in the ARB-treated patients, one can presume that the ARB showed renal benefits "beyond BP control." However, the three-arm study design reduced statistical power, such that it was not possible to show a statistically significant reduction in the incidence of end-stage renal disease, despite a substantial relative decline in this important endpoint (23%, $P = .07$). The patients in IDNT were recruited because of their high risk of the primary renal endpoint, rather than cardiovascular events. However, during follow-up, 644 patients experienced the primary renal endpoint, and 821 patients had cardiovascular events. With the exception of heart failure, which was prevented significantly more effectively by the ARB than by either of the other two initial therapies, no major differences across the groups in the various types of cardiovascular events were reported.[30]

The RENAAL study used the same primary endpoint, but it randomized its 1513 patients to only two treatment arms: losartan in combination with conventional therapy or conventional therapy alone.[31] Neither group was supposed to receive either an ARB or an ACE inhibitor. These patients had slightly higher serum creatinine levels than those in IDNT (1.9 mg/dL on average) and somewhat higher baseline protein excretion rates (~3 g/day, based on the reported urinary albumin-to-creatinine ratios). Their baseline BPs were lower (153/82 mm Hg, on average), and most of those patients in the losartan group required the maximum (100 mg/day) dose. Proteinuria was significantly reduced in the losartan-treated group (by 35% compared with the conventional therapy group). After an average of 3.5 years of follow-up, there were significant reductions in both the primary endpoint (by 16%, $P = .02$) and the incidence of end-stage renal disease (28%, $P = .002$) for the losartan-treated group. These findings were the basis for an FDA-approved indication for losartan to prevent the progression of type 2 diabetic nephropathy. The group randomized to losartan had reduced rates of hospitalization for heart failure (by 32%, $P = .005$),[31] MI (by 28%, $P = .08$), and stroke (by 6%, $P = .78$).[32]

The only long-term study with renal outcomes in non-diabetic renal disease compared the incidence of doubling of serum creatinine or end-stage renal disease in 269 Japanese patients who were given trandolapril (at 3 mg/day, a dose beyond which no further reduction in proteinuria occurred), losartan (100 mg/day, the highest dose approved in Japan at the time), or the combination of the two drugs.[24] BP was no different across the three regimens over more than 3 years of follow-up, but proteinuria was reduced from baseline by about 50% with either monotherapy. With the combination of full-dose ACE inhibitor and ARB, however, proteinuria was reduced about another 50% (or 75% compared with baseline). Similarly, the incidence of the primary endpoint was significantly lower ($P < .02$ overall) in the group given the combination. In a multivariate model, combination therapy was associated with a significant 62% reduction in end-stage renal disease. Only one death was reported during follow-up (in the losartan-treated group), and other adverse effects were no more frequent with the combination than with either monotherapy. So far, these are the best data about the combination of a full-dose ACE inhibitor and a full-dose ARB on renal endpoints.

Cardiac Disorders

The LIFE trial is the lynchpin in the argument that ARBs have cardiac benefits "beyond BP control." After 4 weeks of placebo treatment, 9193 hypertensive patients with very strictly defined electrocardiographic criteria for LVH were randomized to either losartan or atenolol, followed by HCTZ and then other drugs to lower BP to less than 140/90 mm Hg.[33] The primary endpoint was a composite of stroke, MI, or cardiovascular death. After an average of 4.8 years of follow-up, the primary endpoint was significantly less common among those given losartan (by 14.6%, P = .009). In an unusual step, the planners of the study were concerned about possible imbalances in the randomized groups (a concern that turned out to be unwarranted), and therefore they prespecified an adjusted analysis as their preferred outcome of interest. After adjusting for the degree of LVH and for the Framingham Heart Study risk score at baseline, the losartan-treated group still had a significantly lower incidence of the primary endpoint, but only by 13.0% (P = .021). In fact, nearly all the reduction resulted from a reduction in stroke (−25%, P < .001), with much less reduction in cardiovascular death (−11%, P = .21) and an actual *increase* in MI (+7%, P = .49). This finding was especially surprising because the baseline abnormality that increased cardiovascular risk in LIFE patients was a cardiac problem. The losartan-treated group also had significantly fewer adverse effects, a bigger improvement in LVH, fewer new cases of diabetes, and, for the first time with an ARB, a reduction in major cardiovascular events among diabetic patients.[47] Subsequent publications of prespecified subgroups showed a significant advantage of the ARB (over the β-blocker) in preventing cardiovascular events among those with "isolated systolic hypertension" at baseline,[48] as well as a reduction in the urinary albumin-to-creatinine ratio.[49] Unlike many other clinical trials, these benefits were more easily attributed to the specific drug used as initial therapy, rather than the reduction in BP, because the difference in BPs between the two groups during the trial was only 1.3/0.4 mm Hg. In fact, however, few individuals in either group ended up taking only monotherapy, even though the doses were relatively high (82 mg/day for losartan, 79 mg/day for atenolol). Black patients comprised the only subgroup that appeared not to benefit from the ARB; for unclear reasons, the 533 blacks in LIFE had significantly better prevention of the primary endpoint (17 versus 11 events) and stroke (9 versus 5 events) with atenolol as the initial drug. Because LIFE included a month-long placebo run-in period (after which some individuals who would otherwise have qualified for the study were declared ineligible, because their BPs were either too high or too low), the BPs in both groups are likely to have been better matched both at baseline and during follow-up, compared with other trials that "switched" immediately from prerandomization therapy to a blinded study drug. This run-in period also confounds the estimated benefit of treatment, because those who have cardiovascular events during the first month (i.e., prerandomization) are not counted in the final result.[50]

ARBs have been more widely studied in chronic heart failure. Initially, direct comparisons of an ARB and an ACE inhibitor were undertaken with each as first-line therapy, but these comparisons were not as successful as anticipated. Early, short-term studies indicated that ARBs improved symptoms and other surrogate outcomes in chronic heart failure as well as ACE inhibitors, but in the first head-to-head comparison (ELITE), no significant difference was seen in serum creatinine (the primary endpoint) in 772 patients. However, a secondary endpoint in the original protocol, all-cause mortality, was significantly lower in the losartan-treated group

(4.8%, compared with captopril, at 8.7%, P = .035), and so a second, larger study (with 3153 patients) was undertaken with the same study design. Unfortunately, the second trial (ELITE II) showed nonsignificant trends favoring captopril over losartan in total mortality (P = .16) and every other "hard" endpoint, although there were fewer withdrawals from therapy in those receiving losartan.

Perhaps because of the lack of success of head-to-head trials of an ARB versus an ACE inhibitor, several studies were undertaken that added an ARB to an ACE inhibitor in patients with chronic heart failure. The first of these was a small feasibility trial (RESOLVD), which compared 4, 8, and 16 mg/day of candesartan (n = 327) versus 10 mg/day of enalapril (n = 109) versus 4 or 8 mg/day of candesartan in combination with 10 mg/day of enalapril (n = 332) on exercise tolerance, ventricular function, and quality of life for 18 and 43 weeks.[51] Systolic BP was reduced to a much greater extent by the combination therapy, and this may explain the slightly (but not significantly) increased number of hospitalizations or deaths in that group. The combination therapy group also had a greater improvement in left ventricular (LV) function, but other endpoints were not significantly different, perhaps because of the small sample size and the limited duration of follow-up.

The Val-HeFT trial was a much more ambitious comparison. It randomized 5010 patients with New York Heart Association class II to IV heart failure (62%/36%/2%, respectively) to either valsartan 40 mg (titrated to a target of 160 mg) twice daily or matching placebo. This therapy was given in addition to "conventional best treatment" (which included an ACE inhibitor in 92.7%, a diuretic in 86%, digoxin in 67%, a β-blocker in 36%, and spironolactone in 5%). A stratified randomization ensured roughly equal numbers of patients in each treatment group who were initially given a β-blocker. In an unusual step, the study design specified *two* primary endpoints: mortality and a composite endpoint that included either death or hospitalization resulting from heart failure, cardiac arrest, or intravenous administration of a positive inotropic agent. After an average of 23 months, the group receiving valsartan had a nonsignificant 2% increase in mortality, but a highly significant 13.2% reduction in the second primary endpoint that was largely attributable to a 27.5% reduction in heart failure hospitalization.[41] Valsartan-treated patients had more improvements in functional status, ejection fraction, and signs and symptoms of heart failure, but more drug discontinuations, dizziness, and increases in serum potassium, blood urea nitrogen, and creatinine. By the time Val-HeFT was completed, β-blockers had become the recommended second-line therapy for heart failure. The subgroup analysis of 1610 patients who received both an ACE inhibitor and a β-blocker at baseline indicated a significantly higher mortality in the valsartan-treated group than in the placebo group, a finding that raised concerns. A more positive subgroup analysis of the 366 patients who could not tolerate an ACE inhibitor at baseline showed highly significant improvements with valsartan over placebo in mortality (41%), the composite primary endpoint (49%), and hospitalization for heart failure (57%).[52] These data led the U.S. FDA to approve valsartan for heart failure when an ACE inhibitor was contraindicated or not tolerated.

A much more complex trio of studies was launched in CHARM. CHARM-Added was quite similar in study design to

Val-HeFT, and it enrolled 2548 patients who were taking the maximum tolerated dose of an ACE inhibitor. This trial randomized half the patients to placebo and half to candesartan (initially 4 to 8 mg once daily, but titrated to 32 mg once daily if possible). CHARM-Alternative was similar to the subgroup of 366 in Val-HeFT, in that 2028 patients with a LV ejection fraction of less than 40% who could not take an ACE inhibitor were randomized. CHARM-Preserved enrolled 3026 patients with signs and symptoms of heart failure but with a LV ejection fraction greater than 40%; an ACE inhibitor was recommended, but it was not mandatory in this population. The primary endpoint for all three studies was cardiovascular death or heart failure–related hospitalization, but the results of all three were combined to analyze the overall primary endpoint of all-cause mortality. In CHARM-Alternative, about 72% of the patients had a prior history of cough with an ACE inhibitor. After an average of 34 months of follow-up, the primary endpoint was reduced by 23% in the group randomized to candesartan, primarily because of a highly significant 32% reduction in heart failure–related hospitalization.[53] These point estimates are slightly lower than those seen in Val-HeFT, but the adverse effects of hypotension, hyperkalemia, and increased serum creatinine with the ARB were similar. Drug discontinuations were very similar with candesartan or placebo, but only 1 of 39 patients with a prior history of angioedema developed this side effect after randomization to candesartan. In CHARM-Added, more patients were taking diuretics (90%), β-blockers (56%), and spironolactone (17%) than in Val-HeFT. The doses of ACE inhibitor used in CHARM-Added were very similar to those used in Val-HeFT (e.g., ~17 mg/day of lisinopril or enalapril). After an average follow-up of 41 months, the primary endpoint was reduced 15% in the group randomized to candesartan, but in CHARM-Added, both cardiovascular death and heart failure–related hospitalization were significantly reduced.[54] Perhaps more important, the subgroup taking both an ACE inhibitor and a β-blocker at baseline had a significant reduction in the primary endpoint, and no excess mortality was reported in the group randomized to candesartan. The U.S. FDA therefore approved candesartan for heart failure, whether an ACE inhibitor was used or not. Side effects were similar to those seen in CHARM-Alternative. CHARM-Preserved broke new ground in attempting to determine whether candesartan was also beneficial in what has been called "diastolic dysfunction," (i.e., heart failure with preserved LV function). In this study, 3025 patients were randomized; their background antihypertensive therapy was more heterogeneous than those in the other two CHARM studies, but their signs and symptoms of heart failure were essentially identical to those in the other studies.[55] Most patients (75%) took a diuretic, 56% a β-blocker, 19% an ACE inhibitor, and 12% spironolactone, and fully 28% took a digitalis preparation. After an average of 37 months of follow-up, fewer (and barely nonsignificant) primary endpoints were noted in the group given candesartan. The total number of investigator-reported heart failure hospitalizations, but not the time to the initial hospitalization, was significantly lower with candesartan. After multivariate adjustments for imbalances in the randomization, however, the primary endpoint just missed significance ($P = .051$), but the initial hospitalization and other composite endpoints did achieve statistical significance. The authors interpreted their data

conservatively, with a suggestion of benefit of candesartan in this previously unstudied, but moderately prevalent, group of patients with heart failure. Across the three studies in CHARM, the reduction in all-cause mortality with candesartan was significant only after the adjustment for baseline differences, but the reduction in cardiovascular mortality was significant (at 12%, unadjusted $P = .012$). The composite of cardiovascular death or heart failure hospitalization was significantly reduced by 16%, with no significant heterogeneity across the three trials. Importantly, all studies showed a significant benefit of candesartan in reducing this endpoint, whether the patient was or was not taking an ACE inhibitor or a β-blocker at baseline. The CHARM data therefore provide a wealth of information about the benefits of ARBs in heart failure, including diastolic dysfunction.

Two comparative studies of an ARB versus an ACE inhibitor in patients who developed heart failure after an acute MI have been published, but their chosen agents, dosing strategies, and results differ. In OPTIMAAL, 5477 patients who developed heart failure or LV dysfunction within 10 days of diagnosis of an acute MI were randomized at 327 centers in seven European countries to either losartan 12.5 to 50 (mean, 45) mg once daily or captopril 6.25 to 50 (mean, 44) mg three times daily. After a mean follow-up of 2.7 years, all prespecified adverse clinical outcomes favored captopril: death (by 13%, $P = .07$), sudden death (by 19%, $P = .07$), death related to MI or coronary heart disease (by 3%, $P = .72$), hospitalization (by 3%, $P = .37$), and cardiovascular death (by 17%, $P = .032$). Only 17% of patients discontinued losartan, compared with 23% who stopped captopril ($P < .0001$). When the dose of losartan was limited to 50 mg/day (as in OPTI-MAAL, ELITE, and ELITE II), no significant benefit was seen, whereas when higher doses were allowed (RENAAL, LIFE), losartan was extremely beneficial. Whether this is the basis for the difference in the results of OPTIMAAL versus VALIANT is unknown.

In VALIANT, 14,703 patients who developed signs or symptoms of heart failure, or who had evidence of LV dysfunction within 10 days of an acute MI, were randomized to one of three treatments: valsartan (≤160 mg twice daily), captopril (≤50 mg three times daily), or the combination (captopril, ≤50 mg three times daily, in addition to valsartan, 80 mg twice daily). The study was powered not only for a superiority difference in survival between the groups but also for a non-inferiority claim for valsartan versus captopril. After a median of 24.7 months of follow-up, no significant differences in survival were reported across the three groups, but the combination group had more drug-related adverse effects.[43] Importantly, the statistical criteria for "equivalence" of valsartan and captopril were met, thus giving credence to the prior hypothesis that valsartan was certainly not inferior to captopril in this patient population.

Thus, unlike the situation in renal disease, in which ARBs have clear benefits over placebo and a dihydropyridine CCB in patients with type 2 diabetes (in which ACE inhibitors have not been adequately studied), it has been much more difficult to show better than equivalent benefits of ARBs over ACE inhibitors in heart disease. Perhaps this is because ACE inhibitors were first studied against placebo in cardiac disorders, and ARBs could not ethically be compared with placebo when effective therapy had already become "standard of care."

Cerebrovascular Disorders

Two clinical trials have been completed using an ARB in patients with stroke. In ACCESS, 337 German patients with acute cerebral ischemia and very high BPs were randomized on the first day of hospitalization to either candesartan, 4 to 32 mg/day, or 7 days of placebo. After the first week in hospital, candesartan was given to all but 2 of the 166 patients who received the initial placebo. The study was stopped prematurely, not because of a significant difference in the primary endpoint (death and disability at 3 months), but because of a 52% reduction in major adverse cardiovascular events at 1 year ($P < .05$). No BP differences were reported between groups after discharge from hospital, and the number of strokes was similar (19 versus 13, late candesartan versus early candesartan). Candesartan was chosen for this trial because of its relatively slow onset of action and its low propensity to lower BP rapidly in the setting of an acute stroke. At the least, this study shows that lowering very high BP acutely in the setting of an acute ischemic stroke was not harmful; more studies will be needed to convince the general medical and neurologic community that this regimen may be beneficial.

MOSES was a more complex comparative trial in the post-stroke setting, and it suggested that an ARB may be better than the dihydropyridine CCB nitrendipine, which was effective in primary stroke prevention in the Systolic Hypertension in Europe and Systolic Hypertension in China trials.[56,57] In MOSES, 1352 hypertensive German patients who were, on average, about 1 year from the index stroke were given either eprosartan, 600 mg, or nitrendipine, 10 mg, in the morning.[37] These doses could be increased, then a diuretic, β-blocker, α-blocker, and thereafter other drugs were added, to achieve BP lower than 140/90 mm Hg. The average doses of the initial drugs used were 610 mg and 16 mg/day, respectively. Patients were, on average, about 66 years of age, with slightly more men than women in each group. About 61% had a prior stroke, and about 27% had a prior transient ischemic attack. Although 84% were previously treated with antihypertensive drugs, the baseline office BPs were about 151/87 mm Hg in each group and about 140/81 mm Hg for the 24-hour average on ambulatory BP monitoring. The primary endpoint was the total occurrence of cardiovascular events (not a time-to-first-event analysis). During about 3.5 years of follow-up, BPs were reduced in both groups, with the nitrendipine-treated group having about 1.0/0.8 mm Hg lower BP. The total number of events, however, favored eprosartan (206 versus 255, $P = .014$), as was also the case for recurrent stroke (102 versus 134, $P = .02$). Only the latter was significant, however, in a traditional time-to-first-event analysis. Mortality, cause-specific mortality, and functional scores after treatment were no different across the two groups. The authors concluded that an ARB-based treatment prevented more cardiovascular and cerebrovascular events in a post-stroke population than a regimen based on a proven dihydropyridine CCB, despite less of a reduction in BP.

Ongoing Outcomes-Based Trials

The encouraging, but not definitive results of CHARM-Preserved will soon be supplemented by the Irbesartan in Heart Failure with Preserved Systolic Function (I-PRESERVE) trial. This is a double-blind, placebo-controlled trial of irbesartan in 3600 patients drawn from 360 centers in 29 countries, all of whom had symptomatic heart failure during a recent hospitalization for heart failure or other clinical findings consistent with diastolic dysfunction. All patients will have an LV ejection fraction of 45% or higher. Because the efficacy of an ACE inhibitor in this setting is unproven, patients will be allowed to enter I-PRESERVE with or without ACE inhibitor therapy, but such therapy will be limited to one third of the patients, and then those patients already taking an ACE inhibitor will no longer be enrolled. After a 2-week placebo run-in period, randomization will occur between irbesartan (target dose, 300 mg/day) and placebo, but other drugs (excluding an ACE inhibitor or ARB) can be added as needed to control BP. Two primary endpoints will be involved: all-cause mortality, which is unlikely to show a significant difference, because patients in Val-HeFT and even CHARM abandoned their randomized drug after a heart failure–related hospitalization; and cardiovascular mortality or morbidity, including cardiovascular hospitalization, MI, and stroke. The study will end after 1440 patients have achieved one or both primary endpoints, and it is expected to provide about 24 to 28 months of average follow-up.

Valsartan is the primary antihypertensive drug in the second Appropriate Blood Pressure Control in Diabetes (ABCD) trial, in which about 800 patients with type 2 diabetes in Colorado will be randomization to two different levels of BP control. The primary endpoint is the same as that of IDNT and RENAAL, but the accrual rate of this endpoint has been slower than expected. There may well be differences between those patients who were initially normotensive and those who were initially hypertensive, as was the case for the original ABCD trial. These results should be forthcoming soon.

Because of possible beneficial effects of an ARB in atrial fibrillation (discussed earlier), the second randomization in the Atrial Fibrillation Clopidogrel Trial with Irbesartan for Prevention of Vascular Events (ACTIVE) will compare irbesartan and placebo in about 14,000 patients with atrial fibrillation.[58] The first randomization will compare various anticoagulation regimens, and (in a 2 × 2 factorial design), the same patients will be observed for about 3 years to see which therapies are more effective in preventing major cardiovascular events. This trial may confirm the observation that, in 342 patients with baseline atrial fibrillation and LVH in LIFE, losartan was associated with a significantly lower rate of both the primary endpoint and stroke.[59]

The largest outcomes-based study will be the Ongoing Telmisartan Alone and in Combination with Ramipril Global Endpoint Trial (ONTARGET), which has randomized 25,620 patients at high risk for cardiovascular events (aged ≥55 years, but not necessarily hypertensive) to long-term treatment with the ARB telmisartan, 80 mg/day, the ACE inhibitor ramipril, 10 mg/day, or their combination.[60] Eligible patients have a history of coronary disease, stroke, peripheral vascular disease, or diabetes with target organ damage. The primary endpoint is a composite of major cardiovascular events (cardiovascular death, MI, stroke, or hospitalization for heart failure) during an average expected 4.5 years of average follow-up. More than 5775 otherwise eligible patients for ONTARGET who were unable to tolerate an ACE inhibitor were entered into a parallel study of telmisartan versus placebo, the Telmisartan Randomized Assessment Study in

ACE Intolerant Subjects with Cardiovascular Disease (TRANSCEND). Both these trials will study the incidence of type 2 diabetes as a prominent secondary endpoint. These studies are expected to complete their follow-up in 2007 and will probably provide the strongest data regarding outcomes with the combination of a full-dose ACE inhibitor and a full-dose ARB.

Perhaps the most novel of the ARB trials was the Trial of Preventing Hypertension (TROPHY). It was the first clinical trial to attempt to reduce incident hypertension using a BP-lowering drug. Because of excellent tolerability and general lack of side effects, an ARB (candesartan) was selected as the active comparator versus placebo. Eight hundred nine otherwise healthy subjects (59% male, average age 49 ± 8.1 years old) with what was formerly called high-normal BP (130 to 139/85 to 89 mm Hg) but which now falls into the prehypertensive category in JNC 7 were randomized at 71 study sites to either 16 mg daily of candesartan or placebo and were followed for 2 years for the development of hypertension (BP ≥ 140/90 mm Hg at any three office visits, or at the final office visit, BP ≥ 160/100 mm Hg at any visit, or development of target organ damage).[61] During active treatment, the risk of developing hypertension was reduced by nearly two thirds in the group given candesartan, and this group also had fewer side effects, hospitalizations, and cardiovascular events. The second phase of TROPHY involved a 2-year observation period when all patients who were still not hypertensive were treated only with placebo. At the end of the fourth year, there was still significant prevention of hypertension in the group that originally received candesartan (by about 16%). TROPHY showed that it was feasible to treat prehypertensive patients with drugs and that doing so prevented both the development of hypertension and adverse effects, but these findings may not result in an FDA-approved indication for this drug yet.

ADVERSE EFFECTS

ARBs are generally well-tolerated drugs. Possibly for this reason, more people in the United States refill prescriptions for this class of antihypertensive agent than for any other.[61] This is true in both short-term (1-year)[62,63] and long-term (4-year) studies.[64]

As with ACE inhibitors, the most feared adverse effect of ARBs is teratogenicity. Perhaps because ARBs came to market after ACE inhibitors had been associated with craniofacial birth defects and major problems with development of the kidneys (including renal agenesis), more attention has been paid to avoiding ARBs during the second and third trimesters of pregnancy. Although the numbers of affected patients are extremely small, the same "black box warning" appears for ARBs as with ACE inhibitors, because it is assumed that these drugs share this important adverse effect. All ARBs are contraindicated in pregnancy and should be discontinued as soon as pregnancy is detected.[65]

Similarly, the effect of ARBs in patients with bilateral renal artery stenosis or arterial stenosis to a solitary kidney are expected to be very similar to those of ACE inhibitors: acute renal failure, manifested by an acute rise in serum creatinine, blood urea nitrogen, and occasionally hyperkalemia, is usually reversible after the ARB or ACE inhibitor is stopped.[66,67] Several studies were organized to probe the comparative differences in hyperkalemia for an ARB versus an ACE inhibitor in renal artery stenosis, but patient recruitment was difficult, and the studies were never completed. Known or suspected renal artery stenosis is therefore usually also listed as a contraindication for all ARBs.

The most common adverse effect of ACE inhibitors is a nonproductive cough, which is more frequent in Asians, blacks, and women; this side effect is much less common with ARBs (Fig. 21-3). However, the relative risk of cough for ARBs versus ACE inhibitors depends on the population studied. In the six studies that compared cough frequencies in patients who had previously manifested cough when they were given ACE inhibitors, an 8.7-fold (95% CI, 5.0- to 12.2-fold) increase in cough was seen after repeated challenge with an ACE inhibitor, as compared with those patients randomized to an ARB. In the 21 prospective, randomized studies of an ACE inhibitor versus an ARB that examined cough as a primary or secondary endpoint, the increase was only 4.1-fold (95% CI, 2.2- to 5.9-fold).[68] The probable reason for this discrepancy is that the studies in those patients known to cough with an ACE inhibitor have a large expectation bias, and this also explains the approximate 20% incidence of cough in patients randomized to a "negative control" (e.g., placebo or HCTZ).

The relationship between ARBs and angioedema is more controversial. Because angioedema is thought to be in large part the result of bradykinin, which is not generally affected by ARBs, it may be expected that the incidence of angioedema with an ARB should be the same as in the general population.[69] This was indeed the experience in LIFE: 11 of the 4588 patients given atenolol developed angioedema, but only 6 of the 4605 patients randomized to losartan were so affected.[33] In CHARM-Alternative, only 1 of 39 patients with a past history of angioedema developed it again after being given candesartan; none of the 44 patients randomized to placebo were afflicted.[53] The numbers of patients who developed angioedema in other randomized outcome trials in hypertension that involved an ARB have not been reported. In the largest published series of 64 patients who developed angioedema with an ACE inhibitor, only 2 of the 26 who switched to an ARB had recurrent angioedema.[70] Some authors suggest that a history of ACE inhibitor–associated angioedema is a contraindication to the use of an ARB.[71] Given the potential risk of laryngeal edema and death (previously observed with ACE inhibitor therapy), the ethics of a clinical trial to answer this question will be a severe challenge.[72]

In addition to dizziness and diarrhea, many rare and unusual adverse effects have been reported with ARBs. Perhaps the most interesting is anemia in patients with chronic kidney disease (especially those undergoing dialysis), which may result from decreased production of erythropoietin (because it often requires a dose increase) or a direct suppressive effect on burst-forming units for erythrocytes. Psoriasis, dysgeusia, aphthous ulcers of the mouth, pancreatitis, immune thrombocytopenia, and Schönlein-Henoch purpura have all been precipitated or exacerbated with ARBs.

SUMMARY

The ARBs are the newest of the commonly used orally available antihypertensive drugs. They lower BP as well as other

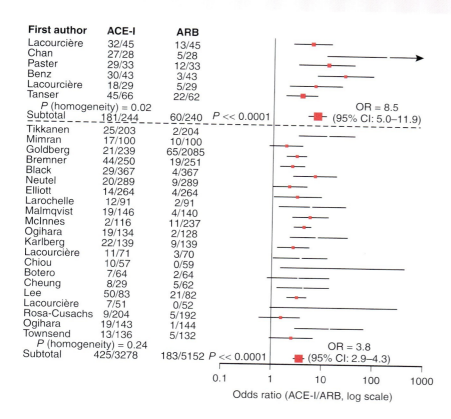

First author	ACE-I	ARB
Lacourcière	32/45	13/45
Chan	27/28	5/28
Paster	29/33	12/33
Benz	30/43	3/43
Lacourcière	18/29	5/29
Tanser	45/66	22/62
P (homogeneity) = 0.02		
Subtotal	181/244	60/240
Tikkanen	25/203	2/204
Mimran	17/100	10/100
Goldberg	21/239	65/2085
Bremner	44/250	19/251
Black	29/367	4/367
Neutel	20/289	9/289
Elliott	14/264	4/264
Larochelle	12/91	2/91
Malmqvist	19/146	4/140
McInnes	2/116	11/237
Ogihara	19/134	2/128
Karlberg	22/139	9/139
Lacourcière	11/71	3/70
Chiou	10/57	0/59
Botero	7/64	2/64
Cheung	8/29	5/62
Lee	50/83	21/82
Lacourcière	7/51	0/52
Rosa-Cusachs	9/204	5/192
Ogihara	19/143	1/144
Townsend	13/136	5/132
P (homogeneity) = 0.24		
Subtotal	425/3278	183/5152

P << 0.0001 OR = 8.5 (95% CI: 5.0–11.9)

P << 0.0001 OR = 3.8 (95% CI: 2.9–4.3)

Odds ratio (ACE-I/ARB, log scale): 0.1 1 10 100 1000

Figure 21–3 Meta-analysis of cough in comparative studies of angiotensin II receptor blockers (ARBs) and angiotensin-converting enzyme inhibitors (ACE-I). The 6 studies at the *top* of the figure involved patients with a known history of ACE inhibitor–associated cough; the 21 studies at the bottom involved patients that were not preselected in this way. In both analyses, there is a significantly higher frequency of cough with ACE inhibitors than with ARBs.

agents, and they have fewer adverse effects. Mechanistically, the ARBs are most similar to ACE inhibitors, but they have a lower incidence of associated cough and angioedema. They have proven benefits in outcomes-based clinical trials in type 2 diabetic nephropathy and LVH, and emerging data show benefits in heart failure and stroke. Emerging data from outcomes-based clinical trials will continue to influence the use of these agents. In JNC VI, ARBs were recommended as a substitute for ACE inhibitors, if the patient developed a cough or was known to be otherwise intolerant to ACE inhibitors. Long appreciated as a very well tolerated class of antihypertensive agents, with all the evidence from many clinical trials, ARBs can now be recommended as a reasonable alternative to ACE inhibitors or even as the preferred initial choice when blockade of the renin-angiotensin-aldosterone system is indicated. When adequate comparative trials are completed in the very near future and when the cost of using these agents is properly analyzed, this issue should be settled.

References

1. Smith RD, Chiu AT, Wong PC, et al. Pharmacology of nonpeptide angiotensin II receptor antagonists. *Annu Rev Pharmacol Toxicol*. 1992;**32**:135-165.
2. Carey RM, Siragy H. Newly recognized components of the renin-angiotensin system: Potential roles in cardiovascular and renal regulation. *Endocr Rev*. 2003;**24**:261-271.
3. de Gasparo M, Catt KJ, Inagami T, et al. International Union of Pharmacology. XXIII. The angiotensin II receptors. *Pharmacol Rev*. 2000;**52**:415-472.
4. Chai SY, Frenando R, Peck G, et al. The angiotensin IV/AT4 receptor. *Cell Mol Life Sci*. 2004;**61**:2728-2737.
5. Mallion J, Siche J, Lacourcière Y. ABPM comparison of the antihypertensive profiles of the selective angiotensin II receptor antagonists telmisartan and losartan in patients with mild-to-moderate hypertension. *J Hum Hypertens*. 1999;**13**:657-664.
6. Mancia G, Dell'Oro R, Turri C, Grassi G. Comparison of angiotensin II receptor blockers: Impact of missed doses of candesartan cilexetil and losartan in systemic hypertension. *Am J Cardiol*. 1999;**84 (Suppl 10A)**:28S-34S.
7. Alderman M, Aiyer KJ. Uric acid: Role in cardiovascular disease and effects of losartan. *Curr Med Res Opin*. 2004;**20**:369-379.
8. Conlin PR, Spence JD, Williams B, et al. Angiotensin II antagonists for hypertension: Are there differences in efficacy? *Am J Hypertens*. 2000;**13**:18-26.
9. Meredith P, Trenkwalder P. Angiotensin II antagonists for hypertension: There are differences in efficacy [letter]. *Am J Hypertens*. 2001;**14**:394-395.
10. Kassler-Taub K, Littlejohn T, Elliott W, et al., for the Irbesartan/Losartan Study Group. Comparative efficacy of two angiotensin II receptor antagonists, irbesartan and losartan, in mild-to-moderate hypertension. *Am J Hypertens*. 1998;**11**:445-453.
11. Andersson OK, Neldam S. The antihypertensive efficacy and tolerability of candesartan cilexetil, a new generation angiotensin II antagonist, in comparison with losartan. *Blood Press*. 1998;**7**:53-59.
12. Oparil S, Guthrie R, Lewin AJ, et al. An elective-titration study of the comparative effectiveness of two angiotensin II-receptor blockers, irbesartan and losartan. Irbesartan/Losartan Study Investigators. *Clin Ther*. 1998;**20**:398-409.
13. Stumpe KO. Olmesartan compared with other angiotensin II receptor antagonists: Head-to-head trials. *Clin Ther*. 2004;**26 (Suppl A)**:A33-A37.
14. Oparil S, Williams D, Chrysant SG, et al. Comparative effects of olmesartan, losartan, valsartan, and irbesartan in the control of essential hypertension. *J Clin Hypertens*. 2001;**3**:283-291.
15. Lacoucière Y, Asmar R. A comparison of the efficacy and duration of action of candesartan cilexetil and losartan as assessed by clinic and ambulatory blood pressure after a missed dose, in truly hypertensive patients: A placebo-controlled,

forced titration study. Candesartan/Losartan Study Investigators. *Am J Hypertens*. 1999;**12**:1181-1187.

16. Hansson L, Smith DH, Reeves R, Lapuerta P. Headache in mild-to-moderate hypertension and its reduction by irbesartan therapy. *Arch Intern Med*. 2000;**160**:1654-1658.

17. Tronvik E, Stovner LJ, Helde G, et al. Prophylactic treatment of migraine with an angiotensin II receptor blocker: A randomized controlled trial. *JAMA*. 2003;**289**:65-69.

18. Madrid AH, Bueno MG, Rebollo JM, et al. Use of irbesartan to maintain sinus rhythm in patients with long-lasting persistent atrial fibrillation: A prospective and randomized study. *Circulation*. 2002;**106**:331-336.

19. Madrid AH, Marin IM, Cervantes CE, et al. Prevention of recurrences in patients with lone atrial fibrillation. The dose-dependent effect of angiotensin II receptor blockers. *J Renin Angiotensin Aldosterone Syst*. 2004;**5**:114-120.

20. Wachtell K, Lehto M, Gerdts E, et al. Angiotensin II receptor blockade reduces new-onset atrial fibrillation and subsequent stroke compared to atenolol: The Losartan Intervention for Endpoint Reduction in Hypertension (LIFE) study. *J Am Coll Cardiol*. 2005;**45**:712-719.

21. Parving H-H, Lehnert H, Brochner-Mortensen J, et al. The effect of irbesartan on the development of diabetic nephropathy in patients with type 2 diabetes. Irbesartan in Patients with Type 2 Diabetes and Microalbuminuria Study Group. *N Engl J Med*. 2001;**345**:870-878.

22. Viberti GC, Wheeldon NM. Microalbuminuria reduction with valsartan in patients with type 2 diabetes: A blood pressure-independent effect. The MARVAL Study Investigators. *Circulation*. 2002;**106**:672-678.

23. Mogensen CE, Neldam S, Tikkanen I, et al. Randomised controlled trial of dual blockade of renin-angiotensin system in patients with hypertension, microalbuminuria, and non-insulin dependent diabetes: The Candesartan and Lisinopril Microalbuminuria (CALM) study. *BMJ*. 2000;**321**:1440-1444.

24. Nakao N, Yoshimura A, Morita H, et al. Combination treatment of angiotensin-II receptor blocker and angiotensin-converting-enzyme inhibitor in non-diabetic renal disease (COOPERATE): A randomised controlled trial. *Lancet*. 2003;**361**:117-124.

25. Barnett AH, Bain SC, Bouter P, et al. Angiotensin-receptor blockade versus converting-enzyme inhibition in type 2 diabetes and nephropathy. *N Engl J Med*. 2004;**351**:1952-1961.

26. Weir MR, Weber MA, Neutel JM, et al. Efficacy of candesartan cilexetil as add-on therapy in hypertensive patients uncontrolled on background therapy: a clinical experience trial: ACTION Study Investigators. *Am J Hypertens*. 2001;**14**:567-572.

27. Narayan P, Man in't Veld AJ. Clinical pharmacology of modern antihypertensive agents and their interaction with alpha-adrenoceptor antagonists. *Br J Urol*. 1998;**81** (**Suppl 1**):6-16.

28. Messerli FH. Vasodilatory edema: A common side effect of antihypertensive therapy. *Curr Cardiol Rep*. 2002;**4**:479-482.

29. Lewis EJ, Hunsicker LG, Clarke WR, et al. Renoprotective effect of the angiotensin-receptor antagonist irbesartan in patients with nephropathy due to type 2 diabetes: Collaborative Study Group. *N Engl J Med*. 2001;**345**:841-860.

30. Berl T, Hunsicker LG, Lewis JB, et al. Cardiovascular outcomes in the Irbesartan Diabetic Nephropathy Trial of patients with type 2 diabetes and overt nephropathy: Irbesartan Diabetic Nephropathy Trial Collaborative Study Group. *Ann Intern Med*. 2003;**138**:542-549.

31. Brenner BM, Cooper ME, de Zeeuw D, et al. Effects of losartan on renal and cardiovascular outcomes in patients with type 2 diabetes and nephropathy: Reduction of Endpoints in Non-Insulin Dependent Diabetes Mellitus with the Angiotensin II Antagonist Losartan (RENAAL) Study Group. *N Engl J Med*. 2001;**345**:861-869.

32. Kowey PR, Dickson TZ, Zhang Z, et al. Losartan and end-organ protection: Lessons from the RENAAL study. *Clin Cardiol*. 2005;**28**:136-142.

33. Dahlöf B, Devereux RB, Kjeldsen SE, et al., for the LIFE Study Group. Cardiovascular morbidity and mortality in the Losartan Intervention for Endpoint Reduction in Hypertension study (LIFE): A randomised trial against atenolol. *Lancet*. 2002;**359**:995-1003.

34. Lithell H, Hansson L, Skoog I, et al. The Study on Cognition and Prognosis in the Elderly (SCOPE): Principal results of a randomized double-blind intervention trial. *J Hypertens*. 2003;**21**:875-886.

35. Schrader J, Luders S, Kulschewski A, et al. The ACCESS study: Evaluation of acute candesartan cilexetil therapy in stroke survivors. *Stroke*. 2003;**34**:1699-1703.

36. Julius S, Kjeldsen S, Weber M, et al. Outcomes in hypertensive patients at high cardiovascular risk treated with regimens based on valsartan or amlodipine: The VALUE randomised trial. *Lancet*. 2004;**363**:2022-2031.

37. Schrader J, Lüders S, Kulschewski A, et al. Morbidity and mortality after stroke, eprosartan compared with nitrendipine for secondary prevention: Principal results of a prospective randomized controlled study (MOSES). *Stroke*. 2005;**36**:1218-1226.

38. Pitt B, Segal R, Martinez FA, et al., for the ELITE Investigators. Results of the Evaluation of Losartan in the Elderly (ELITE) trial. *Lancet*. 1997;**349**:757-762.

39. Pitt B, Poole-Wilson PA, Segal R, et al. Effect of losartan compared with captopril on mortality in patients with symptomatic heart failure: Randomised trial—The Losartan Heart Failure Survival Study ELITE II. *Lancet*. 2000;**355**:1582-1587.

40. McKelvie RS, Yusuf S, Pericak D, et al., RESOLVD Pilot Study Investigators. Comparison of candesartan, enalapril, and their combination in congestive heart failure: Randomized Evaluation of Strategies for Left Ventricular Dysfunction (RESOLVD) pilot study. *Circulation*. 1999;**100**:1056.

41. Cohn JN, Tognoni G, for the Val-HeFT Investigators. A randomized trial of the angiotensin-receptor blocker valsartan in chronic heart failure. *N Engl J Med*. 2001;**345**:1667-1675.

42. Dickstein K, Kjekshus J, and the OPTIMAAL Steering Committee. Effects of losartan and captopril on mortality and morbidity in high-risk patients after acute myocardial infarction: The OPTIMAAL randomised trial. OPTIMAAL Study Group. *Lancet*. 2002;**360**:752-760.

43. Pfeffer MA, McMurray JJV, Velazquez EJ, et al. Valsartan, captopril, or both in myocardial infarction complicated by heart failure, left ventricular dysfunction, or both: VALIANT Investigators. *N Engl J Med*. 2003;**349**:1893-1906.

44. Chobanian AV, Bakris GL, Black HR, et al., and the National High Blood Pressure Education Program Coordinating Committee. The Seventh Report of the Joint National Committee on Prevention, Detection, Evaluation, and Treatment of High Blood Pressure: The JNC 7 Report. *JAMA*. 2003;**289**:2560-2572.

45. Chobanian AV, Bakris GL, Black HR, et al. Seventh Report of the Joint National Committee on Prevention, Detection, Evaluation and Treatment of High Blood Pressure: National High Blood Pressure Education Program Coordinating Committee. *Hypertension*. 2003;**42**:1206-1252.

46. Weber M, Julius S, Kjeldsen KE, et al. Blood pressure dependent and independent effects of antihypertensive treatment on clinical events in the VALUE trial. *Lancet*. 2004;**363**:2049-2051.

47. Lindholm L, Ibsen H, Dahlöf B, et al., for the LIFE Study Group. Cardiovascular morbidity and mortality in patients with diabetes in the Losartan Intervention for Endpoint Reduction in Hypertension study (LIFE): A randomised trial against atenolol. *Lancet*. 2002;**359**:1004-1010.

48. Kjeldsen SE, Dahlöf B, Devereux RB, et al., LIFE (Losartan Intervention for Endpoint Reduction) Study Group. Effects of losartan on cardiovascular morbidity and mortality in patients with isolated systolic hypertension and left ventricular hypertrophy: A Losartan Intervention for Endpoint Reduction (LIFE) substudy. *JAMA*. 2002;**288**:1491-1498.

49. Ibsen H, Wachtell K, Olsen MH, et al. Does albuminuria predict cardiovascular outcome on treatment with losartan versus atenolol in hypertension with left ventricular hypertrophy? A LIFE substudy. *J Hypertens*. 2004;**22**:1805-1811.

50. Pablos-Mendez A, Barr RG, Shea S. Run-in periods in randomized trials: Implications for the application of results in clinical practice. *JAMA*. 1998;**279**:222-225.

51. McKelvie RS, Yusuf S, Pericak D, et al. Comparison of candesartan, enalapril, and their combination in congestive heart failure: Randomized Evaluation of Strategies for Left Ventricular Dysfunction (RESOLVD) pilot study. The RESOLVD Pilot Study Investigators. *Circulation*. 1999;**100**:1056-1064.

52. Maggioni AP, Anand I, Gottlieb SO, et al., Val-HeFT Investigators (Valsartan Heart Failure Trial). Effects of valsartan on morbidity and mortality in patients with heart failure not receiving angiotensin-converting enzyme inhibitors. *J Am Coll Cardiol*. 2002;**40**:1414-1421.

53. Granger CB, McMurray JJV, Yusuf S, et al. Effects of candesartan in patients with chronic heart failure and reduced left-ventricular function intolerant to angiotensin-converting-enzyme inhibitors: The CHARM-Alternative trial. CHARM Investigators and Committees. *Lancet*. 2003;**362**:772-776.

54. McMurray JJV, Östergren J, Swedberg K, et al. Effects of candesartan in patients with chronic heart failure and reduced left-ventricular systolic function taking angiotensin-converting-enzyme inhibitors: The CHARM-Added trial. CHARM Investigators and Committees. *Lancet*. 2003;**362**:767-771.

55. Yusuf S, Pfeffer MA, Swedberg K, et al. Effects of candesartan in patients with chronic heart failure and preserved left-ventricular ejection fraction: The CHARM-Preserved trial. *Lancet*. 2003;**362**:77-781.

56. Staessen JA, Fagard R, Thijs L, et al., for the Systolic Hypertension in Europe (Syst-EUR) Trial Investigators. Morbidity and mortality in the placebo-controlled European Trial on Isolated Systolic Hypertension in the Elderly. *Lancet*. 1997;**360**:757-764.

57. Liu L, Wang J, Gong L, et al., for the Systolic Hypertension in China (Syst-China) Collaborative Group. Comparison of active treatment and placebo in older Chinese patients with isolated systolic hypertension. *J Hypertens*. 1998;**16**:1823-1829.

58. Hohnloser SH, Connolly SJ. Combined antiplatelet therapy in atrial fibrillation: Review of the literature and future research avenues. *J Cardiovasc Electrophysiol*. 2003;**14**:S60-S63.

59. Wachtell K, Hornestam B, Lehto M, et al. Cardiovascular morbidity and mortality in hypertensive patients with a history of atrial fibrillation: The Losartan Intervention for Endpoint Reduction in Hypertension (LIFE) study. *J Am Coll Cardiol*. 2005;**45**:705-711.

60. Teo K, Yusuf S, Anderson C, et al. Rationale, design, and baseline characteristics of 2 large, simple, randomized trials evaluating telmisartan, ramipril, and their combination in high-risk patients: The Ongoing Telmisartan Alone and in Combination with Ramipril Global Endpoint Trial/Telmisartan Randomized Assessment Study in ACE Intolerant Subjects with Cardiovascular Disease (ONTARGET/TRANSCEND) trials. *Am Heart J*. 2004;**148**:52-61.

61. Julius S, Nesbitt S, Egan B, et al. Feasibility of treating prehypertension with an angiotensin receptor blocker. *N Engl J Med*. 2006;**354**:1685-1697.

62. Bloom BS. Continuation of initial antihypertensive medication after one year of therapy. *Clin Ther*. 1998;**20**:671-681.

63. Hasford J, Mimran A, Simons WR. A population-based European cohort study of persistence in newly diagnosed hypertensive patients. *J Hum Hypertens*. 2002;**16**:569-575.

64. Conlin PR, Gerth WC, Fox J, et al. Four-year persistence patterns among patients initiating therapy with the angiotensin II receptor antagonist losartan versus other antihypertensive drug classes. *Clin Ther*. 2001;**23**:1999-2010.

65. Lambot MA, Vermeylen D, Noel JC. Angiotensin-II-receptor inhibitors in pregnancy. *Lancet*. 2001;**357**:1619-1620.

66. Wargo KA, Chong K, Chan EC. Acute renal failure secondary to angiotensin II receptor blockade in a patient with bilateral renal artery stenosis. *Pharmacotherapy*. 2003;**23**:1199-1204.

67. Kiykim AA, Boz M, Ozer C, et al. Two episodes of anuria and acute pulmonary edema in a losartan-treated patient with solitary kidney. *Heart Vessels*. 2004;**19**:52-54.

68. Elliott WJ. Cough with ACE inhibitors or angiotensin II receptor blockers: Meta-analysis of randomized hypertension studies. *J Hypertens*. 2002;**20 (Suppl 4)**:S161.

69. Gavras I, Gavras H. Are patients who develop angioedema with ACE inhibitors at risk of the same problem with AT1 receptor blockers? *Arch Intern Med*. 2003;**163**:240-241.

70. Cicardi M, Zingale LC, Bergamaschini L, Agostoni A. Angioedema associated with angiotensin-converting enzyme inhibitor use: Outcome after switching to a different treatment. *Arch Intern Med*. 2004;**164**:910-913.

71. Howes LG, Tran D. Can angiotensin receptor antagonists be used safely in patients with previous ACE inhibitor-induced angioedema? *Drug Saf*. 2002;**25**:73-76.

72. Dykewicz MS. Cough and angioedema from angiotensin-converting enzyme inhibitors: New insights into mechanism and management. *Curr Opin Allergy Clin Immunol*. 2004;**4**:267-270.

Chapter 22

Calcium Channel Blockers in Hypertension

Alberto Zanchetti

In the years since Fleckenstein's pioneering studies of the 1980s,[1] calcium channel blockers (CCBs) have become important and useful agents for treating hypertension. This chapter discusses the pharmacologic and physiologic mechanisms for their vasodilating action and reviews the large body of clinical outcome studies now available. A summary of the lively debate about the safety of these compounds is provided, with a focus on the methodologic problems encountered and a discussion of how the issue has been resolved by clinical trials. Pharmacologic and clinical differences among subclasses of CCBs and among agents within the same subclass are reviewed. Ancillary properties of CCBs that may make them specifically indicated in some conditions and may limit their usefulness in others are highlighted. Because combination antihypertensive therapy is increasingly needed to achieve desirable blood pressure (BP) goals, the use of CCBs in combination with other BP-lowering agents is also reviewed.

PHYSIOLOGY AND PHARMACOLOGY

Calcium Channels in the Cardiovascular System

Calcium is a ubiquitous intracellular messenger coupling membrane-mediated stimuli with cellular responses.[2,3] In the cardiovascular system, increased intracellular calcium triggers the actin-myosin interaction and the subsequent contraction of myocytes and vascular smooth muscle. Because essential hypertension is characterized by enhanced vasoconstrictive tone, transmembrane calcium exchange in vascular smooth muscle plays an important role in hypertension and is an obvious target for antihypertensive compounds.[3] Physiologically, the extracellular to intracellular calcium ion concentration gradient is positive. Numerous membrane mechanisms maintain this gradient, thus allowing entrance of calcium ions necessary for contraction, but avoiding excess intracellular calcium leading to cell injury. Calcium extrusion from the cell is regulated by the calcium-sodium exchange mechanism, in which one calcium ion is transported out of the cell in exchange for three sodium ions entering the cell, and by an adenosine triphosphate (ATP)–dependent calcium pump, which extrudes calcium with the conversion of ATP to adenosine diphosphate. Calcium inflow occurs through two main sets of channels, the receptor-operated and the voltage-gated calcium channels, as well as through a leak pathway. In addition, at the intracellular level, calcium-binding proteins (including calmodulin) and mechanisms regulating calcium exchange into and out of the sarcoplasmic reticulum and the mitochondria play essential roles.[2]

Receptor-operated channels are often components of messenger-responsive receptors, but the major targets of pharmacologic actions are the voltage-gated channels. Five major subtypes of this family are known: T, L, N, P/Q, and R. Only T and L channels are known to occur in cardiovascular tissue. The T class is activated and inactivated at low membrane potentials, whereas the L-type channel is activated at high membrane potentials. The L-type channel is the dominant one, functionally, in the cardiovascular system, although some role has been ascribed to the T channel as well, particularly in the physiology of sinus node cells. Figure 22-1 shows that the L-type voltage-gated calcium channel is made up of four subunits, α_1 and α_2-δ, β, and γ,[2] but the α_1-subunit appears to be the dominant one at least in cardiovascular tissue, and it is known to be coded by at least 10 different genes.

Mechanism of Action

CCBs (also called calcium antagonists) are pharmacologic agents that inhibit transmembrane calcium inflow through calcium channels.[2] All CCBs used in cardiovascular therapy act on the L channel and specifically on the α_1-subunit, with the exception of mibefradil, which also blocks T channels but is no longer used clinically.

Figure 22-2 shows that different agents bind to different sites on the α_1-subunit, depending on their chemical structure. Thus, 1,4-dihydropyridine CCBs bind at the interface of domains III and IV, with the receptor site localized in transmembrane sequences S_6 of both domains and the S_5-S_6 linker of domain III. The verapamil binding site is in segment S_6 of domain IV and a short segment of the carboxy-terminal intracellular region. The benzothiazepine CCBs have extracellular access, but their binding site overlaps in part with that of verapamil.

Classification

Structure

Several criteria have been used to classify CCBs acting on the cardiovascular system. The simplest classification is based on their chemical structures and subdivides them into 1,4-dihydropyridines, phenylalkylamines, and benzothiazepines (Table 22-1). As pointed out earlier, each group has a specific site of action on the L-channel α_1-subunit. A further widely used subclassification subdivides the compounds within each structural group into first-, second-, and third-generation compounds. Although this scheme roughly follows the historical sequence of introduction of the various compounds, it is obviously arbitrary and variable. The appeal of this classification appears largely to depend on the dubious concept that a later generation is better than the preceding ones. Because pharmacokinetic and pharmacodynamic differences

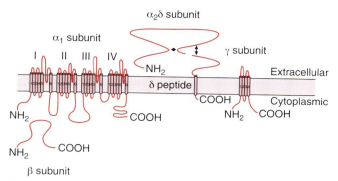

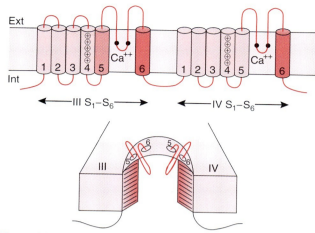

Figure 22–1 Arrangement of the subunits of the L-type voltage-gated calcium channel. The α_1 expresses the major structural and functional properties of the channel, including the permeation machinery and the drug binding sites. (From DeWaard M, Gurnett CA, Campbell KP. Structural and functional diversity of voltage-gated calcium channels. *In:* Narashashi T [ed]. Ion Channels. New York: Plenum Press, 1995, pp 41-87.)

Figure 22–2 *Top,* The α_1-subunit of the voltage-gated calcium channel, depicting the location of the verapamil and nifedipine binding sites on domains III and IV. The phenylalkylamine receptor is located on $IIIS_6$ and IVS_6 *(dark red columns),* and the dihydropyridine receptor is located on $IIIS_5$ *(medium red column).* In addition, it is likely that binding of calcium ions (Ca^{2+}) to glutamate residues in the pore region contributes to the blocking process. *Bottom,* Representation of drug-binding sites, indicating their close proximity to the pore and the channel opening and closing processes. Ext, extracellular; Int, intracellular. (From Triggle DJ. Mechanisms of action of calcium channel antagonists. *In:* Epstein M [ed]. Calcium Antagonists in Clinical Medicine, 3rd ed. Philadelphia: Hanley & Belfus, 2002, pp 1-32.)

across various agents matter clinically, I prefer a classification system based on the vascular selectivity and duration of action of the various compounds.

Vascular Selectivity

CCBs widely differ in terms of selectivity within the cardiovascular system. Phenylalkylamines and benzothiazepines exhibit cardiac depressant properties that are greater than or equal to their vasodilating properties, whereas dihydropyridines are predominantly vasodilators. Within the dihydropyridine subclass, the vascular-to-cardiac selectivity ratio also differs across different agents (see Table 22-1), and it is directly related to the voltage-dependent binding ratio (i.e., the ratio of binding constants of each dihydropyridine compound in polarized versus depolarized cardiac cells). The vascular-to-cardiac selectivity ratio has important clinical consequences: vascular selectivity correlates with greater vasodilatation and more powerful antihypertensive action, whereas a more powerful cardiac action may contribute to a cardioprotective effect and blunt reflex tachycardia.

Pharmacokinetics

The original prototype agents of the three structural groups undergo extensive first-pass hepatic metabolism, and therefore their bioavailability was low and variable. In addition, all these compounds had comparatively short elimination half-lives, and they had to be administered at least three times a day to ensure a constant therapeutic effect.[4] In antihypertensive therapy, once-daily administration is ideal. Therefore, agents with a long duration of action and slow onset have been developed that are suitable for once daily administration and are free of sudden vasodilatation.[4] Three types of long-acting compounds are listed in Table 22-1. The first consists of naturally short-acting agents in galenic preparations or other delivery systems that slow their release and absorption; this group is heterogeneous, because not all these preparations

are equally effective.[4] A second group is represented by amlodipine, a compound with relatively high oral bioavailability, slow absorption, and a very prolonged elimination half-life. A third group is composed of highly lipophilic compounds with relatively short plasma half-lives, but whose long duration and slow onset of action are the result of very strong binding to the lipid bilayer of the vascular smooth muscle cell membrane. Ambulatory BP monitoring studies show that prolonged, smooth BP lowering results when long-acting compounds or preparations are used.[5]

MANAGEMENT OF HYPERTENSION

Blood Pressure–Lowering and Hemodynamic Effects

Demonstration of the antihypertensive effects of verapamil and nifedipine dates back to the late 1970s.[6,7] Since then, many studies have established the CCBs as very effective BP-lowering agents,[8] and they are now considered among the main classes of antihypertensive drugs in all major guidelines.[9-12] Large comparative studies, such as the Treatment of Mild Hypertension Study[13] and the Veterans Affairs Monotherapy Study,[14] have shown CCB monotherapy to be at least equally effective in controlling hypertension as monotherapy with the other major antihypertensive drug

Table 22-1 Classification of Calcium Channel Blockers Active on the Cardiovascular System

Chemical Structure and Site of Action

A. Dihydropyridines (Site: α_1 IIIS$_5$-S$_6$)	B. Phenylalkylamines (Site: α_1 IVS$_6$ intracellular)	C. Benzothiazepines (Site: α_1 IVS$_6$ extracellular)
Nifedipine	Verapamil	Diltiazem
Nicardipine	Gallopamil	
Felodipine	Tiapamil	
Nitrendipine		
Nimodipine		
Nisoldipine		
Amlodipine		
Isradipine		
Lacidipine		
Lercanidipine		
Manidipine		
Barnidipine		

Vascular Cardiac Selectivity

A. Low Selectivity	B. Intermediate Selectivity	C. High Selectivity
Verapamil	Nifedipine	Felodipine
Diltiazem	Amlodipine	Nimodipine
		Nitrendipine
		Nicardipine
		Lacidipine
		Lercanidipine

Duration of Action

A. Short Acting	B. Long Acting		
	a. Special Preparations	b. Long Half-Life	c. Lipophilic Compounds
Verapamil	Verapamil SR	Amlodipine	Lacidipine
Diltiazem	Verapamil COER		Lercanidipine
Nifedipine	Diltiazem SR		Manidipine
Nicardipine	Nifedipine GITS		Barnidipine
Felodipine	Nicardipine SR		
Isradipine	Felodipine ER		

COER, controlled onset, extended release; ER, extended release; GITS, gastrointestinal therapeutic system; SR, sustained release.

classes. The claim that CCBs are more effective in low-renin hypertension, and hence in older patients and in black patients, has only partially been substantiated by the Veterans Affairs study.[14] In that study, CCB monotherapy ranked first (and much higher than angiotensin-converting enzyme [ACE] inhibitors and β-blockers) in controlling BP in black patients, whereas in white patients with hypertension, the ranking of the various monotherapies was not substantially modified by age. A greater antihypertensive response to CCBs than β-blockers and ACE inhibitors in black hypertensive patients has been confirmed by a recent meta-analysis.[15] The concept of the age dependency of the CCB BP-lowering response has also been revived recently, with the suggestion that CCBs and diuretics should be first-choice agents in elderly patients,[16] as recommended by the recent British Hypertension Society guidelines.[17] The antihypertensive effect of CCBs appears to be related to the degree of BP elevation; these drugs have little BP-lowering effect in normotensive subjects.[18]

The BP-lowering action of all CCBs is basically the result of their ability to induce systemic arterial vasodilation. A remarkable series of studies by Lund-Johansen and colleagues investigated the hemodynamic effect at rest and during exercise of a large number of antihypertensive agents and established that all CCBs, including nondihydropyridines, reduce total peripheral resistance with little or no influence on cardiac output both after short-term and during long-term administration.[19] The CCB hemodynamic response is similar to that of the α-blockers and ACE inhibitors, but it differs from that of the β-blockers, which mainly affect BP by reducing cardiac output.[19] Yet long-acting preparations of CCBs differ from other vasodilators, such as hydralazine and minoxidil, by having a more limited sympathetic reflex activation, and they do not result in as much fluid retention. Perhaps for these reasons, CCBs have largely replaced hydralazine and minoxidil in antihypertensive therapy regimens and are well enough tolerated to be given as monotherapy.

Clinical Outcome Studies

Observational Studies

Since the mid-1990s, the role of CCBs in the management of hypertension has been the subject of a lively debate because of concerns that these agents could increase, rather than decrease, the risk of coronary events or at least blunt the coronary protective effect of BP lowering. The main basis of this contention was a meta-analysis of studies in patients with coronary heart disease who were randomly assigned to nifedipine (mostly short-acting preparations with post hoc selection of daily doses of 80 mg or greater),[20] as well as two observational studies (a case-control study[21] and a cohort study[22]) showing that hypertensive subjects receiving treatment with a CCB (mostly short-acting agents) had a much greater risk of a major coronary event than subjects treated with other antihypertensive agents. At the time the debate was most lively, the evidence was reviewed by a World Health Organization–International Society of Hypertension ad hoc committee, which concluded that "the major concern about these observational studies is the large potential for systematic error to affect the results," with confounding by indication representing the most likely bias that is almost impossible to control by statistical adjustments.[23]

The controversy was recently revived by a prospective cohort study of 30,219 older women taking antihypertensive therapy.[24] After 5.9 years of follow-up, monotherapy with CCBs was associated with a 55% greater risk of cardiovascular mortality than diuretic therapy; among women receiving combination therapy, cardiovascular mortality (but not morbidity) was 85% greater in those receiving a diuretic and a CCB than in those receiving a diuretic and a β-blocker. Despite the study's large size, the same comments cited earlier[23] about earlier and smaller observational studies can be applied to this cohort study. Observational studies comparing treated with untreated hypertensive subjects or with normotensive subjects have regularly reported the greatest incidence of events in treated hypertension, an observation that is unanimously ascribed to confounding by indication. Not one of these observational studies has ever been used against the much stronger evidence in favor of BP lowering provided by randomized controlled trials.

Randomized Controlled Trials

In 1997, the World Health Organization–International Society of Hypertension pointed out that "reliable evidence about the safety and efficacy of calcium antagonists requires studies in which both random and systematic errors are minimized concurrently and this can only be provided by large-scale randomized trials."[23] Although no results of randomized trials were available at the time the debate was started, many trials have been completed since then, and reliable evidence is now available to consider the debate substantially closed. Table 22-2 lists all trials that have compared a treatment initiated with a CCB compared with a placebo-initiated treatment[25-30] or a treatment initiated with another active antihypertensive drug class in patients with high BP.[28,31-50]

As illustrated in Table 22-2A, each of the placebo-controlled trials that had cardiovascular events as a primary outcome showed a significant reduction of the primary outcome among CCB-treated patients, a reduction that was particularly remarkable in the two trials in elderly subjects with isolated systolic hypertension.[26,27] In the very large series of trials comparing a CCB with other active antihypertensive drugs (Table 22-2B, C, and D), the incidence of the primary cardiovascular outcome was not significantly different in patients treated with either an initial CCB or a diuretic or β-blocker or in patients treated with an ACE inhibitor or an angiotensin receptor blocker. The much publicized Appropriate Blood Pressure Control in Diabetes–Hypertension (ABCD-HT[46]) and Fosinopril versus Amlodipine Cardiac Events Randomized Trial (FACET[47]) studies, which reported a significant cardiovascular risk with CCBs compared with ACE inhibitors, were carried out in small cohorts of patients (470 and 380, respectively) and were originally designed for investigating changes in renal function,[46] or serum cholesterol,[47] as the primary endpoint.

These trials have been subjected to meta-analyses,[51,52] to increase overall statistical power and to obtain more reliable information on organ-specific outcomes, for which any single study was rarely sufficiently powered. The Blood Pressure Lowering Treatment Trialists' Collaboration meta-analysis[51] has the advantage of prospectively choosing the trials to be included, thus avoiding the most important bias to which meta-analyses are exposed. Figure 22-3 shows that, compared with placebo, CCBs significantly reduced the incidence of stroke (by 38%), coronary events (by 22%), and major cardiovascular events (by 18%), but the reductions in cardiovascular death (by 22%) and total mortality (by 11%) and the increased risk of heart failure (by 21%) were not significant. By comparing CCBs with diuretics or β-blockers, differences in outcomes were all very small, except for a 7% reduction in stroke incidence (of borderline significance) and a significant 33% increase in heart failure. Likewise, comparison with ACE inhibitors showed similar outcomes, except for an 11% significant reduction in stroke and a significant 22% increase in heart failure.

The Blood Pressure Lowering Treatment Trialists' Collaboration meta-analysis includes two small studies not listed in Table 22-2 that were carried out in patients with coronary heart disease,[53,54] and it does not include data from the International Verapamil-Trandolapril (INVEST[44]) or the Valsartan Antihypertensive Long-Term Use Evaluation (VALUE[50]) trials, which were completed subsequently. However, it does not appear that inclusion of INVEST would have changed the conclusions of the comparison of CCBs with β-blockers, and the VALUE results suggest CCBs were not inferior to angiotensin receptor blockers in the treatment of hypertension, except for new-onset heart failure. What the new-onset heart failure diagnosed in antihypertensive treatment trials may mean clinically is still undecided, however. A new diagnosis of heart failure is difficult to make, and most of the studies reporting more heart failure hospitalizations with CCBs have not observed the expected increase in cardiovascular mortality in patients diagnosed with heart failure.[55]

With regard to stroke, another meta-analysis comparing CCB-based treatment with any other type of antihypertensive treatment (diuretics, β-blockers, ACE inhibitors) showed a significant ($P = .002$) 10% reduction in stroke incidence with CCBs. This reduction was still significant when the meta-analysis was limited to trials using a dihydropyridine (-10%, $P = .006$), whereas it fell short of statistical significance (-7%, $P = .390$)

Table 22-2 Trials Comparing Antihypertensive Treatment Initiated by a Calcium Channel Blocker with Placebo Treatment (A) or Treatments Initiated by Another Antihypertensive (B to D)

	Agents Compared (1 vs. 2)	ΔSBP/ΔDBP (1 vs. 2) (mm Hg)	Primary Outcome Difference
A. CCB vs. Placebo			
STONE[25]	Nifedipine SR vs. placebo	–9/–6	–62% (P = .0001) in CV events
Syst-Eur[26]	Nitrendipine vs. placebo	–10/–4,5	–42% (P = .003) in stroke
Syst-China[27]	Nitrendipine vs. placebo	–9/–3	–38% (P = .01) in stroke
IDNT[28]	Amlodipine vs. placebo	–4/–3	Decrease in renal function
ACTION-HT[29]	Nifedipine vs. placebo	–6.6/–3.5	–13% (P ≥ .05) in CV events
FEVER[30]	Felodipine vs. placebo	–4.2/–2.1	–27% (P = .001) in stroke
B. CCB vs. D or BB			
MIDAS[31]	Isradipine vs. HCTZ		Carotid IMT progression
VHAS[32,33]	Verapamil SR vs. chlorthalidone		Carotid IMT progression
STOP-2[34]	Felodipine or isradipine vs. atenolol or pindolol or HCTZ	<1/<1	–3% (NS) in CV death
NICS-EH[35]	Nicardipine vs. trichlormethiazide	0/+2%	–3% (NS) in CV events
NORDIL[36]	Diltiazem vs. β-blocker or diuretic	+3/<1	0% (NS) in CV events
INSIGHT[37]	Nifedipine GITS vs. HCTZ + amiloride	<1/>1	+11% (NS) in CV events
AASK[38,39]	Amlodipine vs. metoprolol	–2/0	Decrease in renal function
ELSA[40]	Lacidipine vs. atenolol	<1/>1	Carotid IMT progression
ALLHAT[41]	Amlodipine vs. chlorthalidone	+1/<1	–2% (NS) in cardiac events
CONVINCE[42]	COER verapamil vs. HCTZ or atenolol	<1/<1	+2% (NS) in CV events
SHELL[43]	Lacidipine vs. chlorthalidone	–1/'	+1% (NS) in CV events
INVEST[44]	Verapamil vs. atenolol	–2/	–2% (NS) in CV events
ASCOT[45]	Amlodipine vs. atenolol	–2.7/–2.1	–10% (NS) in CHD events
C. CCB vs. ACEI			
ABCD-HT[46]	Nisoldipine vs. enalapril	<1/<1	Change in renal function
FACET[47]	Amlodipine vs. fosinopril	+6/0	Change in serum cholesterol
STOP-2[34]	Felodipine ER or isradipine vs. Enalapril or lisinopril	<1/–1.3	–4% (NS) in CV death
AASK[38,39]	Amlodipine vs. ramipril	–2/–1	Decrease in renal function
ABCD-NT[48]	Nisoldipine vs. enalapril	<1/0	Change in renal function
JMCI-B[49]	Nifedipine vs. ACEI	–2/–2	+5% (NS) in cardiac events
ALLHAT[41]	Amlodipine vs. lisinopril	–1.3/<1	–1% (NS) in cardiac events
D. CCB vs. ARB			
IDNT[28]	Amlodipine vs. irbesartan	–1/<1	Decrease in renal function
VALUE[50]	Amlodipine vs. valsartan	–2.6/–1.6	–4% (NS) in cardiac events

ΔDBP, difference in diastolic blood pressure; ΔSBP, difference in systolic blood pressure; AASK, African American Study of Kidney Disease and Hypertension; ABCD-HT, Appropriate Blood Pressure Control in Diabetes–Hypertension; ABCD-NT, Appropriate Blood Pressure Control in Diabetes–Normotension; ACEI, angiotensin-converting enzyme inhibitor; ACTION-HT, A Coronary Disease Trial Investigating Outcome with Nifedipine Gastrointestinal Therapeutic System–Hypertension Subgroup; ALLHAT, Antihypertensive and Lipid-Lowering Treatment to Prevent Heart Attack Trial; ARB, angiotensin receptor blocker; ASCOT, Anglo-Scandinavian Cardiac Outcomes Trial; BB, β-blocker; CCB, calcium channel blocker; CHD, coronary heart disease; COER, controlled onset, extended release; CONVINCE, Controlled Onset Verapamil Investigation of Cardiovascular End Points; CV, cardiovascular; D, diuretic; ELSA, European Lacidipine Study on Atherosclerosis; ER, extended release; FACET, Fosinopril versus Amlodipine Cardiovascular Events Randomized Trial; FEVER, Felodipine Event Reduction study; GITS, gastrointestinal therapeutic system; HCTZ, hydrochlorothiazide; IDNT, Irbesartan Diabetic Nephropathy Trial; IMT, intima-media thickness; INSIGHT, International Nifedipine GITS study: Intervention as a Goal in Hypertension Treatment; INVEST, International Verapamil-Trandolapril Study; JMIC-B, Japan Multicenter Investigation for Cardiovascular Disease-B; MIDAS, Multicenter Isradipine Diuretic Atherosclerosis Study; NICS-EH, National Intervention Cooperative Study in Elderly Hypertensives; NORDIL, Nordic Diltiazem Study; NS, nonsignificant; SHELL, Systolic Hypertension in the Elderly Lacidipine study; SR, sustained release; STONE, Shanghai Trial of Nifedipine in the Elderly; STOP-2, Swedish Trial in Old Patients with Hypertension-2; Syst-China, Systolic Hypertension in China; Syst-Eur, Systolic Hypertension in Europe; VALUE, Valsartan Antihypertensive Long-Term Use Evaluation; VHAS, Verapamil in Hypertension and Atherosclerosis Study.

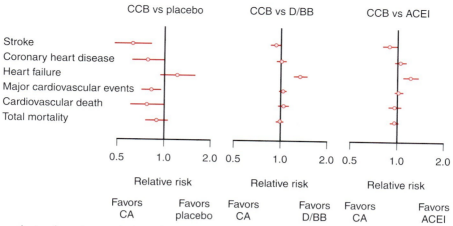

Figure 22–3 Meta-analysis of randomized clinical trials comparing outcomes of blood pressure lowering based on calcium channel blockers (CCB) with placebo treatment *(left column)* with regimens based on diuretics (D) or β-blockers (BB) *(center column)*, and with regimens based on angiotensin-converting enzyme inhibitors (ACEI) *(right column)*. Outcomes are listed on the *left*. The *circles* indicate the relative risks and the *bars* the 95% confidence intervals. (Redrawn from data in Blood Pressure Lowering Treatment Trialists' Collaboration. Effects of different blood-pressure-lowering regimens on major cardiovascular events: Results of prospectively-designed overviews of randomized trials. *Lancet.* 2003;**362**:1527-1535.)

when it was restricted to nondihydropyridine agents.[52] However, the Blood Pressure Lowering Treatment Trialists' Collaboration meta-analysis concerning all types of outcomes does not show significant heterogeneity across trials using dihydropyridines and those using nondihydropyridines.[51]

As the debate about safety of CCBs centered on the claim that they increased the risk of coronary events, it is relevant to stress that not one of the recent meta-analyses indicates any significant additional coronary risk associated with the use of CCBs. In particular, the recent FEVER study[30] found a significant (P = .0153) 32% reduction in coronary events in the felodipine versus the placebo arm and ASCOT[45] a 10% reduction (P = .1050) in the amlodipine-based versus the atenolol-based regimen. Furthermore, two recently completed trials, one carried out specifically in patients with angina (A Coronary Disease Trial Investigating Outcome with Nifedipine Gastrointestinal Therapeutic System [ACTION] trial, comparing nifedipine gastrointestinal therapeutic system [GITS] versus placebo)[30,56] and one in patients with coronary disease and normal BP (Comparison of Amlodipine versus Enalapril to Limit Occurrences of Thrombosis [CAMELOT] trial, comparing amlodipine with placebo or enalapril),[57] both showed a significant reduction in the primary outcome with the CCB, although admittedly this reduction was mostly the result of a reduction in angina-related events.

The final question about the role that differences in achieved BPs between the treatment arms of trials may play in causing or masking some differences in cardiovascular outcomes is difficult to answer in a straightforward manner.[55] Unfortunately, the issue is confounded by the failure of many trials to achieve the same reduction in BP with the two treatment arms (see Table 22-2). On the whole, however, most of the benefits provided by all antihypertensive agents, CCBs included, depend on lowering BP, and according to meta-analyses,[51,52] most of the small differences in organ-specific outcomes can be accounted for by small BP differences. An exception is the increase in new-onset heart failure,[51] as well as a possibly reduced incidence of stroke with CCBs.[52]

Safety

Adverse Effects

Dihydropyridine and nondihydropyridine CCBs have somewhat different side effect profiles. With dihydropyridines vasodilation-dependent adverse effects (flushing, palpitations, ankle edema) predominate, whereas with verapamil and diltiazem, vasodilatation-related symptoms are generally milder, and cardiac conductance and gastrointestinal (mostly constipation) disturbances predominate.[8] Most of these adverse effects are dose dependent[58] and, with the exception of ankle edema, are much more prominent with rapidly acting compounds.

The opinion that CCBs are associated with a markedly greater incidence of adverse effects than other classes of antihypertensive agents was borne out by early studies with the initial fast-onset compounds, but it is not supported by reports from large randomized trials. In the Hypertension Optimal Treatment (HOT) study,[59] in which 18,790 patients received felodipine ER at doses of 5 to 10 mg/day, the adverse event incidence was quite low, even in the group randomized to the lowest BP target and who therefore received a higher average dose of felodipine (peripheral edema, 1.6%). In the HOT study, a careful quality of life investigation was carried out and found that patients randomized to the lowest BP target had improvement rather than worsening in well-being.[60] Table 22-3 lists adverse effects in some of the large randomized trials comparing a CCB-initiated regimen with regimens initiated by different antihypertensive agents. Data in Table 22-3 are from the Verapamil in Hypertension and Atherosclerosis Study (VHAS),[32] the Nordic Diltiazem study (NORDIL),[36] INVEST,[44] the International Nifedipine GITS Study: Intervention as a Goal of Hypertension Treatment (INSIGHT),[37] the Swedish Trial in Old Patients with Hypertension-2 (STOP-2),[34] and VALUE,[50] which have provided detailed information on the most frequent adverse events. Although dihydropyridine compounds have regularly

Table 22-3 Major Adverse Effects (%) Reported in Some Randomized Trials Comparing a Calcium Channel Blocker with a Different Regimen*

Adverse Effect	VHAS[32]		NORDIL[36]			INVEST[44]			INSIGHT[37]			STOP-2[34]			VALUE[50]		
	CCB	D	CCB	D/BB	P	CCB	BB	P	CCB	D	P	CCB	D/BB	ACEI	CCB	ARB	P
Edema	3.1	—	—	—	—	—	—	—	**28**	4.3	<.0001	**25.5**	8.5	8.7	**32.9**	14.9	<.0001
Headache	3.1	3.4	**8.5**	5.7	<.001	—	—	—	**12**	9.2	.0002	**10.0**	5.7	7.7	12.5	**14.7**	<.0001
Flushing	—	—	—	—	—	—	—	—	**4.3**	2.3	<.0001	**9.7**	1.6	2.2	—	—	—
Palpitations	—	—	—	—	—	0.66	**1.26**	<.01	2.5	2.7	NS	**7.9**	2.9	5.3	—	—	—
Bradycardia	—	—	—	—	—	0.73	**1.01**	.03	—	—	—	1.4	**3.7**	0.8	—	—	—
Dyspnea	—	—	2.9	**3.9**	.006	—	—	—	8.0	**10.0**	.006	8.5	**11.8**	7.3	14.3	**16.5**	<.0001
Dizziness	3.5	3.1	9.3	8.9	NS	1.37	1.34	NS	1.5	**2.8**	.0004	24.5	27.8	27.7	1.0	**1.7**	<.0001
Syncope	—	3.1	—	—	—	**1.73**	0.13	<.01	—	—	—	—	—	—	—	—	—
Constipation	**13.7**	—	—	—	—	—	—	—	—	—	—	—	—	—	—	—	—
Fatigue	4.7	**8.4**	4.4	**6.5**	<.001	—	—	—	3.9	**5.7**	.0009	—	—	—	8.9	9.7	NS
Depression	—	—	3.7	3.4	NS	—	—	—	—	—	—	—	—	—	—	—	—
Cough	—	—	5.6	5.4	NS	**1.78**	1.34	0.01	—	—	—	5.7	3.7	30.1	—	—	—

*Trials and regimens as in Table 22-2. The numbers in bold indicate adverse effect with the highest incidence in each trial. VHAS and STOP-2 did not report significance tests for adverse effects.

ACEI, angiotensin-converting enzyme inhibitor; ARB, angiotensin receptor blocker; BB, β-blocker; CCB, calcium channel blocker; D, diuretic; NS, nonsignificant.

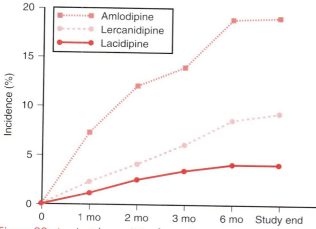

Figure 22–4 Incidence (%) of peripheral edema after 1, 2, 3, and 6 months of treatment and at study end (*n* = 828). Data are separately shown for the lercanidipine *(circles and dashed line),* amlodipine *(squares and dashed line),* and lacidipine *(circles and solid line)* treatment groups. (From Leonetti G, Magnani B, Pessina AC, et al. Tolerability of long-term treatment with lercanidipine versus amlodipine and lacidipine in elderly hypertensives. *Am J Hypertens.* 2002;**15**:932-940.)

induced more peripheral edema and flushing, this was not the case with nondihydropyridine compounds. Verapamil, but not diltiazem, has been associated with more constipation. In contrast, comparative agents (diuretics, β-blockers, ACE inhibitors, angiotensin receptor blockers) have been associated with more dizziness, dyspnea, syncope, and fatigue (see Table 22-3). Different long-acting dihydropyridines may differ in terms of adverse events, especially pedal edema. Several recent studies have concordantly shown that lipophilic compounds, such as lercanidipine, lacidipine, and manidipine, are associated with a lower incidence of ankle edema than amlodipine, despite similar BP reduction[61-63] (Fig. 22-4).

Cancer and Bleeding

In the mid-1990s, a serious allegation raised about the safety of CCBs included not only the claim that these agents were associated with an increase in coronary events,[20-22] but also the claim, made by the same group of authors, that CCBs could be responsible for an increased incidence of cancer and gastrointestinal bleeding.[64-66] These claims have not been confirmed by large randomized trials. In discussing the results of the Antihypertensive and Lipid-Lowering Treatment to Prevent Heart Attack Trial (ALLHAT), some of the principal authors of these claims conceded the following: "A body of literature based on observational studies and secondary CHD prevention trials of short-acting CCBs has suggested that these drugs, especially agents of the DHP-CCB subclass, may increase the risk of cancer, gastrointestinal bleeding, and all-cause mortality. The results of ALLHAT do not support these findings. In fact, the mortality from non-cardiovascular causes was significantly lower in the CCB group."[41] In ALLHAT (the largest of all the CCB trials), the incidence of cancer death was similar in all three arms (amlodipine, 3.4; chlorthalidone, 4.3; and lisinopril, 4.0 per 100 persons over 6

years).[41] No significant difference in cancer incidence was found for those receiving other CCBs in INSIGHT,[37] Controlled Onset Verapamil Investigation of Cardiovascular End Points (CONVINCE),[42] or INVEST.[44] In the placebo-controlled FEVER trial,[30] felodipine was associated with a significantly lower incidence of cancer (−36%, *P* = .017) than placebo. As for gastrointestinal bleeding, ALLHAT reported no difference (amlodipine, 0.4; chlorthalidone, 0.3; and lisinopril, 0.4 per 100 persons in 6 years),[41] whereas CONVINCE found a small but significant excess of bleeding-related hospitalizations with controlled-onset extended-release verapamil.[42] The latter finding, however, was not corroborated in INVEST, despite comparing regimens that included either verapamil or a β-blocker (as did CONVINCE).[44]

Metabolic Effects and New-Onset Diabetes

Not all randomized clinical trials have reported changes in metabolic variables occurring during long-term treatment. Among trials comparing a CCB with another agent, VHAS reported hypokalemia in 5.5% of patients randomized to chlorthalidone, but none with verapamil.[32] The European Lacidipine Study on Atherosclerosis (ELSA) observed a significant difference between lacidipine- or atenolol-treated patients for high-density lipoprotein cholesterol (atenolol, −0.03 ± 0.35; lacidipine, +0.05 ± 0.37 mmol/L; *P* < .0001) and triglycerides (atenolol, 0.26 ± 1.03; lacidipine, 0.09 ± 0.79 mmol/L; *P* <0.001).[40] INSIGHT reported a significantly lower incidence of hypokalemia (*P* < .0001), hyponatremia (*P* < .0001), hyperlipidemia (*P* < .0001), hyperglycemia (*P* = .001), and hyperuricemia (*P* < .0001) in patients randomized to nifedipine GITS rather than to hydrochlorothiazide in combination with amiloride.[37] In ALLHAT, serum potassium at 4 years was significantly higher (*P* < .001) and the prevalence of hypokalemia significantly lower (*P* < .001) in patients randomized to amlodipine (as well as in those randomized to lisinopril) than in patients receiving chlorthalidone.[41] After 4 years of treatment, mean fasting blood glucose was also slightly, though nonsignificantly, lower in the group randomized to amlodipine (as well as to lisinopril) than in the chlorthalidone-treated group.[41]

Perhaps more important, several recent trials have reported different incidences of newly diagnosed diabetes mellitus across groups given different antihypertensive drugs. These data have been reviewed and meta-analyzed.[67-69] In NORDIL,[36] INSIGHT,[37] ALLHAT,[41] and INVEST,[44] there was an 11% to 23% lower risk of developing new-onset diabetes among patients initially receiving a CCB (diltiazem, nifedipine, amlodipine, verapamil) than in those given a diuretic or a β-blocker, with a pooled overall reduction of 16% (95% confidence interval, 9% to 22%).[69] However, when CCBs were compared with agents interfering with the renin-angiotensin system, the incidence of new diabetes was 20% less with the ACE inhibitor lisinopril,[41] and 23% less with the angiotensin receptor blocker valsartan,[50] than with amlodipine. In the placebo-controlled FEVER trial[30] low-dose felodipine was associated with a similar incidence of new diabetes as placebo.

The clinical importance of new-onset diabetes has been debated, and some authors,[41] as well as some guidelines,[9] but not others,[10,11] have minimized the impact of this outcome, on the basis of the argument that "these metabolic differences did not translate into more cardiovascular events" during the average 5-year duration of a trial.[41] However, the recently reported findings of 16-year follow-up of patients enrolled in the Multiple Risk Factor Intervention Trial (MRFIT) indicate that patients who developed new diabetes mellitus during active participation in the study had a significantly higher post-trial mortality than those who did not develop diabetes, although this difference in risk required several years to appear.[70]

On the whole, CCBs, both dihydropyridine and nondihydropyridine compounds, appear to be substantially free of the risk of precipitating overt diabetes in predisposed subjects, a risk that is not negligible with β-blockers and diuretics but that may be even lower with ACE inhibitors and angiotensin receptor blockers.

Combination Therapy

Combination therapy is becoming more frequently used for treating hypertension, because most patients require at least two drugs to achieve target BPs, especially diabetic patients and patients with chronic kidney disease, whose BP target is less than 130/80 mm Hg.[9-11] Indeed, in the HOT study, which recruited patients with BPs higher than 160/100 mm Hg after washout from previous medication, 75% of patients randomized to the lowest BP target required two or more drugs.[59] Multiple-drug therapy was also required to achieve goal BP in the majority of patients in four recent large trials,[41,42,44,50] in which patients were rolled over from previous to randomized treatment. In no trial was combination therapy required more frequently in the group randomized to a CCB than in comparative treatment groups. Accordingly, current guidelines are liberal in recommending use of combination therapy as "step-up" or initial therapy, with the Seventh Report of the Joint National Committee on Prevention, Detection, Evaluation, and Treatment of High Blood Pressure indicating the possibility of starting patients with stage 2 hypertension on two drugs,[9] and the European Society of Hypertension–European Society of Cardiology guidelines recommending combination therapy as an option to be chosen after considering the untreated BP level and the presence or absence of organ damage and other cardiovascular risk factors.[10]

Which agents should best be combined with a CCB is debatable. The agents that have been most widely associated with CCBs in clinical pharmacologic studies have been β-blockers and ACE inhibitors. β-Blockers combine well with dihydropyridine CCBs because of their complementary actions, enhancing efficacy and tolerability.[71] Conversely, combination of a β-blocker with a nondihydropyridine compound such as verapamil and diltiazem should generally be avoided (except for rare specific indications) because of the increased risk of atrioventricular conduction disturbances and cardiac depression.[71] The combination of a CCB, either a dihydropyridine or a nondihydropyridine, with an ACE inhibitor not only is effective, but also reduces the most frequent adverse effect of CCBs, namely ankle edema.[71] The association of a CCB and a diuretic has been considered by some investigators to be less effective, because the antihypertensive actions of the two classes of compounds may not be fully additive.

However, the best evidence of the long-term benefits of combining various antihypertensive drugs comes from

Table 22-4 Drugs Combined with Calcium Channel Blockers in Major Controlled Randomized Trials

Trial	Calcium Channel Blocker	Additional Agent
Syst-Eur[26]	Nitrendipine	ACEI: enalapril
Syst-China[27]	Nitrendipine	ACEI: captopril
VHAS[32,33]	Verapamil	ACEI: captopril
MIDAS[31]	Isradipine	ACEI: enalapril
HOT[59]	Felodipine	ACEI: any (enalapril in United States)
NORDIL[36]	Diltiazem	ACEI: any
INVEST[44]	Verapamil	ACEI: trandolapril
ASCOT[45]	Amlodipine	ACEI: perindopril
HOT[59]	Felodipine	BB: any
STOP-2[34]	Felodipine or isradipine	BB: any
INSIGHT[37]	Nifedipine GITS	BB: atenolol
ALLHAT[41]	Amlodipine	BB: atenolol
ELSA[40]	Lacidipine	D: hydrochlorothiazide
CONVINCE[42]	Verapamil	D: hydrochlorothiazide
VALUE[50]	Amlodipine	D: hydrochlorothiazide
FEVER[30]	Felodipine	D: hydrochlorothiazide

ACEI, angiotensin-converting enzyme inhibitor; ALLHAT, Antihypertensive and Lipid-Lowering Treatment to Prevent Heart Attack Trial; ASCOT, Anglo-Scandinavian Cardiac Outcomes Trial; BB, β-blocker; CONVINCE, Controlled Onset Verapamil Investigation of Cardiovascular End Points; D, Diuretic; ELSA, European Lacidipine Study on Atherosclerosis; FEVER, Felodipine Event Reduction study; GITS, gastrointestinal therapeutic system; HOT, Hypertension Optimal Treatment; INSIGHT, International Nifedipine GITS study: Intervention as a Goal in Hypertension Treatment; INVEST, International Verapamil-Trandolapril Study; MIDAS, Multicenter Isradipine Diuretic Atherosclerosis Study; NORDIL, Nordic Diltiazem Study; STOP-2, Swedish Trial in Old Patients with Hypertension-2; Syst-China, Systolic Hypertension in China; Syst-Eur, Systolic Hypertension in Europe; VALUE, Valsartan Antihypertensive Long-Term Use Evaluation; VHAS, Verapamil in Hypertension and Atherosclerosis Study.

randomized clinical trials in which CCBs, in association with other antihypertensive agents, reduced cardiovascular outcomes better than placebo or as well as combinations of other compounds. Table 22-4 lists the types of drugs that have been successfully combined with a CCB in major trials. Several thousand patients have received a CCB, either a dihydropyridine or a nondihydropyridine compound, in association with an ACE inhibitor, several thousand a dihydropyridine in association with a β-blocker, and very large numbers of patients have also received a dihydropyridine or a nondihydropyridine in association with hydrochlorothiazide. In all randomized trials in which a CCB was combined with a diuretic, there was no suggestion that this combination may have been less effective in reducing morbidity and mortality than comparative agents. These findings indicate that the different conclusions drawn from a nonrandomized cohort study[24] were likely due to confounding by indication. Information on the combination of CCBs with angiotensin receptor blockers is limited to about 20% of the 4937 patients in the Study on Cognition and Prognosis in the Elderly (SCOPE) trial,[72] who received a CCB as third agent in the candesartan arm of that trial, and to a study in diabetic nephropathy in which losartan was added to previous therapy, which often included a CCB.[73]

Fixed-dose combinations of CCBs with β-blockers or with ACE inhibitors are available in both the United States and several European countries. However, the success of these fixed-dose combinations has been more limited in Europe because they are not on the reimbursement list of several national health systems.[71]

ANCILLARY PROPERTIES

Renal Effects

CCBs differ from hydralazine and minoxidil by not having sodium retaining activity and, instead, possessing a distinct natriuretic effect. Repeated administration of felodipine resulted in a negative sodium balance during the first few days, a significant increase in renal plasma flow without any change in glomerular filtration rate (Fig. 22-5), despite increases in plasma renin activity, and, albeit to a smaller extent, in plasma aldosterone concentrations.[74] These findings are consistent with dihydropyridines' inhibition of tubular reabsorption of sodium in the rat. Dihydropyridines and nondihydropyridines differ somewhat in their natriuretic activity: with the same BP decrease, a marked and immediate natriuretic effect occurs with short-acting nifedipine, but that of short-acting verapamil is apparently negligible.[18] However, a negative sodium balance builds up slowly with verapamil, as shown by a reduced body weight and extracellular fluid volume after several weeks of therapy.[6] The negative sodium balance is maintained during long-term dihydropyridine therapy, because transient sodium retention occurs after drug withdrawal.[75] This natriuretic action of CCBs accounts for their long-term effectiveness as monotherapy, without the need of a diuretic, as is typically necessary with hydralazine and minoxidil.

The renal hemodynamic effects of CCBs, consisting of predominant vasodilatation with little or no change in glomerular filtration rate (probably with unchanged intraglomerular pressure resulting from a balancing between the predominantly afferent arteriolar vasodilatation and the con-

spicuous BP decrease), have been the basis for several studies investigating a potential protective effect of CCBs in transplant recipients who are given cyclosporine. Cyclosporine increases BP in nearly 90% of transplant recipients, and this BP increase is associated with both extrarenal and intrarenal vasoconstriction, accompanied by reduced renal plasma flow and reduced sodium excretion.[76] All these effects of cyclosporine can effectively be countered by CCBs.[76] In addition, a "beneficial" drug-drug interaction between cyclosporine and many CCBs allows a reduction in the total daily dose (and cost) of cyclosporine, so CCBs are widely used in transplant recipients.

The predominant site of the renal vasodilating action of CCBs is the afferent arteriole. This characteristic has caused concern about the possibility that the use of these drugs may worsen, rather than improve, long-term renal outcomes in hypertension. This issue is particularly relevant for hypertensive patients with diabetes mellitus and chronic kidney disease and is discussed later in detail in the section on special indications and contraindications of CCBs. In large randomized clinical trials not specifically involving diabetic or renal patients, not one of them indicated a detrimental effect of a

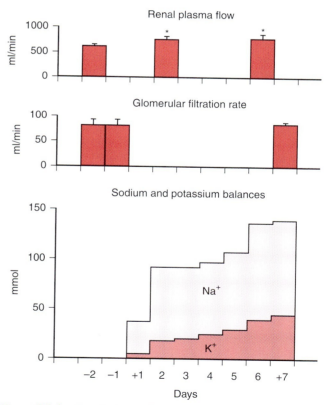

Figure 22–5 Renal plasma flow *(upper)*, glomerular filtration rate *(middle)*, and sodium (Na^+) and potassium (K^+) balances *(lower)* during felodipine therapy. Sodium and potassium balances were calculated by adding daily urinary excretion of sodium (or potassium) minus the excretion during the last day of placebo administration. *$P < .05$ versus placebo. (From Leonetti G, Gradnik R, Terzoli L, et al. Effect of single and repeated doses of the calcium antagonist felodipine on blood pressure, renal function, electrolytes and water balance, and renin-angiotensin-aldosterone system in hypertensive patients. *J Cardiovasc Pharmacol.* 1986;**8**:1243-1248.)

CCB on renal function or proteinuria. In the Systolic Hypertension in Europe (Syst-Eur) trial, patients randomized to nitrendipine had a 64% lower incidence of mild renal dysfunction and a 33% lower incidence of new proteinuria than did placebo-treated patients.[77] Some of this benefit could have been attributed to better BP lowering. Among trials comparing two active antihypertensive regimens and reporting renal function outcomes, INSIGHT found a lower incidence of impaired renal function in patients treated with nifedipine than the diuretic (1.8% versus 4.6%, $P < .0001$),[37] ALLHAT showed a significantly higher estimated glomerular filtration rate during treatment with amlodipine than with chlorthalidone (75.1 versus 70.0 mL/minute/1.73 m^2, $P = .001$) or lisinopril (75.1 versus 70.7 mL/minute/1.73 m^2) and a nonsignificant difference in the incidence of end-stage renal disease with amlodipine, chlorthalidone, and lisinopril (2.1%, versus 1.8%, versus 2.0%, respectively),[41] and VALUE reported very small increases in average serum creatinine concentrations both with amlodipine and with valsartan.[50]

Antiatherogenic Action

In experimental animals, CCBs can protect against the development of atherosclerosis, independent of their antihypertensive effects. Similar evidence has also been obtained in humans, particularly in hypertensive patients. Asymptomatic atherosclerosis can now be detected and quantitatively measured by B-mode ultrasound examination of the carotid arteries, and the resultant measurement, intima-media thickness (IMT), predicts subsequent mortality and morbidity related to myocardial infarction and stroke.[78] Changes at the bifurcations and internal carotid arteries represent a better index of atherosclerosis than changes in the common carotid arteries, where hypertrophy may predominate over atherosclerosis.[78] Recently developed echoreflectivity techniques may provide reliable information from ultrasound scans not only on the thickness but also on the composition of the carotid arterial wall,[79] and they have shown that, in hypertensive patients, carotid lesions are predominantly fibrolipidic.[80]

Five major studies using carotid ultrasound have compared a CCB either with placebo or with other antihypertensive agents (Table 22-5). In the Prospective Randomized Evaluation of Vascular Events with Norvasc Trial (PREVENT) of amlodipine against placebo, a definite BP difference was noted between the two groups, so it is difficult to conclude whether the reduced progression in carotid IMT in the amlodipine-treated group was the result of a specific action of the CCB.[54] The other four studies have all been carried out in hypertensive patients and have compared a treatment based on a CCB with one based on an alternative agent (a diuretic in the Multicenter Isradipine Diuretic Atherosclerosis Study [MIDAS],[31] VHAS,[33] and INSIGHT[81] and a β-blocker in ELSA[40]). MIDAS reported a nonsignificant difference in the primary endpoint, but significant differences in several secondary endpoints, namely, less IMT progression with isradipine, despite a smaller BP reduction. All the other studies found a significantly lower progression of carotid IMT in patients treated with CCBs than in those treated with chlorthalidone,[33] hydrochlorothiazide in combination with amiloride,[81] or atenolol.[40] ELSA, the largest of these studies (2255 patients), found a favorable effect of lacidipine not only on common carotid but also on bifurcation IMT (Fig. 22-6), as well as on the number of plaques per patient.[40] Each of these three studies showed no differences in BP reduction among the treatment groups, and in ELSA achieved ambulatory BP was even lower in the atenolol-treated group than in the lacidipine-treated group. These findings support the conclusion that verapamil, nifedipine GITS, and lacidipine have a specific antiatherosclerotic action, in addition to their antihypertensive effect. This antiatherosclerotic action has been demonstrated on asymptomatic lesions only (in most studies patients with IMTs >4 mm were excluded). This action consists of a significant retardation of progression, rather than regression. ELSA has shown that regression is unlikely when studies include longitudinal quality control protocols to exclude or correct for reading drift or bias.[82] A substudy of INSIGHT also found that nifedipine GITS retarded progression of coronary calcification in hypertensive patients compared with diuretic therapy.[83]

In more advanced atherosclerosis, only three studies in patients with overt coronary heart disease are available. Neither the International Nifedipine Trial on Antiatherosclerotic Therapy (INTACT[84]) nor PREVENT[54] was able to show any difference in lumen changes between CCBs and placebo using quantitative coronary angiography. The more recent CAMELOT trial reported a nonsignificantly slower progression of atheroma by intracoronary ultrasound with amlodipine than with placebo, a finding that correlated with BP changes.[57]

Table 22-5 Studies with Calcium Channel Blockers on Carotid Intima-Media Thickness

Study	Disease	Treatments	IMT Measurement	Patients (n)	Results CCB vs. C mm/yr
PREVENT[54]	CHD	Amlodipine vs. placebo	M$_{max}$	373	−0.0152
MIDAS[31]	HT	Isradipine vs. hydrochlorothiazide	M$_{max}$	833	NS
VHAS[33]	HT	Verapamil vs. chlorthalidone	M$_{max}$	498	−0.0100
INSIGHT[81]	HT	Nifedipine GITS vs. co-amilozide	CC-IMT	324	−0.0081
ELSA[40]	HT	Lacidipine vs. atenolol	CBM$_{max}$	2255	−0.0089

C, control; CBM$_{max}$, mean of maximum intima-media thickness in common carotid and bifurcation; CCB, calcium channel blocker; CC-IMT, intima-media thickness in common carotid; CHD, coronary heart disease; ELSA, European Lacidipine Study on Atherosclerosis; GITS, gastrointestinal therapeutic system; HT, hypertension; IMT, intima-media thickness; INSIGHT, International Nifedipine GITS Study: Intervention as a Goal in Hypertension Treatment; MIDAS, Multicenter Isradipine Diuretic Atherosclerosis Study; M$_{max}$, mean of maximum intima-media thickness in common carotid, bifurcation, and internal carotid; PREVENT, Prospective Randomized Evaluation of the Vascular Effects of Norvasc Trial; VHAS, Verapamil in Hypertension and Atherosclerosis Study.

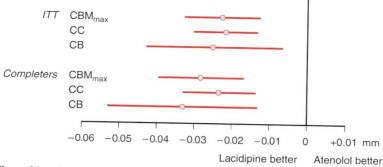

Figure 22–6 Estimated effect of lacidipine versus atenolol on intima-media thickness of far walls of common carotids and bifurcations (CBM$_{max}$), common carotids (CC), and carotid bifurcations (CB), using repeated measurements model analysis. Mean changes over the treatment period (~4 years) are indicated by *circles,* and their 95% confidence intervals are illustrated by *bars.* Values to the *left* of the 0 line indicate less progression with lacidipine. Completers, analysis limited to patients who completed the full course of treatment; ITT, intention-to-treat analysis. (From Zanchetti A, Bond M, Hennig M, et al. Calcium-antagonist lacidipine slows down progression of asymptomatic carotid atherosclerosis. *Circulation.* 2002;**106**:2422-2427.)

Effects on the Endothelium, Endothelial Dysfunction, and Oxidative Stress

In comparative studies, CCBs facilitate endothelium-dependent vasodilation and help to restore impaired endothelial dysfunction in hypertension. An interesting parallelism exists between the observation that lacidipine improves nitric oxide–dependent vasodilation whereas atenolol does not[85] and the findings of the ELSA trial on carotid atherosclerosis.[40] Several CCBs reduce oxidative stress, and this may represent an important mechanism of their antiatherosclerotic action.[40,85]

Regression of Left Ventricular Hypertrophy

Left ventricular hypertrophy (LVH), detected by either electrocardiogram or the more sensitive echocardiogram, is associated with an increased incidence of cardiovascular events, and is considered in some guidelines a cardiovascular risk factor largely independent of BP.[10] Patients who experience regression of LVH during antihypertensive therapy have a lower incidence of cardiovascular events than patients whose hypertrophy does not regress or worsens.[86]

A very large body of echocardiographic studies has assessed the effects of antihypertensive agents on LVH. Unfortunately, considerable numbers of studies claiming superiority of one or another class of antihypertensive agent in causing hypertrophy regression were noncomparative, nonrandomized, or too small.[87] A meta-analysis by Schmieder and colleagues through 1998 summarized 40 studies and reported a reduction of left ventricular mass by 12% for ACE inhibitors, 11% for CCBs, 8% for diuretics, and 5% for β-blockers.[88] Another earlier meta-analysis by Jennings and Wong summarizing 32 studies ranked antihypertensive agents in the following order of decreasing capacity of reducing left ventricular mass: CCBs, ACE inhibitors, diuretics, α-blockers, and β-blockers.[89]

Comparative studies of LVH regression should follow very strict quality criteria to provide sufficiently reliable estimates, with a sufficiently large number of randomized patients to have good power to detect small differences in left ventricular mass, high quality of echocardiograms with central reading by experts, and avoidance of regression to the mean and of readers' bias toward regression.[87] Very few studies have fulfilled all these criteria, but four of these have included a CCB in one treatment arm. Currently, these studies represent the most solid evidence about the comparative ability of CCBs to regress LVH. In three studies, a CCB was compared with an ACE inhibitor, and in the fourth, a CCB was compared with a β-blocker. In the 148 patients in the Effects of Amlodipine and Lisinopril on Left Ventricular Mass and Diastolic Function (ELVERA) study, amlodipine was equally effective as lisinopril in reducing left ventricular mass index over 2 years of treatment.[90] The Prospective Randomized Enalapril Study Evaluating Regression of Ventricular Enlargement (PRESERVE) study showed nifedipine GITS or enalapril to reduce left ventricular mass index by the same extent in 235 patients over 1 year's treatment.[91] The Fosinopril or Amlodipine Multicenter (FOAM) study has found the same left ventricular mass reduction by amlodipine or fosinopril in 144 patients at the end of 9 months' treatment.[92] Finally, an ELSA substudy has reported no significant difference in left ventricular mass index reduction with lacidipine or atenolol after 1 and 4 years of treatment.[93] In all these large comparative studies, BP was reduced to a very similar extent by the drug regimens compared.

In summary, both meta-analyses and large randomized comparative studies indicate that CCBs are not inferior to other antihypertensive agents in regressing LVH. CCBs have not yet been studied to see whether they change excessive cardiac fibrosis, which in some studies is at least as important as regression of cardiac mass in hypertension-related hypertrophy. A decrease in myocardial collagen volume fraction, as detected by echoreflectivity analysis, was seen after treatment with an angiotensin receptor antagonist.[94]

Effects on Large Arteries

Specific effects of antihypertensive agents on large arteries may influence the pulsatile component of BP, a risk factor for cardiovascular events, especially in elderly patients.[95] CCBs can influence large artery function, both directly and indirectly.[96]

Certain dihydropyridine CCBs have been shown to increase the diameter of muscular arteries, such as the brachial artery, but not that of elastic arteries, such as the carotid, acutely and chronically. Both long- and short-term treatment with nitrendipine or isradipine decreases stiffness of large arteries, independent of geometric and BP modifications.[96] In patients with end-stage renal disease, increased aortic distensibility during prolonged administration of nitrendipine was only initially related to the BP decrease, a finding suggesting that arterial structural changes in the long-term may substitute initial functional changes. CCBs reduce pulse-wave velocity, thus decreasing the wave reflection component of systolic BP in the aorta and central arteries, and this is different from β-blockers, which increase pulse-wave velocity.[96]

CCBs thus have a profound effect, not only on arterioles, but also on large arteries. Because increased arterial stiffness and altered wave reflection are the primary physiologic mechanisms of isolated systolic hypertension, the effects of CCBs on these factors may be important contributors to the reduced cardiovascular mortality and morbidity seen with these agents in elderly patients with isolated systolic hypertension.[26,27]

Effect on Cognitive Activity

Loss of cognitive activity is frequent in elderly patients and is at least partly related to previous hypertension. However, only a few large randomized trials have tested the effects of antihypertensive therapy on cognitive function or incident dementia. Data from five studies, all placebo controlled, are currently available. No significant differences in cognitive function were found in the Systolic Hypertension in the Elderly Program (SHEP), which compared a diuretic with placebo in elderly subjects with isolated systolic hypertension,[97] in the Medical Research Council (MRC) study, which compared a diuretic or a β-blocker with placebo in older hypertensives,[98] or in SCOPE, which compared an angiotensin receptor antagonist with placebo (in addition to other antihypertensive therapy) in elderly hypertensive patients.[72] In the Perindopril Protection against Recurrent Stroke Study (PROGRESS), only patients with a recurrent stroke had significant prevention of dementia with an ACE inhibitor plus a diuretic (versus placebo).[99] In Syst-Eur, however, investigators found a significant 55% reduction in incident dementia of elderly patients with isolated systolic hypertension in the group initially given nitrendipine.[100] Whether this is specific to CCBs or an effect of greater BP reduction by active versus placebo treatment (a difference that was comparable to that seen in SHEP, MRC, and PROGRESS, however) remains to be established. Further large studies on the effects of various antihypertensive regimens on cognitive function and dementia prevention are urgently required.

SPECIAL INDICATIONS AND CONTRAINDICATIONS

Diabetes Mellitus and Diabetic Nephropathy

Concerns about CCBs' increasing cardiovascular morbidity and mortality in patients with type 2 diabetes mellitus were raised by two small studies. Each claimed that treatment with an initial CCB was associated with a significantly higher risk of cardiovascular events than ACE inhibitor therapy (ABCD-HT,[46] and FACET[47]). However, a 2002 review of available evidence from major trials reported that three studies that had

compared CCBs with diuretics or β-blockers in type 2 diabetes patients (INSIGHT,[37,101] NORDIL,[36] and STOP-2[102]), no relative advantage had been found for either class on major cardiovascular events, cardiovascular death, or all-cause mortality.[67] Likewise, among trials comparing CCBs and ACE inhibitors, a companion study of ABCD-HT (Appropriate Blood Pressure Control in Diabetics–Normotensive subgroup, ABCD-NT[48]) and STOP-2[102] did not find a statistically significant difference in incident cardiovascular events between patients treated with ACE inhibitors and those treated with CCBs.

In 2005, the effects of different BP-lowering regimens in individuals with and without diabetes mellitus were compared by a prospective meta-analysis of 27 trials.[103] For all comparisons and outcomes, no significant differences were reported in the effects of CCBs in patients with or without diabetes, and for no outcome (except heart failure) did head-to-head comparisons between CCBs and diuretics or β-blockers and ACE inhibitors provide any evidence of substantial differences in the effects of the different drug classes.[103] The analysis of the diabetic cohort in the INVEST study,[104] comparing verapamil-based with atenolol-based treatment, which was not included in the meta-analysis,[103] is totally in line with the results showing no difference in outcome between the two treatment strategies.

The question whether different antihypertensive agents may differently affect another important outcome of diabetes, nephropathy, has been addressed by a very large number of studies. An attempt to reducing confounding (because many studies were done on small cohorts followed only for a short time) restricted data analysis to those studies with at least 90 randomized patients with a minimum follow-up of 2 years.[67] In general, active or more intensive treatment was associated, in most but not all studies, with better preservation of renal function, delay of renal failure, reduction of proteinuria, or a delay in appearance of new proteinuria.[67] However, in only three of these placebo-controlled studies did active treatment start with a CCB: amlodipine failed to show renal protection in diabetic nephropathy in IDNT,[28] as did verapamil in the diabetic patients without nephropathy in the Bergamo Nephrologic Diabetes Complications Trial (BENEDICT),[105] and nitrendipine was associated with only slightly delayed new overt proteinuria in diabetic patients in Syst-Eur.[106] More definite evidence is provided by comparisons of active regimens, starting with different drug classes.[67] Five large studies have compared CCB-based treatment with a diuretic (INSIGHT[101]), an ACE inhibitor (ABCD-HT,[107] ABCD-NT,[48] ENEDICT[105]), or an angiotensin receptor antagonist (IDNT[28]). Only IDNT was able to show a significantly greater incidence of end-stage renal disease in diabetic patients who were treated with amlodipine than with irbesartan,[28] whereas ABCD-HT reported only a significantly greater (but transient) reduction in urinary albumin excretion with enalapril than with nisoldipine.[107] BENEDICT found a significant reduction of new microalbuminuria with trandolapril, but not with verapamil.[105]

In conclusion, the great attention paid to identifying the antihypertensive agent of "first" choice for patients with type 2 diabetes may appear rather questionable in view of the evidence that multiple drugs in combination are required to lower BP to the goal of less than 130/80 mm Hg, recently recommended by all guidelines for diabetic patients.[9-11,17] As summarized by the European guidelines,[10] "it appears reasonable to recommend that all of effective and well tolerated antihypertensive agents can be used (in diabetes mellitus), generally in combination. Available evidence suggests that renoprotection may benefit from the regular inclusion of an angiotensin receptor antagonist in these combinations." To achieve the low BP goal required, very seldom is a CCB absent from an effective combination regimen.

Chronic Kidney Disease

Most current guidelines recommend intensive lowering of BP in patients with nondiabetic chronic kidney disease, to the same level as diabetic patients.[9,10] This target is supported by a recent meta-analysis of 11 randomized, controlled trials.[108] In all these studies, ACE inhibitors were compared with either placebo or non–ACE inhibitor active therapy. The results of these analyses suggest a beneficial role (i.e., retardation of progression of renal disease) of more intensive BP lowering, especially in patients with urine protein excretion greater than 1.0 g/day, but also a beneficial effect of ACE inhibition, independent of its effects on BP and proteinuria.[108] In one of two studies in which an ACE inhibitor was compared with a CCB, renal survival was 50% better with fosinopril than with nifedipine GITS, with a decrease in proteinuria (by 57%) with fosinopril only.[109] However, the other study reported no difference in the progression toward renal insufficiency between captopril and slow-release nifedipine.[110] In African-American hypertensive patients, no difference was found between usual or more aggressive BP lowering in the decline of glomerular filtration rate, but the CCB amlodipine was significantly less effective than the ACE inhibitor ramipril.[38,39]

As is the case with diabetic nephropathy, nondiabetic chronic kidney disease, particularly if accompanied by proteinuria, benefits from more aggressive BP lowering and from an ACE inhibitor. Available data indicate that, when used in combination with either an ACE inhibitor or an angiotensin receptor blocker, CCBs neither hasten progression of renal disease nor worsen proteinuria.

Pregnancy

A limited number of antihypertensive agents can be used during pregnancy. ACE inhibitors and angiotensin receptor antagonists must be absolutely avoided because of fetal toxicity, and the use of diuretics is discouraged because of the low plasma volume characterizing pregnancy-related hypertension. The drugs most widely used in chronic hypertension of pregnancy have been methyldopa, labetalol, other β-blockers (mostly atenolol), and CCBs. A recent meta-analysis of 40 available trials comparing different antihypertensive regimens showed no clear difference in maternal or fetal outcomes,[111] although prior data suggest that β-blockers may increase the probability of small-for-gestational-age infants and may be less effective in lowering BP than CCBs, verapamil, and nicardipine.

For severe hypertension presenting later in pregnancy (usually as preeclampsia), parenteral hydralazine has long been considered the standard therapy, but CCBs play an important adjunctive role.[112] A recent meta-analysis of 21 trials comparing hydralazine with other agents given parenterally showed a higher rate of maternal side effects and

worse maternal and perinatal outcomes than with either labetalol or nifedipine.[113] Disadvantages of nifedipine in this setting include its secretion into breast milk and its propensity to cause weakness, hypotension, fetal distress, and hypocalcemia when it is administered with magnesium sulfate.

Despite these concerns, CCBs play an important role in pregnancy-related hypertension, both for long-term treatment and for acute emergencies. However, the evidence base is small,[111-113] and it includes only a few of the available compounds: nifedipine, nicardipine, verapamil, and nimodipine.

Isolated Systolic Hypertension

As discussed previously in this chapter and in Chapters 14 and 38, the benefits of CCBs, especially dihydropyridines, have been proved in event-based placebo-controlled trials in elderly patients with isolated systolic hypertension.[26,27] These compounds exert a favorable action on large artery function and possibly structure, which are altered in isolated systolic hypertension. CCBs are particularly suitable to treat this type of hypertension and, in general, hypertension in the elderly.

Angina

Three recent large studies evaluated CCBs in patients with stable angina pectoris or angiographically documented coronary disease.[44,56,57] In the ACTION study, patients randomized to nifedipine GITS had less refractory angina, less need of coronary angiography, fewer percutaneous coronary interventions, and less coronary bypass surgery than patients randomized to placebo.[29,56] In the CAMELOT study, patients randomized to amlodipine had fewer hospitalizations for angina and fewer coronary revascularizations than patients randomized to placebo: for these endpoints, amlodipine was also superior to enalapril.[57] In INVEST, which recruited patients with coronary artery disease, there were similar incidences of angina and coronary interventions in the group randomized to long-acting verapamil, compared with those given a well-proven antianginal agent, the β-blocker atenolol.[44] In the recent VALUE study, 46% of enrolled patients had a history of coronary disease; overall, amlodipine-treated patients had significantly less angina and myocardial infarction than valsartan-treated patients.[50]

Heart Failure

CCBs are less effective than other antihypertensive agents (especially diuretics) in the prevention of heart failure.[51] However, when BP is uncontrolled with the multiple drugs used for heart failure (see Chapter 28), a long-acting dihydropyridine CCB is effective in lowering BP, and it does not increase cardiovascular risk more than placebo, as demonstrated with amlodipine in the two Prospective Randomized Amlodipine in Survival Evaluation studies.[114,115]

CONCLUSION

Table 22-6 summarizes the conditions favoring or not favoring the use of CCBs (separately for dihydropyridines and nondihydropyridines) for hypertension, as listed in the European guidelines.[10] Contraindications to these drugs are

Table 22-6 Special Indications and Contraindication for Calcium Channel Blockers

		Contraindications	
Class	Conditions Favoring the Use	Compelling	Possible
Dihydropyridines	Elderly patients Isolated systolic hypertension Angina pectoris Peripheral vascular disease Carotid atherosclerosis Pregnancy		Tachyarrhythmias Heart failure
Nondihydropyridines	Angina pectoris Carotid atherosclerosis Supraventricular tachycardia	Atrioventricular block (grade 2 or 3) Heart failure	

From Guidelines Committee. 2003 European Society of Hypertension–European Society of Cardiology guidelines for the management of arterial hypertension. *J Hypertens.* 2003;**21**:1011-1059.

few, whereas conditions favoring their use are quite common and clinically important. In addition, CCBs are a reasonable choice, either when used alone or in combination therapy, both in patients with uncomplicated hypertension and in patients in whom a lower BP target must be achieved.

References

1. Fleckenstein A. Calcium Antagonism in Heart and Smooth Muscle. New York: Wiley & Sons, 1983.
2. Triggle DJ. Mechanisms of action of calcium channel antagonists. *In:* Epstein M (ed). Calcium Antagonists in Clinical Medicine, 3rd ed. Philadelphia: Hanley & Belfus, 2002, pp 1-32.
3. Godfraind T. Calcium Channel Blockers. Basel, Birkhäuser, 2004.
4. Meredith PA, Elliott HL. Dihydropyridine calcium channel blockers: Basic pharmacological similarities but fundamental therapeutic differences. *J Hypertens.* 2004;**22**:1641-1648.
5. Mancia G, Parati G. Ambulatory blood pressure monitoring in the evaluation of antihypertensive treatment with calcium antagonists. *In:* Epstein M (ed). Calcium Antagonists in Clinical Medicine, 3rd ed. Philadelphia: Hanley & Belfus, 2002, pp 117-137.
6. Leonetti G, Sala C, Bianchini C, et al. Antihypertensive and renal effects of oral administration of verapamil. *Eur J Clin Pharmacol.* 1980;**18**:375-382.
7. Olivari MT, Bartorelli C, Polese A, et al. Treatment of hypertension with nifedipine, a calcium antagonist agent. *Circulation.* 1979;**59**:1056-1062.
8. Epstein M. Calcium antagonists in the management of hypertension. *In:* Epstein M (ed). Calcium Antagonists in Clinical Medicine, 3rd ed. Philadelphia: Hanley & Belfus, 2002, pp 292-313.
9. Chobanian AV, Bakris GL, Black HR, et al., and the National High Blood Pressure Education Program Coordinating Committee. The Seventh Report of the Joint National Committee on Prevention, Detection, Evaluation, and Treatment of High Blood Pressure: The JNC 7 report. *JAMA.* 2003;**289**:2560-2572.
10. Guidelines Committee. 2003 European Society of Hypertension–European Society of Cardiology guidelines for the management of arterial hypertension. *J Hypertens.* 2003;**21**:1011-1059.
11. World Health Organization–International Society of Hypertension Writing Group. World Health Organization– International Society of Hypertension statement on management of hypertension. *J Hypertens.* 2003;**21**:1983-1992.
12. Burlando G, Sanchez RA, Ramos FH, et al. Latin American consensus on diabetes mellitus and hypertension. *J Hypertens.* 2004;**22**:2229-2241.
13. Neaton JD, Grimm RH Jr, Prineas RJ, et al. Treatment of Mild Hypertension Study: Final results. *JAMA.* 1993;**279**:713-724.
14. Materson BJ, Reda DJ, Cushman WC. Department of Veterans Affairs single-drug therapy of hypertension study: Revised figures and new data. *Am J Hypertens.* 1995;**8**:189-192.
15. Brewster LM, van Montfrans GA, Kleijnen J. Systematic review: Antihypertensive drug therapy in black patients. *Ann Intern Med.* 2004;**141**:614-627.
16. Brown MJ, Cruickshank JK, Dominiczak AF, et al. Better blood pressure control: How to combine drugs. *J Hum Hypertens.* 2003;**17**:81-86.
17. Williams B, Poulter NR, Brown MJ, et al. Guidelines for management of hypertension: Report of the fourth working party of the British Hypertension Society, 2004-BHS IV. *J Hum Hypertens.* 2004;**18**:139-185.
18. Leonetti G, Cuspidi C, Sampieri L, et al. Comparison of cardiovascular, renal, and humoral effects of acute administration of calcium channel blockers in normotensive and hypertensive subjects. *J Cardiovasc Pharmacol.* 1982;**4** (**Suppl 3**):19-24.
19. Lund-Johansen P. Hemodynamic effects of calcium antagonists in hypertension. *In:* Epstein M (ed). Calcium Antagonists in Clinical Medicine, 3rd ed. Philadelphia: Hanley & Belfus, 2002, pp 315-335.
20. Furberg C, Psaty B, Meyer J. Nifedipine. Dose-related increase in mortality in patients with coronary heart disease. *Circulation.* 1995;**92**:1325-1331.
21. Psaty B, Heckbert S, Koepsell T, et al. The risk of myocardial infarction associated with antihypertensive drug therapies. *JAMA.* 1995;**274**:620-625.
22. Pahor M, Guralnik J, Corti M, et al. Long-term survival and use of antihypertensive medications in older persons. *J Am Geriatr Soc.* 1995;**43**:1191-1197.
23. Ad Hoc Subcommittee of the Liaison Committee of the World Health Organization and the International Society of Hypertension. Effects of calcium antagonists on the risk of coronary heart disease, cancer and bleeding. *J Hypertens.* 1997;**15**:105-115.
24. Wassertheil-Smoller S, Psaty B, Greenland P, et al. Association between cardiovascular outcomes and antihypertensive drug treatment in older women. *JAMA.* 2004;**292**:2849-2859.
25. Gong L, Zhang W, Zhu Y, et al. Shanghai Trial of Nifedipine in the Elderly (STONE). *J Hypertens.* 1996;**14**:1237-1245.

26. Staessen J, Fagard R, Thijs L, et al. Randomised double-blind comparison of placebo and active treatment for older patients with isolated systolic hypertension in Europe. *Lancet.* 1997;**350**:757-764.

27. Liu L, Wang JG, Gong L, et al. Comparison of active treatment and placebo in older Chinese patients with isolated systolic hypertension (Syst-China). *J Hypertens.* 1998;**16**:1823-1829.

28. Lewis E, Hunsicker L, Clarke W, et al. Renoprotective effect of the angiotensin-receptor antagonist irbesartan in patients with nephropathy due to type 2 diabetes. *N Eng J Med.* 2001;**345**: 851-860.

29. Lubsen J, Wagener G, Kirwan B-A, et al. Effects of long-acting nifedipine on mortality and cardiovascular morbidity in patients with symptomatic stable angina and hypertension: The ACTION trial. *J Hypertens.* 2005;**23**:641-648.

30. Liu L, Zhang Y, Liu G, et al. The Felodipine Event Reduction (FEVER) Study: A randomized long-term placebo-controlled trial in Chinese hypertensive patients. *J Hypertens.* 2005;**23**: 2157-2172.

31. Borhani NO, Mercuri M, Borhani PA, et al. Final outcome results of the Multicenter Isradipine Diuretic Atherosclerosis Study (MIDAS), a randomized controlled trial. *JAMA.* 1996;**276**:785-791.

32. Agabiti-Rosei E, Dal Palù C, Leonetti G, et al., for the VHAS investigators. Clinical results of the Verapamil in Hypertension and Atherosclerosis Study. *J Hypertens.* 1997;**15**:1337-1344.

33. Zanchetti A, Agabiti-Rosei E, Dal Palù C, et al. The Verapamil in Hypertension and Atherosclerosis Study (VHAS): Results of long-term randomised treatment with either verapamil or chlorthalidone on intima-media thickness. *J Hypertens.* 1998; **16**:1667-1676.

34. Hansson L, Lindholm L, Ekbom T, et al. Randomised trial of old and new antihypertensive drugs in elderly patients: Cardiovascular mortality and morbidity—the Swedish Trial in Old Patients with Hypertension-2 study. *Lancet.* 1999;**354**: 1751-1756.

35. National Intervention Cooperative Study in Elderly Hypertensives Study Group. Randomized double-blind comparison of a calcium-antagonist and a diuretic in elderly hypertensives. *Hypertension.* 1999;**34**:1129-1133.

36. Hansson L, Hedner T, Lund-Johansen P, et al. Randomised trial of effects of calcium-antagonists compared with diuretics and β-blockers on cardiovascular morbidity and mortality in hypertension: The Nordic Diltiazem (NORDIL) study. *Lancet.* 2000;**356**:359-365.

37. Brown M, Palmer C, Castaigne A, et al. Morbidity and mortality in patients randomised to double-blind treatment with a long-acting calcium-channel blockers or diuretic in the International Nifedipine GITS study: Intervention as a Goal in Hypertension Treatment (INSIGHT). *Lancet.* 2000;**356**: 366-372.

38. Agodoa LY, Appel L, Bakris GL, et al., for the African American Study of Kidney Disease and Hypertension (AASK) Study Group. Effect of ramipril vs. amlodipine on renal outcomes in hypertensive nephrosclerosis: A randomized controlled trial. *JAMA.* 2001;**285**:2719-2728.

39. Wright JT Jr, Bakris GL, Green T, et al. Effect of blood pressure lowering and antihypertensive drug class on progression of hypertensive kidney disease: Results from the AASK Trial. *JAMA.* 2002;**288**:2421-2431.

40. Zanchetti A, Bond M, Hennig M, et al. Calcium-antagonist lacidipine slows down progression of asymptomatic carotid atherosclerosis. *Circulation.* 2002;**106**:2422-2427.

41. ALLHAT Officers and Coordinators for the ALLHAT Collaborative Research Group. Major outcomes in high-risk hypertensive patients randomized to angiotensin-converting enzyme inhibitor or calcium channel blocker vs diuretic. *JAMA.* 2002;**288**:2981-2997.

42. Black HR, Elliott WJ, Grandis G, et al. Principal results of the Controlled Onset Verapamil Investigation of Cardiovascular End Points (CONVINCE) trial. *JAMA.* 2003;**289**:2073-2082.

43. Malacco E, Mancia G, Rappelli A, et al., for the SHELL Investigators. Treatment of isolated systolic hypertension: The SHELL study results. *Blood Press.* 2003;**12**:160-167.

44. Pepine CJ, Handberg EM, Cooper-De Hoff RM, et al. A calcium antagonist versus a non-calcium antagonist hypertension treatment strategy for patients with coronary artery disease: The International Verapamil-Trandolapril Study (INVEST). A randomized controlled trial. *JAMA.* 2003;**290**: 2805-2819.

45. Dahlöf B, Sever PS, Poulter NR, et al. Role of blood pressure and other variables in the differential cardiovascular event rates noted in the Anglo-Scandinavian Cardiac Outcomes Trial-Blood Pressure Lowering Arm (ASCOT-BPLA). *Lancet.* 2005;**366**:907-913.

46. Estacio R, Jeffers B, Hiatt W, et al. The effect of nisoldipine as compared with enalapril on cardiovascular outcomes in patients with non–insulin dependent diabetes and hypertension. *N Engl J Med.* 1998;**338**:645-652.

47. Tatti P, Pahor M, Byington RD, et al. Outcome results of the Fosinopril versus Amlodipine Cardiovascular Events Randomized Trial (FACET) in patients with hypertension and NIDDM. *Diabetes Care.* 1998;**21**:597-603.

48. Schrier R, Estacio R, Esler A, et al. Effect of aggressive blood pressure control in normotensive type 2 diabetic patients on albuminuria, retinopathy and strokes. *Kidney Int.* 2002;**61**: 1086-1097.

49. Yui Y, Sumiyoshi T, Kodama K, et al. Comparison of nifedipine retard with angiotensin converting enzyme inhibitors in Japanese hypertensive patients with coronary artery disease: The Japan Multicenter Investigation for Cardiovascular Disease-B (JMIC-B) randomized trial. *Hypertens Res.* 2004;**27**: 181-191.

50. Julius S, Kjeldsen SE, Weber M, et al. Outcomes in hypertensive patients at high cardiovascular risk treated with regimens based on valsartan or amlodipine: The VALUE randomised trial. *Lancet.* 2004;**363**:2022-2031.

51. Blood Pressure Lowering Treatment Trialists' Collaboration. Effects of different blood-pressure-lowering regimens on major cardiovascular events: Results of prospectively-designed overviews of randomized trials. *Lancet.* 2003;**362**:1527-1535.

52. Angeli F, Verdecchia P, Reboldi GP et al. Calcium channel blockade to prevent stroke in hypertension: A meta-analysis of 13 studies with 103,793 subjects. *Am J Hypertens.* 2004;**17**: 817-822.

53. Dens J, Desmet W, Coussement P, et al. Usefulness of nisoldipine for prevention of restenosis after percutaneous transluminal coronary angioplasty (results of the NICOLE study). *Am J Cardiol.* 2001;**87**:28-33.

54. Pitt B, Byington R, Furberg C, et al. Effect of amlodipine on the progression of atherosclerosis and the occurrence of clinical events. *Circulation.* 2000;**102**:1503-1510.

55. Zanchetti A. Evidence-based medicine in hypertension: What type of evidence? *J Hypertens.* 2005;**23**:1113-1120.

56. Poole Wilson PA, Lubsen J, Kirwan BA, et al. Effect of long-acting nifedipine on mortality and cardiovascular morbidity in patients with stable angina requiring treatment (ACTION trial): Randomised controlled trial. *Lancet.* 2004;**364**:849-857.

57. Nissen SE, Turzcu EM, Libby P, et al. Effect of antihypertensive agents on cardiovascular events in patients with coronary disease and normal blood pressure: The CAMELOT Study. A randomized controlled trial. *JAMA.* 2004;**292**:2217-2226.

58. Messerli FH. Vasodilatory edema: A common side effect of antihypertensive therapy. *Am J Hypertens.* 2001;**14**:978-979.

59. Hansson L, Zanchetti A, Carruthers S, et al. Effects of intensive blood-pressure lowering and low-dose aspirin in patients with

hypertension: Principal results of the Hypertension Optimal Treatment (HOT) randomised trial. *Lancet*. 1998;**351**: 1755-1762.

60. Wiklund I, Halling K, Ryden-Bergsten T, et al. Does lowering the blood pressure improve the mood? Quality-of-life results from the Hypertension Optimal Treatment (HOT) Study. *Blood Press*. 1997;**6**:357-362.

61. Leonetti G, Magnani B, Pessina AC, et al. Tolerability of long-term treatment with lercanidipine versus amlodipine and lacidipine in elderly hypertensives. *Am J Hypertens*. 2002;**15**:932-940.

62. Lund-Johansen P, Stranden E, Helberg S, et al. Quantification of leg oedema in postmenopausal hypertensive patients treated with lercanidipine or amlodipine. *J Hypertens*. 2003;**21**: 1003-1010.

63. Zanchetti A, Omboni S, La Commare P, et al. Efficacy, tolerability, and impact on quality of life of long-term treatment with manidipine or amlodipine in patients with essential hypertension. *J Cardiovasc Pharmacol*. 2001;**38**: 642-650.

64. Pahor M, Guralnik J, Salive M, et al. Do calcium channel blockers increase the risk of cancer? *Am J Hypertens*. 1996;**9**: 695-699.

65. Pahor M, Guralnik J, Ferrucci L, et al. Calcium channel blockade and incidence of cancer in aged populations. *Lancet*. 1996;**348**:493-497.

66. Pahor M, Guralnik J, Furberg C, et al. Risk of gastrointestinal haemorrhage with calcium antagonists in hypertensive persons over 67 years old. *Lancet*. 1996;**347**:1061-1065.

67. Zanchetti A, Ruilope LM. Antihypertensive treatment in patients with type-2 diabetes mellitus: What guidance from recent controlled randomized trials? *J Hypertens*. 2002;**20**: 2099-2110.

68. Opie LH, Schall R. Old antihypertensives and new diabetes. *J Hypertens*. 2004;**22**:1453-1458.

69. Messerli FH, Grossman E, Leonetti G. Antihypertensive therapy and new onset diabetes. *J Hypertens*. 2004;**22**:1845-1847.

70. Eberly LE, Cohen JD, Prineas R, et al. Impact of incident diabetes and incident non fatal cardiovascular disease on 18-year mortality: The Multiple Risk Factor Intervention Trial experience. *Diabetes Care*. 2003;**26**:848-854.

71. Epstein M, Waeber B. Fixed-dose combination therapy with calcium antagonists. *In*: Epstein M (ed). Calcium Antagonists in Clinical Medicine, 3rd ed. Philadelphia: Hanley & Belfus, 2002, pp 713-730.

72. Lithell H, Hansson L, Skoog I, et al. The Study on Cognition and Prognosis in the Elderly (SCOPE): Principal results of a randomised double-blind intervention trial. *J Hypertens*. 2003; **21**:875-886.

73. Brenner B, Cooper M, De Zeeuw D, et al. Effects of losartan on renal and cardiovascular outcomes in patients with type 2 diabetes and nephropathy. *N Engl J Med*. 2001;**345**:861-869.

74. Leonetti G, Gradnik R, Terzoli L, et al. Effect of single and repeated doses of the calcium antagonist felodipine on blood pressure, renal function, electrolytes and water balance, and renin-angiotensin-aldosterone system in hypertensive patients. *J Cardiovasc Pharmacol*. 1986;**8**:1243-1248.

75. Pevahouse JB, Markandu ND, Cappuccio FP, et al. Long term reduction in sodium balance: Possible additional mechanism whereby nifedipine lowers blood pressure. *BMJ*. 1990;**301**: 580-584.

76. Weir MR. The clinical utility of calcium antagonists in renal transplant recipients. *In*: Epstein M (ed). Calcium Antagonists in Clinical Medicine, 3rd ed. Philadelphia: Hanley & Belfus, 2002, pp 603-628.

77. Voyaki SM, Staessen JA, Thijs L, et al. Follow-up of renal function in treated and untreated older patients with isolated systolic hypertension. *J Hypertens*. 2001;**19**:511-519.

78. Zanchetti A. The antiatherogenic effects of antihypertensive treatment: Trials completed and ongoing. *Curr Hypertens Rep*. 2001;**3**:350-359.

79. Ciulla MM, Paliotti R, Ferrero S, et al. Assessment of carotid plaque composition in hypertensive patients by ultrasonic tissue characterization: A validation study. *J Hypertens*. 2002;**20**:1589-1596.

80. Paliotti R, Ciulla MM, Hennig M, et al. Carotid wall composition in hypertensive patients after 4-year treatment with lacidipine or atenolol. An echoreflectivity study. *J Hypertens*. 2005;**23**:1203-1209.

81. Simon A, Gariépy J, Moyse D, et al. Differential effects of nifedipine and co-amilozide on the progression of early carotid wall changes. *Circulation*. 2001;**103**:2949-2954.

82. Zanchetti A, Bond MG, Hennig M, et al. Absolute and relative changes in carotid intima-media thickness and atherosclerotic plaques during long-term antihypertensive treatment: Further results of the European Lacidipine Study on Atherosclerosis (ELSA). *J Hypertens*. 2004;**22**:1201-1212.

83. Motro M, Shemesh J. Calcium channel blocker nifedipine slows down progression of coronary calcification in hypertensive patients compared with diuretics. *Hypertension*. 2001;**37**:1410-1413.

84. Lichtlen PR, Hugenholtz PG, Raffenbeul W, et al. Retardation of angiographic progression of coronary artery disease by nifedipine: Results of the International Nifedipine Trial on Antiatherosclerotic Therapy (INTACT). *Lancet*. 1990;**335**:1109-1113.

85. Taddei S, Virdis A, Ghiadoni L, et al. Effect of calcium antagonist or beta-blockade treatment on nitric oxide-dependent vasodilation and oxidative stress in essential hypertensive patients. *J Hypertens*. 1998;**16**:1913-1916.

86. Devereux RB, Wachtell K, Gerdts E, et al. Prognostic significance of left ventricular mass change during treatment of hypertension. *JAMA*. 2004;**292**:2396-2398.

87. Cuspidi C, Leonetti G, Zanchetti A. Left ventricular hypertension regression with antihypertensive treatment: Focus on candesartan. *Blood Press*. 2003;**12 (Suppl 2)**:5-15.

88. Schmieder RE, Schlaich MF, Klingbell AU, et al. Update on reversal of left ventricular hypertrophy in essential hypertension (a meta-analysis of all randomized double-blind studies until December 1998). *Nephrol Dial Transplant*. 1998; **13**:564-569.

89. Jennings GL, Wong J. Reversibility of left ventricular hypertrophy and malfunction by antihypertensive treatment. *In*: Hansson L, Birkenhäger WH (eds). Handbook of Hypertension, vol 18: Assessment of Hypertensive Organ Damage. Amsterdam: Elsevier, 1997, pp 184-229.

90. Tepstra WL, May JF, Smith AJ, et al. Long-term effects of amlodipine and lisinopril on left ventricular mass and diastolic function in elderly, previously untreated hypertensive patients: The ELVERA trial. *J Hypertens*. 2001;**19**:303-309.

91. Devereux RB, Palmieri V, Sharpe N, et al. Effects of once-daily angiotensin-converting enzyme inhibition and calcium channel blockade-based antihypertensive treatment regimens on left ventricular hypertrophy and diastolic filling in hypertension: The Prospective Randomized Enalapril Study Evaluating Regression of Ventricular Enlargement (PRESERVE) trial. *Circulation*. 2001;**104**:1248-1254.

92. Zanchetti A, Ruilope LM, Cuspidi C, et al. Comparative effects of the ACE inhibitor fosinopril and the calcium antagonist amlodipine on left ventricular hypertrophy and urinary albumin excretion in hypertensive patients: Results of FOAM, a multicenter European study [abstract]. *J Hypertens*. 2001;**19 (Suppl 2)**:S92.

93. Agabiti-Rosei E, Trimarco B, Muiesan ML, et al,, on behalf of the ELSA echocardiographic substudy group: Cardiac structural and functional changes during long-term antihypertensive

treatment with lacidipine and atenolol in the European Lacidipine Study on Atherosclerosis (ELSA). *J Hypertens.* 2005;**23**:1091-1098.

94. Ciulla MM, Paliotti R, Esposito A, et al. Different effects of antihypertensive therapies based on losartan or atenolol on ultrasound and biochemical markers of myocardial fibrosis: Results of a randomized trial. *Circulation.* 2004;**110**:552-557.

95. Benetos A, Zureik M, Morcet J, et al. A decrease in diastolic blood pressure combined with an increase in systolic blood pressure is associated with a higher cardiovascular mortality in men. *J Am Coll Cardiol.* 2000;**35**:673-680.

96. London GM, Safar ME. Arterial compliance and effect of calcium antagonists. *In:* Epstein M (ed). Calcium Antagonists in Clinical Medicine, 3rd ed. Philadelphia: Hanley & Belfus, 2003, pp 345-362.

97. SHEP Collaborative Research Group. Prevention of stroke by antihypertensive drug treatment in older persons with isolated systolic hypertension: Final results of the Systolic Hypertension in the Elderly Program (SHEP). *JAMA.* 1991;**265**:3255-3264.

98. Prince MJ, Bird AS, Blizard RA, Mann AH. Is the cognitive function of older patients affected by antihypertensive treatment? Results from 54 months of the Medical Research Council's trial of hypertension in older adults. *BMJ.* 1996;**312**:801-805.

99. PROGRESS Collaborative Study Group. Randomised trial of perindopril based blood pressure-lowering regimen among 6108 individuals with previous stroke or transient ischaemic attack. *Lancet.* 2001;**358**:1033-1041.

100. Forette F, Seux ML, Staessen JA, et al. The prevention of dementia with antihypertensive treatment: New evidence from the Systolic Hypertension in Europe (Syst-Eur) Study. *Arch Intern Med.* 2002;**162**:2046-2052.

101. Mancia G, Brown M, Castaigne A, et al. Outcomes with nifedipine GITS or co-amilozide in hypertensive diabetics and non diabetics in Intervention as a Goal in Hypertension (INSIGHT). *Hypertension.* 2003;**41**:431-436.

102. Lindholm LH, Hansson L, Ekbom T, et al. Comparison of antihypertensive treatments in preventing cardiovascular events in elderly diabetics patients: Results from the Swedish Trial in Old Patients with Hypertension-2. STOP Hypertension-2 Study Group. *J Hypertens.* 2000;**18**:1671-1675.

103. Turnbull F, Neal B, Algert C, for the Blood Pressure Lowering Treatment Trialists' Collaboration. Effect of different blood pressure lowering regimens on major cardiovascular events in individuals with and without diabetes: Results of prospectively designed overviews of randomized trials. *Arch Intern Med.* 2005;**165**:1410-1419.

104. Bakris GL, Gaxiola E, Messerli FH, et al. Clinical outcomes in the diabetes cohort of the International Verapamil SR-Trandolapril Study. *Hypertension.* 2004;**44**:637-642.

105. Ruggenenti P, Fassi A, Ilieva AP, et al. Preventing microalbuminuria in type 2 diabetes. *N Engl J Med.* 2004;**351**:1941-1956.

106. Tuomilehto J, Rastenyte D, Birkenhäger WH, et al. Effects of calcium channel blockade in older patients with diabetes and systolic hypertension. *N Engl J Med.* 1999;**340**:677-684.

107. Estacio RO, Jeffers BW, Gifford N, Schrier RW. Effect of blood pressure control on diabetic microvascular complications in patients with hypertension and type 2 diabetes. *Diabetes Care.* 2000;**23** (**Suppl 2**):B54-B64.

108. Jafar TH, Stark PC, Schmid CH, et al. Progression of chronic kidney disease: The role of blood pressure control, proteinuria, and angiotensin-converting enzyme inhibition. A patient-level meta-analysis. *Ann Intern Med.* 2003;**139**:244-252.

109. Marin R, Ruilope LM, Aljama P, et al. A random comparison of fosinopril and nifedipine GITS in patients with primary renal disease. *J Hypertens.* 2001;**19**:1871-1876.

110. Zucchelli P, Zuccalà A, Borghi M, et al. Long-term comparison between captopril and nifedipine in the progression of renal insufficiency. *Kidney Int.* 1992;**42**:452-458.

111. Abalos E, Duley L, Steyn DW, Henderson-Smart DJ. Antihypertensive drug therapy for mild to moderate hypertension during pregnancy. *Cochrane Database Syst Rev.* 2001;1:CD002252.

112. Sibai B, Dekker G, Kupferminc M. Pre-eclampsia. *Lancet.* 2005;**365**:785-799.

113. Magee LA, Cham C, Waterman EJ, et al. Hydralazine for treatment of severe hypertension in pregnancy: Meta-analysis. *BMJ.* 2003;**327**:1-10.

114. Packer M, O'Connor CM, Ghali JK, et al. Effect of amlodipine on morbidity and mortality in severe chronic heart failure: Prospective Randomized Amlodipine in Survival Evaluation Study Group. *N Engl J Med.* 1996;**335**:1107-1114.

115. Cabell CH, Trichon BH, Valzquez EJ, et al. Importance of echocardiography in patients with severe nonischemic heart failure: The second Prospective Randomized Amlodipine Survival Evaluation (PRAISE-2) echocardiographic study. *Am Heart J.* 2004;**147**:151-157.

Chapter 23

α-Blockers

William J. Elliott and James L. Pool

SYMPATHETIC NERVOUS SYSTEM IN BLOOD PRESSURE REGULATION

Two major types of transmembrane receptors, alpha- (α-) and beta- (β-) adrenoceptors, mediate most of the biologic signals generated by the adrenergic system within the human vasculature. Since the discovery of these adrenoceptors by classical pharmacologic techniques in the late 1940s,[1] α-adrenoceptors have been found to play a major role in physiologic regulation of vascular resistance, in hypertension,[2] and in other cardiovascular (CV) abnormalities,[3] including myocardial hypertrophy.[4] Familiarity with the pharmacologic modulation of α-adrenoceptors facilitates a better understanding of how antagonists for these receptors can be useful in hypertension and other diseases. The sympathetic nervous system (SNS) plays a prominent role in the development of hypertension, especially in younger persons, as well as in its maintenance in persons of all ages (see also Chapter 3).[2,5,6]

For tissues to be perfused with an adequate blood flow, arterial blood pressure (BP) must be balanced with an appropriate amount of resistance within the tissue bed. Arterial BP is regulated primarily by cardiac output and peripheral vascular resistance (PVR), the major regulator of which is smooth muscle tone within the blood vessels. The vascular smooth muscle cells that regulate BP control the cross-sectional area of the vessel, which is the major determinant of resistance to blood flow. Smooth muscle tone is regulated primarily by two neurohormonal systems: the autonomic nervous system and the renin-angiotensin-aldosterone system. The peripheral autonomic nervous system consists of three major components: (1) the SNS, which includes the autonomic outflow from both the thoracic and upper lumbar segments of the spinal cord; (2) the parasympathetic nervous system (PNS), which includes the outflow from the cranial nerves and the low lumbar and sacral spinal cord; and (3) the enteric nervous system, which includes the intrinsic neurons in the gut walls. The SNS and PNS neurons also regulate other functions (besides blood vessel diameter) in such diverse tissues as the urinary bladder (micturition), penis (erection), and prostate (ejaculation).[7,8] As discussed later in this chapter, the SNS also influences benign prostatic hyperplasia (BPH) and lower urinary tract symptoms (LUTS), both of which are common among older men with hypertension.

Abnormalities of the Sympathetic Nervous System in Hypertension

Increased SNS activity is one of many abnormalities that have been detected in patients with hypertension (see Chapter 3). This increase results in an increase in both vasoconstriction and PVR. Particularly in younger people with either pre-hypertension and early stage 1 hypertension, increased cardiac

β-adrenergic activity leads commonly to increased cardiac output, faster heart rate, and increased vascular α-adrenergic tone.[9] Longitudinal 20-year follow-up of prehypertensive individuals has shown that these early abnormalities moderate over time as the person becomes frankly hypertensive, cardiac output normalizes, and PVR increases.[10] This transformation is largely controlled by modifications of SNS receptors and α-adrenergic receptors. Early in the transition, β-adrenergic responsiveness in the heart is down-regulated,[11] with resulting alteration of cardiac vascular anatomy and function, followed by a gradual increase in PVR. During the early development of hypertension, the response of blood vessels to adrenergic and nonadrenergic vasoconstrictors is exaggerated.[12]

SUBTYPES OF α-ADRENORECEPTORS

Essentially all vasomotor neurons are adrenergic, because norepinephrine produces vasoconstriction by interacting with a specific type of transmembrane receptor on the vascular smooth muscle (i.e., the α-adrenoceptor). Six major subtypes of α-adrenoceptors are now recognized, and one more minor subtype (α_{1L}) has been identified that may be a close conformational relative of the α_{1B}-adrenoceptor (Table 23-1).[13-15] In addition to the important α-adrenoceptors located on vascular smooth muscle, the vascular endothelium (the second largest body organ by surface area) is host to at least two different subtypes of α-adrenoceptors (α_{2A}, α_{2C}) and three different β-adrenoceptor subtypes (β_1, β_2, and β_3). These receptors also actively participate in the regulation of vascular tone, either directly or indirectly through release of nitric oxide. Unfortunately, the exact roles for each of these various adrenoceptor subtypes in BP regulation are still not well defined, but they remain the subject of intense clinical investigation.[16]

Molecular Mechanisms of α₁-Adrenoceptor Activation

As shown schematically in Figure 23-1, innervation of smooth muscle by sympathetic nerve terminals takes place within a "tight junction" (or synapse) that keeps the two subcellular structures in close proximity. Sympathetic nerve impulses travel down the neuron to the foot process, separated from the smooth muscle cell by a "synaptic cleft" visible only by electron microscopy, that depolarizes the nerve terminal. This then releases norepinephrine from its storage vesicles in the neural end plate by fusing its membrane into the presynaptic neuronal cell membrane. The contents of these vesicles then empty norepinephrine into the synaptic cleft, where it is available to bind to α₁-adrenoceptors, which reside on the

Table 23-1 α₁-Adrenoceptor Subtypes (1994 Classification)

Native Receptor	Cloned Receptor	Located on Human Chromosome No.
α_{1A}	α_{1a}	8
α_{1B}	α_{1b}	5
α_{1D}	α_{1d}*	20

*Historically, the cloned α_{1D} receptor was sometimes called the $\alpha_{1a/d}$ or α_{1a} receptor.
Adapted from Bylund DB, Eikenberg DC, Hieble JP, et al. International Union of Pharmacology nomenclature of adrenoceptors. *Pharmacol Rev.* 1994;**46**:121-136.

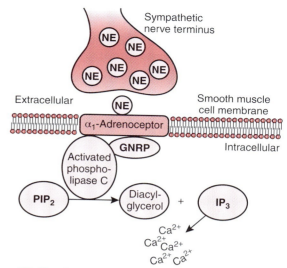

Figure 23–1   Schematic representation of subcellular events, beginning with depolarization of sympathetic nerves, release of norepinephrine (NE) into the synaptic cleft by exocytosis, binding to (and activation of) the α_1-adrenoceptor. After this important event, several enzymes are activated, resulting in smooth muscle cell contraction: activation of the α_1-adrenoceptor couples to a guanine nucleotide–releasing protein (GNRP here, but often abbreviated Gq/G11 in physiology texts), thereby activating phospholipase C, which hydrolyzes phosphatidylinositol 4,5-bisphosphate (PIP_2), generating inositol 1,4,5-trisphosphate (IP_3) and diacylglycerol. IP_3 causes release of intracellularly stored calcium ions (Ca^{2+}); this release activates chloride channels and membrane depolarization that opens voltage-gated calcium channels, thus causing vascular smooth muscle cell contraction. In addition, diacylglycerol transiently activates protein kinase C, which also contributes (through a phosphorylation-dependent process) to opening calcium channels and further increases the probability of vascular smooth muscle contraction.

postsynaptic (i.e., smooth muscle cell) side of the tight junction.

The molecular processes that characterize the activation of the α_1-adrenoceptors are quite complex. The α_1-adrenoceptor spans the width of the cell membrane of the smooth muscle cell, and it has specific features that "recognize" and bind the released norepinephrine from the neuron. The α_1-adrenoceptor complex consists of several working parts, including (1) the α_1-adrenoceptor itself, (2) a contiguous "transducer subunit" consisting of the guanine nucleotide–releasing protein that links the α_1-adrenoceptor with more enzymatic machinery, (3) a "catalytic subunit" that includes phospholipase C (PLC), and (4) two "second messengers"—inositol 1,4,5-triphosphate (IP_3) and diacylglycerol. This closely linked cascade of enzymes is activated when norepinephrine binds to the α_1-adrenoceptor: the activated α_1-adrenoceptor couples with guanine nucleotide–releasing protein, thus activating phospholipase C, which hydrolyzes phosphatidylinositol 4,5-bisphosphate and thereby generates both IP_3 and diacylglycerol. This newly synthesized IP_3 causes a sharp rise in cytoplasmic ionized calcium ions by releasing stored calcium from other organelles. The large but transient increase in calcium ions activates chloride channels and depolarizes the cell membrane, thus opening voltage-gated calcium channels, releasing calcium ions into the cytoplasm, and resulting in contraction of the vascular smooth muscle. Simultaneously, the other newly released "second messenger," diacylglycerol, activates protein kinase C, which activates appropriately selected calcium channels through a phosphorylation-dependent process; this also increases cytoplasmic free calcium ions and assists in cellular depolarization and (eventually) smooth muscle contraction.

Selective Postsynaptic α₁-Adrenoceptor Blockade

As discussed in detail earlier, stimulation of postsynaptic α_1-adrenoceptors in smooth muscle cells leads to constriction of arteries and arterioles and thereby increases PVR and raises BP. In early hypertension, particularly in young individuals, overactivity of the SNS results in excessive stimulation of postsynaptic α_1-adrenoceptors. The notion that the α_1-adrenoceptors could be selectively blocked, without affecting β-adrenoceptors, was a sound therapeutic rationale for developing highly selective α_1-adrenoceptor blockers for the treatment of hypertension. Early studies showed that, especially

acutely, the selective α_1-adrenoceptor blocking agents were very potent in reducing BP, particularly when BP was measured with the patient in the standing position. Even after a year of therapy (see Fig. 23-3), significant BP reductions are observed with little or no change in heart rate, cardiac index, or stroke index.[17] The BP-lowering effects of selective α_1-adrenoceptor blockers are particularly evident during exercise, and this finding distinguishes blockade of this receptor from that of the β-adrenoceptor, which typically reduces heart rate, cardiac index, and exercise tolerance.[17]

CLINICAL PHARMACOLOGY OF α-ADRENOCEPTOR ANTAGONISTS

The first α-adrenoceptor antagonists to be studied and approved for clinical use were phentolamine and phenoxybenzamine. These two compounds are nonselective α-blockers (i.e., antagonists of both α_1- and α_2-adrenoceptors); phentolamine is a competitive antagonist, so its effects can be overcome by repeated injection of an α-agonist (e.g., phenyl-ephrine for priapism after intracavernous injection of phento-lamine and papaverine). Phentolamine can be given only parenterally; its major therapeutic use is to control hyperten-sion in the short term in patients in pheochromocytoma-related crisis (see Chapter 10). As with all α-blockers, rapid or high-dose administration can lead to severe hypotension, par-ticularly when the patient stands. Phenoxybenzamine is an orally administered, nonselective α-blocker that irreversibly alkylates the α-adrenoceptor and renders it unresponsive to its normal ligand. Phenoxybenzamine is used primarily to prepare patients with pheochromocytoma for surgery, or (if the tumor is already metastatic at diagnosis) to blunt the symptomatic swings in BP if surgery is not feasible. Postural hypotension is typically used as the endpoint for dose titra-tion, and it can be debilitating. Nasal stuffiness is another common side effect, particularly for patients who take the drug for more than 2 weeks.

Three selective α₁-adrenoceptor antagonists have been developed and approved for use in hypertension (Fig. 23-2): prazosin, terazosin, and doxazosin. The last drug is available in several European countries as a long-acting preparation containing the gastrointestinal therapeutic system (GITS).[18] This formulation, which provides a true 24-hour delivery and apparently reduces the risk of first-dose hypotension, was recently approved by the U.S. Food and Drug Administration. Prazosin has a relatively short elimination half-life (of ~3 to 4 hours) and is administered twice or three times daily. Terazosin has an elimination half-life of approxi-mately 12 hours and is typically given once daily Although doxazosin has a longer elimination half-life (~20 hours), its BP-lowering effects are greater over the 24-hour period if the dose is taken in the evening; the BP-lowering effects of the GITS preparation do not depend on the time of adminis-tration.[19]

Two "uroselective" α₁A-adrenoceptor antagonists have been widely studied to treat the urologic symptoms of BPH. Although these compounds are allegedly more specific for the α₁A-adrenoceptor, which accounts for approximately 70% of the α-adrenoceptors in the prostate, some studies show a significant dose-dependent increase in orthostatic hypoten-sion in treated hypertensive men with BPH who were given these drugs in clinical trials. No formal studies of the BP-lowering effects of these drugs have been conducted in untreated hypertensive men. A placebo-controlled trial was performed in 12 hypertensive patients taking stable doses of nifedipine, atenolol, or enalapril for 1 week at 0.4 mg/day and for a second week at 0.8 mg/day. No "clinical significant effects on BP or pulse rate" were reported in the eight patients given tamsulosin, compared with the four given placebo. When taken after a meal (as recommended), tamsulosin achieves a peak serum concentration 6 to 7 hours after administration, and it has an elimination half-life of 14 to 15 hours in the target (older) population. Alfuzosin has not been quite as extensively studied, but it is available only in a single 10 mg/day dose form. Because its elimination half-life is only 10 hours, even when it is administered with food (as recom-mended), an extended-release tablet was developed so once-a-day dosing could be accomplished. In a study of eight healthy volunteers given a simultaneous dose of atenolol of 100 mg and of alfuzosin of 2.5 mg (immediate-release formulation), significant reductions in BP and heart rate were seen, com-pared with a single dose of atenolol alone. This may well be the result of a drug-drug interaction, because atenolol's maximal drug concentration and area under the atenolol concentration-time curve were both significantly increased when alfuzosin was co-administered with atenolol. Neither tamsulosin nor alfuzosin is indicated for the treatment of hypertension.

Two currently marketed β-blockers also have some α₁-adrenoceptor antagonist activity: labetalol and carvedilol. The labetalol molecule has two chiral centers, and the marketed product is an equimolar mixture of all four diastereomers. One of these antipodes is a weak selective α₁-adrenoceptor antagonist, with approximately 10% of the activity of phen-tolamine in animals. Two of the diastereomers are phar-macologically inactive, but the fourth is a nonselective β-adrenoceptor antagonist with very weak intrinsic sym-pathomimetic activity. This compound was purified and developed as an antihypertensive drug on its own merits (as dilevalol), until serious hepatotoxicity was detected. Labetalol is a more powerful β- than α-blocker (~3:1 when given orally), but its α-blocker potency increases when it is given intra-venously (to ~7:1). Carvedilol is a molecule with only one chiral center; the marketed product is the racemate. One enantiomer has both nonselective β-blocker activity and selective α₁-adrenoceptor antagonist activity; the other antipode has only α₁-blocking activity. The relative potency of carvedilol in humans is approximately 10:1 (β- to α-blockade). Because these agents have so much more β- than α-blocking activity, they are not discussed further in this chapter (see Chapter 19).

TREATMENT OF HYPERTENSION WITH α₁-ADRENOCEPTOR ANTAGONISTS

Since the early 1970s, many clinical trials of α₁-adrenoceptor blockers have been conducted in hypertensive individuals and have shown a dose-dependent lowering of BP much greater than that of placebo.[18,20] In these studies, α₁-blockers typically had no significant effect on heart rate, cardiac output, or other important central hemodynamic parameters. In normoten-sive individuals with normal sympathetic tone and PVR, α₁-blockers typically have very little BP-lowering effect, and this is one reason that they were such appealing drugs for other conditions, including BPH and Raynaud's phenomenon. Typically, in placebo-controlled trials of α₁-blockers, approxi-mately 50% of patients with baseline BPs in the 140 to 179/90 to 119 mm Hg range achieved seated diastolic BP lower than 90 mm Hg, with a smaller percentage achieving seated systolic BP lower than 140 mm Hg.[21,22] These proportions increase if one considers standing, rather than seated or supine, BPs. The BP-lowering response to α₁-blockers is not influenced by the patient's age, race, gender, or plasma renin activity, although the propensity for orthostatic hypotension in older people may be somewhat exaggerated after an α₁-blocker.

Prazosin, terazosin, and doxazosin are all effective anti-hypertensive agents, whether as monotherapy or in combina-tion with other BP-lowering drugs. Because prazosin has a short duration of action and must be taken several times a day, it has largely been replaced by the other two drugs, which often provide effective 24-hour BP control. Monotherapy with an α₁-blocker is sometimes accompanied by fluid and water

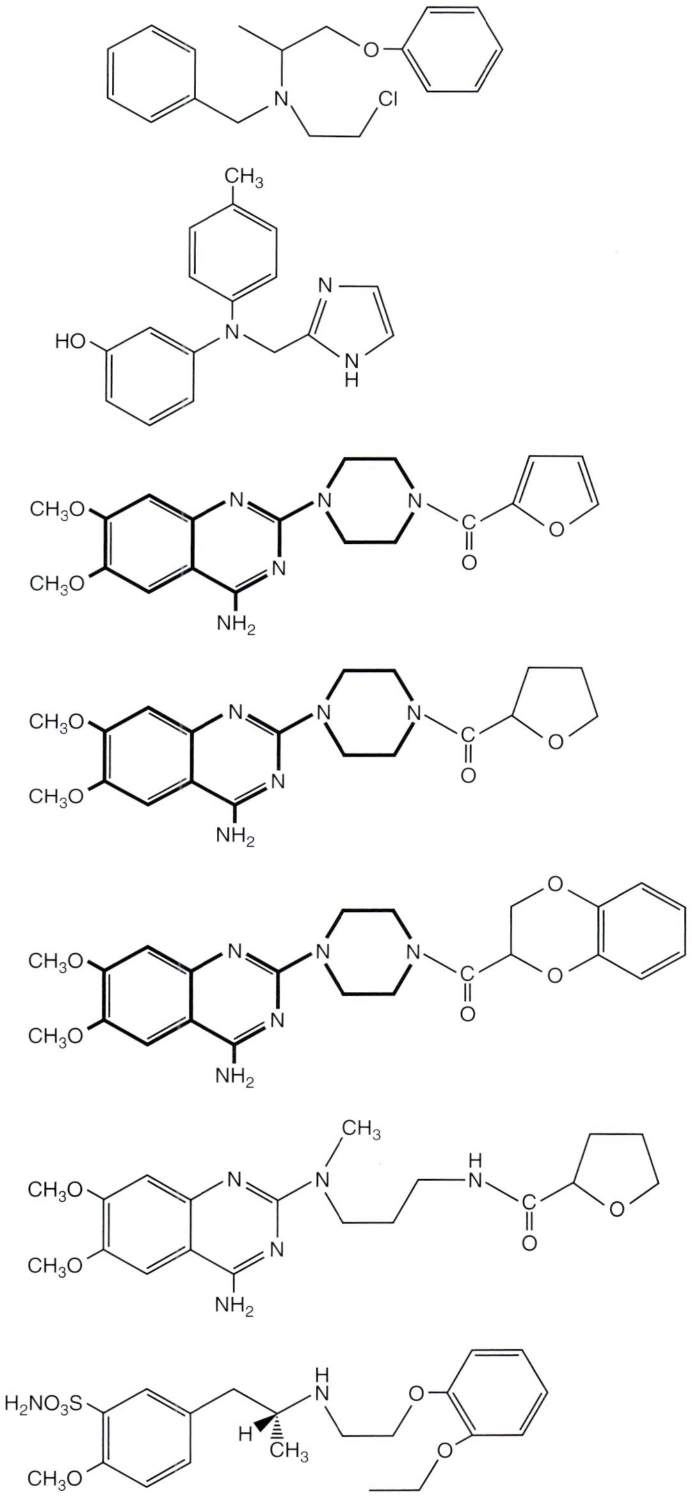

Phenoxybenzamine

Phentolamine

Prazosin

Terazosin

Doxazosin

Alfuzosin

Tamsulosin

Figure 23-2 Chemical structures of the two currently available nonselective α-blockers (phenoxybenzamine and phentolamine), three currently available α_1-selective antagonists (prazosin, terazosin, and doxazosin), and two currently available "uroselective" α_{1A}-selective antagonists (alfuzosin and tamsulosin). The three α_1-blockers commonly used in hypertension share a common quinazoline structure, drawn in *heavier lines*, that differentiates these compounds from the others.

retention, similar to (although less of a problem than with) direct-acting vasodilators (e.g., minoxidil or hydralazine). This complication is most easily overcome by the addition of a small dose of a diuretic, and this is the rationale for the combination of prazosin and polythiazide that was once marketed in the United States.

Cardiovascular Events with an α_1-Blocker in a Long-Term Clinical Trial

Until the double-blind, randomized, multicenter, federally funded Antihypertensive and Lipid-Lowering Treatment to Prevent Heart Attack Trial (ALLHAT), no long-term clinical trial in hypertension had evaluated an α_1-blocker as initial antihypertensive therapy to prevent CV events. In the Treatment of Mild Hypertension Study (TOMHS), doxazosin lowered BP nearly as well or better than other first-line antihypertensive therapies, and it had modest benefits on other CV risk factors (e.g., dyslipidemia, glycemic control) as well.[23] ALLHAT therefore included doxazosin (the longest-acting of the available α_1-blockers) as one of the four first-line randomized antihypertensive therapies and compared its incidence of CV events with that of the well-studied, longest-acting of the thiazide-like diuretics, chlorthalidone, which was given at 12.5 mg/day for the first three "steps" and at 25 mg/day at the fourth "step." The maximum dose of doxazosin used was 8 mg, whereas amlodipine and lisinopril were titrated to maximum approved doses. Of the original 42,448 hypertensive subjects, 55 years of age and older, 9067 were initially given doxazosin, and 15,268 received chlorthalidone. Atenolol, clonidine, or reserpine could be added, followed by hydralazine, if BP was not controlled by the maximum tolerated dose of the randomized drug. During an average follow-up of 3.3 years, seated systolic BP was significantly better controlled by chlorthalidone, by approximately 2.1 mm Hg at 48 months. Diastolic BP, conversely, was not different between the two groups.[24] After review of blinded data by two independent safety committees, the Director of the National Heart, Lung and Blood Institute accepted a recommendation that the doxazosin arm of ALLHAT be terminated because of the futility of showing improved outcomes with doxazosin over chlorthalidone. The primary endpoint (fatal or nonfatal coronary heart disease) was not significantly different between the two randomized arms of the trial (Fig. 23-3). However, stroke and combined CV disease events both were significantly more common among subjects randomized to doxazosin. In addition, ALLHAT reported a more than twofold increase in new heart failure with doxazosin, which, even after considering only fatal or hospitalized heart failure, was highly significant, with a 66% increase in risk. This significant increase in heart failure risk was consistent, seen in every one of the eight prespecified subgroups (based on age, gender, race/ethnicity, and diabetes status). Even though heart failure per se was not originally a prespecified endpoint in ALLHAT, many additional analyses were performed that verified the excess risk.[25-27] These data led the American College of Cardiology and many other groups to recommend that an α_1-blocker should not be used as first-line therapy for hypertension. After the release of the ALLHAT results and shortly after generic α_1-blockers became available, the numbers of prescriptions for α_1-blockers in the United States fell dramatically.[28]

Of course, ALLHAT does not provide answers to many important questions about the optimal use of α_1-blockers in hypertension. Young people, who typically have more active SNS activity, were not included in ALLHAT. Very low-risk hypertensive people who could avoid developing either diabetes or dyslipidemia after beginning an α_1-blocker, rather than a diuretic, were not enrolled in ALLHAT. Combinations of two randomized drugs (e.g., a diuretic and an α_1-blocker) were generally discouraged in ALLHAT. Normotensive men with BPH were not enrolled in ALLHAT. So many good questions about α_1-blockers, besides controversies addressed by the ALLHAT Research Group, still remain.

Perhaps the most important use of α_1-blockers in the post-ALLHAT era is their use as third-, fourth-, or fifth-line anti-

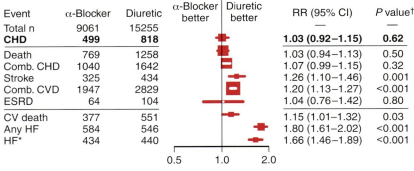

Figure 23–3 Results of the comparison of the doxazosin and chlorthalidone arms in the Antihypertensive and Lipid-Lowering to Prevent Heart Attack Trial (ALLHAT). The various endpoints and the number of patients with each endpoint in the final analysis are shown on the *left*. The relative risk (RR) for each endpoint (*central square,* in proportion to the number of patients with the endpoint) and the 95% confidence limits (95% CI; *ends of horizontal lines*) and numeric values (and *P* values) are given on the *right*. The *first horizontal line* separates coronary heart disease (CHD, the primary endpoint, therefore in boldface) from the prespecified secondary endpoints: Death; Comb. CHD, which represents combined coronary heart disease (CHD death, nonfatal myocardial infarction, coronary revascularization, or hospitalized angina); Stroke; Comb. CVD, which represents combined cardiovascular disease (combined CHD, stroke, treated or hospitalized heart failure, or peripheral arterial disease); and ESRD, end-stage renal disease. The *second horizontal line* separates the prespecified secondary endpoints from others that were analyzed: CV death, cardiovascular death; Any HF, heart failure (fatal, hospitalized, or treated); and HF*, heart failure (fatal or hospitalized cases only). Total n, number of patients in each randomized group. †The prespecified threshold for a "significant" P value for comparison of any endpoint in ALLHAT across the four randomized groups was .0178, which accounted for multiple comparisons and the unbalanced randomization scheme (1.7 to chlorthalidone versus 1 to each of the other three arms of the trial).

hypertensive therapy. α_1-Blockers can be used with diuretics, β-blockers, calcium antagonists, angiotensin-converting enzyme inhibitors, and angiotensin receptor blockers. Many studies in resistant hypertension have shown the benefit of α_1-blockers in lowering BP as part of a multidrug regimen.[29-32] α_1-Adrenoreceptor blockers have been a useful option as "add-on" antihypertensive medication in several recent clinical trials, including the African American Study of Kidney Disease and Hypertension (AASK), the Irbesartan Diabetic Nephropathy Trial (IDNT), and the Reduction of Endpoints in Non–Insulin-Dependent Diabetes Mellitus with the Angiotensin II Antagonist Losartan (RENAAL) study. In the Anglo-Scandinavian Cardiac Outcomes Trial (ASCOT), doxazosin GITS was given as third-line therapy to all patients and was part of the regimen in more than 40% of the subjects studied.

Metabolic Effects of α_1-Blockers

α_1-Adrenoreceptor blockers generally have no clinically important adverse effects on laboratory parameters in hypertensive patients. In large, placebo-controlled studies, very slight decreases in hemoglobin, hematocrit, leukocyte count, serum total protein, and albumin levels have been observed, and these effects were generally attributed to mild fluid retention and resultant hemodilution. Prolonged treatment (e.g., as in ALLHAT) has not led to any long-term concerns about these parameters.

In contrast, α_1-blocker therapy has been associated with small but significant improvements in serum lipid levels. Decreases in total cholesterol (~5%), low-density lipoprotein cholesterol (~5%), and triglycerides (~5%) and increases in high-density lipoprotein cholesterol (~4%) are typical.[24,27,31] These changes occur soon after therapy is begun and are sustained as long as the drug is continued. Several mechanisms are thought to be involved, including an increase in the number of low-density lipoprotein cholesterol receptors and lipoprotein lipase activity and decreases in synthesis of both low-density lipoprotein cholesterol and very-low-density lipoprotein cholesterol, as well as a reduction in the absorption of dietary cholesterol.[33] Additionally, the oxidation of low-density lipoprotein cholesterol can be inhibited by two different hydroxylated metabolites of doxazosin.[34]

Similarly, α_1-blocker therapy has been associated with an improvement in insulin sensitivity in hypertensive patients.[35] This effect is most easily detected by sophisticated glucose-clamping techniques.[36] In ALLHAT, subjects receiving doxazosin therapy experienced a significant decrease ($P < .001$) in their mean fasting glucose (from 122 mg/dL initially to 117 mg/dL at 4 years), whereas the chlorthalidone-treated group experienced an increase from 123 mg/dL at baseline to 125 mg/dL at 4 years.[27]

These metabolic effects of α_1-blocker therapy are most relevant in hypertensive patients with diabetes or the metabolic syndrome. Several studies have shown improvements after α_1-blocker therapy was given to such patients in serum lipids, glycemic control, and endothelial dysfunction.[31,37,38] These intermediate endpoints may be improved by α_1-blocker therapy, but several CV outcomes were worse among diabetic and prediabetic patients who were given doxazosin (rather than chlorthalidone) in ALLHAT.[39] These findings support the concept that results for surrogate endpoints can be mis-leading. Agents that improve what are thought to be reliable immediate endpoints may not necessarily also reduce clinical outcomes.

α_1-BLOCKERS IN OTHER DISEASES

Although many studies in the early 1970s indicated that α_1-blocker therapy improved symptoms, physical signs, and performance characteristics of patients with heart failure more than placebo, other therapies (including nitrates/vasodilators and especially angiotensin-converting enzyme inhibitors) provided better improvements. The only long-term, outcomes-based clinical trial that used an α_1-blocker was the Veterans Administration Cooperative Study on antihypertensive agents, which randomized 642 patients with heart failure to placebo, prazosin, or isosorbide dinitrate in combination with hydralazine.[40] After an average of 2.3 years of follow-up, mortality was least in the isosorbide dinitrate and hydralazine combination group, but it was similar in the prazosin and placebo groups. Changes in left ventricular function over 8 weeks and 1 year showed the same pattern: no difference between the prazosin and placebo groups, but a significant improvement in those given isosorbide dinitrate in combination with hydralazine. The authors concluded that α-blocker therapy did not improve mortality in heart failure.

As alluded to in the discussion of the clinical pharmacology of α-blockers, these drugs are quite effective in the treatment of symptomatic BPH and LUTS.[41] Both terazosin and doxazosin are approved for hypertension or symptoms of BPH, whereas both tamsulosin and alfuzosin are approved only for the latter indication. Because of the high concentrations of α_{1A}-adrenoceptors in the prostate, bladder, and lower urinary tract, the more uroselective compounds are now used successfully by many older men. Several long-term clinical trials have proven the efficacy of terazosin and doxazosin, alone or in combination with other modalities (including finasteride on LUTS). The first of these trials was the Veterans Affairs Cooperative Benign Prostatic Hyperplasia Study, which randomized 1229 men to 1 year of therapy with either terazosin or finasteride or placebo in a 2×2 factorial design.[42] Symptoms and urinary flow rates were significantly improved in those patients who were given terazosin, but treatment with finasteride was no better than placebo. More recently, doxazosin, finasteride, and a combination of the two drugs were compared in 3047 men over 4.5 years; the primary outcome was "overall risk of clinical progression" (a composite of an increase from baseline of four or more points on the American Urology Association's symptom score, acute urinary retention, urinary incontinence, renal insufficiency, or recurrent urinary tract infection).[43] All therapies were better than placebo: doxazosin by 39%, finasteride by 34%, and the combination by 66%. Whereas the combination and finasteride reduced most of the components of the composite endpoint, doxazosin's major improvement was in the symptom score. Such comparative studies have not yet been done with the newer, more uroselective agents.

Before the development of phosphodiesterase-5 inhibitors (e.g., sildenafil), α-blockers were the only class of drug that appeared to have even slightly beneficial effects on erectile dysfunction. This effect was observed first in TOMHS,[23] and it was subsequently confirmed in several other trials.[44] The uroselective α_{1A}-blockers also appear to have beneficial effects on several aspects of male sexual functioning.[45,46]

Many studies from 1970 to 1980 investigated the efficacy of α-blockers on Raynaud's phenomenon; nonselective and α_1-selective α-blockers were tested. Although most studies showed a mild improvement with α-blockers, only two studies were considered of sufficiently high quality to be included in a review by the Cochrane Collaboration; these studies also concluded that α-blockers have a mildly beneficial effect in Raynaud's disease.[47]

ADVERSE EFFECTS OF α_1-BLOCKERS

The α_1-blockers are generally well-tolerated drugs. During trials against placebo, the following adverse effects occurred in more than 5% of the doxazosin-treated hypertensive population: dizziness, 19% (versus 9% with placebo); headache, 14% (versus 16% with placebo); and fatigue or malaise, 12% (versus 6% with placebo). In placebo-controlled trials of prazosin, dizziness (10.3%), headache (7.8%), drowsiness (7.6%), lack of energy (6.9%), weakness (6.5%), and palpitations (5.3%) were reported in more than 5% of patients, but the placebo rates are not available. In placebo-controlled trials of terazosin, 19.3% of patients developed dizziness (versus 7.5% with placebo), 16.3% had headache (versus 15.8% with placebo), 11.3% reported asthenia (versus 4.3% with placebo), 5.9% reported nasal congestion (versus 3.4% with placebo), and 5.5% had peripheral edema (versus 2.4% with placebo). These adverse effects were generally mild and moderated or disappeared during continued administration of the drug. Symptom-specific discontinuation rates were in the 2% to 3% range for dizziness, 1% to 2% for headache, and less than 1% for all others. Dizziness was not always associated with postural hypotension, and the mechanism of this adverse effect is not well understood. The uroselective α_{1A}-blockers have slightly lower percentages of patients affected by these adverse effects, but they still cause more dizziness (6% to 17%), headache (3% to 21%), fatigue (3% to 8%), and symptoms of upper respiratory tract infection (3% to 10%) than placebo.

A major limitation to rapid dose titration and whenever α_1-blocker therapy is started is the *first-dose phenomenon*. This term describes the sudden severe symptomatic orthostatic hypotension (typically with dizziness) that usually occurs within 90 minutes of the first dose or when the dose is increased rapidly. To avoid this problem, the first dose of any α-blocker (typically at the lowest available dose) is given at bedtime; this approach decreases the incidence of syncope to less than 1%. Nonadherent patients are more at risk for this problem, because it can occur after a few doses of long-term medication are missed, and the "new first dose" is taken. Doxazosin GITS appears to be associated with a lower risk of this problem, probably because doxazosin is only slowly released from the tablet.[18]

The most feared complication of syncope, orthostatic hypotension, and dizziness that may be associated with α-blocker therapy is hip fracture. Two studies examined the possible association of α-blocker therapy and these problems. A cohort of 53,824 men with a medical office–generated diagnosis code for LUTS/BPH was followed for 2 years for a medical encounter for hypotension, syncope, dizziness, fractures,

or other injuries. In the first 4 months after a prescription for an α_1-blocker was given, more men had an adverse event, compared with the 4 months before the prescription (1.82 versus 0.02 events per 10,000 person-days).[48] The United Kingdom General Practitioners Research Database was examined for individuals with a hip fracture and prior exposure to α-blocker therapy in a case-control study.[49] A significantly higher risk was found for any α_1-blocker use in general (adjusted odds ratio, 1.9, 95% confidence limits, 1.1 to 3.4), with even higher risk for the first prescription. The uroselective α_{1A}-blockers had a slightly higher associated risk than the α_1-blockers used for hypertension (2.6 versus 1.9), but the numbers of hip fractures with the newer drugs were so small that they did not achieve statistical significance.

Only a few drug-drug interactions with α_1-blockers are clinically important. Hypotension can be precipitated or exacerbated when an α_1-blocker is co-administered with any phosphodiesterase-5 inhibitor, although only tadalafil and vardenafil are specifically contraindicated in this setting. Verapamil and α_1-blockers may produce more orthostatic hypotension and dizziness than either drug alone.

Postmenopausal women with pelvic relaxation syndrome can become incontinent of urine as a result of α_1-blocker–mediated relaxation of the bladder outlet. This can also occur in more unusual types of bladder dysfunction in either gender.

CONCLUSIONS

Although α_1-blockers are effective antihypertensive agents, since ALLHAT, they are no longer recommended as first-line drugs. However, they are particularly useful as "add-on" treatment for patients with resistant hypertension and for those who require multiple antihypertensive drug therapy. The changes in lipid and glucose metabolism associated with long-term use of α_1-blockers are mild, but beneficial. Two α_1-blockers (and two more uroselective α_{1A}-blockers) are now approved in the United States for the treatment of LUTS and BPH, and therefore these are appealing agents for older men. The first-dose phenomenon and dizziness, orthostatic hypotension, and upper respiratory tract infection symptoms are the major concerns.

References

1. Ahlquist RP. A study of the adrenotropic responses. *Am J Physiol.* 1948;**153**:586-600.
2. Somers VK, Anderson EA, Mark AL. Sympathetic neural mechanisms in human hypertension. *Curr Opin Nephrol Hypertens.* 1993;**2**:96-105.
3. Brook RD, Julius S. Autonomic imbalance, hypertension and cardiovascular risk. *Am J Hypertens.* 2000;**13**:112S-122S.
4. Yamazaki T, Komuro I, Yazaki Y. Signaling pathways for cardiac hypertrophy. *Cell Signal.* 1998;**1998**:693-698.
5. Esler M. The sympathetic system and hypertension. *Am J Hypertens.* 2000;**13**:99S-105S.
6. Izzo JL Jr. The sympathetic nervous system in acute and chronic blood pressure elevation. *In:* Oparil S, Weber MA (eds). Hypertension, 2nd ed. A Companion to Brenner and Rector's The Kidney. Philadelphia: Elsevier, 2005, pp 60-76.
7. Andersson KE. Bladder activation: Afferent mechanisms. *Urology.* 2002;**59** (5 Suppl 1):43-50.

8. Andersson KE. Treatment of the overactive bladder: Possible central nervous system drug targets. *Urology*. 2002;**59 (5 Suppl 1)**:18-24.

9. Kim J-R, Kiefe CI, Liu K, et al. Heart rate and subsequent blood pressure in young adults: The CARDIA Study. *Hypertension*. 1999;**33**:640-646.

10. Lund-Johansen P. Central haemodynamics in essential hypertension at rest and during exercise: A 20-year follow-up study. *J Hypertens*. 1989;**7 (Suppl)**:S52-S55.

11. Trimarco B, Volpe M, Ricciardelli B, et al. Studies of the mechanisms underlying impairment of beta-adrenoceptor-mediated effects in human hypertension. *Hypertension*. 1983;**5**:584-590.

12. Sivertsson R, Sannerstedt R, Lundgren Y. Evidence for peripheral vascular involvement in mild elevation of blood pressure in man. *Clin Sci Mol Med*. 1976;**3 (Suppl)**:65S-68S.

13. Bylund DB, Eikenberg DC, Hieble JP, et al. International Union of Pharmacology nomenclature of adrenoceptors. *Pharmacol Rev*. 1994;**46**:121-136.

14. Heible JP, Ruffolo RR Jr. Subclassification and nomenclature of alpha 1- and alpha 2-adrenoceptors. *Prog Drug Res*. 1996;**47**:81-130.

15. Heible JP. Adrenoceptor subclassification: An approach to improved cardiovascular therapeutics. *Pharm Acta Helv*. 2000;**74**:163-171.

16. Piascik MT, Perez DM. Alpha-1 adrenergic receptors: New insights and directions. *J Pharmacol Exp Ther*. 2001;**298**:403-410.

17. Lund-Johansen P, Omvik P. Acute and chronic hemodynamic effects of drugs with different actions on adrenergic receptors: A comparison between alpha blockers and different types of beta blockers, with and without vasodilating effects. *Cardiovasc Drug Ther*. 1991;**6**:605-615.

18. Lund-Johansen P, Kirby RS. Effect of doxazosin GITS on blood pressure in hypertensive and normotensive patients: A review of hypertension and BPH studies. *Blood Press*. 2003;**1 (Suppl)**:5-13.

19. Hermida RC, Calvo C, Ayala DE, et al. Administration-time-dependent effects of doxazosin GITS on ambulatory blood pressure of hypertensive subjects. *Chronobiol Int*. 2004;**21**:277-296.

20. Lund-Johansen P, Hjermann I, Iversen BM, et al. Selective alpha-1 inhibitors: First or second-line antihypertensive agents? *Cardiology*. 1993;**83**:150-159.

21. Materson BJ, Reda DJ, Cushman WC, for the Department of Veterans Affairs Cooperative Study Group on Antihypertensive Agents. Single-drug therapy for hypertension in men. *N Engl J Med*. 1993;**328**:914-921.

22. Materson BJ, Reda DJ, Cushman WC. Department of Veterans Affairs Single-Drug Therapy of Hypertension Study: Revised figures and new data. Department of Veterans Affairs Cooperative Study Group on Antihypertensive Agents. *Am J Hypertens*. 1995;**8**:189-192.

23. Neaton JD, Grimm RH Jr, Prineas RJ, et al. Treatment of mild hypertension study: Final results. *JAMA*. 1993;**270**:713-724.

24. ALLHAT Collaborative Research Group. Major cardiovascular events in hypertensive patients randomized to doxazosin vs. chlorthalidone: The Antihypertensive and Lipid-Lowering Treatment to Prevent Heart Attack Trial (ALLHAT). *JAMA*. 2000;**283**:1967-1975.

25. Validation of heart failure events in the Antihypertensive and Lipid-Lowering treatment to prevent Heart Attack Trial (ALLHAT) participants assigned to doxazosin and chlorthalidone. *Curr Cont Trials Cardiovasc Med*. 2002;**3**:10. Available on the Internet at http://www.cvm.controlled-trials.com/content/3/1/10, accessed 08 JUL 2005 at 20:30 CDT.

26. Davis BR, Cutler JA, Furberg CD, et al. Relationship of antihypertensive treatment regimens and change in blood pressure to risk for heart failure in hypertensive patients randomly assigned to doxazosin or chlorthalidone: Further analyses from the Antihypertensive and Lipid-Lowering Treatment to Prevent Heart Attack Trial. The ALLHAT Collaborative Research Group. *Ann Intern Med*. 2002;**137**:313-320.

27. ALLHAT Officers and Coordinators for the ALLHAT Collaborative Research Group. Diuretic versus alpha-blocker as first-step antihypertensive therapy: Final results from the Antihypertensive and Lipid-Lowering Treatment to Prevent Heart Attack Trial (ALLHAT). *Hypertension*. 2003;**42**:239-246.

28. Stafford RD, Furberg CD, Finkelstein SN, et al. Impact of clinical trial results on national trends in alpha-blocker prescribing, 1996-2002. *JAMA*. 2004;**291**:54-62.

29. Black HR, Sollins JS, Garofalo JL. The addition of doxazosin to the therapeutic regimen of hypertensive patients inadequately controlled with other antihypertensive medications: A randomized, placebo-controlled study. *Am J Hypertens*. 2000;**13**:468-474.

30. Zusman RM. The role of alpha-1 blockers in combination therapy for hypertension. *Int J Clin Pract*. 2000;**54**:36-40.

31. Black HR. Doxazosin as combination therapy for patients with stage 1 and stage 2 hypertension. *J Cardiovasc Pharmacol*. 2003;**41**:866-869.

32. Campo C, Segura J, Roldan C, et al. Doxazosin GITS versus hydrochlorothiazide as add-on therapy in patients with uncontrolled hypertension. *Blood Press*. 2003;**2 (Suppl)**:16-21.

33. Pool JL. Effects of doxazosin on serum lipids: A review of the clinical data and molecular basis for altered lipid metabolism. *Am Heart J*. 1991;**121**:251-259.

34. Chait A, Gilmore M, Kawamura M. Inhibition of low-density lipoprotein oxidation in vitro by the 6- and 7-hydroxy-metabolites of doxazosin, an alpha-1 adrenergic antihypertensive agent. *Am J Hypertens*. 1994;**7**:159-167.

35. Lind L, Pollare T, Berne C, Lithell H. Long-term metabolic effects of antihypertensive drugs. *Am Heart J*. 1994;**128**:1177-1183.

36. Pollare T, Lithell H, Selinus J, Berne C. Application of prazosin is associated with an increase of insulin sensitivity in obese patients with hypertension. *Diabetologia*. 1988;**31**:415-420.

37. Dell'Omo G, Penno G, Pucci L, et al. The vascular effects of doxazosin in hypertension complicated by metabolic syndrome. *Coronary Artery Dis*. 2005;**16**:67-73.

38. Inukai T, Inukai Y, Matsutomo R, et al. Clinical usefulness of doxazosin in patients with type 2 diabetes complicated by hypertension: Effects on glucose and lipid metabolism. *J Internat Med Res*. 2004;**32**:206-213.

39. Barzilay JI, Davis BR, Bettencourt J, et al. Cardiovascular outcomes using doxazosin vs. chlorthalidone for the treatment of hypertension in older adults with and without glucose disorders: A report from the ALLHAT Study. *J Clin Hypertens*. 2004;**6**:116-125.

40. Cohn JN, Archibald DG, Ziesche S, et al. Effect of vasodilator therapy on mortality in chronic congestive heart failure: Results of a Veterans Administration Cooperative Study. *N Engl J Med*. 1986;**314**:1547-1552.

41. Milani S, Djavan B. Lower urinary tract symptoms suggestive of benign prostatic hyperplasia: Latest update on alpha-1 adrenoceptor antagonists. *Br J Urol*. 2005;**95 (Suppl 4)**:29-36.

42. Lepor H, Williford WO, Barry MJ, et al. The efficacy of terazosin, finasteride, or both in benign prostatic hyperplasia: Veterans Affairs Cooperative Studies Benign Prostatic Hyperplasia Study Group. *N Engl J Med*. 1996;**335**:533-539.

43. McConnell JD, Roehrborn CG, Bautista OM, et al. The long-term effect of doxazosin, finasteride, and combination therapy on the clinical progression of benign prostatic hyperplasia. *N Engl J Med*. 2003;**349**:2387-2398.

44. Flack JM. The effect of doxazosin on sexual function in patients with benign prostatic hyperplasia, hypertension, or both. *Int J Clin Pract.* 2002;**56**:527-530.

45. Höffner K, Claes H, De Reijke TM, et al. Tamulosin 0.4 mg once daily: Effect on sexual function in patients with lower urinary tract symptoms suggestive of benign prostatic obstruction. *Eur Urol.* 1999;**36**:335-341.

46. Valllancien G. Sexual function assess by the BSFI is improved with alfuzosin 10 mg once daily [abstract]. *Eur Urol.* 2004;**3 (Suppl)**:91.

47. Pope J, Fenlon D, Thompson A, et al. Prazosin for Raynaud's phenomenon in progressive systemic sclerosis. *Cochrane Database Syst Rev.* 2000;**2**:CD000956.

48. Chrischilles E, Rubenstein L, Chao J, et al. Initiation of nonselective alpha-1 antagonist therapy and occurrence of hypotension-related adverse events among men with benign prostatic hyperplasia: A retrospective cohort study. *Clin Ther.* 2001;**23**:727-743.

49. Souverein PC, van Staa TP, Egberts AC, et al. Use of alpha-blockers and the risk of hip/femur fractures. *J Intern Med.* 2003;**254**:548-554.

Chapter 24

New and Investigational Drugs for Hypertension

Alexander M. M. Shepherd

Several types of agents to lower blood pressure (BP) are either new or investigational. The major classes of drugs discussed in this chapter are as follows:

- Aldosterone antagonists: These agents reduce mortality in heart failure.
- Dopamine-1 (DA1) agonists: These agents cause arterial vasodilation in selected arterial beds.
- Peripheral dopamine-2 (DA2) receptor agonists: These agents reduce norepinephrine and aldosterone release.
- Endothelin antagonists: These agents reduce BP, prevent left ventricular hypertrophy, and preserve myocardial function.
- Central imidazoline agonists: These agents reduce central sympathetic outflow with little sedation.
- Serotonin (5-hydroxytryptamine-1A [5HT1A] antagonists: These agents reduce central sympathetic outflow.
- Neutral endopeptidase (NEP) inhibitors: These agents prevent atrial natriuretic peptide (ANP) breakdown and angiotensin II generation.
- Potassium channel openers: These agents are of limited use because of reflex tachycardia and headache.
- Renin inhibitors: Use of these agents is a specific way to prevent angiotensin II formation.
- Endocannabinoid-1 receptor antagonists: These agents may reduce BP, weight, and several criteria of the "metabolic syndrome."

ALDOSTERONE ANTAGONISTS

Aldosterone plays a central role in causing myocardial and large arterial wall fibrosis. It acts directly on the muscle through mineralocorticoid receptors.[1] In addition, aldosterone may mediate some of the proatherogenic effects of angiotensin II, perhaps by increasing tissue angiotensin-converting enzyme (ACE) activity.[2,3] Drugs that oppose aldosterone action typically reduce oxidative stress and atherogenesis in rats and mice.[4,5] The myocardial effects of aldosterone can be also be prevented in animals by administering aldosterone antagonists, at doses that do not reduce BP. It was originally thought that ACE inhibition would reduce aldosterone levels sufficiently to oppose its deleterious effects in hypertension. However, ACE inhibition depresses circulating aldosterone for only the first few days of therapy.

Two drugs that oppose the actions of aldosterone, spironolactone and eplerenone, have been used in the treatment of hypertension. Both drugs reduce left ventricular hypertrophy in patients with hypertension.[6]

The use of spironolactone is limited by its adverse effects: gynecomastia in men and menstrual irregularities in women caused by the drug's interaction with androgen and progesterone and estrogen receptors. Spironolactone is broken down to several active metabolites, including canrenone, the dethioacetylated (non–sulfur-containing) breakdown product, which accounts for much of spironolactone's therapeutic effect. It exists in equilibrium in plasma with the relatively inactive metabolite canrenoate.[7] Canrenone is water soluble, and this property may permit intravenous administration if a rapid effect is needed.

Canrenoate potassium typically produces its hypotensive effect approximately 1 week after therapy is begun. Oral absorption of both canrenone and canrenoate potassium is greater than 80% after administration. Both drugs are about 85% to 90% bound to plasma proteins, and they have small volumes of distribution (0.5 L/kg for canrenoate potassium and 1.8 L/kg for canrenone).[7,8] Plasma clearance of canrenoate potassium is approximately 1 L/hour, and that of canrenone is approximately 0.3 L/hour.[9] The elimination half-lives of these two drugs are quite variable (4 to 22 hours).

Eplerenone is a newer drug with fewer side effects, because of more potent aldosterone receptor antagonism, and less effect at other steroid receptors. Eplerenone reduces left ventricular mass to an extent similar to that of ACE inhibitor enalapril. When the two drugs are combined, further left ventricular mass reduction is seen. There is a basis, then, for combining ACE inhibition and aldosterone antagonism in patients with high BP and significant cardiac end-organ damage.

Eplerenone is used in doses of 50 to 100 mg/day. Oral bioavailability is approximately 95%, and food has no effect on the extent of absorption. Eplerenone is broken down in the liver by cytochrome P-450 3A4 to inactive metabolites, resulting in potential interactions with drugs that are cytochrome P-450 3A4 inhibitors. Itraconazole and ketoconazole increase the area under the plasma concentration versus time curve by approximately fivefold, and fluconazole, erythromycin, saquinavir, and verapamil approximately double the area under the plasma concentration versus time curve.[10] The plasma half-life of eplerenone is between 4 and 6 hours. Adverse effects occur in less than 1% of patients. No direct comparisons have been made between eplerenone and spironolactone with regard to the ability to reverse target organ damage or safety. The two drugs are approximately equally effective in lowering BP.

Hyperkalemia of greater than 6 mEq/L occurs in about 5% of patients receiving eplerenone, and the likelihood is increased in the setting of impaired renal function. Comparative studies of spironolactone and eplerenone regarding the incidence of hyperkalemia have not yet been published.

DOPAMINE-1 RECEPTOR AGONISTS

The two main dopamine receptors in cardiovascular medicine are the DA1 and DA2 receptors. Stimulation of DA1 receptors results in arterial vasodilation in many arterial beds, including the renal, coronary, cerebral, and mesenteric beds (in decreasing order of DA1-receptor density).

Dopamine itself has different activities at various receptors at different dose levels. At the lowest dose level used clinically, it activates only DA1 and DA2 receptors. At intermediate rates of administration, it also acts as a β_1-receptor agonist, and at higher rates of administration, it has significant nonselective α-adrenergic agonist activity. Dopamine is not useful orally and is given only in acute situations via intravenous infusion.

Several orally absorbed DA1-receptor agonists have been investigated as possible therapies for hypertension. Ibopamine, a DA1-, DA2-, and β- and α-adrenergic receptor agonist, is a prodrug that is de-esterified in the gastrointestinal tract, liver, and blood to form epinine (N-methyldopamine), the active moiety. The elimination half-life is 2.5 hours, and about 60% of the drug is excreted through the kidneys.[11] Most recent work has been directed toward the use of ibopamine as eye drops in open-angle glaucoma, and, because of its multiple actions, particularly β-adrenergic agonism, it is unlikely to be of use in hypertension.

A more selective DA1 agonist, currently available in the United States, is fenoldopam mesylate. It is approximately six to nine times as potent a vasodilator as dopamine. The plasma half-life is approximately 7 minutes, but its antihypertensive effect lasts up to 4 hours.[12] The increased renal plasma flow and stimulation of DA1 receptors in the renal tubules should theoretically cause a natriuretic and diuretic effect. Murphy and colleagues found that in patients with mild to moderate hypertension, renal blood flow increased by 42%, glomerular filtration rate by 6%, and sodium excretion by 300%, but plasma renin and norepinephrine levels also increased, tending to oppose these beneficial effects.[12]

The hemodynamic profile of fenoldopam is appropriate for oral therapy of heart failure and hypertension with vasodilation of renal, coronary, cerebral, and mesenteric arteries. Because oral bioavailability is so low (<6%), the drug is used only intravenously in the management of hypertensive crises. The volume of distribution is approximately 0.5 L/kg, and the drug is extensively metabolized in the liver to the sulfate, glucuronide, and methoxy metabolites.[13]

A further DA1 agonist, dopexamine, is available only as an intravenous agent. It has direct DA1 agonism and also stimulates β_2-adrenergic receptors. It may be useful in heart failure. The recommended dose is an intravenous infusion of 0.5 μg/kg/minute, increased at 10- to 15-minute intervals to a maximum dose of 6 μg/kg/minute.[14] The advantage of dopexamine over dopamine is that its lack of α-adrenergic agonism permits it to be given through a peripheral intravenous line rather than through a central venous catheter. Dopexamine is extensively distributed in human tissues and is broken down in the liver by O-methylation and O-sulfation.[14] The elimination half-life is short, 7 to 11 minutes, resulting in reasonably quick onset and offset of action.

PERIPHERAL DOPAMINE-2 RECEPTOR AGONISTS

Peripheral DA2 receptors are found presynaptically on adrenergic nerve terminals and in sympathetic ganglia. Their activation results in inhibition of norepinephrine release. These receptors are also found in the adrenal cortex, where stimulation results in inhibition of angiotensin II–mediated aldosterone release.[15] Unfortunately, these receptors are also found in the emetic center of the medulla of the brain, stimulation of which typically causes severe nausea and vomiting.

The hemodynamic profile of such drugs may be very beneficial in hypertension because of reduction of norepinephrine and aldosterone secondary to the reduction in angiotensin II. This latter action would affect remodeling of the arteries, the arterioles, and the myocardium. Drugs in this class include bromocriptine, carmoxirole, ropinirole, quinpirole, codergocrine, and cabergoline.[16] Unfortunately, these drugs cross the blood-brain barrier and are associated with very significant side effects, including nausea, vomiting, and prolactin release. The hope is that similar drugs can soon be developed that do not penetrate the central nervous system.[17]

ENDOTHELIN ANTAGONISTS

Endothelins are endogenous vasoconstrictor peptides, approximately 21 amino acids in length, that are important in the control of human BP. These peptides are produced in many tissues, including the vascular endothelium. Stimulation of endothelin A (ETA) receptors causes arterial constriction and myocardial hypertrophy and fibrosis. Stimulation of endothelin B (ETB) receptors in vascular smooth muscle results in vasoconstriction, and in the vascular endothelium, nitric oxide and prostacyclin are released, with consequent vasodilation. Antagonism of ETA and ETB receptors may prevent end-organ damage in hypertension.[18] At least three different endothelins affect the cardiovascular system in hypertension. The main endothelin produced in the vascular endothelium is endothelin-I, which combines with ETA and ETB receptors in vascular smooth muscle to cause vasoconstriction and with ETB receptors in the endothelium to cause vasodilation.

The first orally administered mixed ETA/ETB endothelin antagonist is bosentan. Oral bioavailability of this drug is approximately 50%, plasma protein binding to albumin is 98%, and the volume of distribution is 0.5 L/kg. Bosentan is metabolized by, and induces the activity of, the hepatic isoenzymes cytochrome P-450 2C9 and 3A4. This property will likely result in drug interactions with other drugs metabolized by the same mechanism, including warfarin and ketoconazole. Bosentan may also increase its own metabolism: blood concentrations after multiple doses are only about 50% of those predicted. The half-life is 5 to 8 hours.[19] Approximately 11% of patients given this drug have significant elevations in liver enzyme levels, and approximately 25% of patients have mild to moderate headache. Bosentan-mediated liver injury may be mediated at least partly by intracellular accumulation of cytotoxic bile salts and bile salt–induced liver cell damage.

Bosentan and ACE inhibitors appear to have additive antihypertensive effects.[20] When bosentan is combined with amlodipine, it attenuates diabetic nephropathy in rats by reducing renal protein levels of transforming growth factor-β_1.[21] Bosentan is a pregnancy category X drug because it is fetotoxic.

Tezosentan is also an ETA/ETB antagonist that must be given by the intravenous route. Infusion rates of 20 to 50 mg/hour are effective for treating acute heart failure.[22] The most commonly reported adverse effect is headache. Distribution volume is 16 L/kg, distribution half-life is 6 minutes, elimination half-life is 3 hours, and plasma clearance is 30 L/hour.

Enrasentan (SB209670) is a highly potent nonpeptide mixed endothelin ETA/ETB receptor antagonist with ETA selectivity (affinity constant of ETA, 1.1 nM; affinity constant of ETB, 111 nM).[23] Enrasentan reduces BP, prevents left ventricular hypertrophy, and preserves myocardial function in animals. It may be of clinical use in the treatment of hypertension.[24]

Darusentan is a selective ETA receptor antagonist that protects the kidneys and reverses left ventricular hypertrophy and dysfunction in animals. In patients with moderate hypertension, a dose of 100 mg reduced systolic BP by approximately 11 mm Hg. In several studies, the average pulse rate remained unchanged. Headache, flushing, and peripheral edema are dose-dependent adverse effects.[25-27]

CENTRAL IMIDAZOLINE AGONISTS

The prototype imidazoline agonist is clonidine, which has been used effectively for many years in treating hypertension.

The main symptomatic side effects, sedation and dry mouth, occur in up to 30% of patients taking the drug. The second problem is rebound hypertension, which may occur when doses higher than approximately 0.8 mg/day are stopped abruptly. This situation could easily occur in patients who forget to take their medications or who are unable to obtain a timely refill. Clonidine stimulates central α_2-adrenergic receptors and imidazoline-1 (I-1) receptors. The targets of the imidazoline and α-adrenergic drugs in the central nervous system are shown in Figure 24-1.

Because many adverse effects are caused by stimulation of the central a_2-adrenergic receptors, drugs have been developed that have lower affinity for the α-adrenergic receptor and higher affinity for the I-1 binding site. Imidazolines are compounds with five-membered rings containing two nitrogens. I-1 receptors exist in relatively high concentrations in the brainstem, in the adrenal medulla, and in the kidney. Central α_2-stimulation reduces the respiratory rate and responsiveness to carbon dioxide levels in the blood, and it attenuates respiratory responses to hypoxia. Moxonidine, a drug more selective for I-1 receptors than clonidine, preserves responses to carbon dioxide challenge in cats and has no effect on the respiratory rate in dogs.[28] The more selective I-1 agonists have another advantage in that no rebound hypertension occurs following withdrawal of long-term treatment.[29] The relative and absolute affinities of drugs for the imidazoline and α-adrenergic receptors are shown in Table 24-1.

The second-generation I-1–receptor agonist, moxonidine, has been used safely and effectively in Europe for several years. Blood levels are highest about 2 hours after oral administration,

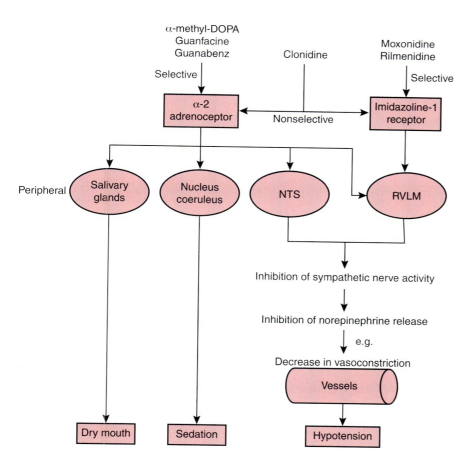

Figure 24–1 Targets of α_2-adrenoceptor and imidazoline (I$_1$)-receptor stimulants in the central nervous system. NTS, nucleus tractus solitarius; RVLM, rostral ventrolateral medulla. (From van Zwieten PA. The renaissance of centrally-acting antihypertensive drugs. *J Hypertens.* 1999;**17 (Suppl)**:S15-S29.)

Table 24-1 Table of the Properties of the Centrally Acting α_2-Adrenergic and Imidazoline Agonist Antihypertensive Drugs

	I_1-Imidazoline Sites		α_2-Adrenergic Sites		
	K_i (nM)*	Efficacy	K_i (nM)	Efficacy	Selectivity Ratio†
Active on I_1- and α_2-receptors					
Moxonidine	2	Agonist	75	Agonist	33
Rilmenidine	6	Agonist	180	Partial agonist	30
Clonidine	1	Agonist	4	Partial agonist	4
Highly selective for α_2-receptors					
Guanfacine	2,500	?	2	Agonist	0.0009
Guanabenz	>10,000	?	7	Agonist	0.0007

?, undetermined.
*Affinity constants (K_i) are ligand concentrations (nM).
†The selectivity ratio is a measure of selectivity for I_1-receptors relative to α_2-receptors and is calculated as the K_i at α_2-adrenergic receptors divided by the K_i at α_2-adrenergic receptors.

oral bioavailability is 90%, plasma protein binding is 7%, distribution volume is 2.5 L/kg, and metabolism in the liver to inactive compounds is minimal (10% to 20%).[30] Because much of the drug is excreted through the kidneys, severe renal impairment requires a reduction in dose. As with many antihypertensive drugs, the short plasma half-life of 2 to 3 hours is coupled with a long duration of action, thus permitting once-daily dosing. The usual initial dose is 200 μg, up to 600 μg/day in two divided doses.

A second central I-1–receptor agonist, rilmenidine, is well absorbed after oral administration and is unaffected by food. Peak blood levels occur 2 hours after an oral dose, protein binding is low, and the distribution volume is 4.5 L/kg. Most of the drug is excreted unchanged in the urine, and the blood half-life is approximately 9 hours. Maintenance clinical doses are generally 1 to 2 mg/day. Although less troublesome than clonidine, both moxonidine and rilmenidine share sedation and dry mouth as common side effects, but the incidence is less than 10% in most studies.

SEROTONIN (OR 5-HYDROXYTRYPTAMINE-1A) AGONISTS

Stimulation of 5HT1A receptors may participate in drug-induced lowering of BP in hypertension in two main sites in the body. Peripheral 5HT1A stimulation participates in the vasodilator action of certain β-blockers through stimulation of 5HT1A receptors in the vascular endothelium, with resulting nitric oxide release. Examples are tertatolol, bopindolol, celiprolol, and nebivolol.[31] Stimulation of 5HT1A receptors in the rostral ventrolateral medulla in the brainstem reduces sympathetic tone and heart rate.[32]

Urapidil is a mixed central 5HT1A receptor stimulant and a peripheral α-adrenergic antagonist. Urapidil is used in Europe, but it is not yet approved for use in the United States as of July 2006. It has desirable pharmacokinetics, rapidly and well absorbed and with a plasma half-life of approximately 3 hours. Plasma clearance is 12 L/hour. The drug is extensively metabolized by the liver to the *para*-hydroxylated (34% in urine), *N*-demethylated (4% in urine), and *O*-demethylated (3% in urine) degradation products.

Elimination is dose linear. Because of the short half-life, the drug is administered as a sustained-release preparation and is given once or twice daily. Adverse effects include headache in 3%, orthostatic hypotension in 1% to 2%, and dizziness in 10% of patients. Biochemical parameters in the blood are not altered.[33] Other 5HT1A agonists have been investigated, but they are not approved for hypertension.

NEUTRAL ENDOPEPTIDASE INHIBITORS

The natriuretic peptides are a family of endogenous substances with three properties: diuretic, natriuretic, and vasodilatory. Three different types are recognized: ANP derived from the cardiac atria, brain natriuretic peptide (BNP) from the ventricles of the heart and the central nervous system, and C-type natriuretic peptide (CNP) from the vascular endothelium. The mechanisms of their release are shown in Figure 24-2.

ANP is a 28-residue peptide that inhibits vasopressin, aldosterone, and renin release. Additional effects include an increase in glomerular filtration rate and reductions in cardiac preload and afterload. Studies to determine potential benefits of exogenous ANP were not successful because the drug, a peptide, was not orally absorbed and was rapidly eliminated.[34]

ANP is broken down by the zinc-dependent, membrane-bound NEP. Its structure is very similar to that of ACE. By inhibiting ANP degradation, the effect of NEP is prolonged, and bradykinin levels increase in the kidney, with resulting diuresis and natriuresis.[35] This effect could also increase bradykinin levels in the heart and be cardioprotective. The NEP inhibitors also decrease circulating endothelin, a potent vasoconstrictor. The drugs that have been studied include UK 69 578 and acetorphan,[36,37] as well as sampatrilat, gemopatrilat, aladotril, MDL 100 240, and Z 13752A (all of which are vasopeptidase inhibitors: NEP inhibitors, combined with some activity in inhibiting ACE).[38] Patients ingesting a high-salt diet typically have much less BP reduction with endopeptidase inhibitors and with vasopeptidase inhibitors.

Omapatrilat combines, in one molecule, an NEP inhibitor and an ACE inhibitor, and it reduces BP in both rats and in humans.[39,40] It has benefits (over and above ACE inhibitors) in heart failure.[41] The Omapatrilat Cardiovascular Treatment

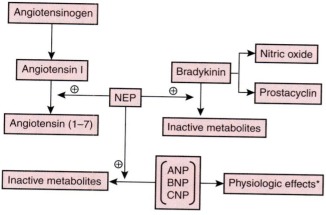

Figure 24–2 Description of the natriuretic peptide system. ANP, atrial natriuretic peptide; BNP, brain natriuretic peptide; CNP, C-type natriuretic peptide; NEP, neutral endopeptidase. (From Burnett JC Jr. Vasopeptidase inhibition: A new concept in BP management. *J Hypertens.* 1999;**17 (Suppl 1)**:S37-S43.)

vs Enalapril (OCTAVE) study found that angioedema occurred in 2.2% of subjects receiving omapatrilat and in 0.7% receiving enalapril. The overall relative risk for omapatrilat versus enalapril was highly significant, at 3.2 (95% confidence interval, 2.5 to 4.1). The average severity of angioedema was also greater with omapatrilat than with enalapril. In black patients, the incidence of angioedema was higher than in whites with both drugs: 5.5% with omapatrilat and 1.6% with enalapril.[42]

The pharmacokinetics of omapatrilat provided no unpleasant surprises: 20% to 30% oral systemic bioavailability with no effect of food ingestion. Plasma protein binding is low, at 80%, and distribution volume is 21 L/kg. Hepatic metabolism is extensive, and the half-life is sufficiently long (14 to 19 hours) to permit once-daily administration.

At this point, clinical development of omapatrilat has ceased, but it may be that some patient populations, with a sufficiently beneficial risk-to-benefit ratio from omapatrilat, will be found. One possibility is in severe heart failure, because the likelihood of angioedema does not appear to be excessively high in this group of patients (as compared with patients with hypertension).

POTASSIUM CHANNEL OPENERS

Adenosine triphosphate (ATP)–sensitive potassium channels in vascular smooth muscle are activated by ATP-dependent potassium channel openers. This process results in hyperpolarization of the plasma membrane and vasodilation of the blood vessel, probably by preventing opening of voltage-activated calcium channels. Several drugs of this type have been investigated, including SKP-450, aprikalim, cromakalim, lemakalim, and nicorandil. Other agents have been in use for some time—diazoxide, pinacidil, and minoxidil. Their major limitation is that vasodilation caused by this mechanism results in reflex tachycardia and fluid retention, which oppose the antihypertensive effect. Diazoxide was used in the emer-

gency treatment of hypertension, and minoxidil is still used in the treatment of stage 2 hypertension, particularly in African Americans and in patients with poor renal function. The main adverse effect is headache, which is caused by cerebral vasodilation, and it may be prevented or reduced in severity by combination with a β-blocker, which is generally necessary to limit reflex tachycardia. KR-30450 is well absorbed when it is given by mouth. Doses of 200 to 300 μg result in arterial vasodilation. Aprikalim may dilate coronary arteries, and cromokalim has been investigated in the treatment of hypertension and asthma. Although this group of drugs may be useful in treating other human diseases, the hemodynamic profile and the symptomatic adverse effects will significantly limit their use in the maintenance therapy of hypertension.

RENIN INHIBITORS

The development of ACE inhibitors was a major advance in the treatment of hypertension, because of the efficacy of these drugs and their low incidence of symptomatic adverse effects. However, ACE inhibitors also promote the breakdown of bradykinin, which may be involved in the pathophysiology of both angioedema and the dry, irritating cough seen in approximately 10% to 15% of patients treated with these drugs. A more specific way to interrupt the renin-angiotensin system would be to block the action of renin and thereby ultimately inhibit the formation of both angiotensin I and angiotensin II. With ACE inhibition, the serum concentration of angiotensin I increases, and it may be converted eventually to angiotensin II by pathways other than the ACE system. A diagram of the renin-angiotensin-aldosterone system is shown in Figure 24-3.

Initial development of renin inhibitors has not been easy. The first group studied consisted of antibodies to renin, but these agents must be given parentally and are antigenic themselves, with resulting symptomatic reactions and loss of efficacy. The most notable of the next several renin inhibitors had a low oral bioavailability. Now orally effective nonpeptide low-molecular-weight renin inhibitors have been developed. The most recent of these is aliskiren.[43,44] Aliskiren is a highly potent and selective renin inhibitor. It has good water solubility and resistance to biodegradation in the intestine, the blood circulation, and the liver. Its half-life is about 24 hours, and maximal reduction of circulating angiotensin II is achieved within 1 hour of drug administration.[45]

In mildly sodium-depleted normotensive volunteers, aliskiren produced strong and prolonged blockade of angiotensin II in the kidney and the adrenals. When it was combined with an angiotensin II receptor antagonist, synergistic effects were seen on hormonal levels. In subjects with mild to moderate hypertension, aliskiren caused a significant decrease in BP with doses of 75 mg/day, and further reduction of BP was reported with doses of 150 and 300 mg/day.[46] The incidence of side effects was very low in these studies, but larger studies are necessary to complete the adverse effect profile of this class of very interesting drugs. Although an interesting class of drugs, their equivalence or superiority to ACE inhibitors and angiotensin II receptor antagonists will need to be demonstrated in morbidity and mortality trials, in view of the large portfolio of such successful studies with ACE inhibitors and angiotensin II receptor antagonists.

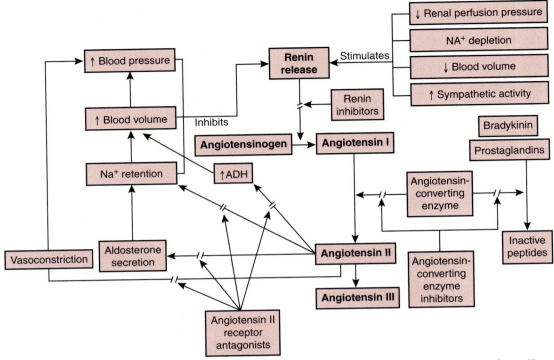

Figure 24–3 Diagram of the renin-angiotensin-aldosterone system. ADH, antidiuretic hormone; Na⁺, sodium. (From Foote EF, Halstenson CE. New therapeutic agents in the management of hypertension: Angiotensin II-receptor antagonists and renin inhibitors. *Ann Pharmacother.* 1993;**27**:1495-1503.)

ENDOCANNABINOID-1 RECEPTOR ANTAGONISTS

A fascinating new set of receptors and antagonists was discovered during research on marijuana. It appears that endocannabinoid-1 receptors are specifically activated by the active ingredient in this illicit substance, which results in acute hunger and BP elevation in the short term and is associated with weight gain and hypertension in the long term. A new class of drugs, the endocannabinoid-1 receptor antagonists, has been shown both to lower BP in animals[47] and in humans over the short term[48] and to result in significant weight loss and improvement in the prevalence of the metabolic syndrome (and many of its components, including waist circumference, high-density lipoprotein cholesterol, triglycerides, and insulin resistance) in humans in a 1-year study.[49] Although early in development, rimonabant, the first of these drugs to be tested in humans, has the potential both to treat the increasing obesity seen in many developed countries and to lower BP in affected obese individuals. This class of drugs holds great promise for the treatment of obesity and its cardiovascular sequelae.

CONCLUSION

Multiple new drug classes have been and are being developed for the treatment of hypertension. The problem is that we currently have effective therapy with a very low likelihood of side effects, and new drugs must be at least equivalent in terms of efficacy and safety. The most likely new drug class on the horizon is that of the renin inhibitors, which appear to combine good efficacy with a low likelihood of side effects. Until recently, vasopeptidase inhibitors were the most promising, but the finding of a significantly increased risk of angioedema, particularly in black patients, may have derailed the development of this class of drugs.

References

1. Lombes M, Farman N, Bonvalet JP, Zennaro MC. Identification and role of aldosterone receptors in the cardiovascular system. *Ann Endocrinol.* 2000;**61**:41-46.
2. Zushida K, Onodera K, Kamei J. Effect of diabetes on pinacidil-induced antinociception in mice. *Eur J Pharmacol.* 2002;**453**: 209-215.
3. Wang J, Yu L, Solenberg PJ, et al. Aldosterone stimulates angiotensin-converting enzyme expression and activity in rat neonatal cardiac myocytes. *J Card Fail.* 2002;**8**:167-174.
4. Virdis A, Neves MF, Amiri F, et al. Spironolactone improves angiotensin-induced vascular changes and oxidative stress. *Hypertension.* 2002;**40**:504-510.
5. Keidar S, Hayek T, Kaplan M, et al. Effect of eplerenone, a selective aldosterone blocker, on blood pressure, serum and macrophage oxidative stress, and atherosclerosis in apolipoprotein E-deficient mice. *J Cardiovasc Pharmacol.* 2003;**41**:955-963.
6. Pitt B, Reichek N, Willenbrock R, et al. Effects of eplerenone, enalapril, and eplerenone/enalapril in patients with essential hypertension and left ventricular hypertrophy: The 4E-left ventricular hypertrophy study. *Circulation.* 2003;**108**:1831-1838.
7. Overdiek HW, Merkus FW. The metabolism and biopharmaceutics of spironolactone in man. *Rev Drug Metab Drug Interact.* 1987;**5**:273-302.

8. Dahlof CG, Lundborg P, Persson BA, Regardh CG. Re-evaluation of the antimineralocorticoid effect of the spironolactone metabolite, canrenone, from plasma concentrations determined by a new high-pressure liquid-chromatographic method. *Drug Metab Disposit.* 1979;**7**:103-107.

9. Krause W, Karras J, Seifert W. Pharmacokinetics of canrenone after oral administration of spironolactone and intravenous injection of canrenoate-K in healthy man. *Eur J Clin Pharmacol.* 1983;**25**:449-453.

10. Krum H, Nolly H, Workman D, et al. Efficacy of eplerenone added to renin-angiotensin blockade in hypertensive patients. *Hypertension.* 2002;**40**:117-123.

11. Azzollini F, De Caro L, Longo A, et al. Ibopamine kinetics after single and multiple dosing in patients with congestive heart failure. *Int J Clin Pharmacol Ther Toxicol.* 1988;**26**:544-551.

12. Murphy MB, Murray C, Shorten GD. Fenoldopam: A selective peripheral dopamine-receptor agonist for the treatment of severe hypertension. *N Engl J Med.* 2001;**345**:1548-1557.

13. Boppana VK, Dolce KM, Cyronak MJ, Ziemniak JA. Simplified procedures for the determination of fenoldopam and its metabolites in human plasma by high-performance liquid chromatography with electrochemical detection: Comparison of manual and robotic sample preparation methods. *J Chromatogr.* 1989;**487**:385-399.

14. Fitton A, Benfield P. Dopexamine hydrochloride: A review of its pharmacodynamic and pharmacokinetic properties and therapeutic potential in acute cardiac insufficiency. *Drugs.* 1990;**39**:308-330.

15. Lokhandwala MF, Hegde SS. Cardiovascular pharmacology of adrenergic and dopaminergic receptors: Therapeutic significance in congestive heart failure. *Am J Med.* 1991;**90**: 2S-9S.

16. Frishman WH, Hotchkiss H. Selective and nonselective dopamine receptor agonists: An innovative approach to cardiovascular disease treatment. *Am Heart J.* 1996;**132**: 861-870.

17. Haeusler G, Lues I, Minck KO, et al. Pharmacological basis for antihypertensive therapy with a novel dopamine agonist. *Eur Heart J.* 1992;**13 (Suppl D)**:129-135.

18. Ram CV. Possible therapeutic role of endothelin antagonists in cardiovascular disease. *Am J Ther.* 2003;**10**:396-400.

19. Dingemanse J, van Giersbergen PL. Clinical pharmacology of bosentan, a dual endothelin receptor antagonist. *Clin Pharmacokinet.* 2004;**43**:1089-1115.

20. Krum H, Viskoper RJ, Lacourciere Y, et al. The effect of an endothelin-receptor antagonist, bosentan, on blood pressure in patients with essential hypertension: Bosentan Hypertension Investigators. *N Engl J Med.* 1998;**338**:784-790.

21. Chen J, Gu Y, Lin F, et al. Endothelin receptor antagonist combined with a calcium channel blocker attenuates renal injury in spontaneous hypertensive rats with diabetes. *Chin Med J.* 2002;**115**:972-978.

22. Dingemanse J, Clozel M, van Giersbergen PL. Pharmacokinetics and pharmacodynamics of tezosentan, an intravenous dual endothelin receptor antagonist, following chronic infusion in healthy subjects. *Br J Clin Pharmacol.* 2002;**53**:355-362.

23. Ohlstein EH, Beck GR Jr, Douglas SA, et al. Nonpeptide endothelin receptor antagonists. II. Pharmacological characterization of SB 209670. *J Pharmacol Exp Ther.* 1996;**271**:762-768.

24. Cosenzi A. Enrasentan, an antagonist of endothelin receptors. *Cardiovasc Drug Rev.* 2003;**21**:1-16.

25. Nakov R, Pfarr E, Eberle S, for the HEAT Investigators. Darusentan: An effective endothelin A receptor antagonist for treatment of hypertension. *Am J Hypertens.* 2002;**15**: 583-589.

26. Rothermund L, Traupe T, Dieterich M, et al. Nephroprotective effects of the endothelin ET(A) receptor antagonist darusentan

27. in salt-sensitive genetic hypertension. *Eur J Pharmacol.* 2003;**468**:209-216.

27. Rothermund L, Vetter R, Dieterich M, et al. Endothelin-A receptor blockade prevents left ventricular hypertrophy and dysfunction in salt-sensitive experimental hypertension. *Circulation.* 2002;**106**:2305-2308.

28. Haxhiu MA, Dreshaj IA, Erokwu B, et al. Effect of I1-imidazoline receptor activation on responses of hypoglossal and phrenic nerve to chemical stimulation. *Ann N Y Acad Sci.* 1995;**763**:445-462.

29. Harron DW. Distinctive features of rilmenidine possibly related to its selectivity for imidazoline receptors. *Am J Hypertens.* 1992;**5**:91S-98S.

30. Theodor R, Weimann HJ, Weber W, Michaelis K. Absolute bioavailability of moxonidine. *Eur J Drug Metab Pharmacokinet.* 1991;**16**:153-159.

31. Kakoki M, Hirata Y, Hayakawa H, et al. Effects of vasodilatory beta-adrenoceptor antagonists on endothelium-derived nitric oxide release in rat kidney. *Hypertension.* 1999;**33**:467-471.

32. Dreteler GH, Wouters W, Saxena PR. Comparison of the cardiovascular effects of the 5-HT1A receptor agonist flesinoxan with that of 8-OH-DPAT in the rat. *Eur J Pharmacol.* 1990;**180**:339-349.

33. Prichard BN, Tomlinson B, Renondin JC. Urapidil, a multiple-action alpha-blocking drug. *Am J Cardiol.* 1989;**64**:11D-15D.

34. Sagnella GA, Markandu ND, Shore AC, MacGregor GA. Raised circulating levels of atrial natriuretic peptides in essential hypertension. *Lancet.* 1986;**1**:179-181.

35. Granger JP. Inhibitors of ANF metabolism: Potential therapeutic agents in cardiovascular disease. *Circulation.* 1990;**82**:313-315.

36. Northridge DB, Jardine AG, Alabaster CT, et al. Effects of UK 69 578: A novel atriopeptidase inhibitor. *Lancet.* 1989;**2**: 591-593.

37. Gros C, Souque A, Schwartz JC, et al. Protection of atrial natriuretic factor against degradation: Diuretic and natriuretic responses after in vivo inhibition of enkephalinase (EC 3.4.24.11) by acetorphan. *Proc Nat Acad Sci U S A.* 1989;**86**:7580-7594.

38. Weber MA. Vasopeptidase inhibitors. *Lancet.* 2001;**358**: 1526-1532.

39. Seymour AA, Sheldon JH, Smith PL, et al. Potentiation of the renal responses to bradykinin by inhibition of neutral endopeptidase 3.4.24.11 and angiotensin-converting enzyme in anesthetized dogs. *J Pharmacol Exp Ther.* 1994;**269**: 263-270.

40. Zanchi A, Maillard M, Burnier M. Recent clinical trials with omapatrilat: New developments. *Curr Hypertens Rep.* 2003;**5**:346-352.

41. Rouleau JL, Pfeffer MA, Isaac DJS, et al. Comparison of vasopeptidase inhibitor, omapatrilat, and lisinopril on exercise tolerance and morbidity in patients with heart failure: IMPRESS randomised trial. *Lancet.* 2000;**356**:615-620.

42. Kostis JB, Packer M, Black HR, et al. Omapatrilat and enalapril in patients with hypertension: The Omapatrilat Cardiovascular Treatment vs. Enalapril (OCTAVE) trial. *Am J Hypertens.* 2004;**17**:103-111.

43. Nussberger J, Wuerzner G, Jensen C, Brunner HR. Angiotensin II suppression in humans by the orally active renin inhibitor aliskiren (SPP100): Comparison with enalapril. *Hypertension.* 2002;**39**:E1-E8.

44. Wood JM, Maibaum J, Rahuel J, et al. Structure-based design of aliskiren, a novel orally effective renin inhibitor. *Biochem Biophys Res Commun.* 2003;**308**:698-705.

45. Dieterle W, Corynen S, Mann J. Effect of the oral renin inhibitor aliskiren on the pharmacokinetics and pharmacodynamics of a single dose of warfarin in healthy subjects. *Br J Clin Pharmacol.* 2004;**58**:433-436.

46. Azizi M, Menard J, Bissery A, et al. Pharmacologic demonstration of the synergistic effects of a combination of the renin inhibitor aliskiren and the AT1 receptor antagonist valsartan on the angiotensin II–renin feedback interruption. *J Am Soc Nephrol.* 2004;**15**:3126-3133.

47. Batkai S, Pacher P, Osei-Hyiaman D, et al. Endocannabinoids acting at cannabinoid-1 receptors regulate cardiovascular function in hypertension. *Circulation.* 2004;**110**:1996-2002.

48. Molecule of the month. Rimonabant hydrochloride. *Drug News Perspect.* 2004;**17**:403.

49. Van Gaal LF, Rissanen AM, Scheen AJ, et al., for the RIO-Europe Study Group. Effects of the cannabinoid-1 receptor blocker rimonabant on weight reduction and cardiovascular risk factors in overweight patients: 1-year experience from the RIO-Europe study. *Lancet.* 2005;**365**:1389-1397.

Outcome Studies

Chapter 25

Design of Outcome Studies

James D. Neaton

The focus of this chapter is on the design and implementation of outcome studies—randomized trials with clinical endpoints that evaluate treatments that lower blood pressure (BP). About 65 million adults in the United States have hypertension,[1] which is associated with an increased risk of heart attacks, strokes, and end-stage renal disease (ESRD).[2-4] The high prevalence of this condition and the consequent significance of even moderately improving clinical outcomes through an improved understanding of treatment make outcome studies a public health imperative. Albert Einstein once said, "Some things you can count don't matter; some things that matter, you can't count." In short-term studies such as those carried out for regulatory approval for marketing of antihypertensives, many things that matter (e.g., myocardial infarctions and strokes) cannot be reliably evaluated because sample sizes are too small and follow-up is too short. If we are to understand fully the consequences of treatments such as BP-lowering drugs, given lifelong to millions of people, randomized outcome studies are needed.

This chapter is organized into two sections. In the first section, selected BP outcome trials are reviewed and some lessons learned from them are given. In the second section, some design and implementation issues that are relevant to future outcome studies are discussed and are illustrated by examples.

HISTORY AND LESSONS LEARNED

The Veterans Affairs (VA; formerly Veterans Administration) landmark trials in the 1960s and 1970s left no doubt about the importance of drug treatment (50 mg hydrochlorothiazide and 0.1 mg reserpine twice daily and 25 mg hydralazine hydrochloride three times daily) for those with persistent diastolic BP 105 mm Hg or higher.[5-7] However, these VA patients were a highly selected group of men, and most had a history of cardiac, central nervous system, or renal abnormalities at entry. There remained uncertainty about the benefits of treating individuals with lower levels of diastolic BP (90 to 104 mm Hg) who account for the majority of persons with hypertension. Thus, numerous BP-lowering trials in the broader population that focused on those with these levels of diastolic BP were initiated in the 2 decades that followed the VA trials. These trials had placebo, no-treatment, or referred care control groups. They were necessarily much larger than trials in more severe hypertension because the target population was at lower absolute risk of stroke and coronary heart disease (CHD) and because it was expected that many participants in the control group would receive BP-lowering treatment.

The first major trial was the Hypertension Detection and Follow-up Program (HDFP).[8-10] In HDFP, 10,940 men and women were enrolled and followed for an average of 6.7 years. The results of HDFP provided convincing evidence that a stepped care program that began with a diuretic (chlorthalidone, 25 to 100 mg/day) resulted in both substantial BP reductions and substantial mortality reductions, compared with those assigned referred care (referral to community sources of medical care for treatment deemed appropriate by local physicians). After 5 years, 78% of stepped care participants and 58% of referred care participants were taking BP-lowering medication, and the diastolic BP difference between treatment groups averaged 4.9 mm Hg.[8] Even though this BP difference between treatment groups was substantially less than the VA reported (~18 mm Hg for those with diastolic BP 90 to 114 mm Hg), after 6.7 years, the stepped care treatment program resulted in an 18.2% reduction in all-cause mortality compared with referred care.[10]

Lesson 1: Intensive BP control in the community is possible, a stepped care treatment program that begins with a diuretic to achieve BP control leads to a substantial reduction in mortality among men and women with diastolic BP 90 mm Hg and higher, and even modest differences in BP reductions among treatment groups can lead to sizable reductions in mortality.

Shortly following HDFP, the results of the Multiple Risk Factor Intervention Trial (MRFIT) were reported. In MRFIT, 8012 men had diastolic BP of 90 mm Hg or higher or were taking antihypertensive drugs at entry.[11,12] At baseline, these hypertensive participants in MRFIT had an average diastolic BP of 95.5 mm Hg, similar to that of participants in the lowest BP stratum in HDFP (96.3 mm Hg).[8] Special intervention (SI) participants were given a diuretic-based antihypertensive regimen that began with either 50 mg chlorthalidone or 50 mg hydrochlorothiazide.[12] After 6 years, diastolic BP averaged 4.5 mm Hg lower in the SI compared with the usual care (UC) group, similar to the treatment difference in the lowest BP stratum in HDFP (4.3 mm Hg). Because the special intervention focused on lipid lowering and smoking cessation as well as BP lowering, more SI than UC men with hypertension quit smoking, and low-density lipoprotein cholesterol after 6 years was 5.6 mg/dL lower in SI compared with UC men. In spite of these favorable risk factor differences between SI and UC, at the end of the trial in 1982, all-cause mortality was 1.1% higher in SI compared with UC hypertensive men; CHD mortality was 3.7% lower, and cardiovascular disease (CVD) mortality was 6.1% higher.[12] These results were in marked contrast to those of HDFP.[8-10]

A few years later, the Medical Research Council (MRC) single-blind trial of mild hypertension was reported.[13] In the MRC trial, 17,354 men and women were enrolled and were followed for an average of 4.9 years.[6] Half the participants were randomized to initial treatment with placebo, and the remainder were randomized to either a diuretic or a β-blocker. Participants assigned placebo were given active treatment (bendrofluazide or propranolol) if their BP increased to 210/115 mm Hg (this cutoff was changed during the trial to 200/110 mm Hg). Both bendrofluazide and propranolol resulted in 5 to 6 mm Hg greater BP reductions than placebo. Like MRFIT, the MRC study found no difference in all-cause mortality among those randomly assigned bendrofluazide (6.0 per 1000 person-years), propranolol (5.5), or placebo (5.9). The MRC did find a substantial benefit of treatment on stroke, but no benefit on CHD.

In 1990, an overview of 14 trials involving nearly 37,000 patients was reported.[14] This overview only included trials focused on BP lowering. MRFIT was not included. Overall, these trials were able to achieve an average difference in diastolic BP between treatment (usually diuretic or a β-blocker) and control (placebo or no treatment) of 5 to 6 mm Hg. Stroke was reduced by 42% (95% confidence interval [CI], 33% to 50%), and CHD was reduced by 14% (4% to 22%) with treatment. Based on epidemiologic analyses involving more than 1 million men and women that take into account regression dilution bias,[4] a 6 mm Hg lower diastolic BP among men and women aged 50 to 59 years (the average age of participants in the overview was 52 years) corresponds to a 48% lower risk of stroke (versus 42% in the overview) and a 33% lower risk of CHD (versus 14% in the overview).

These data raised questions about the optimal approach to lowering BP. In particular, because CHD is more common than stroke among hypertensive patients in the United States, treatments that provided a greater benefit regarding CHD were needed.

Lesson 2: Multiple trials are important to assess reliably the effects of BP-lowering treatment on CHD; very large sample sizes are required to compare different BP-lowering drugs; and research on the optimal approaches for the management of hypertension is needed.

The smaller than expected reduction in CHD based on several overviews,[14-16] including the one mentioned earlier,[14] and the possibility of long-term untoward effects with diuretics (e.g., increased blood glucose, cholesterol, and triglycerides, and decreased potassium) are factors that led to the design of the Treatment of Mild Hypertension Study (TOMHS).[17] TOMHS was based on a new paradigm—BP reduction was important, but it mattered how you did it. This paradigm guided the thinking of many subsequent outcome trials.

In TOMHS, six BP-lowering interventions were compared among 902 men and women (20% black) aged 45 to 69 years, and with diastolic pressure consistently between 90 and 99 mm Hg.[17] The six interventions were nutritional-hygienic advice (i.e., a program that emphasized weight loss, sodium and alcohol restriction, and increased physical activity) in addition to the following: (1) 15 mg/day chlorthalidone, (2) 400 mg/day acebutolol, (3) 1 mg/day doxazosin, (4) 5 mg/day amlodipine, (5) 5 mg/day enalapril, and (6) placebo. A lower dose of the diuretic, chlorthalidone, was used in TOMHS than in previous major BP trials. If BP was not controlled with the initially assigned treatment, chlorthalidone was added unless the participant was randomized to the chlorthalidone group, in which case enalapril was added.

Over a median follow-up of 4.4 years, each of the five classes of drugs, when given with nutritional-hygienic advice, resulted in greater BP reductions than in the group assigned nutritional-hygienic advice alone (an average difference of 3.7 mm Hg in diastolic BP). Furthermore, there was a trend toward fewer major CVD events among those who received an active drug at the first step (relative risk, 0.64; 95% CI, 0.35 to 1.18), and there were only modest and inconsistent differences in intermediate outcomes (BP, quality of life, symptoms, lipids, echocardiographic and electrocardiographic changes) among the five different classes of drug treatments.

Lesson 3: Low doses of diuretics and other classes of drugs are effective in lowering BP among patients with mild hypertension, and differences among classes of drugs when used at low doses may be less than originally suspected for many intermediate outcomes.

TOMHS led to the design and conduct of the Antihypertensive and Lipid-Lowering Treatment to Prevent Heart Attack Trial (ALLHAT),[18-20] in which a low-dose diuretic (chlorthalidone, 12.5 mg/day) was compared for clinical outcomes with a calcium channel blocker (2.5 mg/day amlodipine), an angiotensin-converting enzyme (ACE) inhibitor (10 mg lisinopril), and an α-blocker (1 mg/day doxazosin) in more than 42,000 men and women. Each initial agent was titrated upward to near the usual recommended maximum dose (chlorthalidone, 25 mg; amlodipine, 10 mg; lisinopril, 40 mg; doxazosin, 8 mg). Following the new paradigm of TOMHS, open-label second-step treatment options were identical for each of the treatment groups in ALLHAT, and these treatments were to be used if the preestablished goal (BP <140/90 mm Hg) was not achieved with larger doses of the first-line treatment. Thus, the experimental plan was to achieve equivalent BP lowering in the four treatment groups so comparisons among groups of clinical outcomes would not be confounded by BP differences. Although the achievement of goal BP with the lowest possible dosage of the first-line treatment was the ideal, it was recognized, based on the results of TOMHS, that many participants would require second-step treatments. ALLHAT was powered at 83% to detect a 16% difference in CHD between the treatment groups.

Based on an interim analysis, the α-blocker (doxazosin) group was terminated early in ALLHAT.[19] The BP-lowering strategy that began with doxazosin was associated with a significantly higher risk of the combined CVD outcome, which included heart failure, compared with the strategy that began with chlorthalidone. Furthermore, the doxazosin first-step strategy was not superior to the diuretic first-step strategy for the primary CHD outcome (relative risk [doxazosin/chlorthalidone], 1.03; 95% CI, 0.90 to 1.17) at the time of early termination. In a second report of ALLHAT at the completion of the trial, the principal finding was that there was no evidence of superiority of either amlodipine or lisinopril compared with chlorthalidone for CHD or any other clinical outcome.[20] A recent overview comparing ACE inhibitor treatment and calcium channel blocker with diuretic or β-blocker therapy led to similar conclusions even when the results of ALLHAT, one of the trials in the overview, were excluded.[21]

Lesson 4: Large outcome trials designed to detect small to moderate treatment effects are feasible and necessary to rank order treatments used long term for chronic conditions on many clinical outcomes.

DESIGN AND IMPLEMENTATION ISSUES

Yusuf and colleagues indicated that two general criteria for a good trial were "first and foremost, ask an important question and, secondly, answer it reliably."[22] In this chapter, five design issues that relate to the importance of the question and reliable evaluation of it are reviewed: (1) randomization, (2) choice of control group and superiority versus equivalence versus noninferiority designs, (3) endpoint definition and unbiased assessment of outcomes, (4) sample size and power, and (5) simplicity.

Randomization

It is essential that the comparator groups in a BP outcome study are assigned by a random process. In 1951, Sir Arthur Bradford Hill pointed out the hazards of "imperfect contrasts."[23] Bradford Hill's arguments for randomized studies have been reiterated by many investigators.[24-26] To eliminate the bias, conscious and unconscious, that is associated with comparing treatments that are prescribed by health care providers such as "confounding by indication,"[25] randomization is critical. Randomization is particularly important if the treatment differences, both those intended and unintended, are likely to be small to moderate, such as the differences in clinical outcomes among different treatments to lower BP. MacMahon and Collins made this important point and noted that because of the potential for bias, observational studies are best suited for detecting large effects of treatment, not moderate or small effects.[26] As I noted in 2004, "you need a precision instrument (i.e., a randomized trial) to detect small to moderate effects, but a sledge hammer (i.e., an observational study) might do for large effects."[27]

Nevertheless, as MacMahon and Collins noted, observational studies may be the only source of information when clinical trials are not carried out because of the large sample sizes or the long follow-up required. In the case of BP-lowering drugs, the current U.S. Food and Drug Administration practice is to approve drugs based on BP-lowering effects, not effects on clinical outcomes.[28] Thus, clinical benefit and long-term safety of many agents will have to rely on observational evidence unless this policy changes. Although the results of ALLHAT reinforce the merits of a diuretic-based treatment strategy,[19,20] other BP-lowering drugs will be needed to ensure optimal BP control. The long-term effects of these drugs will be important to understand, and the evidence for long-term benefit and safety should be assessed in randomized trials.

Choice of Control Group and Superiority versus Equivalence versus Noninferiority Designs

Once it has been established that the treatment groups will be assigned by randomization, the specific nature of the groups to be compared must be determined. The importance or relevance of the question is determined in large part by the definition of the comparison groups. Following the completion of trials such as HDFP,[8-10] the MRC study,[13] and the other trials described in overviews,[14-16] it was no longer possible to conduct long-term clinical outcome trials with control groups that did not receive BP-lowering treatment. Based on the

results of these studies and on national guidelines, use of treatments that would lower BP to less than 140/90 mm Hg among participants in the study was essential.[29] Thus, active-controlled trials had to be conducted either to show superiority of new agents to diuretics or β-blockers or to demonstrate equivalence or noninferiority. Such trials had to be much larger because the outcome differences among active treatment groups would likely be much smaller than outcome differences between active drugs and placebos or no treatment.

Diuretics and β-blockers were the logical control treatments to use as first-line agents because substantial evidence existed regarding the long-term effects of drugs in these classes on clinical outcomes. Although some data on clinical outcomes existed on low versus high doses of diuretics,[30] most of the outcome data for low-dose diuretics were for trials in elderly patients.[31-33] In one of these trials, chlorthalidone (12.5 to 25.0 mg/day) was used.[32] The two other studies used 25 mg hydrochlorothiazide in combination with either 2.5 mg amiloride[33] or 50 mg triamterene.[31] The use of lower doses of diuretics in trials such as ALLHAT[18-20] was based on these trials and on smaller trials, such as TOMHS,[17] that documented the BP-lowering effects of low-dose chlorthalidone with minimal metabolic side effects.

An active controlled study may be a superiority trial, a noninferiority trial, or an equivalence trial. ALLHAT was designed as superiority study,[18] to answer the question: "Is there any evidence that other classes of drugs are *better* as first-line treatment than a diuretic?" The primary hypotheses were that the composite outcome of fatal or nonfatal CHD would be lower for those randomized to amlodipine, lisinopril, or doxazosin, as compared with chlorthalidone. The primary hypotheses were evaluated with three separate comparisons, each drug class versus diuretic.

Figure 25-1 illustrates the chlorthalidone and lisinopril comparison in ALLHAT for the primary CHD incidence endpoint (CHD death or nonfatal MI) and for two of the secondary endpoints, fatal or nonfatal CVD and ESRD. The CVD composite outcome includes CHD death, nonfatal MI, stroke, coronary revascularization procedures, hospitalized or treated angina, treated or hospitalized heart failure, and peripheral arterial disease. For the CHD endpoint, the 95% CI for the hazard ratio (lisinopril/chlorthalidone) unadjusted for the three planned comparisons includes 1.00 (0.91 to 1.08). Thus, the superiority of lisinopril over chlorthalidone cannot be supported. Likewise, the superiority of chlorthalidone cannot be supported. For the CVD composite endpoint, the CI excludes 1.00, favoring chlorthalidone (1.05 to 1.16). Thus, the superiority of chlorthalidone over lisinopril can be stated for this endpoint. For the ESRD outcome, the CI is very broad—based on the bounds of the 95% CI, the real risk of ESRD could be 12% lower or 38% higher with lisinopril compared with chlorthalidone. Thus, even though the hazard ratio for ESRD is greater than that for the CVD composite (1.11 versus 1.10), the superiority of chlorthalidone over lisinopril cannot be supported because the CI for this endpoint includes 1.00.

What happens if a superiority study fails to demonstrate superiority of one treatment over the other? Can equivalence or noninferiority be claimed? The ALLHAT study and the Optimal Trial in Myocardial Infarction with the Angiotensin II Antagonist Losartan (OPTIMAAL) illustrate some statistical interpretation issues in this regard.[34] The following points are important to consider:

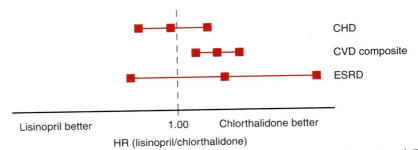

Figure 25–1 Superiority trial. Antihypertensive and Lipid-Lowering Treatment to Prevent Heart Attack Trial: lisinopril versus chlorthalidone for coronary heart disease (CHD) incidence, cardiovascular disease (CVD) composite outcome, and end-stage renal disease (ESRD). HR, hazard ratio. (From ALLHAT Officers and Coordinators for the ALLHAT Collaborative Research Group. Major outcomes in high-risk hypertensive patients randomized to angiotensin-converting enzyme inhibitor or calcium channel blocker vs. diuretic: The Antihypertensive and Lipid-Lowering Treatment to Prevent Heart Attack Trial [ALLHAT]. *JAMA.* 2002;**288**:2981-2997.)

1. The width of the CI depends on the number of events. In ALLHAT, the CI is broader for the ESRD and CHD endpoints than for the CVD composite endpoint (see Fig. 25-1). Because of the large sample and long follow-up period in ALLHAT, many CHD and CVD events occurred, and the difference in the widths of the CIs for these two endpoints was not very great. A much smaller trial may have resulted in the same estimate of the hazard ratio for the CVD composite, but the CI would have included 1.00. The hazard ratio would not have been estimated with the same precision in a smaller trial.

2. The absence of a significant difference among treatment groups does not mean that there is not a clinically relevant difference (i.e., does not imply equivalence). This is illustrated with the ESRD comparison. The lack of a significant difference in ESRD between lisinopril and chlorthalidone ($P = .38$) does not mean that there is not an important difference. *P* values are a function of sample size and the magnitude of the treatment difference. CIs are generally more informative because the precision of the estimate is apparent.

3. In some cases, a claim of noninferiority or equivalence may be of interest in a superiority study. For example, the upper bound of the 95% CI for CHD in ALLHAT is 1.08. Is this close enough to argue noninferiority? Readers of the study report will have to make their own judgment about how "similar" the treatments are with respect to the CHD outcome. Unless a protocol or data analysis plan states criteria for noninferiority or equivalence, claims for such in a superiority trial should not be made. An example of a trial that aimed to assess both superiority and noninferiority is the OPTIMAAL study.[34] The investigators stated their primary hypothesis as "treatment with losartan would be superior or noninferior to captopril at decreasing the risk of all-cause mortality...." These investigators prespecified an upper bound for the hazard ratio (losartan/captopril) of 1.10 for the noninferiority assessment. Secondary hypotheses related to cardiac death and fatal or nonfatal reinfarction were stated as superiority hypotheses only. The CI for all-cause mortality was 0.99 to 1.28. With respect to all-cause mortality, losartan was neither superior nor noninferior to captopril.[34]

Many active controlled trials are designed as equivalence or noninferiority trials.[35-38] An equivalence trial is two-sided. It is designed to show the absence of a clinically meaningful difference *in either direction* between a new treatment and an established control treatment—are the treatments similar and can they be used interchangeably? A noninferiority trial is one-sided. It is designed to show that the new treatment is not *worse* than an established control treatment by some margin—is the new treatment as good as the control treatment? Noninferiority trials are more common than equivalence trials, particularly in a regulatory setting. It is possible that a new treatment, although offering no advantage in terms of increased efficacy, may have fewer side effects or be cheaper. In the case of new BP-lowering drugs, the former was a consideration for some treatments, whereas the latter was not. The Controlled Onset Verapamil Investigation of Cardiovascular End Points (CONVINCE) trial was designed as an equivalence trial.[39,40] CONVINCE will be used as an example to illustrate some important considerations in the planning of equivalence and noninferiority trials.

- For both equivalence and noninferiority trials, the equivalence or noninferiority margin has to be stated a priori (usually negotiated). In other words, how much worse can the new treatment be, compared with the control, to declare the two treatments "similar?" In CONVINCE, it was stated a priori that if the upper bound of the CI for the hazard ratio (verapamil/control) for the composite CVD outcome was greater than 1.16, then the treatments would not be declared "similar." Because CONVINCE was designed as an equivalence trial, a lower bound for the hazard ratio (0.86) was also set. If the lower bound of the 95% CI was less than 0.86, the treatments would not be considered "similar." Conclusions for both equivalence and noninferiority trials should be supported by CIs. The 95% CI for the hazard ratio for the primary endpoint in CONVINCE was 0.88 to 1.18, and the authors stated that equivalence was not demonstrated.[40] This is illustrated in Figure 25-2. Also shown in Figure 25-2 is the CI for the same endpoint for the Captopril Primary Prevention Project (CAPPP).[41] This trial had a slightly smaller number of primary endpoints compared with CONVINCE (698

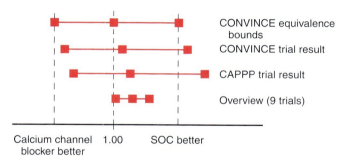

Calcium channel   1.00   SOC better
blocker better

HR (verapamil/SOC) for CONVINCE and overview
HR (captopril/SOC) for CAPPP

Figure 25–2 Interpretation of equivalence trials. CAPPP, Captopril Primary Prevention Project; CONVINCE, Controlled Onset Verapamil Investigation of Cardiovascular End Points; HR, hazard ratio; SOC, standard of care.

versus 729 events, respectively), and the 95% CI for the hazard ratio (captopril versus diuretic or β-blocker) was 0.90 to 1.22. These authors, however, concluded "captopril and conventional treatment did not differ in efficacy." This conclusion is inappropriate in the absence of preestablished bounds for what is similar. As noted earlier, the absence of difference does not mean there is not one. This example also illustrates that "equivalence is in the eyes of the beholder." Even though the data and the thinking used for specifying the equivalence bounds for CONVINCE (see later) could have been used for CAPPP, they apparently were not.

- In equivalence trials, it is possible that the new treatment and control may differ significantly from one another. This is illustrated in Figure 25-2 by plotting the pooled finding for the CVD composite outcome for nine trials that compared a calcium channel blocker with a diuretic or a β-blocker.[21] The hazard ratio (calcium channel blocker treatment versus diuretic or β-blocker treatment) was 1.04 (95% CI, 1.00 to 1.09). Using the bounds established for CONVINCE, these pooled results indicate that calcium channel blockers and diuretics or β-blockers (standard of care [SOC]) are equivalent (the summary confidence bounds lie within the preestablished equivalence bounds for CONVINCE); however, the difference among treatment groups significantly favors the SOC group. In practical terms, the statistical significance may not be considered clinically significant. As noted previously for superiority trials, a given trial, depending on the result, may make a claim of both superiority and equivalence or noninferiority.

- For both equivalence and noninferiority trials, the equivalence or noninferiority margin must be set at a level to be certain that the new treatment is not worse than placebo or no treatment. The comparison with no treatment or placebo has to be done indirectly because the trial does not include a placebo or no-treatment group (the comparison with placebo must be imputed). For the design of CONVINCE, data were gathered from a meta-analysis of trials that compared diuretics and/or β-blockers with placebo or no-treatment control groups,[14] as well as from three trials completed after the meta-analysis.[32,33,42] Based on these trials, it was estimated that the composite CVD

endpoint to be used in CONVINCE would be reduced by 26% with diuretics and/or β-blockers compared with placebo or no treatment. In CONVINCE, control participants could take either hydrochlorothiazide (12.5 mg/day) or atenolol (50 mg/day) as the SOC regimen. It was assumed that 75% of control patients would receive hydrochlorothiazide and 25% would receive atenolol (in fact,[40] 46% received hydrochlorothiazide and 54% received atenolol). The data from the meta-analysis and three trials were weighted with these assumptions, and, as a result, the assumed reduction in the composite CVD outcome with diuretics and/or β-blockers was assumed to be 24% (i.e., the SOC arm in CONVINCE would presumably result in a 24% reduction in CVD compared with placebo or no treatment). The equivalence margin in CONVINCE was set to ensure that there would be no more than a 50% loss of efficacy based on this point estimate. The CI around the estimated efficacy of SOC (24%) was relatively narrow (±5% to 6%), but had the lower bound been used instead of the point estimate, even more stringent criteria for equivalence would have resulted. It is important to consider how reliable the estimate of the efficacy of the active control arm is in planning an equivalence or noninferiority trial. The estimate used in CONVINCE resulted in an upper bound of the CI for the hazard ratio of 1.16 = 0.88 (12% reduction)/0.76 (24% reduction). The CONVINCE trial was not designed to estimate the hazard ratio of verapamil versus no treatment (assumed to be no greater than 0.88) or the hazard ratio of control treatment (diuretic or β-blocker) to no treatment; these values had to be imputed.

- Because the noninferiority or equivalence margin is set by making use of historical data concerning the efficacy of the control treatment, it is important that the patients to be enrolled in the trial are similar to those previously studied. One needs to be certain that the control treatment has efficacy among patients in the trial of the new treatment similar to that in the historical trials used for planning. For example, with CONVINCE, it was assumed that had a no-treatment arm been included, the control arm would have resulted in a 24% reduction in CVD compared with it.

- In superiority trials, nonadherence to the study treatments results in a loss of power, and intention-to-treat analyses are conservative with respect to type 1 error. In equivalence and noninferiority trials, nonadherence can increase the likelihood that the treatments will be considered similar when they are not (it increases the risk of a type 1 error). Thus, intention-to-treat analyses can be anticonservative. It is particularly important in equivalence and noninferiority trials that nonadherence be minimized.

Because a large body of evidence for hypertensive individuals supports the clinical efficacy of diuretics and β-blockers, most BP outcome trials carried out since the early 1990s used a diuretic or a β-blocker, or both, as the first-line active control treatment. Some trials used a diuretic as a control, some used a β-blocker, and some used both. For example, ALLHAT used a diuretic as the first-line control treatment.[18-20] A β-blocker (atenolol, 25 mg/day) was one of the second-line agents that could be used. The African American Study of Kidney Disease and Hypertension (AASK[43]) and the Losartan Intervention for Endpoint Reduction (LIFE) study used a β-blocker as the first-line control arm.[44] AASK used metoprolol (50 to 200 mg/day), and LIFE used atenolol (50 to 100 mg/day). AASK used the diuretic furosemide as the second-line treatment (because all participants had diminished renal function); LIFE used hydrochlorothiazide (12.5 to 25 mg/day) as the second-line treatment (because patients with chronic renal impairment were excluded). As previously noted, in CONVINCE, control participants could take either hydrochlorothiazide (12.5 mg/day) or atenolol (50 mg/day) initially. This was accomplished by prespecifying the control arm choice for each participant before randomization. Participants were then randomized to either verapamil or their SOC choice. In CONVINCE, hydrochlorothiazide was the second-line treatment for those assigned verapamil or atenolol; for patients assigned hydrochlorothiazide as the first-line control treatment, atenolol was the second-line treatment. By giving participants and clinicians the choice of control treatment and still maintaining the randomization, this could more closely mimic clinical practice and increase the enrollment in BP outcome trials. Data from CONVINCE or other trials are not available to assess this issue. However, many would view the question addressed to be more important or clinically relevant if the choice of control treatment used could be optimized for each patient by the participating investigators.

Endpoint Definition and Unbiased Assessment of Relevant Clinical Outcomes

General factors to consider in choosing a primary endpoint have been reviewed.[45-48] Ideally, the primary outcome in a clinical trial should be clinically relevant, easily ascertainable in all patients, capable of unbiased assessment, sensitive to the hypothesized effects of the treatment, and inexpensive to measure. Blinding investigators and patients to the study treatments received helps to ensure unbiased ascertainment of endpoints.

Because outcome trials are typically of many years' duration, unbiased comparisons of treatments are also ensured by excellent follow-up of all patients for all outcomes of interest to the end of the trial. Sloppily conducted trials may yield biased estimates of efficacy and safety and may compromise power. A recent commentator noted that bias resulting from poor follow-up cannot be corrected in the analysis, and widely used analytic procedures to do so depend on assumptions that are usually not defensible.[49] For example, in time-to-event analyses such as those for BP outcome trials, participants lost to follow-up are censored. If this censoring is informative (i.e., depends on the outcomes assessed and is not the same for each treatment group), treatment hazard ratios will be biased. Excellent follow-up is essential in outcome trials. This can be accomplished by choosing endpoints that are easily ascertainable, by educating trial participants on the importance of excellent follow-up as part of the informed consent process and throughout the trial, by investing in staffing at clinical sites to carry out this education, by regularly discussing the importance of good follow-up with trial investigators, and by insisting on high standards.

The selection of a primary endpoint is an important step in a clinical trial. Along with the treatments and the definition of the target population, the primary endpoint defines the research question, its importance, and relevance. Most BP-lowering trials with clinical outcomes have utilized composite endpoints as primary or secondary outcomes. Meinert defined a composite outcome as "an event that is considered to have occurred if any one of several different events or outcomes is observed."[50] Freemantle and associates discussed the pros and cons of composite outcomes.[51] My colleagues and I reviewed composites for human immunodeficiency virus (HIV) and heart failure trials.[47,52] The primary advantage of composite outcomes is that if the treatment affects each of the components of the composite in a similar way, then sample size can be reduced. The principal disadvantage occurs when the treatment effect varies considerably for the components of the composite. In general, a single well-defined, clinically relevant outcome, such as all-cause mortality (as used in HDFP[8-10]), is preferable, but the sample size requirements with use of a single outcome may be too great.

A typical composite outcome is similar to that used in the CONVINCE trial. In CONVINCE, the primary outcome was the first occurrence of (1) fatal or nonfatal myocardial infarction, (2) fatal or nonfatal stroke, or (3) death from another CVD cause.[40] Figure 25-3 illustrates how patients were counted for the composite endpoint used in CONVINCE. The event history of five patients is illustrated. Time zero is randomization. The "X" and "O" in Figure 25-3 denote event and censoring times, respectively, for the time-to-event analysis, and the "&" denotes events that do not count for the composite endpoint analysis. The first patient experienced a myocardial infarction shortly after randomization; the second patient did not experience the composite outcome (was event-free at the end of the trial); the third patient died of CVD without a preceding nonfatal stroke or myocardial infarction; the fourth patient died of a non-CVD cause and is censored at the time (the patient is no longer at risk for the CVD composite endpoint); the fifth patient experienced a myocardial infarction and a stroke and then died of CVD (but only the first event is counted).

These fictitious patients illustrate some characteristics of composite endpoints analyzed with time-to-event methods: (1) although a CVD death would generally be regarded as more serious than a myocardial infarction, the shortest failure time is for the first patient who was hospitalized for a myocar-

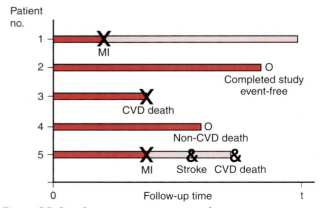

Figure 25–3 Composite outcomes and event counting. X and O denote event and censoring times, respectively, for the time-to-event analysis; & denotes events that do not count for the composite endpoint analysis. CVD, cardiovascular disease; MI, myocardial infarction; t, time.

dial infarction; (2) because non-CVD deaths are treated as censored observations and do not count as events, a priori it would be important to expect no effect of treatment on non-CVD mortality because if there were, the interpretation of the composite would be complicated; and (3) even though the fifth patient had the more severe event history, only the first event was counted, and it occurred after the primary events occurred for the first and third patients.

My colleagues and I reviewed different approaches for handling the varying severity of clinical events that patients could experience and for using all the information on events that occur during a trial.[47] One of those approaches is a marginal model, that is, an approach that yields a pooled hazard ratio, which is a weighted average of hazard ratios for each type or number (e.g., first or second) of events with an estimate of the standard error that takes into account the correlation among different event times.[53] The Wei, Lin, and Weissfeld approach was used in the Second Australian National Blood Pressure study group (ANBP2).[53,54] In ANBP2, 490 patients assigned to the ACE inhibitor–treated group experienced at least one CVD event or died, compared with 529 patients in the diuretic-treated group. The hazard ratio (ACE inhibitor to diuretic) and 95% CI for the first event analysis were 0.89 (0.79 to 1.01). With consideration of all events (695 in the ACE inhibitor–treated group and 736 in the diuretic-treated group), the hazard ratio was identical, and the 95% CI was very similar—0.89 (0.79 to 1.00).[54] Walker and colleagues noted that standard errors with marginal models such as the Wei, Lin, and Weissfeld approach may not be reduced, as was the case in ANBP2, presumably because of the high correlation of event times.[55] In addition, as noted by Hughes, consideration of events after the first could result in a loss of power if patients were more likely to modify their study treatment after an event.[56] Thus, designs that utilize these analyses for composite outcomes will need to consider the possibility that the treatment effects may vary both for different components of the composite and according to the order in which they occur.

In trials with a composite endpoint, patients should be followed to the end of the study for all components of the composite outcome. Continued data collection of all outcomes comprising the composite endpoint will permit a proper intent-to-treat analysis of each component of the composite as well as the composite. This approach has been referred to as the "Consumer Reports" analysis.[57] For example, if the composite outcome includes cardiovascular mortality, nonfatal myocardial infarction, or nonfatal stroke, patients who experience a nonfatal stroke should continue to be followed for a nonfatal myocardial infarction or cardiovascular death. Otherwise, the analysis of individual components of the composite endpoint could be biased. This type of analysis is essential to rank order the treatment on different outcomes so a fully informed assessment can be made on whether the new treatment is better than or as good as the control.

The trial report should also describe the frequency with which each component occurred as the first event for those with endpoints. For example, if 100 patients who were assigned the new treatment experienced the composite outcome described earlier (cardiovascular mortality, nonfatal myocardial infarction, or nonfatal stroke), the trial report should state how many of these 100 events were a result of

cardiovascular mortality and how many were nonfatal myocardial infarction or stroke.

These two analyses will allow the reader (the consumer of your trial report) to assess whether treatment differences for each component of the composite trend in the same direction and whether the first event experienced by those with an endpoint is similar for the treatment groups. Freemantle and Montori and their associates, as well as my colleagues and I, also emphasized the importance of the "Consumer Reports" analysis in trial reports.[47,51,52,58] In addition, Freemantle and colleagues advocated defining each component of the composite endpoint as a secondary outcome.[51] The CONVINCE trial report illustrates the "Consumer Reports" analysis (see Table 25-2).[40]

Sample Size and Power

The power of outcome trials arises from the number of primary events. The number of primary events needed can be determined by specifying the hypothesized treatment difference and the type 1 and 2 errors.[59] The latter are usually set at 0.05 (two-sided) and at 0.10 and 0.20 (or equivalent power of 0.90 or 0.80). This principle is illustrated in Table 25-1, with the number of event determined using Schoenfeld's approach.[59] Relatively few events are needed to rule out large differences across randomized arms of a trial (40% to 50% treatment differences); moderate effects (20% to 30%) require approximately 500 events; and small effects (<20%) require thousands of events. Because the likelihood of large or moderate treatment differences is small and because small differences are important from a public health point of view, trials need to enroll a sufficient number of people and follow them long enough to accrue a few thousand events. Thus, for the ALLHAT's comparison of chlorthalidone and lisinopril mentioned earlier, 2158 CHD events occurred.[20] CONVINCE was designed to accrue 2024 events, and this was later increased to 2246 events.[39,40] The CONVINCE study was stopped early by the sponsor for commercial reasons at a time when only 729 events had occurred. Thus, as executed, CONVINCE had limited statistical power to evaluate equivalence of the two regimens.

As noted earlier, a critical determinant of sample size is the expected treatment difference, sometimes referred to as the minimally important difference that is clinically relevant.

Table 25-1 Number of Primary Events Required to Detect Specified Difference in Hazard (Expressed as Percentage Reduction in Hazard in Control Group) for Type 1 Error of 0.05 (Two-Sided) and Power of 0.80 for Two Treatment Groups of Equal Size

Reduction in Hazard (%)	Required No. of Patients with Endpoint
50	65
40	120
30	250
25	380
20	630
15	1190
10	2825

The treatment difference observed is influenced by nonadherence to the treatments, both "dropouts" (participants that do not adhere to the experimental treatment and use either control treatment or non-study treatment) and "dropins" (participants assigned control who take the experimental treatment), and in some cases by the duration of follow-up (i.e., treatment effects may wane or increase with time).[60,61] Nonadherence to the control arm that reflects missing doses of the regimen may not have to be taken into account in sample size estimation, if the control event rate data being used are based on intention-to-treat analyses of the control treatment.

Table 25-2 illustrates the impact of nonadherence on the realized hazard ratio. This, in turn, has a major impact on the number of events required and the sample size or duration of follow-up. Five different sets of assumptions for nonadherence in the experimental and control groups of a hypothetical trial are considered. These are expressed as the cumulative percentage of participants not adhering to their assigned treatment after 8 years of follow-up. It is assumed that a 9-year study is planned: 2 years of enrollment and 7 years of minimum follow-up, resulting in an average follow-up of 8 years. It is also assumed that the rates of nonadherence in the treatment and control groups are constant over the 8-year average follow-up period. The required number of events was based on Shih's method.[61]

The first line in Table 25-2 corresponds to the second last line in Table 25-1. In the absence of nonadherence, power is 0.80 to detect a hazard ratio of 0.850, and 1190 primary events are needed. If 25% of participants do not adhere to the new treatment and adherence to the control treatment is 100%, then the realized hazard ratio is 0.868 (the treatment effect will be attenuated), and the required number of events to ensure 80% power increases to 1555. These assumptions may be suitable for a study in which it is unlikely that control patients will have access to the new treatment (e.g., the new treatment is not yet marketed).

If nonadherence to both the new treatment and control treatments is likely, but less so in the control arm (10% versus 25% for the new treatment), then the realized hazard ratio is 0.872, and the required number of events is 1685. As the last two lines of Table 25-2 indicate, this attenuation of the hazard ratio is greater if nonadherence to the new treatment is 50% instead of 25%.

To provide some perspective for these estimates, the following statistics were taken from the ALLHAT report comparing lisinopril with chlorthalidone.[20] For lisinopril, the test treatment, 39% of participants were not taking blinded drug after 5 years of follow-up; 24% were taking a diuretic. For chlorthalidone, the control treatment, 30% of participants were not taking blinded drug after 5 years, and 22% were taking either an ACE inhibitor or a calcium channel blocker. In the design of ALLHAT, it was assumed that 24% of participants would cross over to another medication at least once in 6 years.[18] Although this percentage cannot be directly compared with the estimates in Table 25-2, nonadherence needs to be accounted for, because if it is not, power will be lost.

Simplicity

Several years after his article on the clinical trial, Sir Austin Bradford Hill explained that he initially tried to convince clinicians to assign patients alternately to treatments and that he avoided using the term "randomization." He noted, "I was trying to persuade the doctors to come into controlled trials in the very simplest form and I might have scared them off ... I thought it would be better to get doctors to walk first, before I tried to get them to run."[62]

We have been fairly successful in getting doctors to "run." This is no more evident than in the study of BP-lowering drugs, of which numerous large trials have been conducted. However, more cost-efficient approaches for the conduct of clinical trials of BP-lowering drugs and other interventions are very much needed, because the number of treatments to compare with one another continues to grow rapidly. We need to determine how to "run" much faster. By that I do not mean we should take shortcuts in our attempts to understand the real benefits of interventions such as BP lowering, which can have substantial public health benefits. We must insist on randomized studies, excellent long-term follow-up, and both clinically relevant outcomes and comparison groups.

We need more doctors running! How do we accomplish this?

- Simple clinical site registration procedures
- Simple trial procedures
- Simple monitoring procedures

Procedures required to register sites for participation in clinical trials by the National Institutes of Health (NIH) are daunting—Federal Wide Assurances are needed, and a local Institutional Review Board has to exist and be properly constituted. In international trials, sites may have to incorporate elements in the informed consent that differ from local policies. As noted by McNay and colleagues, these requirements are designed to protect the rights and welfare of human study subjects, but they may discourage some investigators from participating in research and may create delays in doing so.[63]

Many practicing physicians will need help with these tasks to participate in multicenter clinical trials. Wood and associates suggested a regional ethics organization as a replace-

Table 25-2   Impact of Nonadherence on Hypothesized Hazard Ratio and Target Number of Events

New Treatment*	Control†	Hazard Ratio‡	Required No. of Primary Events§
0	0	0.850	1190
25	0	0.868	1555
25	10	0.872	1685
50	0	0.888	2205
50	10	0.891	2375

*Discontinuation and crossover to control treatment or non-study treatment.
†Crossover to new treatment.
‡Constant rate of nonadherence to new treatment and control over 9 years (2-year enrollment period; 7 years of minimum follow-up; 8 year average follow-up).
§$\alpha = .05$ (two-sided) and power = 0.80; two treatment groups of equal size.

ment for the current local Institutional Review Board system.[64] Central and regional coordinating centers, like the ones developed to conduct ALLHAT, are needed to assist physicians in the community to enroll their patients in trials.[18,65] This model of support has also been successfully applied in HIV international trials.[66] As I noted elsewhere, some minimal infrastructure funding for participating clinicians will have to be provided. This cannot be too much, because otherwise there would be occasions when one could be paying for staff "dressed up but with no place to go."[27]

Screening and enrollment procedures should be simple in BP outcome studies. This can be accomplished if eligibility criteria are broad and if randomization and drug distribution procedures are "user friendly." Follow-up procedures should also be simple. This can be accomplished with focused data collection (i.e., on major endpoints that are easily ascertainable, not ancillary data).

It is important that participants (whether as investigators or research subjects) understand what they are joining. As noted earlier, ensuring excellent long-term follow-up for outcome trials needs to begin with the informed consent process. Flory and Emanuel's assessment is that many participants do not understand elements of the informed consent, and interventions to improve understanding have had only limited success.[67] More research on the informed consent process is needed, both the consent process before randomization and the later consent process related to protocol amendments or possible safety issues.

Richard Horton, editor of *The Lancet*, summarized public perception of clinical trials in an article entitled, "The Clinical Trial: Deceitful, Disputable, Unbelievable, Unhelpful, and Shameful: What Next?"[68] He argued that trials were deceitful because of fraudulent behavior by investigators. One of his recommendations was to think more critically about the practical methodology of the studies we undertake. Large, long-term trials do not have to be expensive. The simplicity and cost savings achieved by stripping trials of unnecessary regulatory requirements and ancillary data could result in more studies. More research on the practical methodology for conducting studies is needed. It should be possible both to do a better job of protecting the safety of patients in trials and to conduct trials in a more cost-effective manner.[69,70]

SUMMARY

Donald Fredrickson, former director of NIH, stated, "Clinical trials lack glamour, they strain our resources and patience, and they protract to excruciating limits the moment of truth."[71] This is certainly true of BP outcome trials. However, such trials are critical to achieving small to moderate incremental improvements in public health.

In 2003, Tunis and colleagues coined the phrase "practical" clinical trials.[72] These investigators characterized such trials as follows: "(1) select clinically relevant alternative interventions to compare; (2) include a diverse population of study participants; (3) recruit patients from heterogeneous practice settings; and (4) collect data on a broad range of health outcomes." These investigators noted that too few practical clinical trials are carried out and that, as a consequence, health care decision makers do not have adequate-quality information to make well-informed decisions.

Future BP outcome trials must be a partnership among academia, government, and industry. As noted earlier, the regulatory processes need to reconsider the importance of BP outcome trials for licensure. Industry sponsors should be encouraged and rewarded for examining the risks and benefits of new agents. Government sponsors such as NIH need to focus more on strategic or "practical" trials. For example, trials that examine optimal use of available BP-lowering agents and nutritional-hygienic approaches to obtain optimal BP levels with minimal risks will require government sponsorship.

Many lessons learned from the design and implementation of BP outcome trials can be applied to interventions for other risk factors and to multiple CVD risk factors. The lessons are also relevant to the study of interventions in other diseases. Specifically, for many areas, large trials are needed because disease event rates are low and treatment differences are expected to be modest but nevertheless important. Treatments for many trials will have to be practically determined, and certain important, easily ascertainable outcomes will have to be assessed to rank order the interventions compared. Finally, many sites will be required to carry out the trials, and to do so cost-effectively, simplicity will be key.

References

1. American Heart Association. Heart and Stroke Facts: 2005 Statistical Supplement. Dallas, Tex: 2004. Available on the internet at http://www.americanheart.org, accessed 23 MAR 05.
2. Neaton JD, Kuller L, Stamler J, Wentworth DN. Impact of systolic and diastolic blood pressure on cardiovascular mortality. *In:* Laragh JH, Brenner BM (eds). Hypertension: Pathophysiology, Diagnosis, and Management. New York: Raven Press, 1995, pp 127-144.
3. Klag MJ, Whelton PK, Randall BL, et al. Blood pressure and incidence of end-stage renal disease in men. *N Engl J Med.* 1996;**334**:13-18.
4. Prospective Studies Collaboration. Age-specific relevance of usual blood pressure to vascular mortality: A meta-analysis of individual data for one million adults in 61 prospective studies. *Lancet.* 2002;**360**:1903-1913.
5. Veterans Administration Cooperative Study Group on Antihypertensive Agents. Effects of treatment on morbidity in hypertension: Results in patients with diastolic blood pressure averaging 115 through 129 mm Hg. *JAMA.* 1967;**202**:1028-1034.
6. Veterans Administration Cooperative Study Group on Antihypertensive Agents. Effects of treatment on morbidity in hypertension. II: Results in patients with diastolic blood pressure averaging 90 through 114 mm Hg. *JAMA.* 1970;**213**: 1143-1152.
7. Veterans Administration Cooperative Study Group on Antihypertensive Agents. Effects of treatment on morbidity in hypertension. III: Influence of age, diastolic pressure, and prior cardiovascular disease; further analysis of side effects. *Circulation.* 1972;**45**:991-1004.
8. Hypertension Detection and Follow-up Program Cooperative Group. I: Reduction in mortality of persons with high blood pressure, including mild hypertension. *JAMA.* 1979;**242**: 2562-2571.
9. Hypertension Detection and Follow-up Program Cooperative Group. II: Mortality by race-sex and age. *JAMA.* 1979;**242**: 2572-2577.
10. Hypertension Detection and Follow-up Program Cooperative Group. Persistence of reduction in blood pressure and mortality of participants in the Hypertension Detection and Follow-up Program. *JAMA.* 1988;**259**:2113-2122.

11. Multiple Risk Factor Intervention Trial Research Group. Multiple Risk Factor Intervention Trial: Risk factor changes and mortality results. *JAMA*. 1982;**248**:1465-1477.

12. Multiple Risk Factor Intervention Trial Research Group. Mortality after 10 1/2 years for hypertensive participants in the Multiple Risk Factor Intervention Trial. *JAMA*. 1990;**82**:1616-1628.

13. Medical Research Council Working Party. MRC trial of treatment of mild hypertension: Principal results. *BMJ*. 1985;**291**:97-104.

14. Collins R, Peto R, MacMahon S, et al. Blood pressure, stroke, and coronary heart disease. Part 2: Short-term reductions in blood pressure. Overview of randomized trials in their epidemiologic context. *Lancet*. 1990;**335**:827-838.

15. MacMahon SA, Cutler JA, Furberg CD, et al. The effects of drug treatment for hypertension on morbidity and mortality from cardiovascular disease: A review of randomized controlled trials. *Prog Cardiovasc Dis*. 1986;**29 (3 Suppl 1)**:99-119.

16. Holme I. Drug treatment for mild hypertension to reduce the risk of CHD: Is it worthwhile? *Stat Med*. 1988;**7**:1109-1120.

17. Neaton JD, Grimm RH, Prineas RJ, et al. Treatment of Mild Hypertension Study: Final results. *JAMA*. 1993;**270**:713-724.

18. Davis BR, Cutler JA, Gordon DG, et al. Rationale and design for the Antihypertensive and Lipid-Lowering Treatment to Prevent Heart Attack Trial (ALLHAT). *Am J Hypertens*. 1996;**9**:342-360.

19. ALLHAT Officers and Coordinators for the ALLHAT Collaborative Research Group. Major cardiovascular events in hypertensive patients randomized to doxazosin vs. chlorthalidone: The Antihypertensive and Lipid-Lowering Treatment to Prevent Heart Attack Trial (ALLHAT). *JAMA*. 2000;**283**:1967-1975.

20. ALLHAT Officers and Coordinators for the ALLHAT Collaborative Research Group. Major outcomes in high-risk hypertensive patients randomized to angiotensin-converting enzyme inhibitor or calcium channel blocker vs. diuretic: The Antihypertensive and Lipid-Lowering Treatment to Prevent Heart Attack Trial (ALLHAT). *JAMA*. 2002;**288**:2981-2997.

21. Blood Pressure Lowering Treatment Trialists' Collaboration. Effects of different blood-pressure-lowering regimens on major cardiovascular events: Results of prospectively-designed overviews of randomized trials. *Lancet*. 2003;**362**:1527-1535.

22. Yusuf S, Collins R, Peto R. Why do we need large, simple randomized trials? *Stat Med*. 1984;**3**:409-420.

23. Hill AB. The clinical trial. *Br Med Bull*. 1951;**7**:278-282.

24. Armitage P. The role of randomization in clinical trials. *Stat Med*. 1982;**1**:345-352.

25. Miettinen OS. The need for randomization in the study of intended effects. *Stat Med*. 1983;**2**:267-271.

26. MacMahon S, Collins R. Reliable assessment of the effects of treatment on mortality and major morbidity. II: Observational studies. *Lancet*. 2001;**357**:455-462.

27. Neaton JD. Quantitative science. *In:* Mayer KH, Pizer HF (eds). The AIDS Pandemic: Impact on Science and Society. New York: Elsevier Academic Press, 2004, pp 58-89.

28. Temple R. Are surrogate markers adequate to assess cardiovascular disease drugs? *JAMA*. 1999;**282**:790-795.

29. Chobanian AV, Bakris GL, Black HR, et al., and the National High Blood Pressure Education Program Coordinating Committee. The Seventh Report of the Joint National Committee on Prevention, Detection, Evaluation, and Treatment of High Blood Pressure: The JNC 7 report. *JAMA*. 2003;**289**:2560-2572.

30. Psaty BM, Smith NL, Siscovick DS, et al. Health outcomes associated with antihypertensive therapies used as first-line agents: A systematic review and meta-analysis. *JAMA*. 1997;**277**:739-745.

31. Amery A, Birkenhager W, Brixko P, et al. Mortality and morbidity results from the European Working Party on high blood pressure in the elderly trial. *Lancet*. 1985;**1**:1349-1354.

32. SHEP Cooperative Research Group. Prevention of stroke by antihypertensive drug treatment in older persons with isolated systolic hypertension: Final results of the Systolic Hypertension in the Elderly Program (SHEP). *JAMA*. 1991;**265**:3255-3264.

33. MRC Working Party. Medical Research Council trial of treatment of hypertension in older adults: Principal results. *BMJ*. 1992;**304**:405-412.

34. Dickstein K, Kjekshus J, and the OPTIMAAL Steering Committee. Effects of losartan and captopril on mortality and morbidity in high-risk patients after acute myocardial infarction: The OPTIMAAL randomized trial. *Lancet*. 2002;**360**:752-760.

35. Blackwelder WC. "Proving the null hypothesis" in clinical trials. *Cont Clin Trials*. 1982;**3**:345-353.

36. Jones B, Jarvis P, Lewis JA, Ebbutt AF. Trials to assess equivalence: The importance of rigorous methods. *BMJ*. 1999;**313**:36-39.

37. Fleming TR. Evaluation of active control trials in AIDS. *J Acquir Immune Defic Syndr*. 1990;**3**:S82-S87.

38. Pocock S. The pros and cons of noninferiority trials. *Fund Clin Pharmacol*. 2003;**17**:483-490.

39. Black HR, Elliott WJ, Neaton JD, et al. Rationale and design for the Controlled Onset Verapamil Investigation of Cardiovascular End Points (CONVINCE) Trial. *Cont Clin Trials*. 1998;**19**:370-390.

40. Black HR, Elliott WJ, Grandits G, et al. Principal results of the Controlled Onset Verapamil Investigation of Cardiovascular End Points (CONVINCE) Trial. *JAMA*. 2003;**289**:2073-2082.

41. Hansson L, Lindholm LH, Niskanen L, et al. Effect of angiotensin-converting enzyme inhibition compared with conventional therapy on cardiovascular morbidity and mortality in hypertension: The Captopril Prevention Project (CAPPP) randomized trial. *Lancet*. 1999;**353**:611-616.

42. Dahlöf B, Lindholm LH, Hansson L, et al. Morbidity and mortality in the Swedish Trial on Old Patients with Hypertension (STOP-Hypertension). *Lancet*. 1991;**338**:1281-1285.

43. Wright JT, Bakris G, Greene T, et al. Effect of blood pressure lowering and antihypertensive drug class on progression of hypertensive kidney disease: Results from the AASK Trial. *JAMA*. 2002;**288**:2421-2431.

44. Dahlof B, Devereux RB, Kjeldsen SE, et al. Cardiovascular morbidity and mortality in the Losartan Intervention for Endpoint reduction in hypertension study (LIFE): A randomized trial against atenolol. *Lancet*. 2002;**359**:995-1003.

45. Friedman LM, Furberg CD, DeMets DL. Fundamentals of Clinical Trials, 3rd ed. New York: Springer, 1998.

46. Meinert CL. Clinical Trials: Design, Conduct and Analysis. New York: Oxford University Press, 1986.

47. Neaton JD, Wentworth DN, Rhame F, et al. Considerations in choice of a clinical endpoint for AIDS clinical trials. *Stat Med*. 1994;**13**:2107-2125.

48. Pocock SJ. Clinical Trials: A Practical Approach. New York: John Wiley & Sons, 1997.

49. Ware JH. Interpreting incomplete data in studies of diet and weight loss. *N Engl J Med*. 2003;**348**:2136-2137.

50. Meinert CL. Clinical Trials Dictionary. Baltimore: Johns Hopkins Center for Clinical Trials, 1996.

51. Freemantle N, Calvert M, Wood J, et al. Composite outcomes in randomized trials: Greater precision but with greater uncertainty? *JAMA*. 2003;**289**:2554-2559.

52. Neaton JD, Gray G, Zuckerman B, Konstam MA. Key issues in endpoint selection for heart failure trials: Composite end points. *J Card Fail*. 2005;**11**:457-575.

53. Wei LJ, Lin DY, Weissfeld L. Regression analysis of multivariate incomplete failure time data by modeling marginal distributions. *J Am Stat Assoc*. 1989;**84**:1065-1073.

54. Wing LMH, Reid CM, Ryan P, et al. A comparison of outcomes with angiotensin-converting enzyme inhibitors and diuretics for hypertension in the elderly. *N Engl J Med*. 2003;**348**:583-592.

55. Walker AS, Babiker AG, Darbyshire JH. Analysis of multivariate failure-time data from HIV trials. *Cont Clin Trials*. 2000;**21**:75-93.

56. Hughes MD. Power considerations for clinical trials using multivariate time-to-event data. *Stat Med*. 1997;**16**:865-882.

57. Califf RM, Harrelson-Woodlief L, Topol EJ. Left ventricular ejection fraction may not be useful as an endpoint of thrombolytic therapy: Comparative trials. *Circulation*. 1990;**82**:1847-1853.

58. Montori VM, Permanyer-Miralda G, Ferreira-Gonzalez I, et al. Validity of composite end points in clinical trials. *BMJ*. 2005;**330**:594-596.

59. Schoenfeld DA. Sample-size formula for the proportional hazards model. *Biometrics*. 1983;**39**:499-503.

60. Halperin M, Rogot E, Gurian J, et al. Sample sizes for medical trials with special reference to long term therapy. *J Chronic Dis*. 1968;**21**:13-23.

61. Shih J. Sample size calculation for complex clinical trials with survival endpoints. *Cont Clin Trials*. 1995;**16**:395-407.

62. Hill AB. Memories of the British Streptomycin Trial in Tuberculosis. *Cont Clin Trials*. 1990;**11**:77-79.

63. McNay LA, Tavel JA, Oseekey K, et al. Regulatory approvals in a large multinational clinical trial: The ESPRIT experience. *Cont Clin Trials*. 2002;**23**:59-66.

64. Wood A, Grady C, Emanuel EJ. Regional ethics organizations for protection of human research participants. *Nat Med*. 2004;**10**:1283-1288.

65. Wright JT Jr, Cushman WC, Davis BR, et al. The Antihypertensive and Lipid-Lowering Treatment to Prevent Heart Attack Trial (ALLHAT): Clinical center recruitment. *Cont Clin Trials*. 2001;**22**:659-673.

66. Emery S, Abrams DI, Cooper DA, et al. Evaluation of subcutaneous Proleukin (interleukin-2) in a randomized international trial: Rationale, design and methods of ESPRIT. *Cont Clin Trials*. 2002;**23**:198-220.

67. Flory J, Emanuel E. Interventions to improve research participants' understanding in informed consent for research: A systematic review. *JAMA*. 2004;**292**:1593-1601.

68. Horton R. The clinical trial: Deceitful, disputable, unbelievable, unhelpful, and shameful: What next? *Cont Clin Trials*. 2001;**22**:593-604.

69. Emanuel EJ, Wood A, Fleischman A, et al. Oversight of human participants research: Identifying problems to evaluate reform proposals. *Ann Intern Med*. 2004;**141**:282-291.

70. Califf RM, Morse MA, Wittes J, et al. Toward protecting the safety of participants in clinical trials. *Cont Clin Trials*. 2003;**24**:256-271.

71. Fredrickson DS. The field trial: Some thoughts on the indispensable ordeal. *Bull N Y Acad Med*. 1968;**44**:985-993.

72. Tunis SR, Stryer DB, Clancy CM. Practical clinical trials. Increasing the value of clinical research for decision making in clinical and health policy. *JAMA*. 2003;**290**:1624-1632.

Chapter 26

Meta-analyses of Hypertension Trials

Fiona Turnbull and Bruce Neal

Over the last few decades, meta-analyses have been central to the advancement of medicine in a broad range of specialities. The "conscientious, explicit and judicious use" of the evidence provided by this technique now underpins much of clinical practice and allows clinicians to make truly informed decisions about how best to deliver care to many different types of patients.[1] In the cardiovascular field, meta-analyses of the effects of different blood pressure (BP)–lowering regimens have been in the vanguard of this approach. Huge volumes of data derived from multiple large-scale clinical trials have allowed for extensive investigation of the effects of different approaches to BP lowering. As a result, practitioners are now better informed about the implications of their choices of BP-lowering treatment than about almost any other mode of therapy to which they have access. For example, by using meta-analyses, it has been possible to determine whether real differences exist among drug classes in the protection they afford against different types of serious cardiovascular events and to identify whether the benefits obtained vary according to characteristics of patients such as age and the presence or absence of diabetes. This chapter outlines some key features of meta-analysis and reports the main findings from the largest, ongoing series of meta-analyses conducted in the field, those of the Blood Pressure Lowering Treatment Trialists' Collaboration.

META-ANALYSES

The term *meta-analysis* describes the statistical procedure whereby the results of several different studies addressing the same question are combined in an effort to obtain a more precise and more reliable answer to the question under investigation.[2] The technique may be used for data from a range of different study designs (both observational and interventional), but meta-analysis is now most usually identified with systematic overviews of randomized controlled trials. Meta-analyses of randomized controlled trials have been particularly useful because although the individual estimates provided by small trials may be imprecise, their robust design means that the estimate is usually not biased. As such, the combined result of all the relevant randomized controlled trials should give a precise and reliable estimate of the real effect of the intervention under investigation. In addition, in a field in which multiple trials frequently address a given question, a meta-analysis can be a convenient and practical way of summarizing information for clinicians.

Two main methods are used for combining data from randomized controlled trials in a meta-analysis: the fixed-effects model and the random-effects model. The fixed-effects model is based on the assumption that the results of the individual trials are all estimates of one true effect of the intervention, and the differences between the results of each individual trial and that one true effect are solely a consequence of the play of chance.[2] By contrast, the random-effects model works on the assumption that more than just the play of chance may possibly explain the differences in the results of the contributing trials. In practice, differences in the point estimate of the effect obtained with the two methods are not large, unless there are contributing trials with particularly extreme results. However, because the random-effects model allows for the possibility of both random and systematic differences among the results of the contributing trials, the confidence interval obtained with the random-effects model is wider than that obtained with the fixed-effects model.

To fulfill the criteria for a meta-analysis, the trials to be included all need to address the same basic question. However, agreement on what constitutes the basic question and on which trials should or should not be used in a meta-analysis is frequently difficult to achieve. Ultimately, any meta-analysis will have differences in the characteristics of the included trials; for example, trials addressing the effects of different BP-lowering regimens on major cardiovascular events have frequently been combined, but they include quite varied participants and markedly different durations of follow-up. Likewise, many trials have investigated the effects of regimens based on diuretics compared with angiotensin-converting enzyme (ACE) inhibitors, but the specific drugs used and the dosing regimens employed vary markedly among them. Whether such differences in trial characteristics ultimately strengthen or weaken meta-analysis findings has been the topic of considerable discussion. On balance, it appears that the availability of multiple different studies with varying characteristics probably strengthens rather than weakens the conclusions. In particular, exploration of the constancy of treatment effects across different participant subgroups and varying trial groupings can be done if a range of similar, but not identical, trials is included. Systematic and quantitative estimates of the likelihood of interactions between the treatment under study and a range of different trial and patient characteristics can be calculated, and significant insight into the likely efficacy of the treatment for a broad range of different patient groups can be obtained. Such analyses may also greatly increase the perceived generalizability of the study findings, thereby resulting in enhanced care for more patients.

To obtain unbiased estimates of the treatment effect in a meta-analysis of randomized controlled trials, it is essential to include all the trials addressing the question. It is well established that trials with inconclusive or unfavorable results are not published as frequently as trials with positive findings (publication bias), and the systematic exclusion of unpublished neutral or negative trials could cause effect estimates from a meta-analysis to be biased toward a positive result.[3] Meta-analyses based solely on published data and done without the cooperation of industry and lead investigators in the field are relatively easy to conduct, but they may be especially prone to publication bias. By contrast, more resource-intensive meta-analysis projects conducted by large, well-informed collaborative networks are less subject to publication bias.

Prospective, collaborative meta-analysis projects such as those conducted by the Blood Pressure Lowering Treatment Trialists' Collaboration,[4-6] and others,[7,8] are the current standard in the field. In particular, the prospective nature of such projects limits the potential for bias, because all major decisions about analysis and reporting are specified before the results of any of the contributing trials are known, and the broad collaborative group ensures that all relevant trials are identified. With strong collaborative arrangements, there is also considerably enhanced scope for the standardization of outcome definitions and the sharing of individual participant data sets with consequent analytic advantages.

One of the main drivers of meta-analyses in the BP field has been the need for reliable information about the comparability of the effects of the different drug classes. With tens of millions of individuals using BP-lowering treatment and with tens of billions of dollars expended on it each year, even small differences in the effectiveness of drug classes would have profound implications for guidelines. A very large volume of data is required to attain such reliable information. For example, to detect a relative risk difference of 15% among agents requires more than a thousand outcome events. To detect a difference of 10% requires several thousand, and to define the effects reliably in different patient subgroups requires even more. With the exception of one or two very large trials, few studies have recorded sufficient events to enable these types of questions to be addressed. Meta-analyses of the BP-lowering trials have, however, now gone a considerable way toward addressing these questions.

BLOOD PRESSURE LOWERING TREATMENT TRIALISTS' COLLABORATION

The Blood Pressure Lowering Treatment Trialists' Collaboration is an international collaboration of the principal investigators of large randomized trials of BP-lowering regimens. The broad aim of the collaboration is to provide the most reliable evidence possible about the effects of commonly used BP-lowering regimens on major cardiovascular events by means of prospective meta-analyses of randomized trials.

Prespecified Methods for Meta-analyses

The overviews are conducted and reported in accordance with a protocol that, in 1995, prespecified the trial eligibility criteria, primary outcomes, and main treatment comparisons.[4]

Eligible Trials and Their Identification

Trials are eligible for inclusion in the overviews if they satisfy one of the following criteria: (1) random allocation of patients to regimens based on different BP-lowering agents, (2) random allocation of patients to a BP-lowering agent or placebo, or (3) random allocation of patients to various BP goals. In addi-

tion, eligible trials have to have a planned minimum follow-up of 1000 patient-years per treatment arm and could not have published or presented main trial results before July 1995. Although trials with factorial assignment to other interventions, such as cholesterol-lowering treatment, are eligible for inclusion, trials in which additional treatments are jointly assigned with BP-lowering treatment are not eligible, because these other treatments act as potential confounders.

Eligible trials are identified by numerous methods, including computer-aided literature searches, scrutiny of the reference lists of trial reports and review articles, scrutiny of abstracts and meeting proceeding, and enquiry among colleagues, collaborators, and industry. Principal investigators of eligible studies are identified and are invited to join the collaboration on an ongoing basis.

Data Collection

Both individual patient data and summary tabular data are sought from each trial. Although most trials provide tabular data in the first instance, individual patient data facilitate data checking and the conduct of more comprehensive statistical analyses. The data requested include participant characteristics recorded at screening or randomization, selected measurements made during follow-up, and details of the occurrence of all prespecified outcomes during the scheduled follow-up period. All data are reviewed for accuracy and completeness and, once tabulated, are sent to collaborating investigators for checking.

Prespecified Outcomes

The study outcomes chosen for these overviews represent the main cardiovascular outcomes likely to be affected by BP-lowering treatment regimens and the main non–cardiovascular disease outcomes for which questions about the safety of some agents have arisen. The six prespecified primary outcomes are nonfatal stroke or death from cerebrovascular disease (codes 430 to 438 in the ninth revision of the International Classification of Disease [ICD]), nonfatal myocardial infarction or death from coronary heart disease (CHD, ICD 41 to 414), heart failure causing death or requiring hospitalization (ICD 428), total cardiovascular deaths (ICD 396 to 459), total major cardiovascular events (stroke, CHD events, heart failure, other cardiovascular death), and total mortality. The secondary study outcomes include the following: hemorrhagic stroke (ICD 431 to 432); ischemic stroke (ICD 433 to 434); death or hospitalization for renal disease (ICD 189, 403 to 404, 580 to 593); arterial revascularization procedure (ICD 36, 38.0, 38.1, and 38.4); any bone fracture (ICD 800 to 829); death, hospitalization, or transfusion for any noncerebral hemorrhage (ICD 459, 578.9, but not 430 to 432); major site-specific cancer such as lung (ICD 162), large bowel (ICD 153 to 154), breast (ICD 174 to 175), or prostate (ICD 185); and admission to a hospital for any cause.

Prespecified Comparisons and Subgroup Analyses

The comparisons prespecified in the protocol can be broadly divided into two groups. The first group comprises comparisons of active BP-lowering regimens with control regimens: ACE inhibitor–based regimens versus placebo, calcium antagonist–based regimens versus placebo, and regimens targeting different BP goals (more-intensive versus less-intensive BP-lowering regimens). The second group comprises comparisons of different active regimens intended to produce similar BP reductions: ACE inhibitor–based regimens versus diuretic- and/or β-blocker–based regimens, calcium antagonist–based versus diuretic-based or β-blocker–based regimens, and ACE inhibitor–based regimens versus calcium antagonist–based regimens. For each of these comparisons, the null hypothesis of no difference among regimens in their effects on primary outcomes is tested.

Subgroup analyses prespecified in the protocol include analyses by age (less than 65 years old and 65 years old or older), sex, diabetes status, preexisting cardiovascular disease, baseline serum creatinine level, baseline serum cholesterol level, baseline systolic and diastolic BPs, and non-study BP-lowering treatment at study entry.

Statistical Analyses

Analyses for each primary outcome are based on the first relevant event experienced by a participant. Each participant can contribute only one event to the analysis of each outcome but may contribute events to separate analyses of several different outcomes. For each study, the relative risk and 95% confidence interval for each outcome are calculated according to the principle of intention to treat. Overall estimates of effect are calculated with a fixed-effects model, in which the log relative risk for each trial is weighted by the reciprocal of the variance of the log relative risk. The assumption of homogeneity among the treatment effects in different trials is tested with chi-square Q and, more recently, the I^2 statistic.[9] If the assumption of homogeneity is rejected, then additional exploratory analyses are conducted with a random-effects model and by including and excluding trials leading to the heterogeneity. Mean levels of baseline characteristics and mean differences in follow-up BP among randomized comparisons are calculated with estimates from individual trials weighted by the number of individuals in the study.

Main Findings

Since the establishment of the collaboration, two cycles of overviews have been reported.[5,6] The first, published in 2000, included results from 15 trials and nearly 75,000 individuals. More recently, the second cycle reported the results from 30 trials and 160,000 individuals (Table 26-1).

Trials and Participants in Second-Cycle Overviews

Nine trials (25,000 individuals and 3500 major cardiovascular events) provided data from placebo-controlled comparisons of ACE inhibitors and calcium antagonists, and five trials (22,000 individuals and 1200 major cardiovascular events) provided data from trials targeting different BP goals. Sixteen trials (101,000 participants and 10,000 major cardiovascular events) provided data on comparisons on different active regimens based on ACE inhibitors, calcium antagonists, and diuretics and/or β-blockers. For most trials, patients were selected on the basis of high BP and an additional cardiovascular risk factor such as diabetes, renal disease, or increased age. The overall mean age of participants was 65 years, and slightly more than half (52%) were men. The mean duration of follow-up for contributing trials ranged from 2.0 to 8.4 years, resulting in more than 700,000 patient-years of follow-up.

Comparisons of Active Regimens and Controls

Comparisons of active regimens and controls (ACE inhibitor versus placebo, calcium antagonist versus placebo, and more-intensive versus less-intensive BP-lowering regimens) are shown in Figure 26-1.

Stroke, Coronary Heart Disease, and Heart Failure

The second cycle of overviews showed that, compared with placebo, significant reductions in the risk of stroke (28% to 38%) and CHD (22%) could be achieved with regimens based on ACE inhibitors or calcium antagonists. In trials that randomized patient to receive either more-intensive (lower BP targets) or less-intensive BP-lowering regimens, investigators also reported a significant reduction in stroke and a nonsignificant trend for benefit for CHD with more-intensive BP reduction.

Heart failure events were defined as those resulting in death or admission to hospital. The second cycle of overviews demonstrated a protective effect against heart failure from regimens based on ACE inhibitors compared with placebo (18%), a nonsignificant trend toward harm for calcium antagonist–based regimens, and a nonsignificant trend toward benefit for regimens targeting lower BP goals. For both the latter two analyses, the confidence intervals were wide, reflecting the small amount of data available.

Major Cardiovascular Events, Cardiovascular Death, and Total Mortality

More than 17,000 major cardiovascular events (a composite outcome comprising stroke, CHD, and heart failure events, in addition to death from any other cardiovascular cause) contributed to the second cycle of overviews. Significant reductions were reported in the risk of this outcome with active treatment based on either ACE inhibitors (22%) or calcium antagonists (21%) compared with placebo, as well as for more-intensive compared with less-intensive regimens (14%).

For fatal events attributable to cardiovascular causes and to all causes, ACE inhibitor–based regimens reduced the risk of death by 20% and 12%, respectively, compared with placebo. There was also a trend toward fewer cardiovascular deaths with calcium antagonist–based regimens. However, no clear evidence indicated a reduction in risk for fatal cardiovascular events or death from any cause with regimens targeting lower BP goals.

Comparisons of Different Active Regimens

Comparisons of different active regimens (ACE inhibitor versus diuretic/β-blocker, calcium antagonist versus diuretic/β-blocker, and ACE inhibitor versus calcium antagonist) are shown in Figure 26-2.

Stroke, Coronary Heart Disease, and Heart Failure

Greater protective effects of borderline significance were seen for regimens based on calcium antagonists, compared with both conventional therapy (diuretic/β-blockers) and ACE

Table 26-1   Trials Included in Second Cycle of Blood Pressure Lowering Treatment Trialists' Collaboration Overviews

Trials	Main Treatments Compared	Entry Criteria*
Trials Comparing Active Treatment and Control		
AASK	MAP ≤92 mm Hg vs. 102-107 mm Hg	HBP + nephropathy, Afr
ABCD-HT	DBP ≤75 mm Hg vs. ≤90 mm Hg	HBP + DM
ABCD-NT	DBP 10 mm Hg lower than baseline vs. 80-89 mm Hg	DM
HOPE	Ramipril vs. placebo	CHD, CVD, or DM + RF
HOT	DBP ≤80 mm Hg vs. ≤85 or ≤90 mm Hg	HBP
IDNT	Amlodipine vs. placebo	HBP + DM + nephropathy
NICOLE	Nisoldipine vs. placebo	CHD
PART-2	Ramipril vs. placebo	CHD or CVD
PREVENT	Amlodipine vs. placebo	CHD
PROGRESS	Perindopril (with or without indapamide) vs. placebo(s)	Cerebrovascular disease
QUIET	Quinapril vs. placebo	CHD
SCAT	Enalapril vs. placebo	CHD
Syst-Eur	Nitrendipine vs. placebo	HBP, ≥60 yr
UKPDS-HDS	DBP <85 mm Hg vs. <105 mm Hg	HBP + DM
Trials Comparing ARB-Based Regimens and Other Regimens		
IDNT	Irbesartan vs. placebo	HBP + DM + nephropathy
LIFE	Losartan vs. atenolol	HBP + CVD RF
RENAAL	Losartan vs. placebo	DM + nephropathy
SCOPE	Candesartan vs. placebo	HBP, 70-89 yr
Trials Comparing Regimens Based on Different Drug Classes		
AASK	Ramipril vs. metoprolol vs. amlodipine	HBP + nephropathy, Afr
ABCD-HT	Enalapril vs. nisoldipine	HBP + DM
ABCD-NT	Enalapril vs. nisoldipine	DM
ALLHAT	Lisinopril vs. chlorthalidone vs. amlodipine	HBP + R
ANBP2	Enalapril vs. hydrochlorothiazide	HBP, 65-84 yr
CAPPP	Captopril vs. β-blocker or diuretic	HBP
CONVINCE	COER verapamil vs. hydrochlorothiazide or atenolol	HBP+ RF
ELSA	Lacidipine vs. atenolol	HBP
INSIGHT	Nifedipine GITS vs. hydrochlorothiazide + amiloride	HBP + RF
JMIC-B	ACE inhibitor vs. nifedipine	HBP + CHD
NICS-EH	Nicardipine vs. trichlormethiazide	HBP, ≥60 yr
NORDIL	Diltiazem vs. β-blocker or diuretic	HBP
SHELL	Lacidipine vs. chlorthalidone	HBP, ≥60 yr
STOP-2	Enalapril or lisinopril vs. felodipine or isradipine vs. atenolol or metoprolol or pindolol or hydrochlorothiazide + amiloride	HBP, 70-84 yr
UKPDS-HDS	Captopril vs. atenolol	HBP + DM
VHAS	Verapamil vs. chlorthalidone	HBP

*Definitions of high blood pressure and nephropathy varied among studies.
AASK, African American Study of Kidney Disease and Hypertension; ABCD-HT, Appropriate Blood Pressure Control in Diabetes–Hypertension; ABCD-NT, Appropriate Blood Pressure Control in Diabetes–Normotensive Subgroup; ACE, angiotensin-converting enzyme; Afr, African American; ALLHAT, Antihypertensive and Lipid-Lowering Treatment to Prevent Heart Attack Trial; ANBP2, Second Australian National Blood Pressure study; ARB, angiotensin receptor blocker; CAPPP, Captopril Prevention Project; CHD, coronary heart disease; COER, controlled onset-extended release; CONVINCE, Controlled Onset Verapamil Investigation of Cardiovascular End Points; CVD, cardiovascular disease; DB, double-blind; DBP, diastolic blood pressure; DM, diabetes mellitus; ELSA, European Lacidipine Study on Atherosclerosis; GITS, gastrointestinal transport system; HBP, high blood pressure; HOPE, Heart Outcomes Prevention Evaluation; HOT, Hypertension Optimal Treatment; IDNT, Irbesartan Diabetic Nephropathy Trial; INSIGHT, International Nifedipine GITS Study: Intervention as a Goal in Hypertension Treatment; JMIC-B, Japan Multicenter Investigation for Cardiovascular Disease-B; LIFE, Losartan Intervention for Endpoint Reduction in Hypertension; MAP, mean arterial pressure; NICOLE, Nisoldipine in Coronary Artery Disease in Leuven; NICS-EH, National Intervention Cooperative Study in Elderly Hypertensives; NORDIL, Nordic Diltiazem Study; PART-2, Prevention of Atherosclerosis with Ramipril; PREVENT, Prospective Randomized Evaluation of the Vascular Effects of Norvase Trial; PROGRESS, Perindopril Protection against Recurrent Stroke Study; QUIET, Quinapril Ischemic Event Trial; RENAAL, Reduction of Endpoints in Non–Insulin Dependent Diabetes Mellitus with the Angiotensin II Antagonist Losartan; RF, other cardiovascular risk factor; SCAT, Simvastatin/Enalapril Coronary Atherosclerosis Trial; SCOPE, Study on Cognition and Prognosis in the Elderly; SHELL, Systolic Hypertension in the Elderly: Lacidipine Long-Term study; STOP-2, Swedish Trial in Old Patients with Hypertension-2; Syst-Eur, Systolic Hypertension in Europe; UKPDS-HDS, United Kingdom Prospective Diabetes Study–Hypertension in Diabetes study; HDS, Hypertension in Diabetes Study; VHAS, Verapamil in Hypertension and Atherosclerosis Study. Modified from Blood Pressure Lowering Treatment Trialists' Collaboration. Effects of different blood pressure lowering regimens on major cardiovascular events: Second cycle of prospectively designed overviews. *Lancet.* 2003;**362**:1527-1535.

	Trials	Events/participants 1st listed	2nd listed	Mean ΔBP (mm Hg)[1]	Favors 1st listed	Favors 2nd listed	Relative risk (95% CI)
Stroke							
ACE-I vs placebo	5	473/9111	660/9118	−5/−2			0.72 (0.64,0.81) (p homog = 0.33)
CA vs placebo	4	76/3794	119/3688	−8/−4			0.62 (0.47,0.82) (p homog = 0.90)
More vs less	4	140/7494	261/13394	−4/−3			0.77 (0.63,0.95) (p homog = 0.15)
Coronary heart disease							
ACE-I vs placebo	5	667/9111	834/9118	−5/−2			0.80 (0.73,0.88) (p homog = 0.91)
CA vs placebo	4	125/3794	156/3688	−8/−4			0.78 (0.62,0.99) (p homog = 0.34)
More vs less	4	215/7494	261/13394	−4/−3			0.86 (0.72,1.03) (p homog = 0.35)
Heart failure							
ACE-I vs placebo	4	219/8233	269/8246	−5/−2			0.82 (0.69,0.98) (p homog = 0.60)
CA vs placebo	3	104/3382	88/3274	−8/−4			1.21 (0.93,1.58) (p homog = 0.17)
More vs less	4	54/7494	72/13394	−4/−3			0.84 (0.59,1.18) (p homog = 0.11)
Major cardiovascular events							
ACE-I vs placebo	5	1283/9111	1648/9118	−5/−2			0.78 (0.73,0.83) (p homog = 0.42)
CA vs placebo	3	280/3382	337/3274	−8/−4			0.82 (0.71,0.95) (p homog = 0.54)
More vs less	5	493/8034	729/13948	−4/−3			0.86 (0.77,0.96) (p homog = 0.25)
Cardiovascular death							
ACE-I vs placebo	5	488/9111	614/9118	−5/−2			0.80 (0.71,0.89) (p homog = 0.29)
CA vs placebo	5	107/3382	135/3274	−8/−4			0.78 (0.61,1.00) (p homog = 0.43)
More vs less	5	209/8034	271/13948	−4/−3			0.93 (0.77,1.11) (p homog = 0.15)
Total mortality							
ACE-I vs placebo	5	839/9111	951/9118	−5/−2			0.88 (0.81,0.96) (p homog = 0.54)
CA vs placebo	4	239/3794	263/3688	−8/−4			0.89 (0.75,1.05) (p homog = 0.99)
More vs less	5	404/8034	549/13948	−4/−3			0.96 (0.84,1.09) (p homog = 0.09)

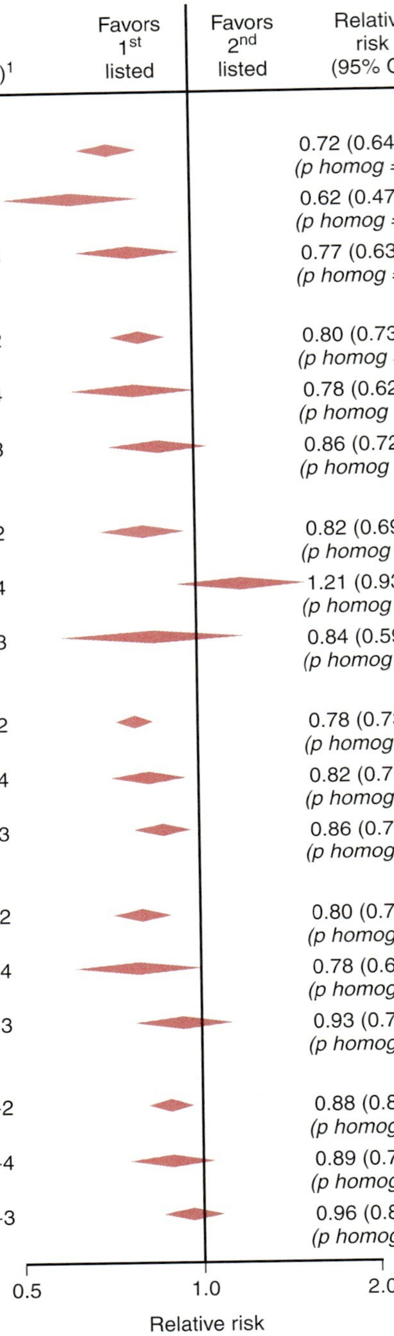

0.5   1.0   2.0

Relative risk

Figure 26–1   Effects of angiotensin-converting enzyme inhibitors (ACE-I) and calcium antagonists (CA) compared with placebo and more-intensive compared with less-intensive blood pressure–lowering regimens on the risks of major vascular outcomes and death. 95% CI, 95% confidence intervals; less, less-intensive blood pressure–lowering regimen; more, more-intensive blood pressure–lowering regimen; p homog, P homogeneity. [1]Overall mean blood pressure difference (systolic/diastolic) during follow-up in the actively treated group compared with the control group, calculated by weighting the difference observed in each contributing trial by the number of individuals in the trial. The negative values indicate lower mean follow-up blood pressure levels in the first-listed treatment groups (i.e., ACE, CA, more). (From Blood Pressure Lowering Treatment Trialists' Collaboration. Effects of different blood pressure lowering regimens on major cardiovascular events: Second cycle of prospectively designed overviews. *Lancet.* 2003;**362**:1527-1535.)

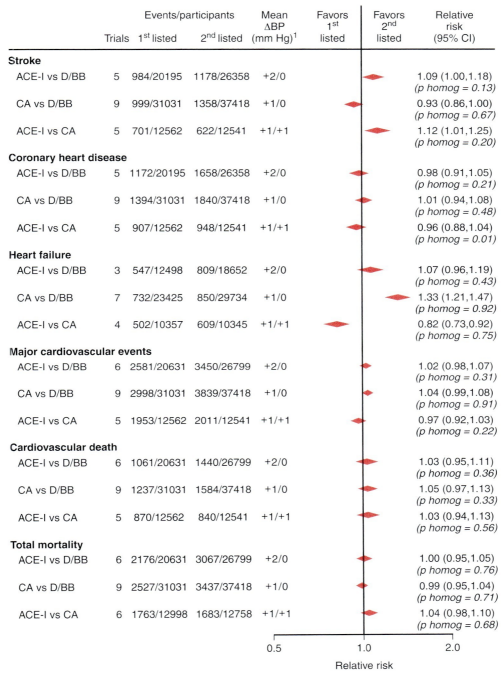

		Events/participants		Mean ΔBP (mm Hg)[1]	Favors 1st listed	Favors 2nd listed	Relative risk (95% CI)
	Trials	1st listed	2nd listed				
Stroke							
ACE-I vs D/BB	5	984/20195	1178/26358	+2/0			1.09 (1.00,1.18) (p homog = 0.13)
CA vs D/BB	9	999/31031	1358/37418	+1/0			0.93 (0.86,1.00) (p homog = 0.67)
ACE-I vs CA	5	701/12562	622/12541	+1/+1			1.12 (1.01,1.25) (p homog = 0.20)
Coronary heart disease							
ACE-I vs D/BB	5	1172/20195	1658/26358	+2/0			0.98 (0.91,1.05) (p homog = 0.21)
CA vs D/BB	9	1394/31031	1840/37418	+1/0			1.01 (0.94,1.08) (p homog = 0.48)
ACE-I vs CA	5	907/12562	948/12541	+1/+1			0.96 (0.88,1.04) (p homog = 0.01)
Heart failure							
ACE-I vs D/BB	3	547/12498	809/18652	+2/0			1.07 (0.96,1.19) (p homog = 0.43)
CA vs D/BB	7	732/23425	850/29734	+1/0			1.33 (1.21,1.47) (p homog = 0.92)
ACE-I vs CA	4	502/10357	609/10345	+1/+1			0.82 (0.73,0.92) (p homog = 0.75)
Major cardiovascular events							
ACE-I vs D/BB	6	2581/20631	3450/26799	+2/0			1.02 (0.98,1.07) (p homog = 0.31)
CA vs D/BB	9	2998/31031	3839/37418	+1/0			1.04 (0.99,1.08) (p homog = 0.91)
ACE-I vs CA	5	1953/12562	2011/12541	+1/+1			0.97 (0.92,1.03) (p homog = 0.22)
Cardiovascular death							
ACE-I vs D/BB	6	1061/20631	1440/26799	+2/0			1.03 (0.95,1.11) (p homog = 0.36)
CA vs D/BB	9	1237/31031	1584/37418	+1/0			1.05 (0.97,1.13) (p homog = 0.33)
ACE-I vs CA	5	870/12562	840/12541	+1/+1			1.03 (0.94,1.13) (p homog = 0.56)
Total mortality							
ACE-I vs D/BB	6	2176/20631	3067/26799	+2/0			1.00 (0.95,1.05) (p homog = 0.76)
CA vs D/BB	9	2527/31031	3437/37418	+1/0			0.99 (0.95,1.04) (p homog = 0.71)
ACE-I vs CA	6	1763/12998	1683/12758	+1/+1			1.04 (0.98,1.10) (p homog = 0.68)

0.5   1.0   2.0

Relative risk

Figure 26–2 Effects of blood pressure (BP)–lowering regimens based on different drug classes on the risks of major vascular outcomes and death. 95% CI, 95% confidence intervals ACE-I, angiotensin converting enzyme inhibitor–based regimen; CA, calcium antagonist–based regimen; D/BB, diuretic- or β-blocker–based regimen; p homog, P homogeneity. [1]Overall mean blood pressure difference (systolic/diastolic) during follow-up in the group assigned the first-listed treatment compared with the group assigned the second-listed treatment, calculated by weighting the difference observed in each contributing trial by the number of individuals in the trial. The positive values indicate a higher mean follow-up blood pressure in the first-listed treatment group compared with the second-listed treatment group (i.e., for all except diastolic blood pressure in the comparison of calcium antagonists with diuretics/β-blockers). (From Blood Pressure Lowering Treatment Trialists' Collaboration. Effects of different blood pressure lowering regimens on major cardiovascular events: Second cycle of prospectively designed overviews. *Lancet.* 2003;**362**:1527-1535.)

inhibitors despite minimal BP differences among randomized groups. Although a similar borderline protective effect was seen for regimens based on diuretics/β-blockers compared with ACE inhibitors, the mean 2 mm Hg lower BP in the diuretic/β-blocker group probably accounted for this finding.

No evidence indicated any differences among active regimens in the protection afforded against CHD. Some evidence indicated heterogeneity across the trials contributing to the pooled estimate for the comparison of ACE inhibitors versus calcium antagonists for this outcome. This was attributable to one trial,[10] but neither exclusion of this trial from the fixed-effects model nor the use of a random-effects model altered the conclusions for this outcome. These data provide substantial support for prior reports,[11,12] and they refute claims of large increases in coronary risk in hypertensive patients treated with calcium antagonists.

Compared with regimens based on calcium antagonists, those based on diuretics and/or β-blockers and on ACE inhibitors produced greater reductions in the risk of heart failure. These differences could not be attributed to different effects of the regimens on BP control and appear to be mediated through some alternate mechanism. Likewise, because heart failure events were restricted to those that resulted in death or hospitalization, minor side effects of calcium antagonists, such as peripheral edema, do not account for this finding. Separate analyses of the trials that used dihydropyridine agents and those that used nondihydropyridine agents did not result in different conclusions for this outcome.

Major Cardiovascular Events, Cardiovascular Death, and Total Mortality

No significant differences were reported among regimens based on any of the active agents (ACE inhibitors, calcium antagonists, or diuretics and/or β-blockers) for any of the composite outcomes. The confidence intervals around the estimates of treatment effect were tight, reflecting the many thousands of events available for these analyses.

Trials of Angiotensin Receptor Blockers

By the end of 2003, data from four angiotensin receptor blocker (ARB) trials were included in the second cycle of overviews (Fig. 26-3). These trials were the Irbesartan Diabetic Nephropathy Trial (IDNT),[13] the Reduction of Endpoints in Non–Insulin Dependent Diabetes Mellitus with the Angiotensin II Antagonist Losartan (RENAAL) study,[14] the Study on Cognition and Prognosis in the Elderly (SCOPE),[15] and the Losartan Intervention for Endpoint Reduction in Hypertension (LIFE) trial.[16] The first three were specified as placebo-controlled trials.[13,15] However, each of the three placebo-controlled studies had substantial and differential use of other BP-lowering regimens in the placebo control arm. In SCOPE, this resulted from protocol-driven initiation of active treatment in a large proportion of the placebo-treated group early in follow-up, and in IDNT and RENAAL, it resulted from an attempt to achieve comparable BP reductions in all active and control arms of the trials. As such, although LIFE was the only trial specifically designed as a head-to-head comparison between agents (an ARB and a β-blocker), all trials randomized patients to an ARB and were therefore combined in a single overview.

In these meta-analyses, significant reductions (10% to 20%) were noted in the risk of stroke, heart failure, and total major cardiovascular events with regimens based on ARBs, compared with control regimens, reductions that were probably in large part attributable to the lower follow-up BP levels in the ARB-treated groups compared with the groups receiving conventional therapy. For the remaining outcomes, no significant differences were reported.

	Trials	Events/participants ARB	Events/participants Control	Mean ΔBP (mm Hg)[1]	Favors ARB	Favors control	Relative risk (95% CI)
Stroke	4	396/8412	500/8379	−2/−1			0.79 (0.69, 0.90) (p homog = 0.46)
Coronary heart disease	4	435/8412	450/8379	−2/−1			0.96 (0.85, 1.09) (p homog = 0.43)
Heart failure	3	302/5935	359/5919	−2/−1			0.84 (0.72, 0.97) (p homog = 0.26)
Major cardiovascular events	4	1135/8412	1268/8379	−2/−1			0.90 (0.83, 0.96) (p homog = 0.78)
Cardiovascular death	4	491/8412	511/8379	−2/−1			0.96 (0.85, 1.08) (p homog = 0.34)
Total mortality	4	887/8412	943/8379	−2/−1			0.94 (0.86, 1.02) (p homog = 0.59)

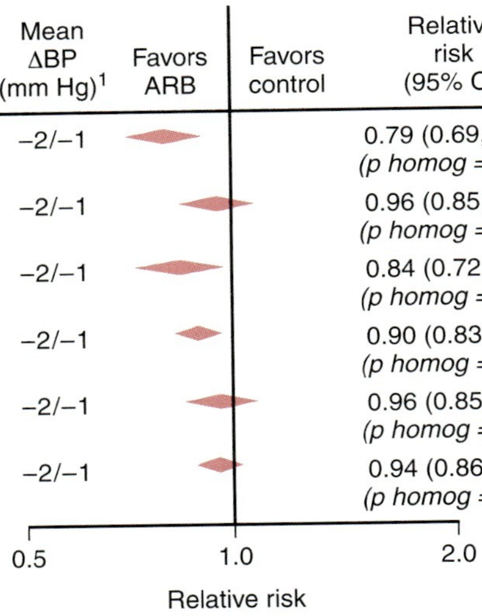

0.5   1.0   2.0
Relative risk

Figure 26–3 Effects of angiotensin receptor blocker (ARB)–based regimens compared with control regimens on the risks of major vascular outcomes and death. 95% CI, 95% confidence intervals; BP, blood pressure; p homog, P homogeneity. [1]Overall mean blood pressure difference (systolic/diastolic) during follow-up in the ARB-treated group compared with the control group, calculated by weighting the difference observed in each contributing trial by the number of individuals in the trial. The negative values indicate lower mean follow-up blood pressure levels in the ARB-treated group. (From Blood Pressure Lowering Treatment Trialists' Collaboration. Effects of different blood pressure lowering regimens on major cardiovascular events: Second cycle of prospectively designed overviews. Lancet. 2003;**362**:1527-1535.)

Blood Pressure and Risk

Large observational studies have demonstrated the direct and continuous relationship of BP and cardiovascular risk, a benefit that appears to extend to levels traditionally regarded as normotensive. In the second cycle of overviews, the weighted mean BP differences among the randomized groups of each treatment comparison were plotted against the pooled relative risks for each outcome. This approach showed a direct and continuous association between the magnitude of the BP difference and the size of the risk difference (Fig. 26-4). The association was consistent for all cardiovascular outcomes, with the exception of heart failure, a finding that may be attributable to BP-independent adverse effects of calcium antagonist–based regimens on this outcome.

Findings in Patients with and without Diabetes

Subgroup analyses prespecified in the original protocol for the Blood Pressure Lowering Treatment Trialists' Collaboration are intended to identify whether important differences exist in the effects of different BP-lowering regimens in particular patient groups. To date, the collaboration has reported on the

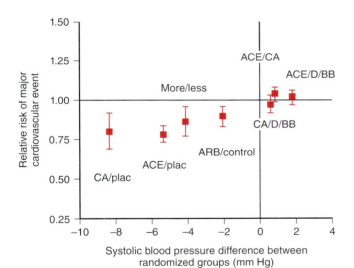

Figure 26–4 Association of blood pressure differences between randomized groups and the risk of major cardiovascular events. Results are calcium antagonist (CA) versus placebo (plac), angiotensin-converting enzyme (ACE) inhibitor versus placebo, more-intensive (more) versus less-intensive (less) blood pressure lowering, angiotensin receptor blocker (ARB) versus control, ACE inhibitor versus calcium antagonist, calcium antagonist (CA) versus diuretic (D)/β-blocker (BB), and ACE inhibitor versus diuretic/β-blocker. The boxes are plotted at the point estimate of effect for the relative risk of the event and the mean follow-up blood pressure in the first-listed group compared with the second-listed group. The *vertical bars* represent 95% confidence intervals. (Modified from Blood Pressure Lowering Treatment Trialists' Collaboration. Effects of different blood pressure lowering regimens on major cardiovascular events: Second cycle of prospectively designed overviews. *Lancet.* 2003;**362**:1527-1535.)

subgroup analyses for patients with and without diabetes. Twenty-two of the 29 trials (33,395 individuals with and 125,314 individuals without diabetes) contributing to the second-cycle main results were able to provide data for these analyses. The results showed that the short- to medium-term effects (average follow-up times, 2 to 5 years) on major cardiovascular events of the BP-lowering regimens studied were highly comparable for patients with and without diabetes for most outcomes studied. The few exceptions were the comparisons of ARB-based regimens with other regimens, in which ARBs may provide lesser protection against stroke among patients with diabetes compared with patients without diabetes (*P* homogeneity = .05) and, conversely, greater protection to patients with diabetes compared with patients without diabetes for the outcome of heart failure (*P* homogeneity = .005). However, whether these differences are real or a consequence of differential BP reductions in the two subgroups, BP-independent effects in one subgroup or the other, or simply the play of chance is unclear.

Current Status and Future Plans

Since the publication of the second cycle of overviews, several trials participating in the collaboration[17-22] have reported their findings. A third cycle of overviews by the collaboration is planned to include these new data. Of particular importance are the recent trials of ARBs, which, once incorporated, will allow for standard and separate treatment comparisons of this class of agent not previously possible. Other planned subgroup analyses (age, sex, baseline BP, and renal impairment) are also under way.

SUMMARY AND CONCLUSIONS

Meta-analyses such as those conducted by the Blood Pressure Lowering Treatment Trialists' Collaboration provide clinicians and their patients with uniquely reliable information about the relative benefits and risks of widely used classes of BP-lowering drugs. The results are applicable to a broad population of hypertensive and nonhypertensive individuals at high risk of cardiovascular disease.

These overviews show that treatment with any commonly used regimen reduces the risk of total major cardiovascular events, and larger reductions in BP produce larger reductions in risk. For some outcomes, important differences among regimens appear to be independent of BP lowering. In particular, regimens based on ACE inhibitors and on diuretics and/or β-blockers are more effective at preventing heart failure than are regimens based on calcium antagonists, and these results are broadly consistent with other trials of ACE inhibitors[23] and calcium antagonists[24] in patients with established heart failure. Although different drug regimens may have different effects on stroke, this remains less clear.

Acknowledgments

We would like to thank members of the Blood Pressure Lowering Treatment Trialists' Collaboration: L. Agodoa, C. Baigent, H. Black, J-P. Boissel, B. Brenner, M. Brown, C. Bulpitt, R. Byington, J. Chalmers, R. Collins, J. Cutler, B. Dahlof, B. Davis, J. Dens, R. Estacio, R. Fagard, K. Fox, L.

Hansson (deceased), R. Holman, L. Hunsicker, Y. Imai, J. Kostis, K. Kuramoto, E. Lewis, L. Lindholm, J. Lubsen, S. MacMahon, E. Malacco, G. Mancia, B. Neal, C. Pepine, M. Pfeffer, B. Pitt, P. Poole-Wilson, G. Remuzzi, A. Rodgers, P. Ruggenenti, R. Schrier, P. Sever, P. Sleight, J. Staessen, K. Teo, R. Turner (deceased), P. Whelton, L. Wing, Y. Yui, S. Yusuf, A. Zanchetti.

References

1. Sackett D, Rosenberg W, Gray J, et al. Evidence based medicine: What it is and what it isn't. *BMJ*. 1996;**312**:71-72.

2. Egger M, Smith G, Phillips AN. Meta-analysis: Principles and procedures. *BMJ*. 1997;**315**:1533-1537.

3. Blettner M, Sauerbrei W, Schlehofer B, et al. Traditional reviews, meta-analyses and pooled analyses in epidemiology. *Int J Epidemiol*. 1999;**28**:1-9.

4. World Health Organization–International Society of Hypertension Blood Pressure Lowering Treatment Trialists' Collaboration. Protocol for prospective collaborative overviews of major randomized trials of blood-pressure lowering treatments. *J Hypertens*. 1998;**16**:127-137.

5. Blood Pressure Lowering Treatment Trialists' Collaboration. Effects of ACE inhibitors, calcium antagonists and other blood pressure lowering drugs: Results of prospectively designed overviews of randomised trials. *Lancet*. 2000;**355**:1955-1964.

6. Blood Pressure Lowering Treatment Trialists' Collaboration. Effects of different blood pressure lowering regimens on major cardiovascular events: Second cycle of prospectively designed overviews. *Lancet*. 2003;**362**:1527-1535.

7. Antithrombotic Trialists' Collaboration. Collaborative meta-analysis of randomised trials of antiplatelet therapy for prevention of death, myocardial infarction and stroke in high risk pateints. *BMJ*. 2002;**324**:71-86.

8. Cholesterol Treatment Trialists' (CTT) Collaboration. Protocol for a prospective collaborative overview of all current and planned randomized trials of cholesterol treatment regimens. *Am J Cardiol*. 1995;**75**:1130-1134.

9. Higgins J, Thompson S. Quantifying heterogeneity in a meta-analysis. *Stat Med*. 2002;**21**:1539-1558.

10. Estacio R, Jeffers B, Hiatt W, et al. The effect of nisoldipine as compared with enalapril on cardiovascular outcomes in patients with non-insulin dependent diabetes and hypertension. *N Engl J Med*. 1998;**338**:645-652.

11. Ad Hoc Subcommittee of the Liaison Committee of the World Health Organization and the International Society of Hypertension. Effects of calcium antagonists on the risks of coronary heart disease, cancer and bleeding. *J Hypertens*. 1997;**15**:105-115.

12. MacMahon S, Collins R, Chalmers J. Reliable and unbiased assessment of the effects of calcium antagonists: Importance of minimizing both systematic and random errors. *J Hypertens*. 1997;**15**:1201-1204.

13. Lewis E, Hunsicker L, Clarke W, et al. Renoprotective effect of the angiotensin-receptor antagonist irbesartan in patients with nephropathy due to type 2 diabetes. *N Engl J Med*. 2001;**345**:851-860.

14. Brenner B, Cooper M, De Zeeuw D, et al. Effects of losartan on renal and cardiovascular outcomes in patients with type 2 diabetes and nephropathy. *N Engl J Med*. 2001;**345**:861-869.

15. Lithell H, Hansson L, Skogg I, et al. The Study on Cognition and Prognosis in the Elderly (SCOPE): Principal results of a randomised double-blind intervention trial. *J Hypertens*. 2003;**21**:875-886.

16. Dahlof B, Devereux R, Kjeldsen S, et al. Cardiovascular morbidity and mortality in the Losartan Intervention for Endpoint reduction in hypertension study (LIFE): A randomised trial against atenolol. *Lancet*. 2002;**359**:995-1003.

17. Poole-Wilson P, Lubsen J, Kirwan B, et al. Effect of long-acting nifedipine on mortality and cardiovascular morbidity in patients with stable angina requiring treatment (ACTION trial): Randomised controlled trial. *Lancet*. 2004;**364**:849-857.

18. Pepine C, Handberg E, Cooper-DeHoff R, et al. A calcium antagonist vs a non-calcium antagonist hypertension treatment strategy for patients with coronary artery disease: The International Verapamil-Trandolapril Study (INVEST). A randomized controlled trial. *JAMA*. 2003;**290**:2805-2816.

19. Fox K, European Trial on Reduction of Cardiac Events with Perindopril in Stable Coronary Artery Disease Investigators. Efficacy of perindopril in reduction of cardiovascular events among patients with stable coronary artery disease: Randomised, double-blind, placebo-controlled, multicentre trial (the EUROPA study). *Lancet*. 2003;**362**:782-788.

20. Braunwald E, Domanski M, Fowler S, et al. Angiotensin-converting-enzyme inhibition in stable coronary artery disease. *N Engl J Med*. 2004;**351**:2058-2068.

21. Marre M, Lievre M, Chatellier G, et al. Effects of low dose ramipril on cardiovascular and renal outcomes in patients with type 2 diabetes and raised excretion of urinary albumin: Randomised, double blind, placebo controlled trial (the DIABHYCAR study). *BMJ*. 2004;**328**:495.

22. Ruggenenti P, Fassi A, Ilieva A, et al. Preventing microalbuminuria in type 2 diabetes. *N Engl J Med*. 2004;**351**:1941-1951.

23. Garg R, Yusuf S. Overview of randomized trials of angiotensin-converting enzyme inhibitors on mortality and morbidity in patients with heart failure. *JAMA*. 1995;**273**:1450-1456.

24. Cohn J, Ziesche S, Smith R, et al. Effect of calcium antagonist felodipine as supplementary vasodilator therapy in patients with chronic heart failure treated with enalapril: V-HeFT III. Vasodilator-Heart Failure Trial (V-HeFT) study group. *Circulation*. 1997;**96**:856-863.

Hypertension and Concomitant Diseases

SECTION CONTENTS

Chapter 27

Ischemic Heart Disease in Hypertension

Clive Rosendorff

A strong association exists between hypertension and coronary artery disease (CAD).[1,2] Patients with hypertension are at much higher risk of developing all types of occlusive vascular disease, including CAD. CAD may limit myocardial perfusion and therefore oxygen supply. Myocardial oxygen demand is increased for two reasons: first, because of the increased output impedance to left ventricular (LV) ejection; and second, because hypertension can cause LV hypertrophy. This combination of decreased oxygen supply and increased oxygen demand is particularly pernicious and explains why hypertensive patients are more likely than normotensive people to develop angina, to have a myocardial infarction (MI) or other major coronary event, and to be at higher risk of dying following MI.

This chapter is divided into (1) a brief review of the epidemiologic and functional relationship between hypertension and CAD; (2) strategies for the primary and secondary prevention of coronary events in patients with hypertension; (3) the management of hypertension in patients with established CAD and stable angina; and (4) the management of hypertension in patients with acute coronary syndromes, unstable angina, or acute MI. In all these situations, the recurring theme consists of β-blockers, angiotensin-converting enzyme (ACE) inhibitors (and angiotensin receptor antagonists), and calcium antagonists as critical elements in management.

RELATIONSHIP BETWEEN HYPERTENSION AND CORONARY ARTERY DISEASE

Many epidemiologic studies, especially the Framingham Heart Study,[2] have established the major risk factors for the development of CAD (Table 27-1). All the major cardiovascular risk factors contribute in a powerful and independent way to the development of CAD. Hypertension is well documented as a major risk factor for the development of CAD, cardiac failure, atherothrombotic brain infarction, and peripheral artery disease. Over all ages and genders, systolic blood pressure (SBP) has been shown to have a greater impact on all atherosclerotic cardiovascular disease outcomes than diastolic BP (DBP). Isolated systolic hypertension is more prevalent in women than in men, and it increases in both sexes with age. A correlation also exists between hypertension and body mass, and both factors are strongly correlated with CAD. Hypertension and abdominal obesity are components of a larger risk factor constellation for cardiovascular risk that also includes characteristic dyslipidemia (high triglycerides and low high-density lipoprotein cholesterol), insulin resistance, or frank type 2 diabetes mellitus, referred to as the *metabolic syndrome*.

The association of hypertension with arteriosclerotic arterial disease, including CAD, has led to a vigorous controversy about causality. Does the hypertension produce arteriosclerosis, or vice versa? The classical view, during the 1970s and 1980s, was that the initial pathophysiologic abnormality in hypertension in young people is increased cardiac output, with a variable autoregulatory increase in peripheral resistance ("labile hypertension"). The physiologic vasoconstriction then progresses to structural changes in the resistance vessels that perpetuate the hypertension, even though cardiac output returns to normal. We now know that arteriosclerotic disease is the consequence of a complex interaction of inflammatory cells, cytokines, free radicals, growth factors, lipids, and endocrine and paracrine factors. Many of these substances adversely affect endothelial function and have, as a final common pathway, hypertrophy and reduced compliance of large and medium-sized arteries and arterioles (Fig. 27-1). These changes are frequently present in the vasculature of young individuals before they develop hypertension, especially in the children of hypertensive parents, a finding supporting the idea of a genetic component. In addition, however, and significantly, the hypertension is also a consequence of the vasculopathy. Then a positive feedback develops whereby the hypertension exacerbates the arteriosclerosis and its complications, and this process is significantly slowed or reduced by aggressive antihypertensive treatment. Hypertension causes fragmentation and fracture of elastin fibers and collagen deposition in arteries, changes that contribute to thickening and stiffening of those arteries. Hypertension also induces endothelial dysfunction, thus reducing endothelium-dependent vasodilator capacity.

One of the hallmarks of hypertension is stiff arteries. *Compliance* of an artery is defined as the change of lumen diameter (ΔD), or of cross-sectional area (ΔA), during each cardiac cycle, as a function of the change of distending pressure (ΔP). The change in the distending pressure over one cardiac cycle is the difference between the SBP and DBP, or the pulse pressure. Compliance is represented by the slope of $\Delta D/\Delta P$ (or $\Delta A/\Delta P$). In arteriosclerotic disease, ΔD is diminished because of the structural rigidity of the vessels. Pulse pressure is a function both of the stroke volume, which is usually normal in patients with established or stable hypertension, and of the stiffness of large arteries, increased in hypertension. More recently, an additional mechanism for increasing pulse pressure has been recognized (Fig. 27-2). A pressure wave is generated with each ejection of blood from the left ventricle. The stiffer the large arteries, the greater is the pulse-wave velocity. That wave is reflected back from any point of discontinuity or increased resistance in the arterial tree, particularly at the level of small arteries and arterioles, and the reflected wave returns to the aorta and the left ventricle. In younger persons, this reflected wave reaches the

Table 27-1 Risk of Coronary Heart Disease According to Standard Risk Factors: Framingham Heart Study 36-Year Follow-up

Factors	Age 35-64 yr				Age 65-94 yr			
	Age-Adjusted Biennial Rate per 1000		Age-Adjusted Relative Risk*		Age-Adjusted Biennial Rate per 1000		Age-Adjusted Relative Risk*	
	Men	Women	Men	Women	Men	Women	Men	Women
High cholesterol (>240 mg/dL)	34	15	1.9[†]	1.9[‡]	59	39	1.2[§]	2.0[†]
Hypertension (>140/90 mm Hg)	45	21	2.0[†]	2.2[†]	73	44	1.6[†]	1.9[†]
Diabetes	39	42	1.5[†]	3.7[†]	79	62	1.6[†]	2.1[†]
Electrocardiographic left ventricular hypertrophy	79	55	3.0[†]	4.6[†]	134	94	2.7[†]	3.0[†]
Smoking	33	13	1.5[‡]	1.1	53	38	1.0	1.2

*Relative risk for persons with a given trait versus those without it. For cholesterol >240 mg/dL compared with <200 mg/dL.
[†]$P < .001$.
[‡]$0.001 < P < .01$.
[§]$0.01 < p < .05$.
From Kannel WB. Multivariate Evaluation of Persons at Risk for Cardiovascular Disease. *In:* Rosendorff C (ed). Essential Cardiology: Principles and Practice. Philadelphia, WB Saunders, 2001, p 2.

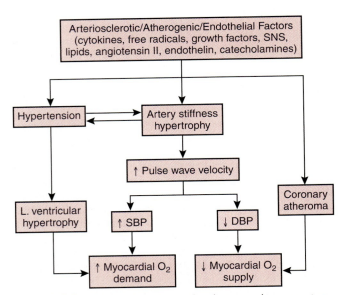

Figure 27–1 Schematic relationship between hypertension and coronary artery disease. See the text for a detailed explanation. DBP, diastolic blood pressure, SBP, systolic blood pressure; SNS, sympathetic nervous system.

are the characteristics of isolated systolic hypertension, common in older individuals with poorly compliant arteries causing high SBP, normal or low DBP, and elevated pulse pressure (Fig. 27-3) (see Chapter 14). Thus, increased myocardial oxygen *demand* results both from the increased resistance to LV ejection and from LV hypertrophy. The myocardial oxygen *supply* is diminished, not only because of the atherosclerotic CAD, but also because of the decreased coronary filling pressure associated with the lower than normal DBP. This combination of increased oxygen demand and reduced supply in the myocardium (which, unlike the brain, is unable to compensate for a decreased blood flow by increasing the extraction of oxygen from the coronary blood) gives us a clear understanding of the pernicious effect of hypertension on cardiac function.

PRIMARY PREVENTION OF CORONARY ARTERY DISEASE IN PATIENTS WITH HYPERTENSION

In all individuals who are at risk of developing CAD (i.e., just about everybody), we should promote risk-reducing healthy lifestyles, including smoking cessation, management of lipids, diabetes, and weight, and a suitable exercise regimen. In addition, daily aspirin reduces the risk of cardiovascular events in a broad category of individuals at risk. In patients with hypertension, vigorous antihypertensive therapy has had a remarkable effect in reducing all cardiovascular disasters, including stroke, acute MI, and peripheral vascular disease. The real issue is whether this is a function of BP lowering alone or whether certain classes of antihypertensive drugs are better than others by virtue of additional actions independent of BP lowering. The next section examines this question in the context of CAD prevention.

aortic valve after closure, leads to a higher DBP, and enhances coronary perfusion pressure. In older individuals with stiffer arteries and arterioles, the retrograde pressure wave has a greater velocity, and it may reach the aortic valve before closure, thereby leading to a higher SBP and afterload and a lower DBP with decreased coronary perfusion pressure. These

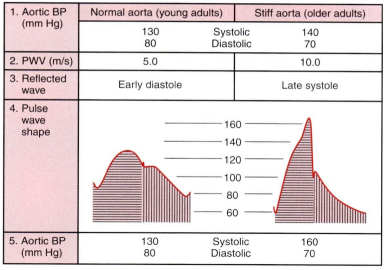

1. Aortic BP (mm Hg)	Normal aorta (young adults)		Stiff aorta (older adults)
	130	Systolic	140
	80	Diastolic	70
2. PWV (m/s)	5.0		10.0
3. Reflected wave	Early diastole		Late systole
4. Pulse wave shape			
5. Aortic BP (mm Hg)	130	Systolic	160
	80	Diastolic	70

Figure 27–2 Change in aortic pressure profile resulting from age-related vascular stiffening and increased pulse-wave velocity (PWV). *1,* Increased systolic blood pressure (SBP) and decreased diastolic blood pressure (DBP) owing to decreased aortic distensibility. *2,* Increased PWV as a result of decreased aortic distensibility and increased distal (arteriolar) resistance. *3,* Return of the reflected primary pulse to the central aorta in systole rather than in diastole as a result of faster wave travel. *4,* Change in aortic pulse wave profile because of early wave reflection. Note the summation of antegrade and retrograde pulse waves to produce a large SBP. This increases left ventricular stroke work and therefore myocardial oxygen demand. Note also the reduction in the diastolic pressure time (integrated area under the DBP curve). This reduction in coronary perfusion pressure increases the vulnerability of the myocardium to hypoxia. *5,* The aortic BP resulting from decreased aortic distensibility and early reflected waves. (Modified from Smulyan H, Safar ME. The diastolic blood pressure in systolic hypertension. *Ann Intern Med.* 2000;**132**:233-237.)

Which Antihypertensive Drug to Use for the Primary or Secondary Prevention of Coronary Artery Disease?

Diuretics and β-Blockers

Early clinical trials (Hypertension Detection and Follow-up Program [HDFP],[3] Medical Research Council trial [MRC],[4] Systolic Hypertension in the Elderly Program [SHEP],[5] Swedish Trial in Old Patients with Hypertension [STOP-Hypertension],[6] and Medical Research Council trial in the elderly [MRC-elderly][7]) used diuretics or β-blockers. In general, these studies showed a significant benefit of treatment for reducing stroke morbidity and mortality in all age groups (Table 27-2). However, the reduction in ischemic heart disease risk with treatment was less than half that for stroke, except in older patients, in whom the benefit was still not as great as it was for stroke. Many explanations were advanced for the dissociation between the favorable stroke outcomes and the mediocre outcomes in ischemic heart disease, one being the potential arrhythmogenic effect of diuretic-induced hypokalemia.

Calcium Antagonists

Since the mid-1990s, several trials of calcium antagonists and of ACE inhibitors for the primary prevention of cardiovascular complications of hypertension have been conducted. The calcium antagonist trials (Systolic Hypertension in Europe [Syst-Eur],[8] Systolic Hypertension in China [Syst-China],[9] Prospective Randomized Evaluation of the Vascular Effects of Norvasc Trial [PREVENT],[10] Multicenter Isradipine Diuretic Atherosclerosis Study [MIDAS],[11] Nordic Diltiazem study [NORDIL],[12] and International Nifedipine GITS study: Intervention as a Goal in Hypertension Treatment [INSIGHT][13]) tended to show a significant degree of prevention of stroke, usually compared with placebo or with a diuretic or β-blocker alone or in combination. The absolute risk reduction in ischemic heart disease deaths or nonfatal coronary events was much less impressive, with the exception of the Syst-Eur study. However, in Syst-Eur, the reference drug was placebo, and a significant number of patients in the active treatment group received one of the add-on agents, including enalapril, which may have improved the results. The International Verapamil-Trandolapril (INVEST) study, in which verapamil sustained-release (SR) was compared with atenolol, was also complicated by the fact that, at study end, most subjects were taking a combination of verapamil SR in combination with trandolapril or atenolol in combination with hydrochlorothiazide, so the equivalent study outcomes tell us little about the selective ability of calcium antagonists to prevent cardiovascular events.[14] The Controlled Onset Verapamil Investigation of Cardiovascular End Points (CONVINCE) trial did not show that verapamil was equivalent to atenolol or hydrochlorothiazide in preventing cardiovascular disease events.[15] In a selective meta-analysis of trials of calcium antagonists versus low-dose diuretics, Psaty and colleagues showed a significantly greater CAD risk reduction in the diuretic cohort.[16] A more extensive meta-analysis, by the Blood Pressure Lowering Treatment Trialists' Collaboration (BPLTTC), provided strong support for the benefits of ACE

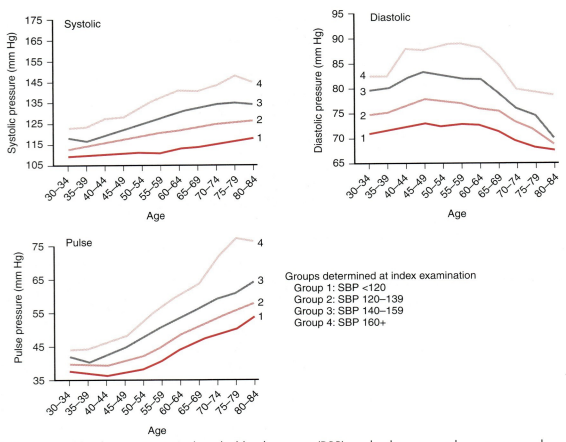

Figure 27–3 Systolic blood pressure (SBP), diastolic blood pressure (DBP), and pulse pressure by age, grouped according to SBP at the index examination in a population-based cohort from the Framingham Heart Study. Note the progressive increase in SBP in all groups throughout the whole age range, with a progressive decrease in DBP starting around 50 years of age and a consequent increase in pulse pressure with age. MAP, mean arterial pressure. (Modified from Franklin SS, Gustin W, Wong ND, et al. Hemodynamic patterns of age-related changes in blood pressure. *Circulation.* 1997;**96**:308.)

inhibitors or calcium antagonists over placebo and for regimens that targeted lower BP goals, but this group found that when calcium antagonists were compared with diuretics or β-blockers, there was a significant lowering of stroke risk, but no difference in CAD and a 33% increase in heart failure.[17] ACE inhibitors were better than calcium antagonists for heart failure prevention and were better than diuretics, β-blockers or calcium antagonists for CAD prevention. By contrast, the recent Anglo-Scandinavian Cardiac Outcomes Trial (ASCOT) was terminated early because the amlodipine-based treatment (with, as needed, perindopril and doxazosin) was superior to an atenolol-based regimen (with, as needed, bendroflumethiazide and doxazosin) in preventing CAD events in high-risk hypertensive patients.[18] However, on the basis of most of the published trials, it can be concluded that calcium antagonists have not been shown to be superior to other antihypertensive agents, particularly ACE inhibitors, in the prevention of coronary events.

Angiotensin-Converting Enzyme Inhibitors

In animal models of hypertension, ACE inhibitors prevent or reverse myocardial and vascular hypertrophy, and they retard atherogenesis.[19] Recently, much attention has focused on trials of ACE inhibitors in patients, hypertensive or nonhypertensive, who have established CAD or who are at high risk for CAD. In the Heart Outcomes Prevention Evaluation (HOPE) study, after 4.5 years the relative risk for death from cardiovascular causes in the ramipril-treated group versus the placebo-treated group was 0.74, for MI it was 0.80, for revascularization procedures it was 0.85, for cardiac arrest it was 0.63, and for heart failure it was 0.77, all highly significant findings.[20] The results applied equally to hypertensive and nonhypertensive patients and to patients with known ischemic heart disease and those without coronary vascular disease. HOPE was a convincing demonstration of the protective effect of an ACE inhibitor for MI and stroke in high-risk patients, almost half of whom were hypertensive. Substudies of HOPE revealed that ACE inhibition reduced progression of atherosclerosis and improved myocardial remodeling. A smaller trial, the Prevention of Atherosclerosis with Ramipril Trial (PART-2), of ramipril versus placebo in high-risk patients, showed, in the treated group, a relative risk for fatal CAD of 0.43, but no difference in the rate of MI or unstable angina.[21] In the BPLTTC meta-analysis, which included not only HOPE and PART-2, but also two studies of patients with established heart disease, Simvastatin/Enalapril Coronary Atherosclerosis Trial (SCAT)[22] and Quinapril Ischemic

Table 27-2 Which Antihypertensive Drugs Prevent Coronary Events?

Trial/Study Acronym*	Report	Duration (yr)	Treatment	Patients	Mean Age	Total Coronary Events/ 1000 Patients/yr	
						Active	Control/ Reference
Diuretics or Blockers vs. Placebo							
HDFP	1979	5	Diuretics ± (reserpine/methyldopa ± hydralazine ± guanethidine) vs. referred care	10,940	51	6	7
MRC	1985	5	Bendrofluazide or propanolol vs. placebo	17,354	51	5	4
SHEP	1991	4.5	Chlorthalidone (± atenolol) vs. placebo	4,736	72	15[†]	20
STOP	1992	2	3 β-blockers + HCTZ vs. placebo	1,627	76	17[†]	25
MRC-Elderly	1992	5.8	Atenolol or HCTZ + amiloride vs. placebo	4,396	70	7 (diuretic)[†] 12 (β-blocker)	13
Calcium Channel Blockers vs. Placebo							
Syst-Eur	1997	2	Nitrendipine(± enalapril ± HCTZ) vs. placebo	4,695	70	34[†]	44
Syst-China	1998	2	Nitrendipine (± captopril ± HCTZ) vs. placebo	2,394	67	5	7
PREVENT	2000	3	Amlodipine vs. placebo	825	57	21[†]	25
ACE Inhibitors vs. Placebo							
HOPE	2000	5	Ramipril vs. placebo	9,297	67	93[†]	104
PART-2	2000	4	Ramipril vs. placebo	617	61	56	61
EUROPA	2003	4	Perindopril vs. placebo	13,655	60	19	24
PEACE	2004	5	Trandolapril vs. placebo	8,290	64	17	18
Calcium Channel Blockers vs. Other Agents							
MIDAS	1996	3	Isradipine vs. HCTZ	883	59	14	8
NORDIL	2000	5	Diltiazem (± ACEI ± diuretic or α-blocker) vs. diuretic + β-blocker (±ACEI or α-blocker)	10,881	60	6	7
INSIGHT	2000	4	Nifedipine (± atenolol or enalapril) vs. co-amilozide (HCTZ + amiloride) (± atenolol or enalapril)	6,321	65	16	17
ALLHAT	2000	4.9	Amlodipine (+ atenolol, clonidine, reserpine, hydralazine) vs. chlorthalidone (+ atenolol, etc.)	24,303	67	19	19
INVEST	2003	2	Verapamil SR (+ trandolapril + HCTZ) vs. atenolol (+ trandolapril + HCTZ)	22,576	67	23	23
ACE Inhibitors vs. Other Agents							
UKPDS	1998	9	Captopril (± furosemide ± nifedipine ± methyldopa ± prazosin) vs. atenolol (± furosemide ± nifedipine ± methyldopa ± prazosin)	758	56	26	23
CAPPP	1999	6	Captopril vs. β-blockers ± diuretics	10,985	53	13	13
STOP-2	1999	6	ACEIs vs. calcium antagonists or diuretic and/or β-blocker	6,614	76	13	14 (diuretics/ β-blocker) 17 (calcium antagonists)

continued

Table 27–2   Which Antihypertensive Drugs Prevent Coronary Events?—cont'd

Trial/Study Acronym*	Report	Duration (yr)	Treatment	Patients	Mean Age	Total Coronary Events/ 1000 Patients/yr Active	Control/ Reference
ACE Inhibitors vs. Other Agents—cont'd							
ABCD	1998	5	Enalapril (± metoprolol ± HCTZ) vs. nisoldipine (± metoprolol ± HCTZ)	470	58	4[†]	21
ALLHAT	2002	4.9	Lisinopril vs. amlodipine vs. chlorthalidone	23,056	67	19	19
ANBP-2	2003	4.1	Enalapril (+ others) vs.HCTZ (+ others)	6,083	72	14	16
Angiotensin Receptor Blockers vs. Other Agents							
LIFE	2002	4.8	Losartan vs. atenolol	9,193	67	16	15
VALUE	2004	4.2	Valsartan (+ HCTZ + others) vs. amlodipine (+ HCTZ + others)	15,245	67	11.4	9.6

*See text for explanations of trial/study acronyms.
[†]$P < 0.05$.
ACEI, angiotensin-converting enzyme inhibitor; HCTZ, hydrochlorothiazide; SR, sustained release.

Event Trial (QUIET),[23] the relative risk ratios for the ACE inhibitor–treated group were 0.80 for CAD, 0.82 for heart failure, 0.78 for major cardiovascular events, and 0.80 for cardiovascular mortality.[17]

Both HOPE and PART-2 were trials of an ACE inhibitor versus placebo. Trials of ACE inhibitors versus other antihypertensive therapy (including the Captopril Prevention Project [CAPPP][24] and the United Kingdom Prospective Diabetes Study [UKPDS][25]) were not as impressive as HOPE. In CAPPP and UKPDS (ACE inhibitors versus diuretics/β-blockers), ACE inhibitors lowered overall cardiovascular morbidity and mortality, especially stroke, but failed to demonstrate a clear-cut benefit over diuretics or β-blockers for the prevention of acute coronary events. However, STOP-2 did show that, for the prevention of MI, ACE inhibitors were better than "conventional therapy" (a diuretic or a β-blocker), although this did not achieve statistical significance.[26] The BPLTTC group included CAPPP, UKPDS, and STOP-2 in their meta-analysis of ACE inhibitors versus diuretics/β-blockers and found the relative risk in the ACE inhibitor–treated patients was 0.98 for CAD, 1.07 for heart failure, 1.02 for major cardiovascular events, and 1.03 for cardiovascular death.[17]

Two trials, STOP-2[26] and Appropriate Blood Pressure Control in Diabetes (ABCD),[27] compared ACE inhibitors with calcium antagonists. In STOP-2 and ABCD, there were highly significant reductions in the ACE inhibitor–treated patients for the relative risk of CAD (0.81), heart failure (0.82), and major cardiovascular events (0.92), but no difference in stroke (1.02) or cardiovascular death (1.04).

The Antihypertensive and Lipid-Lowering Treatment to Prevent Heart Attack Trial (ALLHAT) was a huge (>42,000 subjects) study comparing outcomes in high-risk patients treated with a thiazide-like diuretic (chlorthalidone), an ACE inhibitor (lisinopril), an α-blocker (doxazosin), or a calcium antagonist (amlodipine) as first-line therapy for hypertension.[28,29] The results showed superiority of the diuretic chlorthalidone over lisinopril or doxazosin in preventing stroke and over lisinopril, doxazosin, or amlodipine in preventing heart failure. However, no significant differences were reported among chlorthalidone, lisinopril, or amlodipine in combined fatal CAD or nonfatal MI (the primary outcome of the study), in combined CAD (the primary outcome, coronary revascularization, or hospitalization for angina), or in all-cause mortality. The ALLHAT authors concluded, "thiazide-type diuretics are superior in preventing one or more major forms of cardiovascular disease, and ... should be preferred for first step antihypertensive therapy." The results of ALLHAT are controversial.[30,31] Criticisms have included the following: (1) the diuretic used in the trial was not superior to the other drugs in preventing the primary outcome; (2) the "add-on" drugs (primarily a β-blocker) favored chlorthalidone so the BP was slightly but significantly lower in the diuretic-treated group; (3) the superiority of chlorthalidone over doxazosin in preventing heart failure could have been the result of a masking effect of the diuretic in patients with heart failure and peripheral edema; and (4) long-term diuretic therapy increases the risk of developing diabetes.[32] These issues are discussed more fully in Chapters 18, 23, 28, 34, and 43. Soon after the ALLHAT results were published, the Second Australian National Blood Pressure study group (ANBP-2) reported the results of a prospective, randomized, open-label study in patients aged 65 to 84 years of age with hypertension; this study showed better outcomes with ACE inhibitors than with diuretic agents, despite similar reductions of BP.[33]

Angiotensin Receptor Blockers

The use of angiotensin receptor blockers (ARBs) for the treatment of hypertension in patients with CAD has a solid foundation in animal studies and surrogate endpoint studies in humans. One such study in human subjects with hypertension showed that irbesartan reduced LV mass more than atenolol, despite similar reductions in BP.[34] The Losartan Intervention for Endpoint Reduction (LIFE) study was the first large (>9000 patients) study to evaluate the effects of an ARB on cardiovascular outcomes.[35] Losartan was significantly better than atenolol in reducing stroke, but there were no significant differences for cardiovascular mortality or MI. In the Valsartan Antihypertensive Long-Term Use Evaluation (VALUE), no significant difference was seen in the primary endpoint (a composite of nine cardiovascular events) between a valsartan-based and an amlodipine-based treatment regimen in high-risk patients, but this result (like many of the other clinical trials already cited) is difficult to interpret because nearly all the subjects were receiving other therapy, mainly diuretics (~25%), other combinations of study drugs (about 20%), or no study drug (~25%) at the end of the study and also because amlodipine lowered BP more than valsartan, especially during the early months of treatment.[36]

In yet another meta-analysis, Staessen and colleagues came to a very conservative conclusion, namely that it may not matter which antihypertensive drug is used; the beneficial effect on cardiovascular outcomes is simply a function of the amount of BP reduction.[37] This conclusion does not confirm data from animal and smaller human studies that suggest cardioprotective and vasculoprotective effects of ACE inhibitors and, to a lesser extent, calcium antagonists.

Many of the trials noted earlier seem to support the use of ACE inhibitors, rather than calcium antagonists, as first-line drugs for the treatment of hypertension to prevent CAD, although evidence that ACE inhibitors are superior to diuretics or β-blockers in this regard remains insufficient. Although compelling evidence exists for the benefits of ACE inhibitors and β-blockers (and calcium antagonists and diuretics in ALLHAT) in preventing MI in high-risk subjects, we are still unsure of how much of the benefit is the result of BP lowering and how much is caused by specific drug actions.

How Far Should the Blood Pressure Be Lowered?

The coronary vascular bed, like most others, is capable of autoregulating its flow in the presence of quite large changes in perfusion pressure. The relationship of coronary blood flow F, perfusion pressure P, and coronary vascular resistance R, is $F \propto P/R$. In a rigid tube with a fixed resistance, it is $F \propto P$. The coronary circulation, however, can alter its resistance, such that an increase in perfusion pressure P causes coronary vasoconstriction (increased R), so if ventricular work is kept constant, flow will remain relatively constant, up to a level at which the vasoconstriction is maximal (the upper limit of coronary vascular autoregulation). Conversely, a fall in perfusion pressure stimulates vasodilatation so flow will remain relatively constant, down to a level of perfusion pressure at which vessels are maximally dilated (the lower limit of coronary vascular autoregulation). Below that limit, any further decline in perfusion pressure will result in decreased flow. Because nearly all coronary blood flow occurs in diastole, the perfusion pressure referred to here is the mean DBP. The instantaneous coronary flow is a function of DBP, and the total flow per cardiac cycle is proportional to both DBP and the duration of diastole, assessed by the integrated area under the pressure curve during diastole.

It is theoretically possible that, in hypertensive patients, DBP could be reduced by therapy to levels lower than the lower limit of coronary vascular autoregulation, with a consequent reduction in coronary blood flow. The problem is that we do not have very good data on the exact DBP level at which this occurs in the intact human coronary circulation. In addition, the presence of any significant occlusive coronary atherosclerotic disease shifts the lower limit of autoregulation upward and makes patients less tolerant of low DBPs, especially if these patients have additional myocardial oxygen demand from LV hypertrophy.

Further considerations are the effects of myocardial hypertrophy and exercise. At any given perfusion pressure, coronary reserve is the difference between autoregulated and maximally dilated coronary flow.[38] In Figure 27-4, curve A_1 represents coronary blood flow over a wide range of perfusion pressures, and the perfusion pressure P_1 is at the lower limit of autoregulation. If the coronary vessels are maximally dilated, a steep, linear pressure-flow relationship will exist between pressure and flow (line D_1). The difference between autoregulated and maximally vasodilated flow at any given perfusion pressure represents the coronary flow reserve (R_1). If myocardial

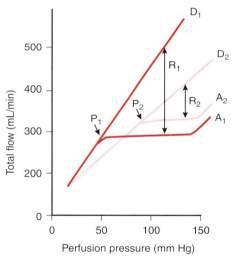

Figure 27–4 Autoregulation of coronary blood flow and myocardial flow reserve in the presence of left ventricular hypertrophy. A_1 represents total coronary blood flow over a range of perfusion pressures (diastolic blood pressure), P_1 is the lower limit of the autoregulatory range, and D_1 is the pressure-flow relationship in the maximally dilated coronary bed. At any given perfusion pressure, the coronary flow reserve is R_1. A_2, P_2, D_2, and R_2 represent corresponding values in patients with hypertension and left ventricular hypertrophy. At any given perfusion pressure, the coronary flow reserve is less in the hypertensive/hypertrophied hearts, thus increasing the vulnerability of the myocardium to ischemia especially during exercise or any other situation requiring increased coronary flow. Moreover, the lower limit of coronary autoregulation is shifted to the right (P_1 to P_2) in the hypertensive heart, thereby increasing the vulnerability to a severe drop in perfusion pressure (diastolic blood pressure). (Modified from Hoffman JIE. A critical view of coronary reserve. *Circulation.* 1987;**75 [Suppl I]**:I6.)

hypertrophy is present, total coronary flow will be greater, with a higher autoregulatory line (curve A_2) and a rightward shift of the lower limit of autoregulation. However, the pressure-flow relation at maximal vasodilatation is less steep (line D_2), so the coronary flow reserve (R_2) any given perfusion pressure is less. Moreover, the point at which coronary flow reserve is exhausted (point P_2) in the hypertrophied heart coincides with a higher perfusion pressure than normal (point P_1). The clear message is that, in patients with hypertension and LV hypertrophy, the lower limit of autoregulation is set at a higher level of perfusion pressure (and therefore DBP), and at any level of perfusion pressure, or DBP, the coronary flow reserve is less than it would be in the normal ventricle.[38]

These considerations have generated the concept of the "J-curve."[39] Many epidemiologic studies and clinical trials have shown a continuous relationship between DBP and the risk of a coronary event: the lower the DBP, the lower the risk. However, investigators have suggested that there is a lower DBP limit of about 85 mm Hg below which the MI rate begins to climb, thus producing a J-shaped curve to describe the relationship between DBP and CAD risk. A 2004 analysis of the Framingham Heart Study data showed that, in the general population, a clearly demonstrable increase in cardiovascular risk is present when the DBP is less than 80 mm Hg, but only in those subjects whose SBPs are higher than 140 mm Hg.[40] This finding makes sense, because the low DBP may reduce coronary perfusion pressure, and the higher SBP increases myocardial oxygen demand and may increase intramyocardial wall tension, thus further limiting perfusion. These data were obtained in a general population; in patients with occlusive CAD, the perfusion pressure downstream of the stenosis would be even further reduced, and the elevated LV SBP and the presence of LV hypertrophy would further increase myocardial oxygen demand. These considerations are consistent with epidemiologic data that both pulse pressure and the presence of LV hypertrophy are strongly predictive of coronary events.

The Hypertension Optimal Treatment (HOT) trial was designed to answer prospectively the question whether aggressive lowering of DBP would increase cardiovascular events.[41] Only among diabetic patients with the lowest DBP target was the cardiovascular risk the lowest; overall, there was a small increase in major cardiovascular events, MI, and cardiovascular mortality (but not for stroke or renal failure) at DBPs at or lower than 80 mm Hg. This finding suggests a unique myocardial susceptibility to low diastolic perfusion pressures, because, in contrast to the cerebral circulation, there is maximal oxygen extraction by the myocardium, which therefore cannot compensate for a reduced flow by increasing oxygen extraction. This concept would seem to be supported by the notion that whereas stroke morbidity and mortality are best correlated with the level of mean BP, the best predictor of coronary events in the Framingham Heart Study seems to be pulse pressure.[42] Pulse pressure is usually greatest in isolated systolic hypertension, in which the DBP is "normal" and is often lower than 80 mm Hg, even before treatment. All of this is fine in theory, but it seems to have little support from the data of many large clinical trials, and not in a meta-analysis that included nearly a million subjects from 61 prospective observational studies.[43] In elderly patients with isolated systolic hypertension and low DBP, no J-shaped curve has been described with antihypertensive therapy, even though

DBP may be reduced even further. In fact, the three outcome trials in elderly patients with isolated systolic hypertension (SHEP,[5] Syst-Eur,[8] and Syst-China[9]) together showed decreases in 25% in MI, including sudden death, in the active treatment group compared with those who received placebo. Diabetic patients benefited significantly from aggressive BP lowering in the HOT,[41] ABCD,[27] and UKPDS[25] trials, so current recommendations are to lower BP in diabetic patients to less than 130/80 mm Hg. A recent meta-analysis has provided convincing data that the increased mortality of patients with very low DBP (<65 mm Hg) was not related to antihypertensive treatment and was not specific to BP-related events.[44] Poor health, including poor LV function, leading to low BP, and increased risk of death seem to provide alternative explanations for the J-shaped curve.

There is no question that aggressive BP lowering to less than target values is lifesaving. Nevertheless, it seems prudent to lower the BP slowly in patients with significant occlusive CAD and elevated pretreatment DBP, and caution is advised in inducing falls of BP below 70 mm Hg if the patient is older than 60 years. One of the therapeutic challenges of the next few years will be to find a pharmacologic agent that selectively lowers SBP in patients with isolated systolic hypertension. Nevertheless, it seems prudent to lower the BP slowly in patients with significant occlusive CAD and elevated pretreatment DBP, and caution is advised in inducing falls of BP below 70 mm Hg in those patients older than 60 years.

MANAGEMENT OF HYPERTENSION IN PATIENTS WITH CORONARY ARTERY DISEASE AND STABLE ANGINA

Hypertension enhances the risk of an acute coronary event in patients with chronic stable angina because of the enhanced myocardial oxygen demand created by elevations in BP, especially SBP, and LV hypertrophy, if present.

The diagnostic workup for patients with chronic stable angina, with or without hypertension, starts with a detailed symptom history, a focused physical examination, and directed risk factor assessment, including cigarette smoking, hypertension, diabetes, dyslipidemia, and a family history of premature CAD.[45,46] Initial laboratory tests should include at least the hemoglobin and hematocrit values, fasting glucose concentration, and a fasting lipid panel of total cholesterol, high-density lipoprotein cholesterol, triglycerides, and calculated low-density lipoprotein cholesterol. A resting 12-lead electrocardiogram (ECG) should be performed in patients without an obvious noncardiac cause of chest pain or in any patient during an episode of chest pain; however, the ECG will be normal in up to half of patients with chronic stable angina. Evidence of LV hypertrophy on an ECG, as in many patients with hypertension, increases the probability that chest discomfort is angina pectoris. A chest radiograph is informative in patients with signs or symptoms of congestive heart failure, valvular heart disease, pericardial disease, or aortic dissection or thoracic aneurysm.

If the patient has an intermediate pretest probability of CAD based on age, gender, and symptoms, including those patients with complete right bundle branch block or less than 1 mm of rest ST-segment depression, then an exercise ECG should be ordered. The diagnostic utility of the exercise ECG in patients with a high or low pretest probability of CAD is very much less. A positive exercise test is one in which there is more than 1 mm of horizontal or down-sloping ST-segment depression or elevation for 60 to 80 milliseconds after the end of the QRS complex. Exercise myocardial perfusion imaging or exercise echocardiography should be performed if the patient with an intermediate pretest probability has the pre-excitation (Wolff-Parkinson-White) syndrome, or more than 1 mm of rest ST-segment depression. If the patient has a pacemaker or has left bundle-branch block, or if the patient is unable to exercise, adenosine or dipyridamole myocardial perfusion imaging or dobutamine echocardiography would be a better choice.

Coronary angiography should be done for all patients who have survived sudden cardiac death. It is probably also indicated in all patients in whom noninvasive testing is contraindicated, in whom it is unlikely to be adequate as a result of illness, disability, or physical characteristics, and in whom noninvasive testing is abnormal but not clearly diagnostic, as well as when a revascularization procedure is considered.

The treatment of patients with symptomatic CAD is directed toward preventing MI and death and reducing the symptoms of angina and the occurrence of ischemia. Treatment of risk factors includes, besides BP control, smoking cessation, management of diabetes, exercise training, lipid lowering (low-density lipoprotein cholesterol to <100 mg/dL and preferably to 70 mg/dL, triglycerides to <150 mg/dL, and elevating high-density lipoprotein cholesterol), and weight reduction in obese patients. Less well established are folate and vitamin B_6 supplements for patients with elevated homocysteine levels. There is compelling evidence for the use of antiplatelet agents, aspirin if not contraindicated, and otherwise clopidogrel. Other important therapies are short- or long-acting nitrates (but *not* with sildenafil or other phosphodiesterase-5 inhibitors.) The role of revascularization procedures is outside the scope of this review.

β-Blockers reduce angina symptoms, improve mortality, and lower BP, and they should be the drugs of first choice in hypertensive patients with CAD and stable angina. β-Blockers reduce cardiac inotropy and slow heart rate and atrioventricular conduction. The reduced inotropy and heart rate lower myocardial oxygen demand, and the slowing of the heart rate prolongs the diastolic perfusion time of the coronary arteries, thus enhancing myocardial blood flow. The reduced cardiac output lowers BP, although there is also a significant BP-lowering effect from the blockade of β-adrenoreceptors on the cells of the renal juxtaglomerular apparatus, the major source of circulating renin. Diabetes is not a contraindication to the use of β-blockers, although the patient should be aware that the symptoms of hypoglycemia may be masked. In stable LV failure, β-blockers (especially carvedilol or metoprolol) may be used as a component of the anti–heart failure therapy, but they should be started at a very low dose and titrated up very slowly.

When contraindications to the use of β-blockers exist, such as obstructive airways disease, severe peripheral vascular disease, or severe bradyarrhythmias (e.g., a high degree of atrioventricular block or the sick sinus syndrome), *calcium antagonists*, either long-acting dihydropyridine agents (e.g., amlodipine, felodipine, or a long-acting formulation of nifedipine) or nondihydropyridine drugs (e.g., verapamil or diltiazem) are appropriate therapeutic agents for angina and

hypertension. Short-acting dihydropyridine calcium antagonists have the potential to enhance the risk of adverse cardiac events and should be avoided. Calcium antagonists decrease peripheral resistance, thus reducing BP and LV wall tension and decreasing myocardial oxygen consumption. These drugs also lower coronary resistance, thereby enhancing myocardial oxygen supply, and they are especially useful if there is coronary spasm, as in variant (Prinzmetal's) angina. Nondihydropyridine calcium antagonists have the additional benefit of decreasing heart rate.

One study, the Total Ischaemic Burden European Trial (TIBET[47]), has shown equal efficacy of β-blockers and calcium antagonists in controlling stable angina, but most studies (e.g., Angina Prognosis Study in Stockholm [APSIS][48] and Total Ischemic Burden Bisoprolol Study [TIBBS][49]) have shown β-blockers to be superior. Long-term outcomes in INVEST were equivalent, whether the antihypertensive regimen began with verapamil or with atenolol.[14] Combining a β-blocker with a dihydropyridine calcium channel blocker enhances antianginal and antihypertensive efficacy. Because of the increased risk of severe bradycardia or heart block if β-blockers are used together with verapamil or diltiazem, long-acting dihydropyridine calcium antagonists are preferred for combination therapy. In A Coronary Disease Trial Investigating Outcome with Nifedipine Gastrointestinal Therapeutic System (ACTION), the addition of nifedipine gastrointestinal therapeutic system (GITS) to conventional treatment of angina pectoris had no effect on major cardiovascular event-free survival,[50] whereas in the Comparison of Amlodipine versus Enalapril to Limit Occurrences of Thrombosis (CAMELOT) study, the administration of amlodipine to patients with CAD (most of whom were receiving a β-blocker) significantly reduced adverse cardiovascular events, compared with placebo.[51]

Cardiovascular outcome studies using *ACE inhibitors* in patients with established CAD but with preserved ventricular function have produced conflicting results. The QUIET study included only patients with demonstrated CAD, half of whom were hypertensive, and showed no difference between patients treated with quinapril or placebo in coronary events or angiographic evidence of new coronary lesions or progression of existing lesions.[23] The Prevention of Events with Angiotensin-Converting Enzyme Inhibition (PEACE) trial included patients with stable CAD and normal or slightly reduced LV function, almost half of whom were hypertensive. In this trial, the addition of trandolapril to the subjects' other therapy did not provide further benefit in terms of death from cardiovascular causes, MI, or coronary revascularization.[52] In contrast, in HOPE, which included about 80% of patients with CAD, slightly less than half of whom were hypertensive, there were significant improvements in coronary outcomes with ramipril.[20] Similarly, in the European Trial on Reduction of Cardiac Events with Perindopril in Stable Coronary Artery Disease (EUROPA), perindopril significantly improved outcomes.[53] On the basis of HOPE and EUROPA, it is entirely reasonable to include an ACE inhibitor in the management of all patients with symptomatic CAD. To resolve the discrepancy among HOPE, EUROPA, and PEACE, some investigators have pointed to the large differences in how well treated other risk factors were in the latter study, compared with the two former studies. When patients receive all other appropriate therapies (e.g., aspirin, β-blockers, statins), their absolute risk may be so low that the addition of an ACE inhibitor prevents very few events.

MANAGEMENT OF HYPERTENSION IN PATIENTS WITH ACUTE CORONARY SYNDROMES

Unstable Angina and Non–ST-Segment Myocardial Infarction

Patients with *unstable angina* (defined as rest angina, new-onset angina, increasing frequency or intensity of previously stable angina, or angina within 6 weeks of a MI, but with normal cardiac markers of ischemia) or with *non–ST-segment elevation MI* (characterized by elevated markers of myocardial injury, such as troponin I or T, or the MB isoenzyme of creatine phosphokinase [CK-MB], but without ST-segment elevation) should be admitted to a hospital, preferably to a specialized coronary care unit.[54] Anti-ischemic therapy includes bed rest, continuous ECG monitoring, intravenous nitroglycerin, supplemental oxygen, morphine sulfate, and a β-blocker. Cardioselective β-blocker therapy (metoprolol or atenolol) should be initiated intravenously (especially if it can be administered within 12 hours of symptom onset) or orally. This should be followed by oral β-blockers without intrinsic sympathomimetic activity (e.g., atenolol, metoprolol, timolol, carvedilol). Carvedilol or metoprolol should be used if the patient has LV dysfunction (ejection fraction <40%).

BP should be treated to a goal of less than 140/90 mm Hg and to less than 130/80 mm Hg for patients with diabetes or chronic kidney disease. The drugs of choice are *β-blockers*, *ACE inhibitors,* and *diuretics*. Most patients require two or more drugs to reach this goal, and because all three classes of drugs have also been shown to reduce long-term cardiovascular risk in these patients, the use of all three drugs from the outset is not unreasonable. An ACE inhibitor (or an angiotensin receptor antagonist, if ACE inhibitors are not tolerated) should certainly be added to the β-blocker if there is LV systolic dysfunction or heart failure, as well as in patients with diabetes. Use ACE inhibitors with caution in the acute phase of MI in patients with a history of hypertension but low SBP (<120 mm Hg) at presentation, in whom critical hypotension is more prone to develop after such treatment.[55] A thiazide diuretic would be another add-on option for BP control, and an aldosterone antagonist such as eplerenone can be added as well if the patient has heart failure.[56] Patients taking an ACE inhibitor, a thiazide diuretic, or eplerenone should have frequent measurements of serum potassium. If β-blockers are contraindicated, a nondihydropyridine calcium channel antagonist (e.g., verapamil or diltiazem) can be prescribed for angina control if no LV dysfunction is present. Verapamil or diltiazem should not be added to β-blocker therapy because of the risk of bradycardia or heart block. The second-generation dihydropyridine calcium channel antagonists such as amlodipine and felodipine have not been studied in acute MI. Nevertheless, these agents are frequently used as add-on therapy in patients with an acute MI when hypertension is not adequately controlled by β-blockers, ACE inhibitors, and thiazide diuretics.

Antiplatelet therapy usually means aspirin (or clopidogrel, or both, if an early noninterventional approach is planned).

Anticoagulant therapy can consist of intravenous unfractionated heparin or subcutaneous low-molecular-weight heparin, to which should be added a platelet glycoprotein IIb/IIIa receptor antagonist (e.g., intravenous abciximab or oral eptifibatide or tirofiban) in patients with continuing ischemia or other high-risk features and in patients in whom percutaneous coronary intervention is planned. Because of the increased risk of hemorrhagic stroke in patients with uncontrolled hypertension who are given antiplatelet or anticoagulant therapy, the hypertension should be treated aggressively. In general, the indications for percutaneous coronary interventions and coronary artery bypass grafting are similar to those in stable angina. High-risk patents with recurrent angina or ischemia at rest or with low-level activities despite intensive anti-ischemic therapy, elevated troponin T or I levels, recurrent angina or ischemia with congestive heart failure symptoms, and S_1 gallop, pulmonary edema, worsening rales, new or worsening mitral regurgitation, high-risk findings on noninvasive testing, new ST-segment depression, LV systolic dysfunction, hemodynamic instability, percutaneous coronary intervention within 6 months, or prior coronary artery bypass graft should be evaluated for an early invasive strategy (percutaneous coronary intervention or coronary artery bypass graft) on an individual basis. Follow-up BP should be controlled with a goal BP of less than 130/80 mm Hg, although no data from randomized clinical trials are available to support this goal.

ST-Segment Elevation Myocardial Infarction

The management of *ST-segment elevation MI* is similar to that for unstable angina and non–ST-segment elevation MI, except that primary percutaneous transluminal angioplasty or fibrinolytic therapy and arrhythmia control are definitely indicated.[57] In addition, in the absence of contraindications, all patients with acute MI, whether they are hypertensive or not, should have a β-blocker and an ACE inhibitor, and both drugs should be continued over the long term. Quite frequently, a thiazide diuretic is also needed for BP control.

β-Blockers diminish myocardial oxygen consumption by reducing heart rate, myocardial contractility, and systemic arterial pressure. In addition, prolongation of diastole caused by the reduction in heart rate helps to augment perfusion to the injured myocardium. Intravenous β-blocker therapy should be started within 12 hours of the onset of chest pain, followed by an oral β-blocker within the first 2 days.

Some large, randomized clinical trials (Survival and Ventricular Enlargement [SAVE] trial, with captopril,[58] Acute Infarction Ramipril Efficacy [AIRE] study, with ramipril,[59] Trandolapril Cardiac Evaluation [TRACE] study, with trandolapril[60]) have shown a significant morbidity and mortality benefit of *ACE inhibitors* started early in the course of acute MI complicated by LV dysfunction. In these three studies combined, the odds ratio for death was 0.74, that for reinfarction was 0.80, and that for readmission for heart failure was 0.73. ACE inhibitors should be initiated early after an MI and continued indefinitely. The patient's creatinine and electrolyte levels should be checked before the initiation of therapy and regularly thereafter until the highest tolerated dose has been administered and renal function is stable. In heart failure (Studies of Left Ventricular Dysfunction [SOLVD][61]), treatment with ACE inhibitors reduced complications (odds ratio for reinfarction, 0.78; readmission for heart failure, 0.63) and mortality (odds ratio, 0.87); they also improved endothelial function, were antithrombotic and prothrombolytic, and had beneficial effects on ventricular and vascular remodeling.

Two large outcome studies in patients with acute MI and LV systolic dysfunction compared an *ARB* with a dose of captopril (50 mg thrice daily), previously proven to be effective in reducing mortality in SAVE.[58] In the Optimal Trial in Myocardial Infarction with the Angiotensin II Antagonist Losartan (OPTIMAAL), there was a nonsignificant trend toward superiority of captopril over losartan (50 mg once a day) in all endpoints, including death and new MI.[62] In the Valsartan in Acute Myocardial Infarction Trial (VALIANT), valsartan (80 mg twice daily) was equivalent to captopril in reducing mortality and other prespecified secondary clinical outcomes.[63] Also in VALIANT, mortality and other endpoints were not reduced by combination (valsartan in combination with captopril) treatment compared with captopril alone, although the combination did lower BP (and increase adverse events) more than captopril. These results confirm the utility of valsartan as an alternative therapy in those patients intolerant to an ACE inhibitor because of side effects, of which a dry cough is the most frequent.

A *thiazide diuretic* should be added to the regimen if BP control is not achieved with a β-blocker and an ACE inhibitor (or an angiotensin receptor antagonist). Many clinicians would argue, on the basis of the ALLHAT data,[28] that a diuretic should always be prescribed. An aldosterone antagonist may be indicated in patients with an ejection fraction of 40% or less, who have symptomatic heart failure or diabetes mellitus, and who have a serum creatinine level of 2.5 mg/dL or less in men or 2.0 mg/dL or less in women and a serum potassium level of 5 mEq/L or less. Close monitoring of serum potassium levels is required.

Calcium antagonists do not reduce mortality rates in the setting of acute MI, based on the Danish Verapamil Infarction Trial (DAVIT)[64] and the Multicenter Diltiazem Postinfarction Trial (MDPIT),[65] and they can increase mortality if there is depressed LV function or pulmonary edema. These drugs should not be used except when β-blockers are contraindicated or are inadequate to control angina or supraventricular tachycardia, or as adjunct therapy for BP control, but never in patients with impaired LV function.

CONCLUSION

In primary and secondary prevention of CAD in patients with arterial hypertension, aggressive BP lowering is critical, especially in diabetic patients, but care should be exercised in lowering the DBP too severely or too quickly in patients with significant occlusive CAD. Although some, but not all, of the recent trials have shown the superiority of ACE inhibitors over other classes of drugs for the reduction of overall cardiovascular morbidity and mortality, especially stroke, the evidence for better CAD outcomes is far from clear. It seems reasonable to recommend the use of an ACE inhibitor, usually with a thiazide diuretic, as first-line therapy in the primary prevention of coronary events in patients with hypertension. Treatment choices for the patient with hypertension and established CAD are more straightforward. β-Blockers are effective in the management of hypertension with angina. Long-acting calcium antagonists are an appropriate alternative if β-blockers are contraindicated or not tolerated. If both classes of drug are needed for angina or hypertension control, then a long-acting dihydropyridine calcium antagonist should be used with the β-blocker. An ACE inhibitor is also a reasonable option. In acute coronary syndromes, therapy of the hypertension should include β-blockers with an ACE inhibitor (especially if there is LV dysfunction). An ARB may be used as an alternative to ACE inhibitors in all situations, although the clinical trial data for ARBs are not as extensive as those for ACE inhibitors. A thiazide diuretic or a dihydropyridine calcium channel blocker could be added for BP control. Verapamil and diltiazem may be used as alternatives to β-blockers in unstable angina, but they should not be used together with β-blockers, in the presence of depressed LV function, or in acute MI.

References

1. Wilson PW. Established risk factors and coronary artery disease: The Framingham study. *Am J Hypertens*. 1994;**7**:7S-12S.
2. Kannel WB. Framingham study insights into the hypertensive risk of cardiovascular disease. *Hypertens Res*. 1995;**18**:181-196.
3. Hypertension Detection and Follow-up Program Cooperative Group. Five-year findings of the Hypertension Detection and Follow-up Program. I: Reduction in mortality of persons with high blood pressure, including mild hypertension. *JAMA*. 1979;**242**:2562-2571.
4. Medical Research Council Working Party. MRC trial of mild hypertension: Principal results. *BMJ*. 1985;**291**:97-104.
5. SHEP Cooperative Research Group. Prevention of stroke by antihypertensive drug treatment in older persons with isolated systolic hypertension: Final results of the Systolic Hypertension in the Elderly Program. *JAMA*. 1991;**265**:3255-3264.
6. Dahlof B, Lindholm LH, Hansson L, et al. Morbidity and mortality in the Swedish Trial in Old Patients with Hypertension (STOP-Hypertension). *Lancet*. 1991;**338**:1281-1285.
7. MRC Working Party. Medical Research Council trial of treatment of hypertension in older adults: Principal results. *BMJ*. 1992;**304**:405-412.
8. Staessen JA, Fagard R, Lutgarde T, et al. Randomised double-blind comparison of placebo and active treatment for older patients with isolated systolic hypertension. *Lancet*. 1997;**350**:757-764.
9. Liu L, Wang JG, Gong L et al. Comparison of active treatment and placebo in older Chinese patients with isolated systolic hypertension: Systolic Hypertension in China (Syst-China) Collaborative Group. *J Hypertens*. 1998;**16**:1823-1829.
10. Pitt B, Byington RP, Furberg CD, et al. Effect of amlodipine on the progression of atherosclerosis and the occurrence of clinical events. *Circulation*. 2000;**102**:1503-1510.
11. Borhani NO, Mercuri M, Borhani PA, et al. Final outcome results of the Multicenter Isradipine Diuretic Atherosclerosis Study (MIDAS). *JAMA*. 1996;**276**:785-791.
12. Hansson L, Hedner T, Lund-Johansen P, et al. Randomised trial of effects of calcium antagonists compared with diuretics and β-blockers on cardiovascular morbidity and mortality in hypertension: The Nordic Diltiazem (NORDIL) study. *Lancet*. 2000;**356**:359-365.
13. Brown MJ, Palmer CR, Castaigne A, et al. Morbidity and mortality in patients randomised to double-blind treatment with a long-acting calcium-channel blocker or diuretic in the International Nifedipine GITS study: Intervention as a Goal on Hypertension Treatment (INSIGHT). *Lancet*. 2000;**356**:366-372.

14. Pepine CJ, Handberg EM, Cooper-DeHoff RM, et al. A calcium antagonist vs. a non–calcium antagonist hypertension treatment strategy for patients with coronary artery disease: The International Verapamil-Trandolapril Study (INVEST). A randomized controlled trial. *JAMA.* 2003;**290**:2805-2816.

15. Black HR, Elliott WJ, Grandits G, et al. Principal results of the Controlled Onset Verapamil Investigation of Cardiovascular End Points (CONVINCE) trial. *JAMA.* 2003;**289**:2073-2082.

16. Psaty BM, Lumley T, Furberg CD, et al. Health outcomes associated with various antihypertensive therapies used as first line agents: A network meta-analysis. *JAMA.* 2003;**289**: 2534-2544.

17. Blood Pressure Lowering Treatment Trials' Collaboration. Effects of different blood-pressure–lowering regimens on major cardiovascular events: Results of prospectively-designed overviews of randomised trials. *Lancet.* 2003;**362**:1527-1535.

18. Dahlöf B, Sever PS, Poulter NR, et al. Prevention of cardiovascular events with an antihypertensive regimen of amlodipine adding perindopril as required versus atenolol adding bendroflumethiazide as required, in the Anglo-Scandinavian Cardiac Outcomes Trial–Blood Pressure Lowering Arm (ASCOT-BPLA): A multicentre randomised controlled trial. *Lancet,* 2005;**366**:895-906.

19. Rosendorff C. The renin-angiotensin system and vascular hypertrophy. *J Am Coll Cardiol.* 1996;**28**:803-812.

20. Heart Outcomes Prevention Evaluation Study Investigators. Effects of an angiotensin-converting-enzyme inhibitor, ramipril, on cardiovascular events in high-risk patients. *N Engl J Med.* 2000;**342**:145-153.

21. MacMahon S, Sharpe N, Gamble G, et al. Randomized, placebo-controlled trial of the angiotensin-converting enzyme inhibitor, ramipril, in patients with coronary or other occlusive arterial disease: PART-2 Collaborative Research Group. Prevention of Atherosclerosis with Ramipril. *J Am Coll Cardiol.* 2000;**36**:438-443.

22. Teo K, Burton J, Buller C, et al. Long-term effects of cholesterol lowering and angiotensin-converting enzyme inhibition on coronary atherosclerosis: The Simvastatin/Enalapril Coronary Atheroscrerosis Trial (SCAT). *Circulation.* 2000;**102**:1748-1754.

23. Cashin-Hemphill L, Holmvang G, Chan RC, et al. Angiotensin-converting enzyme inhibition as antiatherosclerotic therapy: No answer yet. *Am J Cardiol.* 1999;**83**:42-47.

24. Hansson L, Lindholm L, Niskanen L, et al. Effect of angiotensin-converting-enzyme inhibition compared with conventional therapy on cardiovascular morbidity and mortality in hypertension: The Captopril Prevention Project (CAPPP) randomised trial. *Lancet.* 1999;**353**;611-616.

25. UK Prospective Diabetes Study Group. Efficacy of atenolol and captopril in reducing risk of macrovascular and microvascular complications in type 2 diabetes: UKPDS 39. *BMJ.* 1998;**317**:713-720.

26. Hansson L, Lindholm LH, Ekbom T, et al. Randomised trial of old and new antihypertensive drugs in elderly patients: Cardiovascular mortality and morbidity the Swedish Trial in Old Patients with Hypertension-2 study. *Lancet.* 1999;**354**: 1751-1756.

27. Estacio R, Jeffers B, Hiatt W, et al. The effect of nisoldipine as compared with enalapril on cardiovascular outcomes in patients with non–insulin dependent diabetes and hypertension. *N Engl J Med.* 1998;**338**:645-652.

28. ALLHAT Officers and Coordinators for the ALLHAT Collaborative Research Group. Major outcomes in high risk hypertensive patients randomized to angiotensin-converting enzyme inhibitor or calcium channel blocker vs. diuretic. *JAMA.* 2002;**288**:2981-2997.

29. ALLHAT Officers and Coordinators for the ALLHAT Collaborative Research Group. Diuretic versus α-blocker as first step antihypertensive therapy: Final results from the Antihypertensive and Lipid-Lowering Treatment to prevent Heart Attack Trial (ALLHAT). *Hypertension.* 2003;**42**: 239-246.

30. Weber MA. The ALLHAT report: A case of information and misinformation. *J Clin Hypertens.* 2003;**5**:9-13.

31. Davis BR, Furberg CD, Wright. JT Jr, et al. ALLHAT: Setting the record straight. *Ann Intern Med.* 2004;**141**:39-46.

32. Opie LH, Schall R. Old antihypertensives and new diabetes. *J Hypertens.* 2004;**22**:1453-1458.

33. Wing LMH, Reid CM, Ryan P, et al. A comparison of outcomes with angiotensin-converting-enzyme inhibitors and diuretics for hypertension in the elderly. *N Engl J Med.* 2003;**348**: 583-592.

34. Malmqvist K, Öhman KP, Lind L, et al. Long-term effects of irbesartan and atenolol on the renin-angiotensin-aldosterone system in human primary hypertension: The Swedish Irbesartan Left Ventricular Hypertrophy Investigation versus Atenolol (SILVHIA). *J Cardiovasc Pharmacol.* 2003;**42**:719-726.

35. Dahlöf B, Devereux RB, Kjeldsen SE, et al. Cardiovascular morbidity and mortality in the Losartan Intervention for Endpoint reduction in hypertension study (LIFE): A randomised trial against atenolol. *Lancet.* 2002;**359**:995-1003.

36. Julius S, Kjeldsen SE, Weber M, et al. Outcomes in hypertensive patients at high cardiovascular risk treated with regimens based on valsartan or amlodipine: The VALUE randomized trial. *Lancet.* 2004;**363**:2022-2031.

37. Staessen JA, Wang J-G, Thijs L. Cardiovascular protection and blood pressure reduction: A quantitative overview updated until 1 March 2003. *J Hypertens.* 2003;**21**:1055-1076.

38. Hoffman JIE. A critical view of coronary reserve. *Circulation.* 1987;**75**:I6-I11

39. Cruickshank JM, Thorp JM, Zacharias FJ. Benefits and potential harm of lowering high blood pressure. *Lancet.* 1987;**1**:581-583.

40. Kannel WB, Wilson PWF, Nam B-H, et al. A likely explanation for the J-curve of blood pressure cardiovascular risk. *Am J Cardiol.* 2004;**94**:380-384.

41. Hansson L, Zanchetti A, Carruthers SG, et al. Effects of intensive blood-pressure lowering and low dose aspirin in patients with hypertension: Principal results of the Hypertension Optimal Treatment (HOT) randomised trial. *Lancet.* 1998;**351**:1755-1762.

42. Franklin SS, Khan SA, Wong ND, et al. Is pulse pressure useful in predicting risk for coronary artery disease? The Framingham Heart Study. *Circulation.* 1999;**100**:354-360.

43. Prospective Studies Collaborative. Age-specific relevance of usual blood pressure to vascular mortality: A meta-analysis of individual data for one million adults in 61 prospective studies. *Lancet.* 2002;**360**:1903-1913.

44. Boutitie F, Gueyffier F, Pocock S, et al. J-shaped relationship between blood pressure and mortality in hypertensive patients: New insights from a meta-analysis of individual-patient data. *Ann Intern Med.* 2002;**136**:438-448.

45. ACC/AHA/ACP-ASIM Guidelines for the management of patients with chronic stable angina. *Circulation.* 1999;**99**: 2829-2848.

46. Gibbons RJ, Abrams J, Chatterjee K, et al. ACC/AHA 2002 guideline update for the management of patients with chronic stable angina: Summary article. *Circulation.* 2003;**107**:149-158.

47. Dargie HJ, Ford I, Fox KM. Total Ischaemic Burden European Trial (TIBET): Effects of ischaemia and treatment with atenolol, nifedipine SR and their combination on outcome in patients with chronic stable angina. *Eur Heart J.* 1996;**17**:104-112.

48. Held C, Hjemdahl P, Rehnqvist N, et al. Fibrinolytic variables and cardiovascular prognosis in patients with stable angina pectoris treated with verapamil or metoprolol: Results from the Angina Prognosis Study in Stockholm. *Circulation.* 1997;**95**:2380-2386.

49. Von Arnim T. Medical treatment to reduce total ischemic burden: Total ischemic burden bisoprolol study (TIBBS), a multicenter trial comparing bisoprolol and nifedipine. The TIBBS Investigators. *J Am Coll Cardiol*. 1995;**25**:231-238.

50. Poole-Wilson PA, Lubsen J, Kirwan B-A, et al. Effect of long-acting nifedipine on mortality and cardiovascular morbidity in patients with stable angina requiring treatment (ACTION trial): A randomized controlled trial. *Lancet*. 2004;**364**:849-857.

51. Nissen SE, Tuzcu EM, Libby P, et al. Effect of antihypertensive agents on cardiovascular events in patients with coronary disease and normal blood pressure: The CAMELOT study. A randomized controlled trial. *JAMA*. 2004;**292**:2217-2225.

52. Braunwald E, Domanski MJ, Fowler SE, et al., for the PEACE Trial Investigators. Angiotensin-converting-enzyme inhibition in stable coronary artery disease. *N Engl J Med*. 2004;**351**: 2058-2068.

53. Fox KM, for the European Trial on Reduction of Cardiac Events with Perindopril in Stable Coronary Artery Disease Investigators. Efficiency of perindopril in reduction of cardiovascular events among patients with stable coronary artery disease: Randomized, double-blind, placebo-controlled, multicenter trial (the EUROPA study). *Lancet*. 2003;**362**: 782-788.

54. Braunwald E, Antman EM, Beasley JW, et al. ACC/AHA 2002 guideline update for the management of patients with unstable angina and non–ST-segment elevation myocardial infarction. *Circulation*. 2002;**106**:1893-1900.

55. Avanzini F, Ferrario G, Santoro L, et al. Risks and benefits of early treatment of myocardial infarction with an angiotensin-converting enzyme inhibitor in patents with a history of arterial hypertension: An analysis of the GISSI-3 database. *Am Heart J*. 2002;**144**:1018-1025.

56. Pitt B, Remme W, Zannad E, et al. Eplerenone, a selective aldosterone blocker, in patients with left ventricular dysfunction, after myocardial infarction. *N Engl J Med*. 2003;**348**:1309-1321.

57. Antman EM, Anbe DT, Armstrong PW, et al. ACC/AHA guidelines for the management of patients with ST-elevation myocardial infarction: Executive summary. A report of the ACC/AHA Task Force on Practice Guidelines. *Circulation*. 2004;**110**:588-636.

58. Pfeffer MA, Braunwald E, Moyé LA, et al. Effect of captopril on mortality and morbidity in patients with left ventricular dysfunction after myocardial infarction: Results of the Survival and Ventricular Enlargement (SAVE) trial. *N Engl J Med*. 1992;**327**:669-677.

59. AIRE Investigators. Effect of ramipril on mortality and morbidity of survivors of acute myocardial infarction with clinical evidence of heart failure: The Acute Infarction Ramipril Efficacy (AIRE) Study. *Lancet*. 1992;**342**:821-828

60. Kober L, Torp-Pedersen C, Carlsen JE, et al. A clinical trial of the angiotensin-converting-enzyme inhibitor trandolapril in patients with left ventricular dysfunction after myocardial infarction: Trandolapril Cardiac Evaluation (TRACE) Study Group. *N Engl J Med*. 1995;**333**:1670-1676.

61. SOLVD Investigators. Effect of enalapril on mortality and the development of heart failure in symptomatic patients with reduced left ventricular ejection fractions. *N Engl J Med*. 1992;**327**:685-691.

62. Dickstein K, Kjekshus J, for the OPTIMAAL Steering Committee of the OPTIMAAL Study Group. Effects of losartan and captopril on mortality and morbidity in high risk patients after acute myocardial infarction: The OPTIMAAL randomized trial. Optimal Trial in Myocardial Infarction with Angiotensin II Antagonist Losartan. *Lancet*. 2002;**360**:752-760

63. Pfeffer MA, McMurray JJV, Velasquez EJ, et al. Valsartan, captopril, or both in myocardial infarction complicated by heart failure, left ventricular dysfunction, or both. *N Engl J Med*. 2003;**349**:1893-1906.

64. Danish Study Group on Verapamil in Myocardial Infarction. Effect of verapamil on mortality and major events after acute myocardial infarction (the Danish Verapamil Infarction Trial II—DAVIT II). *Am J Cardiol*. 1990;**66**:779-785.

65. Multicenter Diltiazem Postinfarction Trial Research Group. The effect of diltiazem on mortality and reinfarction after myocardial infarction: The Multicenter Diltiazem Postinfarction Trial Research Group. *N Engl J Med*. 1988;**319**:385-392.

Chapter 28

Heart Failure in Hypertension

Ronald S. Freudenberger and John B. Kostis

Since the 1970s, age-adjusted mortality from cardiovascular disease has decreased by approximately 50% in men and women. Death from acute myocardial infarction has also decreased with the advent of thrombolytic therapy, percutaneous interventions, and adjunctive pharmacologic therapy. These factors, as well as the relatively poor control of hypertension in the community and the aging of the general population, have resulted in an increased incidence of left ventricular (LV) systolic and diastolic dysfunction and heart failure (HF).[1] HF is currently the single most frequent Medicare discharge diagnosis from acute care hospitals in the United States. Although therapeutic advances have had a favorable impact on the long-term outlook for many patients with HF, mortality rates among hospitalized patients with HF are high,[2] and the usual clinical course is still characterized by repeated hospitalizations, progressive deterioration, and elevated risk of sudden death. In the 2002 mortality statistics from the United States, more deaths were caused by HF than by all forms of cancer combined, and so prevention of HF is a critical public health concern. HF is a syndrome characterized by decreased exercise tolerance in the presence of cardiac dysfunction. Fatigue, dyspnea, edema, pulmonary rales, orthopnea, and nocturia are usually present, and increased central venous pressure, a fourth or third heart sound, and possibly a cardiac murmur of mitral regurgitation may be detected on physical examination. HF represents the last stage in the progression of cardiovascular disease, which begins with the presence of risk factors such as hypertension.[3]

EPIDEMIOLOGY

The incidence of HF shows a graded relationship with age, with most events occurring after the age of 60 years and with a very high incidence after the age of 80 years.[4] The incidence of HF in the United States did not decline significantly between 1979 and 2000, but survival after the onset of HF has increased overall, with less improvement among women and elderly persons.[5] The number of HF deaths also shows similar trends.[6] The number of persons aged 55 to 64 years in the United States is projected to increase by 73% between 2000 and 2020, and the number of those who are more than 65 years old will grow by 54%.[7] Although the aging of the population is more pronounced in developed countries, similar trends of increased life expectancy and lower birth rates are observed worldwide. LV dysfunction, both systolic and diastolic, has a strong relationship with the subsequent development of HF, and it become more frequent with increasing age and is associated with higher mortality.[8] Mild diastolic dysfunction is present in more than 50% of persons who are more than 75 years old, moderate diastolic dysfunction is

present in about 15%, and depressed ejection fraction occurs in about 12%.[9]

PATHOPHYSIOLOGY

LV dysfunction and HF in most people result from two overlapping but distinct pathways: hypertension and coronary artery disease.

Hypertension and Aging

Uncontrolled hypertension and aging interact in the development of HF, especially in the presence of obesity or diabetes, which further contribute to increased LV mass, LV wall thickness, and abnormal diastolic LV filling patterns. Impaired LV filling may cause the syndrome of diastolic HF with symptoms related to high pulmonary venous pressure and decreased cardiac output when the diastolic filling abnormalities are severe. Impairment of systolic function is initially compensated by increased LV thickness, but ultimately, LV remodeling associated with neurohormonal activation, increased wall tension, apoptosis, myocyte loss, fibrosis, chamber dilatation, and depressed systolic function leads to HF with depressed ejection fraction.[10]

Hypertension accelerates and enhances the age-related decrease in arterial compliance and leads to increases in systolic blood pressure (BP), afterload, and LV mass. These changes result from increased myocyte size as well as collagen deposition, and they cause impairment of myocardial relaxation and decreased rapid filling phase, as well as decreased LV compliance and elevated filling pressures. The concentric hypertrophy induced by hypertension is associated with changes in the myosin heavy chain toward β or embryonic chain with different (slower) contractile characteristics.[11] The concentration of calcium at end diastole is increased in response to changes in calcium adenosine triphosphatase of the sarcoplasmic reticulum. The increase in collagen and other matrix proteins is associated with a rise in the number of fibroblasts, and this pathway may be stimulated by activation of the renin-angiotensin-aldosterone system. The degree of LV hypertrophy (LVH) induced by hypertension depends on the patient's demographics (more in men and in blacks), on the severity and duration of hypertension, and on factors such as angiotensin II and norepinephrine that stimulate hypertrophic growth.[12] The cardiac changes described previously decrease cardiac reserve during exercise and ultimately may result in the syndrome of HF with preserved LV function, termed by some as *diastolic HF* or HF caused by LV diastolic dysfunction. Persistence of LVH with elevated diastolic pressures, as described earlier, results in atrial hypertension, atrial dilatation, and atrial pathophysiologic changes, often leading to atrial fibrillation.

The prevalence of LVH in hypertensive populations depends on the technique used for diagnosis and the diagnostic criteria. The electrocardiogram and chest radiograph are not as sensitive as the echocardiogram and magnetic resonance imaging. A fourth heart sound on physical examination and the presence of left atrial enlargement on the electrocardiogram are also suggestive of this condition. Among the many electrocardiographic criteria used for diagnosing LVH, the Sokolow criteria (a sum of S in V_1 and R in V_5 or V_6 greater than 35 mV) and the Cornell criteria (the product of the QRS duration and the sum of the R wave in aVL and S wave in V_3 greater than 2440 mV/millisecond) are the most commonly used. Echocardiographic LVH is thought to be present if LV free wall thickness is greater than or equal to 11 mm or if calculated LV mass is high (>100 g/m^2 in women or 131 g/m^2 in men).

When LV systolic overload is sustained, sensitivity of the myocardium to neurohormones is impaired. The result is suboptimal sympathetic increase of contractility in response to the increased afterload, and LV systolic dysfunction ensues. Persistence of hypertension and increased afterload over a period of years worsens the subtle decrease of systolic function observed early in the disease and results in eccentric hypertrophy, with additional sarcomeres, myocyte elongation and slippage, apoptosis, myocyte loss, fibrosis, progressive LV dilation, and HF with low ejection fraction and impaired systolic function. This cascade is enhanced by neurohormonal activation including the renin-angiotensin system and the sympathetic nervous system, and the results are progressive LV dilatation, LV failure, mitral regurgitation, pulmonary hypertension, and right ventricular failure.[12] In the Cardiovascular Health Study, LV systolic dysfunction in the absence of HF was associated in a graded fashion with higher incidence of future clinical HF, as well as with a higher death rate.[13]

Coronary Artery Disease

The second pathway leading to cardiac damage in hypertension is mediated through the effect of hypertension as an important risk factor for coronary artery disease. Myocardial infarction, especially ST-segment elevation myocardial infarction, results in the death of significant numbers of myocytes. The infarcted myocardial segment and the heart as a whole undergo progressive remodeling, resulting in hypokinesis, akinesis or dyskinesis of the involved segment, LV dilatation, and ultimately impaired LV global systolic function. Although the noninfarcted segments are initially hypercontractile, the continuing activation of the sympathetic and renin-angiotensin systems results in progressive ventricular dilatation, HF with depressed ejection fraction, mitral regurgitation, and right-sided HF.

The two types of HF (with preserved versus with low ejection fraction or systolic function) represent the extremes of a spectrum and share many characteristics in that both are associated with varying degrees of impairment of systolic and diastolic ventricular function and both are associated with increased LV mass, myocyte hypertrophy, interstitial fibrosis, and abnormal calcium handling.[14] The major differences are that one type is characterized by a low ejection fraction and

large ventricular volumes, and the other is characterized by normal ejection fraction and normal volumes. Both types of HF are associated with high mortality, a high rate of hospitalization, and impairment of functional capacity. HF with impaired systolic function has a higher mortality than HF with preserved systolic function. Sudden cardiac death, end-stage HF, and possibly thromboembolism are common causes of mortality in HF. In addition, LVH without overt HF and LV systolic dysfunction without overt HF are associated with increased mortality and the subsequent development of HF.

Congestive HF is associated with neurohormonal activation involving the sympathetic, endothelin, vasopressin, and renin-angiotensin systems, which maintain and worsen the myocardial changes described earlier while at the same time contribute to inadequate peripheral circulatory adaptation and physical deconditioning. Physical deconditioning in itself aggravates the circulatory abnormalities resulting from HF and low cardiac output and leads to wasting and abnormalities in skeletal muscle metabolism.[15] In end-stage HF, blood flow to end organs is compromised, and the associated endothelial dysfunction may cause dysfunction of peripheral organs (muscles, kidney, brain). Coronary blood flow reserve is reduced in patients with either dilated ventricles or concentric hypertrophy, in part because of impaired nitric oxide production and endothelial dysfunction.

PREVENTION OF HEART FAILURE IN PATIENTS WITH HYPERTENSION

Prevention of HF, a major objective of antihypertensive therapy, should include lifestyle changes and pharmacologic treatment. Antihypertensive therapy may prevent 30% to 50% of HF events, and better BP control results in better outcomes.[11,12] Controlling hypertension helps to prevent LVH and acute myocardial infarction and thus to reduce the incidence of HF. Achieving the latter goal requires attention to the total risk profile of the patient and includes interventions aimed at encouraging physical activity, controlling diabetes, avoiding smoking and overweight, achieving optimum cholesterol control, and, in high-risk patients, taking aspirin.

In large, placebo-controlled randomized clinical trials, BP control results in a marked decrease in the rate of developing HF. In the Systolic Hypertension in the Elderly (SHEP) trial, chlorthalidone-based stepped care therapy resulted in a 50% decrease in the occurrence of HF. A quantitative overview of all large controlled clinical trials available in 2003 indicated a reduction of the occurrence of HF by all major classes of antihypertensive agents. Better control of BP was associated with larger decrease in risk with the exception of calcium channel blockers as initial therapy. These agents had a major impact in preventing stroke, myocardial infarction, and cardiovascular events but were not associated with significant effects in preventing HF.[16] In the Antihypertensive and Lipid-Lowering Treatment to Prevent Heart Attack (ALLHAT) trial, a calcium antagonist, an ACE inhibitor, and an α-blocker were compared with a diuretic with respect to cardiovascular outcomes. The α-blocker limb of the study was discontinued early, because doxazosin was associated with a 25% higher risk for major cardiovascular events, including doubling of the risk for HF, compared with chlorthalidone. In ALLHAT, the calcium antagonist amlodipine was associated with a 38% higher incidence of HF, whereas angiotensin-converting enzyme (ACE) inhibition was associated with a 19% higher incidence of HF than chlorthalidone. BP differences may in part account for the latter difference. This beneficial effect of the diuretic was also observed among the more than 11,000 ALLHAT participants who also had diabetes. ACE inhibitors have been shown to prevent the occurrence of HF among patients with LV systolic dysfunction and hypertension.[17]

In the Losartan Intervention for Endpoint Reduction in Hypertension (LIFE) study in patients with hypertension and LVH, the angiotensin receptor blocker (ARB) losartan and the β-blocker atenolol achieved similar BP reductions (when used with a diuretic as second-line therapy), but losartan was superior in causing regression of LVH and in decreasing clinical morbid and mortal events. This difference was more pronounced in patients with diabetes.[18,19]

CLASSIFICATION

The American College of Cardiology/American Heart Association guidelines for the evaluation and management of chronic HF in the adult classify HF in four stages: stage A, patients at high risk for HF without structural heart disease or symptoms of HF; stage B, those with structural heart disease without symptoms of HF; stage C, those with structural heart disease with prior or current symptoms of HF; and stage D, patients with refractory HF requiring specialized interventions (Fig. 28-1). An echocardiogram and, in some cases, cardiac catheterization and magnetic resonance imaging are important diagnostic techniques, and an elevated serum level of brain natriuretic peptide may be used as an adjunct to diagnosis and follow-up of HF.

TREATMENT OF HYPERTENSION AND SYSTOLIC DYSFUNCTION

The treatment of patients with hypertension and LV systolic dysfunction, with or without overt HF, should alleviate symptoms, prevent hospitalization, slow or reverse progressive LV remodeling, and decrease mortality.

Effective treatment of HF may require lowering BP to values lower than currently recommended targets. Very low BP is a desirable outcome for these patients because the lower the systolic BP, the lower the afterload and the better the myocardial performance will be. There are no specific threshold BP levels as long as the patient has no functional impairment. Some patients, especially those with intervening large myocardial infarctions, develop marked LV dilatation, severe LV dysfunction, and low systolic BP (<100 mm Hg). In such patients, β-blockers, ACE inhibitors, and digitalis should still be administered while carefully titrating diuretics. When symptomatic hypotension limits the ability to titrate β-blockers and ACE inhibitors, a lower dose of both drugs rather than a high dose of one is often necessary. In stage D HF, hypotension rather than hypertension is associated with a worse prognosis. Current recommendations for therapy are based on the new American College of Cardiology/American Heart Association staging system.

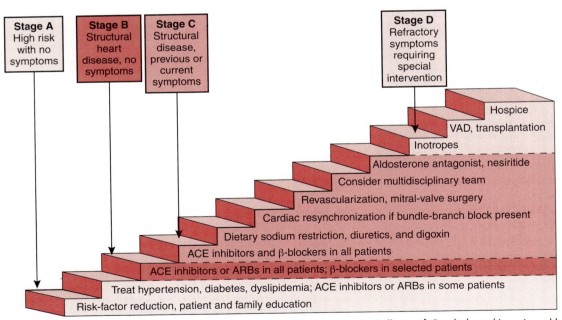

Figure 28–1 Classification of heart failure: relationship between the American College of Cardiology/American Heart Association classification of heart failure (by stages) and the New York Heart Association's functional classes. ACE, angiotensin-converting enzyme; ARB, angiotensin receptor blocker; VAD, ventricular assist device. (Modified from Hunt SA, Baker DW, Chin MH, et al. ACC/AHA guidelines for the evaluation and management of chronic heart failure in the adult: Executive summary. A report of the American College of Cardiology/American Heart Association Task Force on Practice Guidelines [Committee to revise the 1995 Guidelines for the Evaluation and Management of Heart Failure]. *J Am Coll Cardiol.* 2001;**38**:2101-2112.)

Stage A ("At Risk")

Therapy includes the following: control of systolic and diastolic BP; treatment of lipid abnormalities; avoidance of behaviors that may increase the risk of HF (e.g., smoking, alcohol consumption, and illicit drug use); ACE inhibition in patients with atherosclerotic disease, diabetes mellitus, or hypertension, and associated cardiovascular risk factors; control of ventricular rate in patients with supraventricular tachyarrhythmias; and treatment of thyroid disorders.

Stage B ("Asymptomatic")

Therapy includes ACE inhibition and β-blockade in the following patients: those with a history of myocardial infarction regardless of ejection fraction; those with a reduced ejection fraction, whether or not they have experienced a myocardial infarction; and those with a recent myocardial infarction, regardless of ejection fraction, as well as valve replacement or repair for patients with hemodynamically significant disease.

Stages C and D ("Symptomatic")

Therapy includes (unless contraindicated) diuretics in patients with fluid retention, ACE inhibition in all patients, β-adrenergic blockade in all stable patients, digitalis, withdrawal of drugs known to affect the clinical status of HF patients adversely (e.g., nonsteroidal anti-inflammatory drugs, most antiarrhythmic drugs, and most calcium channel blocking drugs), and spironolactone.

Specific Drugs

Diuretics

Diuretics have no proven mortality benefit in patients with established HF. However, diuretic therapy is preventive and is also an essential adjunct to β-blocker and ACE inhibitor therapy to decrease congestive symptoms and signs of HF (pulmonary congestion, hepatomegaly, and edema). A particularly useful strategy is to teach the patient to adjust the amount of loop diuretic based on daily weights. In early LV dysfunction, thiazide or thiazide-like diuretics such as hydrochlorothiazide or chlorthalidone can be used, but as cardiac or renal function deteriorates, loop diuretics become increasingly important. The combination of loop and thiazide or thiazide-like diuretics can be helpful in patients with hyperkalemia.

Angiotensin-Converting Enzyme Inhibitors and Angiotensin Receptor Blockers

Most studies with ACE inhibitors have shown a decreases in mortality, rates of hospitalization, and myocardial infarction in patients with HF and LV systolic dysfunction of all degrees of severity. The recommendation that ACE inhibitors should be used in patients with hypertension and all stages of LV systolic dysfunction is supported by post hoc analyses of the hypertensive subsets of large controlled clinical trials, including the Studies of Left Ventricular Dysfunction (SOLVD),[19] the Acute Infarction Ramipril Efficacy (AIRE)

study,[20] and the Trandolapril Cardiac Evaluation (TRACE) study.[21] These studies showed a significant decrease in total mortality, HF hospitalizations, ischemic endpoints, and cost savings because hospitalizations are costlier than medication.

ACE inhibitor use in all stages of HF has been shown to improve survival (Fig. 28-2). The SOLVD and Survival and Ventricular Enlargement (SAVE) trials provided evidence for mortality reduction in patients with mild HF.[22,23] The Veterans Affairs Vasodilator-Heart Failure (V-HeFT) trial provided evidence of improved survival in moderate HF.[24] The Cooperative North Scandinavian Enalapril Survival Study I (CONSENSUS-I) provided evidence for class IV HF patients.[25]

More recently, several studies evaluating the use of ARBs in patients with HF have been published. ARBs may be beneficial either in conjunction with ACE inhibitors or in lieu of ACE inhibitors. The use of ACE inhibitors in conjunction with ARBs may be important, given the effects of ACE inhibitors on inhibiting the breakdown of bradykinin (Fig. 28-3).

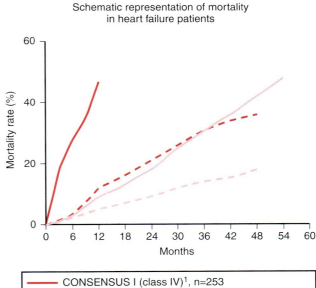

Schematic representation of mortality in heart failure patients

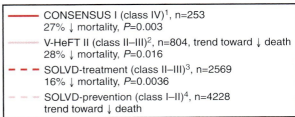

Figure 28–2   Survival curves for placebo-treated patients with heart failure in early clinical trials of angiotensin-converting enzyme (ACE) inhibitors demonstrating the increased mortality with increasing New York Heart Association class. The mortality benefits in the ACE inhibitor–treated groups are shown with each curve. CONSENSUS I, Cooperative North Scandinavian Enalapril Survival Study I; V-HeFT II, Veterans Affairs Vasodilator–Heart Failure Trial II; SOLVD-Treatment, Study of Left Ventricular Dysfunction, Treatment trial; SOLVD-Prevention, Study of Left Ventricular Dysfunction, Prevention trial. (Data from references 22, 24, 25, and *N Engl J Med.* 1992;**327**:685-693.)

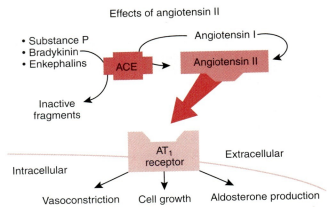

Effects of angiotensin II

Figure 28–3 Biochemical and pharmacologic pathways for angiotensin II formation and binding to extracellular receptors that are important in heart failure. ACE, angiotensin converting-enzyme; AT_1 receptor, angiotensin II subtype 1 receptor.

Several studies have been published examining these issues. The Valsartan Heart Failure Trial (Val-HeFT) evaluated 5010 New York Heart Association (NYHA) class II, III, or IV HF patients who were randomly assigned to receive 160 mg valsartan or placebo twice daily.[26] The two primary outcomes were mortality and the composite endpoint of mortality and morbidity, defined as the incidence of cardiac arrest with resuscitation, hospitalization for HF, or receipt of intravenous inotropic or vasodilator therapy for at least 4 hours. A marked benefit of the ARB was observed among 366 patients who were not receiving background ACE inhibitor therapy. In this study, now-standard therapy with β-blockers was not mandated, resulting in a relatively low usage rate (35%). A subgroup analysis suggested that the combination of ACE inhibitors, ARBs, and β-blockers increased mortality. This finding was confirmed in subsequent studies (e.g., Candesartan in Heart Failure: Assessment of Reduction in Morbidity and Mortality [CHARM]).

The CHARM study was a randomized, double-blind, controlled, clinical trial that compared candesartan with placebo in three distinct HF populations: patients with LV ejection fraction of 40% or less who were not receiving ACE inhibitors because of previous intolerance; patients who were currently receiving ACE inhibitors; and patients with LV ejection fraction higher than 40%.[27] Most patients in the first group were intolerant of ACE inhibitors as a result of cough. In these patients, candesartan was generally well tolerated and reduced cardiovascular mortality and morbidity.[27] The addition of candesartan to an ACE inhibitor reduced each of the components of the primary outcome significantly, as well as the total number of hospital admissions for HF.[28] The benefits of candesartan were similar in all predefined subgroups, including patients receiving baseline β-blocker treatment (i.e., contrary to the results of the much smaller group treated with all three agents in Val-HeFT).[28] Clear superiority of ARBs over ACE inhibitors in treating HF has not been demonstrated, and current guidelines recommend that ARBs be administered to patients with HF who cannot tolerate ACE inhibitors, but this may change as the results of CHARM-Added are more widely appreciated and other studies are completed. The addition of an ARB to an ACE inhibitor results in better hemodynamic and renal effects, but no convincing evidence indicates that this combination results in lower mortality. A large clinical trial on this issue is now being conducted.

β-Blockers

β-Blocker therapy reduces mortality in otherwise appropriately treated patients with HF and coronary artery disease. Despite their intrinsic negative inotropic effects, β-blockers exert beneficial effects in HF by reducing heart rate, controlling BP, controlling supraventricular and ventricular arrhythmias, and exerting anti-ischemic effects. In a meta-analysis of controlled trials using carvedilol or bisoprolol, β-blocker use was associated with a 30% reduction in mortality and a 40% reduction in hospitalizations in patients with class II and III HF. β-Blockers (except those with partial agonist activity or intrinsic sympathomimetic activity) have been shown to reduce cardiac mortality and morbidity in patients with coronary artery disease in the majority of more than 40 clinical trials.

Aldosterone Antagonists

Aldosterone is elevated in patients with HF. The effects of aldosterone include vasoconstriction, fibrosis, sodium retention, potassium excretion, and endothelial dysfunction.[29] All these properties would likely worsen HF in patients with systolic LV dysfunction. Two studies have examined the use of aldosterone antagonists in patients with HF. In the Randomized Aldactone Evaluation Study (RALES), patients with NYHA class III or IV HF were randomized to receive the aldosterone antagonist, spironolactone, 25 mg/day, or placebo. The primary outcome was all-cause mortality. After a mean follow-up of 24 months, the study was stopped early because of a lower mortality in the group receiving spironolactone (relative risk of death, 0.70; 95% confidence interval, 0.60 to 0.82; $P < .001$).[30]

The Eplerenone Post–Myocardial Infarction Heart Failure Efficacy and Survival Study (EPHESUS) compared the use of the selective aldosterone antagonist, eplerenone, versus placebo in 6632 patients who were within 7 days of a myocardial infarction and had signs or symptoms of HF.[31] Patients randomized to eplerenone had a 15% improvement in survival versus placebo. Hyperkalemia may be produced by the aldosterone antagonists used in HF, especially when these drugs are co-administered with ACE inhibitors, potassium supplements, or potassium-sparing diuretics. Low doses and careful monitoring are important.[32]

Aldosterone blockade is beneficial in patients with hypertension and isolated systolic hypertension in terms of lowering BP, reducing microalbuminuria, and reducing LVH.[33,34]

Electrical Therapy

This therapy includes pacing for chronotropic incompetence, for the prevention of arrhythmias, improving atrioventricular (AV) synchrony, for the prevention of out-of-hospital arrhythmic death, and for cardiac resynchronization (interventricular synchrony).

Since the early 1990s, the role of pacing to improve the hemodynamic status of subjects with dilated cardiomyopathy, but without a standard bradycardia pacing indication, has been the subject of considerable interest and investigation. Hochleitner and colleagues first reported that pacing from the right ventricular apex with a short AV delay could improve symptoms of HF.[35] These investigators evaluated 16 patients with end-stage cardiomyopathy and observed a marked improvement in functional status and LV ejection fraction with VDD (ventricular/dual/dual) dual-chamber pacing and an AV delay of 100 milliseconds. Subsequent acute echocardiographic studies, in patients with dilated cardiomyopathy, suggested that the hemodynamic improvement seen in pacing may be apparent only in those subgroups with mitral regurgitation or first-degree AV block.[36] Later, controlled studies failed to show a benefit of right ventricular pacing with a short AV delay in patients with dilated cardiomyopathy.[37] Gold and colleagues performed a randomized double-blind study of 12 patients with chronic NYHA class III or IV HF; VDD pacing with a 100-millisecond delay was compared with VVI (ventricular/ventricular/inhibited) pacing, and each patient served as his or her control. Neither acute nor chronic hemodynamic or functional benefit was observed, despite the high prevalence (75%) of first-degree AV block.[38]

Given the disappointing results with pacing from the right ventricular apex, alternative stimulation sites were explored, including the RV outflow tract, which yielded similarly unsatisfactory findings. However, more encouraging results have been obtained using biventricular pacing in an effort to improve ventricular synchronization. In a study of patients with dilated cardiomyopathy and left bundle branch block, Blanc and associates evaluated the acute hemodynamic effects of right ventricular apex, right ventricular outflow tract, or LV endocardial pacing. No changes were observed with right ventricular pacing, but marked hemodynamic improvements were noted with LV pacing either alone or with simultaneous right ventricular pacing.[39] More recently, the European Multisite Stimulation in Cardiomyopathy (MUSTIC) study was conducted. In this randomized study comparing biventricular pacing with no pacing at all, biventricular pacing improved exercise capacity in patients with prolonged QRS duration.[40] The MIRACLE trial evaluated 453 patients with moderate to severe symptoms of HF associated with an ejection fraction of 35% or less and a QRS interval of 130 milliseconds or more, who were randomly assigned to cardiac resynchronization therapy (228 patients) or to control treatments that did not include a pacemaker (225 patients) for 6 months while conventional therapy for HF was maintained. The primary endpoints were the NYHA functional class, quality of life, and the distance walked in 6 minutes. As compared with the control group, patients assigned to cardiac resynchronization experienced an improvement in the distance walked in 6 minutes (+39 versus +10 m, P = .005), functional class (P < .001), quality of life score (−18.0 versus −9.0 points, P = .001), time on the treadmill during exercise testing (+81 versus +19 seconds, P = .001), and ejection fraction (+4.6% versus −0.2%, P < .001).[41] A quantitative overview of four randomized trials of cardiac resynchronization therapy demonstrated a statistically and clinically significant decrease in mortality related to progressive HF, with a significant difference in all-cause mortality.[42]

The public health impact of these findings is significant and may provide improvement in functional parameters for a large segment of the population. Freudenberger and colleagues found that fully 21% of patients referred for heart transplantation were eligible for biventricular pacing for HF indications. This finding suggests that in addition to a multidrug regimen for HF, 21% of patients may benefit from additional therapy with pacing devices.[43]

Several studies have examined the impact of ventricular pacing in patients with LV dysfunction. In the Dual Chamber and VVI Implantable Defibrillator (DAVID) trial, permanent pacing increased the combined endpoint of death or hospitalization for HF compared with backup bradycardia pacing.[44] These results are also consistent with a post hoc analysis of the Mode Selection Trial (MOST), a trial of pacemaker therapy for sick sinus syndrome that demonstrated that the cumulative percentage of right ventricular apical pacing, calculated from stored pacemaker data, was a strong predictor of HF hospitalization.[45] Moreover, Freudenberger and colleagues conducted a cohort study of patients undergoing initial permanent pacemaker insertion (n = 11,426). Subjects without a current or prior diagnosis of HF who underwent permanent pacemaker insertion were compared with a matched cohort of patients without pacemakers or a diagnosis of HF (n = 11,656). Both cohorts were followed by record linkage with 1997 to 2001 files to determine the incidence of new HF hospitalization or death (median follow-up of 33 months). Cox regression models adjusted for age, gender, diabetes, myocardial infarction, hypertension, atrial fibrillation, AV block, and sick sinus syndrome were used to compare differences. Patients with pacemakers experienced significantly more new HF hospitalizations (n = 2314) compared with the controls (n = 1459). Single-chamber pacemaker implantation (27% of the insertions) was associated with significantly higher risk of HF hospitalization or HF death compared with controls than was observed with dual-chamber pacemakers. The adjusted risk of fatal or nonfatal HF was significantly higher with single-chamber pacing versus dual-chamber pacing. Within the paced group, single-chamber pacing was significantly worse than dual-chamber pacing. Thus, permanent pacemakers (particularly single-chamber devices) implanted in patients without HF increased the risk of subsequent HF or death.[46]

Surgical Treatments

Mitral Valve Surgery

Progressive ventricular dilation often leads to mitral and tricuspid annular dilation with resultant regurgitation. Mitral insufficiency leads to increasing volume overload of the dilated left ventricle, with consequent progression of annular dilatation, worsening of mitral valve regurgitation, and volume overload. The resulting mitral valve insufficiency is often refractory to medical therapy and predicts a poor survival in this patient group. Investigators have hypothesized that this cycle could be interrupted by correction of the mitral valve insufficiency. Mitral valve reconstruction in patients with HF may lead to clinical and functional improvement; however, the procedure is often believed to be associated with substantial perioperative risk. In general, mitral valve repair is thought to be superior to mitral valve replacement because of the preservation of the annular (chordal) papillary muscle continuity.[47] Since the mid-1990s, studies have found that mitral annuloplasty with undersizing of the ring leads to acceptable short-term prognosis and improved long-term prognosis.[48,49]

There is much current interest in surgical ventricular restoration (SVR), which includes operative methods that reduce LV volume and restore ventricular elliptical shape.[50,51] This operation is also referred to as the Dor procedure. The international Reconstructive Endoventricular Surgery, Returning Torsion Original Radius Elliptical Shape to the Left Ventricle (RESTORE) team published their report on the RESTORE SVR registry with 5-year follow-up of 1198 postinfarction patients who underwent this procedure. Concomitant procedures included coronary artery bypass grafting (CABG) in 95%, mitral valve repair in 22%, and mitral valve replacement in 1%. Overall 30-day mortality after SVR was 5.3% (8.7% with mitral repair versus 4.0% without repair; $P < .001$). Perioperative mechanical support was uncommon (<9%). Global systolic function improved postoperatively. Ejection fraction increased from 29.6% ± 11.0% preoperatively to 39.5% ± 12.3% postoperatively ($P < .001$). Overall 5-year survival was 68.6% ± 2.8%.

The Surgical Treatment for Ischemic Heart Failure (STICH) study is sponsored by the U.S. National Institutes of Health. STICH is a prospective randomized study that will include 2800 patients from 100 centers. Patients with LV dysfunction and coronary artery disease amenable to CABG will be randomized to combinations of three different treatment strategies: CABG, SVR, and intensive medical therapy (MED). Two primary hypotheses will be considered: (1) CABG combined with MED improves long-term survival when compared with MED alone, and (2) SVR provides an additional long-term survival benefit when combined with CABG and MED alone. Secondary endpoints of the trial include cardiac morbidity and mortality rates, economic impact of the various treatments, patient quality of life, and utility of biochemical and imaging modalities for predicting optimal treatment strategy. Patients will be included in the trial on the basis of an ejection fraction less than 35%, coronary anatomy suitable for revascularization, and age older than 18 years.[52]

Ventricular Assist Devices

The ventricular assist device (VAD) is a blood pump designed to assist or replace the function of either the right or left ventricle. A right VAD supports the pulmonary circulation, whereas a left VAD provides systemic perfusion, in the absence of adequate right or LV ejection, respectively. Implantable VADs are positioned intracorporeally, under the anterior abdominal wall or within the thorax or abdomen. Extracorporeal VADs may be located in a paracorporeal position, on the patient's anterior abdomen, or externally, at the patient's bedside. Five pulsatile VAD systems have approval by the U.S. Food and Drug Administration (FDA) for clinical use. The total artificial heart is an orthotopically positioned cardiac replacement device.[53] The pneumatic total artificial heart is used infrequently, and only with FDA approval, as a mechanical bridge to cardiac transplantation. Completely implantable electric VADs and artificial hearts that do not employ a percutaneous drive line have been successfully implanted in experimental animals and are expected to reach the clinical arena in the near future.

If the cumulative experience of the bridge patients is reviewed, approximately two thirds of patients requiring VAD support survive to heart transplantation.[54] More important, 86% of patients who require VAD support and who undergo successful heart transplantation survive to hospital discharge.[55,56]

LVADs have also been used as a bridge to recovery with temporary support followed by explantation. In the settings of myocarditis and dilated cardiomyopathy, LVAD support is accompanied by marked hemodynamic, neurohormonal, physiologic, cellular, and molecular changes indicative of recovery. Despite these changes, experience and clinical successes with the device are limited.[57] Whether these observations can be attributed to the natural history of myocarditis or to true reverse remodeling resulting from unloading of the ventricle is unknown.

LVAD as destination therapy appears to be a reasonable alternative to heart transplantation in select patients. The Randomized Evaluation of Mechanical Assistance for the Treatment of Congestive Heart Failure (REMATCH) trial compared "optimal medical therapy" with LVAD placement for patients with end-stage cardiomyopathy. One hundred twenty-nine patients ineligible for heart transplantation were randomized to medical therapy or LVAD placement.[58] The rates of survival at 1 year were 52% in the device group and 25% in the medical therapy group ($P = .002$), and the rates at 2 years were 23% and 8% ($P = .09$), respectively. The frequency of serious adverse events in the device group was 2.35 (95% confidence interval, 1.86 to 2.95) times that in the medical therapy group, with a predominance of infection, bleeding, and malfunction of the device. Despite the substantial survival benefit, the morbidity and mortality associated with the use of the LVAD were considerable. In particular, infection and mechanical failure of the device were major factors in the 2-year survival rate of only 23%. The optimal medical therapy group had a β-blocker usage rate of only 20%.[58] Optimal candidates for destination therapy have yet to be defined. Many contraindications to heart transplantation may also significantly limit the benefits of LVAD support.

Heart Transplantation

In general, patients with advanced HF, NYHA class III or IV, who are receiving maximal medical therapy are candidates for heart transplantation. Patients with increasing medication requirements, frequent hospitalizations, or overall deterioration of clinical status should also be considered for evaluation for cardiac transplantation. In addition to these clinical characteristics, ejection fraction and hemodynamic parameters are generally obtained to risk stratify patients further. Patients with low ejection fraction tend to have a poor prognosis. However, when the ejection fraction is less than 20%, this index of ventricular function has limited ability to provide further prognostic information. In such patients, bicycle ergometry with gas exchange to determine the oxygen consumption at maximal exercise has proved to be a useful tool. In general, a maximal oxygen consumption of more than 14 mL/kg/minute predicts a good prognosis. In contrast, patients with a maximal oxygen consumption of less than 14 mL/kg/minute have a poor prognosis and should be considered for cardiac transplantation.[58a]

Exclusion Criteria

In 1992, a group of transplant surgeons, cardiologists, nurses, and representatives from the United Network of Organ Sharing

Table 28-1 Contraindications to Heart Transplantation

- Advanced age (>70 yr)
- Severe peripheral vascular or cerebrovascular disease
- Insulin-requiring diabetes mellitus with end-organ damage
- Active infection
- Recent cancer with uncertain status
- Psychiatric illness, poor medical compliance
- Systemic disease that would significantly limit survival or rehabilitation
- Pulmonary hypertension with pulmonary vascular resistance
- >6 Wood units or 3 Wood units after treatment with vasodilators
- Significant irreversible hepatic disease (total bilirubin >2.5 mg/dL)
- Significant irreversible renal disease (creatinine concentration >2.5 mg/dL, creatinine clearance <35 mL/min)
- Cachexia or obesity
- Severe osteoporosis
- Current cigarette smoking
- Recent (<2 yr previously) drug or alcohol abuse

Data from International Society for Heart and Lung Transplantation [ISHLT] Transplant Registry Quarterly Reports for Heart in North America. ISHLT 2004. Electronic citation. Found on the Internet at http://www.ishlt.org/registries/quarterlyDataReport.asp, accessed 20 MAY 05 at 12:01 CDT.

(UNOS) met to discuss various aspects of cardiac transplantation, including criteria for exclusion (Table 28-1).[59]

Irreversible pulmonary hypertension creates a high risk of postoperative right ventricular failure. A pulmonary vascular resistance index higher than 6 to 8 Wood units/m^2, a pulmonary artery systolic pressure greater than 50 to 60 mm Hg, and a transpulmonic gradient greater than 15 mm Hg that does not decrease by 50% with the use of vasodilators are all considered contraindications to cardiac transplantation. Various pharmacologic agents, including dobutamine, nitroglycerin, prostacyclin, and nitric oxide, have been used to assess the reversibility of these pressures. Coexisting medical illness with a poor prognosis remains a contraindication to transplantation, because the patient is likely to have a poor short-term survival or a difficult postoperative course.

Physiology of the Transplanted Heart

Soon after transplantation, cardiac output is often depressed, and maintenance of a high central venous pressure and inotropic medication is important for maintaining cardiac output. This effect is probably the result of an early restrictive type of physiology caused by ischemia and the damaging effects of hypothermic preservation techniques and abnormal atrial dynamics. Because of the midatrial anastomosis between donor and recipient hearts, varying proportions of the donor and recipient atria are present. Furthermore, the recipient atria do not contract synchronously with the donor atria, because recipient sinus node electrical activity does not pass through anastomotic suture lines. This results in an approximately 80% loss of the normal atrial contribution to the total stroke volume of the heart.

Many patients have normal resting intracardiac pressures after transplantation. The pressures can increase with exercise as a result of an early restrictive hemodynamic pattern. When this situation is present early after transplantation, it usually resolves. More recently, investigators have recognized that a subclinical, latent, restrictive component is present and is unmasked by volume challenge. This may be confounded by post-transplantation hypertension with resultant LVH and by bouts of rejection.

The transplanted heart displays a unique response to exercise. During early exercise, cardiac output increases by augmentation of end-diastolic volume and stroke volume. At more intense exercise levels, heart rate and contractility are increased by circulating catecholamines. The heart rate response is blunted in these individuals because of vagal denervation. The maximal cardiac output achieved is generally lower than that of physiologically normal individuals because of a blunted heart rate response and a lower peak stroke volume.

Denervation of the heart leads to resting tachycardia (95 to 115 beats/minute) because of the loss of vagal input. Moreover, the heart rate does not respond to carotid sinus massage or to drugs that depend on intact innervation of the heart, such as atropine. High levels of circulating catecholamines affect the blunted heart rate response to exercise that occurs relatively late. Administration of quinidine and disopyramide (agents that have vagolytic effects in the innervated heart) tends to increase AV conduction time as a result of the direct depressant AV nodal effects of these drugs.

Following transplantation, there is a 16% 1-year mortality rate and an approximately 7% mortality rate per year for each year thereafter.[59] Acute and chronic rejection remains a significant problem in these patients, although the risk decreases with time. A report from the Cardiac Transplant Research Database Group demonstrated that the risk of acute rejection in patients receiving heart transplants peaked at approximately 1 month after transplantation and then rapidly declined.[60] That study also found a mean of 1.25 episodes of acute rejection per patient during the first year, 0.18 episodes per patient in the second year, and 0.13 and 0.02 episodes per patient in the third and fourth years, respectively. This finding implies that a degree of immune tolerance develops over time after orthotopic heart transplantation.

Complications

The most common causes of death in the first year after heart transplantation are rejection and infection. Both occur most frequently in the first 2 months after transplantation. Therefore, the most intensive follow-up after transplantation is within this initial period, during which patients are instructed to remain in close proximity to the medical center. Patients are seen twice weekly as outpatients to be examined for evidence of infection, rejection, or graft dysfunction. They undergo endomyocardial biopsy weekly during the first 6 to 8 weeks and at gradually lower frequencies thereafter.

One third of all transplant recipients develop an infection that requires intravenous antibiotics during the first year following transplantation. Infection is the most common cause of death in this period.

Acute cellular rejection, the most common form of rejection, occurs at least once in approximately half of heart transplant recipients.[61,62] Even though the propensity toward allograft rejection decreases over time and nearly half of the rejection episodes occur in the first 2 to 3 months, late rejection can and does occur. Humoral rejection may be manifest by otherwise unexplained cardiac allograft dysfunction with or without distinct histologic characteristics. Histologic findings are scant cellular infiltrate with abundant co-localized immunoglobulin and complement components in the allograft microvasculature seen on one or more biopsy specimens. In addition, humoral rejection may be manifest only histologically in the absence of allograft dysfunction.[61] Humoral rejection is often detected early after transplantation and has been linked to hemodynamic compromise, graft arteriopathy, and subsequent poor patient survival. Humoral rejection is more difficult to treat than acute cellular rejection and is more often accompanied by hemodynamic compromise or instability, a worse prognosis, and nearly tenfold the risk of cardiac allograft vasculopathy (CAV).[61]

Clinically, most rejection episodes are detected by surveillance endomyocardial biopsies and manifest no signs or symptoms. If the episode is symptomatic, the most frequent symptom is fatigue. Later in the rejection process, exercise intolerance or frank HF symptoms may occur. Surveillance for allograft rejection generally centers on the routine use of endomyocardial biopsy.

Long-term graft survival has not improved appreciably since the early 1980s, in large part because of poor understanding of the mechanisms of chronic graft failure. Chronic graft failure in heart transplantation results from CAV, also referred to as chronic rejection. After the first few years following transplantation, CAV is the leading cause of death and the cause of significant morbidity.[63-65] Even with newer immunosuppression regimens, no significant decline in the incidence of CAV has occurred.[66] The prevalence of angiographically detectable CAV approaches 50% to 60% at 5 years. The prevalence of disease detected by intravascular ultrasonography or at autopsy is greater. Thus far, the improvements in immunosuppression have not greatly affected the incidence and morbidity associated with CAV development. CAV is not a homogeneous disease and can change over time. Early CAV is characterized by diffuse and distal involvement, whereas later-onset coronary artery disease is more proximal, focal, and eccentric. Although many factors have been suggested for increasing the risk of CAV, little is known about contributive changes in gene expression over time.

CAV has been observed as an incidental finding at autopsy as early as 3 months after cardiac transplantation.[67] Significant coronary disease may produce arrhythmias, myocardial infarction, sudden death, or impaired LV function with HF.[68] Angina pectoris is rare because the cardiac allograft remains essentially denervated, so patients may present with sudden and severe cardiac dysfunction. The disease tends to be diffuse and concentric, and coronary angiograms must be closely inspected and compared with previous studies to appreciate the reduction in coronary diameter.

Immunosuppressed transplant recipients have a 1% to 2% risk per year of developing a malignancy. Solid organ transplant patients are not at higher risk of developing the common tumors such as cancer of the lung, prostate, breast, and colon. Rather, they are at a higher risk of developing squamous cell carcinoma of the skin, lymphoma, Kaposi's sarcoma, carcinoma of the vulva or perineum, carcinoma of the kidney, and hepatobiliary tumors. Cutaneous malignancy is the most common malignant disease seen in this setting. A unique type of lymphoma, referred to as post-transplant lymphoproliferative disease, is a non-Hodgkin's B-cell lymphoma.

Survival

Overall, heart transplant recipients experience a general improvement both in quality of life and survival. Data from the Cardiac Transplant Research Database indicate that the 1-year survival rate in major North American transplant centers is 85%. It is estimated that the 5-year survival rate in major North American transplant centers is 75%. Several studies have addressed the quality of life in addition to the duration of life. The National Transplantation Study examined quality of life in detail and analyzed data from 85% of transplantation programs in the United States. This study found that 80% to 85% of patients were physically active, and 90% of the patients who were analyzed described themselves as normal or stated that they had minimal signs or symptoms of disease. Only 7.2% rated their health status as poor, and 9% of patients needed assistance. Thus, despite its limitations, cardiac transplantation offers a viable option for improving both quality and quantity of life in selected patients.

References

1. Gottdiener JS, McClelland RL, Marshall R, et al. Outcome of congestive heart failure in elderly persons: Influence of left ventricular systolic function. The Cardiovascular Health Study. *Ann Intern Med.* 2002;**137**:631-639.
2. MacIntyre K, Capewell S, Stewart S, et al. Evidence of improving prognosis in heart failure: Trends in case fatality in 66,547 patients hospitalized between 1986 and 1995. *Circulation.* 2000;**102**:1126-1131.
3. Jessup M, Brozena S. Heart failure. *N Engl J Med.* 2003;**348**:2007-2018.
4. Senni M, Tribouilloy CM, Rodeheffer RJ, et al. Congestive heart failure in the community: Trends in incidence and survival in a 10-year period. *Arch Intern Med.* 1999;**159**:29-34.
5. Roger VL, Weston SA, Redfield MM, et al. Trends in heart failure incidence and survival in a community-based population. *JAMA.* 2004;**292**:344-350.
6. Massie BM, Shah NB. Evolving trends in the epidemiologic factors of heart failure: Rationale for preventive strategies and comprehensive disease management. *Am Heart J.* 1997;**133**:703-712.
7. Dickerson P, Johnson P. U. S. Census Bureau: International Data Base (IDB). IDB summary demographic data for United States. Found on the internet at www.census.gov/cgi-bin/ipc/idbsum?cty=US, accessed 01 SEP 05 at 09:14 CDT.
8. Aurigemma GP, Gottdiener JS, Shemanski L, et al. Predictive value of systolic and diastolic function for incident congestive heart failure in the elderly: The Cardiovascular Health Study. *J Am Coll Cardiol.* 2001;**37**:1042-1048.
9. Redfield MM, Jacobsen SJ, Burnett JC Jr, et al. Burden of systolic and diastolic ventricular dysfunction in the community: Appreciating the scope of the heart failure epidemic. *JAMA.* 2003;**289**:194-202.
10. Lakatta EG. Age-associated cardiovascular changes in health: Impact on cardiovascular disease in older persons. *Heart Fail Rev.* 2002;**7**:29-49.
11. Izzo JL Jr, Levy D, Black HR. Clinical Advisory Statement: Importance of systolic blood pressure in older Americans. *Hypertension.* 2000;**35**:1021-1024.

12. Izzo JL Jr. Systolic hypertension, arterial stiffness, and vascular damage: Role of the renin-angiotensin system. *Blood Press Monit*. 2000;**5 (Suppl 2)**:S7-S11.

13. Gottdiener JS, McClelland RL, Marshall R, et al. Outcome of congestive heart failure in elderly persons: Influence of left ventricular systolic function. The Cardiovascular Health Study. *Ann Intern Med*. 2002;**137**:631-639.

14. Zile MR, Baicu CF, Gaasch WH. Diastolic heart failure: Abnormalities in active relaxation and passive stiffness of the left ventricle. *N Engl J Med*. 2004;**350**:1953-1959.

15. Ennezat PV, Malendowicz SL, Testa M, et al. Physical training in patients with chronic heart failure enhances the expression of genes encoding antioxidative enzymes. *J Am Coll Cardiol*. 2001;**38**:194-198.

16. Turnbull F, for the Blood Pressure Lowering Treatment Trialists' Collaboration. Effects of different blood-pressure–lowering regimens on major cardiovascular events: Results of prospectively-designed overviews of randomised trials. *Lancet*. 2003;**362**:1527-1535.

17. Kostis JB, Davis BR, Cutler J, et al. Prevention of heart failure by antihypertensive drug treatment in older persons with isolated systolic hypertension: SHEP Cooperative Research Group. *JAMA*. 1997;**278**:212-216.

18. ALLHAT Collaborative Research Group. Major cardiovascular events in hypertensive patients randomized to doxazosin vs. chlorthalidone: The Antihypertensive and Lipid-Lowering treatment to present Heart Attack Trial (ALLHAT). *JAMA*. 2000;**283**:1967-1975.

19. Kostis JB. The effect of enalapril on mortal and morbid events in patients with hypertension and left ventricular dysfunction. *Am J Hypertens*. 1995;**8**:909-914.

20. Spargias K, Ball S, Hall A. The prognostic significance of a history of systemic hypertension in patients randomised to either placebo or ramipril following acute myocardial infarction: Evidence from the AIRE study. Acute Infarction Ramipril Efficacy. *J Hum Hypertens*. 1999;**13**:511-516.

21. Gustafsson F, Torp-Pedersen C, Kober L, Hildebrandt P. Effect of angiotensin converting enzyme inhibition after acute myocardial infarction in patients with arterial hypertension. Trandolapril Cardiac Event (TRACE) Study Group. *J Hypertens*. 1997;**15**:793-798.

22. SOLVD Investigators. Effect of enalapril on survival in patients with reduced left ventricular ejection fractions and congestive heart failure: The SOLVD Investigators. *N Engl J Med*. 1991;**325**:293-302.

23. Pfeffer MA, Braunwald E, Moye LA, et al. Effect of captopril on mortality and morbidity in patients with left ventricular dysfunction after myocardial infarction: Results of the survival and ventricular enlargement trial. The SAVE Investigators. *N Engl J Med*. 1992;**327**:669-677.

24. Loeb HS, Johnson G, Henrick A, et al. Effect of enalapril, hydralazine plus isosorbide dinitrate, and prazosin on hospitalization in patients with chronic congestive heart failure: The V-HeFT VA Cooperative Studies Group. *Circulation*. 1993;**87 (6 Suppl)**:V178-V187.

25. CONSENSUS Trial Study Group. Effects of enalapril on mortality in severe congestive heart failure: Results of the Cooperative North Scandinavian Enalapril Survival Study (CONSENSUS). *N Engl J Med*. 1987;**31**:1429-1435.

26. Cohn JN, Tognoni G. A randomized trial of the angiotensin-receptor blocker valsartan in chronic heart failure. *N Engl J Med*. 2001;**345**:1667-1675.

27. Granger CB, McMurray JJ, Yusuf S, et al. Effects of candesartan in patients with chronic heart failure and reduced left-ventricular systolic function intolerant to angiotensin-converting-enzyme inhibitors: The CHARM-Alternative trial. *Lancet*. 2003;**362**:772-776.

28. McMurray JJ, Ostergren J, Swedberg K, et al. Effects of candesartan in patients with chronic heart failure and reduced left-ventricular systolic function taking angiotensin-converting-enzyme inhibitors: The CHARM-Added trial. *Lancet*. 2003;**362**:767-771.

29. Farquharson CA, Struthers AD. Spironolactone increases nitric oxide bioactivity, improves endothelial vasodilator dysfunction, and suppresses vascular angiotensin I/angiotensin II conversion in patients with chronic heart failure. *Circulation*. 2000;**101**:594-597.

30. Pitt B, Zannad F, Remme WJ, et al. The effect of spironolactone on morbidity and mortality in patients with severe heart failure: Randomized Aldactone Evaluation Study Investigators. *N Engl J Med*. 1999;**341**:709-717.

31. Pitt B, Remme W, Zannad F, et al. Eplerenone, a selective aldosterone blocker, in patients with left ventricular dysfunction after myocardial infarction. *N Engl J Med*. 2003;**348**:1309-1321.

32. Juurlink DN, Mamdani MM, Lee DS, et al. Rates of hyperkalemia after publication of the Randomized Aldactone Evaluation Study. *N Engl J Med*. 2004;**351**:543-551.

33. Pitt B, Reichek N, Willenbrock R, et al. Effects of eplerenone, enalapril, and eplerenone/enalapril in patients with essential hypertension and left ventricular hypertrophy: The 4E-left ventricular hypertrophy study. *Circulation*. 2003;**108**:1831-1838.

34. Weinberger MH, Roniker B, Krause SL, Weiss RJ. Eplerenone, a selective aldosterone blocker, in mild-to-moderate hypertension. *Am J Hypertens*. 2002;**15**:709-716.

35. Hochleitner M, Hortnagl H, Ng CK, et al. Usefulness of physiologic dual-chamber pacing in drug-resistant idiopathic dilated cardiomyopathy. *Am J Cardiol*. 1990;**66**:198-202.

36. Hochleitner M, Hortnagl H, Hortnagl H, et al. Long-term efficacy of physiologic dual-chamber pacing in the treatment of end-stage idiopathic dilated cardiomyopathy. *Am J Cardiol*. 1992;**70**:1320-1325.

37. Linde C, Gadler F, Edner M, et al. Results of atrioventricular synchronous pacing with optimized delay in patients with severe congestive heart failure. *Am J Cardiol*. 1995;**75**:919-923.

38. Gold MR, Feliciano Z, Gottlieb SS, Fisher ML. Dual-chamber pacing with a short atrioventricular delay in congestive heart failure: A randomized study. *J Am Coll Cardiol*. 1995;**26**:967-973.

39. Blanc JJ, Etienne Y, Gilard M, et al. Evaluation of different ventricular pacing sites in patients with severe heart failure: Results of an acute hemodynamic study. *Circulation*. 1997;**96**:3273-3277.

40. Cazeau S, Leclercq C, Lavergne T, et al. Effects of multisite biventricular pacing in patients with heart failure and intraventricular conduction delay. *N Engl J Med*. 2001;**344**:873-880.

41. Abraham WT, Fisher WG, Smith AL, et al. Cardiac resynchronization in chronic heart failure. *N Engl J Med*. 2002;**346**:1845-1853.

42. Bradley DJ, Bradley EA, Baughman KL, et al. Cardiac resynchronization and death from progressive heart failure: A meta-analysis of randomized controlled trials. *JAMA*. 2003;**289**:730-740.

43. Freudenberger R, Sikora JA, Fisher M, et al. Electrocardiogram and clinical characteristics of patients referred for cardiac transplantation: Implications for pacing in heart failure. *Clin Cardiol*. 2004;**27**:151-153.

44. Wilkoff BL, Cook JR, Epstein AE, et al. Dual-chamber pacing or ventricular backup pacing in patients with an implantable defibrillator: The Dual Chamber and VVI Implantable Defibrillator (DAVID) Trial. *JAMA*. 2002;**288**:3115-3123.

45. Sweeney MO, Hellkamp AS, Ellenbogen KA, et al. Adverse effect of ventricular pacing on heart failure and atrial fibrillation among patients with normal baseline QRS duration in a clinical trial of pacemaker therapy for sinus node dysfunction. *Circulation*. 2003;**107**:2932-2937.

46. Freudenberger RS, Wilson AC, Lawrence-Nelson J, et al. Myocardial Infarction Data Acquisition System Study Group (MIDAS 9): Permanent pacing is a risk factor for the development of heart failure. *Am J Cardiol.* 2005;**95**:671-674.

47. Pitarys CJ, Forman MB, Panayiotou H, Hansen DE. Long-term effects of excision of the mitral apparatus on global and regional ventricular function in humans. *J Am Coll Cardiol.* 1990;**15**:557-563.

48. Bach DS, Bolling SF. Improvement following correction of secondary mitral regurgitation in end-stage cardiomyopathy with mitral annuloplasty. *Am J Cardiol.* 1996;**78**:966-969.

49. Bolling SF, Pagani FD, Deeb GM, Bach DS. Intermediate-term outcome of mitral reconstruction in cardiomyopathy. *J Thorac Cardiovasc Surg.* 1998;**115**:381-386.

50. Di Donato M, Sabatier M, Dor V, et al. Effects of the Dor procedure on left ventricular dimension and shape and geometric correlates of mitral regurgitation one year after surgery. *J Thorac Cardiovasc Surg.* 2001;**121**:91-96.

51. Jatene AD. Left ventricular aneurysmectomy: Resection or reconstruction. *J Thorac Cardiovasc Surg.* 1985;**89**:321-331.

52. Joyce D, Loebe M, Noon GP, et al. Revascularization and ventricular restoration in patients with ischemic heart failure: The STICH trial. *Curr Opin Cardiol.* 2003;**18**:454-457.

53. McCarthy PM, James KB, Savage RM, et al. Implantable left ventricular assist device: Approaching an alternative for end-stage heart failure. Implantable LVAD Study Group. *Circulation.* 1994;**90**:II83-II86.

54. McCarthy PM, Wang N, Vargo R. Preperitoneal insertion of the HeartMate 1000 IP implantable left ventricular assist device. *Ann Thorac Surg.* 1994;**57**:634-637.

55. Kormos RL, Murali S, Dew MA, et al. Chronic mechanical circulatory support: Rehabilitation, low morbidity, and superior survival. *Ann Thorac Surg.* 1994;**57**:51-57.

56. Sapirstein JS, Pae WE Jr, Rosenberg G, Pierce WS. The development of permanent circulatory support systems. *Semin Thorac Cardiovasc Surg.* 1994;**6**:188-194.

57. Kumpati GS, McCarthy PM, Hoercher KJ. Left ventricular assist device as a bridge to recovery: Present status. *J Card Surg.* 2001;**16**:294-301.

58. Rose EA, Gelijns AC, Moskowitz AJ, et al. Long-term mechanical left ventricular assistance for end-stage heart failure. *N Engl J Med.* 2001;**345**:1435-1443.

58a. Mancini DM, Eisen H, Kussmaul W, et al. Value of peak oxygen consumption for optimal timing of cardiac transplantation in ambulatory patients with heart failure. *Circulation.* 1991;**83**:778-786.

59. International Society for Heart and Lung Transplantation [ISHLT] Transplant Registry Quarterly Reports for Heart in North America. ISHLT 2004. Electronic citation. Found on the Internet at http://www.ishlt.org/registries/quarterlyDataReport.asp, accessed 20 MAY 05 at 12:01 CDT.

60. Kubo SH, Naftel DC, Mills RM Jr, et al. Risk factors for late recurrent rejection after heart transplantation: A multi-institutional, multivariable analysis. Cardiac Transplant Research Database Group. *J Heart Lung Transplant.* 1995;**14**:409-418.

61. Ma H, Hammond EH, Taylor DO, et al. The repetitive histologic pattern of vascular cardiac allograft rejection: Increased incidence associated with longer exposure to prophylactic murine monoclonal anti-CD3 antibody (OKT3). *Transplantation.* 1996;**62**:205-210.

62. Humar A, Payne WD, Sutherland DE, Matas AJ. Clinical determinants of multiple acute rejection episodes in kidney transplant recipients. *Transplantation.* 2000;**69**:2357-2360.

63. Hosenpud JD, Bennett LE, Keck BM, et al. The Registry of the International Society for Heart and Lung Transplantation: Seventeenth official report—2000. *J Heart Lung Transplant.* 2000;**19**:909-931.

64. Weis M, von Scheidt W. Cardiac allograft vasculopathy: A review. *Circulation.* 1997;**96**:2069-2077.

65. Costanzo MR, Naftel DC, Pritzker MR, et al. Heart transplant coronary artery disease detected by coronary angiography: A multi-institutional study of preoperative donor and recipient risk factors. Cardiac Transplant Research Database. *J Heart Lung Transplant.* 1998;**17**:744-753.

66. Grattan MT, Moreno-Cabral CE, Starnes VA, et al. Eight-year results of cyclosporine-treated patients with cardiac transplants. *J Thorac Cardiovasc Surg.* 1990;**99**:500-509.

67. Rickenbacher PR, Pinto FJ, Chenzbraun A, et al. Incidence and severity of transplant coronary artery disease early and up to 15 years after transplantation as detected by intravascular ultrasound. *J Am Coll Cardiol.* 1995;**25**:171-177.

68. Gao SZ, Schroeder JS, Hunt SA, et al. Acute myocardial infarction in cardiac transplant recipients. *Am J Cardiol.* 1989;**64**:1093-1097.

Kidney Disease in Hypertension

Kenneth L. Choi and George L. Bakris

Chronic kidney disease (CKD) is traditionally defined as the presence of long-standing injury to the kidney, as confirmed by kidney biopsy or markers of damage, or a glomerular filtration rate (GFR) of less than 60 mL/minute/1.73 m² for longer than 3 months.[1] Clinically, this condition is manifested as an elevation in serum creatinine concentration higher than the normal range (≥1.2 mg/dL in women or ≥1.4 mg/dL in men). This decrease in renal function and the presence of microalbuminuria (>30 mg/day and <300 mg/day) or the development of albuminuria (≥300 mg/day) clearly indicate the presence of renal dysfunction. Stages of CKD are based on the level of GFR (Table 29-1).[1]

CKD has become a worldwide public health problem. The incidence and prevalence of kidney failure treated by dialysis and kidney transplantation continue to increase in the United States (Fig. 29-1).[2] The number of patients with kidney failure in 2002 was 431,284, and the incidence of kidney failure has increased to 333 new cases per every million people, nearly a quadrupling since 1980.[2]

PATHOPHYSIOLOGY

The key components of hypertension in patients with kidney disease include inappropriately elevated sympathetic nervous activity, activation of the renin-angiotensin-aldosterone system (RAAS), increased arterial stiffness, and impaired salt and water excretion by the kidney. An increase in sympathetic activity contributes to efferent arteriolar vasoconstriction (mediated through α-receptors), thus causing a greater fraction of plasma to traverse the glomerulus and be filtered.[3] This relative increase in filtration of plasma leaves a greater concentration of proteins present when plasma finishes its course through the glomerulus and then enters the network of capillaries surrounding the proximal tubule. Because of this protein enrichment, this plasma has a greater oncotic pressure, so it can recover more sodium filtered at the glomerulus while it passes through the peritubular capillaries and tubules. This process leads to overall sodium retention, primarily obtained from glomerular filtrate.

The sympathetic nerves also stimulate renin release through activation of β-receptors. Release of renin initiates the well-known cascade of the RAAS, which results in an increase in angiotensin II. Angiotensin II increases both efferent arteriolar vascular tone and the filtration fraction, thereby rendering plasma enriched with protein and more capable of sodium recovery. Several processes other than direct sympathetic β₁-receptor stimulation also enhance renin release. As sodium absorption in the proximal renal tubule increases, the amount of sodium present in the distal parts of the nephron diminishes. This fall in distal nephron sodium concentration is an additional stimulus of renin release.

Afferent arteriolar stretch also falls as kidney perfusion diminishes in the presence of falling cardiac output, and this fall in afferent arteriolar tone represents another renin-release signal.

In addition to effects on efferent arteriolar tone, angiotensin II also stimulates proximal tubule cells to recover filtered sodium directly through enhancement of activity in the sodium/hydrogen antiporter on the luminal side of the epithelium. Angiotensin II is a potent stimulus to aldosterone production and release, and angiotensin II indirectly stimulates distal tubule sodium recovery by stimulating aldosterone, which primary acts to resorb sodium at these distal sites.

Aldosterone is produced and released under several regulatory pathways. Corticotropin (formerly adrenocorticotropic hormone [ACTH]) from the pituitary gland is a major regulator of aldosterone production; however, angiotensin II is probably more potent in its effects on aldosterone production and release. Increases in potassium intake and falls in sodium levels are additional factors that increase aldosterone production and release. Aldosterone stimulates the activity of the sodium-potassium adenosine triphosphatase enzyme on the basolateral side of the epithelium and thereby prompts transporting epithelial cells, such as those in the distal nephron and the cortical collecting duct of the kidney, to increase sodium reabsorption. As aldosterone increases sodium uptake into cells, potassium or hydrogen ions are extruded into the urinary lumen to replace the recovered sodium and to balance the residual negative charges, and this process leads to hypokalemia and alkalosis.

As kidney disease progresses, the ability of the kidney to excrete salt and water becomes impaired. As previously mentioned, overactivity of the sympathetic nervous system results in activation of the RAAS, which also impairs the ability of the kidney to excrete salt and water. Multiple other physiologic factors may play a role in impaired salt and water excretion including insulin resistance, altered endothelin function, reduction of nitric oxide synthesis, and altered prostaglandin production. The resultant increase in extracellular volume plays a role in the exacerbation of high blood pressure (BP) in kidney disease.

Several nonhemodynamic effects of angiotensin II also contribute to kidney disease. Angiotensin II stimulates mesangial cell proliferation, induces expression of transforming growth factor-β, and stimulates production of plasminogen activator inhibitor-1, all of which enhance kidney inflammation and lead to glomerular and tubulointerstitial fibrosis.[4]

Increased arterial stiffness also plays a role in hypertension in kidney disease. Both vasoconstriction and the inability to vasodilate through complex neurohumoral and metabolic mediators can mediate this effect. Factors that lead to excess vasoconstriction include overactivity of the sympathetic

Table 29-1 Stages and Prevalence of Chronic Kidney Disease in the United States in 2002

			Prevalence	
Stage	Description	GFR (mL/min/1.73 m²)	N (1000s)	(%)
1	Kidney damage with normal or ↑ GFR	≥90	5900	3.3
2	Kidney damage with mild ↓ GFR	60-89	5300	3.0
3	Moderately ↓ GFR	30-59	7600	4.3
4	Severely ↓ GFR	15-29	400	0.2
5	Kidney failure	<15 or dialysis	300	0.1

↑, increased; ↓, decreased; GFR, glomerular filtration rate; N, number of people (in thousands); % refers to the percentage of the U.S. population.
Modified from Kidney Disease Outcomes Quality Initiative. K/DOQI clinical practice guidelines on hypertension and antihypertensive agents in chronic kidney disease. *Am J Kidney Dis.* 2004;**43 (5 Suppl 2)**:1-290.

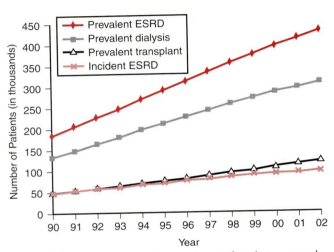

Figure 29–1   Incidence and prevalence of end-stage renal disease (ESRD) in the United States, by modality. (Modified U.S. Renal Data System. USRDS 2004 Annual Data Report: Atlas of End-Stage Renal Disease in the United States, National Institutes of Health, National Institute of Diabetes and Digestive and Kidney Disease, Bethesda, MD, 2004. Found on the Internet at http://www.usrds.org/adr.htm, accessed 13 FEB 05.)

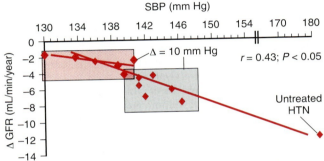

Figure 29–2   Relationship between achieved blood pressures and decline in glomerular filtration rate (GFR) in clinical trials of diabetic and nondiabetic kidney disease. HTN, hypertension; SBP, systolic blood pressure. (Modified from Bakris GL, Williams M, Dworkin L, et al. Preserving renal function in adults with hypertension and diabetes: A consensus approach. National Kidney Foundation Hypertension and Diabetes Executive Committees Working Group. *Am J Kidney Dis.* 2000;**36**:646-661.)

nervous system, activation of the RAAS, and smooth muscle hypertrophy mediated by angiotensin II and potent vasoconstrictors including endothelin. Impaired ability to vasodilate is often mediated by endothelial dysfunction and prostaglandin deficiency.

GOALS OF TREATMENT

Hypertension is both a cause and a complication of CKD. Clinical data support the role of hypertension as a renal risk factor. Data from the Third National Health and Nutrition Examination Survey (NHANES III) estimate that 3% of the civilian population has elevated serum creatinine levels (≥1.6 mg/dL for men and ≥1.4 mg/dL for women) Seventy percent of those with elevated serum creatinine have hypertension.[5] In the 332,544 middle-aged men screened for the Multiple Risk Factor Intervention Trial (MRFIT), BP was a strong predictor of the development of end-stage renal disease

(ESRD) during the 16 years of follow-up.[6] Interventions that lower BP in patients with kidney disease have been shown to slow the progression of that disease. Analysis of long-term clinical trials in diabetic and nondiabetic kidney disease showed that lower achieved BPs result in greater preservation of kidney function (Fig. 29-2).[7] Patients with kidney disease are also at increased risk for cardiovascular events, compared with patients with normal kidney function.[8] Therefore, the goals of antihypertensive therapy in CKD based on the National Kidney Foundation (NKF)–Kidney Disease Outcomes Quality Initiative (K/DOQI) Working Group are to lower BP, to slow the progression of CKD, and to reduce the risk of cardiovascular events.[1]

Blood Pressure Goal

Based on the Seventh Report of the Joint National Committee on Prevention, Detection, Evaluation and Treatment of High Blood Pressure (JNC 7), the BP goal for patients with uncomplicated hypertension is less than 140/90 mm Hg, and if CKD is present, the BP goal is less than 130/80 mm Hg.[9] Two recent trials that randomized hypertensive patients to different levels of BP, the Hypertension Optimal Treatment (HOT) trial and the United Kingdom Prospective Diabetes Study (UKPDS), demonstrated a significant reduction in cardiovascular mortality in diabetic patients assigned to the lower levels of BP.[10,11] In UKPDS, after 9 years of follow-up of 1148 patients with type 2 diabetes, those randomized to "tight BP control" (<150/85 mm Hg) had 24% fewer diabetes-related events (including 44% fewer strokes and 32% fewer deaths) than the group assigned to "less tight control" (<180/105 mm Hg). The initial medication assignment (captopril versus atenolol) did not affect clinical outcomes.[11] Likewise, in the HOT trial of 18,790 people with hypertension, the subgroup of diabetic patients randomized to the lowest BP group (≤80 mm Hg, diastolic) had a highly significant 51% reduction in major cardiovascular events, relative to the group assigned to a diastolic BP of 90 mm Hg or less. Such benefit was not seen, however, for the study as a whole. Thus, with adequate BP reduction, one can prevent or slow the development of cardiovascular events and kidney disease progression.

For patients with CKD, JNC 7 recommends a BP goal of less than 130/80 mm Hg.[10] Achievement of recommended BP goals in CKD is imperative if one is to reduce the rate of kidney disease progression, as well as cardiovascular events. In a meta-analysis of nondiabetic kidney disease studies by the ACE Inhibition in Progressive Renal Disease (AIPRD) study group, the BP associated with the lowest risk of kidney disease progression was a systolic BP range of 110 to 129 mm Hg, which was particularly evident in patients with urinary protein excretion greater than 1 g/day (Fig. 29-3).[12] Table 29-2

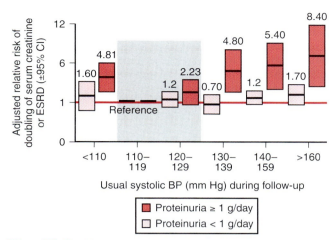

Figure 29–3 Relative risk for kidney disease progression based on in-treatment level of systolic blood pressure (BP) and urine protein excretion (dichotomized by ≥ or <1 g/day), based on a meta-analysis of 11 randomized controlled trials. The reference group for each was a systolic blood pressure of 110 to 119 mm Hg. CI, confidence interval; ESRD, end-stage renal disease. (Modified from Jafar TH, Stark PC, Schmid CH, et al. Progression of chronic kidney disease: The role of blood pressure control, proteinuria, and angiotensin-converting enzyme inhibition. A patient-level meta-analysis. *Ann Intern Med.* 2003;**139**:244-252.)

Table 29-2 Long-Term Outcome Studies with Primary Renal Endpoints

		No. of Patients	Baseline GFR	Follow-up	Favorable Therapy
No Diabetes					
MDRD,[13] 1995	Usual vs. low BP goal	840	40	2.2 yr	Low BP goal in patients with proteinuria
AIPRI,[54] 1996	Benazepril vs. placebo	583	52	3 yr	Benazepril
REIN,[29] 1997	Ramipril vs. placebo	166	56 (39)	16 mo	Ramipril
AASK,[14] 2002	Metoprolol vs. amlodipine vs. ramipril Low vs. usual BP control	1094	46	3-6.4 yr	Ramipril
COOPERATE,[31] 2003	Losartan vs. trandolapril vs. combination	263	38	2.9 yr	Combination
Diabetes					
Captopril Trial,[47] 1993	Captopril vs. placebo	409	68	3 yr	Captopril
Bakris et al.,[49] 1996	Lisinopril vs. nondihydropyridine CCB vs. atenolol	52	59	6 yr	Lisinopril and nondihydropyridine CCB
Bakris et al.,[50] 1997	Verapamil SR vs. atenolol	34	62	54 mo	Verapamil SR
IDNT,[19] 2001	Irbesartan vs. amlodipine vs. placebo	1715	59	2.6 yr	Irbesartan
RENAAL,[18] 2001	Losartan vs. placebo	1513	54	3.4 yr	Losartan
ABCD,[55] 2000	Moderate vs. intensive BP control	470	84	5 yr	No difference

AASK, African American Study of Kidney Disease and Hypertension; ABCD, Appropriate Blood Pressure Control in Diabetes; AIPRI, Angiotensin-Converting Enzyme Inhibition in Progressive Renal Insufficiency; BP, blood pressure; CCB, calcium channel blocker (or antagonist); COOPERATE, Combination Treatment of Angiotensin II Receptor Blocker and Angiotensin-Converting Enzyme Inhibitor in Non-Diabetic Renal Disease; IDNT, Irbesartan Diabetic Nephropathy Trial; MDRD, Modification of Diet in Renal Disease; REIN, Ramipril Efficacy in Nephropathy; RENAAL, Reduction of Endpoints in Non–Insulin-Dependent Diabetes Mellitus with the Angiotensin II Antagonist Losartan; SR, sustained-release.

summarizes long-term clinical trials with primary renal outcomes, including studies that randomized patients to intensive versus regular BP goals. The first trial that randomized patients with advanced nephropathy to two different levels of BP was the Modification of Diet in Renal Disease (MDRD) study. In this study, patients with CKD and high rates of protein excretion who were assigned to the lower BP group (mean arterial pressure [MAP] goal ≤92 mm Hg) had a significantly slower reduction in GFR decline, compared with patients assigned to the higher BP group (MAP ≤107 mm Hg).[13] However, the evidence for this lower BP goal is not as strong in patients with lower levels of proteinuria (i.e., <1 g/day).[13] The African American Study of Kidney Disease and Hypertension (AASK) was another trial that did not show a benefit of a lower BP goal in patients with predominantly microalbuminuria (rather than proteinuria). African American patients with hypertensive kidney disease (GFR between 20 and 65 mL/minute/1.73 m²) and an average urine protein excretion of less than 1 g/day were randomized to a usual BP goal (MAP goal of 102 to 107 mm Hg) or a lower BP goal (MAP goal ≤92 mm Hg). No benefit of the lower BP goal was noted in reducing the decline in GFR, compared with the usual BP goal.[14] These findings are further supported by a meta-analysis by the AIPRD study group, in which no significant relationship was found between the level of achieved systolic BP and the risk of kidney disease progression in patients with less than 1.0 g/day of proteinuria (see Fig. 29-3).[12]

The current BP goals are achieved by 34% of the general population and by 36% of those with diabetes.[15,16] In clinical trials, the percentage of people achieving such goals is roughly double that seen in routine clinical practice, yet in neither setting is it more than 75%. In patients with stage 1 or 2 hypertension (by JNC VI criteria) in the Antihypertensive and Lipid-Lowering Treatment to Prevent Heart Attack Trial (ALLHAT), two medications, on average, were needed to achieve a mean BP of 135/75 mm Hg.[17] Achievement of BP goals is even more difficult in patients with kidney disease, and it requires even more antihypertensive agents to achieve target BP. Data from NHANES III demonstrated that BP control rates in patients with kidney disease were even lower than in the general population, because only 11% of hypertensive patients with elevated serum creatinine had BPs of less than 130/85 mm Hg.[5] To achieve these lower levels of BP control in patients with CKD will require an average of 3.5 to 4.2 different antihypertensive agents in moderate to high doses (Fig. 29-4).[14,18] In the Irbesartan Diabetic Nephrology Trial (IDNT), the study participants, all of whom had diabetic nephropathy (median urinary protein excretion, 2.9 g/day) and renal insufficiency (mean serum creatinine, 1.67 mg/dL), required 4.0 different antihypertensive medications (on average), including the randomized study medication, to reduce mean BP from 159/87 mm Hg at baseline to 140/70 mm Hg at the end of the study.[19]

Although all agents that lower BP reduce cardiovascular risk, certain antihypertensive agents may have an advantage in reducing risk of kidney disease progression in the presence of advanced nephropathy. Both JNC 7 and the K/DOQI-BP guidelines clearly state that compelling and specific indications exist for the use of angiotensin-converting enzyme (ACE) inhibitors and angiotensin receptor blockers (ARBs) to lower BP in patients with either diabetes or kidney disease.[1,9] These guidelines also emphasize that arterial pressure should

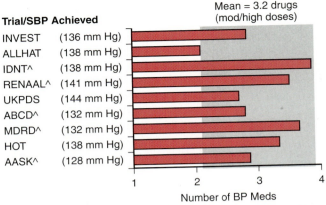

Figure 29–4 Number of blood pressure medications (BP Meds) needed to achieve systolic blood pressure in large clinical trials. The *circumflex* (^) denotes trials with renal endpoints. AASK, African American Study of Kidney Disease and Hypertension; ABCD, Appropriate Blood Pressure Control in Diabetes; ALLHAT, Antihypertensive and Lipid-Lowering Treatment to Prevent Heart Attack Trial; BP, blood pressure; HOT, Hypertension Optimal Treatment; IDNT, Irbesartan Diabetic Nephrology Trial; INVEST, International Verapamil-Trandolapril Study; MDRD, Modification of Diet in Renal Disease; mod/high, moderate to high; RENAAL, Reduction of Endpoints in Non–Insulin-Dependent Diabetes Mellitus with the Angiotensin II Antagonist Losartan; SBP, systolic blood pressure; UKPDS, United Kingdom Prospective Diabetes Study.

be reduced to less than 130/80 mm Hg in such patients, especially in the presence of proteinuria. Once a person has established nephropathy, defined as a serum creatinine of more than 1.4 mg/dL (>123 mmol/L), the most important intervention to slow progression of CKD is aggressive arterial pressure reduction.

Microalbuminuria

The NKF-K/DOQI guidelines define microalbuminuria as a urinary albumin excretion between 30 and 300 mg/day, if measured in a 24-hour urine collection, or 30 to 300 mg/g, if measured by the currently preferred method of spot albumin-to-creatinine ratio (Table 29-3).[1] JNC 7 identified microalbuminuria as a cardiovascular risk factor.[9] People with microalbuminuria in the general population,[20] with or without other cardiovascular risk factors,[5,21,22] are at increased risk for cardiovascular events. As shown in Figure 29-5, higher levels of urinary albumin excretion are associated with an increased risk for adverse cardiovascular disease (CVD) outcomes.[5,20]

Reduction of microalbuminuria is best achieved with agents that block the RAAS system. In the Irbesartan Microalbuminuria for Type 2 Diabetes Mellitus in Hypertensive Patients (IRMA-2) study, which included hypertensive patients with type 2 diabetes and a range of urinary albumin excretion rates from 53.4 to 58.3 μg/minute, treatment with the ARB irbesartan, at 300 mg/day, was associated with a 68% reduction in development of proteinuria resulting from progression of diabetic nephropathy, when compared

Table 29-3   Definitions of Proteinuria and Albuminuria

	Urine Collection Method	Normal	Microalbuminuria	Albuminuria or Clinical Proteinuria
Total Protein	24-Hr excretion	<300 mg/day	NA	>300 mg/day
	Spot urine dipstick	<30 mg/dL	NA	>30 mg/dL
	Spot urine protein-to-creatinine ratio	<200 mg/g	NA	>200 mg/g
Albumin	24-Hr excretion	<30 mg/day	30-300 mg/day	>300 mg/day
	Spot urine albumin-specific dipstick	<3 mg/dL	>3 mg/dL	NA
	Spot urine albumin-to-creatinine ratio	<30 mg/g	30-300 mg/g	>300 mg/g
	Spot urine albumin-to-creatinine ratio (gender-specific definition)	<17 mg/g (men) <25 mg/g (women)	17-250 mg/g (men) 25-355 mg/g (women)	>250 mg/g (men) >355 mg/g (women)

NA, not applicable.
Modified from Kidney Disease Outcomes Quality Initiative. K/DOQI clinical practice guidelines on hypertension and antihypertensive agents in chronic kidney disease. *Am J Kidney Dis.* 2004;**43 (5 Suppl 2)**:1-290.

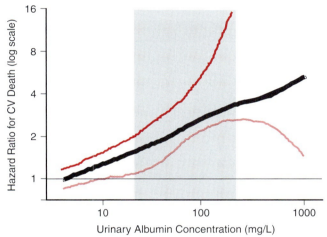

Figure 29-5   Albuminuria as a risk factor for cardiovascular (CV) death in individuals without diabetes. The *black line* in the center corresponds to the mean; the *red and orange lines* correspond to the 95% confidence limits. The *shaded area* between 20 and 200 mg/L denotes the then-current definition of microalbuminuria. (Modified from Hillege HL, Fidler V, Diercks GF, et al. Urinary albumin excretion predicts cardiovascular and noncardiovascular mortality in general population: Prevention of Renal and Vascular End Stage Disease [PREVEND] Study Group. *Circulation.* 2002;**106**:1777-1782.)

with placebo during a 24-month follow-up.[23] Whether reduction of microalbuminuria results in a reduction in cardiovascular endpoints is still uncertain, although the results of the Losartan Intervention for Endpoint Reduction in Hypertension (LIFE) study, the only trial to measure microalbuminuria prospectively in a group at risk for CVD, demonstrated that the group with the lowest event rate had the greatest reduction in microalbuminuria from baseline.[24]

In the Prevention of Renal and Vascular Endstage Disease Intervention Trial (PREVEND IT), 864 inhabitants of the Dutch city, Groningen, who had microalbuminuria (urine albumin excretion of 15 to 300 mg/day) were randomized to fosinopril, 20 mg/day, and/or pravastatin, 40 mg/day, or placebo in a 2 × 2 factorial design.[25] Fosinopril reduced urine

albumin excretion by 26% during a mean follow-up of 46 months; however, the reduction in cardiovascular mortality or cardiovascular hospitalization in patients treated with fosinopril was not statistically significant.[25] The conclusions of this study, however, were limited by the small number of cardiovascular events, as well as by submaximal doses of the ACE inhibitor. The use of adequate doses of agents that block the RAAS is imperative in providing maximal protective effects to the kidney, as demonstrated by IRMA-2, in which only the high dose of irbesartan (300 mg versus 150 mg/day) was clearly associated with reduced progression to albuminuria.[23]

Microalbuminuria, a marker for inflammation, can be prevented by a RAAS blocker in prehypertensive patients with type 2 diabetes. In the Bergamo Nephrologic Diabetes Complications Trial (BENEDICT), diabetic patients with normal urinary albumin excretion were randomized to placebo, the nondihydropyridine calcium antagonist verapamil (240 mg/day), the ACE inhibitor trandolapril (2 mg/day), or their combination (at 180/2 mg/day).[26] There was a significant reduction of progression to microalbuminuria in the subjects treated with trandolapril or the combination (6.0% or 5.7%, respectively), compared with verapamil or placebo (11.9% or 10.0%, respectively).[26]

Proteinuria

The NKF-K/DOQI guidelines define proteinuria as more than 300 mg/day of urinary protein or albumin excretion (see Table 29-3).[1] Elevated levels of urinary albumin excretion, as well as increased stage of kidney disease, are associated with increased risk of CVD or progression to kidney failure.[1] The goal of therapy in patients with proteinuria is to reduce the risk of CVD and the progression to kidney failure. As shown in the MDRD study and the meta-analysis of the AIPRD study group, reduction of BP in patients with proteinuria slows the progression to kidney failure.[12,13] Additionally, reductions in proteinuria correlate not only with preservation of kidney function, but also with reductions in cardiovascular mortality.[27] The only classes of drugs that fail to reduce proteinuria (i.e., dihydropyridine calcium antagonists, α-blockers, hydralazine, and minoxidil) have also failed either to slow the progression of kidney disease or to reduce mortality in the absence of either ACE inhibitors or some other agents that reduce proteinuria.[28]

ACE inhibitors and ARBs are the antihypertensive agents that most consistently reduce proteinuria in diabetic and non-diabetic kidney disease. The use of ACE inhibitors to reduce proteinuria in nondiabetic kidney disease was supported by the Ramipril Efficacy in Nephropathy (REIN) study, AASK, and the 2001 meta-analysis of the AIPRD study group. In REIN, nondiabetic patients with an average creatinine of 2.4 mg/dL and 24-hour urinary protein excretion of greater than 3 g/day were randomized to ramipril, 5 mg/day, or placebo. Patients treated with ramipril had a significant reduction in the decline of GFR and urine protein excretion compared with placebo, with a 55% reduction in median urine protein excretion compared with baseline.[29] In the AASK trial, African American patients with hypertensive nephrosclerosis, mean serum creatinine 2.2 mg/dL, and 24-hour urine protein 0.6 g/day were randomized to ramipril, amlodipine, or metoprolol. Patients treated initially with ramipril had a 22% reduction in the secondary composite outcome of a 50% reduction of GFR, ESRD, or death, compared with metoprolol and a 36% reduction compared with amlodipine.[14] A meta-analysis of nondiabetic kidney disease by the AIPRD study group showed that regimens including an ACE inhibitor were associated with a 31% reduction in progression to ESRD and a 30% reduction in the combined endpoint of doubling of serum creatinine or progression to ESRD.[30] Two randomized controlled trials have shown that ARBs are effective in reducing proteinuria and in slowing the progression of CKD in type 2 diabetic nephropathy. The important secondary endpoint of ESRD alone was significantly lower in the ARB group in the Reduction of Endpoints in Non–Insulin-Dependent Diabetes Mellitus with the Angiotensin II Antagonist Losartan (RENAAL) study, but not in IDNT. This could be because the follow-up time was shorter in IDNT than RENAAL, or the IDNT may have been underpowered for this endpoint because it split enrollment into three randomized groups, rather than two, as in RENAAL. In RENAAL, diabetic patients with nephropathy (mean creatinine, 1.9 mg/dL, and median urine albumin-to-creatinine ratio, 1237 mg/g) were randomized to losartan or placebo. Treatment with losartan resulted in a 16% reduction in the primary endpoint of doubling of serum creatinine, progression to ESRD, or death. Treatment with losartan also resulted in a 35% reduction in the urinary albumin-to-creatinine ratio, whereas patients in the placebo group tended to have an increase in this parameter.[18] In IDNT, diabetic patients with nephropathy (mean serum creatinine, 1.65 to 1.69 mg/dL, and median urinary protein excretion, 2.9 g/day) were randomized to initial treatment with irbesartan, amlodipine, or placebo. Patients treated with irbesartan had a 19% reduction compared with placebo and a 24% reduction compared with amlodipine in the primary composite outcome of doubling of serum creatinine, ESRD, serum creatinine greater than 6.0 mg/dL, or death from any cause. Proteinuria was reduced by 33%, or 1.1 ± 1.7 g/day, in the irbesartan-treated group versus 6%, or 0.1 ± 2.9 g/day, in the amlodipine-treated group and 10%, or 0.3 ± 4.3 g/day, in the placebo group.[19] These trials support the use of ACE inhibitors or ARBs in diabetic and nondiabetic kidney disease with proteinuria.

Dual blockade of the RAAS with ACE inhibitors and ARBs for kidney protection has not been as well studied. However, initial data show that dual blockade of the RAAS can reduce proteinuria and can slow kidney disease progression more than either agent alone. In the Combination Treatment of Angiotensin II Receptor Blocker and Angiotensin-Converting Enzyme Inhibitor in Nondiabetic Renal Disease (COOPERATE) trial, patients with nondiabetic kidney disease and mean urinary protein excretion of 2.5 g/day were randomized to an ARB (losartan, 100 mg/day), an ACE inhibitor (trandolapril, 3 mg daily), or a combination of the two drugs at the same doses.[31] The patients treated with the combined therapy had a 60% to 62% reduction in the primary composite outcome of time to doubling of serum creatinine or ESRD during the 3-year follow-up, compared with either the losartan- or trandolapril-treated group. Urinary protein excretion was reduced significantly more with combined therapy (75.6%), compared with losartan (44.1%) or trandolapril (44.3%) alone.[31] Moreover, these findings were independent of BP differences, because both the office and 24-hour ambulatory BP reductions were similar across all three groups.[32] Larger studies are needed to confirm these findings, given that only 263 patients were randomized in this trial.

Further blockade of the RAAS with aldosterone antagonists may be beneficial in patients already taking an ACE inhibitor or an ARB. Blockade of the RAAS with ACE inhibitors does not necessarily result in decreased plasma aldosterone levels.[33,34] A preliminary study showed that hypertensive patients treated with losartan, 50 mg/day, had no change in plasma aldosterone levels at 12 months.[35] Levels of plasma aldosterone are also elevated in patients with CKD and may play a role in kidney injury.[36,37] Blockade of aldosterone in patients already treated with ACE inhibitors may have beneficial effects in hypertension, CKD, and CVD.[38] Preliminary data suggest that blockade of aldosterone with spironolactone reduces urinary protein excretion in patients with CKD.[39,40] Future studies of aldosterone blockade in combination with an ACE inhibitor or ARB are needed in larger populations of patients to demonstrate kidney function preservation.

Finally, early reductions in proteinuria are predictive of long-term renal outcomes. In a 2005 analysis of the AASK trial, a reduction in proteinuria by more than 50% over the first 6 months yielded a relative risk reduction of ESRD at 5 years by 72%.[41] These data, coupled with similar observations of reductions in microalbuminuria that were associated with fewer cardiovascular events in the LIFE trial,[42] add new importance to assessing albumin-to-creatinine ratios not only initially, but also during follow-up.

Cardiovascular Disease

Patients with decreased GFR are at increased risk for CVD events, compared with patients with normal kidney function, and the risk increases progressively as GFR decreases.[8,43] Dialysis-treated patients have a risk of cardiovascular death approximately 50 to 500 times higher than that of the general population.[1,44] A significant correlation between cardiovascular outcomes and mortality and progressively decreasing GFR has also been demonstrated in patients after a myocardial infarction.[45] Based on the NKF-K/DOQI guidelines, patients with CKD should be considered to be in the highest risk category for CVD.[1]

Because of the slow rate of decline of kidney function and the high death rate associated with CKD, most patients with CKD will not develop kidney failure, but instead will die of complications of CVD. Modification of cardiovascular risk factors is imperative in the treatment of CKD to reduce morbidity and mortality. Therapeutic approaches include risk factor reduction, antiplatelet therapy (e.g., aspirin), aggressive lipid management, BP control, correction of anemia (hematocrit <30%), and possibly coronary revascularization.

MANAGEMENT OF HYPERTENSION IN KIDNEY DISEASE

As mentioned earlier, the ability to achieve the goal BP of less than 130/80 mm Hg in patients with CKD has proved difficult and requires multiple medications. The selection of agents to lower BP is based on the pathophysiology of hypertension in kidney disease, including impaired salt and water excretion and increased vasoconstriction resulting from activation of both the RAAS and the sympathetic nervous system. Therefore, agents that affect these mechanisms, when used in concert, counteract the effects of these systems and thereby help to control BP levels and, consequently, reduce organ injury.

As a result of the increased salt and water retention that accompany worsening kidney function, diuretics typically need to be included in the antihypertensive regimen of patients with CKD. Because thiazide diuretics become less effective when GFR falls to less than 30 to 50 mL/minute/1.73 m^2, adequate BP control in patients with impaired renal function will likely need to include a loop diuretic as part of the antihypertensive regimen.

In patients with CKD and proteinuria, agents that block the RAAS, such as ACE inhibitors or ARBs, are preferred.[1] Based on RENAAL and IDNT, both of which showed a slowing in the decline of GFR, as well as a delay in ESRD, ARBs are the agents of choice for type 2 diabetic nephropathy.[18,19] However, the results of the Diabetics Exposed to Telmisartan and Enalapril (DETAIL) trial tend to corroborate what the K/DOQI guidelines say: either ACE inhibitors or ARBs could be used to manage BP in patients with type 2 diabetes to preserve kidney function.[46] In patients with type 1 diabetic nephropathy, ACE inhibitors are the agents of choice, based on the Captopril in Diabetic Nephropathy trial.[47] This trial

randomized 409 patients with type 1 diabetes and with baseline serum creatinine levels lower than 2.5 mg/dL (average, 1.3 mg/dL) and 24-hour urinary protein excretion of 500 mg/day or higher (average, 2500 to 3000 mg/day) to either captopril 25 mg three times/day or placebo. Patients treated with captopril had a 50% reduction in the combined endpoint of death, need for dialysis, or transplantation compared with placebo.[47] In patients with nondiabetic kidney disease and proteinuria, ACE inhibitors are the agents of choice, based on the REIN study and AASK.[14,29] According to NKF-K/DOQI guidelines, an ACE inhibitor and a diuretic should be the antihypertensive agents of choice in patients with kidney disease, because two or more antihypertensive agents are necessary to achieve BP goal, and ACE inhibitors and ARBs are the preferred agents in kidney disease with proteinuria.[1] Table 29-4 is a summary of the antihypertensive agents of choice in diabetic and nondiabetic kidney disease.

Calcium antagonists (or calcium channel blockers, CCBs) are effective antihypertensive agents in patients with CKD; however, the subclasses of these agents have different antiproteinuric properties beyond their BP-lowering effects in patients with proteinuric kidney disease.[48] As shown in Table 29-2, nondihydropyridine CCBs reduce proteinuria,[49,50] whereas dihydropyridine CCBs do not, unless they are used with a RAAS blocker.[51,52] Additionally, dihydropyridine CCBs are less efficacious in slowing kidney disease progression. In IDNT, patients with proteinuria resulting from type 2 diabetes who were treated with irbesartan had a 24% reduction in the primary endpoint, compared with amlodipine, as well as a significant reduction in urinary protein excretion.[19] Similar findings with ACE inhibitors compared with nondihydropyridine CCBs have been observed in patients with nondiabetic kidney disease with proteinuria. In the AASK trial, African American patients with hypertensive nephrosclerosis who were treated with ramipril had a 36% reduction in the composite outcome of 50% reduction of GFR, ESRD, or death, compared with patients treated with amlodipine.[14] Dihydropyridine CCBs are effective in lowering BP; however, they should not be used in diabetic or nondiabetic kidney disease with proteinuria in the absence of an ACE inhibitor or an ARB.

Table 29-4 Recommendations on Hypertension and Antihypertensive Agents in Chronic Kidney Disease

Type of Kidney Disease	Blood Pressure Target (mm Hg)	Preferred Agents for CKD, with (or without) Hypertension	Other Agents to Reduce CVD Risk and Reach Blood Pressure Target
Diabetic kidney disease	<130/80	ACE inhibitor or ARB	Diuretic preferred, then BB or CCB
Nondiabetic kidney disease with spot urine total protein-to-creatinine ratio ≥200 mg/g	<130/80	ACE inhibitor or ARB	Diuretic preferred, then BB or CCB
Nondiabetic kidney disease with spot urine total protein-to-creatinine ratio <200 mg/g	<130/80	None preferred	Diuretic preferred, then ACE inhibitor, ARB, BB, or CCB

ACE, angiotensin-converting enzyme; ARB, angiotensin II receptor blocker; BB, β-blocker; CCB, calcium channel blocker (or antagonist); CKD, chronic kidney disease; CVD, cardiovascular disease.
Modified from Kidney Disease Outcomes Quality Initiative. K/DOQI clinical practice guidelines on hypertension and antihypertensive agents in chronic kidney disease. *Am J Kidney Dis.* 2004;**43 (5 Suppl 2)**:1-290.

The antihypertensive effects of β-blockers have been well established; however, no evidence indicates that these agents provide additional renoprotective effects. Evidence regarding whether β-blockers are associated with increased risk of progression of kidney disease is conflicting. In a study of non–insulin-dependent diabetes and proteinuria, patients were titrated to atenolol, 100 mg/day, versus sustained-release verapamil, 480 mg/day. Patients treated with verapamil had a significant reduction in creatinine rise and proteinuria, compared with the β-blocker group at 54 months.[50] However, in UKPDS, patients with type 2 diabetes were randomized to captopril or atenolol. No significant difference was reported in the percentage of patients with doubling of serum creatinine concentration, development of proteinuria, or urine albumin concentration greater than 50 mg/L.[11] These findings suggest that any renoprotective effect of atenolol was the result of lowering of BP.

Despite the large body of evidence from long-term clinical trials demonstrating the renal protective effects of ACE inhibitors and ARBs for patients with CKD, some clinicians hesitate to prescribe these agents in patients with serum creatinine levels greater than 1.4 mg/dL, because these levels often rise after the drug is given. The most common cause of increased creatinine following blockade of the RAAS is decreased arterial blood volume, often resulting from volume depletion or low cardiac output. With kidney dysfunction, the autoregulatory ability of the kidney to maintain renal arterial pressure diminishes. This results in a direct relationship between BP and GFR; therefore, an abrupt decrease in BP often causes a pressure-related drop in GFR, manifesting as an increase in serum creatinine. Analysis of long-term clinical trials has confirmed that ACE inhibitor–induced reduction in kidney function plateaus within 2 months.[53] If the serum creatinine level increases by more than 30%, or if it continues to rise after 3 months of therapy, volume depletion, unsuspected left ventricular dysfunction, or bilateral renal artery stenosis should be considered. In addition to these potential problems with increases in serum creatinine, ACE inhibitors and ARBs are often discontinued because of rises in serum potassium levels. This should be worrisome only if serum potassium rises 0.5 mEq/L or more and the baseline level is already greater than 5 mEq/L. Otherwise, elevations in serum potassium can often be managed, typically with dietary education about potassium-containing foods. In the COOPERATE trial, only 8% (7 of 88) of the patients receiving combination treatment with an ACE inhibitor and an ARB developed hyperkalemia. All these patients were successfully treated with dietary education or potassium binders for their hyperkalemia.[32] Therefore, ACE inhibitors should be withdrawn only when the rise in serum creatinine exceeds 30% more than baseline within the first 2 months of therapy or when hyperkalemia (serum potassium >5.6 mEq/L) occurs.

CONCLUSION

Because of the rising prevalence of CKD in the population, slowing the progression of renal dysfunction has become increasingly important in preventing kidney failure. The goals of therapy in patients with CKD are to control BP, to slow the progression of renal dysfunction, and to reduce cardiovascular risk. Strong evidence now indicates that BP should be reduced to less than 130/80 mm Hg in patients with CKD, especially if proteinuria is present. ACE inhibitors or ARBs are effective in reducing proteinuria and in slowing the progression of renal dysfunction. Based on these observations, as well as the need for multiple antihypertensive agents to control BP, patients with hypertension and proteinuria should be initially managed with a diuretic and ACE inhibitor or ARB, with other classes of antihypertensive agents added to reach goal BP.

References

1. Kidney Disease Outcomes Quality Initiative. K/DOQI clinical practice guidelines on hypertension and antihypertensive agents in chronic kidney disease. *Am J Kidney Dis.* 2004;**43** (**5 Suppl 2**):1-290.
2. U.S. Renal Data System. USRDS 2004 Annual Data Report: Atlas of End-Stage Renal Disease in the United States, National Institutes of Health, National Institute of Diabetes and Digestive and Kidney Disease, Bethesda, Md, 2004. Found on the Internet at http://www.usrds.org/adr.htm, accessed 13 FEB 05.
3. Joles JA, Koomans HA. Causes and consequences of increased sympathetic activity in renal disease. *Hypertension.* 2004;**43**: 699-706.
4. Taal MW, Brenner BM. Renoprotective benefits of RAS inhibition: From ACEI to angiotensin II antagonists. *Kidney Int.* 2000;**57**:1803-1817.
5. Coresh J, Wei GL, McQuillan G, et al. Prevalence of high blood pressure and elevated serum creatinine level in the United States: Findings from the third National Health and Nutrition Examination Survey (1988-1994). *Arch Intern Med.* 2001;**161**:1207-1216.
6. Klag MJ, Whelton PK, Randall BL, et al. Blood pressure and end-stage renal disease in men. *N Engl J Med.* 1996;**334**:13-18.
7. Bakris GL, Williams M, Dworkin L, et al. Preserving renal function in adults with hypertension and diabetes: A consensus approach. National Kidney Foundation Hypertension and Diabetes Executive Committees Working Group. *Am J Kidney Dis.* 2000;**36**:646-661.
8. Go AS, Chertow GM, Fan D, et al. Chronic kidney disease and the risks of death, cardiovascular events, and hospitalization. *N Engl J Med.* 2004;**351**:1296-1305.
9. Chobanian AV, Bakris GL, Black HR, et al. Seventh Report of the Joint National Committee on Prevention, Detection, Evaluation, and Treatment of High Blood Pressure. *Hypertension.* 2003;**42**:1206-1252.
10. Hansson L, Zanchetti A, Carruthers SG, et al. Effects of intensive blood-pressure lowering and low-dose aspirin in patients with hypertension: Principal results of the Hypertension Optimal Treatment (HOT) randomised trial. HOT Study Group. *Lancet.* 1998;**351**:1755-1762.
11. UK Prospective Diabetes Study Group. Tight blood pressure control and risk of macrovascular and microvascular complications in type 2 diabetes: UKPDS 38. *BMJ.* 1998;**317**:703-713.
12. Jafar TH, Stark PC, Schmid CH, et al. Progression of chronic kidney disease: The role of blood pressure control, proteinuria, and angiotensin-converting enzyme inhibition. A patient-level meta-analysis. *Ann Intern Med.* 2003;**139**:244-252.
13. Peterson JC, Adler S, Burkart JM, et al. Blood pressure control, proteinuria, and the progression of renal disease: The Modification of Diet in Renal Disease study. *Ann Intern Med.* 1995;**123**:754-762.
14. Wright JT Jr, Bakris G, Greene T, et al. Effect of blood pressure lowering and antihypertensive drug class on progression of hypertensive kidney disease: Results of the AASK trial. *JAMA.* 2002;**288**:2421-2431.

15. Cheung BMY, Ong KL, Man YB, et al. Prevalence, awareness, treatment and control of hypertension: United States National Health and Nutrition Examination Survey, 2001-2002. *J Clin Hypertens*. 2006;**8**:93-98.

16. Saydah SH, Fradkin J, Cowie CC. Poor control of risk factors for vascular disease among adults with previously diagnosed diabetes. *JAMA*. 2004;**291**:335-342.

17. ALLHAT Officers and Coordinators for the ALLHAT Collaborative Research Group. Major outcomes in high-risk hypertensive patients randomized to angiotensin-converting enzyme inhibitor or calcium channel blocker vs diuretic: The Antihypertensive and Lipid-Lowering Treatment to Prevent Heart Attack Trial (ALLHAT). *JAMA*. 2002;**288**:2981-2997.

18. Brenner BM, Cooper ME, de Zeeuw D, et al. Effects of losartan on renal and cardiovascular outcomes in patients with type 2 diabetes and nephropathy. *N Engl J Med*. 2001;**345**:861-869.

19. Lewis EJ, Hunsicker LG, Clarke WR, et al. Renoprotective effect of the angiotensin-receptor antagonist irbesartan in patients with nephropathy due to type 2 diabetes. *N Engl J Med*. 2001;**345**:851-860.

20. Hillege HL, Fidler V, Diercks GF, et al. Urinary albumin excretion predicts cardiovascular and noncardiovascular mortality in general population: Prevention of Renal and Vascular End Stage Disease (PREVEND) Study Group. *Circulation*. 2002;**106**:1777-1782.

21. Gerstein HC, Mann JF, Yi Q, et al. Albuminuria and risk of cardiovascular events, death, and heart failure in diabetic and nondiabetic individuals. *JAMA*. 2001;**286**:421-426.

22. Wachtell K, Ibsen H, Olsen MH, et al. Albuminuria and cardiovascular risk in hypertensive patients with left ventricular hypertrophy: The LIFE study. *Ann Intern Med*. 2003;**139**:901-906.

23. Parving HH, Lehnert H, Brochner-Mortensen J, et al. The effect of irbesartan on the development of diabetic nephropathy in patients with type 2 diabetes. *N Engl J Med*. 2001;**345**:870-878.

24. Ibsen H, Wachtell K, Olsen MH, et al. Does albuminuria predict cardiovascular outcome on treatment with losartan versus atenolol in hypertension with left ventricular hypertrophy? A LIFE substudy. *J Hypertens*. 2004;**22**:1805-1811.

25. Asselbergs FW, Diercks GF, Hillege HL, et al. Effects of fosinopril and pravastatin on cardiovascular events in subjects with microalbuminuria. *Circulation*. 2004;**110**:2809-2816.

26. Ruggenenti P, Fassi A, Ilieva AP, et al. Preventing microalbuminuria in type 2 diabetes. *N Engl J Med*. 2004;**351**:1941-1951.

27. Bakris GL. Microalbuminuria: Prognostic implications. *Curr Opin Nephrol Hypertens*. 1996;**5**:219-223.

28. Makrilakis K, Bakris G. Diabetic hypertensive patients: Improving their prognosis. *J Cardiovasc Pharmacol*. 1998;**31** (**Suppl 2**):S34-S40.

29. GISEN Group (Gruppo Italiano di Studi Epidemiologici in Nefrologia). Randomised placebo-controlled trial of effect of ramipril on decline in glomerular filtration rate and risk of terminal renal failure in proteinuric, non-diabetic nephropathy: The GISEN Group (Gruppo Italiano di Studi Epidemiologici in Nefrologia). *Lancet*. 1997;**349**:1857-1863.

30. Jafar TH, Schmid CH, Landa M, et al. Angiotensin-converting enzyme inhibitors and progression of nondiabetic renal disease: A meta-analysis of patient-level data. *Ann Intern Med*. 2001;**135**:73-87.

31. Nakao N, Yoshimura A, Morita H, et al. Combination treatment of angiotensin II receptor blocker and angiotensin converting-enzyme inhibitor in non-diabetic renal disease (COOPERATE): A randomised controlled trial. *Lancet*. 2003;**361**:117-124.

32. Nakao N, Seno H, Kasuga H, et al. Effects of combination treatment with losartan and trandolapril on office and ambulatory blood pressures in non-diabetic renal disease: A COOPERATE-ABP substudy. *Am J Nephrol*. 2004;**24**:543-548.

33. Sato A, Saruta T. Aldosterone breakthrough during angiotensin-converting enzyme inhibitor therapy. *Am J Hypertens*. 2003;**16**:781-788.

34. Sato A, Saruta T. Aldosterone escape during angiotensin-converting enzyme inhibitor therapy in essential hypertensive patients with left ventricular hypertrophy. *J Int Med Res*. 2001;**29**:13-21.

35. Grossman E, Peleg E, Carroll J, et al. Hemodynamic and humoral effects of the angiotensin II antagonist losartan in essential hypertension. *Am J Hypertens*. 1994;**7**:1041-1044.

36. Hene RJ, Boer P, Koomans HA, Mees EJ. Plasma aldosterone concentrations in chronic renal disease. *Kidney Int*. 1982;**21**:98-101.

37. Hollenberg NK. Aldosterone in the development and progression of renal injury. *Kidney Int*. 2004;**66**:1-9.

38. Hostetter TH, Ibrahim HN. Aldosterone in chronic kidney and cardiac disease. *J Am Soc Nephrol*. 2003;**14**:2395-2401.

39. Chrysostomou A, Becker G. Spironolactone in addition to ACE inhibition to reduce proteinuria in patients with chronic renal disease. *N Engl J Med*. 2001;**345**:925-926.

40. Sato A, Hayashi K, Naruse M, Saruta T. Effectiveness of aldosterone blockade in patients with diabetic nephropathy. *Hypertension*. 2003;**41**:64-68.

41. Lea J, Greene T, Hebert L, et al. The relationship between magnitude of proteinuria reduction and risk of end-stage renal disease: Results of the African American Study of Kidney Disease and Hypertension. *Arch Intern Med*. 2005;**165**:947-953.

42. Ibsen H, Olsen MH, Wachtell K, et al. Reduction in albuminuria translates to reduction in cardiovascular events in hypertensive patients: Losartan Intervention For Endpoint Reduction in Hypertension Study. *Hypertension*. 2005;**45**:198-202.

43. Manjunath G, Tighiouart H, Ibrahim H, et al. Level of kidney function as a risk factor for atherosclerotic cardiovascular outcomes in the community. *J Am Coll Cardiol*. 2003;**41**:47-55.

44. Sarnak MJ, Levey AS. Cardiovascular disease and chronic renal disease: A new paradigm. *Am J Kidney Dis*. 2000;**35** (**4 Suppl 1**):S117-S131.

45. Anavekar NS, McMurray JJ, Velazquez EJ, et al. Relation between renal dysfunction and cardiovascular outcomes after myocardial infarction. *N Engl J Med*. 2004;**351**:1285-1295.

46. Barnett AH, Bain SC, Bouter P, et al. Angiotensin-receptor blockade versus converting-enzyme inhibition in type 2 diabetes and nephropathy. *N Engl J Med*. 2004;**351**:1952-1961.

47. Lewis EJ, Hunsicker LG, Bain RP, Rohde RD. The effect of angiotensin-converting-enzyme inhibition on diabetic nephropathy: The Collaborative Study Group. *N Engl J Med*. 1993;**329**:1456-1462.

48. Bakris GL, Weir MR, Secic M, et al. Differential effects of calcium antagonist subclasses on markers of nephropathy progression. *Kidney Int*. 2004;**65**:1991-2002.

49. Bakris GL, Copley JB, Vicknair N, et al. Calcium channel blockers versus other antihypertensive therapies on progression of NIDDM associated nephropathy. *Kidney Int*. 1996;**50**:1641-1650.

50. Bakris GL, Mangrum A, Copley JB, et al. Effect of calcium channel or beta-blockade on the progression of diabetic nephropathy in African Americans. *Hypertension*. 1997;**29**:744-750.

51. Smith AC, Toto R, Bakris GL. Differential effects of calcium channel blockers on size selectivity of proteinuria in diabetic glomerulopathy. *Kidney Int*. 1998;**54**:889-896.

52. Bakris GL, Weir MR, Shanifar S, et al. Effects of blood pressure level on progression of diabetic nephropathy: Results from the RENAAL study. *Arch Intern Med*. 2003;**163**:1555-1565.

53. Bakris GL, Weir MR. Angiotensin-converting enzyme inhibitor-associated elevations in serum creatinine: Is this a cause for concern? *Arch Intern Med*. 2000;**160**:685-693.

54. Maschio G, Alberti D, Janin G, et al. Effect of the angiotensin-converting-enzyme inhibitor benazepril on the progression of chronic renal insufficiency: The Angiotensin-Converting Enzyme Inhibition in Progressive Renal Insufficiency Study Group. *N Engl J Med*. 1996;**334**:939-945.

55. Estacio RO, Jeffers BW, Gifford N, Schrier RW. Effect of blood pressure control on diabetic microvascular complications in patients with hypertension and type 2 diabetes. *Diabetes Care*. 2000;**23 (Suppl 2)**:B54-B64.

Chapter 30

Transplant Hypertension

Sandra J. Taler

Hypertension is a common feature in solid organ transplantation, as a result of preexisting disease and the vascular effects of immunosuppressive medications. Transplant recipients frequently carry a heavy burden of atherosclerotic disease involving multiple vascular beds. Hypertension may be a cause or a complication of native kidney disease or renal allograft injury. Regardless of which manifests first, hypertension may accelerate further renal decline, particularly when proteinuria is present. Thus, transplant recipients are at high cardiovascular (CV) risk at the time of transplantation, and they require treatment to attempt to reduce this risk, including blood pressure (BP) control.

Hypertension occurs regularly following solid organ transplantation in heart, liver, kidney, and bone marrow recipients. In the pre–calcineurin inhibitor (CNI) era before 1985, the incidence of hypertension after renal transplant was estimated to be 45% to 55%; it increased with adoption of cyclosporine-based and then tacrolimus-based immunosuppression to current rates of 70% to 90%.[1] CNIs are also associated with hypertension in nontransplant settings.[2,3] Hypertension after transplantation may be a continuation of pretransplant hypertension, or it may be related to immunosuppressive medications (CNIs, corticosteroids) or sodium and volume retention. In kidney transplant recipients, worsening or de novo hypertension may result from reduced renal function caused by graft rejection, chronic allograft nephropathy, or hypoperfusion related to transplant renal artery stenosis. De novo hypertension may occur when a normotensive recipient receives a kidney from a hypertensive donor. As immunosuppressive medication doses are reduced with time after transplant, the severity of hypertension declines, resulting in improved control rates. Even so, current control rates are suboptimal, and treatment can be challenging.

As outcomes of solid organ transplantation continue to improve, the premature death of a patient with a functioning graft, often as a result of CV disease, has become a major cause of transplant failure.[4,5] Frequently, other CV risk factors (e.g., weight, lipid levels) also worsen.[6,7] Clinicians caring for transplant recipients must understand the impact of hypertension on CV risk, on renal insufficiency, and, for renal transplant recipients, on long-term success of the renal allograft. Nonimmunologic factors such as hypertension are major determinants of long-term kidney graft survival.[8,9] Levels of BP 1 year after renal transplant predict allograft survival over subsequent years.[10] Whether effective BP control can reduce renal allograft injury and improve survival is not yet proven.

PATHOGENESIS

Immunosuppressive Therapy

Post-transplant hypertension results from a combination of factors, including preexisting disease, effects of calcineurin inhibition and corticosteroids, and underlying renal dysfunction. These effects result in the new appearance or exacerbation of hypertension in virtually every clinical situation in which CNIs are used. Improved survival rates with cyclosporine, as compared with previous regimens, led to broad expansion of solid organ transplantation, including liver, heart, lung, and kidney-pancreas combinations.[11] Tacrolimus shares the final common pathway of calcineurin inhibition, but it differs from cyclosporine in potency and side effects. Whereas the rate of rise in BP and accelerated CV risk are more prominent with cyclosporine, tacrolimus causes greater nephrotoxicity and glucose intolerance. Prevalence rates of post-transplant hypertension with cyclosporine and tacrolimus are similar by 1 year after transplant.[12] Vasoconstriction in the kidney results in decreased renal blood flow and glomerular filtration rate (GFR) within hours of CNI administration.[13-16] Studies in physiologically normal subjects indicate a rise in arterial BP within days to weeks of cyclosporine administration, before changes in renal function or sodium balance can be detected.[1,17] With addition of corticosteroids, BP may increase further over the first weeks or months.[16,18]

Hypertension prevalence rates for heart and liver transplant recipients who are treated with the combination of CNIs and corticosteroids range from 70% to 100%.[1] Following liver transplantation, hypertension typically occurs de novo in previously normotensive individuals. Serial studies in liver transplant recipients indicate that the rise in BP progresses to clinically significant levels over several weeks, sometimes rising 40 to 50 mm Hg and requiring initiation of antihypertensive therapy.[1] Hemodynamic measurements document a transition from hyperdynamic to normal cardiac output and a progressive rise in systemic vascular resistance from lower than normal levels to widespread vasoconstriction. Early volume expansion resolves gradually by pressure-induced natriuresis, despite reduced renal blood flow and GFR. Renal transplant recipients present a special challenge in isolating the hypertensive and nephrotoxic effects of CNIs. Most patients with renal failure are hypertensive before transplantation. Transplant complications such as rejection, organ preservation injury, and transplant renal artery stenosis can impair renal function and worsen hypertension. Nevertheless, direct aggravation of hypertension by CNIs has been confirmed by BP reductions seen with later conversion to a non–CNI-based immunosuppressive regimen.[19] This phenomenon occurs despite equally severe renal dysfunction in patients whose hypertension "resolves."

Although multiple factors may be responsible for CNI-induced vasoconstriction, careful mechanistic studies are lacking, because animal models fail to reflect findings in humans. The hemodynamic basis for elevated arterial pressure during CNI administration is increased systemic vascular resistance. Plasma renin activity is low early after transplantation and then rises gradually, perhaps related to renal parenchymal injury and arteriolar disease.[20,21] Local production of vasoactive mediators, such as nitric oxide, prostacyclin, and endothelin, may profoundly alter vasomotor tone. Endothelin and thromboxane are increased in the systemic and renal circulations,[22,23] whereas prostacyclin and nitric oxide levels fall, indicating impaired vasodilatation.[20,24-26] It is likely that CNIs alter function of the endothelium by shifting the relative balance of vasoconstrictive and vasodilatory pathways.

The role of the sympathetic nervous system in post-transplant hypertension remains uncertain. Microneurographic studies of adrenergic nerve traffic in cardiac transplant recipients indicate that cyclosporine enhances nerve activity, although circulating catecholamine levels are normal.[27] Other studies have not confirmed these results.[28] Renal transplant recipients demonstrate CNI-induced vasoconstriction and hypertension immediately after transplantation, despite surgical denervation. Studies in liver transplant recipients report a decrease in sympathetic nerve activity during cyclosporine administration.[29]

Hypertension and renal dysfunction attributed to CNIs commonly coexist. Although both conditions reflect vasoconstriction, CNI nephrotoxicity alone does not explain CNI-induced hypertension. CNIs produce transient, intense vasoconstriction within the kidney shortly after administration that leads to reductions in renal blood flow, GFR, and sodium excretion.[30] These changes may reverse if treatment is discontinued or reduced. Sustained administration of CNIs results in vascular and interstitial changes that eventually become irreversible. CNI nephrotoxicity may cause end-stage renal failure in up to 10% of cardiac and liver transplant recipients, and it leads to consideration of second transplants in individual cases. As with other types of renal failure, worsening hypertension is a characteristic feature as renal function deteriorates.

Azathioprine and mycophenolate mofetil have not been associated with hypertension. The effects of sirolimus on BP are less clear, but reports of BP lowering with conversion from cyclosporine to sirolimus support either less or no hypertensive effects.[31]

Corticosteroids

Although the magnitude of the effect is not well documented, corticosteroids are associated with hypertension in nontransplant settings.[32,33] Multiple studies have demonstrated reductions in BP with dose reduction or discontinuation of corticosteroids, even in patients taking prednisone doses as low as 5 mg/day.[34] Estimates suggest that up to 15% of cases of post-transplant hypertension may be explained by corticosteroid effect, and this complication adds substantial cost to the management of transplant recipients.[35] Glucocorticoids can cause hypertension, even in the absence of a mineralocorticoid effect. At doses usually used after transplantation, some activation of mineralocorticoid receptors occurs, manifested by potassium wasting, especially with high sodium intake. Glucocorticoid effects include increased cardiac output and enhanced pressor responses to epinephrine, angiotensin II, and other pressure stimuli.[36]

The role of corticosteroids in CNI-induced hypertension is complex. Although glucocorticoids alone rarely have major effects on BP in physiologically normal subjects, corticosteroids administered in immunosuppressive doses to patients with impaired renal function commonly aggravate hypertension. The association of higher hypertension incidence rates with higher steroid dosage in liver transplant recipients receiving tacrolimus suggests that higher steroid doses profoundly affect the rate and severity of BP change.[12] Experience with steroid withdrawal indicates that BP falls, despite continued CNI administration.[34,37] Hence, it is likely that CNIs, steroids, and their combination are major elements in the prevalence and severity of post-transplant hypertension.

CLINICAL FEATURES

Hypertension developing after organ transplantation is characterized by abnormal circadian BP rhythm (Fig. 30-1), with absence or reversal of the normal 10% to 20% nocturnal fall commonly seen in physiologically normal subjects and in those with essential hypertension. The magnitude of this fall is blunted after transplantation, and some patients develop a paradoxical rise in BP, with the highest pressures in the overnight hours. In the nontransplant setting, loss of a nocturnal BP fall is associated with accelerated target organ damage, including left ventricular hypertrophy, lacunar stroke, and microalbuminuria.[38-40] Thus, nocturnal BP elevations may predispose transplant recipients to accelerated atherosclerotic complications. Patients may present with nocturnal headaches and profound nocturia associated with accelerated hypertension, producing retinal hemorrhages and central nervous system symptoms. This phenomenon is best documented using overnight ambulatory BP monitoring. Circadian reversal has been observed following heart, liver, and kidney transplantation, most commonly in the first year.[41] In a study of 241 renal transplant recipients at a median ambulatory BP monitoring–transplant interval of 14 weeks, abnormal systolic diurnal variation correlated positively with age, serum creatinine, and blood cyclosporine trough level and negatively with GFR and the time interval from transplantation.[42] In this series, 21% of patients had isolated nocturnal hypertension with normal daytime pressures. Only age and GFR were independent predictors of abnormal systolic diurnal variation.

Serial studies in cardiac and liver transplant recipients suggest that some patients will regain more normal circadian BP patterns within the first year after transplantation.[43,44] Steroids have been associated with loss of nocturnal BP fall in other situations, such as Cushing's syndrome.[45,46] Because steroid doses are routinely tapered at later times after transplantation, it is difficult to separate the effects of steroid dose

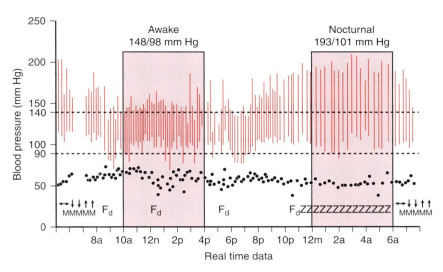

Figure 30–1 Example of reversed circadian blood pressure (BP) rhythm following liver transplantation. The magnitude of the normal nocturnal BP fall may be blunted, and some patients develop a paradoxical rise in BP, with highest pressures in the overnight hours. This is sometimes associated with nocturia, headache, and disrupted sleep. F_d indicates food intake; M, indicates manual calibration measurements in the ↔ supine, ↓↓ seated, and ↑↑ standing positions; z indicates sleep; • indicates heart rate.

from the effects of other time-related mechanisms after transplant. In some patients, this phenomenon represents exaggeration of disturbed autonomic nervous system control associated with diabetes or obstructive sleep apnea.

Primarily reported with cyclosporine, CNI-associated hypertension may progress to an accelerated phase with vascular injury, including microangiopathic hemolysis, encephalopathy, and seizures.[1] Intracranial hemorrhage has occurred. The most severe manifestations occur in children and in patients who were previously normotensive. Distinguishing between the effects of high BP and direct vascular toxicity from cyclosporine may be difficult.

EVALUATION

The diagnosis of hypertension in transplant recipients follows criteria published in the Seventh Report of the Joint National Committee on Prevention, Detection, Evaluation and Treatment of High Blood Pressure.[47] Elevated office BP measurements should be verified by standardized nurse-administered measurements, ambulatory BP monitoring, or home self-measurement. For recipients of nonrenal allografts, post-transplant hypertension is primarily related to the effects of immunosuppression, including volume retention and nephrotoxicity. Following kidney transplantation, BP alterations may provide clues to subclinical acute rejection, hypoperfusion, or chronic allograft nephropathy. Causes of post-transplant hypertension occurring within the first 3 months after transplant generally differ from causes of late or persistent hypertension (Table 30-1). This distinction is useful when considering possible causes and choosing appropriate treatment.

Severe hypertension during the early postoperative period is more common in patients with severe hypertension before transplantation, in African Americans, and in patients with delayed graft function. Primary mediators include hypervolemia, high CNI and glucocorticoid doses, withdrawal of preoperative antihypertensive medications, and postoperative pain. In a recent series of deceased donor kidney recipients, postoperative systolic hypertension was associated with an increased risk for acute rejection, perhaps related to the

Table 30-1 Causes of Post-transplant Hypertension

Within the First 3 Months
Pretransplant hypertension
African-American race
Renal allograft dysfunction
Renal outflow obstruction
Hypervolemia
High-dose calcineurin inhibitors
High-dose corticosteroids
Postoperative pain
Discontinuation of pretransplant antihypertensive medications

During Long-Term Care
Donor variables
Increased donor age
African-American donor
Hypertensive donor

Recipient variables
Older age
African-American race
Male gender
Obesity
Diabetes mellitus
Pretransplant hypertension
Native kidney disease
Renal allograft dysfunction
Recurrent primary renal disease
Immunosuppressive medications
   Calcineurin inhibitors
   Corticosteroids
Transplant renal artery stenosis

inability of donor kidneys to autoregulate, with consequent augmented graft inflammation and injury.[10,48] Beyond the first 3 months, hypertension may relate to donor variables, because donor age and donor hypertension are strongly associated with graft function. A well-functioning renal allograft frequently improves and may even normalize BP in the recipient. Many features of post-transplant hypertension are similar to those of the general population with hypertension, including higher prevalence in African Americans, in male recipients, and in those at higher weight or body mass index. Recipients with preexisting diabetes are more likely to be hypertensive, with primarily systolic hypertension and widened pulse pressures.[49] Studies in nontransplant populations implicate arterial stiffening as the cause for this pattern, which is associated with greater CV risk.

In evaluating patients with post-transplant hypertension, hypertension is both a sign of kidney disease and a cause of kidney dysfunction. Renal transplant recipients with lower renal function (creatinine clearance <60 mL/minute in the first year) are more likely to develop post-transplant hypertension.[50] Alternatively, hypertension is associated with reduced renal allograft survival, independent of renal function.[8] Worsening hypertension suggests an acute or chronic graft pathologic process that may be otherwise clinically silent. A kidney allograft biopsy often provides clinically useful information, including the presence of subclinical acute rejection, recurrent or de novo glomerulopathies, CNI toxicity, viral infections, or other pathologic changes that require modifications in treatment. Hypertension is likely to worsen with declining allograft function, and it may be particularly severe in patients with chronic transplant glomerulopathy or focal segmental glomerulosclerosis developing late after transplant.

Transplant renal artery stenosis may present as de novo or worsening hypertension or as a decline in renal function precipitated by BP treatment, particularly with use of angiotensin-converting enzyme (ACE) inhibitors or angiotensin receptor blockers (ARBs). Anastomotic stenosis is most likely in recipients of pediatric deceased donor kidneys related to smaller donor vessels and in recipients of living donor kidneys related to the nature of the anastomotic technique without use of a donor aortic patch. Risk factors include older recipient age, male sex, a history of smoking, and preexisting diabetes. Stenosis of the iliac artery is likely the result of atherosclerotic disease, and it may be associated with other symptoms of peripheral vascular disease. Stenosis of the allograft artery may result from atherosclerotic disease of donor origin or, more often, progressive stenosis at the surgical anastomotic site. Low-pitched systolic bruits are common over the surgical anastomotic site without stenosis; even systolic-diastolic bruits may result from an arteriovenous fistula caused by allograft biopsy. Several Doppler ultrasound series report arterial stenosis prevalence rates of 9% to 12%, but the technique requires operator expertise because of the variability in angles required to visualize the artery.[51] Magnetic resonance angiography has been reported to give a high proportion of false-positive results, although visualization is superior. Treatment by endovascular repair with angioplasty or stenting can provide recovery of blood flow with improvement or stabilization of renal function.[52] Restenosis is common and may require surgical correction of the stenotic segment.

TREATMENT

Current hypertension treatment guidelines advise target BP levels lower than 130/80 mm Hg in all high-risk groups, especially patients with diabetes or proteinuric renal disease.[53]

For kidney transplant recipients, as for patients with chronic kidney disease, there may be additional benefits of lowering BP to these targets. During the first few months after transplant, rapid changes in immunosuppression, volume shifts, and changes in renal function require close monitoring of serum creatinine as a marker of renal function. Concurrent rapid changes in antihypertensive treatment may affect creatinine levels and may implicate antihypertensive agents as the cause of renal function loss, with resulting dose reductions and inadequate control long term. Thus, early after transplantation, it has been suggested that BP be lowered gradually to less than 150/90 mm Hg, with further refinement later.

Nonpharmacologic Therapy

Although efficacy has not been demonstrated in the renal transplant population, lifestyle modification has demonstrated value in BP lowering in patients with essential hypertension and in elderly populations.[54,55] Because these interventions are not harmful and may provide other health benefits, they should be recommended to transplant recipients as well. As in the general U.S. and world populations, obesity is increasingly common in the transplant population; most recipients gain weight after transplantation. Weight gain is often associated with worsening hypertension, and even modest weight loss may produce measurable BP reductions. Alcohol in excess has a pressor effect on BP and provides a rich source of calories contributing to obesity. Regular alcohol use may be a factor in nonadherence.

Increased plasma volume occurs commonly as a compensatory response to antihypertensive therapy, and it may manifest as fluid retention (weight gain, edema) or a poor response to increased BP medication. High sodium intake and obesity contribute to increased plasma volume. Hence, sodium restriction enhances the antihypertensive efficacy of most BP medications and minimizes diuretic-induced potassium wasting. Because renal transplant recipients are more sensitive to hypovolemia, extreme sodium restriction should be avoided. Regular exercise decreases BP primarily by facilitating weight loss. The use of the Dietary Approaches to Stop Hypertension (DASH)[56] diet may benefit transplant recipients, but it should be introduced with caution, because the emphasis on vegetable-based foods may cause hyperkalemia in patients receiving CNIs.

Pharmacologic Therapy

Most treatment principles relevant to treating essential hypertension apply to transplant recipients as well. Treatment may require three or more antihypertensive agents to achieve recommended target BP levels lower than 130/80 mm Hg. Transplant recipients are exposed to complex drug regimens with a high potential for serious drug interactions. Particular attention should be paid to selection of calcium channel blockers (CCBs) metabolized through the cytochrome P-450 pathways, in which enhancement or blunting of CNI metabolism may induce major changes in CNI levels and may trigger rejection or drug toxicity. Transplant recipients may develop unique side effects and have a higher incidence of known side effects that occur less commonly in other hypertensive populations. Antihypertensive agents may affect kidney function, and agent and dose changes require close monitoring.

Table 30-2 Drug Treatment of Post-transplant Hypertension

Drug Class	Adverse Effects	Comments
β-Blockers Atenolol Metoprolol Others	Negative cardiac inotropic and chronotropic effects, bronchospasm, hyperglycemia, fatigue	Recommended for cardiac protection in patients with coronary disease
Calcium Channel Blockers Nifedipine Amlodipine Isradipine Nicardipine Diltiazem Verapamil	 Edema, palpitations, headache, flushing Same Same Same Negative cardiac inotropic and chronotropic effects, constipation Similar to diltiazem, more constipation	Use extended-release preparations only Minimal effect on CSA levels Increases CSA levels Increases CSA levels, used at some centers to reduce CSA doses Increases CSA levels, used at some centers to reduce CSA doses
Angiotensin-Converting Enzyme Inhibitors Captopril Enalapril Lisinopril Ramipril Others	Cough, angioedema, anemia, hyperkalemia, azotemia	Slow loss of renal function (especially if proteinuria is present), prevent diabetes, reduce cardiovascular risk in nontransplant settings
Angiotensin Receptor Blockers Losartan Irbesartan Candesartan Telmisartan Others	Anemia, hyperkalemia, azotemia	Slow loss of renal function (especially if proteinuria present), prevent diabetes, reduce cardiovascular risk in nontransplant settings
Thiazide and Thiazide-like Diuretics Hydrochlorothiazide Chlorthalidone Indapamide Metolazone Others	Prerenal azotemia, hyponatremia, hypokalemia, hypomagnesemia, hypercalcemia, hypercalcemia, hyperglycemia, hyperuricemia	Potentiate effectiveness of other antihypertensive agents, ineffective at GFR <30 mL/min
Loop Diuretics Furosemide Bumetanide Torsemide	Prerenal azotemia, hypokalemia, hypomagnesemia, hyperuricemia	Potentiate effectiveness of other antihypertensive agents, effective in azotemic patients, can be used in place of thiazide for patients with hyponatremia or hypercalcemia
α-Blockers Terazosin Doxazosin	Orthostatic hypotension Urinary incontinence	Useful as secondary agent
Centrally Acting Sympathetic Agents	Dry mouth, sedation	Lack of trial data in transplant setting
Direct vasodilators	Edema, tachycardia	Lack of trial data in transplant setting

CSA, cyclosporine; GFR, glomerular filtration rate.

Lacking prospective data testing the efficacy and safety of each agent in transplant recipients, treatment recommendations are based on clinical experience.[57] Transplant-specific comments and adverse effects of hypertension drug classes are listed in Table 30-2. Several principles merit emphasis. The choice of antihypertensive agent should take into account the reduced GFR and renal vasoconstriction universally present. Uric acid levels are elevated, sometimes profoundly. CNIs partially inhibit renal potassium and hydrogen ion excretion and thereby predispose patients to hyperkalemic metabolic acidosis. Diuretic therapy is often avoided, to prevent worsening of azotemia and hyperuricemia. Potassium-sparing agents must be used with caution. ACE inhibitors and ARBs, when used alone, have limited efficacy and may aggravate both hyperkalemia and acidosis.

High CV risk and CV event rates in patients with renal failure and in renal transplant recipients support close attention to cardioprotection. β-Blockers are underused in the general hypertension population and in the transplant setting. For patients with coronary artery disease, β-blockade should be started preoperatively to reduce surgical mortality and then continued to blunt the reflex tachycardia often seen with vasodilatory or peripherally active agents (vasodilators, dihydropyridine CCBs, or α-blockers). Combination α- and β-blocking agents are preferred for their increased potency and minimal drug interactions in this setting. Fatigue, bradycardia, worsening glucose tolerance, and bronchospasm may limit use and dosage.

Compared with dihydropyridine CCBs, verapamil and diltiazem are less commonly used after transplantation because of their effects on gastrointestinal motility and CNI blood levels. At some centers, these agents have been used as cyclosporine dose-sparing agents to provide cost savings and improved patient survival.[58] Diltiazem may offer protection from early graft failure in renal transplant recipients,[59] and it may slow development of the atypical coronary vascular lesions observed after cardiac transplantation.[60] The vasodilatory effects of dihydropyridine CCBs directly counter the vasoconstrictive effects of CNIs but produce significant side effects, including peripheral edema, headache, and reflex tachycardia. Edema may be severe and is a frequent cause of drug discontinuation. Nifedipine, isradipine, and felodipine have negligible effects on cyclosporine disposition, and they have been used successfully in transplant settings.[58] Amlodipine has minor effects on cyclosporine levels and has been utilized in renal transplant recipients with good results.[61-63] Recipients taking CCB-based treatment have higher GFRs, both immediately and at 2 years after transplantation, compared with patients using other agents.[64] Experimental studies suggest that CCBs have minor immunosuppressive properties and may blunt interstitial fibrosis. On the negative side, CCB-treated patients have higher levels of urinary protein excretion, a finding raising concern that, as in the nontransplant setting, increased glomerular pressure caused by arterial vasodilation and increased proteinuria may accelerate renal decline.

ACE inhibitors and ARBs are widely used in patients with chronic kidney disease for BP control, cardiac and renal protection, and proteinuria reduction. In the transplant setting, several concerns merit close attention. Early after transplantation, patients are at risk for swings in volume status, often with volume excess. The renin-angiotensin system is frequently suppressed, and inhibitors are generally ineffective for BP control. In the setting of marginal renal function, ACE inhibitors and ARBs increase the risk of hyperkalemia, already a risk because of renal insufficiency, CNI use, and the common use of trimethoprim-sulfamethoxazole. Beyond the first few months after transplant, as volume shifts become less pronounced and renal function is more clearly defined, ACE inhibitors and ARBs may provide renal benefits similar to those in patients with native kidney disease. These agents are indicated for patients with proteinuria and those at risk for developing proteinuria or glomerular diseases such as diabetic nephropathy, because these drugs lower glomerular pressures and protein excretion. A recent study in renal transplant recipients compared treatment with losartan with captopril and amlodipine, by using prestudy and poststudy renal allograft biopsies. Treatment with losartan reduced plasma transforming growth factor-β_1 levels and 24-hour urine protein excretion.[65] Further, the rate of histologic scarring was lower in the losartan-treated group. Although unproven, ACE inhibitors may slow progression of chronic allograft nephropathy by reducing intraglomerular pressure and thus hyperfiltration. Evidence for reductions in CV events in patients with normal renal function who are not transplant recipients and in those with mild renal impairment (serum creatinine, 1.4 to 2.4 mg/dL) support use of these agents in the renal transplant recipient.[66] Several trials indicate that ACE inhibitors may be used safely, particularly when they are combined with diuretics.[67,68]

The benefits of ACE inhibitors and ARBs for renal and CV protection must be balanced against two major disadvantages: anemia and acute reductions in graft function. ACE inhibitors or ARBs in renal transplant recipients cause a predictable decline in hemoglobin of 1.0 to 1.5 g/dL. This effect may be less common with ARBs, or it may reflect less clinical experience with these agents in the transplant setting. Although this side effect has been used to treat post-transplant erythrocytosis, it may require treatment with erythropoietin injections in some patients. ACE inhibitors and ARBs can precipitate functional acute renal failure in patients with marginal arterial flow to the allograft, similar to the picture seen clinically in patients with native kidney bilateral renal artery stenosis. A similar pattern may result from small vessel disease. Risk factors include higher baseline serum creatinine levels, higher doses or levels of CNIs, and higher plasma renin levels. ACE inhibitors or ARBs should be started at very low doses, with close monitoring of serum potassium and creatinine over the first several weeks, after which slow dose titration is recommended.

Diuretics are commonly withheld after transplantation because of concerns that they may impair renal function. Diuretics counter the sodium-retaining effects of corticosteroids, β-blockers, ACE inhibitors and ARBs, and CNIs, thus allowing the kidney to maintain sodium balance at lower BP levels. Control of volume expansion improves the BP response to other agents. In the patient with renal insufficiency and sodium and volume retention, loop diuretics are often required to achieve lower BP targets. Disadvantages of diuretic therapy center on the expected rise in serum creatinine associated with their use. This is more likely in patients with compromised renal blood flow, including small vessel disease associated with allograft dysfunction, or in the setting of contracted intravascular volume. Most thiazide diuretics are ineffective at GFRs lower than 30 mL/minute, and in this setting, a loop diuretic such as furosemide, bumetanide, or torsemide should be considered.

Although few data from controlled trials are available, other agents may be used to treat post-transplant hypertension. Peripheral α-blockers may be used as second-line agents.[69] Although these agents may improve bladder outflow in men, women may develop urinary incontinence. It is important to monitor for pronounced postural BP changes, particularly in patients with autonomic dysfunction. These agents magnify sodium retention and may require diuretic therapy to maintain their BP-lowering effect. Centrally acting sympatholytic agents are reserved for third- or fourth-line treatment because of their more pronounced side effects. Clonidine is effective in patch or oral form, but its use is limited by the side effects of fatigue and dry mouth. Although direct vasodilators are very effective, they must be used in combination with diuretics and either β-blockers or central sympatholytic agents to counteract edema and reflex tachycardia, respectively.

Modification of Immunosuppressive Regimen

Modifications in immunosuppressive regimen may provide substantial benefits to BP control. Transitioning from cyclosporine to tacrolimus, or from a CNI to sirolimus, may effectively lower BP and simplify management. Immunologic suppression must be maintained as first priority when changes in immunosuppression are considered primarily for BP benefit. Current trends to steroid-free immunosuppression may also benefit BP control.

Native Nephrectomy

For patients with severe hypertension before transplant, BP may remain resistant, even in the setting of a functioning allograft. Native kidney nephrectomy has been used successfully to reduce hypertension severity in select cases.[70,71] Since the advent of pharmacologic renin-angiotensin blockade, this procedure has become uncommon, although interest has increased with the availability of laparoscopic nephrectomy techniques.[72] Reports of lower BP in transplant recipients undergoing pretransplant bilateral nephrectomy support a role for native kidney disease in the maintenance of post-transplant hypertension. Particularly in the setting of a well-functioning allograft, removal of atrophic or infarcted native kidneys offers potential improvement in BP control, with the use of fewer medications in patients at low surgical risk.

CONCLUSIONS

Development of hypertension occurs commonly during CNI-based immunosuppression, in both transplant and nontransplant settings. Particularly in the transplant recipient, the underlying mechanism of altered vascular reactivity and systemic and renal vasoconstriction results in impaired glomerular filtration and sodium retention, magnified by the effects of corticosteroids. Hypertension after transplantation represents a major risk factor for CV disease and affects long-term function of the allograft. Management of this disease may be difficult and requires attention to drug-drug interactions and to the effects of antihypertensive therapy on native or renal allograft function. Therapy should include nonpharmacologic and pharmacologic modalities. Target BP levels should recognize the increased CV and renal risks of these patients.

References

1. Textor SC, Canzanello VJ, Taler SJ, et al. Cyclosporine-induced hypertension after transplantation. *Mayo Clin Proc*. 1994;**69**: 1182-1193.
2. Brown AL, Thomas TH, Levell N, et al. The effect of short-term low-dose cyclosporin on renal function and blood pressure in patients with psoriasis. *Br J Dermatol*. 1993;**128**:550-555.
3. Charnick SB, Nedelman JR, Chang C-T, et al. Description of blood pressure changes in patients beginning cyclosporin A therapy. *Ther Drug Monit*. 1997;**19**:17-24.
4. Dimeny EM. Cardiovascular disease after renal transplantation. *Kidney Int*. 2002;**61 (Suppl 80)**:S78-S84.
5. Kasiske BL, Guijarro C, Massy ZA, et al. Cardiovascular disease after renal transplantation. *J Am Soc Nephrol*. 1996;**7**:158-165.
6. Peschke B, Scheuermann EH, Geiger H, et al. Hypertension is associated with hyperlipidemia, coronary artery disease, and chronic graft failure in kidney transplant recipients. *Clin Nephrol*. 1999;**51**:290-295.
7. Canzanello VJ, Schwartz L, Taler SJ, et al. Evolution of cardiovascular risk after liver transplantation: A comparison of cyclosporine A and tacrolimus (FK506). *Liver Transplant Surg*. 1997;**3**:1-9.
8. Mange KC, Feldman HI, Joffe MM, et al. Blood pressure and the survival of renal allografts from living donors. *J Am Soc Nephrol*. 2004;**15**:187-193.
9. Cosio FG, Falkenhain ME, Pesavento TE, et al. Relationships between arterial hypertension and renal allograft survival in African-American patients. *Am J Kidney Dis*. 1997;**29**: 419-427.
10. Cosio FG, Pelletier RP, Pesavento TE, et al. Elevated blood pressure predicts the risk of acute rejection in renal allograft recipients. *Kidney Int*. 2001;**59**:1158-1164.
11. Faulds D, Goa KL, Benfield P. Cyclosporin. A review of its pharmacodynamic and pharmacokinetic properties, and therapeutic use in immunoregulatory disorders. *Drugs*. 1993;**45**:953-1040.
12. Taler SJ, Textor SC, Canzanello VJ, et al. Role of steroid dose in hypertension early after liver transplantation with tacrolimus (FK506) and cyclosporine. *Transplantation*. 1996;**62**:1588-1592.
13. Bennett WM, Pulliam JP. Cyclosporine nephrotoxicity. *Ann Intern Med*. 1983;**99**:851-854.
14. Porter GA, Bennett WM, Sheps SG. Cyclosporine-associated hypertension: National High Blood Pressure Education Program. *Arch Intern Med*. 1990;**150**:280-283.
15. U.S. Multicenter FK506 Liver Study Group. A comparison of tacrolimus (FK506) and cyclosporine for immunosuppression in liver transplantation. *N Engl J Med*. 1994;**331**:1110-1115.
16. Textor SC, Wiesner R, Wilson DJ, et al. Systemic and renal hemodynamic differences between FK506 and cyclosporine in liver transplant recipients. *Transplantation*. 1993;**55**: 1332-1339.
17. Sturrock NDC, Lang CC, Struthers AD. Cyclosporin-induced hypertension precedes renal dysfunction and sodium retention in man. *J Hypertens*. 1993;**11**:1209-1216.
18. Textor SC. De novo hypertension after liver transplantation. *Hypertension*. 1993;**22**:257-267.
19. Hilbrands LB, Hoitsma AJ, van Hamersvelt HW, et al. Acute effects of nifedipine in renal transplant recipients treated with cyclosporine or azathioprine. *Am J Kidney Dis*. 1994;**24**: 838-845.
20. Textor SC, Wilson DJ, Lerman A, et al. Renal hemodynamics, urinary eicosanoids, and endothelin after liver transplantation. *Transplantation*. 1992;**54**:74-80.
21. Bantle JP, Boudreau RJ, Ferris TF. Suppression of plasma renin activity by cyclosporine. *Am J Med*. 1987;**83**:59-64.
22. Textor SC, Burnett JC, Romero JC, et al. Urinary endothelin and renal vasoconstriction with cyclosporine or FK506 after liver transplantation. *Kidney Int*. 1995;**47**:1426-1433.
23. Perico N, Ruggenenti P, Gaspari F, et al. Daily renal hypoperfusion induced by cyclosporine in patients with renal transplantation. *Transplantation*. 1992;**54**:56-60.
24. Petric R, Freeman D, Wallace C, et al. Effect of cyclosporine on urinary prostanoid excretion, renal blood flow, and glomerulotubular function. *Transplantation*. 1988;**45**: 883-889.
25. Gaston RS, Schlessinger SD, Sanders PW, et al. Cyclosporine inhibits the renal response to L-arginine in human kidney transplant recipients. *J Am Soc Nephrol*. 1995;**5**:1426-1433.
26. Richards NT, Poston L, Hilston PJ. Cyclosporin A inhibits endothelium-dependent, prostanoid-induced relaxation in human subcutaneous resistance vessels. *J Hypertens*. 1990;**8**:159-163.
27. Sander M, Victor RG. Hypertension after cardiac transplantation: Pathophysiology and management. *Curr Opin Nephrol Hypertens*. 1995;**4**:443-451.
28. Kaye D, Thompson J, Jennings G, Esler M. Cyclosporine therapy after cardiac transplantation causes hypertension and renal vasoconstriction without sympathetic activation. *Circulation*. 1993;**88**:1101-1109.

29. Floras JS, Legault L, Morali GA, et al. Increased sympathetic outflow in cirrhosis and ascites: Direct evidence from intraneural recordings. *Ann Intern Med.* 1991;**114**:373-380.

30. Conte G, Dal Canton A, Sabbatini M, et al. Acute cyclosporine dysfunction reversed by dopamine infusion in healthy subjects. *Kidney Int.* 1989;**36**:1086-1092.

31. Johnson RW, Kreis H, Oberbauer R, et al. Sirolimus allows early cyclosporine withdrawal in renal transplantation resulting in improved renal function and lower blood pressure. *Transplantation.* 2001;**72**:777-786.

32. Sato A, Funder JW, Okubo M, et al. Glucocorticoid-induced hypertension in the elderly; relation to serum calcium and family history of essential hypertension. *Am J Hypertens.* 1995;**8**:823-828.

33. Whitworth JA. Mechanisms of glucocorticoid-induced hypertension. *Kidney Int.* 1987;**31**:1213-1224.

34. Hricik DE, Lautman J, Bartucci MR, et al. Variable effects of steroid withdrawal on blood pressure reduction in cyclosporine-treated renal transplant recipients. *Transplantation.* 1992;**53**:1232-1235.

35. Veenstra DL, Best JH, Hornberger J, et al. Incidence and long-term cost of steroid-related side effects after renal transplantation. *Am J Kidney Dis.* 1999;**33**:829-839.

36. Whitworth JA. Studies on the mechanisms of glucocorticoid hypertension in humans. *Blood Press.* 1994;**3**:24-32.

37. Hollander AAMJ, Hene RJ, Hermans J, et al. Late prednisone withdrawal in cyclosporine-treated kidney transplant patients: A randomized study. *J Am Soc Nephrol.* 1997;**8**:294-301.

38. Verdecchia P, Schillaci G, Guerrieri M, et al. Circadian blood pressure changes and left ventricular hypertrophy in essential hypertension. *Circulation.* 1990;**81**:528-536.

39. Shimada K, Kawamoto A, Matsubayashi K, et al. Diurnal blood pressure variations and silent cerebrovascular damage in elderly patients with hypertension. *J Hypertens.* 1992;**10**:875-878.

40. Bianchi S, Bigazzi R, Baldari G, et al. Diurnal variations of blood pressure and microalbuminuria in essential hypertension. *Am J Hypertens.* 1994;**7**:23-29.

41. Taler SJ, Textor SC, Canzanello VJ, et al. Loss of nocturnal blood pressure fall after liver transplantation during immunosuppressive therapy. *Am J Hypertens.* 1995;**8**:598-605.

42. Haydar AA, Covic A, Jayawardene S, et al. Insights from ambulatory blood pressure monitoring: Diagnosis of hypertension and diurnal blood pressure in renal transplant recipients. *Transplantation.* 2004;**77**:849-853.

43. van de Borne P, Leeman M, Primo G, Degaute JP. Reappearance of a normal circadian rhythm of blood pressure after cardiac transplantation. *Am J Cardiol.* 1992;**69**:794-801.

44. von Polnitz A, Bracht C, Kemkes B, Hofling B. Circadian pattern of blood pressure and heart rate in the longer term after heart transplantation. *J Cardiovasc Pharmacol.* 1990;**16** (**Suppl**):S86-S89.

45. Imai Y, Abe K, Sasaki S, et al. Exogenous glucocorticoid eliminates or reverses circadian blood pressure variations. *J Hypertens.* 1989;**7**:113-120.

46. Imai Y, Abe K, Sasaki S, et al. Altered circadian blood pressure rhythm in patients with Cushing's syndrome. *Hypertension.* 1988;**12**:11-19.

47. Chobanian AV, Bakris GL, Black HR, et al. Seventh Report of the Joint National Committee on Prevention, Detection, Evaluation and Treatment of High Blood Pressure. National High Blood Pressure Education Program Coordinating Committee. *Hypertension.* 2003;**42**:1206-1252.

48. Thomas MC, Mathew TH, Russ GR, et al. Perioperative blood pressure control, delayed graft function, and acute rejection after renal transplantation. *Transplantation.* 2003;**75**:1989-1995.

49. Cosio FG, Pesavento TE, Kim S, et al. Patient survival after renal transplantation. IV: Impact of post-transplant diabetes. *Kidney Int.* 2002;**62**:1440-1446.

50. Fernandez-Fresnedo G, Palomar R, Escallada R, et al. Hypertension and long-term renal allograft survival: Effect of early glomerular filtration rate. *Nephrol Dial Transplant.* 2001;**16** (**Suppl 1**):105-109.

51. Bruno S, Ferrari S, Remuzzi G, Ruggenenti P. Doppler ultrasonography in posttransplant renal artery stenosis: A reliable tool for assessing effectiveness of revascularization? *Transplantation.* 2003;**76**:16-17.

52. Ruggenenti P, Mosconi L, Bruno S, et al. Post-transplant renal artery stenosis: The hemodynamic response to revascularization. *Kidney Int.* 2001;**60**:309-318.

53. Chobanian AV, Bakris GL, Black HR, et al., and the National High Blood Pressure Education Program Coordinating Committee. The Seventh Report of the Joint National Committee on Prevention, Detection, Evaluation, and Treatment of High Blood Pressure: The JNC 7 report. *JAMA.* 2003;**289**:2560-2572.

54. Whelton PK, Appel LJ, Espeland MA, et al. Sodium reduction and weight loss in the treatment of hypertension in older persons. *JAMA.* 1998;**279**:839-848.

55. Trials of Hypertension Prevention Collaborative Research Group. The effects of nonpharmacologic interventions on blood pressure of persons with high normal levels: Results of the Trials of Hypertension Prevention, phase I. *JAMA.* 1992;**267**:1213-1220.

56. Sacks FM, Svetkey LP, Vollmer WM, et al. Effects on blood pressure of reduced dietary sodium and the Dietary Approaches to Stop Hypertension (DASH) diet. *N Engl J Med.* 2001;**344**:3-10.

57. EBPG Expert Group on Renal Transplantation. European best practice guidelines for renal transplantation. Section IV: Long-term management of the transplant recipient IV: 5.2. Arterial hypertension. *Nephrol Dial Transplant.* 2002;**17** (**Suppl 4**):25-26.

58. van den Dorpel MA, Zietse R, Ijzermans JN, et al. Effect of isradipine on cyclosporin A related hypertension. *Blood Press.* 1994;**1**:50-53.

59. Neumayer HH, Kunzendorf U, Schreiber M. Protective effects of calcium antagonists in human renal transplantation. *Kidney Int.* 1992;**41** (**Suppl 36**):87s-93s.

60. Schroeder JS, Gao SZ, Alderman EL, et al. A preliminary study of diltiazem in the prevention of coronary artery disease in heart-transplant recipients. *N Engl J Med.* 1993;**328**:164-170.

61. Sennesael J, Lamote J, Violet I, et al. Comparison of perindopril and amlodipine in cyclosporine-treated renal allograft recipients. *Hypertension.* 1995;**26**:436-444.

62. Toupance O, Lavoud S, Canivet E, et al. Antihypertensive effect of amlodipine and lack of interference with cyclosporine metabolism in renal transplant recipients. *Hypertension.* 1994;**24**:297-300.

63. Pesavento TE, Jones PA, Julian BA, Curtis JJ. Amlodipine increases cyclosporine levels in hypertensive renal transplant patients: Results of a prospective study. *J Am Soc Nephrol.* 1996;**7**:831-835.

64. Textor SC, Schwartz L, Wilson DJ, et al. Systemic and renal effects of nifedipine in cyclosporine-associated hypertension. *Hypertension.* 1994;**23** (**Suppl I**):I220-I224.

65. el-Agroudy AE, Hassan NA, Foda MA, et al. Effect of angiotensin II receptor blocker on plasma levels of TGF-beta 1 and interstitial fibrosis in hypertensive kidney transplant patients. *Am J Nephrol.* 2003;**23**:300-306.

66. Heart Outcomes Prevention Evaluation Study Investigators. Effects of an angiotensin-converting enzyme inhibitor, ramipril, on cardiovascular events in high-risk patients. *N Engl J Med.* 2000;**342**:145-153.

67. Brozena SC, Johnson MR, Ventura H, et al. Effectiveness and safety of diltiazem or lisinopril in treatment of hypertension after heart transplantation. *J Am Coll Cardiol.* 1996;**27**:1707-1712.

68. Midtvedt K, Ihlen H, Hartmann A, et al. Reduction of left ventricular mass by lisinopril and nifedipine in hypertensive renal transplant recipients: A prospective randomized double-blind study. *Transplantation.* 2001;**72**:107-111.

69. ALLHAT Collaborative Research Group. Major cardiovascular events in hypertensive patients randomized to doxazosin vs chlorthalidone: The Antihypertensive and Lipid-Lowering Treatment to Prevent Heart Attack Trial (ALLHAT). *JAMA.* 2000;**283**:1967-1975.

70. Vanrenterghem Y, Waer M, Christiaens MR, Michielsen P. Bilateral nephrectomy of the native kidneys reduces the incidence of arterial hypertension and erythrocytosis in kidney graft recipients treated with cyclosporin: Leaven Collaborative Group for Transplantation. *Transplant Int.* 1992;**5** (**Suppl 1**): S35-S37.

71. Curtis JJ, Luke RG, Diethelm AG, et al. Benefits of removal of native kidneys in hypertension after renal transplantation. *Lancet.* 1985;**2**:739-742.

72. Fricke L, Doehn C, Steinhoff J, et al. Treatment of posttransplant hypertension by laparoscopic bilateral nephrectomy. *Transplantation.* 1998;**65**:1182-1187.

Obesity in Hypertension

F. Xavier Pi-Sunyer and Panagiotis Kokkoris

Obesity is a major health problem in the United States. According to the Third National Health and Nutrition Examination Survey (NHANES III), approximately 59.4% of men and 50.7% of women in the United States are obese or overweight (defined as body mass index [BMI] >25 kg/m^2).[1] By the year 2000, the prevalence of obesity had increased by 7.6% since the time the NHANES III was conducted in 1988 to 1994.[2]

Obesity has been associated with increased morbidity and mortality. In the Nurses' Health Study, mortality from all causes was greater in obese or overweight women, compared with women of normal weight, and this result was more obvious when smokers were excluded from the study.[3] Similar results were found in the Framingham Heart Study in both men and women.[4] In a prospective study from the Netherlands, individuals who were obese at the age of 40 years had an average decrease in life expectancy of 7.1 years for women and 5.8 years for men.[5]

Many serious disorders are much more common in obese individuals. These disorders include diabetes mellitus, dyslipidemia, stroke, heart failure, myocardial infarction, gallbladder disease, osteoarthritis, sleep apnea, end-stage renal disease, some cancers, and hypertension.[6-8]

Hypertension is very common among obese individuals. The Framingham Heart Study showed that obese persons have an almost twofold increase in the prevalence of hypertension, and for every 10% increase in body weight, there is a 6.5 mm Hg increase in systolic blood pressure (BP). Obesity or weight gain was responsible for 70% of cases of recently diagnosed hypertension.[4] Weight loss of as little as 5 kg can reduce BP or can even prevent hypertension in a significant proportion of obese individuals.[4,9] It is estimated that for every kilogram of weight loss, BP decreases by 0.45 mm Hg.[10]

ASSESSMENT OF FAT BURDEN

It is important to know the total fat burden and fat distribution for the evaluation and treatment of an obese individual. A simple and relatively accurate tool to assess total fat burden is the BMI. The BMI is calculated as (weight in kilograms)/(height in meters squared) (Table 31-1) and correlates well with total fat, except in very muscular individuals.[11] A BMI of 18.5 to 24.9 kg/m^2 is defined as normal, whereas a BMI of 25 to 29.9 kg/m^2 is now defined as overweight and a BMI greater than 30 kg/m^2 as obesity, with different classes of obesity (Table 31-2).

Central fat distribution (also called abdominal or visceral obesity) is particularly associated with an increased risk of morbid conditions, such as diabetes mellitus, cardiovascular disease, and hypertension. Central obesity can be evaluated by measuring the waist circumference or the waist-to-hip ratio. The waist circumference should be less than 102 cm (40 in) in men and less than 88 cm (35 in) in women.[12] Waist circumference is very useful in estimating additional cardiovascular disease risk in patients with a BMI of 25 to 34.9 kg/m^2, because individuals with a BMI greater than 35 kg/m^2 are considered to be at very high risk already, regardless of their waist circumference.[12] A waist-to-hip ratio greater than 1.0 in men and 0.85 in women is also considered abnormal.

BLOOD PRESSURE MEASUREMENT

Special care should be taken for the measurement of BP in obese individuals (see Chapter 5). The patient should rest for at least 5 minutes before the measurement, and the final BP should be the average of two or more readings. A common error is the use of a cuff that is not wide or long enough and so gives a falsely high BP measurement.

MECHANISMS OF OBESITY-RELATED HYPERTENSION

Several mechanisms are probably involved in the pathogenesis of hypertension in obese individuals. However, the interactions and relative importance of these mechanisms are not completely clear. Some possible causes are abnormal renal function, sympathetic nervous system overactivity, hormonal changes, including insulin and leptin, and alterations in the activity of the renin-angiotensin-aldosterone system (Fig. 31-1).

Renal Mechanisms

The increased renal sodium reabsorption in obese individuals can contribute to sodium retention and to an increase in extracellular and blood volume. The increase in blood volume is necessary to maintain sodium balance, but this results in elevation of BP.[13,14] Another renal factor contributing to the development of obesity-related hypertension is compression of the kidneys caused by visceral fat accumulation. The result is increased intrarenal pressure, which leads to increased renal sodium reabsorption, water retention, and, finally, elevated BP. Additionally, fat tissue not only compresses the kidney, but also may penetrate the renal capsule and thus elevate intrarenal pressure further.[15,16]

Sympathetic Nervous System Activity

The sympathetic nervous system plays an important role in the pathogenesis of hypertension in obesity. Fasting suppresses sympathetic nervous system activity, whereas over-

Table 31-1 Methods of Body Mass Index Calculation

If kilograms and meters are used:
BMI = weight (kg)/height squared (m²)

If pounds and inches are used:
BMI = weight (pounds) × 703/height squared (inches²)

BMI, body mass index.

Table 31-2 Classification of Obesity and Overweight by Body Mass Index

Classification	Body Mass Index (kg/m²)
Underweight	<18.5
Normal weight	18.6-24.9
Overweight	25.0-29.9
Obesity (class I)	30.0-34.9
Obesity (class II)	35.0-39.9
Extreme obesity (class III)	≥40

feeding increases it. Obese individuals have elevated plasma levels of norepinephrine.[17,18] It seems likely that increased sympathetic nervous activity raises BP, both directly by causing vasoconstriction and indirectly by increasing renal sodium reabsorption through activation of renal nerves.[19]

Hormonal Factors

Insulin

Insulin resistance and hyperinsulinemia are characteristics of the metabolic syndrome, which is very common among obese individuals. Although the exact mechanisms are still unclear, hyperinsulinemia seems to play a role in raising BP in obese persons. It is believed that insulin raises BP by increasing sympathetic nervous system activity,[20,21] increasing renal sodium reabsorption,[22,23] and stimulating vascular smooth muscle hypertrophy.[13] However, the presence of hyperinsulinemia alone probably is not adequate to elevate BP, because patients with an insulinoma do not have a higher incidence of hypertension than do appropriate control groups.[24,25]

Leptin

Leptin is a peptide hormone secreted from adipocytes that decreases appetite and increases energy expenditure in experi-

mental animals. However, in humans, obesity is associated with elevated serum leptin levels, a finding indicating resistance to leptin action.[26] Serum leptin levels are elevated in hypertensive individuals compared with normotensive persons, independent of BMI and body fat pattern.[27] Leptin seems to have different effects when it is administered on a short-term basis or a long-term basis in rats. Acute infusion of leptin does not elevate BP, even though sympathetic nervous system activity increases, probably because nitric oxide (which is stimulated by leptin) counteracts this effect.[28] In contrast, long-term administration of leptin in rats increases BP.[29] Long-term infusion studies have not been done in humans, but subcutaneous injection in obese persons for 4 to 24 weeks did not result in any changes in vital signs.[30]

Renin-Angiotensin-Aldosterone System

The activity of the renin-angiotensin-aldosterone system is enhanced in obesity, despite increased sodium retention and blood volume expansion. Plasma renin activity is increased in obese individuals and declines with weight loss.[31,32] BP decreases with weight loss and correlates well with reduced plasma renin activity.[33] Apart from the systemic renin-angiotensin-aldosterone system activity and its role in obesity, there seems to be a local renin-angiotensin system in adipose tissue, because adipose tissue has all the necessary components

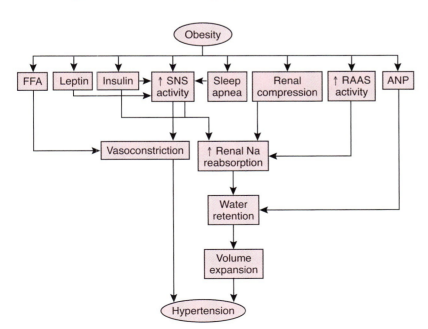

Figure 31–1   Possible mechanisms of obesity induced hypertension. ANP, atrial natriuretic peptide; FFA, free fatty acids; Na, sodium; RAAS, renin-angiotensin-aldosterone system; SNS, sympathetic nervous system.

and can produce angiotensin II. This angiotensin II, locally produced by the adipose tissue, probably also contributes to the pathogenesis of hypertension in obesity. Another argument for the role of the renin-angiotensin-aldosterone system in the pathogenesis of obesity-related hypertension is that angiotensin-converting enzyme (ACE) inhibitors and angiotensin II receptor blockers are effective treatments of hypertension in obese patients.[34]

Additional Factors

Free Fatty Acids

Obese individuals have high levels of free fatty acids,[35] and this may be another factor contributing to obesity-related hypertension. Free fatty acids are correlated with increased BP, probably as a result of their vasoconstrictive effect. This effect is produced through an increased activity of the α_1-adrenergic agonists, because the use of α_1-adrenergic receptor blockers prevents the BP increase.[36,37]

Natriuretic Peptides

Natriuretic peptides play an important role in BP regulation. They are produced mainly in the heart, the brain, and the kidneys, and they decrease the vascular sympathetic tone and increase natriuresis. Increased natriuresis decreases plasma volume and as a result lowers BP. Levels of atrial natriuretic peptide have been found to be low in obese hypertensive patients.[38,39]

Sleep Apnea Syndrome

Obese patients with sleep apnea have a higher incidence of hypertension than obese persons without sleep apnea.[40] The reason could be the increased sympathetic nervous system activity that is observed in this group of patients.[41]

Cardiac Alterations

Obesity combined with hypertension results in elevation of both cardiac preload and afterload, which can lead to significant left ventricular hypertrophy (LVH). The pattern of LVH in obese hypertensive patients is eccentric, whereas in nonobese hypertensive patients, it is most commonly concentric.[42] Because LVH is a risk factor for heart failure and sudden death, obese hypertensive patients are at higher risk of developing one of these complications compared with nonobese hypertensive patients.[43]

EFFECT OF WEIGHT LOSS ON BLOOD PRESSURE

Overview

Weight loss plays an important role in BP regulation in obese hypertensive patients. Weight loss is a difficult and time-consuming process that may include diet, exercise, drug treatment, or even weight loss surgery, but appropriate patient motivation is a prerequisite for any attempt at weight loss. Behavioral modification targets include changing eating habits, increasing exercise, altering attitudes toward food, and developing support systems. Before starting a weight loss program, both the patient and the physician have to consider the following questions:

1. Is the patient determined to lose weight?
2. Does the patient know the health hazards associated with obesity?
3. Does the patient have support from his or her family and social environment in the attempt to lose weight?
4. Can the patient increase physical activity along with diet?

It is very important for the physician or any other health care provider involved in the weight loss process to build a strong partnership with the patient, so the patient will trust the physician. They have to set a reasonable target for weight loss. Many obese patients have unrealistic expectations and become rapidly disappointed when they do not reach their target. An achievable goal is to lose 10% of initial weight and to maintain this loss over time. If a patient is successful, a new goal can be set, but the weight loss process has to be gradual.

Another significant requirement is to identify and control the stimuli that affect eating behavior. The patient has to recognize the situations that are associated with overeating, such as watching television, and learn to control these situations. Another technique that helps is setting small rewards as specific goals are achieved. This motivates the patient and helps in continuing the effort. Stress is another very important factor that needs to be controlled. Stress drives some people to overeat, and stress management can prevent overeating. Finally, support from the patient's environment (e.g., family, friends, colleagues) helps the patient to continue his or her efforts and to remain motivated.

A hypocaloric diet, combined with increased physical activity, is the cornerstone of a successful weight loss program. The typical U.S. diet consists of 14% protein, 40% fat, and 46% carbohydrates, of which 28% are complex and 18% are simple.[44] Consumption of fat and sugar should be decreased, whereas intake of fiber should be encouraged. Total fat should not exceed 30% of total calories, with saturated fatty acids not more than 10% of total daily calories. Monounsaturated and polyunsaturated fatty acids should offer the rest of the calories from fat. Protein should be of high biologic value. Carbohydrates should be approximately 55% of total daily caloric intake and should contain at least 20 to 30 g of fiber from fruits, vegetables, whole grains, and legumes (Table 31-3). A weight loss diet should include the necessary amount of vitamins and micronutrients. Alcohol should be avoided because it contains 7 calories/g. Portion sizes should be reduced. A caloric deficit of 500 to 1000 calories/day, combined with increased physical activity, could achieve a reasonable weight loss of 0.5 to 1 kg/week.[12] Very-low-calorie diets (<800 calories/day) should be avoided because they are stressful and are not more effective than low-calorie diets (500- to 1000-kcal deficit) in long-term weight loss.[45]

Effect of Diet

Several studies have indicated the beneficial effect of dietary modifications, with or without weight loss, on BP, either in improving or preventing hypertension. The Dietary Approaches to Stop Hypertension (DASH) trial evaluated the effect of specific dietary intakes on BP without any change in weight (Table 31-4). In this trial, 459 adults with systolic BP less than 160 mm Hg and diastolic BP between 80 and 95 mm Hg were fed for 3 weeks with a control diet low in fruits, vegetables, and dairy products and with a fat content typical of the average U.S. diet. After this introductory period, the participants were randomly assigned to one of three different groups. The first group continued the control diet for 8 more weeks; the second group received a diet rich in fruits and vegetables; and the third group received a combination diet rich in fruits, vegetables, and low-fat dairy products, with reduced saturated and total fat (the DASH diet). Body weight and sodium intake were stable during the study in all three groups. At the end of the study, compared with the control group, there was a reduction in systolic and diastolic BP by 5.5 and 3.0 mm Hg, respectively, in the combination diet group, whereas the reduction in the fruits and vegetables group was 2.8 and 1.1 mm Hg, respectively. In the subgroup of participants with hypertension (systolic BP ≥140 mm Hg and/or diastolic BP ≥90 mm Hg), the effects were more prominent. The systolic and diastolic BPs were reduced by 11.4 and 5.5 mm Hg, respectively, in the combination diet group, compared with the control group (Fig. 31-2).[46]

A subsequent study, the DASH-Sodium trial, examined the effect on BP of reducing dietary sodium in conjunction with the DASH diet. In this study, a total of 412 participants underwent a 2-week introductory phase, in which they all received a control diet high in sodium. They were then randomly assigned into two main groups, one following a typical U.S. diet and the other following the DASH diet. Within each group were three subgroups, with high, intermediate, and low sodium intake. The study lasted for 30 days, and the weight

Table 31-3 Recommended Daily Nutrient and Caloric Intake for Losing Weight

Recommended Daily Nutrient Intake	
Nutrient	Recommended Intake
Calories	500-1000 kcal/day less from usual intake
Proteins	15% of total calories
Carbohydrates	55% of total calories
Total fat	<30% of total calories
Saturated fatty acids	<10% of total calories
Monounsaturated fatty acids	Up to 15% of total calories
Polyunsaturated fatty acids	Up to 10% of total calories
Cholesterol	<300 mg/day
Sodium	<2.4 g/day (or <6 g sodium chloride/day)
Calcium	1000-1500 mg/day
Fiber	20-30 g/day

Table 31-4 Nutrient Targets and Average Daily Number of Servings for Experimental Diet in the Dietary Approaches to Stop Hypertension Study

	Control Diet	Fruits and Vegetables	DASH Diet
Nutrients			
Fat (% of total calories)	37	37	27
Saturated fat	16	16	6
Monounsaturated fat	13	13	13
Polyunsaturated fat	8	8	8
Carbohydrates (%)	48	48	55
Protein (%)	15	15	18
Cholesterol (mg/day)	300	300	150
Fiber (g/day)	9	9	31
Potassium (mg/day)	1700	4700	4700
Magnesium (mg/day)	165	500	500
Calcium (mg/day)	450	450	1240
Sodium (g/day)	3	3	3
Food Groups (Servings/Day)			
Fruits and juices	1.6	5.2	5.2
Vegetables	2.0	3.3	4.4
Grains	8.2	6.9	7.5
Low-fat dairy	0.1	0	2.0
Regular-fat dairy	0.4	0.3	0.7
Nuts, seeds, legumes	0	0.6	0.7
Beef, pork, ham	1.5	0.8	0.5
Poultry	0.8	0.4	0.6
Fish	0.2	0.3	0.5
Fat and oil	5.8	5.3	2.5
Snacks and sweets	4.1	1.4	0.7

DASH, Dietary Approaches to Stop Hypertension.
Modified from Appel LJ, Moore TJ, Obarzanek E, et al. A clinical trial of the effects of dietary patterns on blood pressure: DASH Collaborative Research Group. *N Engl J Med.* 1997;**336**:1117-1124.

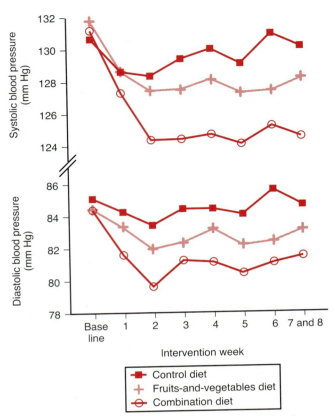

Figure 31-2   Changes in systolic and diastolic blood pressures during the intervention period according to diet in the Dietary Approaches to Stop Hypertension (DASH) study. (From Appel LJ, Moore TJ, Obarzanek E, et al. A clinical trial of the effects of dietary patterns on blood pressure: DASH Collaborative Research Group. *N Engl J Med.* 1997;**336**:1117-1124.)

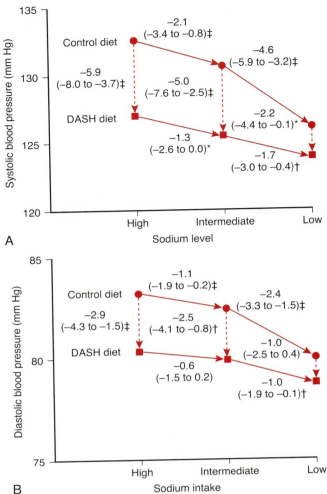

Figure 31-3   Effect of the Dietary Approaches to Stop Hypertension (DASH) diet on systolic (**A**) and diastolic (**B**) blood pressure according to the level of sodium intake. *Asterisks* (*P*<.05), *daggers* (*P*<.01), and *double daggers* (*P*<.001) indicate significant differences in blood pressure between groups or between dietary sodium categories. (From Sacks FM, Svetkey LP, Vollmer WM, et al. DASH-Sodium Collaborative Research Group: Effects on blood pressure of reduced dietary sodium and the Dietary Approaches to Stop Hypertension [DASH] diet. DASH-Sodium Collaborative Research Group. *N Engl J Med.* 2001;**344**:3-10.)

of the participants did not change. At the end of the study, the results were the following: (1) in each of the sodium intake levels, the reduction of BP was greater in the DASH diet group compared with the control diet group; (2) reduction of sodium intake from high to intermediate or low decreased BP in both the DASH and the control diets (Fig. 31-3); and (3) the most significant difference, when subgroups were compared, was observed between the DASH diet–low-sodium group and the control diet–high-sodium group. There was a reduction in systolic and diastolic BP of 11.5 and 5.7 mm Hg, respectively, in the DASH–low-sodium diet, compared with the control–high-sodium diet in the hypertensive participants. The reduction in the normotensive participants was 7.1 mm Hg in systolic BP and 3.7 mm Hg in diastolic BP.[47]

The Diet, Exercise, and Weight Loss Intervention Trial (DEW-IT) was a smaller trial that enrolled 45 overweight hypertensive adults on a single BP medication, to examine the results of lifestyle modifications on BP. The participants were randomized into two groups: a control group and a lifestyle intervention group that was fed a hypocaloric, low-sodium DASH diet and did moderate-intensity exercise. At the end of the 9-week study, the intervention group had a mean weight loss of 4.9 kg and a mean reduction in 24-hour ambulatory

systolic and diastolic BP of 9.5 and 5.3 mm Hg, respectively, compared with the control group.[48]

The PREMIER trial examined the effects of lifestyle modifications over a longer period (6 months). In this trial, 810 mostly (95%) overweight adults with systolic BP 120 to 159 mm Hg and diastolic BP 80 to 95 mm Hg who were not taking antihypertensive medication were randomly assigned to three different groups. Group 1 had the "established" recommendations for lowering BP (weight loss, increased physical activity, and low sodium intake), group 2 had the "established" recommendations in addition to the DASH diet, and group 3 was the "advice-only" comparison group. After subtracting change in the advice-only group, the mean net reductions of systolic and diastolic BP were 3.7 and 1.7 mm Hg, respectively, for the established group and 4.3 and 2.6 mm Hg for the established plus DASH group. The difference between these two groups was 0.6 mm Hg for systolic and 0.9 mm Hg for diastolic BP. Compared with the overall prevalence of hypertension at baseline of 37.5%, at the end of the study, only 26% of the advice-only group, 17% of the established group, and 12% of the established plus DASH group had hypertension.[49]

The Trial of Nonpharmacologic Interventions in the Elderly (TONE) investigated the effect of dietary modifications or weight loss on older people (60 to 80 years old) who had systolic BP less than 145 mm Hg and diastolic BP less than 85 mm Hg while they were receiving a single antihypertensive medication. A total of 975 persons participated in this study, of whom 585 were obese. The obese participants were randomized into four different groups. Group 1 was instructed on a low sodium intake, group 2 was assigned to a weight loss program using diet and exercise, group 3 had both a weight loss program and reduced sodium intake, and group 4 was the control group. The nonobese participants were assigned to either a low-sodium-intake group or a control group. Withdrawal of antihypertensive medication was attempted after 3 months of intervention, and the participants were followed for a further 30 months. The systolic and diastolic BPs decreased by 3.4 and 1.9 mm Hg, respectively, compared with baseline in the sodium reduction group, by 4.0 and 1.1 mm Hg in the weight loss group, by 5.3 and 3.4 mm Hg in the weight loss and low-sodium group, and by only 0.8 and 0.8 in the control group. The likelihood of remaining free of elevated BP, antihypertensive drug therapy, and cardiovascular events for the obese participants at the end of the study was 34% for the sodium reduction group, 37% for the weight loss group, 44% for the weight loss plus low sodium group, and 16% for the control group.[50]

In the Treatment of Mild Hypertension Study (TOMHS), 902 participants with "mild" hypertension (diastolic BP <100 mm Hg) were all advised to lose weight, to decrease alcohol and sodium consumption, and to increase physical activity, and they were then assigned to one of six different treatment groups (chlorthalidone, acebutolol, doxazosin, amlodipine, enalapril, or placebo). At 4 years after randomization, both systolic and diastolic BPs were reduced in all treatment groups compared with baseline. Although participants in the drug treatment groups had significantly greater BP reductions compared with the placebo group (−13.4/−11.1 versus −8.8/−8.8 mm Hg, respectively), there was also a significant decrease in BP in the placebo group compared with baseline, a finding indicating that lifestyle interventions play an important role in BP regulation.[51]

The Hypertension Control Program was a 4-year study that examined the possibility for patients with modestly elevated BP to discontinue antihypertensive medication by using nutritional means. In this study, participants were randomized to one of three groups. In group 1, patients discontinued antihypertensive medications and modified their diets, by reducing salt and losing weight. In group 2, patients discontinued medications without any dietary changes; in group 3, patients continued taking their usual treatment. At the end of the study, 39% of the patients in group 1 remained normotensive without drug therapy, whereas only 5% in group 2 remained free of medication.[52]

In the Trial of Antihypertensive Interventions and Management (TAIM), the effect of weight loss alone or in combination with antihypertensive drugs on diastolic BP was examined. In this study, 529 obese or overweight participants were randomized to one of three drug treatment groups (placebo, chlorthalidone, or atenolol). Within each of these groups, participants were also randomized to a usual diet or a weight reduction diet. At 6 months of the study, BP reduction in the placebo with weight reduction diet group was 11.6 mm Hg for participants who lost at least 4.5 kg (10 lb), and it was not statistically different from the reduction achieved with the usual diet and 25 mg chlorthalidone (−11.1 mm Hg) or 50 mg atenolol (−12.4 mm Hg). For participants in the placebo with weight reduction diet group who lost less than 2.25 kg (5 lb), the reduction in BP was smaller (−7 mm Hg). In this study, effective weight loss (>10 lb in a 6-month period) lowered BP similarly to low-dose drug therapy.[53]

The Trials of Hypertension Prevention Phases I and II (TOHP I and TOPH II) examined the effect of weight loss in the prevention of hypertension. In TOHP I, 564 participants who were obese or overweight (body weight 15% to 65% greater than desirable for height) and who had a diastolic BP between 80 and 89 mm Hg were assigned to either an 18-month weight loss intervention with nutrition counseling and an increase in physical activity or a usual care control condition. The average weight losses in the intervention group at 6, 12, and 18 months of follow-up were 6.5, 5.6, and 4.7 kg for men and 3.7, 2.7, and 1.6 kg for women, respectively. The mean change in BPs at the end of the study, compared with the usual care group, were −3.1/−2.8 mm Hg for men and −2.0/−1.1 mm Hg for women, respectively. BP reduction was greater for those participants who lost more weight.[54]

TOHP II examined the effects of dietary interventions in preventing hypertension over a longer period in obese or overweight individuals with systolic BP less than 140 mm Hg and diastolic BP of 83 to 89 mm Hg. The participants were randomized into four different groups: a usual care group, a sodium reduction group, a weight loss group, and a combined intervention group. Compared with the usual care group, the reduction in systolic and diastolic BPs at 6 months was 2.9/1.6 mm Hg for the sodium reduction group, 3.7/2.7 mm Hg for the weight loss group, and 4.0/2.8 mm Hg for the combined intervention group. At 36 months, the reductions were 1.2/0.7 mm Hg for the sodium reduction group, 1.3/0.9 mm Hg for the weight loss group, and 1.1/0.6 mm Hg for the combined intervention group. Through 48 months, the incidence of hypertension was significantly less in each intervention group, compared with the usual care group.[55] The mean weight loss from baseline for the weight loss group was 4.4, 2.0, and 0.2 kg at 6, 18, and 36 months of the study. In the usual care group, there was an *increase* in body weight of 0.1, 0.7, and 1.8 kg at the same time points (Fig. 31-4). BP was significantly lower in the weight loss group than in the usual care group at all time points. Participants who lost at least 4.5 kg at 6 months and who maintained this weight for the next 30 months had a 65% lower risk of developing hypertension (Fig. 31-5).[56]

All the previously mentioned studies indicate the importance of lifestyle modifications, including diet and sodium

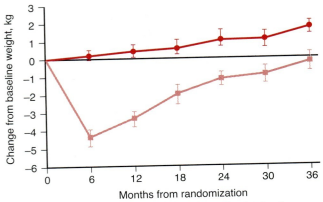

Figure 31–4 Mean change in weight in the Trials of Hypertension Prevention Phase II (TOHP II) (*orange line,* weight loss group; *red line,* control group). (From Stevens VJ, Obarzanek E, Cook NR, et al., Trials for the Hypertension Prevention Research Group. Long-term weight loss and changes in blood pressure: Results of the Trials of Hypertension Prevention, Phase II. *Ann Intern Med.* 2001;**134**:1-11.)

restriction, in preventing or improving hypertension. A summary of the studies indicating the effects of diet and weight loss on BP is presented in Table 31-5.

Effect of Exercise

Physical activity plays a very important role in BP regulation in obese hypertensive individuals. Increased physical activity should be a major component of any weight loss and maintenance plan, along with diet, to decrease BP or to prevent hypertension. Exercise increases energy expenditure, which, in conjunction with decreased caloric intake, results in weight loss. It also improves insulin sensitivity in obese subjects. In a study of sedentary overweight individuals with BPs 130 to 180/85 to 110 mm Hg while they were not taking antihypertensive medications, 133 participants were randomized into three different groups. Group 1 had a weight reduction program including diet and exercise; group 2 had only aerobic exercise; and group 3 was the control group. After 6 months, clinic BPs dropped by 7.4/5.6, 4.4/4.3, and 0.9/1.4 mm Hg in the weight loss, exercise only, and control groups, respectively. Ambulatory BP monitoring showed similar differences across the three groups. This study showed that diet and exercise have an additive effect in decreasing BP.[57] However, exercise seems to have a beneficial effect on BP even in the absence of weight loss.[58] The Seventh Report of the Joint National Committee on Prevention, Detection, Evaluation, and Treatment of High Blood Pressure (JNC 7) strongly suggests that hypertensive individuals perform regular physical activity at least 30 minutes/day, most days of the week.[59] Sedentary obese hypertensive patients should start with low-intensity aerobic exercise and should gradually increase to more vigorous activity. The exact mechanism by which exercise has an antihypertensive effect is not completely understood. A possible mechanism is a reduction in norepinephrine levels after exercise.[60] Another possible mechanism may be

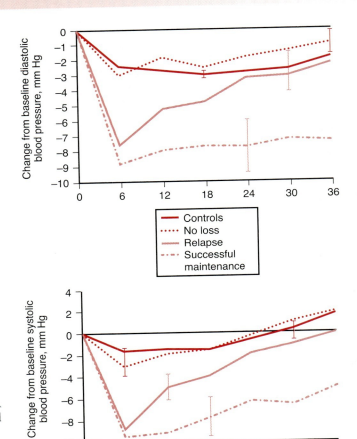

Figure 31–5 Mean changes in diastolic (*top*) and systolic (*bottom*) blood pressures during the intervention period in the Trials of Hypertension Prevention Phase II (TOHP II). (From Stevens VJ, Obarzanek E, Cook NR, et al., Trials for the Hypertension Prevention Research Group. Long-term weight loss and changes in blood pressure: Results of the Trials of Hypertension Prevention, Phase II. *Ann Intern Med.* 2001;**134**:1-11.)

increased endothelial nitric oxide release, which, in turn, causes vasodilation.[61,62]

Effects of Weight Loss Medications

Two drugs are approved in the United States for long-term use, orlistat and sibutramine. If lifestyle modifications are tried for a period of 6 months and are unsuccessful in reducing weight, it is possible to add a weight loss drug, in an effort to lower not only weight but also BP.

Orlistat

Orlistat is the drug of choice for weight loss in hypertensive patients. It is an inhibitor of pancreatic lipase. With its use, about one third of the triglycerides that are eaten are not hydrolyzed, cannot be absorbed through the gut, and are therefore excreted in the stool. Numerous studies have shown the efficacy of orlistat in weight loss. The European

Table 31-5   Studies Indicating the Effects of Weight Loss on Blood Pressure

Study	Participant Characteristics	Study Duration	Treatment Groups	Weight Change	Blood Pressure Change (mm Hg)
DASH	459 adults with hypertension	8 wk	1. Control diet 2. Fruits/vegetables 3. Fruits/vegetables and low-fat diet (DASH)	−0.1* −0.3* −0.4*	 −2.8/−1.1[†] −5.5/−3.0[†]

DASH-Low sodium	412 adults (41% with hypertension)	30 days	1. Control diet
			  a. High-sodium
			  b. Intermediate-sodium
			  c. Low-sodium
			2. DASH diet
			  a. High-sodium
			  b. Intermediate-sodium
			  c. Low-sodium
					
					−5.9/−2.9[†]
					−5.0/−2.5[†]
					−2.2/−1.0[†]

DEW-IT	45 hypertensive obese adults	9 wk	1. Control diet 2. Hypocaloric low-salt DASH diet and exercise	−0.6* −5.5*	 −9.5/−5.3[†]
PREMIER	810 overweight adults with mild hypertension	6 mo	1. Control diet 2. Hypocaloric low-salt diet and exercise 3. Hypocaloric low-salt DASH diet and exercise	−1.1* −4.9* −5.8*	 −3.7/−1.7[†] −4.3/−2.6[†]
TONE	975 elderly patients receiving a blood pressure medication (585 obese)	29 mo average	1. Control diet 2. Low-salt diet 3. Hypocaloric diet 4. Low-salt and hypocaloric diet	−0.9 for groups 1 and 2* −3.8 for groups 3 and 4*	−0.8/−0.8* −3.4/−1.9* −4.0/−1.1* −5.3/−3.4*
TOHP I	564 adults with high-normal blood pressure	18 mo	1. Control group 2. Diet and exercise	0 −4.7 (men)*	−2.5/−3.9* −5.4/−6.2*
TOHP II	1191 obese adults	36 mo	1. Control group 2. Intervention group	+1.8* −0.2*	 −1.3/−0.9[†]

*From baseline.
[†]Compared with control.
DASH, Dietary Approaches to Stop Hypertension; DEW-IT, Diet, Exercise, and Weight Loss Intervention Trial; TONE, Trial of Nonpharmacologic Interventions in the Elderly; TOHP I and TOHP II, Trials of Hypertension Prevention Phases I and II.

Multicenter Orlistat Study Group reported on a placebo-controlled randomized trial in 681 obese persons. After 1 year, the average weight loss in the orlistat group was 10.2%, versus 6.1% for the placebo group.[63] A similar study was done in the United States, randomizing 892 obese volunteers to an orlistat group or a placebo group. After 1 year, participants receiving orlistat had lost 8.76 ± 0.37 kg, and the placebo group had lost 5.81 ± 0.67 kg.[64] During the second year, both groups regained weight, but the gain was greater in the placebo group than in the orlistat group (3.2 ± 0.45 versus 5.63 ± 0.42 kg).

A randomized controlled study of the effect of orlistat and diet versus placebo and diet on BP in hypertensive obese patients has also been reported.[65] In this study, the BMI changes at 1 year were 1.9 kg/m^2 versus 0.9 kg/m^2, and the diastolic BP drop was 11.4 versus 8.4 mm Hg. A similar study involving 628 obese hypertensive patients showed decreases in both systolic and diastolic BPs that were greater for the orlistat group than for the placebo group (9.4/7.7 versus 4.6/5.6 mm Hg).[66]

Sibutramine

Sibutramine is a serotonin and norepinephrine reuptake inhibitor that works centrally to reduce food intake. Because of its norepinephrine action, it does not have the BP-lowering effect that one would expect for a given amount of weight loss. Although most patients decrease their BP while taking the drug, some may increase it, in which case the drug must be stopped.

Numerous randomized controlled studies of sibutramine have investigated its weight loss effect. In a dose-ranging study in the United States, 1047 obese volunteers took various doses of the drug or placebo for 6 months. Weight loss was 2.7% of the baseline weight with placebo, 3.9% with 5 mg/day, 6.1% with 10 mg/day, and 7.4% with 25 mg/day.[67] In a second study, a very low-calorie diet was used with sibutramine or placebo.[68] After 6 months, 86% of participants in the sibutramine group lost at least 5% of their baseline weight, whereas 55% in the placebo group did so. At 12 months, 75% of the sibutramine group maintained their weight loss, compared with only 42% of the placebo group.

Another randomized controlled trial with a different design was the Sibutramine Trial of Weight Reduction and Maintenance (STORM).[69] In this trial, 605 patients were placed on a very low-calorie diet and sibutramine 10 mg/day for 6 months. Those who lost at least 5% of baseline weight were then randomized to continue sibutramine at 10 mg/day or to take placebo for another 18 months. Of the completers, 80% of the sibutramine group maintained their weight loss, compared with only 16% of the placebo group.

The most important side effect of sibutramine is cardiovascular. The drug can increase heart rate and can elevate BP. As a result, it should not be used in patients with coronary heart disease, arrhythmias, or heart failure. Some studies have tested sibutramine for weight loss in obese hypertensive patients. Generally, BP drops slightly but not as much as would be expected for the level of weight loss.[70,71] The drug should not be used for patients with uncontrolled hypertension. BP and heart rate should be monitored regularly in all patients.

For neither drug are long-term data available on morbidity and mortality. Both drugs, as stated, have significant side effects. As a result, the best strategy is to emphasize lifestyle changes.

Effects of Obesity Surgery

According to National Institutes of Health guidelines, obesity surgery is an option for weight loss for patients with a BMI greater than 40 kg/m² or a BMI greater than 35 kg/m² with co-morbidities.[72] The Swedish Obese Subjects (SOS) study is the largest investigation of the effects of weight loss after surgical therapy of obesity on co-morbid conditions. At 2 years after surgery, weight loss was 28 kg (versus 0.5 kg for the control group), and at 8 years after surgery, it was 20 kg (versus 0.7 kg weight gain for the control). There was a significant reduction in diabetes mellitus and hypertension incidence 2 years after the operation, but, surprisingly, at 8 years postoperatively, the beneficial effect of weight loss on BP was lost, whereas the beneficial effects of weight loss in diabetes mellitus was maintained.[73-76] A cautionary note about bariatric surgery is in order. The risk-to-benefit ratio can be high. Besides the acute risk of the surgery, certain long-term adverse effects are possible. These include anemia from vitamin B_{12} and iron deficiency, metabolic bone disease with low calcium and vitamin D, and protein-calorie malnutrition.

ANTIHYPERTENSIVE TREATMENT IN OBESITY

Weight loss is the treatment of choice in obese hypertensive individuals. However, if they do not lose weight or if they lose weight but BP is still elevated, an antihypertensive medication should be added. Selection of the appropriate antihypertensive drug has to be made. The physician needs to take into account the pathophysiology and the hemodynamic changes characteristic of obesity-related hypertension and the effect the drug may have on these mechanisms. For example, hypertension in obesity is associated with enhanced sympathetic nervous system activity, increased activity of the renin-angiotensin-aldosterone system, sodium retention, insulin resistance, and a specific type of LVH. Pharmacokinetic factors probably also play a role in the action of specific antihypertensive drugs, depending on their lipophilic or hydrophilic nature. Because obese individuals have excessive body fat, the pharmacokinetics of lipophilic drugs can be affected. Moreover, other conditions that often coexist in obese hypertensive individuals, such as diabetes mellitus, hyperlipidemia, and elevated serum uric acid levels, should be considered when one chooses an antihypertensive drug. Surprisingly, not many large-scale studies have investigated the effect of antihypertensive drugs in obese patients. The Antihypertensive and Lipid-Lowering Treatment to Prevent Heart Attack Trial (ALLHAT) included many overweight or obese patients and can give some useful information about the four antihypertensive drugs that were compared (a diuretic, an α-blocker, an ACE inhibitor, and a calcium channel blocker).[77,78] The role of each class of antihypertensive drugs in obesity is discussed in the following sections.

Diuretics

Diuretics have their effect on BP through their ability to reduce renal sodium and water reabsorption and to decrease intravascular volume and cardiac output (see Chapter 18).[79] However, diuretics can increase the activity of both the sympathetic nervous system and the renin-angiotensin-aldosterone system,[80] and when these drugs are used as monotherapy at high doses, they may adversely affect insulin resistance and dyslipidemia.[81]

The Treatment in Obese Patients with Hypertension study compared the effect of the diuretic hydrochlorothiazide with the ACE inhibitor lisinopril on BP and metabolic parameters in 232 obese hypertensive patients. Hydrochlorothiazide was as effective as lisinopril in lowering BP; however, usually a higher dose of diuretic was necessary to achieve an antihypertensive effect comparable to that of the low-dose ACE inhibitor. Although neither medication significantly affected insulin levels or lipid profiles, there was an increase in blood glucose after 12 weeks of treatment with hydrochlorothiazide. An interesting finding in this study was that hydrochlorothiazide was more effective in lowering BP in black obese hypertensive patients, whereas lisinopril was more effective in white patients.[82] Another study also compared the effectiveness of a low-dose diuretic (12.5 mg hydrochlorothiazide) with an ACE inhibitor (lisinopril, 20 mg) in controlling BP. Although there was a significant fall in BP with the diuretic, lisinopril was more effective. Hydrochlorothiazide had marginal negative effects on glucose, insulin, lipids, and lipoproteins.[83]

Because many obese patients have insulin resistance, diuretics should be used with caution in these patients. However, diuretics in low doses alone or in combination with other agents (e.g., ACE inhibitors and ARBs) can be used in the treatment of obesity-related hypertension.[59]

α-Blockers

α-Blockers are generally safe in controlling BP in obese hypertensive patients, because these drugs usually do not have unfavorable metabolic effects (see Chapter 23). They decrease the early insulin response and improve insulin sensitivity.[84,85] They also have a favorable effect on the lipid profile, with decreases in triglyceride and low-density lipoprotein cholesterol levels. Theoretically, α-blockers could be used for obese hypertensive patients with glucose intolerance or lipid abnormalities. However, in ALLHAT, patients who received the α-blocker doxazosin had higher BPs and an 80% increased risk of heart failure compared with patients who received the diuretic chlorthalidone.[86] Most authorities agree that α-blockers are not appropriate first-line antihypertensive drugs because of these data, despite the favorable metabolic effects of these agents.

β-Blockers

β-Blockers achieve their BP-lowering effect, in part, by decreasing cardiac output and reducing plasma renin activity (see Chapter 19). Because obese hypertensive patients have increased cardiac output,[87] and an activated renin-angiotensin-aldosterone system, these agents may be considered antihypertensive drugs in the obese population. β-Blockers also have an antiarrhythmic effect, and they prevent sudden death. They are useful as second-line drugs for treatment of heart failure, a condition commonly seen in obese hypertensive patients.[88] However, β-blockers have some unfavorable metabolic effects with respect to glucose and lipids that limit the use of these drugs. β-Blockers are associated with impaired glucose tolerance, increased levels of triglycerides, and decreased levels of high-density lipoprotein cholesterol.[89,90] Another limitation to the use of β-blockers is that they can either cause weight gain or prevent loss of weight, a particularly undesirable feature for obese or overweight patients.[91] Therefore, β-blockers may be the drug of choice for obese hypertensive patients with arrhythmias or heart failure, but another drug should be selected for obese patients who do not have these complications.

Calcium Channel Blockers

Calcium channel blockers achieve their antihypertensive action through a peripheral vasodilator effect and an increase in natriuresis (see Chapter 22).[92] Because obese hypertensive patients have increased intravascular volume, calcium channel blockers are effective in decreasing BP. Calcium channel blockers are metabolically neutral: their use seems to have neither a negative nor a positive effect on glucose metabolism or lipid profile,[93-95] and they can be used without any problem in obese hypertensive diabetic patients. A possible disadvantage of these drugs use is their association with lower extremity edema, which may be particularly troublesome for obese individuals. This adverse effect is ameliorated with the addition of an ACE inhibitor. Unlike dihydropyridine calcium channel blockers, the nondihydropyridine calcium channel blockers, verapamil and diltiazem, decrease heart rate and can be used in obese hypertensive patients if β-blockers are contraindicated.[96]

Angiotensin-Converting Enzyme Inhibitors

ACE inhibitors are probably, along with the ARBs, the drugs of choice for the treatment of hypertension in obese individuals (see Chapter 20). Their BP-lowering effect is achieved primarily through inhibition of the renin-angiotensin system, but they also have an inhibitory action on sympathetic nervous system activity.[97] Another possible mechanism of action is through the accumulation of bradykinin, which stimulates nitric oxide release and promotes vasodilatation.[98,99] ACE inhibitors do not have any negative metabolic effects with respect to glucose or lipid metabolism. They improve insulin sensitivity,[81] and they also prevent the development of type 2 diabetes mellitus.[100] These drugs are also effective in regression of LVH and in prevention of heart failure (in some studies). Finally, ACE inhibitors are effective in preventing the onset and progression of albuminuria in obese diabetic patients.[101] The Treatment in Obese Patients with Hypertension study has shown the effectiveness of the ACE inhibitor lisinopril in obese hypertensive patients.[82]

Angiotensin II Receptor Blockers

Angiotensin II receptor blockers have mechanisms of antihypertensive action similar to those of the ACE inhibitors (see Chapter 21). ARBs also have an inhibitory effect on the renin-angiotensin system, and they decrease sympathetic nervous system activity.[102] A difference is that ARBs do not increase bradykinin levels.[103] These drugs also improve insulin sensitivity and prevent or decrease albuminuria,[104] so they can be used in obese hypertensive diabetic patients. A study in obese hypertensive individuals compared the efficacy of the ARB candesartan with that of hydrochlorothiazide. The two drugs had similar effects in reducing BP after 12 weeks of treatment; however, candesartan decreased sympathetic nervous system activity and increased insulin sensitivity, whereas hydrochlorothiazide did not have these effects.[105] ARBs have a preventive effect in the development of diabetes, similar to that of ACE inhibitors.[106]

Centrally Acting Drugs

Because sympathetic nervous system activity is increased in obesity, centrally acting drugs offer theoretical benefits in treating obese hypertensive patients in that these agents reduce sympathetic nervous activity and plasma levels of norepinephrine.[107] Decreased sympathetic nervous activity results in reduced sodium reabsorption and decreased extracellular volume.[108] Clonidine, the most commonly used drug of this class, stimulates central α$_2$-adrenergic receptors. Centrally acting drugs do not have negative metabolic effects[109]; however, they may promote weight gain, which is undesirable for obese patients.

In conclusion, a summary of the advantages and disadvantages of different classes of antihypertensive medications in the treatment of hypertension in obese patients is presented in Table 31-6. The choice of drugs for the treatment of obesity-related hypertension is difficult and should be individualized for each particular patient, depending on the presence of other co-morbid conditions. However, ACE inhibitors and ARBs seem to be effective in controlling BP, and they may protect against incident diabetes. Low-dose diuretics or calcium channel blockers can also be used as monotherapy or in combination with ACE inhibitors. β-Blockers can be used for patients with arrhythmias or heart failure.

Table 31-6 Advantages and Disadvantages of Antihypertensive Medications for Treating Obesity-Related Hypertension

Medication	Advantages	Disadvantages
Diuretics	↓ Renal sodium reabsorption ↓ Intravascular volume	↑ SNS activity ↑ RAAS activity ↑ Insulin resistance Dyslipidemia (in high doses)
α-Blockers	↑ Insulin sensitivity ↓ Triglycerides and low-density lipoprotein cholesterol	↑ Risk of heart failure
β-Blockers	↓ RAAS activity ↓ Cardiac output Protection from congestive heart failure	Impaired glucose metabolism ↑ Triglycerides ↓ High-density lipoprotein cholesterol Weight gain
Calcium channel blockers	Peripheral vasodilation ↑ Natriuresis ↓ Intravascular volume Neutral metabolic effects ↓ Heart rate (verapamil only)	Lower extremity edema
ACE inhibitors	↓ RAAS activity ↓ SNS activity Peripheral vasodilation ↑ Insulin sensitivity Prevention of microalbuminuria No effects on lipids Regression of LVH	None
Angiotensin receptor blockers	Same as ACE inhibitors	None
Centrally acting drugs	↓ SNS activity ↓ Renal sodium reabsorption Neutral metabolic effects	Weight gain

↑, increase; ↓, decrease; ACE, angiotensin-converting enzyme; LVH, left ventricular hypertrophy; RAAS, renin-angiotensin-aldosterone system; SNS, sympathetic nervous system.

SUMMARY

Obesity is a common problem in the United States that affects much of the population. Hypertension is a condition very often seen in obese individuals. The cause of obesity-related hypertension is multifactorial, but it has been clearly shown that weight loss improves BP. Weight loss can be achieved with diet, with physical activity, or with the assistance of the weight reduction drugs orlistat and sibutramine. If weight loss is not sufficient to control BP, addition of an antihypertensive drug should be considered, based on the metabolic and other characteristics of each patient.

References

1. Kuczmarski RJ, Carroll MD, Flegal KM, Troiano RP. Varying body mass index cutoff points to describe overweight prevalence among U.S. adults: NHANES III (1988 to 1994). *Obes Res.* 1997;**5**:542-548.
2. Flegal KM, Carroll MD, Ogden CL, Johnson CL. Prevalence and trends in obesity among US adults, 1999-2000. *JAMA.* 2003;**288**:1723-1727.
3. Manson JE, Willett WC, Stampfer MJ, et al. Body weight and mortality among women. *N Engl J Med.* 1995;**333**:677-685.
4. Corrigan SA, Raczynski JM, Swencionis C, Jennings SG. Weight reduction in the prevention and treatment of hypertension: A review of representative clinical trials. *Am J Health Promot.* 1991;**5**:208-214.
5. Peeters A, Barendregt JJ, Willekens F, et al., for NEDCOM, the Netherlands Epidemiology and Demography Compression of Morbidity Research Group. Obesity in adulthood and its consequences for life expectancy: A life-table analysis. *Ann Intern Med.* 2003;**138**:24-32.
6. Pi-Sunyer FX. A review of long-term studies evaluating the efficacy of weight loss in ameliorating disorders associated with obesity. *Clin Ther.* 1996;**18**:1006-1035.
7. Pi-Sunyer FX. Health implications of obesity. *Am J Clin Nutr.* 1991;**53**:1595S-1603S.
8. Pi-Sunyer FX. Medical hazards of obesity. *Ann Intern Med.* 1993;**119**:655-660.
9. He J, Whelton PK, Appel LJ, et al. Long-term effects of weight loss and dietary sodium reduction on incidence of hypertension. *Hypertension.* 2000;**35**:544-549.
10. Reisin E, Frohlich ED, Messerli FH, et al. Cardiovascular changes after weight reduction in obesity hypertension. *Ann Intern Med.* 1983;**98**:315-319.
11. Gallagher D, Visser M, Sepulveda D, et al. How useful is body mass index for comparison of body fatness across age, sex, and ethnic groups? *Am J Epidemiol.* 1996;**143**:228-239.
12. National Institutes of Health. Clinical guidelines on the identification, evaluation, and treatment of overweight and obesity in adults: The evidence report. *Obes Res.* 1998;**6** (**Suppl 2**):51S-209S.

13. Hall JE, Louis K. Dahl Memorial Lecture: Renal and cardiovascular mechanisms of hypertension in obesity. *Hypertension*. 1994;**23**:381-394.

14. Hall JE, Brands MW, Henegar JR. Mechanisms of hypertension and kidney disease in obesity. *Ann N Y Acad Sci*. 1999;**18**:91-107.

15. Hall JE, Jones DW, Kuo JJ, et al. Impact of the obesity epidemic on hypertension and renal disease. *Curr Hypertens Rep*. 2003;**5**:386-392.

16. Hall JE, Henegar JR, Dwyer TM, et al. Is obesity a major cause of chronic kidney disease? *Adv Ren Replace Ther*. 2004;**11**:41-54.

17. Sowers JR, Whitfield LA, Catania RA, et al. Role of the sympathetic nervous system in blood pressure maintenance in obesity. *J Clin Endocrinol Metab*. 1982;**54**:1181-1186.

18. Tuck ML, Sowers JR, Dornfeld L, et al. Reductions in plasma catecholamines and blood pressure during weight loss in obese subjects. *Acta Endocrinol (Copenh)*. 1983;**102**:252-257.

19. Mikhail N, Golub MS, Tuck ML. Obesity and hypertension. *Prog Cardiovasc Dis*. 1999;**42**:39-58.

20. Landsberg L. Hyperinsulinemia: Possible role in obesity-induced hypertension. *Hypertension*. 1992;**19** (**1 Suppl**):I61-I66.

21. Landsberg L. Insulin resistance, energy balance and sympathetic nervous system activity. *Clin Exp Hypertens A*. 1990;**12**:817-830.

22. Rocchini AP, Katch V, Kveselis D, et al. Insulin and renal sodium retention in obese adolescents. *Hypertension*. 1989;**14**:367-374.

23. Gupta AK, Clark RV, Kirchner KA. Effects of insulin on renal sodium excretion. *Hypertension*. 1992;**19** (**1 Suppl**):I78-I82.

24. O'Brien T, Young WF Jr, Palumbo PJ, et al. Hypertension and dyslipidemia in patients with insulinoma. *Mayo Clin Proc*. 1993;**68**:141-146.

25. Sawicki PT, Baba T, Berger M, Starke A. Normal blood pressure in patients with insulinoma despite hyperinsulinemia and insulin resistance. *J Am Soc Nephrol*. 1992;**3** (**4 Suppl**):S64-S68.

26. Considine RV, Sinha MK, Heiman ML, et al. Serum immunoreactive-leptin concentrations in normal-weight and obese humans. *N Engl J Med*. 1996;**334**:292-295.

27. Barba G, Russo O, Siani A, et al. Plasma leptin and blood pressure in men: Graded association independent of body mass and fat pattern. *Obes Res*. 2003;**11**:160-166.

28. Lembo G, Vecchione C, Fratta L, et al. Leptin induces direct vasodilation through distinct endothelial mechanisms. *Diabetes*. 2000;**49**:293-297.

29. Shek EW, Brands MW, Hall JE. Chronic leptin infusion increases arterial pressure. *Hypertension*. 1998;**31**:409-414.

30. Heymsfield SB, Greenberg AS, Fujioka K, et al. Recombinant leptin for weight loss in obese and lean adults. *JAMA*. 1999;**282**:1568-1575.

31. Hall JE, Brands MW, Dixon WN, Smith MJ Jr. Obesity-induced hypertension: Renal function and systemic hemodynamics. *Hypertension*. 1993;**22**:292-299.

32. Engeli S, Sharma AM. The renin-angiotensin system and natriuretic peptides in obesity-associated hypertension. *J Mol Med*. 2001;**79**:21-29.

33. Tuck ML, Sowers J, Dornfeld L, et al. The effect of weight reduction on blood pressure, plasma renin activity, and plasma aldosterone levels in obese patients. *N Engl J Med*. 1981;**304**:930-933.

33. Weir MR, Reisin E, Falkner B, et al. Nocturnal reduction of blood pressure and the antihypertensive response to a diuretic or angiotensin converting enzyme inhibitor in obese hypertensive patients: TROPHY Study Group. *Am J Hypertens*. 1998;**11**:914-920.

35. Jensen MD. Diet effects on fatty acid metabolism in lean and obese humans. *Am J Clin Nutr*. 1998;**67** (**3 Suppl**):531S-534S.

36. Stepniakowski KT, Goodfriend TL, Egan BM. Fatty acids enhance vascular alpha-adrenergic sensitivity. *Hypertension*. 1995;**25**:774-778.

37. Grekin RJ, Dumont CJ, Vollmer AP, et al. Mechanisms in the pressor effects of hepatic portal venous fatty acid infusion. *Am J Physiol*. 1997;**273**:R324-R330.

38. Dessi-Fulgheri P, Sarzani R, Serenelli M, et al. Low calorie diet enhances renal, hemodynamic, and humoral effects of exogenous atrial natriuretic peptide in obese hypertensives. *Hypertension*. 1999;**33**:658-662.

39. Dessi-Fulgheri P, Sarzani R, Tamburrini P, et al. Plasma atrial natriuretic peptide and natriuretic peptide receptor gene expression in adipose tissue of normotensive and hypertensive obese patients. *J Hypertens*. 1997;**15**:1695-1699.

40. Pickering TG. Sleep apnea and hypertension. *J Clin Hypertens (Greenwich)*. 2002;**4**:437-440.

41. Phillips BG, Narkiewicz K, Pesek CA, et al. Effects of obstructive sleep apnea on endothelin-1 and blood pressure. *J Hypertens*. 1999;**17**:61-66.

42. Frohlich ED, Apstein C, Chobanian AV, et al. The heart in hypertension. *N Engl J Med*. 1992;**327**:998-1008.

43. Kenchaiah S, Evans JC, Levy D, et al. Obesity and the risk of heart failure. *N Engl J Med*. 2002;**347**:305-315.

44. Bialostosky K, Wright JD, Kennedy-Stephenson J, et al. Dietary intake of macronutrients, micronutrients, and other dietary constituents: United States 1988-94. *Vital Health Stat 10*. 2002;**245**:1-158.

45. Wadden TA, Foster GD, Letizia KA. One-year behavioral treatment of obesity: Comparison of moderate and severe caloric restriction and the effects of weight maintenance therapy. *J Consult Clin Psychol*. 1994;**62**:165-171.

46. Appel LJ, Moore TJ, Obarzanek E, et al. A clinical trial of the effects of dietary patterns on blood pressure: DASH Collaborative Research Group. *N Engl J Med*. 1997;**336**:1117-1124.

47. Sacks FM, Svetkey LP, Vollmer WM, et al., DASH-Sodium Collaborative Research Group. Effects on blood pressure of reduced dietary sodium and the Dietary Approaches to Stop Hypertension (DASH) diet: DASH-Sodium Collaborative Research Group. *N Engl J Med*. 2001;**344**:3-10.

48. Miller ER 3rd, Erlinger TP, Young DR, et al. Results of the Diet, Exercise, and Weight Loss Intervention Trial (DEW-IT). *Hypertension*. 2002;**40**:612-618.

49. Appel LJ, Champagne CM, Harsha DW, et al., Writing Group of the PREMIER Collaborative Research Group. Effects of comprehensive lifestyle modification on blood pressure control: Main results of the PREMIER clinical trial. *JAMA*. 2003;**289**:2083-2093.

50. Whelton PK, Appel LJ, Espeland MA, et al. Sodium reduction and weight loss in the treatment of hypertension in older persons: A randomized controlled trial of nonpharmacologic interventions in the elderly (TONE). TONE Collaborative Research Group. *JAMA*. 1998;**279**:839-846.

51. Neaton JD, Grimm RH Jr, Prineas RJ, et al. Treatment of Mild Hypertension Study: Final results. Treatment of Mild Hypertension Study Research Group. *JAMA*. 1993;**270**:713-724.

52. Stamler R, Stamler J, Grimm R, et al. Nutritional therapy for high blood pressure: Final report of a four-year randomized controlled trial—the Hypertension Control Program. *JAMA*. 1987;**257**:1484-1491.

53. Wassertheil-Smoller S, Blaufox MD, Oberman AS, et al. The Trial of Antihypertensive Interventions and Management (TAIM) study: Adequate weight loss, alone and combined with drug therapy in the treatment of mild hypertension. *Arch Intern Med*. 1992;**152**:131-136.

54. Stevens VJ, Corrigan SA, Obarzanek E, et al. Weight loss intervention in Phase 1 of the Trials of Hypertension Prevention: The TOHP Collaborative Research Group. *Arch Intern Med*. 1993;**153**:849-858.

55. Trials of Hypertension Prevention Collaborative Research Group. Trials of Hypertension Prevention, Phase II: Effects of weight loss and sodium reduction intervention on blood pressure and hypertension incidence in overweight people with high-normal blood pressure. *Arch Intern Med.* 1997;**157**: 657-667.

56. Stevens VJ, Obarzanek E, Cook NR, et al., Trials for the Hypertension Prevention Research Group. Long-term weight loss and changes in blood pressure: Results of the Trials of Hypertension Prevention, Phase II. *Ann Intern Med.* 2001; **134**:1-11.

57. Blumenthal JA, Sherwood A, Gullette EC, et al. Exercise and weight loss reduce blood pressure in men and women with mild hypertension: Effects on cardiovascular, metabolic, and hemodynamic functioning. *Arch Intern Med.* 2000;**160**: 1947-1958.

58. Carroll JF, Kyser CK. Exercise training in obesity lowers blood pressure independent of weight change. *Med Sci Sports Exerc.* 2002;**34**:596-601.

59. Chobanian AV, Bakris GL, Black HR, et al. Joint National Committee on Prevention, Detection, Evaluation, and Treatment of High Blood Pressure, National Heart, Lung and Blood Institute, National High Blood Pressure Education Program Coordinating Committee. Seventh Report of the Joint National Committee on Prevention, Detection, Evaluation, and Treatment of High Blood Pressure. *Hypertension.* 2003;**42**:1206-1252.

60. Nelson L, Jennings GL, Esler MD, Korner PI. Effect of changing levels of physical activity on blood-pressure and haemodynamics in essential hypertension. *Lancet.* 1986;**2**:473-476.

61. Kingwell BA, Sherrard B, Jennings GL, Dart AM. Four weeks of cycle training increases basal production of nitric oxide from the forearm. *Am J Physiol.* 1997;**272**:H1070-H1077.

62. Goto C, Higashi Y, Kimura M, et al. Effect of different intensities of exercise on endothelium-dependent vasodilation in humans: Role of endothelium-dependent nitric oxide and oxidative stress. *Circulation.* 2003;**108**:530-535.

63. Sjostrom L, Rissanen A, Anderse T, et al. Randomized placebo-controlled trial of orlistat for weight loss and prevention of weight regain in obese patients: European Multicenter Orlistat Study Group. *Lancet.* 1998;**352**:167-172.

64. Davidson MH, Hauptman J, DiGirolamo M, et al. Weight control and risk factor reduction in obese subjects treated for 2 years with orlistat: A randomized controlled trial. *JAMA.* 1999;**281**:235-242.

65. Bakris G, Calhoun D, Egan B, et al. Orlistat improves blood pressure control in obese subjects with treated but inadequately controlled hypertension: Orlistat and Resistant Hypertension Investigators. *J Hypertens.* 2002;**20**:2257-2267.

66. Sharma AM, Golay A. Effect of orlistat-induced weight loss on blood pressure and heart rate in obese patients with hypertension. *J Hypertens.* 2002;**20**:1873-1878.

67. Bray GA, Blackburn GL, Ferguson JM, et al. Sibutramine produces dose-related weight loss. *Obes Res.* 1999;**7**:189-198.

68. Apfelbaum M, Vague P, Ziegler O, et al. Long-term maintenance of weight loss after a very-low-calorie diet: A randomized blinded trial of the efficacy and tolerability of sibutramine. *Am J Med.* 1999;**106**:179-184.

69. Hansen D, Astrup A, Toubro S, et al. Predictors of weight loss and maintenance during 2 years of treatment by sibutramine in obesity: Results from the European multicenter STORM trial (Sibutramine Trial of Weight Reduction and Maintenance). *Int J Obes Relat Metab Disord.* 2001;**25**:496-501.

70. McMahon FG, Weinstein SP, Rowe E, et al. Sibutramine is safe and effective for weight loss in obese patients whose hypertension is well controlled with angiotensin-converting enzyme inhibitors. *J Hum Hypertens.* 2002;**16**:5-11.

71. Sramek JJ, Leibowitz MT, Weinstein SP, et al. Efficacy and safety of sibutramine for weight loss in obese patients with hypertension is well controlled with angiotensin-converting enzyme inhibitors. *J Hum Hypertens.* 2002;**16**:13-19.

72. National Institutes of Health conference. Gastrointestinal surgery for severe obesity: Consensus Development Conference Panel. *Ann Intern Med.* 1991;**115**:956-961.

73. Sjostrom CD, Lissner L, Wedel H, Sjostrom L. Reduction in incidence of diabetes, hypertension and lipid disturbances after intentional weight loss induced by bariatric surgery: The SOS Intervention Study. *Obes Res.* 1999;**7**:477-484.

74. Sjostrom CD, Peltonen M, Sjostrom L. Blood pressure and pulse pressure during long-term weight loss in the obese: The Swedish Obese Subjects (SOS) Intervention Study. *Obes Res.* 2001;**9**:188-195.

75. Sjostrom CD, Peltonen M, Wedel H, Sjostrom L. Differentiated long-term effects of intentional weight loss on diabetes and hypertension. *Hypertension.* 2000;**36**:20-25.

76. Torgerson JS, Sjostrom L. The Swedish Obese Subjects (SOS) study: Rationale and results. *Int J Obes Relat Metab Disord.* 2001;**25 (Suppl 1)**:S2-S4.

77. Grimm RH Jr, Margolis KL, Papademetriou V, et al. Baseline characteristics of participants in the Antihypertensive and Lipid-Lowering Treatment to Prevent Heart Attack Trial (ALLHAT). *Hypertension.* 2001;**37**:19-27.

78. Oparil S. Antihypertensive and Lipid-Lowering Treatment to Prevent Heart Attack Trial (ALLHAT): Practical implications. *Hypertension.* 2003;**41**:1006-1009.

79. Sharma AM, Pischon T, Engeli S, Scholze J. Choice of drug treatment for obesity-related hypertension: Where is the evidence? *J Hypertens.* 2001;**19**:667-674.

80. Tuck ML. Obesity, the sympathetic nervous system, and essential hypertension. *Hypertension.* 1992;**19 (1 Suppl)**:I67-I77.

81. Pollare T, Lithell H, Berne C. A comparison of the effects of hydrochlorothiazide and captopril on glucose and lipid metabolism in patients with hypertension. *N Engl J Med.* 1989;**321**:868-873.

82. Reisin E, Weir MR, Falkner B, et al. Lisinopril versus hydrochlorothiazide in obese hypertensive patients: A multicenter placebo-controlled trial. Treatment in Obese Patients with Hypertension (TROPHY) Study Group. *Hypertension.* 1997;**30**:140-145.

83. Reaven GM, Clinkingbeard C, Jeppesen J, et al. Comparison of the hemodynamic and metabolic effects of low-dose hydrochlorothiazide and lisinopril treatment in obese patients with high blood pressure. *Am J Hypertens.* 1995;**8**:461-466.

84. Lehtonen A. Doxazosin effects on insulin and glucose in hypertensive patients: The Finnish Multicenter Study Group. *Am Heart J.* 1991;**121**:1307-1311.

85. Pollare T, Lithell H, Selinus I, Berne C. Application of prazosin is associated with an increase of insulin sensitivity in obese patients with hypertension. *Diabetologia.* 1988;**31**: 415-420.

86. ALLHAT Officers and Coordinators for the ALLHAT Collaborative Research Group. Diuretic versus α-blocker as first-step antihypertensive therapy: Final results from the Antihypertensive and Lipid-Lowering treatment to prevent Heart Attack Trial (ALLHAT). *Hypertension.* 2003;**42**: 239-246.

87. Rocchini AP. Cardiovascular regulation in obesity-induced hypertension. *Hypertension.* 1992;**19 (1 Suppl)**:I56-I60.

88. Koch R, Sharma AM. Obesity and cardiovascular hemodynamic function. *Curr Hypertens Rep.* 1999;**1**:127-130.

89. Morel Y, Gadient A, Keller U, et al. Insulin sensitivity in obese hypertensive dyslipidemic patients treated with enalapril or atenolol. *J Cardiovasc Pharmacol.* 1995;**26**:306-311.

90. MacMahon SW, Macdonald GJ, Bernstein L, et al. Comparison of weight reduction with metoprolol in treatment of hypertension in young overweight patients. *Lancet.* 1985;**1**:1233-1236.

91. Sharma AM, Pischon T, Hardt S, et al. Hypothesis: Beta-adrenergic receptor blockers and weight gain. A systematic analysis. *Hypertension*. 2001;**37**:250-254.

92. Tuck ML. Metabolic considerations in hypertension. *Am J Hypertens*. 1990;**3**:355S-365S.

93. de Courten M, Ferrari P, Schneider M, et al. Lack of effect of long-term amlodipine on insulin sensitivity and plasma insulin in obese patients with essential hypertension. *Eur J Clin Pharmacol*. 1993;**44**:457-462.

94. Pollare T, Lithell H, Morlin C, et al. Metabolic effects of diltiazem and atenolol: Results from a randomized, double-blind study with parallel groups. *J Hypertens*. 1989;**7**: 551-559.

95. Elliott WJ, Stein PP, Black HR. Drug treatment of hypertension in patients with diabetes mellitus. *Diabetes Care*. 1995;**18**:477-509.

96. Pischon T, Sharma AM. Recent developments in the treatment of obesity-related hypertension. *Curr Opin Nephrol Hypertens*. 2002;**11**:497-502.

97. Crozier IG, Teoh R, Kay R, Nicholls MG. Sympathetic nervous system during converting enzyme inhibition. *Am J Med*. 1989;**87** (**Suppl 6B**):29S-32S.

98. Hornig B, Kohler C, Drexler H. Role of bradykinin in mediating vascular effects of angiotensin-converting enzyme inhibitors in humans. *Circulation*. 1997;**95**:1115-1118.

99. Gainer JV, Morrow JD, Loveland A, et al. Effect of bradykinin-receptor blockade on the response to angiotensin-converting-enzyme inhibitor in normotensive and hypertensive subjects. *N Engl J Med*. 1998;**339**:1285-1292.

100. Elliott WJ. Differential effects of antihypertensive agents on incident diabetes? *Curr Hypertens Rep*. 2005;**7**:249-256.

101. Aneja A, El-Atat F, McFarlane SI, Sowers JR. Hypertension and obesity. *Recent Prog Horm Res*. 2004;**59**:169-205.

102. Moan A, Risanger T, Eide I, Kjeldsen SE. The effect of angiotensin II receptor blockade on insulin sensitivity and sympathetic nervous system activity in primary hypertension. *Blood Press*. 1994;**3**:185-188.

103. Goossens GH, Blaak EE, van Baak MA. Possible involvement of the adipose tissue renin-angiotensin system in the pathophysiology of obesity and obesity-related disorders. *Obes Rev*. 2003;**4**:43-55.

104. Parving HH, Lehnert H, Brochner-Mortensen J, et al. Irbesartan in Patients with Type 2 Diabetes and Microalbuminuria Study Group: The effect of irbesartan on the development of diabetic nephropathy in patients with type 2 diabetes. *N Engl J Med*. 2001;**345**:870-878.

105. Grassi G, Seravalle G, Dell'Oro R, et al. CROSS Study. Comparative effects of candesartan and hydrochlorothiazide on blood pressure, insulin sensitivity, and sympathetic drive in obese hypertensive individuals: Results of the CROSS study. *J Hypertens*. 2003;**21**:1761-1769.

106. Dahlöf B, Devereux RB, Kjeldsen SE, et al., LIFE Study Group. Cardiovascular morbidity and mortality in the Losartan Intervention For Endpoint reduction in hypertension study (LIFE): A randomised trial against atenolol. *Lancet*. 2002;**359**:995-1003.

107. Jarrott B, Conway EL, Maccarrone C, Lewis SJ. Clonidine: Understanding its disposition, sites and mechanism of action. *Clin Exp Pharmacol Physiol*. 1987;**14**:471-479.

108. Campese VM, Romoff M, Telfer N, et al. Role of sympathetic nerve inhibition and body sodium-volume state in the antihypertensive action of clonidine in essential hypertension. *Kidney Int*. 1980;**18**:351-357.

109. Nilsson-Ehle P, Ekberg M, Fridstrom P, et al. Lipoproteins and metabolic control in hypertensive type II diabetics treated with clonidine. *Acta Med Scand*. 1988;**224**:131-134.

Chapter 32

Peripheral Arterial Disease in Hypertension

Michael H. Criqui and Matthew A. Allison

EPIDEMIOLOGY

Peripheral arterial disease (PAD) is a chronic disease of the large conduit arteries in the lower extremities that is primarily caused by a significant atherosclerotic burden resulting in luminal obstruction. This condition is often associated with considerable functional limitations.[1] The clinical diagnosis of PAD can be confirmed using noninvasive methods. Clinically, patients usually present with intermittent claudication (IC), which is defined as pain in the calf during exertion. The thigh or the buttock may also be affected. The pain may be described as a dull ache, cramp, or fatigue and is relieved by rest. Notably, fewer than 50% of patients with significant occlusive disease are symptomatic, and many symptomatic patients present atypically.

A method for detection of subclinical PAD and for confirmation of symptomatic PAD is available for office use. Briefly, systolic blood pressures (SBPs) in both ankles and both arms are obtained, preferably using a Doppler probe for both. The ratio of the systolic pressure at each ankle to the higher systolic in the two arms is the *ankle-brachial index* (ABI) for that leg. A significant reduction in flow in the lower extremity results in a lowering of the systolic ankle pressure, thereby reducing the ABI. The diagnosis of PAD is made in patients with an ABI of less than 0.9 in either leg. Recent evidence suggests that ABIs greater than 1.40 may also suggest PAD and are a result of stiff peripheral arteries.[2] Such elevated ABIs are most common in diabetic patients.

Prevalence

The prevalence of PAD depends on the definition used. Estimates of the overall prevalence of PAD based on the diagnosis of IC range from 1.1% to 2.4%.[3-5] Studies limited to patients who are more than 60 years old estimate the prevalence of IC at 3% to 6%.[6] However, a symptom-based definition of PAD tends to underestimate the prevalence of significant lower extremity arterial obstructive disease, because most cases of PAD are asymptomatic or are atypically symptomatic.[5] For example, in patients with PAD diagnosed using ABI criteria, only 6.3% reported symptoms of IC in the Rotterdam study. When the definition of PAD is based on the presence of subclinical (i.e., ABI) and clinical disease, the overall prevalence of this condition increases to 4.5%, or about 5 million persons in the United States (using the 2000 Census).[7] More refined estimates that also account for prior surgery for lower extremity occlusive disease increase this number to 6.1%, or 7.1 million U.S. residents (Fig. 32-1).[8]

Prevalence rates have been reported to vary somewhat by ethnicity. Both male and female African Americans have the highest rates, followed by Hispanics, Native Americans, non-Hispanic Whites, and Asian Americans.[7,8] Within each ethnic group, the rates are higher in men and increase exponentially with age, whereby prevalence roughly doubles during each decade of life.

Patients with coronary heart disease (CHD) have a high prevalence of PAD. In one study, 22% of subjects with angiographically documented CHD had lower extremity vascular occlusive disease diagnosed using the ABI or plethysmography, with the prevalence of PAD correlated with the severity of CHD.[9] In another study, 40% of hospitalized subjects with a history of CHD had concomitant PAD.[10]

Risk Factors

The risk factors for IC are, in general, similar to those for an abnormal ABI. In the Framingham Offspring Study, every 10-year increase in age was associated with a more than 2.5 times higher risk for PAD after adjustment for the standard risk factors.[4] Similar results were found in the National Health and Nutrition Examination Survey (NHANES), 1999 to 2000.[7] The risk for PAD in African Americans is twice that in non-Hispanic whites, and it has been reported to be independent of traditional cardiovascular disease (CVD) risk factors.[11]

Of the major risk factors for CVD, diabetes, cigarette smoking, and hypertension (HTN) have the largest magnitude of associations with PAD. Patients with diabetes have two to four times the prevalence[12] and risk,[7,13] whereas an impaired fasting glucose has been associated with a 20% increase in risk after adjustment for other CVD risk factors.[14] The risk associated with cigarette smoking ranges from 2.0 to 4.5.[4,7] High cholesterol is also associated with an increased risk, but these associations have not always been statistically significant. However, individuals with familial hypercholesterolemia have a substantially higher prevalence of PAD than controls.[15] The risk of PAD in patients with documented CHD is more than twice that for persons without this condition.[4] In addition, a diagnosis of PAD in patients with CHD has been associated with a 2.5 times higher risk for CVD morbidity.[16]

The relationship between the ABI and cardiovascular risk factors is nonlinear, and it may be described as a backward J or U-shape.[2] In other words, the prevalence and mean values of risk factors such as cigarette smoking, fasting plasma glucose, and waist circumference are highest in persons with an ABI of less than 0.9, lowest for those with an ABI of 1.0 to 1.39, and intermediate in those with an ABI greater than 1.4. This "stiff artery" high-ABI group is also characterized by a high prevalence of patients with type 2 diabetes as well as markers for this condition, such as fasting serum insulin levels and body mass index.

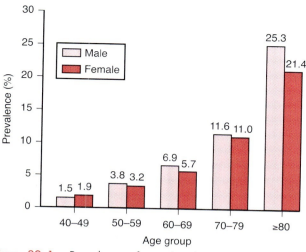

Figure 32–1 Prevalence of peripheral arterial disease by age group. (Modified from Allison MA, Criqui MH, Ho E, Jo D. The estimated ethnic specific prevalence of peripheral arterial disease in United States, 2000. *Circulation.* 2004;**110**:e817.)

Outcomes

Patients with PAD have a significantly increased risk for future CVD events, including myocardial infarction, stroke, and CVD-associated mortality. For example, after 10 years of follow-up, men and women with PAD had a 2.5- and 5-fold increase in risk, respectively, for a composite CVD endpoint.[17] Over the same time frame, the risk for mortality from total CVD and CHD causes has been reported to be 3.1, 5.9, and 6.6, respectively.[18] Patients with PAD and CAD have a 25% higher risk of mortality compared with those with CAD alone.[19] Further, the ABI predicts fatal myocardial infarction independently of traditional CVD risk factors.

CAUSES OF PERIPHERAL ARTERIAL DISEASE

Symptoms or subclinical manifestations of obstruction to blood flow in the large or medium-sized arteries of the lower extremities may be caused by numerous clinical syndromes. By far the most common cause is atherosclerosis. In this disease process, atherosclerotic plaques develop in characteristic stages from fatty streaks to lesions with large fatty deposits to complex fibrous atheromas with evidence of inflammation and thrombosis. Lesions tend to develop earlier in the iliac vessels and may progress sufficiently to cause flow-limiting stenoses and hence the signs and symptoms of PAD. Atherosclerotic plaques occur preferentially at sites of injury to the endothelium and arterial branch points, which are sites of increased turbulence and altered shear stress. Involvement of the distal vasculature is most common in elderly men, diabetic patients, or heavy smokers. The most common location for plaque development is the femoral artery, particularly in the adductor canal, and the popliteal artery (80% to 90% of patients with PAD). Other less common sites of involvement include the tibial and peroneal arteries (40% to 50% of patients) and the iliac arteries (30% of symptomatic patients).

Other conditions associated with PAD include arteriosclerosis obliterans, thromboangiitis obliterans (Buerger's disease), and various arteritides.[20] Buerger's disease is a nonatherosclerotic, inflammatory vascular occlusive disease that involves the medium-sized or small arteries and eventually results in perivascular fibrosis and recanalization. The typical clinical description is that of a man less than 40 years old who is a heavy smoker and who presents with IC of the arch of the foot or the calf. Involvement of the small arteries of the hand and wrist is common. Connective tissue disorders that cause vascular inflammation (systemic lupus erythematosus and scleroderma) may also be associated with PAD. In systemic lupus erythematosus and scleroderma, the occlusive disease is usually limited to the distal arteries, but it may occur in the larger arteries in the former disease.

HYPERTENSION AS A CONTRIBUTING FACTOR TO PERIPHERAL ARTERIAL DISEASE

It is generally accepted that the "big three" modifiable risk factors for CHD are cigarette smoking, dyslipidemia, and elevated BP (HTN). Age and male sex are also major risk factors for CHD, but they are not modifiable. The prevalence of PAD increases with age, and the rates are higher in men. Similarly, SBPs are usually higher in these groups. Other important risk factors include diabetes, obesity, and physical inactivity. Because each of the foregoing is thought to influence atherosclerosis, these risk factors should be related to PAD as well as to CHD. However, cigarette smoking and diabetes appear to be the most important risk factors for PAD. The association of HTN with PAD is examined later, with the evidence stratified by different definitions of PAD.

Intermittent Claudication Prevalence

IC is the classic symptom of PAD, defined as ambulatory leg pain that is not present at rest and is relieved by rest. By definition, this criterion excludes asymptomatic and presumably less severe PAD. However, studies of the relationship between HTN and IC produced conflicting results; some studies showed a positive association, whereas others failed to demonstrate a relationship. Typically, this relationship has been stronger for SBP than for diastolic BP (DBP).

Cross-sectional studies of IC could be biased by numerous factors. First, IC is an imprecise endpoint for PAD. Although IC reflects symptomatic and thus usually significant obstruction, surprisingly nearly half of the patients reporting IC in a population study had no demonstrable reduction in arterial flow on extensive noninvasive testing.[5] Such misclassification would result in a reduced correlation between HTN and PAD. Second, a similarly reduced HTN-PAD correlation could also be introduced by diet, lifestyle, or pharmacologic interventions after the diagnosis of IC. Additionally, it seems possible that cross-sectional studies could produce a spuriously high correlation by an increase in peripheral resistance secondary to PAD. In this instance, PAD could cause HTN rather than vice versa (see Chapter 8 for a discussion of PAD in the renal arterial bed).

Ankle-Brachial Index Prevalence

In general, an ankle pressure that is less than 90% of the brachial pressure is considered indicative of PAD. Studies using this criterion or a more conservative one, such as an ABI of less than 0.8 (or even <0.75), have generally found an association with elevated BP. In NHANES 1999 to 2000, the prevalence of PAD in patients with HTN was 6.9% compared with 2.2% in those without HTN, and this equated to a multivariable odds ratio (OR) of 1.75 for PAD in patients with HTN.[7] In the Framingham Offspring Study, investigators noted a significant trend for increasing prevalence of HTN and decreasing levels of the ABI. Further, HTN was associated with over twice the risk (OR = 2.2) for PAD (ABI <0.9) on multivariable analysis.[4] In the Atherosclerosis Risk in Communities (ARIC) study, an inverse and graded relationship was shown between ABI categories and the proportion of subjects with an SBP of 140 mm Hg or more.[21] In a study of only women, Yeh and associates found that, after adjusting for age, the mean SBP was higher in those with an ABI of less than 0.8 (144.4 versus 139.7 mm Hg), whereas the DBP was significantly lower (73.6 versus 74.3 mm Hg; $P < .01$ for both).[22] Similarly, the prevalence of HTN was 75.5% compared with 55.4%. The OR for an ABI of less than 0.8 was 94% higher in patients with HTN after age adjustment. Further, on multivariable logistic regression, each 1 mm Hg increase in SBP was associated with a 16% increase in risk for PAD.[22]

In several studies, the association with SBP appeared to be stronger than the association with DBP. In the Cardiovascular Health Study (CHS), a highly significant gradation of effect was noted, with an inverse relationship between the ABI and the percentage of patients who reported HTN (SBP >160 mm Hg, DBP >95 mm Hg, or self-report of this condition along with use of antihypertensive medications) and SBP. In other words, after adjustment for age and sex, as the ABI decreased, the prevalence of persons reporting HTN and the relative risk of developing HTN increased, as did the mean SBP. Conversely, DBP did not differ significantly with varying levels of ABI. Moreover, the association of SBP (but not DBP) and HTN was more prevalent in patients with PAD (ABI <0.9) in a German cohort.[23] Other studies have shown a similar association between ABI and HTN. However, these studies may have the limitations of cross-sectional studies and the use of the ABI as the only criterion for PAD, an approach that results in some false-negative results, although almost no false-positive results.

Prevalence by Multiple Noninvasive Tests

A study in an older, free-living population in the United States used ratios of SBPs at several levels of the lower extremity to the systolic brachial pressure, as well as flow velocity measurements in the femoral and posterior tibial arteries, to define PAD.[5] In addition, a few patients who had previous surgery for PAD were included. Of the nonsurgical patients, only 20% had ambulatory leg pain, and, overall, approximately 33% of the patients were asymptomatic. Of all 66 patients (including 6 with revascularization), only 10.6% had classic IC, 16.7% had atypical exertional leg pain, 18.2% had pain that at least sometimes began at rest, and 54.5% denied exertional leg pain. This investigation resulted in a broader spectrum of disease, with many more mild cases of PAD than usually

Table 32-1   Age-Adjusted Mean Levels of Blood Pressure by Peripheral Arterial Disease Status

PAD Status	Men	Women	Men and Women (Sex-Adjusted)
Normal (N)	(183)	(225)	(408)
SBP	131.2	128.2	129.2
DBP	77.2	73.9	75.4
Moderate PAD (N)	(22)	(27)	(49)
SBP	138.9*	125.4	131.4
DBP	80.0	71.6	75.2
Severe PAD (N)	(12)	(6)	(18)
SBP	140.4*	141.9*	140.9†
DBP	78.2	74.8	77.2

*$P \le .05$; compared with the normal group.
†$P \le .01$; compared with the normal group.
DBP, diastolic blood pressure; N, number of patients; PAD, peripheral arterial disease; SBP, systolic blood pressure. From Criqui MH, Fronek A, Barrett-Connor E, et al. The prevalence of peripheral arterial disease in a defined population. *Circulation*. 1985;**71**:510-515.

Table 32-2   Age- and Sex-Adjusted Percentages of Hypertensive Patients by Peripheral Arterial Disease Status*

PAD Status	Men	Women	Men and Women (Sex-Adjusted)
Normal (N)	(183)	(225)	(408)
HTN1 (%)	39.5	46.6	41.6
HTN2 (%)	24.3	32.8	26.9
Moderate PAD (N)	(22)	(27)	(49)
HTN1 (%)	65.4†	58.5	60.3‡
HTN2 (%)	54.2‡	43.8	46.5‡
Severe PAD (N)	(12)	(6)	(18)
HTN1 (%)	74.5†	90.0†	81.2§
HTN2 (%)	53.8†	61.8	55.7†

*Using two different definitions of hypertension: HTN1, antihypertensive drugs or SBP ≥140 or DBP ≥90 mm Hg; HTN2, antihypertensive drugs or SBP ≥160 or DBP ≥95 mm Hg.
†$P \le .05$; compared with the normal group.
‡$P \le .01$; compared with the normal group.
§$P \le .001$; compared with the normal group.
DBP, diastolic blood pressure; N, number of patients; PAD, peripheral arterial disease; SBP, systolic blood pressure. From Criqui MH, Fronek A, Barrett-Connor E, et al. The prevalence of peripheral arterial disease in a defined population. *Circulation*. 1985;**71**:510-515.

found in epidemiologic studies. In this study, the extensive use of noninvasive testing minimized the number of false-negative cases. Patients with moderate PAD showed a small increase in SBP, but the difference was not statistically significant. Patients with severe PAD showed a significant increase in SBP (11.7 mm Hg), but the increase in DBP (1.8 mm Hg) was not statistically significant (Table 32-1).

We also evaluated this association in this population including information on any use of antihypertensive medications (Table 32-2). HTN was defined either liberally, as an SBP

Table 32-3 Adjusted Odds Ratios* with 95% Confidence Intervals for Systolic Blood Pressure Greater than 140 mm Hg with the Presence of Isolated Arterial Lesions

	Male		Female	
	OR	(95% CI)	OR	(95% CI)
Aortoiliac	3.0	(1.6-5.4)	5.1	(1.6-16.0)
Femoropopliteal	2.3	(1.3-4.3)	2.4	(1.2-4.9)
Tibioperoneal	0.9	(0.5-1.9)	5.0	(1.7-14.4)

*Adjusted for age, status as current smoker or former smoker, diabetes, history of angina, ischemic heart disease, stroke, and congestive heart failure.
CI, confidence interval; OR, odds ratio.
From Vogt MT, Wolfson SK, Kuller LH. Segmental arterial disease in the lower extremities: Correlates of disease and relationship to mortality. *J Clin Epidemiol.* 1993;**46**: 1267-1276.

of 140 mm Hg or higher or a DBP of 90 mm Hg or higher or the use of antihypertensive medications ("HTN1"), or more conservatively, by changing the BP criterion to an SBP of 160 mm Hg or higher or a DBP of 95 mm Hg or higher or the use of antihypertensive medications ("HTN2"). By either definition, both sexes had a stepwise increase in the proportion of hypertensive patients, from no PAD to moderate PAD to severe PAD. For men and women combined, subjects with moderate PAD had an increase in HTN of at least 50%, whereas subjects with severe PAD had nearly twice as much HTN as did subjects free of PAD. These findings were highly statistically significant and suggest a stronger relationship between HTN and PAD when antihypertensive medication use is included in the definition.

In a study of subjects from a vascular laboratory, which used segmental pressures to assess PAD, an SBP greater than 140 mm Hg was highly associated with PAD at all levels in the lower extremity in women and in the two proximal levels in men (Table 32-3).[24] In the San Luis Valley Diabetes Study, Hiatt, using the two-vessel criteria (both the dorsalis pedis and the posterior tibial artery meeting ABI criteria), found that the ORs of HTN for a low ABI were progressively higher with progressively lower ABIs.[25] At the fifth ABI percentile, the HTN OR was 1.6; at the 2.5th percentile, it was 2.2; and at the first percentile, it was 3.1. All results were significant at $P < .05$.

Prevalence by Angiography

In these studies, PAD was confirmed by angiography or by angiography in combination with other tests or symptoms. Thus, the diagnosis of PAD in these studies is highly reliable, and most patients have disease severe enough to be symptomatic. Nonetheless, in studies for which prevalent PAD was defined as IC, the results are mixed, ranging from no association to strong associations. An Italian study found a statistically significant, more than fivefold increase in the prevalence of HTN in patients with PAD, compared with age- and sex-matched control subjects.[26] When matching patients with PAD and controls by mean arterial pressure, Safar and col-

leagues found that patients with PAD had increased SBP and decreased DBP and thus increased pulse pressure.[27] Pulse pressure was inversely correlated with arterial compliance, presumably because of changes in viscoelastic properties of the arterial wall. Again, data in these studies are subject to the usual cross-sectional study limitations. Furthermore, unlike population-based epidemiologic studies, angiographic studies use clinical samples, which may not be representative of the general population.

Incidence Studies

These studies have the distinct advantage of BP measurements made before the development of the PAD endpoint of interest. The Framingham Heart Study showed a steep, more or less linear gradient between the baseline level of SBP and the 26-year incidence of IC (Fig. 32-2).[28] For baseline DBP, the data suggest a threshold effect, beginning at the fourth quintile (87 to 94 mm Hg) in women and the fifth quintile (≥95 mm Hg) in men. For the fifth quintile of SBP (≥180 mm Hg) compared with the first (≤119 mm Hg), the relative risk was 2.7 in men and 5.2 in women. The attributable (or excess) risk for the fifth versus the first quintile was the same in both men and women (8/1000 biennial rate). The misclassification inherent in defining PAD by IC would suggest that these strong associations could be underestimates.

Progression

Palumbo and colleagues reported on the prospective progression of PAD as defined by the rate of change in the postexercise ABI over 4 years, as well as the occurrence of clinical events, such as PAD-related surgery (including amputation). In multivariable analysis, SBP was independently and significantly predictive of PAD progression.[29]

Randomized Controlled Trials

The only definitive way to test whether HTN is a causal factor in the pathogenesis of PAD would be a randomized controlled trial. Unfortunately, only limited data are available. In the Prevention of Atherosclerotic Complications with Ketanserin (PACK) study, nearly 4000 patients with IC and an ABI of less than 0.85 were randomized, and 46% had HTN defined as a SBP higher than 160 or a DBP higher than 95 mm Hg. Above-ankle amputations were reduced by 47% (17 versus 32) in the ketanserin-treated group.[30] Although this finding is consistent with a causal association between HTN and PAD, it does not represent definitive proof because ketanserin, in addition to being an antihypertensive agent, also inhibits platelet aggregation and has hematorheologic effects.

Outcomes Studies of Peripheral Arterial Disease and Hypertension

In ARIC, the rate of incident stroke was significantly higher in patients with an abnormal ABI and an SBP of 140 mm Hg or higher (23%), compared with those with a normal ABI and an SBP lower than 140 mm Hg (15%; relative risk, 1.5) after approximately 7 years of follow-up.[21] The relative risk for those taking compared with those not taking antihypertensive agents was similar (1.6).

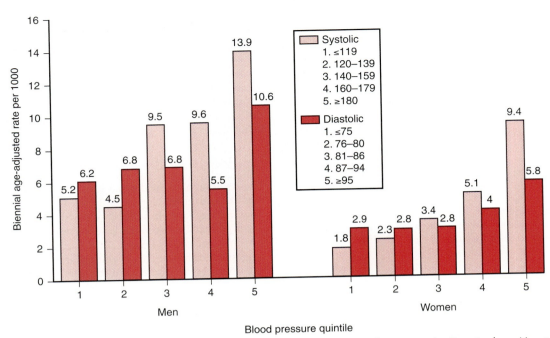

Figure 32–2   Baseline blood pressure and 26-year incidence of intermittent claudication in the Framingham Heart Study. (Modified from Kannel WB, McGee DL. Update on some epidemiologic features of intermittent claudication: The Framingham Study. *J Am Geriatr Soc.* 1985;**33**:13-18.)

Conclusions

Most studies addressing the association of HTN and PAD find a positive association, which is typically stronger for SBP than for DBP. Some studies are flawed by inexact definitions of PAD, whereas cross-sectional studies have the inherent limitation of being unable to determine whether any observed BP differences preceded or followed the development of PAD. Despite this disadvantage, in general, cross-sectional studies with better methodology tend to show more consistent relationships between HTN and PAD. Results from the limited number of available prospective (incidence) studies suggest a rather strong relationship between HTN and PAD. Although currently available data are not definitive, we conclude that HTN is likely to be an important causal factor in the pathogenesis of PAD.

TREATMENT OF HYPERTENSION FOR PATIENTS WITH PERIPHERAL ARTERIAL DISEASE

Principles

Patients with PAD are at significantly increased risk for morbidity and mortality from CVD. Moreover, approximately 30% to 50% of those diagnosed with PAD already have CHD. Therefore, it is imperative that patients with PAD receive aggressive risk factor reduction therapies. Such strategies should include smoking cessation, exercise programs, dietary counseling, and weight reduction, as well as dyslipidemia and antiplatelet therapies as appropriate. Indeed, management of

these risk factors has favorable effects on outcomes in patients with PAD. In addition, the subset of patients with IC may benefit from therapies directed at improving walking distance, such as supervised exercise and cilostazol.

However, treatment of HTN in the patient with PAD is complex. Because BP reduction is associated with reduced flow distal to stenotic atherosclerotic lesions in the peripheral vasculature, treatment with antihypertensive agents could in theory exacerbate the symptoms of IC. In the next sections, we review the results of studies on lifestyle and pharmacologic therapies for patients with HTN and concomitant PAD.

Nonpharmacologic Treatment

Exercise Programs

Endurance-based exercise programs lower BP in adults with HTN or normal BP. Results from many studies of exercise as a treatment for HTN continue to indicate that exercise training decreases BP in approximately 75% of individuals with HTN. Furthermore, a meta-analysis of 54 randomized trials conducted from 1966 to 2000 found overall reductions of 4.9 and 3.7 mm Hg for SBP and DBP, respectively, in subjects with HTN.[31]

During exercise, peripheral vasodilatation occurs distal to sites of significant arterial obstruction and results in a decrease in perfusion pressure, often to levels less than those generated in the interstitial tissue by the exercising muscle. Thus, leg exercise, such as walking, typically leads to the onset of IC symptoms. Nonetheless, several studies have demonstrated that regular exercise of mild to moderate intensity improves physical functioning as well as self-reported health-related quality of life in patients with clinical or sub-clinical PAD.

Various forms of exercise have been shown to be beneficial, including walking, "pole-striding" (akin to cross-country skiing), and upper extremity ergometry, with 24 weeks of training more effective than 12 weeks.[32] These improvements in exercise capacity and symptoms of IC have been associated with decreases in plasma and muscle short-chain acylcarnitine concentrations,[33] as well as a concomitant decrease in serum amyloid A protein and C-reactive protein.[34] Conversely, strength training exercises have been associated with mild improvements in peak walking times but not time to onset of claudication.[35]

Dietary Therapy

The Dietary Approaches to Stop Hypertension (DASH) diet emphasizes fruits, vegetables, and low-fat dairy foods; it includes whole grains, poultry, fish, and nuts; and it contains smaller amounts of red meat, sweets, and sugar-containing beverages than the typical diet in the United States. In a trial comparing three different levels of sodium intake within the DASH diet, investigators noted a graded decrease in both SBP and DBP with decreasing dietary sodium intake, a relationship seen across all demographic subgroups.[36] PAD status was not determined in this trial. To our knowledge, no randomized studies have been conducted on the potential effect of dietary modifications on walking distance or symptoms of IC in patients with PAD.

Pharmacologic Therapy

In general, studies that have examined the effects of pharmacologic therapy for elevated BP in patients with PAD or the treatment of this condition with antihypertensive drugs are limited. Furthermore, most of the trials conducted have small sample sizes. Despite these limitations, the Seventh Report of the Joint National Committee on Prevention, Detection, Evaluation, and Treatment of High Blood Pressure (JNC 7) recommends the use of "any class of antihypertensive drugs ... in most PAD patients."[36a] The following are summaries, restricted to randomized, placebo-controlled trials, of the available literature on this subject by drug class.

Angiotensin-Converting Enzyme Inhibitors

Angiotensin-converting enzyme inhibitors block the activation of the renin-angiotensin system in the plasma as well as in the vascular wall. In the Heart Outcomes Prevention Evaluation (HOPE) trial, 9297 subjects (44% with PAD) were randomized to receive the angiotensin-converting enzyme inhibitor ramipril or placebo, in addition to whatever other medications were indicated. After an average of 4.5 years of follow-up, treatment with ramipril was associated with a significant risk reduction for the primary composite outcome of myocardial infarction, stroke, and cardiovascular death (relative risk, 0.78; $P < .001$).[36] The benefit for the primary outcome was actually somewhat greater in patients with PAD compared with those without PAD. Furthermore, an ancillary study to HOPE of 38 subjects with PAD determined that ambulatory BPs were significantly reduced, primarily because of BP lowering at night.[37] However, it is not clear to what

extent the marked benefits from therapy in HOPE were directly attributable to BP reduction.

β-Blockers

All β-adrenergic antagonists compete with catecholamines for binding at sympathetic receptor sites in multiple tissues. These drugs block sympathetic stimulation mediated by β_1-adrenergic receptors in the heart and β_2-receptors in vascular smooth muscle, with resulting decreases in heart rate and arterial resistance, respectively. Increases in peripheral blood flow are the consequence of this diminished resistance unless significant obstruction to flow exists and thereby decreases flow distally. Theoretically, in patients with PAD, nonselective β-blockers would be associated with such a decrease in flow, with a resulting increase in the probability for either the onset or worsening of claudication symptoms. Conversely, β-blockers that are selective for cardiac tissue (β_1) would be expected to be associated with less of a reduction in peripheral flow and thereby less severe symptoms.

The potential benefit of this class of medications has been examined in several studies of either selective or nonselective β-blockers as well as those without intrinsic sympathomimetic activity in subjects with PAD. In a small study directly comparing propranolol (a nonselective agent) and metoprolol (a β_1-selective agent), neither drug decreased the time to initial symptoms of IC or intolerable pain.[38] In 1991, Radack and Deck conducted a meta-analysis of the available randomized controlled trials studying β-adrenergic blockers in patients with mild to moderate PAD. After pooling 11 available treatment comparisons from six trials, the results showed no significant difference in pain-free walking distance. Only one study reported that certain β-blockers were associated with worsening of IC.[39]

More recently, celiprolol, atenolol, and isosorbide dinitrate were compared in a placebo-controlled trial in 56 patients with chronic ischemic heart disease and stage IIb PAD. Patients receiving 50 mg/day atenolol (a β_1-selective agent) showed a significant reduction in both pain-free and maximal walking distance compared with the controls, whereas those in the celiprolol (β_1-selective agent with intrinsic sympathomimetic activity) or isosorbide dinitrate arms of the trial demonstrated significant increases in pain-free and maximal walking distance compared with the control group.[40]

Calcium Antagonists

Calcium antagonists, also known as calcium channel blockers (CCBs), inhibit the influx of extracellular calcium across the myocardial and vascular smooth muscle cell membranes. Calcium channels in vascular smooth muscle cell membranes are selective and allow a slow inward flow of calcium. These drugs inhibit this influx and cause in a decrease in intracellular calcium, which inhibits the contractile processes of the smooth muscle cells and results in dilation of the systemic arteries. These actions decrease total peripheral resistance and thus systemic BP.

Several small studies have been conducted to determine whether CCBs are beneficial in the treatment of PAD. Two randomized studies compared verapamil with placebo in patients with IC. In the first study, 4 weeks of treatment with this CCB resulted in a 7% increase in walking distance despite no change in the ABI.[41] The second was a randomized, placebo-controlled, double-blind crossover trial that also found no differences in systolic ankle pressure or the ABI, but the investigators found a significant increase in the mean pain-free and maximum walking distances by 29% and 49%, respectively.[42] Conversely, in a study of isradipine versus placebo, treatment with the former was not associated with a significant increase in the distance to initial claudication symptoms.[43] These results suggest that CCBs do not significantly change the ABI or symptoms of IC. However, larger studies are needed.

Comparisons of Multiple Classes of Antihypertensive Agents

Numerous studies have examined the effects of different classes of antihypertensive drugs on PAD. In a study comparing placebo with captopril, atenolol, labetalol, and pindolol, 20 subjects receiving 1 month of any of the β-blockers had significant decreases in pain-free and maximum walking distances as well as postexercise calf blood flow availability, whereas these reductions were not evident in the captopril-treated group.[44] In a study of 10 normotensive men with PAD that compared captopril, nicardipine, and placebo, neither active therapy modified the duration of exercise compared with placebo.[45] Treatment with either class of these medications has been associated with a reduction in cardiovascular event rates for patients with PAD and type 2 diabetes mellitus.[46]

In a placebo-controlled comparison of atenolol and nifedipine in 49 patients, neither medication significantly affected claudication or walking distance, but the combination of these two medications was associated with a small but significant (9%) reduction in walking distance.[47] Similar results of no change in walking capacity were found for before and after comparisons of metoprolol (a β_1-selective agent) and methyldopa compared with placebo in 14 patients with IC.[48]

Conclusions

Dietary modifications and exercise programs are effective in reducing BP in hypertensive patients with PAD. Additionally, exercise is beneficial in reducing the symptoms associated with PAD while improving the functional status of these patients. To maximize benefit in this group of patients, these training programs should be as long as possible and may target different anatomic locations. Furthermore, these exercise programs should preferably be aerobic, because the results of anaerobic (strength) training are limited. The best results appear to occur in supervised settings.

The limited data available support the concept that treatment of HTN in patients with PAD is effective in reducing cardiovascular events,[36,46] as would be expected, given the extensive results in other patients with CVD. However, concern exists about the potential effect of antihypertensive therapy with specific drugs on walking distance and IC in patients with PAD. With respect to studies on walking distance and IC, evidence is limited for angiotensin-converting enzyme inhibitors. Notably, renal function should be assessed before, and after, instituting this therapy because of the relatively high concordance between PAD and renal artery stenosis (~39%).

The results from studies of β-blockers (including those with intrinsic sympathomimetic activity) and CCBs are mixed. In general, these drug classes do not appear to reduce walking distance or to worsen the symptoms of IC significantly. As in any clinical situation, use of antihypertensive medications should be monitored to ensure efficacy in BP reduction as well as any effects on patients' symptoms.

References

1. McDermott MM, Greenland P, Ferrucci L, et al. Lower extremity performance is associated with daily life physical activity in individuals with and without peripheral arterial disease. *J Am Geriatr Soc.* 2002;**50**:247-255.
2. Resnick HE, Lindsay RS, McDermott MM, et al. Relationship of high and low ankle brachial index to all-cause and cardiovascular disease mortality: The Strong Heart Study. *Circulation.* 2004;**109**:733-739.
3. Jensen SA, Vatten LJ, Romundstad PR, Myhre HO. The prevalence of intermittent claudication: Sex-related differences have been eliminated. *Eur J Vasc Endovasc Surg.* 2003;**25**: 209-212.
4. Murabito JM, Evans JC, Nieto K, et al. Prevalence and clinical correlates of peripheral arterial disease in the Framingham Offspring Study. *Am Heart J.* 2002;**143**:961-965.
5. Criqui MH, Fronek A, Barrett-Connor E, et al. The prevalence of peripheral arterial disease in a defined population. *Circulation.* 1985;**71**:510-515.
6. Dormandy J, Heeck Land Vig S. Intermittent claudication: A condition with underrated risks. *Semin Vasc Surg.* 1999;**12**: 96-108.
7. Selvin E, Erlinger TP. Prevalence of and risk factors for peripheral arterial disease in the United States: Results from the National Health and Nutrition Examination Survey, 1999-2000. *Circulation.* 2004;**110**:738-743.
8. Allison MA, Criqui MH, Ho E, Jo D. The estimated ethnic specific prevalence of peripheral arterial disease in United States, 2000. *Circulation.* 2004;**110**:e817.
9. Atmer B, Jogestrand T, Laska J, Lund F. Peripheral artery disease in patients with coronary artery disease. *Int Angiol.* 1995;**14**: 89-93.
10. Dieter R, Tomasson J, Gudjonsson T, et al. Lower extremity peripheral arterial disease in hospitalized patients with coronary artery disease. *Vasc Med.* 2003;**8**:233-236.
11. Criqui M, Vargas V, Ho E, et al. Ethnicity and peripheral arterial disease: The San Diego Population Study. *Circulation.* 2002;**105**:e113.
12. Gregg EW, Sorlie P, Paulose-Ram R, et al. Prevalence of lower-extremity disease in the U.S. adult population ≥40 years of age with and without diabetes: 1999-2000 National Health and Nutrition Examination Survey. *Diabetes Care.* 2004;**27**: 1591-1597.
13. Newman AB, Siscovick DS, Manolio TA, et al. Ankle-arm index as a marker of atherosclerosis in the Cardiovascular Health Study: Cardiovascular Heart Study (CHS) Collaborative Research Group. *Circulation.* 1993;**88**:837-845.
14. Beks PJ, Mackaay AJ, de Neeling JN, et al. Peripheral arterial disease in relation to glycaemic level in an elderly Caucasian population: The Hoorn study. *Diabetologia.* 1995;**38**: 86-96.
15. Kroon A, Ajubi N, van Asten W, Stalenhoef A. The prevalence of peripheral vascular disease in familial hypercholesterolaemia. *J Intern Med.* 1995;**238**:451-459.
16. Criqui MH, Denenberg JO. The generalized nature of atherosclerosis: How peripheral arterial disease may predict adverse events from coronary artery disease. *Vasc Med.* 1998;**3**:241-245.

17. Criqui MH, Langer RD, Fronek A, Feigelson HS. Coronary disease and stroke in patients with large-vessel peripheral arterial disease. *Drugs.* 1991;**42 (Suppl 5)**:16-21.

18. Criqui MH, Langer RD, Fronek A, et al. Mortality over a period of 10 years in patients with peripheral arterial disease. *N Engl J Med.* 1992;**326**:381-386.

19. Eagle KA, Rihal CS, Foster ED, et al., The Coronary Artery Surgery Study (CASS) Investigators. Long-term survival in patients with coronary artery disease: Importance of peripheral vascular disease. *J Am Coll Cardiol.* 1994;**23**:1091-1095.

20. Spittel J. Some uncommon types of occlusive peripheral arterial disease. *Curr Probl Cardiol.* 1983;**8**:1-35.

21. Tsai AW, Folsom AR, Rosamond WD, Jones DW. Ankle-brachial index and 7-year ischemic stroke incidence: The ARIC study. *Stroke.* 2001;**32**:1721-1724.

22. Yeh ST, Morton DJ, Barrett-Connor E. Lower extremity arterial disease in older women: The Rancho Bernardo Study. *J Womens Health Gend Based Med.* 2000;**9**:373-380.

23. Diehm C, Schuster A, Allenberg JR, et al. High prevalence of peripheral arterial disease and co-morbidity in 6880 primary care patients: Cross-sectional study. *Atherosclerosis.* 2004;**172**:95-105.

24. Vogt MT, Wolfson SK, Kuller LH. Segmental arterial disease in the lower extremities: Correlates of disease and relationship to mortality. *J Clin Epidemiol.* 1993;**46**:1267-1276.

25. Hiatt WR, Hoag S, Hamman RF. Effect of diagnostic criteria on the prevalence of peripheral arterial disease: The San Luis Valley Diabetes Study. *Circulation.* 1995;**91**:1472-1479.

26. Strano A, Novo S, Avellone G, et al. Hypertension and other risk factors in peripheral arterial disease. *Clin Exp Hypertens.* 1993;**15 (Suppl 1)**:71-89.

27. Safar ME, Laurent S, Asmar RE, et al. Systolic hypertension in patients with arteriosclerosis obliterans of the lower limbs. *Angiology.* 1987;**38**:287-295.

28. Kannel WB, McGee DL. Update on some epidemiologic features of intermittent claudication: The Framingham Study. *J Am Geriatr Soc.* 1985;**33**:13-18.

29. Palumbo PJ, O'Fallon WM, Osmundson PJ, et al. Progression of peripheral occlusive arterial disease in diabetes mellitus. What factors are predictive? *Arch Intern Med.* 1991;**151**:717-721.

30. Prevention of Atherosclerotic Complications with Ketanserin Trial Group. Prevention of atherosclerotic complications: Controlled trial of ketanserin. *BMJ.* 1989;**298**:424-430.

31. Petrella R. How effective is exercise training for the treatment of hypertension? *Clin J Sport Med.* 1998;**8**:224-231.

32. Regensteiner J, Steiner J, Hiatt W. Exercise training improves functional status in patients with peripheral arterial disease. *J Vasc Surg.* 1996;**23**:104-115.

33. Hiatt W, Regensteiner J, Hargarten M, et al. Benefit of exercise conditioning for patients with peripheral arterial disease. *Circulation.* 1990;**81**:602-609.

34. Tisi P, Hulse M, Chulakadabba A, et al. Exercise training for intermittent claudication: Does it adversely affect biochemical markers of the exercise-induced inflammatory response? *Eur J Vasc Endovasc Surg.* 1997;**14**:344-350.

35. Hiatt W, Wolfel E, Meier R, Regensteiner J. Superiority of treadmill walking exercise versus strength training for patients with peripheral arterial disease: Implications for the mechanism of the training response. *Circulation.* 1994;**90**:1866-1874.

36. Yusuf S, Sleight P, Pogue J, et al. Effects of an angiotensin-converting-enzyme inhibitor, ramipril, on cardiovascular events in high-risk patients: The Heart Outcomes Prevention Evaluation Study Investigators. *N Engl J Med.* 2000;**342**:145-153.

36a. Chobanian AV, Bakris GL, Black HR, et al. Seventh report of the Joint National Committee on Prevention, Detection, Evaluation, and Treatment of High Blood Pressure. *Hypertension.* 2003;**42**:1206-1252.

37. Svensson P, de Faire U, Sleight P, et al. Comparative effects of ramipril on ambulatory and office blood pressures: A HOPE substudy. *Hypertension.* 2001;**38**:28e-32e.

38. Bogaert M, Clement D. Lack of influence of propranolol and metoprolol on walking distance in patients with chronic intermittent claudication. *Eur Heart J.* 1983;**4**:203-204.

39. Radack K, Deck C. Beta-adrenergic blocker therapy does not worsen intermittent claudication in subjects with peripheral arterial disease: A meta-analysis of randomized controlled trials. *Arch Intern Med.* 1991;**151**:1769-1776.

40. Schweizer J, Kaulen R, Nierade A, Altmann E. Beta-blockers and nitrates in patients with peripheral arterial occlusive disease: Long-term findings. *Vasa.* 1997;**26**:43-46.

41. Kimose H, Bagger J, Aagaard M, Paulsen P. Placebo-controlled, double-blind study of the effect of verapamil in intermittent claudication. *Angiology.* 1990;**41**:595-598.

42. Bagger J, Helligsoe P, Randsbaek F, et al. Effect of verapamil in intermittent claudication: A randomized, double-blind, placebo-controlled, cross-over study after individual dose-response assessment. *Circulation.* 1997;**95**:411-414.

43. Catalano M, Tomasini M, Scandale G, et al. Isradipine in the treatment of peripheral occlusive vascular disease of the lower limbs: A pilot study. *J Int Med Res.* 1992;**20**:323-330.

44. Roberts D, Tsao Y, McLoughlin G, Breckenridge A. Placebo-controlled comparison of captopril, atenolol, labetalol, and pindolol in hypertension complicated by intermittent claudication. *Lancet.* 1987;**2**:650-653.

45. Bernardi D, Bartoli P, Ferreri A, et al. Assessment of captopril and nicardipine effects on chronic occlusive arterial disease of the lower extremity using Doppler ultrasound. *Angiology.* 1988;**39**:942-952.

46. Mehler PS, Coll JR, Estacio R, et al. Intensive blood pressure control reduces the risk of cardiovascular events in patients with peripheral arterial disease and type 2 diabetes. *Circulation.* 2003;**107**:753-756.

47. Solomon S, Ramsay L, Yeo W, et al. Beta blockade and intermittent claudication: Placebo controlled trial of atenolol and nifedipine and their combination. *BMJ.* 1991;**303**:1100-1104.

48. Lepantalo M, von Knorring J. Walking capacity of patients with intermittent claudication during chronic antihypertensive treatment with metoprolol and methyldopa. *Clin Physiol.* 1984;**4**:275-282.

Chapter 33

Cerebrovascular Disease in Hypertension

Neil Chapman, Craig Anderson, and John Chalmers

Cerebrovascular disease, manifest predominantly as stroke and dementia, constitutes a major proportion of the global disease burden. Worldwide, stroke is the second most common cause of death and is a leading cause of adult disability, whereas dementia is the eighth leading cause of death and disability. The burden of disease associated with both stroke and dementia is projected to rise substantially in the first quarter of the 21st century as a result of demographic restructuring and lifestyle changes in populations.

Elevated blood pressure (BP) is the most important modifiable risk factor for stroke and is associated with vascular, as well as other forms of, dementia. Strong evidence from randomized controlled trials indicates that BP lowering reduces the risk of stroke, deaths from stroke, and the burden of physical and mental disability associated with stroke. This chapter reviews the associations between BP and cerebrovascular disease, the proposed mechanisms that underlie these associations, and current evidence on the benefits of BP-lowering therapy in relation to this disease.

STROKE

Despite advances in technology, stroke remains essentially a clinical diagnosis made on the basis of the temporal profile of clinical features. *Stroke* is defined by the World Health Organization as "rapidly developing clinical signs of focal (or global) disturbance of cerebral function with symptoms lasting 24 hours or longer (or leading to death), with no apparent cause other than vascular origin."[1] If symptoms (and signs) resolve within 24 hours, the syndrome is termed a *transient ischemic attack* (TIA). This time-cut definition is quite arbitrary and was established before the widespread use of radiologic (computed tomography or magnetic resonance imaging) brain imaging. It is now accepted that TIAs may be associated with neuronal lesions, and the frequency with which a lesion is evident on brain imaging increases with the duration of symptoms (Fig. 33-1).[2] Moreover, with the advent of thrombolytic treatment for acute ischemic stroke, clinical decision making is now focused on the first few hours after the onset of symptoms in the hope that early intervention may reduce the size of the evolving ischemic lesion. Thus, TIAs should not be considered a benign condition but rather part of the spectrum of cerebrovascular disease that carries the same prognosis of death and permanent disability as that of a minor ("completed") stroke (Fig. 33-2).[3] Despite these caveats, it is often useful, both clinically and epidemiologically, to consider TIAs separately from stroke.

Pathologically, stroke occurs as a result of a heterogeneous group of disorders that are not necessarily related to atherosclerosis, have different patterns of occurrence and outcome, and may require different management. Broadly speaking, two major pathologic categories are recognized: ischemic stroke and hemorrhagic stroke (Fig. 33-3).[2,4] Ischemic stroke, accounting for approximately 80% of stroke cases in white populations, may occur through various mechanisms including cardioembolism (e.g., secondary to atrial fibrillation or valvular heart disease), large vessel atherosclerosis (e.g., in situ occlusion of intracerebral arteries, or artery-to-artery embolism from carotid stenosis or aortic plaques), small vessel disease (lacunar stroke), and, more rarely, arterial dissection, hematologic disease, or other disorders. However, it is often difficult to assign an exact single etiologic mechanism in individual ischemic strokes because of nonspecific or overlapping risk factors and other features. Hemorrhagic stroke includes primary intracerebral hemorrhage (mainly from spontaneous rupture of an intracerebral vessel) and subarachnoid hemorrhage (mainly from rupture of an intracranial aneurysm). Both types of hemorrhagic stroke are associated with a risk of death or permanent disability greater than that from ischemic stroke.

Global Burden and Epidemiology

Worldwide, approximately 20 million strokes occur each year. Therefore, cerebrovascular disease is the sixth leading cause of disease burden, a burden predicted to rise substantially by 2020 (Fig. 33-4).[5] Approximately one fourth of all strokes are fatal, thus making stroke the second most common cause of death (after ischemic heart disease) and accounting for more than 5 million deaths (almost 10% of all deaths) each year.[6] Among patients who survive, at least one third will suffer long-term disability,[7] and approximately one in five will have a further stroke within the next 5 years.[8]

The incidence of, and mortality from, stroke varies across different countries and regions. In Asia, where the burden of stroke is particularly high, mortality from stroke is proportionally greater than that from myocardial infarction. This pattern is the reverse of that seen in Western countries,[9] possibly the result of a greater proportion of intracerebral hemorrhage. Among populations studied as part of the World Health Organization Multinational Monitoring of Trends and Determinants in Cardiovascular Disease (MONICA) project, age- and sex-standardized stroke incidence rates varied from 63 in 100,000 in Italian women to 438 in 100,000 in Russian men.[10] Analyses of other population-based studies with more rigorous methodologic criteria have found less geographic variation,[11,12] although high stroke rates are consistently observed in Eastern Europe in line with higher rates of cardiovascular disease in general in this region. In many populations, stroke incidence and mortality declined in the latter part of the 20th century,[12-14] although, with some exceptions, this decline appears to have reached a plateau, or even reversed, since 1990 (Fig. 33-5). In a few populations, how-

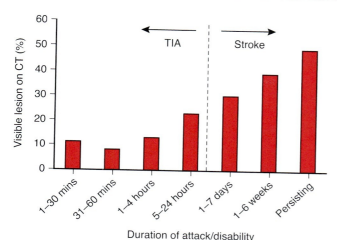

Figure 33–1   Duration of stroke symptoms (stroke versus transient ischemic attack [TIA]) and frequency of lesion visible on a computed tomography (CT) scan. (From Koudstaal PJ, van Gijn J, Frenken CW, et al. TIA, RIND, minor stroke: A continuum, or different subgroups? Dutch TIA Study Group. *J Neurol Neurosurg Psychiatry.* 1992;**55**: 95-97.)

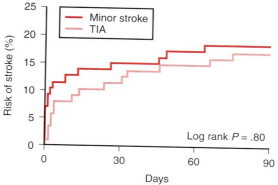

Figure 33–2   Cumulative risk of stroke after a transient ischemic attack (TIA) or a minor stroke. (From Coull AJ, Lovett JK, Rothwell PM. Population based study of early risk of stroke after transient ischaemic attack or minor stroke: Implications for public education and organisation of services. *BMJ.* 2004;**328**:326.)

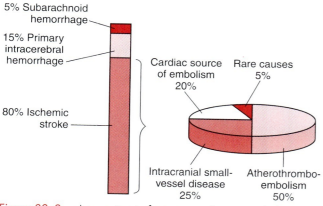

Figure 33–3   Approximate frequency of main pathologic types of stroke (in white populations) and of main subtypes of ischemic stroke as shown from population-based studies. (From Warlow C, Sudlow C, Dennis M, Sandercock P. *Stroke. Lancet.* 2003;**362**:1211-1224.)

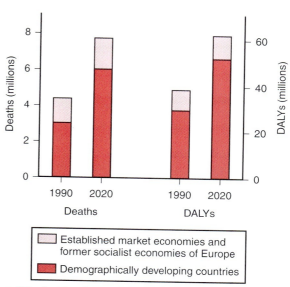

Figure 33–4   Deaths and disability-adjusted life-years (DALYs) attributed to stroke in 1990 with projections to 2020. (Data from the World Health Organization. Global Burden of Disease: A Comprehensive Assessment of Mortality and Disability from Diseases, Injuries and Risk Factors in 1990 and Projected to 2020. Boston: Harvard School of Public Health, 1996.)

ever, notably in Eastern Europe, stroke incidence and mortality have consistently increased.[10,13]

Although age-adjusted stroke incidence and mortality may have declined in many regions, the absolute number of people experiencing strokes and the rates of mortality and dependence from stroke continue to increase. This apparent paradox is mainly the result of the rapid increase in the number of individuals surviving to middle and old age and the steep rise in stroke incidence with age. As a result of these factors, and the associated epidemiologic transition from infectious to chronic diseases in middle- and lower-income countries, cerebrovascular diseases are predicted to remain the

second most common cause of death worldwide until 2020, when it is estimated that 7.7 million deaths annually will result from stroke (see Fig. 33-4).[5]

Worldwide, the standardized annual incidence of intracerebral hemorrhage varies between 26 and 60 in 100,000 population in persons aged 45 to 84 years.[11,12] In the United States, this number equates to approximately 70,000 cases annually, but in China, where this type accounts for up to 30% of all strokes, the number is estimated to be at least 300,000. The annual incidence of subarachnoid hemorrhage varies among different populations but is approximately 6 to 8 in 100,000 population.[15,16] Although it accounts for a minority

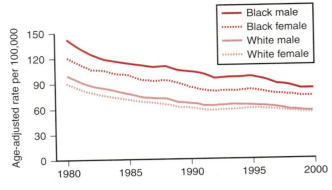

Age adjusted to the 2000 Standard Population

Figure 33–5 Decline in stroke mortality in the United States from 1980 to 2000. (From National Center for Health Statistics. Available at: http://www.cdc.gov/nchs/howto/howto.htm.)

Table 33-1 Important Risk Factors and Predictors of Stroke

Variable	Relative Risk	Absolute Risk
Older age	+++	+++
Male sex	++	++
Nonwhite race	++	++
Family history of stroke	+	+
Elevated blood pressure	+++	+++
Cigarette smoking	+++	+++
Excessive alcohol intake	+++	+
Raised body mass	++	++
Diabetes mellitus	++	++
Elevated serum cholesterol	++	++
Moderate to severe carotid artery stenosis	+++	+
Nonvalvular atrial fibrillation	+++	+++
Other forms of heart disease	+++	+

+, low; ++, intermediate; +++, high.

of all strokes, subarachnoid hemorrhage is responsible for a disproportionately high economic burden because of the high case fatality and associated disability, as well as its occurrence predominantly in people of working age.[17]

Blood Pressure as a Risk Factor

Stroke is associated with numerous identified modifiable and nonmodifiable risk factors (Table 33-1). High BP is the most important modifiable risk factor for stroke; worldwide, it is estimated that 62% of cases of cerebrovascular disease are attributable to suboptimal BP (systolic BP >115 mm Hg).[6]

BP is a major determinant of both initial (primary) stroke and recurrent (secondary) stroke.[18-20] Observational studies have demonstrated a strong and continuous relationship between the risk of stroke and the usual level of BP (Fig. 33-6). The association exists not only in patients with hypertension, but also among those with average or below-average levels of BP, with no threshold level of BP below which the risk of stroke does not continue to fall. The association becomes attenuated with increasing age, although it remains strongly positive for all age groups. Thus, a 10 mm Hg lower usual systolic BP is associated with a 40% to 50% lower risk of stroke among persons less than 60 years of age, a 30% to 40% lower risk among those age 60 to 69 years, and a 20% to 30% lower risk among those 70 years old and older.[21-23] The association is consistent in men and women, in non-Asian and Asian populations, and for both fatal and nonfatal events. The association between BP and different stroke subtypes also appears to be broadly similar, although some evidence indicates that the relationship between BP and hemorrhagic stroke is steeper than that observed with ischemic stroke (Fig. 33-7).[24]

Elevated BP is a significant risk factor for intracerebral hemorrhage and subarachnoid hemorrhage.[25,26] This factor accounts for up to one third of such strokes among people whose BP is poorly controlled.[27] In addition, extracranial carotid artery atherosclerosis is an important risk factor for ischemic stroke, and studies have shown an association between the extent of carotid atheroma and BP levels.[28] Finally, disturbances of the normal diurnal variation in BP, including the absence of a nocturnal drop in BP levels ("nondipping") and an excessive early morning acceleration

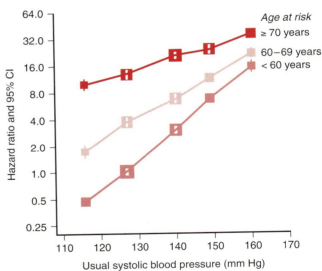

Figure 33–6 Risk of stroke against usual systolic blood pressure by age group. CI, confidence interval. (From Asia Pacific Cohort Studies Collaboration. Blood pressure and cardiovascular disease in the Asia Pacific region. *J Hypertens*. 2003;**21**:707-716.)

in BP ("morning surge"), are associated with strokes and other manifestations of cerebrovascular disease.[29]

Blood Pressure Lowering and Primary Prevention

Benefits of Blood Pressure–Lowering Treatment

Early trials demonstrated that BP lowering was remarkably effective at prolonging life in subjects with malignant hypertension.[30] The benefit of treating severe, but nonmalignant, hypertension was proven in the landmark Veterans Administration Cooperative Study on Antihypertensive Agents, in which antihypertensive treatment significantly reduced

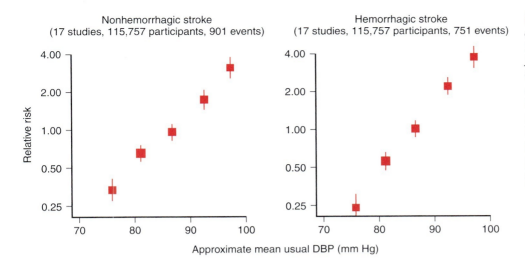

Nonhemorrhagic stroke
(17 studies, 115,757 participants, 901 events)

Hemorrhagic stroke
(17 studies, 115,757 participants, 751 events)

Figure 33–7 Relative risk of hemorrhagic and nonhemorrhagic stroke in Japanese and Republic of China cohorts according to approximate usual diastolic blood pressure (DBP). (From Eastern Stroke and Coronary Heart Disease Collaborative Research Group. Blood pressure, cholesterol, and stroke in eastern Asia. *Lancet.* 1998;**352**:1801-1807.)

hypertension-related morbidity. In this study, more strokes and deaths than myocardial infarctions were prevented.[31]

By the early 1990s, evidence was available from a series of randomized controlled trials conducted among mainly middle-aged subjects with mild to moderate hypertension and using a variety of different drugs, particularly diuretics, β-blockers, and adrenergic blocking drugs, as initial treatment. A meta-analysis of 14 trials, published in 1990, demonstrated significant reductions in the risks of stroke, coronary heart disease, and vascular death among those patients

assigned active BP-lowering therapy (Fig. 33-8).[32] Subsequent trials extended evidence of the benefits of BP-lowering therapy to include older subjects with either essential or systolic hypertension. Updated meta-analyses (including 17 trials and >47,000 individuals) demonstrated that the risk of stroke was reduced by 38%, and that of coronary heart disease by 16%, with similar reductions in both fatal and nonfatal strokes.[33] These benefits were achieved with average differences in BP between actively treated participants and controls of 10 to 12 mm Hg systolic and 5 to 6 mm Hg diastolic. The observed reduction in stroke risk, achieved with just a few years treatment, was consistent with the full benefit predicted from observational studies.[18,19] In contrast, the observed reduction in the risk of coronary heart disease was only approximately two thirds of that predicted from the epidemiologic data.

More recently, randomized controlled trials have confirmed that the benefits of BP lowering extend to newer classes of antihypertensive drugs such as angiotensin-converting enzyme (ACE) inhibitors and calcium channel blockers (Fig. 33-9). Most of these trials were conducted among high-risk individuals and included participants irrespective of their baseline level of BP. Meta-analyses of placebo-controlled trials of ACE inhibitors (conducted primarily among patients with coronary disease or diabetes) demonstrated reductions in the risk of stroke of approximately 28%.[34,35] Meta-analyses of placebo-controlled trials of calcium channel blockers (mainly elderly participants with isolated systolic hypertension) demonstrated reductions in stroke risk of approximately 38%.[34,35]

Three placebo-controlled trials of angiotensin receptor blocker (ARB) therapy completed to date differ somewhat from those involving ACE inhibitors or calcium channel blockers. In two trials conducted among patients with diabetic nephropathy, the randomized groups had identical BP targets to be achieved by the use of non-study medications; neither study was powered to detect effects of treatment on stroke or other cardiovascular outcomes.[36,37] In the third study of elderly hypertensive patients, active antihypertensive treatment was recommended and initiated, for ethical reasons, in a large proportion of subjects in the placebo group at an early point in the study.[38] In none of these three trials was any beneficial effect of active treatment observed on stroke.

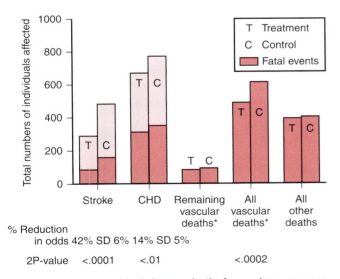

% Reduction in odds 42% SD 6% 14% SD 5%

2P-value <.0001 <.01 <.0002

* Includes any deaths from unknown causes

Figure 33–8 Crudely summated results of unconfounded randomized trials of blood pressure–lowering therapy. Data are from 14 trials that included 37,000 patients, with mean diastolic blood pressure at entry of 99 mm Hg and mean diastolic blood pressure difference during follow-up of 5 to 6 mm Hg. CHD, coronary heart disease. (From Collins R, Peto R, MacMahon S, et al. Blood pressure, stroke, and coronary heart disease: Part 2. Short-term reductions in blood pressure: Overview of randomised drug trials in their epidemiological context. *Lancet.* 1990;**335**:827-838.)

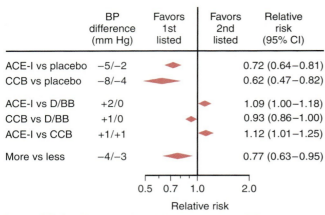

	BP difference (mm Hg)	Favors 1st listed	Favors 2nd listed	Relative risk (95% CI)
ACE-I vs placebo	−5/−2			0.72 (0.64−0.81)
CCB vs placebo	−8/−4			0.62 (0.47−0.82)
ACE-I vs D/BB	+2/0			1.09 (1.00−1.18)
CCB vs D/BB	+1/0			0.93 (0.86−1.00)
ACE-I vs CCB	+1/+1			1.12 (1.01−1.25)
More vs less	−4/−3			0.77 (0.63−0.95)

Figure 33–9 The benefits of blood pressure (BP)–lowering therapy on the risk of stroke from meta-analyses of trials comparing angiotensin-converting enzyme inhibitors (ACE-I) with placebo, calcium channel blockers (CCB) with placebo, more intensive (more) and less intensive (less) BP-lowering regimens, and trials comparing different classes of BP-lowering drug. *Diamonds* represent the 95% confidence intervals (CI) for each comparison and are centered on the pooled relative risk. Blood pressure differences (systolic/diastolic) are weighted mean differences during follow-up between actively treated groups and placebo, groups randomized to more intensive or less intensive therapy, or groups randomized to different active treatment groups. Positive values indicate higher BP in the first-listed treatment group. D/BB, diuretics and/or β-blockers. (Data from Blood Pressure Lowering Treatment Trialists' Collaboration. Effects of different blood-pressure–lowering regimens on major cardiovascular events: Results of prospectively-designed overviews of randomised trials. *Lancet.* 2003;**362**:1527-1535.)

Effects on Stroke Risk in Patient Subgroups

The benefits of BP lowering are consistent across a wide range of patient characteristics (Fig. 33-10).[23] BP lowering reduces stroke risk in subjects with isolated systolic hypertension and in elderly persons.[23,39] However, the relative benefit of BP lowering is less than in younger subjects, in keeping with the observed attenuation of the relationship between BP and stroke with increasing age. Despite this attenuation, the absolute benefits of BP lowering are greater among older individuals because of the much greater absolute stroke risk in elderly persons.

Most randomized controlled trials of BP lowering to date have recruited participants from among predominantly white populations in North America, Europe, and Australasia. Relatively few data are available from black and Asian populations, among whom the risk of stroke is particularly high. However, the available evidence suggests that the effects of BP lowering on stroke risk are similar among white and Asian populations.[40,41]

Relative Benefits of Different Drug Regimens

The few randomized trials that have directly compared the effects of BP-lowering regimens based on diuretics with those based on β-blockers failed to detect any significant difference in the effects of these drugs on stroke risk; however, even when the data from these trials are combined, the statistical power

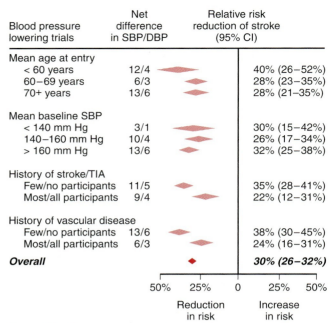

Blood pressure lowering trials	Net difference in SBP/DBP	Relative risk reduction of stroke (95% CI)
Mean age at entry		
< 60 years	12/4	40% (26−52%)
60−69 years	6/3	28% (23−35%)
70+ years	13/6	28% (21−35%)
Mean baseline SBP		
< 140 mm Hg	3/1	30% (15−42%)
140−160 mm Hg	10/4	26% (17−34%)
> 160 mm Hg	13/6	32% (25−38%)
History of stroke/TIA		
Few/no participants	11/5	35% (28−41%)
Most/all participants	9/4	22% (12−31%)
History of vascular disease		
Few/no participants	13/6	38% (30−45%)
Most/all participants	6/3	24% (16−31%)
Overall		***30% (26−32%)***

Figure 33–10 Relative risk of stroke in randomized controlled trials comparing blood pressure (BP)–lowering drugs with placebo (or no treatment) by subgroup. *Diamonds* are centered on the pooled estimate of effect and represent 95% confidence intervals (CI). The *bold red diamond* represents the pooled relative risk and 95% CI for all contributing trials. DBP, diastolic BP; SBP, systolic BP; TIA, transient ischemic attack. (From Lawes CMM, Bennett DA, Feigin VL, Rodgers A. Blood pressure and stroke: An overview of published studies. *Stroke.* 2004;**35**:776-785.)

to detect modest differences reliably is limited. More recently, some completed randomized trials have compared the effects of BP-lowering regimens based on newer classes of antihypertensive drugs. Although meta-analyses of these trials have failed to detect any differences among regimens on combined major cardiovascular events (stroke, coronary heart disease, heart failure, or cardiovascular death), some, albeit inconclusive, evidence indicates modest differences in their effects on cause-specific outcomes, including stroke.[35] Investigators noted trends toward greater reductions in stroke risk with regimens based on diuretics or β-blockers compared with those based on ACE inhibitors and with regimens based on calcium channel blockers compared with those based on diuretics or β-blockers or with those based on ACE inhibitors (see Fig. 33-9).[35] These modest trends may be related, at least partly, to the small differences in BP (of 1 to 2 mm Hg) achieved by the different regimens. In the more recently published International Verapamil-Trandolapril Study (INVEST), investigators reported a nonsignificant trend toward lower risk of nonfatal stroke among participants assigned initial treatment with a calcium channel blocker compared with those initially assigned a β-blocker.[42] The Anglo-Scandinavian Cardiac Outcomes Trial (ASCOT) compared the effects of a calcium channel blocker (amlodipine), adding an ACE inhibitor as required, with a β-blocker (atenolol), adding a thiazide diuretic as required, in more than 19,000 subjects with hypertension and other cadiovascular risk factors. The calcium channel blocker–based regimen was associated with a 23% lower risk of stroke compared with that of the β-blocker–based regimen.[42a] Inclusion of these results in updated meta-analyses comparing regimens based on calcium channel blockers with those based on diuretics or β-blockers demonstrates that calcium channel blockers confer a modest, but significant, reduction in stroke risk.

The largest single randomized trial to date that compared the effects of different BP-lowering regimens was the Antihypertensive and Lipid-Lowering Treatment to Prevent Heart Attack Trial (ALLHAT), which compared the effects of a diuretic (chlorthalidone) with those of an ACE inhibitor (lisinopril), a calcium channel blocker (amlodipine), and an α-adrenergic blocker (doxazosin) in more than 40,000 high-risk hypertensive participants.[43] The doxazosin limb of the trial was discontinued early after interim analyses showed higher rates of several outcomes, including stroke, among subjects assigned the α-blocker as initial therapy compared with subjects assigned initial treatment with a diuretic.[44] The remaining limbs of the trial contributed substantial data to the meta-analyses of trials comparing different regimens described earlier and illustrated in Figure 33-9.[35] No differences were noted among the diuretic, ACE inhibitor, and calcium channel blocker limbs of the trial for the primary outcome (fatal coronary heart disease or nonfatal myocardial infarction), nor was any difference seen between the diuretic and calcium channel blocker groups in the risk of stroke. However, the diuretic group had a 15% lower risk of stroke compared with the ACE inhibitor group, largely because of a 40% lower risk of stroke among black participants assigned the diuretic; no difference was reported among nonblack participants. This observation may largely be accounted for by differences in BP among the groups.[45] Overall, participants assigned a diuretic had 2 mm Hg lower systolic BP than those in the ACE inhibitor group, but this difference was 4 mm Hg among black participants.[43]

Two trials have, by design, compared an ARB with other classes of drug. In the Losartan Intervention for Endpoint Reduction in Hypertension study (LIFE), losartan was associated with a 25% lower risk of stroke than treatment with atenolol, despite similar BP reductions in each randomized group.[46] However, a 2004 meta-analysis of four trials involving approximately 7000 participants raised doubts about the efficacy of atenolol in the prevention of cardiovascular events, particularly stroke, possibly as a result of inferior non–BP-lowering mechanisms.[47] In the Valsartan Antihypertensive Long-Term Use Evaluation (VALUE) trial, valsartan was compared with a calcium channel blocker in high-risk hypertensive participants; no significant differences were reported between the randomized groups for either the primary endpoint (cardiac mortality and morbidity) or stroke (a secondary endpoint), but the trends for both these endpoints favored the group with the lower achieved BP.[48]

Blood Pressure Differences and Reduction in Risk of Stroke

The continuous relationship between BP and stroke risk suggests that greater BP reductions may be expected to lower the risk of stroke. A meta-analysis of four trials (two of which were conducted solely among subjects with diabetes) that randomized participants to more intensive or less intensive BP-lowering regimens demonstrated that more intensive BP lowering (with mean achieved BP 4/3 mm Hg lower than in the less intensive group) reduced the relative risk of stroke by 23% (see Fig. 33-9).[35]

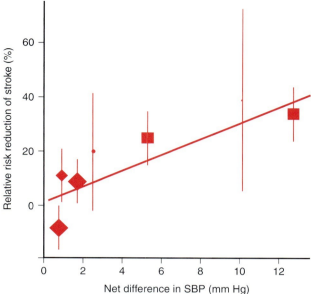

Figure 33–11 Meta-regression demonstrating the direct relationship between the net reduction in systolic blood pressure (SBP) and relative risk reduction in stroke for each of seven meta-analyses of BP-lowering therapy. From *left* to *right*, the *diamonds* represent the meta-analyses for (1) β-blockers and/or diuretics versus calcium channel blockers, (2) calcium channel blockers versus angiotensin-converting enzyme (ACE) inhibitors, and (3) β-blockers and/or diuretics versus ACE inhibitors; (4) the *circle* represents comparisons between more intensive versus less intensive BP-lowering regimens; and the *squares* are (5) ACE inhibitors versus placebo, (6) calcium channel blockers versus placebo, and (7) β-blockers and/or diuretics versus placebo or no treatment. The sizes of the *diamonds, circle,* and *squares* are larger where more strokes occurred; *vertical lines* represent 95% confidence intervals. (From Lawes CMM, Bennett DA, Feigin VL, Rogers A. Blood pressure and stroke: An overview of published studies. *Stroke.* 2004;**35**:776-785.)

The association between net BP reduction and observed differences in stroke risk in meta-analyses of randomized trials has been explored using meta-regression.[23,35] A linear relationship appears to exist between BP differences and reduction in stroke risk; the slope of the regression line suggests that a 10 mm Hg lower BP is associated with a 31% lower risk of stroke (Fig. 33-11),[23] a finding that is broadly consistent with the risk reduction predicted using age-specific data from observational cohort studies.[21,22]

Blood Pressure Lowering and Prevention of Secondary Stroke

Limited data available from observational studies suggest that the association between BP and risk of recurrent (secondary) stroke is similar to that observed in the general population (Fig. 33-12).[20] Until about 1998, however, little conclusive evidence on the benefits of BP lowering in this group was available. An early overview of four trials with published results failed to establish any benefit conclusively.[49] A further meta-analysis, which included results from subgroups of patients with

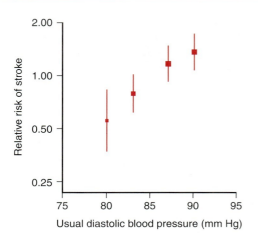 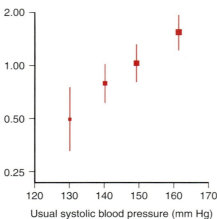

Figure 33–12 Relationship between usual diastolic and systolic blood pressure and the risk of recurrent stroke in the United Kingdom Transient Ischaemic Attack study. (From Rodgers A, MacMahon S, Gamble G, et al. Blood pressure and risk of stroke in patients with cerebrovascular disease. The United Kingdom Transient Ischaemic Attack Collaborative Group. *BMJ.* 1996;**313**:147.)

cerebrovascular disease drawn from larger trials of BP-lowering therapy, concluded that antihypertensive treatment reduced stroke risk by approximately 30% among hypertensive stroke survivors; however, the meta-analysis was unable to address the effects of this treatment in normotensive individuals.[50]

Two large randomized controlled trials recently addressed the question. The Post-stroke Antihypertensive Treatment Study (PATS) compared the diuretic indapamide with placebo in 5665 Chinese patients with a history of stroke or TIA. Although the results have been published only in preliminary form, active treatment lowered BP by 5/2 mm Hg and decreased the relative risk of recurrent stroke during 2 years of follow-up by 29%.[51]

The Perindopril Protection against Recurrent Stroke Study (PROGRESS) assigned 6105 participants with prior stoke or TIA to the ACE inhibitor perindopril (alone or in combination with indapamide) or placebo.[52] During an average of 4 years of follow-up, the relative risk of stroke was reduced by 28% among actively treated participants. The reduction in stroke was significantly greater among those treated with combination therapy (43%) than among those treated with perindopril alone (nonsignificant 5% reduction), a finding likely to be explained by the greater BP difference achieved with combination therapy (12/5 versus 5/3 mm Hg). Notably, the benefit was particularly great among the subgroup of participants with prior hemorrhagic stroke, a group in whom, before PROGRESS, no therapy had proved beneficial. The benefits were similar across a wide range of subgroups, including those with normal levels of BP.

Updating previous meta-analyses, to include the results of PATS, PROGRESS, and the subgroup of patients with prior cerebrovascular disease in the Heart Outcomes Prevention Evaluation (HOPE) study,[53] reveals that BP lowering reduces the risk of recurrent stroke by 24% (Fig. 33-13). This observation is consistent with the findings of a recent systematic review that also demonstrated a significant relationship between the size of the BP difference among randomized groups and the reduction in the risk of recurrent stroke.[54]

One randomized trial, the Morbidity and Mortality After Stroke—Eprosartan vs. Nitrendipine for Secondary Prevention (MOSES), demonstrated that an ARB reduced the risk of cerebrovascular events by 25% compared with a calcium channel blocker.[54a] However, other than this single study, published data are currently insufficient to determine reliably whether any class of BP-lowering drug is superior to others in the prevention of recurrent stroke.[45]

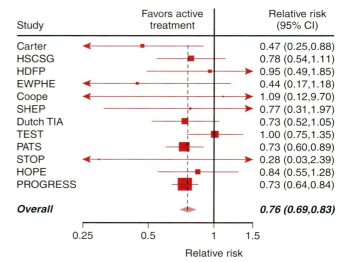

Figure 33–13 Updated meta-analysis of the risk of recurrent stroke in randomized trials of blood pressure (BP)–lowering therapy in participants with prior cerebrovascular disease or of subgroups of participants with cerebrovascular disease drawn from larger trials of BP-lowering therapy. *Boxes* and *horizontal lines* represent relative risk and 95% confidence intervals (CI) for each trial. Box size is larger where more events occurred. The *diamond* represents the 95% CI for the pooled estimate of effect and is centered on the pooled relative risk. EWPHE, European Working Party on Hypertension in the Elderly; HDFP, Hypertension Detection and Follow-up Program; HOPE, Heart Outcomes Prevention Evaluation; HSCSG, Hypertension-Stroke Cooperative Study Group; PATS, Post-stroke Antihypertensive Treatment Study; PROGRESS, Perindopril Protection against Recurrent Stroke Study; SHEP, Systolic Hypertension in the Elderly Program; STOP, Swedish Trial in Old Patients with Hypertension; TEST, Tenormin after Stroke and Transient Ischemic Attack; TIA, transient ischemic attack. (Data from references 49 to 53.)

Blood Pressure and Blood Pressure Lowering in Acute Stroke

Elevated BP is commonly observed in the acute phase of stroke and occurs in approximately three fourths of patients with ischemic stroke.[55,56] BP tends to fall over the subsequent week but remains elevated in a significant proportion of these patients. High BP occurs in approximately 80% of patients with intracerebral hemorrhage, and levels tend to be higher than among patients with ischemic stroke.[57,58] In the context of acute stroke, BP elevation is likely to result from a combination of factors including preexisting hypertension, activation of neuroendocrine (sympathetic, glucocorticoid, and mineralocorticoid) systems, increased cardiac output, and the Cushing reflex.

Observational studies of the association between BP and outcome after acute stroke have produced conflicting results, partly because many studies did not differentiate between ischemic and hemorrhagic stroke. A systematic review of 32 observational studies (including >10,000 patients) concluded that, among all patients with stroke, high systolic or diastolic BP (defined using a variety of different criteria) was associated with 1.5- to fivefold increases in the risks of death or combined death or dependence.[59] Among participants with ischemic stroke in the first International Stroke Trial, a U-shaped relationship was found between baseline BP and both early death and late death or dependence.[60] The best outcomes occurred among patients with modestly raised or high-normal BP (optimum systolic BP ~150 mm Hg). High BP was independently associated with an increased risk of death from presumed cerebral edema, whereas low BP was associated with severe clinical stroke syndromes and an excess of deaths from coronary heart disease.

It remains unclear whether acute interventions to alter BP in acute stroke have any benefit.[61] Under normal circumstances, autoregulation maintains cerebral perfusion across a wide range of systemic BPs. Autoregulation becomes dysfunctional during the acute phase of stroke, and perfusion depends on systemic pressure.[62] Theoretically, under these circumstances, acute interventions to raise or lower BP could result in further changes in cerebral blood flow and could worsen ischemic brain injury. One randomized trial, the Acute Candesartan Cilexetil Therapy in Stroke Survivors (ACCESS) trial, compared an ARB with placebo among patients with acute ischemic stroke and severely raised BP.[63] The trial was terminated early because of a large, significant, 52% reduction in the frequency of a composite secondary endpoint (combined death, cerebrovascular and cardiovascular events) in the actively treated group. However, interpretation of this result is difficult because the finding for the secondary outcome could be the consequence of chance, and no significant effect was noted on the primary outcome of total death and disability at 3 months. In addition, no significant difference in achieved BP was reported between the two treatment groups. As a result, the study does not provide the level of evidence required to recommend the routine use of BP-lowering therapy in acute ischemic stroke, and it has not resulted in widespread change in clinical practice.

Despite the persisting uncertainty, a strong rationale exists for believing that BP lowering may confer real benefits for patients in the acute phase of stroke. It is hoped that studies currently under way (e.g., Efficacy of Nitric Oxide in Stroke [ENOS], Control of Hypertension and Hypotension Immediately Post-stroke [CHHIPS], Continue or Stop Post-stroke Antihypertensives Collaborative Study [COSSACS]),[64] and others in the planning stages, will provide definitive evidence to guide clinical practice, as well as addressing the important unresolved question whether usual antihypertensive agents should be continued during the acute phase of stroke.

Meanwhile, on the basis of available evidence, various guidelines currently recommend that antihypertensive agents should be avoided unless the systolic BP is higher than 180 to 220 mm Hg or the diastolic BP is higher than 110 to 120 mm Hg, depending on whether the stroke is hemorrhagic, ischemic, or of unknown type. The guidelines recommend that when BP lowering is required, the use of sublingual nifedipine and other agents that may lower BP precipitously should be avoided.[65]

Other Interventions for the Prevention of Stroke

This section briefly summarizes the evidence for interventions other than BP lowering in the prevention of stroke, to put the latter in context (Table 33-2).[66] Because stroke is heterogeneous, interventions should be considered in the context of the individual patient.[67]

Antiplatelet Therapy

Meta-analyses have demonstrated that, compared with control results, antiplatelet therapy (mainly aspirin) reduces the relative risk of nonfatal stroke by one fourth. The relative risk of ischemic stroke (fatal and nonfatal) is reduced by 30%, whereas the risk of hemorrhagic stroke is increased by 22%.[68] Among hypertensive patients who have no associated cardiovascular risk factors, antiplatelet therapy should be considered only once BP is adequately controlled,[68,69] because uncontrolled hypertension is associated with increased risk of hemorrhagic stroke. Antiplatelet drugs should probably be avoided in survivors of intracerebral hemorrhage.

Therapies other than aspirin may also have a role. Randomized trials have shown that the thienopyridine clopidogrel reduced vascular events to a modestly greater extent than did aspirin among a broad range of high-risk "atherosclerotic" patients,[70] and the combination of aspirin and dipyridamole reduced the risk of recurrent major strokes to a greater extent than did aspirin alone.[71] Although trials of combined antiplatelet therapy with clopidogrel and aspirin have demonstrated benefits in patients with acute coronary syndromes,[72] the Management of Atherothrombosis with Clopidogrel in High-Risk Patients (MATCH) study, conducted among patients with recent cerebrovascular events, demonstrated that the modest additional benefits of such therapy are offset by an increased long-term risk of major bleeding complications in this group of patients.[73]

Anticoagulant Therapy

Atrial fibrillation secondary to rheumatic heart disease is associated with a very high relative risk of cardioembolic stroke, but it is an uncommon cause of stroke in predominantly white populations. Nonvalvular atrial fibrillation, conversely, predisposes to intracardiac thrombus formation and is a leading cause of cardioembolic stroke worldwide.[74] Individuals with nonvalvular atrial fibrillation are approximately five times as likely to suffer a stroke as those without this arrhythmia, and these strokes are frequently large and are more likely to lead to death or permanent disability than other forms of ischemic stroke. Overall, the annual risk of stroke among persons with nonvalvular atrial fibrillation is approximately 5%, but the rate varies from less than 2% to more than

Table 33-2 Stroke Prevention Strategies: Absolute Benefits of Treatment

	NNT
I. Standard Stroke Preventives	
A. Antiplatelet agents vs. aspirin*	
1. Aspirin 50 mg/day vs. aspirin 50 mg plus extended-release dipyridamole 400 mg/day	33 to save 1 stroke at 2 yr
2. Aspirin 1300 mg/day vs. ticlopidine 500 mg/day	40 to save 1 stroke at 2 yr
3. Aspirin 325 mg/day vs. clopidogrel 75 mg/day	125 to save 1 stroke at 2 yr
B. Carotid endarterectomy plus medical management vs medical management alone: symptomatic patients	
1. 70% to 99% carotid stenosis	8 to save 1 stroke at 2 yr
2. 50% to 69% carotid stenosis	20 to save 1 stroke at 2 yr
3. <50% carotid stenosis	67 to save 1 stroke at 2 yr
C. Carotid endarterectomy plus medical management vs. medical management alone: asymptomatic patients	
1. ≥50% carotid stenosis	48 to save 1 stroke at 2 yr
2. ≥60% carotid stenosis	83 to save 1 stroke at 2 yr
D. Warfarin in symptomatic (prior cerebral ischemic event) atrial fibrillation	12 to save 1 stroke at 1 year
E. Aspirin in acute stroke treatment	100 to save 1 stroke at 6 mo
II. Newer Stroke Preventives	
A. Perindopril-based therapy	
1. Overall	23 to prevent 1 stroke at 5 yr (≈1% reduction/yr)
2. Combination perindopril plus indapamide therapy	14 to prevent 1 stroke at 5 yr
B. Ramipril-based therapy	67 to prevent 1 stroke at 5 yr
C. Pravastatin vs. placebo after myocardial infarction	83 to prevent 1 stroke at 5 yr
III. Antihypertensive Agents for First Stroke Prevention	
A. 90-110 mm Hg diastolic blood pressure	118 to prevent 1 stroke at 5 yr
B. ≤115 mg Hg diastolic blood pressure	52 to prevent 1 stroke at 5 yr
C. >115 mm Hg diastolic blood pressure	29 to prevent 1 stroke at 5 yr

*NNT favors nonaspirin intervention.
NNT, number needed to treat.
From Gorelick PB. Stroke prevention therapy beyond antithrombotics: Unifying mechanisms in ischemic stroke pathogenesis and implications for therapy. *Stroke.* 2002;**33**:862-875.

10%, depending on the presence of elevated BP, cardiac hypertrophy, and other risk factors. In unselected patients with nonvalvular atrial fibrillation, anticoagulation with warfarin (adjusted to an international normalized ratio of 2 to 3) reduces the risk of stroke by approximately 65%, aspirin reduces the risk (mainly of smaller noncardioembolic strokes) by approximately 20%, and warfarin reduces the risk by approximately 45% compared with aspirin.[75] However, the relative and absolute benefits of warfarin vary widely according to background level of risk. Validated risk stratification schemes are available to identify patients who are most likely to benefit.[76]

3-Hydroxy-3-methylglutaryl–Coenzyme A Reductase Inhibitors (Statins)

Cholesterol has opposing effects on the risk of different pathologic stroke types; the association is positive for ischemic stroke and negative for hemorrhagic stroke. Although several randomized trials of statin therapy in secondary or high-risk primary prevention have reported relative reductions in stroke risk of approximately one fifth to one fourth, other studies have failed to demonstrate significant benefits, probably, at least partly, because of the insufficient differences in cholesterol levels achieved among study arms. Meta-analyses of trials of statins in primary or secondary prevention have demonstrated a relative stroke risk reduction of approximately one fifth,[77,78] with the greatest benefit occurring in patients with known vascular disease who are at greatest risk of ischemic, rather than hemorrhagic, stroke.

Carotid Revascularization

Elevated BP is an important risk factor for carotid stenosis,[28] and severe carotid stenosis affects 3% to 5% of all patients with stroke. In symptomatic patients with severe stenosis, the annual risk of stroke is 10% to 20%. Although the usual relationship between BP and stroke risk holds for patients with mild or unilateral carotid stenosis, in those with severe bilateral disease, an inverse relationship exists between BP and stroke risk.[79] Therefore, it is currently recommended that aggressive BP lowering should be avoided in this group of patients until after they undergo carotid endarterectomy.

In large-scale randomized trials among patients with symptomatic carotid stenosis, endarterectomy resulted in large (>10%) absolute reductions in the risk of stroke or death, compared with medical therapy alone.[80,81] Likewise, endarterectomy confers substantial benefits (absolute 5-year stroke risk reduction ~5% to 6%) in asymptomatic patients with severe carotid stenosis.[82]

VASCULAR DEMENTIA

Dementia is a clinical syndrome characterized by chronic or progressive impairment of memory and of other cognitive functions (language, orientation, constructional abilities, abstract thinking, problem solving, and praxis) in an alert person that is of sufficient severity to interfere with occupational or social performance and that is often accompanied by disturbances of mood, behavior, and personality.[83] Several different forms of dementia are recognized, of which *Alzheimer's disease* and *vascular dementia* are the most prevalent. Alzheimer's disease is more common than vascular dementia in developed countries,[84] but cerebrovascular disease is the leading cause of dementia in developing countries. An insidious onset, followed by gradually progressive cognitive decline with few or no focal neurologic symptoms and signs and with typical degenerative neuropathologic features, has been regarded as the hallmark of Alzheimer's disease. In contrast, vascular dementia is more likely to be characterized by an abrupt deterioration in cognition, or a fluctuating, stepwise progression of cognitive deficits. However, because of the convergence of different lines of evidence—genetic, clinical, morphologic, functional—it is becoming increasingly clear that the dementias are heterogeneous in terms of clinical pattern, disease progression, and, possibly, response to treatment. It is also increasingly apparent that the different forms of dementia share common risk factors and pathologic features, and it is now thought that cerebrovascular disease may play an important role in the origin (or time to presentation) of Alzheimer's disease and of vascular dementia.[85-91]

Modern neuroimaging has led to a greater understanding of the complex interactions among the different types of cerebral vascular lesions and cognitive impairments and has allowed the identification and refinement of the etiologic and pathologic factors that influence vascular dementia. Vascular dementia can be classified into at least eight subtypes, of which multi-infarct dementia and subcortical small vessel disease dementia are the most common; rarer forms include Binswanger's disease, genetically determined cerebral autosomal dominant arteriopathy with subcortical infarcts and leukoencephalopathy (CADASIL), familial amyloid angiopathy, and coagulopathy. In addition, before the development of overt dementia, patients may have a prodromal stage of mild cognitive impairment, in which the cognitive impairment is focal or memory is relatively spared or the symptoms are not sufficiently severe to cause functional impairment. Mild cognitive impairment is probably more prevalent than dementia and is often associated with vascular risk factors or features.

Blood Pressure as a Risk Factor

The major risk factors for vascular dementia are age, male sex, high BP, coronary heart disease, diabetes, atherosclerosis, smoking, hyperlipidemia, and history of stroke, as well as genetic associations.[92,93] Most longitudinal studies have demonstrated an association between BP and cognitive decline and both vascular dementia and Alzheimer's disease.[90,94-96] The inconsistent results observed in certain short-term studies probably reflect the finding that the asso-

ciation appears to be strongest for BP measured 10 to 20 years before the development of dementia, whereas BP measured at the time of diagnosis tends to be similar or lower than among persons who do not develop dementia.[95] Other major cardiovascular risk factors that tend to cluster with elevated BP, such as raised cholesterol, obesity, and diabetes mellitus, also appear to be associated with mild cognitive impairment and dementia.[88,90] In studies using magnetic resonance imaging, elevated BP is associated with the extent of cerebral atrophy and white matter lesions independent of age.[97-99]

The incidence of dementia de novo, and as a progression from mild cognitive impairment, is higher than expected in patients with stroke.[100-106] Outcome studies suggest that approximately one fourth of patients meet diagnostic criteria for dementia 3 months after acute ischemic stroke (although some of these patients have preexisting Alzheimer's disease), and patients who are cognitively intact at an early stage after stroke are at increased risk of subsequent dementia.[101,102] The development of dementia following stroke appears to depend on both the volume and the site of brain tissue loss, and it independently and adversely influences long-term survival after stroke.[107]

Blood Pressure–Lowering Treatment and Prevention of Dementia

Nonrandomized studies of the effects of BP-lowering treatments on cognitive function or the development of dementia have produced conflicting results. In some trials, antihypertensive treatment resulted in improved cognitive function among hypertensive patients or in patients with multi-infarct dementia,[108,109] and this therapy reduced the risk of cognitive decline in elderly persons.[110] Conversely, other studies have observed adverse associations between BP-lowering therapy and the extent of white matter lesions detected on magnetic resonance imaging and on measures of cognitive function in elderly persons.[111,112]

To date, five large randomized controlled trials of BP-lowering treatment have included dementia or measures of cognitive function as an outcome. The Medical Research Council (MRC) trial in older patients with moderate hypertension included cognitive assessments in a substantial subset of trial participants in view of concerns that BP lowering could adversely affect cognitive function; however, compared with placebo, no beneficial or harmful effect of treatment with diuretics or β-blockers was detected.[113]

The Systolic Hypertension in the Elderly Program (SHEP) compared the effects of a diuretic with placebo on dementia in elderly subjects with systolic hypertension. No significant effect was observed, although the number of cases of dementia was small (37 versus 44 cases in the active and placebo groups, respectively).[114] However, follow-up was incomplete, and it has been suggested that differential dropout rates between persons who developed dementia and those who did not may have biased the results toward the null.[115]

The Systolic Hypertension in Europe (Syst-Eur) trial compared the effects of active treatment with a calcium channel blocker with placebo on the risk of dementia in elderly patients. In a subset of elderly trial participants, active treatment reduced the risk of incident (mainly Alzheimer's) dementia by 50% after a median follow-up of 2 years.[116] Once again, however, the number of cases was small ($n = 32$), and

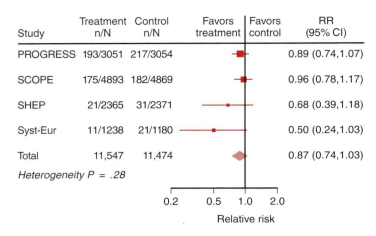

Study	Treatment n/N	Control n/N	Favors treatment	Favors control	RR (95% CI)
PROGRESS	193/3051	217/3054			0.89 (0.74,1.07)
SCOPE	175/4893	182/4869			0.96 (0.78,1.17)
SHEP	21/2365	31/2371			0.68 (0.39,1.18)
Syst-Eur	11/1238	21/1180			0.50 (0.24,1.03)
Total	11,547	11,474			0.87 (0.74,1.03)

Heterogeneity P = .28

Figure 33–14 Results of a meta-analysis of trials of blood pressure–lowering treatment on prevention of dementia and/or cognitive decline. *Boxes* and *horizontal lines* represent relative risk and 95% confidence intervals (CI) for each trial. Box size is larger where more events occurred. The *diamond* represents the 95% CI for the pooled estimate of effect and is centered on the pooled relative risk. PROGRESS, Perindopril Protection against Recurrent Stroke Study; SCOPE, Study on Cognition and Prognosis in the Elderly; SHEP, Systolic Hypertension in the Elderly Program; Syst-Eur, Systolic Hypertension in Europe. (From Feigin V, Ratnasabapathy Y, Anderson C. Does blood pressure lowering treatment prevent dementia or cognitive decline in patients with cardiovascular and cerebrovascular disease? *J Neurol Sci.* 2005;**229-230**:151-155.)

the confidence intervals (CIs) around the estimate of effect were large (95% CI, 0% to 76%). After completion of the double-blind phase of the trial, all participants (from both active and placebo arms) were offered open-label active treatment and were followed for a further 2 years. During this extended follow-up period, the number of cases of dementia doubled, but the relative risk remained similar, with a 55% reduction of dementia among those participants who had received active treatment from the beginning of the study.[117]

More recently, the PROGRESS study showed that active treatment resulted in an overall nonsignificant 12% (95% CI, –1% to 28%) reduction in the risk of dementia.[118] Among those who received combination therapy with both perindopril and indapamide (in whom the BP reduction was greater), investigators noted a borderline significant 23% reduction in the risk of dementia. The benefit appeared to be mainly the result of preventing dementia as a consequence of recurrent stroke. This study differed from those that preceded it in that a large number (*n* = 410) of cases of dementia occurred, thus making it the largest trial of dementia prevention to date.

Finally, dementia outcomes were also evaluated in the Study on Cognition and Prognosis in the Elderly (SCOPE), which compared the effects of an ARB with placebo in elderly participants with hypertension.[38] Although active treatment failed to show any benefit on dementia, few outcome events occurred. In addition, as discussed previously, widespread use of non-study BP-lowering medication led to small BP differences between the randomized groups, so the study had little power to detect an effect.

A meta-analysis of the results of the four randomized trials for which numbers of events are available in the literature showed a trend toward reduced risks of dementia and cognitive impairment with active antihypertensive treatment (Fig. 33-14),[119] although this trend was not significant. Therefore, whether BP-lowering treatment has a beneficial effect on dementia and cognitive function and whether certain agents (e.g., calcium channel blockers) have greater effects than others remain uncertain.

SUMMARY AND CONCLUSIONS

BP is a major risk factor for cerebrovascular disease and the main modifiable risk factor for stroke. An increasing body of evidence indicates that BP-lowering therapy results in sub-

stantial reductions in the risk of both primary and secondary stroke and is the only intervention proven effective in secondary prevention after hemorrhagic stroke. On the basis of current evidence, modest differences may exist among different classes of antihypertensive drugs relative to stroke risk, but this remains to be confirmed. There is still no clear evidence that interventions affecting BP in the context of acute stroke have any significant effect (either beneficial or harmful) on outcomes. BP is also associated with both vascular and Alzheimer's dementias, although whether BP-lowering therapy reduces the risk of dementia and cognitive decline has still not been established conclusively. Programs to detect and treat high BP, at both an individual and a population level, have the capacity to reduce the burden of BP-related cerebrovascular disease greatly.

Acknowledgments

We would like to thank Sam Colman and Beverley Mullane for their assistance with the figures.

References

1. World Health Organization Task Force on Stroke and Other Cerebrovascular Disorders. Stroke 1989: Recommendations on stroke prevention, diagnosis and therapy. Report of the WHO Task Force on Stroke and other Cerebrovascular Disorders. *Stroke.* 1989;**20**:1407-1431.
2. Warlow C, Dennis M, van Gijn J, et al. Stroke: A Practical Guide to Management. Oxford: Blackwell Science, 1996.
3. Coull AJ, Lovett JK, Rothwell PM. Population based study of early risk of stroke after transient ischaemic attack or minor stroke: Implications for public education and organisation of services. Oxford Vascular Study. *BMJ.* 2004;**328**:326.
4. Warlow C, Sudlow C, Dennis M, et al. Stroke. *Lancet.* 2003;**362**:1211-1224.
5. World Health Organization. Global Burden of Disease: A Comprehensive Assessment of Mortality and Disability from Diseases, Injuries and Risk Factors in 1990 and Projected to 2020. Boston: Harvard School of Public Health, 1996.
6. World Health Organization. The World Health Report 2002: Reducing Risks, Promoting Healthy Life. Geneva: World Health Organization, 2002.
7. Hankey GJ, Jamrozik K, Broadhurst RJ, et al. Long-term disability after first-ever stroke and related prognostic factors in the Perth Community Stroke Study, 1989-1990. *Stroke.* 2002;**33**:1034-1040.

8. Hankey GJ, Warlow CP. Treatment and secondary prevention of stroke: Evidence, costs and effects on individuals and populations. *Lancet*. 1999;**354**:1457-1463.

9. World Health Organization. WHO Statistics Annual 1994. Geneva: World Health Organization, 1995.

10. Sarti C, Stegmayr B, Tolonen H, et al. Are changes in mortality from stroke caused by changes in stroke event rates or case fatality? Results from the WHO MONICA Project. *Stroke*. 2003;**34**:1833-1840.

11. Sudlow CL, Warlow CP. Comparable studies of the incidence of stroke and its pathological types: Results from an International Collaboration. International Stroke Incidence Collaboration. *Stroke*. 1997;**28**:491-499.

12. Feigin VL, Lawes CM, Bennett DA, Anderson CS. Stroke epidemiology: A review of population-based studies of incidence, prevalence, and case-fatality in the late 20th century. *Lancet Neurol*. 2003;**2**:43-53.

13. Sarti C, Rastenyte D, Cepaitis Z, Tuomilehto J. International trends in mortality from stroke, 1968 to 1994. *Stroke*. 2000;**31**:1588-1601.

14. Muntner P, Garrett E, Klag MJ, Coresh J. Trends in stroke prevalence between 1973 and 1991 in the US population 25 to 74 years of age. *Stroke*. 2002;**33**:1209-1213.

15. Linn FH, Ringel GJ, Algra A, van Gijn J. Incidence of subarachnoid hemorrhage: Role of region, year, and rate of computed tomography. A meta-analysis. *Stroke*. 1996;**27**:625-629.

16. Ingall T, Asplund K, Mahonen M, Bonita R. A multinational comparison of subarachnoid hemorrhage epidemiology in the WHO MONICA Stroke Study. *Stroke*. 2000;**31**:1054-1061.

17. Hop JW, Rinkel GJ, Algra A, van Gijn J. Case-fatality rates and functional outcome after subarachnoid hemorrhage: A systematic review. *Stroke*. 1997;**28**:660-664.

18. MacMahon S, Peto R, Cutler J, et al. Blood pressure, stroke, and coronary heart disease: Part 1. Prolonged differences in blood pressure: Prospective observational studies corrected for the regression dilution bias. *Lancet*. 1990;**335**:765-774.

19. Prospective Studies Collaboration. Cholesterol, diastolic blood pressure, and stroke: 13,000 strokes in 450,000 people in 45 prospective cohorts. *Lancet*. 1995;**346**:1647-1653.

20. Rodgers A, MacMahon S, Gamble G, et al. Blood pressure and risk of stroke in patients with cerebrovascular disease: The United Kingdom Transient Ischaemic Attack Collaborative Group. *BMJ*. 1996;**313**:147.

21. Prospective Studies Collaboration. Age-specific relevance of usual blood pressure to vascular mortality: A meta-analysis of individual data for one million adults in 61 prospective studies. *Lancet*. 2002;**360**:1903-1913.

22. Asia Pacific Cohort Studies Collaboration. Blood pressure and cardiovascular disease in the Asia Pacific region. *J Hypertens*. 2003;**21**:707-716.

23. Lawes CMM, Bennett DA, Feigin VL, Rodgers A. Blood pressure and stroke: An overview of published studies. *Stroke*. 2004;**35**:776-785.

24. Eastern Stroke and Coronary Heart Disease Collaborative Research Group. Blood pressure, cholesterol, and stroke in eastern Asia. *Lancet*. 1998;**352**:1801-1807.

25. Woo D, Sauerbeck LR, Kissela BM, et al. Genetic and environmental risk factors for intracerebral hemorrhage: Preliminary results of a population-based study. *Stroke*. 2002;**33**:1190-1195.

26. Kissela BM, Sauerbeck L, Woo D, et al. Subarachnoid hemorrhage: A preventable disease with a heritable component. *Stroke*. 2002;**33**:1321-1326.

27. Woo D, Haverbusch M, Sekar P, et al. Effect of untreated hypertension on hemorrhagic stroke. *Stroke*. 2004;**35**:1703-1708.

28. Su TC, Jeng JS, Chien KL, et al. Hypertension status is the major determinant of carotid atherosclerosis: A community-based study in Taiwan. *Stroke*. 2001;**32**:2265-2271.

29. Kario K, Pickering TG, Umeda Y, et al. Morning surge in blood pressure as a predictor of silent and clinical cerebrovascular disease in elderly hypertensives: A prospective study. *Circulation*. 2003;**107**:1401-1406.

30. Harington M, Kincaid-Smith P, McMichael J. Results of treatment of malignant hypertension: A seven-year experience in 94 cases. *BMJ*. 1959;**5158**:969-980.

31. Veterans Administration Cooperative Study Group on Antihypertensive Agents. Effects of treatment on morbidity in hypertension: Results in patients with diastolic blood pressure averaging 115 through 129 mm Hg. *JAMA*. 1967;**202**:1028-1034.

32. Collins R, Peto R, MacMahon S, et al. Blood pressure, stroke, and coronary heart disease: Part 2. Short-term reductions in blood pressure: Overview of randomised drug trials in their epidemiological context. *Lancet*. 1990;**335**:827-838.

33. Collins R, MacMahon S. Blood pressure, antihypertensive drug treatment and the risks of stroke and of coronary heart disease. *Br Med Bull*. 1994;**50**:272-298.

34. Blood Pressure Lowering Treatment Trialists' Collaboration. Effects of ACE inhibitors, calcium antagonists, and other blood-pressure-lowering drugs: Results of prospectively designed overviews of randomised trials. *Lancet*. 2000;**356**:1955-1964.

35. Blood Pressure Lowering Treatment Trialists' Collaboration. Effects of different blood-pressure-lowering regimens on major cardiovascular events: Results of prospectively-designed overviews of randomised trials. *Lancet*. 2003;**362**:1527-1535.

36. Lewis EJ, Hunsicker LG, Clarke WR, et al. Renoprotective effect of the angiotensin-receptor antagonist irbesartan in patients with nephropathy due to type 2 diabetes. *N Engl J Med*. 2001;**345**:851-860.

37. Brenner BM, Cooper ME, de Zeeuw D, et al. Effects of losartan on renal and cardiovascular outcomes in patients with type 2 diabetes and nephropathy. *N Engl J Med*. 2001;**345**:861-869.

38. Lithell H, Hansson L, Skoog I, et al. The Study on Cognition and Prognosis in the Elderly (SCOPE): Principal results of a randomized double-blind intervention trial. *J Hypertens*. 2003;**21**:875-886.

39. Staessen JA, Gasowski J, Wahg JG, et al. Risks of untreated and treated isolated systolic hypertension in the elderly: Meta-analysis of outcome trials. *Lancet*. 2000;**355**:865-872.

40. Liu L, Wang JG, Gong L, et al. Comparison of active treatment and placebo in older Chinese patients with isolated systolic hypertension: Systolic Hypertension in China (Syst-China) Collaborative Group. *J Hypertens*. 1998;**16**:1823-1829.

41. Staessen JA, Fagard R, Thijs L, et al. Randomised double-blind comparison of placebo and active treatment for older patients with isolated systolic hypertension: The Systolic Hypertension in Europe (Syst-Eur) Trial Investigators. *Lancet*. 1997;**350**:757-764.

42. Pepine CJ, Handberg EM, Cooper-DeHoff RM, et al. A calcium antagonist vs a non-calcium antagonist hypertension treatment strategy for patients with coronary artery disease: The International Verapamil-Trandolapril Study (INVEST). A randomized controlled trial. *JAMA*. 2003;**290**:2805-2816.

42a. Dahlöf B, Sever PS, Poulter NR, et al. Prevention of cardiovascular events with an antihypertensive regimen of amlodipine adding perindopril as required versus atenolol adding bendroflumethiazide as required in the Anglo-Scandinavian Cardiac Outcomes Trial-Blood Pressure Lowering Arm (ASCOT-BPLA): A multicentre randomised controlled trial. *Lancet*. 2005;**366**:895-906.

43. ALLHAT Officers and Coordinators for the ALLHAT Collaborative Research Group. Major outcomes in high-risk hypertensive patients randomized to angiotensin-converting enzyme inhibitor or calcium channel blocker vs diuretic. *JAMA*. 2002;**288**:2981-2997.

44. ALLHAT Officers and Coordinators for the ALLHAT Collaborative Research Group. Major cardiovascular events in hypertensive patients randomized to doxazosin vs chlorthalidone: The Antihypertensive and Lipid-Lowering Treatment to Prevent Heart Attack Trial (ALLHAT). *JAMA*. 2000;**283**:1967-1975.

45. Chalmers J, Todd A, Chapman N, et al., International Society of Hypertension Writing Group. International Society of Hypertension (ISH): Statement on blood pressure lowering and stroke prevention. *J Hypertens*. 2003;**21**:651-663.

46. Dahlöf B, Devereux RB, Kjeldsen SE, et al. Cardiovascular morbidity and mortality in the Losartan Intervention for Endpoint reduction in hypertension study (LIFE): A randomised trial against atenolol. *Lancet*. 2002;**359**:995-1003.

47. Carlberg B, Samuelsson O, Lindholm LH. Atenolol in hypertension: Is it a wise choice? *Lancet*. 2004;**364**:1684-1689.

48. Julius S, Kjeldsen SE, Weber M, et al. Outcomes in hypertensive patients at high cardiovascular risk treated with regimens based on valsartan or amlodipine: The VALUE randomised trial. *Lancet*. 2004;**363**:2022-2031.

49. Rodgers A, Neal B, MacMahon S. The effects of blood pressure lowering in cerebrovascular disease. *Neurol Rev Int*. 1997;**2**:12-15.

50. Gueyffier F, Boissel JP, Boutitie F, et al. Effect of antihypertensive treatment in patients having already suffered from stroke: Gathering the evidence. The INDANA Project Collaborators. *Stroke*. 1997;**28**:2557-2562.

51. PATS Collaborating Group. Post-stroke antihypertensive treatment study: A preliminary result. *Chin Med J*. 1995;**108**:710-717.

52. PROGRESS Collaborative Group. Randomised trial of a perindopril-based blood-pressure–lowering regimen among 6105 individuals with previous stroke or transient ischaemic attack. *Lancet*. 2001;**358**:1033-1041.

53. Bosch J, Yusuf S, Pogue J, et al. Use of ramipril in preventing stroke: Double blind randomised trial. *BMJ*. 2002;**324**:699-702.

54. Rashid P, Leonardi-Bee J, Bath P. Blood pressure reduction and secondary prevention of stroke and other vascular events: A systematic review. *Stroke*. 2003;**34**:2741-2748.

54a. Schrader J, Lüders S, Kulschewski A, et al. Morbidity and mortality after stroke, eprosartan compared with nitrendipine for secondary prevention. Principal results of a prospective randomized controlled study (MOSES). *Stroke*. 2005;**34**:1218-1226.

55. Wallace JD, Levy LL. Blood pressure after stroke. *JAMA*. 1981;**246**:2177-2180.

56. Morfis L, Schwartz RS, Poulos R, Howes LG. Blood pressure changes in acute cerebral infarction and hemorrhage. *Stroke*. 1997;**28**:1401-1405.

57. Lip GY, Zarifis J, Farooqi IS, et al. Ambulatory blood pressure monitoring in acute stroke: The West Birmingham Stroke Project. *Stroke*. 1997;**28**:31-35.

58. Jorgensen HS, Nakayama H, Christensen HR, et al. Blood pressure in acute stroke: The Copenhagen Stroke Study. *Cerebrovasc Dis*. 2002;**13**:204-209.

59. Willmot M, Leonardi-Bee J, Bath PM. High blood pressure in acute stroke and subsequent outcome: A systematic review. *Hypertension*. 2004;**43**:18-24.

60. Leonardi-Bee J, Bath PM, Phillips SJ, Sandercock PA. Blood pressure and clinical outcomes in the International Stroke Trial: IST Collaborative Group. *Stroke*. 2002;**33**:1315-1320.

61. Bath P, Chalmers J, Powers W, et al., for the International Society of Hypertension Writing Group. International Society of Hypertension (ISH): Statement on the management of blood pressure in acute stroke. *J Hypertens*. 2003;**21**:665-672.

62. Meyer JS, Shimazu K, Fukuuchi Y, et al. Impaired neurogenic cerebrovascular control and dysautoregulation after stroke. *Stroke*. 1973;**4**:169-186.

63. Schrader J, Luders S, Kulschewski A, et al. The ACCESS Study: Evaluation of Acute Candesartan Cilexetil Therapy in Stroke Survivors. *Stroke*. 2003;**34**:1699-1703.

64. Robinson TG, Potter JF. Blood pressure in acute stroke. *Age Ageing*. 2004;**33**:6-12.

65. Adams HP Jr, Adams RJ, Brott T, et al. Guidelines for the early management of patients with ischemic stroke: A Scientific Statement from the Stroke Council of the American Stroke Association. *Stroke*. 2003;**34**:1056-1083.

66. Gorelick PB. Stroke prevention therapy beyond antithrombotics: Unifying mechanisms in ischemic stroke pathogenesis and implications for therapy. *Stroke*. 2002;**33**:862-875.

67. Gorelick PB, Broder MS, Crowell R, et al. Determining the appropriateness of selected surgical and medical management options in recurrent stroke prevention: A guideline for primary care physicians from the National Stroke Association Work Group on Recurrent Stroke Prevention. *J Stroke Cerebrovasc Dis*. 2004;**13**:196-207.

68. Antithrombotic Trialists' Collaboration. Collaborative meta-analysis of randomised trials of antiplatelet therapy for prevention of death, myocardial infarction, and stroke in high risk patients. *BMJ*. 2002;**324**:71-86.

69. Chobanian AV, Bakris GL, Black HR, et al., and the National High Blood Pressure Education Program Coordinating Committee. The Seventh Report of the Joint National Committee on Prevention, Detection, Evaluation, and Treatment of High Blood Pressure: The JNC 7 Report. *JAMA*. 2003;**289**:2560-2572.

70. CAPRIE Steering Committee. A randomised, blinded, trial of clopidogrel versus aspirin in patients at risk of ischemic events (CAPRIE). *Lancet*. 1996;**348**:1329-1339.

71. ESPRIT Study Group; Halkes PH, van Gijn J, et al. Aspirin plus dipyridamole versus aspirin alone after cerebral ischaemia of arterial origin (ESPRIT): Randomised controlled trial. *Lancet*. 2006;**367**:1665-1773.

72. Yusuf S, Zhao F, Mehta, et al., for the Clopidogrel in Unstable Angina to Prevent Recurrent Events (CURE) Trial Investigators. Effects of clopidogrel in addition to aspirin in patients with acute coronary syndromes without ST-segment elevation. *N Engl J Med*. 2001;**345**:494-502.

73. Diener HC, Bogousslavsky J, Brass LM, et al. Aspirin and clopidogrel compared with clopidogrel alone after recent ischaemic stroke or transient ischaemic attack in high-risk patients (MATCH): Randomised, double-blind, placebo-controlled trial. *Lancet*. 2004;**364**:331-337.

74. Hart RG, Halperin JL. Atrial fibrillation and stroke: Concepts and controversies. *Stroke*. 2001;**32**:803-808.

75. van Walraven C, Hart RG, Singer DE, et al. Oral anticoagulants vs aspirin in nonvalvular atrial fibrillation: An individual patient meta-analysis. *JAMA*. 2002;**288**:2441-2448.

76. Hart RG, Halperin JL, Pearce LA, et al. Lessons from the Stroke Prevention in Atrial Fibrillation trials. *Ann Intern Med*. 2003;**138**:831-838.

77. Baigent C, Keech A, Kearney PM, et al. Efficacy and safety of cholesterol-lowering treatment: Prospective meta-analysis of data from 90,056 participants in 14 randomised trials of statins. *Lancet*. 2005;**366**:1267-1278.

78. Law MR, Wald NJ, Rudnicka AR. Quantifying effect of statins on low density lipoprotein cholesterol, ischaemic heart disease, and stroke: Systematic review and meta-analysis. *BMJ*. 2003;**326**:1423.

79. Rothwell PM, Howard SC, Spence JD, for the Carotid Endarterectomy Trialists' Collaboration. Relationship between blood pressure and stroke risk in patients with symptomatic carotid occlusive disease. *Stroke*. 2003;**34**:2583-2590.

80. European Carotid Surgery Trialists' Collaborative Group. Randomised trial of endarterectomy for recently symptomatic

carotid stenosis: Final results of the MRC European Carotid Surgery Trial (ECST). *Lancet.* 1998;**351**:1379-1387.

81. Paciaroni M, Eliasziw M, Sharpe BL, et al. Long-term clinical and angiographic outcomes in symptomatic patients with 70% to 99% carotid artery stenosis. *Stroke.* 2000;**31**:2037-2042.

82. Halliday A, Mansfield A, Marro J, et al., for the MRC Asymptomatic Carotid Surgery (ACST) Collaborative Group. Prevention of disabling and fatal strokes by successful carotid endarterectomy in patients without recent neurological symptoms: A randomised controlled trial. *Lancet.* 2004;**363**:1491-1502.

83. Ritchie K, Lovestone S. The dementias. *Lancet.* 2002;**360**: 1759-1766.

84. Rocca WA, Hofman A, Brayne C, et al. The prevalence of vascular dementia in Europe: Facts and fragments from 1980-1990 studies. EURODEM-Prevalence Research Group. *Ann Neurol.* 1991;**30**:817-824.

85. Jellinger K, Danielczyk W, Fischer P, et al. Clinicopathological analysis of dementia disorders in the elderly. *J Neurol Sci.* 1990;**95**:239-258.

86. Victoroff J, Mack WJ, Lyness SA, Chui HC. Multicenter clinicopathological correlation in dementia. *Am J Psychiatry.* 1995;**152**:1476-1484.

87. Hofman A, Ott A, Breteler MM, et al. Atherosclerosis, apolipoprotein E, and prevalence of dementia and Alzheimer's disease in the Rotterdam Study. *Lancet.* 1997;**349**:151-154.

88. Skoog I, Gustafson D. Hypertension, hypertension-clustering factors and Alzheimer's disease. *Neurol Res.* 2003;**25**:675-680.

89. Snowdon DA, Greiner LH, Mortimer JA, et al. Brain infarction and the clinical expression of Alzheimer disease: The Nun Study. *JAMA.* 1997;**277**:813-817.

90. Kivipelto M, Helkala EL, Laakso MP, et al. Midlife vascular risk factors and Alzheimer's disease in later life: Longitudinal, population based study. *BMJ.* 2001;**322**:1447-1451.

91. Kalmijn S, Foley D, White L, et al. Metabolic cardiovascular syndrome and risk of dementia in Japanese-American elderly men: The Honolulu-Asia Aging Study. *Arterioscler Thromb Vasc Biol.* 2000;**20**:2255-2260.

92. Skoog I. Status of risk factors for vascular dementia. *Neuroepidemiology.* 1998;**17**:2-9.

93. Gorelick PB. Risk factors for vascular dementia and Alzheimer disease. *Stroke.* 2004;**35 (Suppl I)**:2620-2622.

94. Farmer ME, Kittner SJ, Abbott RD, et al. Longitudinally measured blood pressure, antihypertensive medication use, and cognitive performance: The Framingham Study. *J Clin Epidemiol.* 1990;**43**:475-480.

95. Skoog I, Lernfelt B, Landahl S, et al. 15-Year longitudinal study of blood pressure and dementia. *Lancet.* 1996;**347**:1141-1145.

96. Launer LJ, Ross GW, Petrovitch H, et al. Midlife blood pressure and dementia: The Honolulu-Asia aging study. *Neurobiol Aging.* 2000;**21**:49-55.

97. Longstreth WT Jr, Manolio TA, Arnold A, et al. Clinical correlates of white matter findings on cranial magnetic resonance imaging of 3301 elderly people: The Cardiovascular Health Study. *Stroke.* 1996;**27**:1274-1282.

98. Dufouil C, de Kersaint-Gilly A, Besancon V, et al. Longitudinal study of blood pressure and white matter hyperintensities: The EVA MRI cohort. *Neurology.* 2001;**56**:921-926.

99. Wiseman RM, Saxby BK, Burton EJ, et al. Hippocampal atrophy, whole brain volume, and white matter lesions in older hypertensive subjects. *Neurology.* 2004;**63**:1892-1897.

100. Tatemichi TK, Desmond DW, Mayeux R, et al. Dementia after stroke: Baseline frequency, risks, and clinical features in a hospitalized cohort. *Neurology.* 1992;**42**:1185-1193.

101. Tatemichi TK, Paik M, Bagiella E, et al. Risk of dementia after stroke in a hospitalized cohort: Results of a longitudinal study. *Neurology.* 1994;**44**:1885-1891.

102. Kokmen E, Whisnant JP, O'Fallon WM, et al. Dementia after ischemic stroke: A population-based study in Rochester, Minnesota (1960-1984). *Neurology.* 1996;**46**:154-159.

103. Henon H, Pasquier F, Durieu I, et al. Preexisting dementia in stroke patients: Baseline frequency, associated factors, and outcome. *Stroke.* 1997;**28**:2429-2436.

104. Censori B, Manara O, Agostinis C, et al. Dementia after first stroke. *Stroke.* 1996;**27**:1205-1210.

105. Zhu L, Fratiglioni L, Guo Z, et al. Incidence of dementia in relation to stroke and the apolipoprotein E epsilon 4 allele in the very old: Findings from a population-based longitudinal study. *Stroke.* 2000;**31**:53-60.

106. Solfrizzi V, Panza F, Colacicco AM, et al. Vascular risk factors, incidence of MCI, and rates of progression to dementia. *Neurology.* 2004;**63**:1882-1891.

107. Tatemichi TK, Paik M, Bagiella E, et al. Dementia after stroke is a predictor of long-term survival. *Stroke.* 1994;**25**:1915-1919.

108. Starr JM, Whalley LJ, Deary IJ. The effects of antihypertensive treatment on cognitive function: Results from the HOPE study. *J Am Geriatr Soc.* 1996;**44**:411-415.

109. Meyer JS, Judd BW, Tawaklna T, et al. Improved cognition after control of risk factors for multi-infarct dementia. *JAMA.* 1986;**256**:2203-2209.

110. Tzourio C, Dufouil C, Ducimetiere P, Alperovitch A. Cognitive decline in individuals with high blood pressure: A longitudinal study in the elderly. EVA study group: Epidemiology of Vascular Aging. *Neurology.* 1999;**53**:1948-1952.

111. Heckbert SR, Longstreth WT Jr, Psaty BM, et al. The association of antihypertensive agents with MRI white matter findings and with modified Mini-Mental State Examination in older adults. *J Am Geriatr Soc.* 1997;**45**:1423-1433.

112. Maxwell CJ, Hogan DB, Ebly EM. Calcium-channel blockers and cognitive function in elderly people: Results from the Canadian Study of Health and Aging. *Can Med Assoc J.* 1999;**161**:501-506.

113. Prince MJ, Bird AS, Blizard RA, Mann AH. Is the cognitive function of older patients affected by antihypertensive treatment? Results from 54 months of the Medical Research Council's trial of hypertension in older adults. *BMJ.* 1996;**312**:801-805.

114. SHEP Cooperative Research Group. Prevention of stroke by antihypertensive drug treatment in older persons with isolated systolic hypertension: Final results of the Systolic Hypertension in the Elderly Program (SHEP). *JAMA.* 1991;**265**:3255-3264.

115. Di Bari M, Pahor M, Franse LV, et al. Dementia and disability outcomes in large hypertension trials: Lessons learned from the Systolic Hypertension in the Elderly Program (SHEP) Trial. *Am J Epidemiol.* 2001;**153**:72-78.

116. Forette F, Seux ML, Staessen JA, et al. Prevention of dementia in randomised double-blind placebo-controlled Systolic Hypertension in Europe (Syst-Eur) trial. *Lancet.* 1998;**352**: 1347-1351.

117. Forette F, Seux ML, Staessen JA, et al. The prevention of dementia with antihypertensive treatment: New evidence from the Systolic Hypertension in Europe (Syst-Eur) study. *Arch Intern Med.* 2002;**162**:2046-2052.

118. Tzourio C, Anderson C, Chapman N, et al., for the PROGRESS Collaborative Group. Effects of blood pressure lowering with perindopril and indapamide therapy on dementia and cognitive decline in patients with cerebrovascular disease. *Arch Intern Med.* 2003;**163**:1069-1075.

119. Feigin V, Ratnasabapathy Y, Anderson C. Does blood pressure lowering treatment prevent dementia or cognitive decline in patients with cardiovascular and cerebrovascular disease? *J Neurol Sci.* 2005;**229-230**:151-155.

Chapter 34

Hypertension and Diabetes Mellitus

Maryann N. Mugo, Craig S. Stump, Priya G. Rao, and James R. Sowers

Diabetes mellitus (DM) is the sixth leading cause of death in adults in the United States. This debilitating disease affects 6.3% of the population, or approximately 18.2 million individuals.[1] Among adults who are more than 60 years of age, 8.6 million are affected, a number representing 18.3% of this age group (Fig. 34-1). Although the prevalence of DM is highest in persons who are more than 65 years of age, younger individuals (<45 years) have experienced the greatest increase in DM in the last decade.[2] Although the United States has the leading proportion of afflicted individuals, the rapid rise in the prevalence of DM is occurring globally, and soon more than 300 million persons worldwide will be affected. In the United States, DM is now the leading cause of end-stage renal disease (ESRD) and nontraumatic amputations. Cardiovascular disease (CVD), however, is the major cause of premature mortality in patients with type 2 DM. Coexistent hypertension (HTN) is a major contributor to the development of CVD and renal disease in these patients.[3]

HTN is more common in persons with type 2 DM, and individuals with HTN are 2.5 times more likely to develop DM than are persons who have normal blood pressures (BPs).[4] HTN affects approximately 58 million individuals in the United States, and it is the primary diagnosis in approximately 35 million office visits annually. Accumulating evidence indicates that the intensive treatment of HTN and of other cardiovascular risk factors such as dyslipidemia and hyperglycemia considerably lessens the burden of CVD and renal disease in patients with DM.[5]

HYPERTENSION IN PATIENTS WITH TYPE 1 DIABETES MELLITUS

Patients with type 1 DM currently make up about 6% to 8% of the total diabetic population in the United States.[5] In contrast to patients with type 2 DM, those with type 1 DM typically develop renal disease before they develop HTN.[3,6] However, the development of HTN accelerates the course of microvascular and macrovascular disease in these patients.[3] Therefore, patients with type 1 DM and microalbuminuria should be treated with an angiotensin-converting enzyme (ACE) inhibitor even before they develop HTN.[7] Furthermore, β-blockers should not be used as first-line antihypertensive therapy in patients with type 1 DM because of the propensity of these drugs to promote hypoglycemia and to reduce the patient's ability to perceive and manifest hypoglycemic symptoms appropriately, as well as to respond physiologically to hypoglycemia.[7] Other aspects of antihypertensive therapy are similar to those for patients with type 2 DM (see later).

HYPERTENSION IN THE METABOLIC (CARDIOMETABOLIC) SYNDROME

The National Cholesterol Education Program (NCEP) Adult Treatment Panel III (ATP III) defined the metabolic syndrome as the presence of any three or more of the following: BP, 130/85 mm Hg or higher; waist circumference, larger than 40 inches in men or larger than 35 inches in women; triglycerides, 150 mg/dL or higher; high-density lipoprotein, less than 40 mg/dL in men or less than 50 mg/dL in women; and fasting glucose, 110 mg/dL or higher.[8] The American Diabetes Association (ADA) lowered the impaired fasting glucose threshold from 110 to 100 mg/dL, and this change has not yet been incorporated into the ATP criteria. The syndrome is a clustering of maladaptive characteristics that confers an increased risk of CVD; thus, we prefer the term "cardiometabolic" syndrome. These factors are summarized in Table 34-1.

In the National Health and Nutrition Examination Survey (NHANES) conducted from 1999 to 2000, the overall prevalence of the metabolic syndrome was 26.7%, an increase from the NHANES III (1988 to 1994) survey measurement of 23.1%. Further, an age-dependent increase in prevalence is apparent in both men (10.7%, 33.0%, and 39.7%) and women (18.0%, 30.6%, and 46.1%) for ages 20 to 39 years, 40 to 59 years, and more than 60 years, respectively.[9] The Framingham Heart Study demonstrated the synergistic action of these cardiovascular risk factors in mediating cardiovascular events. Indeed, the coexistence of HTN, the metabolic syndrome, and DM markedly increases the risk of developing macrovascular disease, which includes cerebrovascular, cardiovascular, and peripheral vascular diseases.[3] Even mild hyperglycemia (i.e., impaired fasting glucose), when associated with modest HTN (systolic BP [SBP], 140 to 149 mm Hg), significantly increases CVD mortality. Another key risk factor is obesity, specifically central or visceral obesity, which is associated with insulin resistance and premature CVD. A rising body mass index is independently associated with a linear increase in SBP, diastolic BP (DBP), and pulse pressure.

Insulin resistance is likely a primary contributor to the pathophysiology of the metabolic syndrome. Hypertensive patients have a high prevalence of insulin resistance and a substantially higher risk of developing type 2 DM.[4] Insulin resistance is characterized by impaired ability of insulin to stimulate glucose uptake in insulin-sensitive tissues, in particular skeletal muscle. Factors contributing to the development of insulin resistance in patients with HTN include altered composition of skeletal muscle, decreased blood flow and delivery of insulin to skeletal muscle, and post–insulin receptor abnormalities in metabolic signaling (Table 34-2).

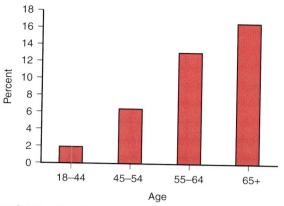

Figure 34–1 Prevalence of diagnosed diabetes mellitus in adults older than 18 years of age in the United States in 2003. (From early release of selected estimates based on data from the 2003 National Health Interview Survey. Available on the Internet at: http://www.cdc.gov/nchs/data/nhis/earlyrelease/200406_14.pdf, accessed 27 MAR 05 at 18:38 CST.)

Table 34-1 Cardiometabolic Syndrome Factors Associated with Risk for Cardiovascular Disease

Hypertension
Central or visceral obesity
Hyperinsulinemia or insulin resistance
Impaired glucose tolerance
Endothelial dysfunction
Microalbuminuria
Low high-density lipoprotein cholesterol levels
High triglyceride levels
Small, dense low-density lipoprotein cholesterol particles
Increased apolipoprotein B levels
Increased fibrinogen levels
Increased plasminogen activator inhibitor 1 and decreased plasminogen activator levels
Increased C-reactive protein level and other inflammatory markers
Absent nocturnal dipping of blood pressure and heart rate
Salt sensitivity
Left ventricular hypertrophy
Premature or excess coronary artery disease, stroke, and peripheral vascular disease

Table 34-2 Mechanisms of Insulin Resistance in Hypertension

Decreased Nonoxidative Glucose Metabolism by Skeletal Muscle	Decreased Delivery of Insulin and Glucose to Skeletal Muscle
Postreceptor Defect	
Decreased signaling through the phosphatidylinositol 3-kinase–Akt pathway	Increased reactive oxygen species
Decreased glucose transporter-4 content and translocation	Reduced generation of nitric oxide
Decreased glycogen synthase activity	Vascular rarefaction
Increased oxidative stress	Vascular hypertrophy
	Increased vasoconstriction
Altered Skeletal Muscle Fiber Type	
Decreased insulin-sensitive slow-twitch skeletal muscle fibers	
Increased fat deposition	

HYPERTENSION AND CARDIOVASCULAR DISEASE IN TYPE 2 DIABETES MELLITUS

HTN markedly increases the risk for CVD in patients with type 2 DM.[3] The Multiple Risk Factor Intervention Trial (MRFIT) followed more than 5000 men with DM and 350,000 nondiabetic men for 12 years to evaluate the impact of various CVD risk factors. The study confirmed that HTN, elevated cholesterol levels, and cigarette smoking were independent CVD risk factors in men with DM, and the impact of these factors was greater in these patients than in nondiabetic persons.[10] In the United Kingdom Prospective Diabetes Study (UKPDS), lowering SBP improved CVD risk in patients with type 2 DM (Fig. 34-2).[11]

In the UKPDS, patients assigned to "tight" BP control (<150/85 mm Hg target versus 144/82 mm Hg achieved) compared with "less tight" (<180/105 mm Hg with 154/87 mm Hg achieved) exhibited significant reductions in DM-related endpoints, including death, stroke, and microvascular disease, especially diabetic retinopathy.[11] Furthermore, the relative benefit on CVD risk factors was more powerful for "tight" BP control than for intensive blood glucose control. The Hypertension Optimal Treatment (HOT) trial reported that, in a diabetic subgroup (n = 1501), major CVD events were reduced by 51% in those randomized to a DBP of less than 80 mm Hg compared with a DBP goal of less than 90 mm Hg.[12] No benefit of more aggressive management was evident in the nondiabetic patients in the HOT trial.

In the Systolic Hypertension in Europe (Syst-Eur) trial, a placebo-controlled trial of treatment of isolated systolic HTN, the 492 patients with DM were reported in a post hoc analysis to have significant reductions in CVD mortality, in all CVD events, and in stroke when mean SBPs were reduced from 175 to 153 mm Hg.[13] These data are consistent with those of the Systolic Hypertension in the Elderly Program (SHEP), in which elderly persons with type 2 DM derived more CVD reduction with active antihypertensive therapy, compared with placebo, relative to what was gained by persons without DM.

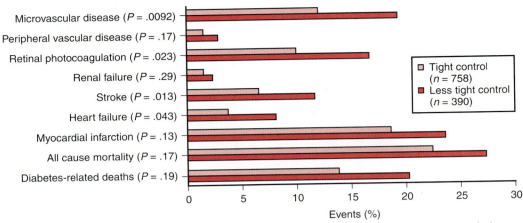

Figure 34–2   Effects of blood pressure control on mortality and vascular events in patients with type 2 diabetes mellitus: The United Kingdom Prospective Diabetes Study 38. (From United Kingdom Prospective Diabetes Study Group. Tight blood pressure control and risk of macrovascular and microvascular complications in type 2 diabetes: UKPDs 38. *BMJ.* 1998;**317**:703-713.)

STROKE IN PATIENTS WITH DIABETES AND HYPERTENSION

In 2002, 57 stroke-related deaths occurred in the United States per 100,000 people. Stroke is currently ranked as the third leading cause of death in the United States.[14] There are more than 700,000 strokes annually and more than 4.5 million stroke survivors. As the prevalence of DM increased, it became a well-documented, independent, modifiable stroke risk factor.[14] Indeed, the incidence of stroke among patients with DM is up to three times that in the general population.[15,16] Both short-term mortality and long-term mortality are increased in patients with DM following stroke, and admission glucose levels are a predictor of poor outcomes in these patients.[14,16]

Prevention of stroke in patients with DM is paramount because of the higher incidence and poorer outcomes in these patients. HTN, heart failure, and cigarette and alcohol use are modifiable risk factors for stroke in patients with and without DM. Intervention trials have provided compelling support for intensive BP control in patients with DM to prevent stroke.[5] In the UKPDS, for combined fatal and nonfatal stroke, achieving a mean BP of 144/82 mm Hg resulted in a marked 44% relative risk reduction compared with the less aggressive control group, whose subjects had a mean BP of 154/87 mm Hg. Additional data from the Syst-Eur trial, with nitrendipine-based antihypertensive therapy, showed that the excess risk of stroke associated with DM was abolished by antihypertensive treatment in older patients with type 2 DM and isolated HTN. In the Microalbuminuria, Cardiovascular, and Renal Outcomes in the Heart Outcomes Prevention Evaluation (MICRO-HOPE), 3577 patients with DM who were treated with ramipril showed a reduction of primary combined endpoints of myocardial infarction, stroke, and CVD death by 25% and of stroke alone by 33%.[17]

Recent studies have shown the beneficial effects of an angiotensin receptor blocker (ARB) and diuretic or an ACE inhibitor and diuretic combination in reducing the incidence of primary and secondary strokes in high-risk patients, including those with DM.[5,18,19] The Antihypertensive and Lipid-Lowering Treatment to Prevent Heart Attack Trial (ALLHAT) also showed that treatments using a diuretic and lowering SBP were very important strategies to reduce stroke incidence in patients with DM.[20] These data support recent guidelines recommending a BP of less than 130/80 mm Hg in patients with DM and HTN.[3]

PATHOPHYSIOLOGY OF HYPERTENSION IN DIABETES MELLITUS

Emerging evidence suggests an important relationship between insulin resistance and HTN.[21] Further, DM and HTN are both associated with insulin resistance and accompanying hyperinsulinemia. Insulin resistance occurs in up to 50% of the 58 million patients with essential HTN in the United States.[22] Untreated patients with essential HTN have higher fasting and postprandial insulin levels than age- and sex-matched normotensive persons regardless of body mass.[5] Normotensive first-degree relatives of patients with HTN also have insulin resistance and dyslipidemia. However, this link does not dictate causality, because a genetic predisposition may contribute to the occurrence of both disorders (see Chapter 2). Furthermore, not all hypertensive patients have insulin resistance and hyperinsulinemia. For example, the relationship between insulin levels and HTN does not occur in secondary HTN.[21,22]

In addition to genetic predispositions, cellular abnormalities in insulin signaling and associated homodynamic and metabolic derangements appear to predispose to the development of HTN.[21,22] Indeed, HTN in DM is the consequence of the interaction of multiple maladaptive pathways that involve not only insulin resistance and hyperinsulinemia, but also vascular and endothelial dysfunction, sodium retention, increased sympathetic nervous system activity, and an overactive tissue renin-angiotensin-aldosterone system (RAAS).[21] Moreover, hyperinsulinemia and insulin resistance elevate the intracellular calcium concentration in vascular smooth muscle cells, thus leading to vasoconstriction, as well as the proliferation of vascular smooth muscle cells, with resulting

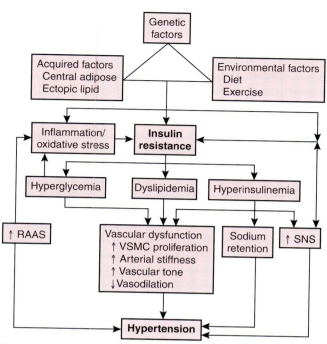

Figure 34–3 Summary of putative pathophysiologic mechanisms in the development of hypertension in diabetes mellitus. RAAS, renin-angiotensin-aldosterone system; SNS, sympathetic nervous system; VSMC, vascular smooth muscle cell.

growth and hypertrophy.[21] Other likely contributors include increased inflammation, oxidative stress, and deranged adipocyte differentiation and fat storage. These factors are summarized later and in Figure 34-3. This issue may be important because the various classes of antihypertensive medications have disparate effects on insulin sensitivity in patients with essential HTN.[4,23]

NEPHROPATHY IN PATIENTS WITH HYPERTENSION AND DIABETES

Diabetic nephropathy has become the leading cause of ESRD in the United States.[24,25] Approximately 35% of persons with DM will develop diabetic nephropathy characterized by proteinuria, decreased glomerular filtration rate, and increased BP.[24] Development of diabetic nephropathy often predates or occurs simultaneously with the evolution of HTN in patients with type 1 DM.[24] Diabetic nephropathy is thus thought to be a powerful promoter of HTN in patients with type 1 DM. In patients with type 2 DM, the incidence of nephropathy is approximately 20%. Nevertheless, because up to 95% of diabetic patients have type 2 DM, more than half of ESRD cases in DM occur in patients with type 2 DM. The prevalence and incidence of ESRD are approximately twice what they were 10 years ago.[25] If the trends of the past 2 decades persist, approximately 175,000 new cases of ESRD will be diagnosed in 2010. This is partly because of the expectation that the incidence of type 2 DM will double in the years up to 2020 and the finding that patients with DM are living longer and are thus more likely to develop chronic problems, including

ESRD. The cost associated with the management of ESRD is expected to exceed $28 billion by 2010.[25]

Microalbuminuria, which heralds the onset of nephropathy, is defined as albuminuria detected in urine at levels of 30 to 299 mg/day. Albumin excretion exceeding these parameters is macroalbuminuria or overt proteinuria. The appearance of clinically detectable, dipstick-positive proteinuria signals the onset of the relentless progression of diabetic nephropathy, which is typically followed by deterioration to ESRD over a period of 10 to 15 years. Furthermore, both macroalbuminuria and microalbuminuria are major independent risk factors for CVD.[26] Microalbuminuria represents an increased permeability of the glomerulus and parallels vascular endothelial dysfunction. Microalbuminuria also predicts the development of CVD and stroke, as well as progression of diabetic nephropathy.[24,26,27] Microalbuminuria has been associated with insulin resistance and hyperinsulinemia,[5] atherogenic dyslipidemia, and the absence of a nocturnal drop in SBP and DBP, and it has been identified as part of the cardiometabolic syndrome.[3] For these reasons, it is not surprising that diabetic glomerulosclerosis parallels the process of diabetic atherosclerosis and is a powerful risk factor for CVD and stroke.[3] Even after adjustment for renal function, microalbuminuria remained a strong risk factor for CVD in a subanalysis of the HOPE trial.[27] In the HOPE trial, the presence of albuminuria doubled the risk for the composite endpoint of myocardial infarction, stroke, or CVD death and all-cause mortality. The risk of heart failure was 3.7 times greater in patients with type 2 DM and microalbuminuria compared with those without albuminuria.[27] Furthermore, these risks were significantly reduced by treatment with the ACE inhibitor ramipril.[27] Medications that interrupt the RAAS, such as ACE inhibitors and ARBs, are increasingly important in slowing the progression of nephropathy in these patients. Chronic kidney disease and the presence of either microalbuminuria or proteinuria dictate lowering BP to a goal of less than 130/80 mm Hg and reducing proteinuria by at least 30% to 50%.[5,28]

HYPERTENSION TREATMENT STRATEGIES IN PATIENTS WITH DIABETES

Nonpharmacologic Treatment

The current recommendations of the Seventh Report of the Joint National Committee on Prevention, Detection, Evaluation, and Treatment of High Blood Pressure (JNC 7) emphasize the need for the adoption of a healthy lifestyle for the prevention and treatment of HTN. Indeed, aggressive nonpharmacologic interventions are pivotal and indispensable in the therapeutic outcome in all hypertensive populations.

Diet and Weight Loss

Several randomized controlled trials have documented the value of modest weight loss in decreasing the risk of HTN.[30,31] Several studies have also shown that modest weight loss can lower or even abrogate the need for antihypertensive medication.[31] In addition, a diet that is high in fiber and potassium and lower in saturated fat, refined carbohydrates, and salt can improve glycemic control, lipid profile, and BP. In the Dietary Approaches to Stop Hypertension (DASH) study, a diet abundant in fruits and vegetables, as well as low-fat dairy products, with or without sodium restriction, substantially reduced BP in hypertensive patients.[30]

Exercise

Physical activity is also beneficial for lowering BP and for improving insulin sensitivity. The Finnish Diabetes Prevention Study showed that overweight subjects with glucose intolerance who received intensified lifestyle intervention, consisting of diet and moderate exercise for at least 30 minutes/day, had not only a marked reduction in the risk of developing type 2 DM, but also a significant drop in BP (4 mm Hg for SBP and 2 mm Hg for DBP compared with control subjects).[32] A prospective study of 8302 Finnish men and 9139 women showed that regular physical activity was associated with a significantly reduced risk for HTN in men and women, independent of age, education, smoking habits, alcohol intake, and history of DM, body mass index, and SBP at baseline.[33] Overweight and obesity were also associated with an increased risk of HTN, and the protective effect of physical activity was consistent in both overweight and normal-weight subjects.[33] Most studies have shown that more benefit is derived from aerobic than from nonaerobic exercise.[34] Data on effects of the intensity of physical activity on HTN are conflicting, however. The most recent data show that high physical activity, defined as a combination of vigorous occupational activity for more than 30 minutes/day and leisure time physical activity for more than 4 hours/week, is associated with a lower risk of HTN, independent of baseline body mass index.[33]

Patients should also be counseled on smoking cessation to reduce their overall CVD risk. Motivating patients to maintain realistic and meaningful lifestyle changes remains a challenge but is extraordinarily important for diabetic patients and those who are likely to develop DM.

Pharmacologic Treatment

Once the decision to begin pharmacologic therapy is made, clinicians are left with a wide choice of antihypertensive agents. Patients with type 2 DM characteristically have multiple CVD risk factors, and the coexistence of CVDs (angina, heart failure, peripheral vascular disease, and dyslipidemia) needs to be considered before drug therapy is initiated. On average, 3.1 antihypertensive agents are required to reach a goal BP of less than 130/85 mm Hg, and the addition of antihypertensive agents to current therapy should be based on the benefits of these agents in diabetic patients and their coexisting illnesses.[35] Recommended nonpharmacologic and pharmacologic approaches are outlined in Figure 34-4.

Angiotensin-Converting Enzyme Inhibitors

The RAAS plays a role in almost every step in the progression of atherosclerosis and HTN. Multiple clinical trials have demonstrated the pleiotropic effects of the ACE inhibitors. In addition to being effective antihypertensive agents, ACE inhibitors have been proven to offer additional benefits in patients with DM.

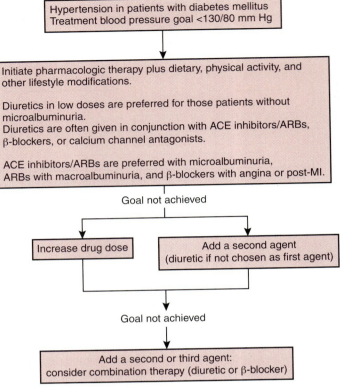

Figure 34–4 Treatment algorithm for antihypertensive therapy in the patient with diabetes. In patients with a serum creatinine level of 1.8 mg/dL or greater (≥159 µmol/L), thiazide diuretics are not effective, and loop diuretics should be substituted. ACE, angiotensin-converting enzyme; ARBs, angiotensin receptor blockers; MI, myocardial infarction.

The HOPE trial studied 9541 patients, 3577 of whom were diabetic.[36] Ramipril use was associated with a significant 25% risk reduction in myocardial infarction, stroke, or cardiovascular death after a median follow-up period of 4.5 years.[36] This benefit was said to be independent of any BP-lowering effect. Furthermore, the MICRO-HOPE substudy also showed that ramipril treatment was associated with a decreased risk of development of proteinuria in patients with type 2 DM and microalbuminuria.[17] Only 18 patients with DM in MICRO-HOPE developed ESRD, but ramipril was associated with a *nonsignificant* 30% reduction in this important endpoint, possibly because of the small number of events.

Of the 10,985 patients in the Captopril Prevention Project (CAPPP), 309 patients in the captopril group and 263 in the conventional therapy group were diabetic. Overall, captopril treatment markedly lowered the risk for fatal and nonfatal myocardial infarction, stroke, and cardiovascular deaths, compared with conventional therapy, which consisted of β-blocker or diuretic therapy. The effects of the two regimens in the diabetic subpopulation showed a clear difference in the risk of developing a primary endpoint in favor of a captopril-based regimen.[37]

In addition to lowering BP, ACE inhibitors also decrease membrane permeability to albumin and decrease intraglomerular pressure. By reducing microalbuminuria, ACE

Table 34-3 Trial Results in which the Risk of Diabetes Development Has Been Reduced with Antihypertensive Treatment

Study* (Reference)	No. of Patients	Patient Group, Disease, Age, Sex	Intervention Treatment	Control Treatment	Absolute Risk Reduction (%)	Relative Risk Reduction (%)
CAPPP[62]	10,985	Diastolic hypertension, men and women 25-66 yr	Captopril	β-Blocker, diuretics	0.8	11
HOPE[36]	9,297	CVD, men and women >55 yr	Ramipril	Placebo	1.8	33
ALLHAT[64]	15,573	Hypertension and at risk for CVD, men and women ≥55 yr	Lisinopril	Chlorthalidone or amlodipine	3.5 and 1.7	30 and 17
SOLVD[66]	291	Left ventricular dysfunction, men and women 18-80 yr	Enalapril	Placebo	16.5	74
LIFE[19]	7998	Hypertension and left ventricular hypertrophy, men and women 55-80 yr	Losartan	Atenolol	2.0	25
CHARM[70]	3023	Heart failure grades II-IV, men and women >18 yr	Candesartan	Placebo	2.0	39
ALPINE[72]	392	Newly detected hypertension, mostly women 18-75 yr	Candesartan	Hydrochlorothiazide	3.6	88
VALUE[73]	10,419	Hypertension and at high risk for CVD, men and women ≥50 yr	Valsartan	Amlodipine	3.3	23
INVEST[50]	16,176	Hypertension and CVD, men and women ≥50 yr	Verapamil SR, adding, in order, trandolapril, hydrochlorothiazide	Atenolol, adding, in order, hydrochlorothiazide, trandolapril	1.2	15
PEACE[67]	6904	Stable CVD, men and women >50 yr	Trandolapril	Placebo	1.7	17
SCOPE[71]	4330	Hypertension, men and women 70-89 yr	Candesartan	Placebo	1.0	19 ($P = .09$)

*See text for study acronyms.
CVD, cardiovascular disease; SR, sustained release.

inhibitors can help to prevent progression to nephropathy. Meta-analyses have shown that this antiproteinuric effect is independent of the changes in BP.[30] In patients with type 1 DM, ACE inhibitors have been shown to prevent the progression of diabetic nephropathy to ESRD. In patients with type 2 DM, the effect of these agents on ESRD is still unclear, but ACE inhibitors slow the progression of nephropathy in microalbuminuric, normotensive patients compared with other antihypertensive patients.[38,39] Volume depletion is an important cause for a slight rise in serum creatinine levels after the initiation of ACE inhibitor therapy, and this change is usually reversible.[40] However, renal function should be carefully monitored because a rise in serum creatinine levels by more than 30% or a continual rise during the first 2 months

of therapy should alarm the physician to the possibility of renal artery stenosis or significant volume depletion.[24,40]

A recent meta-analysis of several long-term trials indicates that ACE inhibitors and ARBs, both of which inhibit the RAAS, also reduce the incidence of new-onset DM.[41] These studies are reviewed later and in Table 34-3.

Angiotensin Receptor Blockers

These agents specifically block the angiotensin II type 1 (AT₁) receptor and theoretically offer more complete blockade of the RAAS. ARBs have antihypertensive efficacy equivalent to that of ACE inhibitors, with fewer side effects, particularly cough and angioedema. This profile may clinically translate to improved adherence with an ARB compared with an ACE inhibitor. Similar to ACE inhibitors, ARBs offer additional benefits in diabetic patients.

The Losartan Intervention for Endpoint Reduction in Hypertension (LIFE) trial with losartan showed a significant 13% reduction in the composite primary endpoint (cardiovascular death, myocardial infarction, or stroke), most of which resulted from a significant 25% decrease in stroke compared with treatment with atenolol.[18] The diabetic patients in this study had an even more significant reduction (24%) in the primary endpoint, as well as in cardiovascular mortality (37%) and total mortality (39%), when compared with atenolol.

Based on the current evidence and because of their tolerability, ARBs are recommended as first-line therapy for patients with DM, HTN, and significant proteinuria.[42] The Reduction of Endpoints in Non–Insulin-Dependent Diabetes Mellitus with the Angiotensin II Antagonist Losartan (RENAAL) trial and the Irbesartan Diabetic Nephropathy Trial (IDNT) showed that ARBs reduce proteinuria, diminish the time to creatinine doubling, and slow the progression of renal disease.[5,43] The Irbesartan Microalbuminuria for Type 2 Diabetes Mellitus in Hypertensive Patients (IRMA-2) study also showed a reduction in progression from microalbuminuria to proteinuria.[5] Again, the beneficial effects of ARBs on nephropathy were said to be independent of the changes in BP.

The Candesartan and Lisinopril Microalbuminuria (CALM) trial showed a numerically greater reduction in both BP and albuminuria when both ARBs and ACE inhibitors were used in combination at half-maximal doses than when either class of agent was used alone.[44] In nondiabetic patients with HTN and the nephrotic syndrome, combination therapy has been shown to be more effective in reducing proteinuria than therapy with an ACE inhibitor or ARB alone. Furthermore, this antiproteinuric effect was not dependent on changes in BP or creatinine clearance.[30] Although this finding appears promising, more data are needed before the combination of these two agents to block the RAAS completely can be recommended.

Thiazide Diuretics

The thiazide diuretics, which are the oldest of the currently available antihypertensive agents, still have an important role in the management of HTN in the diabetic population. Although diuretics may worsen insulin resistance, they have also consistently demonstrated their ability to reduce the cardiovascular mortality in patients with DM. ALLHAT, one of the largest antihypertensive trials, concluded that thiazide diuretics comparably reduced combined fatal and nonfatal coronary artery disease and all-cause mortality when these drugs were compared with an ACE inhibitor and calcium channel blocker (CCB). More importantly, thiazide diuretics prevented heart failure significantly better than any other initial therapy, in both diabetic and nondiabetic patients.[45]

ALLHAT and other studies have a short follow-up period of less than 10 years, and the true impact of new-onset DM may not be fully appreciated on cardiovascular outcomes. In a 2004 analysis of an observational registry of morbidity and mortality in initially untreated individuals with essential HTN, patients who were treated with diuretics and β-blockers

had an increased propensity to develop type 2 DM.[46] The occurrence of new-onset DM in treated hypertensive patients carried a risk for subsequent CVD events that was not statistically different from that of patients who already had DM and HTN at the onset of the study. However, both groups had a much higher risk than did those patients who remained free of DM. Even though electrolyte disturbances and adverse effects on lipid and carbohydrate metabolism are uncommon with low-dose thiazide therapy, these recent observations suggest that thiazide diuretics and β-blockers should be initiated cautiously in hypertensive patients with elevated fasting glucose levels (i.e., >100 mg/dL).[47] Nevertheless, diuretics continue to play an important role in the management of HTN in patients with DM, especially as an adjunct to ACE inhibitors and ARBs. A review of long-term mortality data from the SHEP (mean, 14.3 years) showed that development of DM in patients treated with the diuretic chlorthalidone was not associated with increased cardiovascular or total mortality rates.[48] Moreover, diuretic treatment in diabetic subjects was strongly associated with lower long-term cardiovascular and total mortality rates. Further research is required to define fully the long-term risk-to-benefit profiles of commonly used thiazide diuretics in hypertensive patients with impaired fasting glucose levels, especially because hydrochlorothiazide has been more widely accepted in clinical practice than has chlorthalidone.

Calcium Channel Blockers

At least 65% of hypertensive patients require two or more drugs to achieve BPs of less than 130/80.[5,35] CCBs are effective antihypertensive agents but probably should be viewed as adjuncts to ACE inhibitors and ARBs in patients with DM.[5] CCBs not only lower BP effectively in diabetic patients, but also they are intermediate between ACE inhibitors and ARBs (which reduce the risk of incidence DM) and thiazide diuretics or β-blockers (which increase it).[5,45,49,50] A post hoc analysis of RENAAL suggested no difference in the primary renal endpoint between dihydropyridine and nondihydropyridine CCBs as second-line agents after an ARB.[43,45] In addition, the nondihydropyridine CCBs verapamil and diltiazem can further reduce proteinuria when they are added to RAAS blocker therapy.[30]

The Syst-Eur trial with nitrendipine (versus placebo) demonstrated that intensive antihypertensive therapy for older patients with type 2 DM and isolated systolic HTN eliminated the additional risk for CVD events and stroke associated with DM.[51] However, in ALLHAT, the group receiving an initial CCB had a significantly higher incidence of heart failure compared with the group receiving an initial diuretic but fewer strokes than those receiving an ACE inhbitor.[45]

β-Blockers

The effectiveness of β-blockers in HTN, coronary artery disease, and heart failure management has been proven in multiple clinical trials.[28] Despite their adverse effects on glucose tolerance and the peripheral vasculature, β-blockers play a significant role in the management of HTN in diabetic patients, especially in those with associated microvascular and macrovascular complications. In UKPDS, atenolol was comparable to captopril in reducing BP and CVD outcomes.[52]

However, when comparing atenolol with other agents in many other trials, atenolol has been consistently and significantly worse than other therapies with which it has been compared.[53]

β-Blockers have adverse effects on glucose and lipid profiles and have also been implicated in new-onset DM in obese patients.[4,5] β-Blockade can worsen the symptoms of peripheral vascular disease. However, nonselective β-blockers, such as carvedilol, reduce CVD mortality and microalbuminuria without adversely affecting glucose or lipid profiles, although this may be a BP-lowering effect.[54] When used with renin-angiotensin system (RAS) blockade, carvedilol and atenolol have also been shown to reduce albuminuria.[55] In addition, carvedilol slows the progression of nephropathy and improves insulin sensitivity.[54] Therefore, these agents play a useful role in antihypertensive therapy of diabetic patients, specifically those with coronary artery disease and heart failure.

α-Antagonists

The selective α_1-blockers, such as prazosin, terazosin, and doxazosin, are the only class of antihypertensive agents that may have the combined effect of lowering low-density lipoprotein cholesterol, raising high-density lipoprotein cholesterol levels, and improving insulin sensitivity.[56] They can be useful add-on drugs to reach target BP.[30] However, α-blockers have relatively bothersome side effects, including dizziness (although rarely inducing syncope), headache, and weakness. In a prospective trial in which six different antihypertensive drugs were compared, the α-blocker prazosin had the highest incidence of side effects.[30] Since ALLHAT, α-blockers are not considered first-line therapy for HTN.

Other Agents

Hydralazine, a direct-acting vasodilator, can be recommended for patients with coexistent systolic heart failure and HTN who cannot tolerate an ACE inhibitor or ARB or who have contraindications to the foregoing agents.

Clonidine, an α_2-agonist, can also be helpful in patients with supine HTN associated with orthostatic hypotension, but side effects (primarily central nervous system effects, sexual dysfunction, and dry mouth) limit its use.[30] α_2-Agonists do not have adverse lipid effects, but they do have the potential to inhibit pancreatic β-cell insulin secretion and thereby impair glucose metabolism.[30]

Additional Considerations

In addition to these considerations for antihypertensive therapy in diabetic patients, several other characteristics need to be factored into therapeutic planning. The propensity to develop dysautonomia resulting in disturbances in BP patterns (nondipping BP), a tendency for isolated systolic HTN, and diabetic cardiomyopathy may each confound therapeutic options for treatment of patients with DM.

Dysautonomia

Autonomic neuropathy is common in diabetic patients. It affects 5% to 10% of patients with long-term DM and as many as 35% of those patients with subclinical peripheral neuropathy. Once autonomic neuropathy becomes clinically apparent, it compromises BP regulation.[30] In patients with DM and autonomic dysfunction, excessive venous pooling can cause orthostatic hypotension. Postural hypotension, a decrease in SBP of more than 20 mm Hg on standing from a supine position, is usually associated with hypoadrenergic or hyperadrenergic signs and symptoms, such as lightheadedness, dizziness, dimming of vision, nausea, diaphoresis, and syncope. Because of the increased propensity of diabetic patients to manifest increased orthostatic BP changes, measurements should be performed with patients in both supine and standing positions.[28] Another effective tool is ambulatory BP monitoring, which can be useful in determining the presence of drug resistance, hypotensive symptoms, episodic HTN, or autonomic dysfunction.

Nondipping Blood Pressure and Pulse Pattern

In normotensive and most hypertensive patients, the circadian BP rhythm demonstrates higher BP readings when patients are awake and lower BP readings when they are asleep. This effect is referred to as "dipping," and the expected drop is approximately 10% to 15%. "Nondippers" have less than the usual 10% decline at night, a condition more frequent among diabetic patients, as demonstrated by ambulatory BP monitoring. Loss of nocturnal dipping of BP and heart rate is characteristic of HTN associated with DM. This loss of nocturnal dipping in BP and heart rate appears to be caused, in part, by dysautonomia, which is often present in diabetic patients.[30] The nondipping pattern of BP in patients with DM is associated with microalbuminuria, proteinuria, and left ventricular hypertrophy, thereby conferring a higher risk of CVD morbidity and mortality to patients who have it.[30,57] Reduced vascular compliance further contributes to elevations in SBP, increases in pulse pressure, and associated CVD risk.

Diabetic Cardiomyopathy

Diabetic cardiomyopathy is increasingly recognized as a specific entity in patients with type 2 DM.[58] The development of diabetic cardiomyopathy is most likely multifactorial. Putative mechanisms include metabolic disturbances, such as defective glycolysis and glucose oxidation, myocardial fibrosis, small vessel disease, and autonomic dysfunction. Abnormalities of calcium handling that can lead to subsequent diabetic cardiomyopathy have also been demonstrated.[58] Existence of this condition in a diabetic patient may have several therapeutic implications, including the following: improvement in glycemic control; use of CCBs, ACE inhibitors, and ARBs; exercise training; lipid-lowering therapy; and use of antioxidant and insulin-sensitizing drugs.[58]

CCBs may reverse the intracellular calcium defects and may prevent DM-induced myocardial changes. Verapamil significantly improves the depressed rate of contraction and the rate of relaxation, lowers peak left ventricular systolic pressure, and elevates left ventricular diastolic pressure.[3] ACE inhibitors may improve fibrosis in the myocardium and may improve endothelial dysfunction.[58] Clinically, ACE inhibitors reduce CVD in diabetic patients, particularly patients with HTN.[5,22,59,60] ARBs and aldosterone antagonists may also have effects similar to those of ACE inhibitors on myocardial fibrosis in diabetic patients.

ANTIHYPERTENSIVE AGENTS AND THE DEVELOPMENT OF TYPE 2 DIABETES MELLITUS

As noted earlier, antihypertensive medications appear to have disparate effects on insulin sensitivity in patients with essential HTN. This finding may have important implications for the development of DM in patients with increased risk for the disease. Both diuretics and β-blockers accelerate the appearance of new-onset DM in hypertensive patients.[4,21,46,61] In reports comparing diuretics and β-blockers with ACE inhibitors, the greater incidence of DM associated with the former may have reflected, in part, the beneficial effects of ACE inhibitors on glucose metabolism.[50,62-64] Alternatively, CCBs are generally considered to be metabolically neutral. When diuretics and β-blockers are compared with CCBs, the former have been associated with more cases of new-onset DM.[63,64] For example, in ALLHAT,[64] the diuretic chlorthalidone not only was 43% more likely to be associated with the progression of fasting glucose to 126 mg/dL or higher after 4 years than the ACE inhibitor lisinopril, but also was 18% more likely than the CCB amlodipine. The actual rates were 11.4% (chlorthalidone) versus 8.1% (lisinopril) versus 9.8% (amlodipine) over 4 years.

Overcoming insulin resistance with antihypertensive agents that interrupt the RAAS may prevent or delay the emergence of type 2 DM in patients with essential HTN (see Table 34-3).[20,65] CAPPP was the first controlled clinical trial to show that an ACE inhibitor reduces the incidence of DM in hypertensive patients.[62] This trial was designed to compare the effect of ACE inhibition with conventional antihypertensive agents (β-blockers, diuretics, or both) on CVD morbidity and mortality. The number of patients with newly diagnosed DM was 14% lower in the patients randomized to captopril, compared with those receiving conventional therapy. These findings were confirmed in the HOPE trial in which a fixed dose of ramipril was added to whatever other therapy was prescribed (i.e., β-blockers, CCBs, and diuretics).[36] Overall, 39% of ramipril-treated patients received a β-blocker, the same percentage as in the placebo group. During the 4.5 years of follow-up in HOPE, 5.4% of the 4652 patients in the placebo (control) group developed DM compared with only 3.6% of the 4645 patients in the ramipril-treated group, a difference of 35%.

In the Studies of Left Ventricular Dysfunction (SOLVD) trial, a retrospective analysis of data from one site that followed 292 patients over a 2.9-year study period showed that 5.9% of patients taking enalapril developed DM, as compared with 22.4% of those taking placebo; the result was a relative risk reduction of 74%.[66] In the International Verapamil-Trandolapril Study (INVEST), analysis of add-on medications to groups treated initially with verapamil sustained release (CCB strategy) or atenolol (non-CCB strategy) suggested that the ACE inhibitor trandolapril conferred protection against development of DM that was 7.0% of 8098 patients in the CCB group versus 8.2% of 8078 patients in the non-CCB group. Likewise, trandolapril was associated with a decrease in the incidence of DM compared with placebo in post hoc analysis of the recent Prevention of Events with Angiotensin-Converting Enzyme Inhibition (PEACE) trial.[67] In the PEACE trial, 11.5% of 3472 patients developed DM while they were taking placebo, whereas 9.8% of 3432 patients developed DM while they were taking trandolapril over a median 4.8-year follow-up.

Several clinical trials have now indicated that ARBs also have beneficial effects on glucose metabolism.[68-70] The LIFE study showed that losartan reduced the relative risk of developing DM by 25% compared with the β-blocker atenolol.[68] However, the study included no placebo-treated control group. Consequently, it is likely that the reduction in incident DM reflects the net result of both increased insulin sensitivity in the group taking losartan and increased insulin resistance in the group taking atenolol. Similar findings were reported in the Candesartan in Heart Failure: Assessment of Reduction in Mortality and Morbidity (CHARM) study,[70] the Study on Cognition and Prognosis in the Elderly (SCOPE),[71] and the Antihypertensive Treatment and Lipid Profile in a North of Sweden Efficacy Evaluation (ALPINE),[72] all of which, unlike LIFE, were placebo controlled. The Valsartan Antihypertensive Long-Term Use Evaluation (VALUE) trial demonstrated the advantage of an ARB over a CCB in reducing new-onset DM in hypertensive patients aged 50 years or older and at high risk of cardiac events.[73] In VALUE, patients were randomized to either valsartan or amlodipine and were followed for a mean of 4.2 years, during which investigators noted a relative risk reduction in new-onset DM by 23% in the valsartan group. Because amlodipine is considered neutral in its effects on insulin sensitivity, and it was substantially better than a thiazide in this regard in ALLHAT,[64] drugs in the ARB class may independently improve insulin sensitivity and may have a role in protecting high-risk hypertensive patients from developing DM.

The possibility that an ARB can prevent the transition from impaired glucose tolerance, which is a quite common in patients with essential HTN, to DM is being explored in the Nateglinide and Valsartan in Impaired Glucose Tolerance Outcomes Research (NAVIGATOR) study.[74] Furthermore, in the Diabetes Reduction Approaches with Medication (DREAM) study, patients with impaired fasting glucose are being randomized to ramipril or rosiglitazone versus placebo.[65] In addition, the Ramipril Global Endpoint Trial (ONTARGET) with telmisartan, ramipril, or telmisartan in combination with ramipril will determine the effect of one or both agents on a composite endpoint of CVD disease (myocardial infarction, stroke, or hospitalization for heart failure) over a 5.5-year follow-up.[75] Patients who are unable to tolerate an ACE inhibitor will be entered into a parallel study of telmisartan versus placebo, the Telmisartan Randomized Assessment Study in ACE Intolerant Subjects with Cardiovascular Disease (TRANSCEND).[76] The incidence of DM is a secondary endpoint in both these studies. Collectively, these ongoing studies should clarify the extent to which inhibitors of RAAS can reduce the incidence of new-onset DM in patients with impaired fasting glucose, a group that includes many of the 65 million U.S. residents with essential HTN.[65]

SUMMARY

Insulin resistance and compensatory hyperinsulinemia are not consequences of HTN but may instead represent a genetic predisposition that results in the maladaptive characteristics, including HTN, seen in certain patients. When combined with an enabling milieu (obesity, inactivity, poor diet), insulin resistance can result in the synergistic occurrence of CVD risk factors seen clinically. Additionally, insulin resistance is often a progressive disease.

The approach to treatment of these patients absolutely entails consideration of these underlying pathophysiologic mechanisms and their incorporation into the treatment strategy. Moreover, the presence of peripheral vascular disease, heart failure, coronary artery disease, orthostatic hypotension, dyslipidemia, and diabetic nephropathy all influence the choice of antihypertensive agents. Merely treating the elevated BP, without considering the foregoing conditions, may temporarily control BP levels without impeding the progression of the underlying disease and the worsening of complications propagated by insulin resistance and accompanying compensatory hyperinsulinemia. Reversal of the essential condition with therapy would be ideal, and strategies such as interruption of the RAAS may have this effect. When this is not possible, an approach that targets specific complications, slows progression, or delays the onset of target organ damage should be used.

Quality of life, adverse effects of antihypertensive medications, and other co-morbid conditions all play a role in the successful management of HTN and in the adherence to treatment regimens. More importantly, the health care team should work closely with each individual patient prudently, but aggressively, to achieve and maintain the goal BP of less than 130/80 mm Hg.

References

1. American Diabetes Association National Diabetes Fact Sheet. Available at http://www.diabetes.org/uedocuments/NationalDiabetesFactSheetRev.pdf
2. Ogden CL, Flegal KM, Carroll MD, Johnson CL. Prevalence and trends in overweight among U.S. children and adolescents, 1999-2000. *JAMA*. 2002;**288**:1728-1732.
3. Sowers JR, Epstein M, Frohlich ED. Diabetes, hypertension, and cardiovascular disease: An update. *Hypertension*. 2001;**37**:1053-1059.
4. Gress TW, Nieto FJ, Shahar E, et al. Hypertension and antihypertensive therapy as risk factors for type 2 diabetes mellitus: Atherosclerosis Risk in Communities Study. *N Engl J Med*. 2000;**342**:905-912.
5. Sowers JR. Treatment of hypertension in patients with diabetes. *Arch Intern Med*. 2004;**164**:1850-1857.
6. Perkins BA, Ficociello LH, Silva KH, et al. Regression of microalbuminuria in type 1 diabetes. *N Engl J Med*. 2003;**348**:2285-2293.
7. Sowers JR, Williams M, Epstein M, et al. Hypertension in patients with diabetes: Strategies for drug therapy to reduce complications. *Postgrad Med*. 2000;**107**:47-54, 60.
8. Grundy SM, Brewer HB Jr, Cleeman JI, et al. Definition of metabolic syndrome: Report of the National Heart, Lung, and Blood Institute/American Heart Association conference on scientific issues related to definition. *Circulation*. 2004;**109**:433-438.
9. Ford ES, Giles WH, Mokdad AH. Increasing prevalence of the metabolic syndrome among U.S. Adults. *Diabetes Care*. 2004;**27**:2444-2449.
10. Stamler J, Stamler R, Neaton JD. Blood pressure, systolic and diastolic, and cardiovascular risks. US population data. *Arch Intern Med*. 1993;**153**:598-615.
11. United Kingdom Prospective Diabetes Study Group. Tight blood pressure control and risk of macrovascular and microvascular complications in type 2 diabetes: UKPDS 38. *BMJ*. 1998;**317**:703-713.
12. Hansson L, Zanchetti A, Carruthers SG, et al. Effects of intensive blood-pressure lowering and low-dose aspirin in patients with hypertension: Principal results of the Hypertension Optimal Treatment (HOT) randomised trial. HOT Study Group. *Lancet*. 1998;**351**:1755-1762.
13. Tuomilehto J, Rastenyte D, Birkenhager WH, et al. Effects of calcium-channel blockade in older patients with diabetes and systolic hypertension: Systolic Hypertension in Europe Trial Investigators. *N Engl J Med*. 1999;**340**:677-684.
14. Sowers JR. Stroke in patients with diabetes. *J Clin Hypertens*. 2004;**6**:63-63.
15. Bell DS. Stroke in the diabetic patient. *Diabetes Care*. 1994;**17**:213-219.
16. Sacco RL. Reducing the risk of stroke in diabetes: What have we learned that is new? *Diabetes Obes Metab*. 2002;**4 (Suppl 1)**:S27-S34.
17. Heart Outcomes Prevention Evaluation Study Investigators. Effects of ramipril on cardiovascular and microvascular outcomes in people with diabetes mellitus: Results of the HOPE study and MICRO-HOPE substudy. *Lancet*. 2000;**355**:253-259.
18. Dahlof B, Devereux RB, Kjeldsen SE, et al. Cardiovascular morbidity and mortality in the Losartan Intervention for Endpoint Reduction in Hypertension study (LIFE): A randomised trial against atenolol. *Lancet*. 2002;**359**:995-1003.
19. Lindholm LH, Ibsen H, Dahlof B, et al. Cardiovascular morbidity and mortality in patients with diabetes in the Losartan Intervention for Endpoint Reduction in Hypertension study (LIFE): A randomised trial against atenolol. *Lancet*. 2002;**359**:1004-1010.
20. ALLHAT Officers and Coordinators for the ALLHAT Collaborative Research Group. The Antihypertensive and Lipid-Lowering Treatment to Prevent Heart Attack Trial. Major outcomes in high-risk hypertensive patients randomized to angiotensin-converting enzyme inhibitor or calcium channel blocker vs diuretic: The Antihypertensive and Lipid-Lowering Treatment to Prevent Heart Attack Trial (ALLHAT). *JAMA*. 2002;**288**:2981-2997.
21. Sowers JR. Insulin resistance and hypertension. *Am J Physiol*. 2004;**286**:H1597-H1602.
22. McFarlane SI, Banerji M, Sowers JR. Insulin resistance and cardiovascular disease. *J Clin Endocrinol Metab*. 2001;**86**:713-718.
23. Padwal R, Laupacis A. Antihypertensive therapy and incidence of type 2 diabetes: A systematic review. *Diabetes Care*. 2004;**27**:247-255.
24. Bakris GL, Williams M, Dworkin L, et al. Preserving renal function in adults with hypertension and diabetes: A consensus approach. National Kidney Foundation Hypertension and Diabetes Executive Committees Working Group. *Am J Kidney Dis*. 2000;**36**:646-661.
25. US Renal Data System. USRDS 2005. Annual Data Report: Atlas of End-Stage Renal Disease in the United States. Bethesda, MD: National Institute of Health, National Institute of Diabetes and Digestive and Kidney Disease.
26. Eknoyan G, Hostetter T, Bakris GL, et al. Proteinuria and other markers of chronic kidney disease: A position statement of the National Kidney Foundation (NKF) and the National Institute of Diabetes and Digestive and Kidney Diseases (NIDDK). *Am J Kidney Dis*. 2003;**42**:617-622.
27. Gerstein HC, Mann JF, Pogue J, et al. Prevalence and determinants of microalbuminuria in high-risk diabetic and nondiabetic patients in the Heart Outcomes Prevention Evaluation Study: The HOPE Study Investigators. *Diabetes Care*. 2000;**23 (Suppl 2)**:B35-B39.
28. Sowers JR, Haffner S. Treatment of cardiovascular and renal risk factors in the diabetic hypertensive. *Hypertension*. 2002;**40**:781-788.

29. Chobanian AV, Bakris GL, Black HR, et al., and the National High Blood Pressure Education Program Coordinating Committee. The Seventh Report of the Joint National Committee on Prevention, Detection, Evaluation, and Treatment of High Blood Pressure: The JNC 7 Report. *JAMA.* 2003;**289**:2560-2572.

30. Sowers JR. Obesity as a cardiovascular risk factor. *Am J Med.* 2003;**115 (Suppl 8A)**:37S-41S.

31. Wassertheil-Smoller S, Blaufox MD, Oberman AS, et al. The Trial of Antihypertensive Interventions and Management (TAIM) study: Adequate weight loss, alone and combined with drug therapy in the treatment of mild hypertension. *Arch Intern Med.* 1992;**152**:131-136.

32. Tuomilehto J, Lindstrom J, Eriksson JG, et al. Prevention of type 2 diabetes mellitus by changes in lifestyle among subjects with impaired glucose tolerance. *N Engl J Med.* 2001;**344**:1343-1350.

33. Hu G, Barengo NC, Tuomilehto J, et al. Relationship of physical activity and body mass index to the risk of hypertension: A prospective study in Finland. *Hypertension.* 2004;**43**:25-30.

34. Whelton SP, Chin A, Xin X, et al. Effect of aerobic exercise on blood pressure: A meta-analysis of randomized, controlled trials. *Ann Intern Med.* 2002;**136**:493-503.

35. McFarlane SI, Jacober SJ, Winer N, et al. Control of cardiovascular risk factors in patients with diabetes and hypertension at urban academic medical centers. *Diabetes Care.* 2002;**25**:718-723.

36. Yusuf S, Sleight P, Pogue J, et al. Effects of an angiotensin-converting-enzyme inhibitor, ramipril, on cardiovascular events in high-risk patients: The Heart Outcomes Prevention Evaluation Study Investigators. *N Engl J Med.* 2000;**342**:145-153.

37. Niskanen L, Hedner T, Hansson L, et al. Reduced cardiovascular morbidity and mortality in hypertensive diabetic patients on first-line therapy with an ACE inhibitor compared with a diuretic/beta-blocker-based treatment regimen: A subanalysis of the Captopril Prevention Project. *Diabetes Care.* 2001;**24**:2091-2096.

38. Bakris GL, Smith AC, Richardson DJ, et al. Impact of an ACE inhibitor and calcium antagonist on microalbuminuria and lipid subfractions in type 2 diabetes: A randomised, multicentre pilot study. *J Hum Hypertens.* 2002;**16**:185-191.

39. Ravid M, Lang R, Rachmani R, et al. Long-term renoprotective effect of angiotensin-converting enzyme inhibition in non–insulin-dependent diabetes mellitus: A 7-year follow-up study. *Arch Intern Med.* 1996;**156**:286-289.

40. Bakris GL, Weir MR. Angiotensin-converting enzyme inhibitor–associated elevations in serum creatinine: Is this a cause for concern? *Arch Intern Med.* 2000;**160**:685-693.

41. Scheen AJ. Renin-angiotensin system inhibition prevents type 2 diabetes mellitus: Part 1. A meta-analysis of randomised clinical trials. *Diabetes Metab.* 2004;**30**:487-496.

42. Sowers JR, Treatment of hypertension in patients with diabetes. *Arch Intern Med.* 2004;**164**:1850-1857.

43. Bakris GL, Weir MR, Shanifar S, et al. Effects of blood pressure level on progression of diabetic nephropathy: Results from the RENAAL study. *Arch Intern Med.* 2003;**163**:1555-1565.

44. Mogensen CE, Neldam S, Tikkanen I, et al. Randomised controlled trial of dual blockade of renin-angiotensin system in patients with hypertension, microalbuminuria, and non-insulin dependent diabetes: The Candesartan and Lisinopril Microalbuminuria (CALM) study. *BMJ.* 2000;**321**:1440-1444.

45. ALLHAT Officers and Coordinators for the ALLHAT Collaborative Research Group. Major outcomes in high-risk hypertensive patients randomized to angiotensin-converting enzyme inhibitor or calcium channel blocker vs. diuretic. *JAMA.* 2002;**288**:2981-2997.

46. Verdecchia P, Reboldi G, Angeli F, et al. Adverse prognostic significance of new diabetes in treated hypertensive subjects. *Hypertension.* 2004;**43**:963-969.

47. Bakris GL, Sowers JR. When does new onset diabetes resulting from antihypertensive therapy increase cardiovascular risk? *Hypertension.* 2004;**43**:941-942.

48. Kostis JB, Lawrence-Nelson J, Ranjan R, et al. Association of increased pulse pressure with the development of heart failure in SHEP: Systolic Hypertension in the Elderly (SHEP) Cooperative Research Group. *Am J Hypertens.* 2001;**14**:798-803.

49. Black HR, Elliott WJ, Neaton JD, et al. Baseline characteristics and early blood pressure control in the CONVINCE trial. *Hypertension.* 2001;**37**:12-18.

50. Pepine CJ, Handberg EM, Cooper-DeHoff RM, et al. A calcium antagonist vs. a non-calcium antagonist hypertension treatment strategy for patients with coronary artery disease: The International Verapamil-Trandolapril Study (INVEST). A randomized controlled trial. *JAMA.* 2003;**290**:2805-2816.

51. Birkenhager WH, Staessen JA, Gasowski J, et al. Effects of antihypertensive treatment on endpoints in the diabetic patients randomized in the Systolic Hypertension in Europe (Syst-Eur) trial. *J Nephrol.* 2000;**13**:232-237.

52. Adler AI, Stratton IM, Neil HA, et al. Association of systolic blood pressure with macrovascular and microvascular complications of type 2 diabetes (UKPDS 36): Prospective observational study. *BMJ.* 2000;**321**:412-419.

53. Carlberg B, Samuelsson O, Lindholm LH. Atenolol in hypertension: Is it a wise choice? *Lancet.* 2004;**364**:1684-1689.

54. Jacob S, Balletshofer B, Henriksen EJ, et al. Beta-blocking agents in patients with insulin resistance: Effects of vasodilating beta-blockers. *Blood Press.* 1999;**8**:261-268.

55. Fassbinder W, Quarder O, Waltz A. Treatment with carvedilol is associated with a significant reduction in microalbuminuria: A multicentre randomised study. *Int J Clin Pract.* 1999;**53**:519-522.

56. Khoury AF, Kaplan NM. Alpha-blocker therapy of hypertension: An unfulfilled promise. *JAMA.* 1991;**266**:394-398.

57. Ohkubo T, Hozawa A, Yamaguchi J, et al. Prognostic significance of the nocturnal decline in blood pressure in individuals with and without high 24-h blood pressure: The Ohasama study. *J Hypertens.* 2002;**20**:2183-2189.

58. Fang ZY, Prins JB, Marwick TH. Diabetic cardiomyopathy: Evidence, mechanisms, and therapeutic implications. *Endocr Rev.* 2004;**25**:543-567.

59. Sowers JR. Insulin and insulin-like growth factor in normal and pathological cardiovascular physiology. *Hypertension.* 1997;**29**:691-699.

60. Sowers JR. Insulin resistance and hypertension. *Mol Cell Endocrinol.* 1990;**74**:C87-C89.

61. Savage PJ, Pressel SL, Curb JD, et al. Influence of long-term, low-dose, diuretic-based, antihypertensive therapy on glucose, lipid, uric acid, and potassium levels in older men and women with isolated systolic hypertension: The Systolic Hypertension in the Elderly Program. SHEP Cooperative Research Group. *Arch Intern Med.* 1998;**158**:741-751.

62. Hansson L, Lindholm LH, Niskanen L, et al. Effect of angiotensin-converting-enzyme inhibition compared with conventional therapy on cardiovascular morbidity and mortality in hypertension: The Captopril Prevention Project (CAPPP) randomised trial. *Lancet.* 1999;**353**:611-616.

63. Black HR, Elliott WJ, Grandits G, et al. Principal results of the Controlled Onset Verapamil Investigation of Cardiovascular End Points (CONVINCE) trial. *JAMA.* 2003;**289**:2073-2082.

64. Barzilay JI, Pressel S, Davis BR. Risks and impact of incident glucose disorder in hypertensive older adults treated with an ACE inhibitor, a diuretic, or a calcium channel blocker: A report from the ALLHAT trial [abstract]. *Am J Hypertens.* 2004;**17**:1A.

65. McFarlane SI, Kumar A, Sowers JR. Mechanisms by which angiotensin-converting enzyme inhibitors prevent diabetes and cardiovascular disease. *Am J Cardiol.* 2003;**91**:30H-37H.

66. Vermes E, Ducharme A, Bourassa mg, et al. Enalapril reduces the incidence of diabetes in patients with chronic heart failure: Insight from the Studies of Left Ventricular Dysfunction (SOLVD). *Circulation*. 2003;**107**:1291-1296.

67. Braunwald E, Domanski MJ, Fowler SE, et al. Angiotensin-converting-enzyme inhibition in stable coronary artery disease. *N Engl J Med*. 2004;**351**:2058-2068.

68. Lindholm LH, Ibsen H, Borch-Johnsen K, et al. Risk of new-onset diabetes in the Losartan Intervention for Endpoint Reduction in Hypertension study. *J Hypertens*. 2002;**20**:1879-1886.

69. Pfeffer MA, Swedberg K, Granger CB, et al. Effects of candesartan on mortality and morbidity in patients with chronic heart failure: The CHARM-Overall programme. *Lancet*. 2003;**362**:759-766.

70. Yusuf S, Pfeffer MA, Swedberg K, et al. Effects of candesartan in patients with chronic heart failure and preserved left-ventricular ejection fraction: The CHARM-Preserved trial. *Lancet*. 2003;**362**:777-781.

71. Lithell H, Hansson L, Skoog I, et al. The Study on Cognition and Prognosis in the Elderly (SCOPE): Principal results of a randomized double-blind intervention trial. *J Hypertens*. 2003;**21**:875-886.

72. Lindholm LH, Persson M, Alaupovic P, et al. Metabolic outcome during 1 year in newly detected hypertensives: Results of the Antihypertensive Treatment and Lipid Profile in a North of Sweden Efficacy Evaluation (ALPINE study). *J Hypertens*. 2003;**21**:1563-1574.

73. Julius S, Kjeldsen SE, Weber M, et al. Outcomes in hypertensive patients at high cardiovascular risk treated with regimens based on valsartan or amlodipine: The VALUE randomised trial. *Lancet*. 2004;**363**:2022-2031.

74. Califf RM, Holman R. People at increased risk of cardiovascular disease screened for the NAVIGATOR trial subsequently have undiagnosed diabetes or impaired glucose tolerance [abstract]. *J Am Coll Cardiol*. 2003;**21**:531.

75. Yusuf S. From the HOPE to the ONTARGET and the TRANSCEND studies: Challenges in improving prognosis. *Am J Cardiol*. 2002;**89**:18A-26A.

76. Teo K, Yusuf S, Anderson C, et al. Rationale, design, and baseline characteristics of 2 large, simple, randomized trials evaluating telmisartan, ramipril, and their combination in high-risk patients: The Ongoing Telmisartan Alone and in Combination with Ramipril Global Endpoint Trial/Telmisartan Randomized Assessment Study in ACE Intolerant Subjects with Cardiovascular Disease (ONTARGET/TRANSCEND) trials. *Am Heart J*. 2004;**148**:52-61.

Chapter 35

Dyslipidemia in Hypertension

John C. LaRosa

High blood pressure and abnormalities of circulating lipids and lipoproteins (dyslipidemia) occur frequently in the same individual.[1-3] Because both these disorders are strongly implicated in the prediction and development of atherosclerosis and the often disastrous clinical sequelae, their combined occurrence is a matter of great interest. Because this concurrence first became evident in population studies, possible genetic linkages were hypothesized. Some of the early speculation was directed to the possibility of a single gene disorder.[4,5] Such single gene determinants, however, probably account for only a small percentage of patients. The largest numbers of cases are likely to be the result of combinations of genetic susceptibilities and acquired conditions, particularly obesity.[6]

It is also possible that the presence of one condition could enhance the development of the other. Hypertension and dyslipidemia may also interact synergistically to enhance the atherosclerotic process. Conversely, the treatment of one disorder may affect the severity of the other, either through pathophysiologic mechanisms or by the effects of the drugs used.

Clinical trials have demonstrated the value of treating both hypertension and dyslipidemia in preventing myocardial infarction and stroke. Data have indicated that these benefits are at least additive.[7-11] This finding, in turn, has led to suggestions that, in addition to therapeutic lifestyle changes including dietary compositional changes, exercise, and weight loss,[12] prescription of multiple drugs in a single pill may be useful in facilitating adherence to the long-term regimens necessary to treat these conditions. Because of the high level of concurrence of hypertension and dyslipidemia, their asymptomatic nature, which requires screening for detection, and their potentially catastrophic effects, a better understanding of the interactions of these two disorders is imperative.

ASSOCIATION BETWEEN HYPERTENSION AND DYSLIPIDEMIA

The rate of concurrence between hypertension and dyslipidemia in population studies is remarkably high. In a large, managed care population (Fig. 35-1), half the patients with hypertension also had some form of dyslipidemia, defined as an elevation of circulating triglycerides and cholesterol or a low level of high-density lipoprotein cholesterol (HDL-C). The converse is also true. About half the patients with dyslipidemia had hypertension.[3] In another study, men were more likely than women and blacks were more likely than whites to demonstrate this association.[13] As reflected in Figure 35-1, each of these conditions is strongly related to diabetes mellitus. These associations suggest the likelihood of a common antecedent. Likely candidates include excess body fat (particularly in intra-abdominal fat), insulin resistance, and genetic susceptibility.[14,15]

The recognition that hypertension, dyslipidemia, insulin resistance, and truncal obesity occur so often in a cluster has led to two major changes in our thinking about atherosclerotic risk factors. First, this clustering deserves identification as a genuine syndrome. This "metabolic syndrome" has become increasingly recognized as obesity has become a worldwide problem.[14,15] Second, recognition of risk factor clustering has led to recommendations that the introduction of lipid-lowering drugs be based on estimates of "global risk," that is, the total risk for an atherosclerotic clinical event, rather than focusing solely on elevated lipid levels.[16]

Many definitions of the metabolic syndrome have been proposed, and its origins have been thoroughly discussed. A very useful definition is presented in the most recent iteration of the National Cholesterol Education Program guidelines for the treatment of hyperlipidemia in adults (the Adult Treatment Panel III or ATP III guidelines),[16] as summarized in Table 35-1. This definition has the advantage of requiring only measurements made easily in any medical office. These measurements include waist circumference, blood pressure, and fasting blood levels of triglycerides, HDL-C, and fasting glucose. They do not include any direct measurement of insulin resistance or blood insulin levels. This limitation of the definition does not appear, however, to affect the ability to predict total and cardiac mortality, which is as good as or slightly better with the ATP III definition than with definitions that include insulin-related criteria.[17]

Whether hyperinsulinemia is a consequence or a direct cause of the metabolic syndrome and the role it may play in the development of the individual components of the syndrome are not settled issues. For most patients with the metabolic syndrome, the presence of excess intra-abdominal fat, even in the absence of an increased body mass index, is a key issue, not only in diagnosis, but also in treatment. Reduction of body weight, leading to reduction in abdominal fat content and decreased waist circumference, is beneficial in correcting lipid abnormalities and in lowering blood pressure, as well as in enhancing the susceptibility of these conditions to dietary and pharmacologic treatments.[18]

Current interest in the metabolic syndrome has overshadowed earlier attempts to link a combination of dyslipidemia and hypertension to specific gene disorders. This approach was pioneered by the late Roger Williams and his colleagues.[4,5] These investigators emphasized the strong familial grouping of this combination and suggested possible genetic linkages, including those related to insulin resistance and to hyperinsulinemia. Even in these early studies, however, it is clear that individuals with these two conditions had a greater tendency toward obesity and glucose intolerance. The possible role of genetics in producing this syndrome was

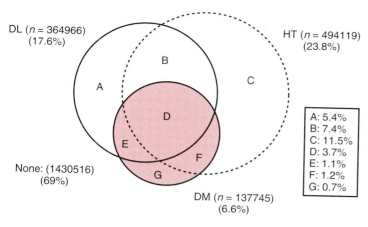

Figure 35–1 Prevalence and concurrence of hypertension (HT), dyslipidemia (DL), and diabetes mellitus (DM) (Kaiser Permanente members, n = 2.1 million adults). (From Selby JV, Peng T, Karter AJ, et al. High rates of co-occurrence of hypertension, elevated low-density lipoprotein cholesterol, and diabetes mellitus in a large managed care population. Am J Manag Care. 2004;10:163-170.)

DL (n = 364966)
(17.6%)

HT (n = 494119)
(23.8%)

None: (1430516)
(69%)

DM (n = 137745)
(6.6%)

A: 5.4%
B: 7.4%
C: 11.5%
D: 3.7%
E: 1.1%
F: 1.2%
G: 0.7%

Table 35-1 Estimated Number* of Adults in the United States Who Need Lifestyle Changes and Drug Treatment

	TLC	Drug Therapy
CHD and CHD risk equivalents		
10-yr risk >20% 2+ risk factors	24.1	20.7
10-yr risk 10%-20% 2+ risk factors	10.9	8.3
10-yr risk <10%	14.6	2.8
0-1 risk factor	15.6	4.7
Total	65.2	36.5

*In millions
CHD, coronary heart disease; TLC, therapeutic lifestyle changes.
From National Cholesterol Education Program Expert Panel. Executive summary of the third report of the National Cholesterol Education Program (NCEP) Expert Panel on detection, evaluation and treatment of high blood cholesterol in adults (Adult Treatment Panel III). JAMA. 2001;**285**:2486-2497.

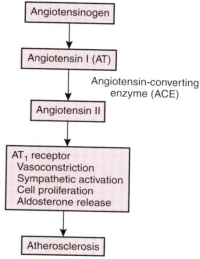

Role of Renin-Angiotension System in Atherogenesis

Angiotensinogen

Angiotensin I (AT)

Angiotensin-converting enzyme (ACE)

Angiotensin II

AT$_1$ receptor
Vasoconstriction
Sympathetic activation
Cell proliferation
Aldosterone release

Atherosclerosis

Figure 35–2 Role of the renin-angiotensin system in atherogenesis. (From Nickenig G. Should angiotensin II receptor blockers and statins be combined? Circulation. 2004;**110**:1013-1020.)

further supported by observations made in the National Heart, Lung, and Blood Institute twin study, demonstrating that concurrence was three times higher in monozygotic twins than in dizygotic pairs.[19] Low HDL-C was also a prominent feature of the syndrome in these subjects, as were obesity and glucose intolerance.

Interaction of Hypertension and Dyslipidemia on the Vascular Wall

It is beyond the scope of this chapter to review the pathophysiology of atherogenesis. Both hypertension and dyslipidemia, however, have adverse effects on the blood vessel wall, with resulting endothelial dysfunction, decreased bioavailability of nitric oxide, increased oxidative stress, and inflammation. Investigators have postulated that the renin-angiotensin system may also promote atherogenesis. Angiotensin II, through stimulation of the angiotensin type 1 receptor (AT$_1$), has been shown to increase lipid uptake in cells, vasoconstriction, and free radical production (Fig. 35-2) and to foster both hypertension and atherosclerosis.[20]

Microalbuminuria has been identified in hypertensive patients as a marker of incipient glomerular dysfunction and as a predictor of coronary artery disease.[21,22] Microalbuminuria has also been associated with lipid abnormalities including high levels of low-density lipoprotein cholesterol (LDL-C) and triglycerides, low levels of HDL-C, and elevated levels of lipoprotein(a),[23] a lipoprotein species made up of an LDL-C molecule linked through a disulfide bond to a peptide that is a fibrinogen analogue. Insulin resistance has also been described in hypertensive patients with microalbuminuria. This area will merit further attention because it suggests a possible role for circulating lipoproteins in the small vessel organ damage associated with hypertension.

Interactions in the Treatment of Hypertension and Dyslipidemia

It is intuitive that simultaneous treatment of two or more risk factors should provide at least additive benefits in preventing atherosclerotic vascular events. Most attempts at documenting the benefits of multiple risk factor interventions, however, have been unsuccessful because of trial design or failure to gain adequate adherence to trial regimens. Recently, the results of two large studies attempting to modify both hypertension and dyslipidemia simultaneously have been reported. The first of these is the Antihypertensive and Lipid-Lowering Treatment to Prevent Heart Attack Trial (ALLHAT; Table 35-2).[9] This study enrolled more than 40,000 patients, 55 years old or older, in a trial designed primarily to test four different antihypertensive drugs, including a calcium channel blocker, an angiotensin-converting enzyme (ACE) inhibitor, an α-adrenergic blocking agent, and a thiazide-like diuretic. Ten thousand subjects in the antihypertensive trial were further randomized either to a group receiving 40 mg/day pravastatin (an LDL-C–lowering drug of the hepatic 3-hydroxy-3-methylglutaryl–coenzyme A reductase inhibitor or "statin" group) or "usual care." The latter group may or may not have included individuals treated with cholesterol-lowering drugs, including statins. In both in the pravastatin and the usual care groups, beginning LDL-C levels were approximately 129 mg/dL, whereas blood pressures in both groups were, on average, 145/84 mm Hg. Unfortunately, over the 5 years of the study, the LDL-C level decreased by 27.7% in the pravastatin group, but it also declined by 11% in the usual care group. The LDL-C differential of 16.7% did not produce a statistically significant difference in death (the primary endpoint), fatal or nonfatal CHD events, or strokes.

The magnitude of the decline in coronary events was similar to that seen with similar degrees of cholesterol lowering in earlier, pre-statin clinical trials. However, the trend was toward reduced event rates for both coronary and cerebrovascular events. Strictly speaking, these results were not strong support for cholesterol lowering as a means of reducing the risk of death, coronary events, or cerebral events in patients with treated hypertension.

Results of the lipid-lowering arm of the Anglo-Scandinavian Cardiac Outcomes Trial (ASCOT-LLA), a study with a very similar design, became public about a year after ALLHAT's publication.[10] ASCOT enrolled more than 19,000 patients with hypertension, 40 to 79 years old, who were treated with an antihypertensive regimen that began with either a calcium channel blocker or a β-blocker. To be randomized into ASCOT-LLA, patients had to have total a cholesterol level equal to or less than 260 mg/dL (subjects with higher values could not ethically be assigned a placebo), as well as three other coronary risk factors. Half of the eligible patients were then randomized to either atorvastatin, 10 mg/day, or placebo, without any attempt to titrate the volunteers to a cholesterol goal. The primary outcome was combined fatal and nonfatal myocardial infarction. Although

Table 35-2 Comparison of Antihypertensive and Lipid-Lowering Treatment to Prevent Heart Attack Trial–LLT and Anglo-Scandinavian Cardiac Outcomes Trial–Lipid Lowering Arm

	ALLHAT-LLT	ASCOT-LLA
Study groups	Pravastatin 20-40 mg/day vs. "usual" care	Atorvastatin 10 mg/day vs. placebo
Sample size	10,355 men and women	10,305 men and women
Mean follow-up	4.8 yr	3.3 yr
Mean blood pressure (mm Hg)		
At baseline	146/84	164/95
At last follow-up	134/74	138/80
Total cholesterol difference	9.6%	20%
LDL-C difference	16.7%	30%
Hazard ratios		
Fatal and nonfatal MI	0.91 (P = .08)	0.64 (P = .0005)
Fatal and nonfatal stroke	0.91 (P = .16)	0.73 (P < .03)
Total mortality	0.99 (P = .80)	0.87 (P = .16)

ALLHAT-LLT, Antihypertensive and Lipid-Lowering Treatment to Prevent Heart Attack Trial–Lipid Lowering Trial; ASCOT-LLA, Anglo-Scandinavian Cardiac Outcomes Trial–Lipid Lowering Arm; LDL-C, low-density lipoprotein cholesterol; MI, myocardial infarction.
ALLHAT-LLT data from ALLHAT Officers and Coordinators for the ALLHAT Collaborative Research Group. Major outcomes in moderately hypercholesterolemic, hypertensive patients randomized to pravastatin vs. usual care: The Antihypertensive and Lipid-Lowering Treatment to Prevent Heart Attack Trial (ALLHAT-LLT). *JAMA.* 2002;**288**:2998-3007; ASCOT-LLA data from Sever PS, Dahlof B, Poulter NR, et al., for the ASCOT Investigators. Prevention of coronary and stroke events with atorvastatin in hypertensive patients who have average or lower-than-average cholesterol concentrations, in the Anglo-Scandinavian Cardiac Outcomes Trial–Lipid Lowering Arm (ASCOT-LLA): A multicentre randomized controlled trial. *Lancet.* 2003;**361**:1149-1158.

follow-up was planned for 5 years, the lipid-lowering arm of the trial was terminated after a median of 3.3 years because of a highly significant reduction in the primary outcome in the treated group compared with placebo.

The major differences from ALLHAT were a dramatically greater decline in total and LDL-C levels between randomized groups and a much smaller drop among those randomized to the control arm of the trial. In ASCOT-LLA, total cholesterol declined by 23% and LDL-C levels declined by 32% in the atorvastatin group. Investigators reported a 5% drop in each one of these parameters in the placebo group. Thus, instead of a 16.7% differential in LDL-C levels achieved in ALLHAT, there was a 27% difference in ASCOT. This was accompanied by a 36% reduction in the risk of the primary outcome events and a 27% reduction in strokes. The reduction in outcome events cannot be explained by a difference in blood pressure, because the blood pressure was 138/80 mm Hg in both groups at the end of follow-up. Thus, the lipid-lowering effects were *additive* to the benefits of blood pressure control. This finding is particularly promising in the case of stroke prevention. The ASCOT results clearly illustrate that LDL-C lowering provides a substantial benefit in stroke reduction even in the presence of adequate blood pressure control.

Stroke reduction with cholesterol lowering has been demonstrated in other statin clinical trials and in meta-analyses of these trials,[24] but never so dramatically as in the ASCOT-LLA. These findings came as a surprise, because the lack of association between circulating lipid levels and stroke in older observational studies implied that lipid lowering would be of little value in stroke prevention. Those older observational studies did not distinguish between hemorrhagic and atherothrombotic stroke. When stroke is separated by modern diagnostic techniques into hemorrhagic and ischemic varieties, the former are negatively associated and the latter are positively associated with circulating cholesterol levels.[25] Recent clinical trial data, then, do not present results that are in conflict with observational studies. In the Heart Protection Study (HPS), a very large study of the long-term effects of cholesterol lowering on coronary events, thrombotic, but not hemorrhagic, strokes were prevented by cholesterol lowering, a finding supporting the very different pathophysiology of these two forms of cerebrovascular damage.[26]

Either cholesterol lowering or the statin drugs that produce it may have some independent effect on blood pressure levels. In a study of patients taking an ACE inhibitor (enalapril or lisinopril), the degree of systolic blood pressure lowering was doubled, and the degree of diastolic blood pressure lowering increased by 25%, when a statin (either lovastatin or pravastatin) was added to the regimen.[7] Because mean cholesterol levels fell by 38%, these results could be attributed to a direct statin effect or to cholesterol lowering.[27] Such differences in blood pressure between patients treated with lipid-lowering therapies and those given a control intervention were not seen in HPS, ASCOT, ALLHAT, and several other large clinical trials. Whether blood pressure–lowering drugs have any effect on circulating lipid levels has been the subject of intense debate for many years. In the case of thiazide diuretics, adverse effects, if they occur at all, appear to be transient and disappear within a year of therapy when they are analyzed by the intent-to-treat approach.

In the case of β-blockers, however, adverse effects, particularly decreases in HDL-C and increases in triglycerides, often associated with weight gain, are more lasting, although there is little evidence of significant long-term clinical effects.[28] All other things being equal, it would be best to choose a blood pressure–lowering medication that has no effect or a beneficial effect on lipid levels. This can be ascertained in an individual patient by serial lipid measurements when blood pressure agents are being introduced.

SPECIAL ASPECTS OF THE TREATMENT OF DYSLIPIDEMIA IN HYPERTENSIVE PATIENTS

Diet

The composition and quantity of food intake are important factors in prevention and treatment of both hypertension and dyslipidemia. Much pessimism has been expressed about the value of dietary intervention in the prevention of these chronic disorders. This pessimism is not the result of the ineffectiveness of dietary intervention, but rather of the difficulty in maintaining it. Diets that are low in saturated and total fat and are rich in fruits, vegetables, and fiber are beneficial in preventing the onset and progression of obesity as well as in lowering LDL-C and blood pressure.[29] When combined with caloric restrictions sufficient to induce weight loss, these diets can, for many patients, be effective enough to eliminate the need for drug therapies. Unfortunately, these recommendations often run counter to the culture, lifestyle, pace, and preferences of modern developed countries in the Americas, Europe, and, increasingly, parts of Asia. When combined with sedentary lifestyles that exclude regular exercise, such factors predispose populations to the epidemic of obesity that has become prevalent in these parts of the world. These trends are not easily interdicted by physicians or resisted by patients.

In the long run, the problem of adult weight gain can probably be addressed only by its prevention. None of this discussion, however, should obscure the truth that dietary intervention is highly effective, very safe, and available to most patients at low cost. When begun early in adult life and combined with a lifetime of regular exercise, a proper diet can prevent, or postpone for many years, the onset and sequelae of many chronic conditions including hypertension, dyslipidemia, and diabetes mellitus, and, eventually, atherosclerosis. The key, however, is early intervention. Trying to change dietary habits and to lose weight in middle age and beyond is much less effective and much more difficult.

Not only do hypertension and dyslipidemia respond to the same dietary alterations, but also interesting evidence indicates that dietary responses in both conditions may be related to genetic makeup. In a study of 44 volunteers, 21 with the apoprotein (apo) E4 phenotype (E4, E3 or E4, E4) had significantly greater blood pressure reduction when they were given a low-fat diet than did volunteers with the apo E3 (E4, E3) phenotype.[30] Patients with the apo E4 phenotype are also known to have higher levels of blood cholesterol related to a diet high in saturated fat,[31] although, in this study, the cholesterol reduction response was not different between the two groups. Undoubtedly, we have much to learn about the genetic determinants of response to diet in both hypertension and dyslipidemia.

Metabolic Syndrome

As previously noted, the constellation of truncal obesity (even in the presence of normal body mass index), hypertension, dyslipidemia (particularly low HDL-C or elevated triglycerides), and hyperglycemia constitutes a cluster of conditions known as the metabolic syndrome. Insulin resistance and hyperinsulinemia are also an integral part of this syndrome. Less well appreciated in such patients is the presence of hypercoagulability, reflected in elevations of plasminogen activator inhibitor-1 and fibrinogen, as well as chronic inflammation reflected in elevations of high-sensitivity C-reactive protein (hs-CRP). Some experts regard hypercoagulability as an indication for aspirin therapy in such patients.[18] The significance of CRP elevations is not entirely clear, but, again, some clinicians consider elevated CRP levels to be indications for more aggressive treatment with both aspirin and lipid-lowering agents, particularly statins. In the metabolic syndrome, significant elevations of LDL-C are less common than are low HDL-C and high triglyceride levels.

Table 35-3 is a summary of suggested guidelines for treatment of the metabolic syndrome that focuses mainly on drug interventions.[18] Without question, however, intervention with low-calorie diets and regular exercise alone can be remarkably effective in reducing truncal obesity and in improving all associated conditions, including hypercoagulability and inflammation.

Although the treatment of patients with so many simultaneous disorders can be demanding, a study from the Steno Diabetes Center in Copenhagen in 160 patients with type 2 diabetes who were at high risk for cardiovascular disease indicates that such treatment can be rewarding.[32] These middle-aged patients were treated with either conventional therapy or an intensive intervention consisting of ACE inhibitors or angiotensin receptor blockers for hypertension, statins or fibrates for dyslipidemia, insulin for diabetes, smoking cessation, and weight reduction over an 8-year period. The benefits were dramatic not only in terms of blood pressure, lipid lowering, and blood glucose lowering, but also in terms of cardiovascular events. Of 118 cardiovascular events, 85 occurred in 35 (of the 80) patients randomized to conventional therapy, whereas only 33 occurred in 19 (of the 80) patients in the intensive therapy group. Although these numbers are derived from a small patient sample, they are nevertheless suggestive of the possible benefit of long-term, focused therapy in patients with multiple risk factors. How many of these patients satisfied the definition of metabolic syndrome is not clear, but the study provides additional evidence of the benefit of aggressive, multiple risk factor interventions.

Table 35-3 Therapy for Metabolic Syndrome and Its Components

Component	Risk Status*	TLC	Medications	Comment
Metabolic syndrome	<10%	Yes	None	Emphasis on TLC
	10%-20%	Yes	Consider	Use of statin, ACE inhibitor/ARB, ASA to reduce risk
	>20%	Yes	Yes	Use of statin, ACE inhibitor/ARB, ASA to reduce risk
Waist circumference >35 inches in women; >40 inches in men		Yes	Consider if multiple factors	Waist circumferences cut-points should be 10% lower in Asian patients
Dyslipidemia: high TG >150 mg/dL; low HDL-C <40 mg/dL in men; <50 mg/dL in women	Increases risk at any level of LDL-C	Yes	Statins, fibrates, niacin	Consider combination therapy with statin/fibrate or statin/niacin in high-risk cases
Hypertension: >130/85 mm Hg		Yes	Yes	ACE inhibitor and ARB reduce risk of type 2 DM, clinical endpoints
Glucose intolerance (impaired glucose tolerance)		Yes	Yes	Metformin best studied; glitazones promising, unproven
Hypercoagulability; plasminogen activator inhibitor-1, fibrinogen not routinely measured		Yes	Yes	Consider low-dose ASA if global risk >10%; some recommend higher doses in DM
Inflammation; elevated hs-CRP		Yes	Increased CRP predicts those who benefit most from ASA, statins	Elevated CRP >3 increases CHD risk; may alter assessment of global risk

*Global risk as calculated in the National Cholesterol Education Program Adult Treatment Panel III guidelines.[16]
ACE inhibitor/ARB, angiotensin-converting enzyme inhibitor/angiotensin receptor blocker; ASA, acetylsalicylic acid; CHD, coronary heart disease; CRP, C-reactive protein; DM, diabetes mellitus; HLD-C, high-density lipoprotein cholesterol; hs-CRP, high-sensitivity C-reactive protein; LDL-C, low-density lipoprotein cholesterol; TG, triglycerides; TLC, therapeutic lifestyle change.
From Wagh A, Stone NJ. Treatment of metabolic syndrome. *Expert Rev Cardiovasc Ther.* 2004;**2**:213-228.

SPECIFIC TREATMENT OF DYSLIPIDEMIA IN HYPERTENSIVE PATIENTS

The guidelines for the treatment of dyslipidemia, both in the United States and in Europe, are complex and beyond the scope of this chapter. They are presented in detail in the literature.[16] However, several principles underlying these guidelines bear emphasis:

1. The thresholds for beginning treatment, as well as the targets for treatment, are influenced heavily by the patient's global risk. *Global risk* is defined as the 10-year risk of having a coronary event based on projections, for example, from the Framingham Heart Study observational data, of the risk contributed by individual risk factors. Numerous clinical trials completed in the last decade have firmly established the value of LDL-C lowering. Statins are the drugs of first choice for prevention of both coronary events and stroke. These guidelines are therefore based primarily on lowering LDL-C levels. Although many observational data identify low HDL-C and high triglycerides as independent predictors of risk, one clinical trial—the Veterans Affairs High-Density Lipoprotein Cholesterol Intervention Trial (VA-HIT) (using gemfibrozil, a fibric acid derivative)—established the value of HDL-C raising and triglyceride lowering in patients whose LDL-C did not change appreciably.[33]

2. Patients with clinically apparent coronary disease or any other clinical form of atherosclerosis, including stroke and abdominal aneurysm, as well as patients with diabetes, are considered to be at high risk and are immediate candidates for interventions to lower LDL-C levels at least to 100 mg/dL. In the United Kingdom, the target for such patients has been set (by the British Hypertension Society) at approximately 80 mg/dL.[34] A recent statement from the National Cholesterol Education Program has opened the option (although it is not formally recommended) of adopting an LDL-C target of 70 mg/dL for selected patients at "very" high risk (i.e., with coronary disease and other active risk factors such as continued smoking).[35] Firm clinical trial evidence for LDL-C targets much lower than 100 mg/dL is not yet complete, however.

3. Although clinical trials have emphasized LDL-C as a target, the most recent U.S. guidelines have introduced the possibility that "non–HDL-C" (i.e., total cholesterol minus HDL-C) should also be considered a target, particularly in patients with high triglycerides. This number reflects all circulating atherogenic lipoproteins. It takes into account high triglycerides as a marker for cholesterol-rich lipoproteins other than LDL-C. These lipoproteins, richer in triglycerides than LDL-C, are nevertheless similar to LDL-C in that they are taken up by arterial endothelium and become the nidus for plaque formation.

4. Because statins are the most thoroughly studied and have a strong history of demonstrated benefit, they are the drugs of first choice in treating dyslipidemia. Their major effect is in lowering LDL-C. Statins are variably potent in raising HDL-C and in lowering triglycerides. As more potent HDL-C–raising drugs are developed, the value of that intervention will become clearer. At present, evidence is insufficient to recommended HDL-C as a primary target for intervention, although it is a powerful risk factor to be considered in decisions about how aggressively to treat patients with high LDL-C levels.

5. Postmenopausal women and elderly patients respond well to statins and have a progressively higher risk of atherosclerotic events as they age. In calculations of global risk, age is by far the greatest determinant of risk. Although clinical trials have not definitively established the benefit of cholesterol lowering on overall mortality in postmenopausal women or in elderly patients, there is much to be said for aggressive lipid lowering to prevent nonfatal events. A reasonable way to regard these issues is to aim for a maximum of disability-free years. The surprisingly strong benefit of LDL-C lowering in preventing strokes makes this approach doubly important in the treatment of patients with hypertension (or diabetes) who are already at a very high risk of cerebrovascular and coronary events.

Recommendations for the treatment of dyslipidemia have focused on high-risk patients (i.e., patients with multiple risk factors, diabetes, or clinically apparent coronary disease). Even the most generous interpretation of LDL-C–lowering trials, however, indicates that the benefit of preventing recurring events within the 5- to 7-year period of most of these trials is approximately 30%. In other words, roughly two thirds of events will still occur even in the presence of fairly aggressive LDL-C lowering. This situation could, of course, reflect the presence of other risk factors, the need for even more aggressive LDL-C lowering, or the burden of atherosclerosis that has accumulated over the preceding decades and that cannot be reversed or attenuated completely, at least not during the clinical trial.

Assuming that the overall burden of atherosclerosis is responsible for at least some treatment failures, the issue of primary prevention, which has been largely untested and unaddressed in lower-risk populations, looms large. Recommendations for very early drug interventions to prevent development of atherosclerosis are not likely to be practical, affordable, or popular. This situation leads, once again, to the necessity of developing effective programs to change lifestyle factors such as diet and exercise to prevent obesity. In addition, we must find ways of identifying individuals early in life who are at particular risk of developing atherosclerosis as they age.

ADHERENCE ISSUES IN HYPERTENSION AND DYSLIPIDEMIA

The strong links among dyslipidemia, hypertension, and, in some patients, diabetes, has led to the resurrection of the concept of the combination pill. Preparations that include both a statin and an antihypertensive agent are now increasingly available.[36] The rationale for such combinations is usually long-term adherence. Adherence is inversely proportional to the number of pills that must be taken, as well as the frequency of administration.[37] A antilipidemic, antihypertensive regimen that could be taken once a day would be more easily remembered and therefore would have a better chance of actually having a beneficial effect. This is no small consideration. Investigators have repeatedly shown that patients with long-term drug regimens tend to drift away from regular drug use after a period of months. Partly to provoke discussion, a cardioprotective "poly pill" was recently suggested by Wald and Law, based on an analysis of more than 750 clinical trials.[38] The proposed formulation would have six components: a statin; three blood pressure–lowering drugs including a thiazide diuretic, a β-blocker, and an ACE inhibitor (each at one-half maximal dose); folic acid; and low-dose aspirin. At this point, no clinical trial evidence indicates that folic acid is protective against atherosclerosis, but the other recommendations are well grounded in clinical trial evidence. Although such a pill is unlikely ever to be produced, it does bring attention to the problem of polypharmacy. Particularly in elderly patients, the large numbers of drugs that are often prescribed lead to confusion, poor adherence, and, ultimately, therapeutic failures.

SUMMARY

Hypertension and dyslipidemia occur together quite often. Roughly 50% of patients with dyslipidemia also are hypertensive, and roughly 50% of hypertensive patients also have some form of dyslipidemia. Often, these two risk factors occur in the presence of the metabolic syndrome, in combination with truncal obesity and diabetes mellitus.

Treatment of dyslipidemia not only prevents coronary events, but also is second only to blood pressure lowering in preventing strokes. Indeed, some evidence indicates that cholesterol-lowering drugs or even cholesterol lowering itself may have a slight, but measurable, effect in reducing blood pressure. Both these risk factors are aggravated by weight gain, particularly when it results in an increase in abdominal fat. At a time when obesity is an increasingly prevalent problem, even among young people, hypertension and dyslipidemia often become management problems in the same patient.

Dietary interventions that lower blood pressure (i.e., diets low in saturated fat and calories and rich in fruit and vegetables) also lower LDL-C and generally improve lipid profiles. Whereas cholesterol-lowering drugs may favorably affect blood pressure, some blood pressure–lowering drugs, particularly thiazide diuretics and some β-blocking agents, may aggravate dyslipidemia, particularly in the short term. Studies have demonstrated that, even in the presence of reasonably well managed blood pressure, the treatment of dyslipidemia, particularly LDL-C lowering, has favorable effects on both coronary and cerebrovascular event rates over and above the benefits of blood pressure lowering itself. Although management of these disorders in high-risk patients usually requires both dietary and pharmacologic intervention, long-term prevention in lower-risk patients is likely to be related to the prevention of obesity, changes in both the quantity and quality of dietary components, and the adoption of regular exercise programs early in life.

The combined problems of an aging population and poor adherence to complex drug regimens requiring the taking of many different pills have led to a reconsideration of combination pills, particularly as they relate to the treatment of hypertension and dyslipidemia. Whether this approach will succeed in improving adherence to drug regimens remains to be seen. The strong concurrence of hypertension and dyslipidemia requires that patients found to have one disorder always be tested for the other. Family screening of patients with these disorders will likely have a rich yield of additional patients requiring treatment. Long-term prevention of atherosclerosis as the major contributor to death and disability requires control of hypertension and dyslipidemia not only with drugs but also by major changes in lifestyle, including dietary and exercise habits.

References

1. Ames RP. Hyperlipidemia in hypertension: Causes and prevention. *Am Heart J*. 1991;**122**:1219-1224.
2. Zanchetti A. Hyperlipidemia in the hypertensive patient. *Am J Med*. 1994;**96 (Suppl 6A)**:3S-8S.
3. Selby JV, Peng T, Karter AJ, et al. High rates of co-occurrence of hypertension, elevated low-density lipoprotein cholesterol, and diabetes mellitus in a large managed care population. *Am J Manag Care*. 2004;**10**:163-170.
4. Williams RR, Hunt SC, Hopkins PN, et al. Familial dyslipidemic hypertension: Evidence from 58 Utah families for a syndrome present in approximately 12% of patients with essential hypertension. *JAMA*. 1988;**259**:3579-3586.
5. Williams RR, Hunt SC, Hopkins PN, et al. Evidence for single gene contributions to hypertension and lipid disturbances: Definition, genetics, and clinical significance. *Clin Genet*. 1994;**46**:80-87.
6. Schmidt MI, Watson RL, Duncan BB, et al., for the Atherosclerosis Risk in Communities Study Investigators. Cluster of dyslipidemia, hyperuricemia, diabetes, and hypertension and its association with fasting insulin and central and overall obesity in a general population. *Metabolism*. 1996;**45**:699-706.
7. Sposito AC, Mansur AP, Coelho OR, et al. Additional reduction in blood pressure after cholesterol-lowering treatment by statins (lovastatin or pravastatin) in hypercholesterolemic patients using angiotensin-converting enzyme inhibitors (enalapril or lisinopril). *Am J Cardiol*. 1999;**83**:1497-1499.
8. Borghi C. Interactions between hypercholesterolemia and hypertension: Implications for therapy. *Curr Opin Nephrol Hypertens*. 2002;**11**:489-496.
9. ALLHAT Officers and Coordinators for the ALLHAT Collaborative Research Group. Major outcomes in moderately hypercholesterolemic, hypertensive patients randomized to pravastatin vs. usual care: The Antihypertensive and Lipid-Lowering Treatment to Prevent Heart Attack Trial (ALLHAT-LLT). *JAMA*. 2002;**288**:2998-3007.
10. Sever PS, Dahlof B, Poulter NR, et al., for the ASCOT Investigators. Prevention of coronary and stroke events with atorvastatin in hypertensive patients who have average or lower-than-average cholesterol concentrations, in the Anglo-Scandinavian Cardiac Outcomes Trial–Lipid Lowering Arm (ASCOT-LLA): A multicentre randomized controlled trial. *Lancet*. 2003;**361**:1149-1158.
11. Chapman N. New evidence in hypertension and hyperlipidaemia. *Heart*. 2004;**90 (Suppl IV)**:IV14-IV17.
12. Franklin BA, Kahn JK, Gordon NF, Bonow RO. A cardioprotective "polypill?" Independent and additive benefits of lifestyle modification. *Am J Cardiol*. 2004;**94**:162-166.
13. O'Meara JG, Kardia SLR, Armon JJ, et al. Ethnic and sex differences in the prevalence, treatment, and control of dyslipidemia among hypertensives adults in the GENOA study. *Arch Intern Med*. 2004;**164**:1313-1318.
14. Reaven GM, Lithell H, Landsberg L. Hypertension and associated metabolic abnormalities: The role of insulin resistance and the sympathoadrenal system. *N Engl J Med*. 1996;**334**:374-381.
15. Hall JE, Brands MW, Zappe DH, Galicia MA. Insulin resistance, hyperinsulinemia, and hypertension: Causes, consequences, or merely correlations? *Proc Soc Exp Biol Med*. 1995;**208**:317-329.

16. National Cholesterol Education Program Expert Panel. Executive summary of the third report of the National Cholesterol Education Program (NCEP) Expert Panel on detection, evaluation and treatment of high blood cholesterol in adults (Adult Treatment Panel III). *JAMA.* 2001;**285**:2486-2497.

17. Hunt KJ, Resendez RG, Williams K, et al. National Cholesterol Education Program versus World Health Organization metabolic syndrome in relation to all-cause and cardiovascular mortality in the San Antonio Heart Study. *Circulation.* 2004;**110**:1251-1257.

18. Wagh A, Stone NJ. Treatment of metabolic syndrome. *Expert Rev Cardiovasc Ther.* 2004;**2**:213-228.

19. Selby JB, Newman B, Quiroga J, et al. Concordance for dyslipidemic hypertension in male twins. *JAMA.* 1991;**265**:2079-2084.

20. Nickenig G. Should angiotensin II receptor blockers and statins be combined? *Circulation.* 2004;**110**:1013-1020.

21. Campese VM, Bianchi S, Bigazzi R. Association between hyperlipidemia and microalbuminuria in essential hypertension. *Kidney Int.* 1999;**56 (Suppl 71)**:S10-S13.

22. Mitchell TH, Nolan B, Henry M, et al. Microalbuminuria in patients with non–insulin-dependent diabetes mellitus relates to nocturnal systolic blood pressure. *Am J Med.* 1997;**102**: 531-535.

23. Sechi LA, Kronenberg F, De Carli S, et al. Association of serum lipoprotein(a) levels and apolipoprotein(a) size polymorphism with target-organ damage in arterial hypertension. *JAMA.* 1997;**277**:1689-1695.

24. Blauw GJ, Lagaay AM, Smelt AH, Westendorp RG. Stroke, statins, and cholesterol: A meta-analysis of randomized, placebo-controlled, double-blind trials with HMG-CoA reductase inhibitors. *Stroke.* 1997;**28**:946-950.

25. Iso H, Jacobs DR, Wentworth D, et al. Serum cholesterol levels and six-year mortality from stroke in 350,977 men screened for the multiple risk factor intervention trial. *N Engl J Med.* 1989;**320**:904-910.

26. Heart Protection Study Collaborative Group. Effects of cholesterol-lowering with simvastatin on stroke and other major vascular events in 20,536 people with cerebrovascular disease or other high-risk conditions. *Lancet.* 2004;**363**:757-767.

27. Wierzbicki AS. Lipid lowering: Another method of reducing blood pressure? *J Hum Hypertens.* 2002;**16**:753-760.

28. Brook RD. Mechanism of differential effects of antihypertensive agents on serum lipids. *Curr Hypertens Rep.* 2000;**2**:370-377.

29. Appel LJ, Moore TJ, Obarzanek E, et al., for the DASH Collaborative Research Group. A clinical trial of the effects of dietary patterns on blood pressure. *N Engl J Med.* 1997;**336**:1117-1124.

30. Rantala M, Savolainen MJ, Kervinen K, Kesaniemi YA. Apolipoprotein E phenotype and diet-induced alteration in blood pressure. *Am J Clin Nutr.* 1997;**65**:543-550.

31. Tikkanen MJ, Huttunen JK, Ehnholm C, Pietinen P. Apolipoprotein E4 homozygosity predisposes to serum cholesterol elevation during high fat diet. *Arteriosclerosis.* 1990;**10**:285-288.

32. Gaede P, Vedel P, Larsen N, et al. Multifactorial intervention and cardiovascular disease in patients with type 2 diabetes. *N Engl J Med.* 2003;**348**:383-393.

33. Rubins HB, Robins SJ, Collins D, et al., for the Veterans Affairs High-Density Lipoprotein Cholesterol Intervention Trial Study Group. Gemfibrozil for the secondary prevention of coronary heart disease in men with low levels of high-density lipoprotein cholesterol. *N Engl J Med* 1999;**341**:410-418.

34. Williams B, Poulter NR, Brown MJ, et al., the BHS guidelines working party, for the British Hypertension Society. British Hypertension Society guidelines for hypertension management 2004 (BHS-IV): Summary. *BMJ.* 2004;**328**:634-640.

35. Grundy SM, Cleeman JI, Merz CNB, et al., for the Coordinating Committee of the National Cholesterol Education Program. Implications of recent clinical trials for the National Cholesterol Education Program Adult Treatment Panel III Guidelines. *Circulation.* 2004;**110**:227-239.

36. Sica DA. Fixed-dose combination therapy: Is it time for this approach to hypertension and dyslipidemia management? *J Clin Hypertens.* 2004;**6**:164-167.

37. LaRosa JH, LaRosa JC. Enhancing drug compliance in lipid-lowering treatment. *Arch Fam Med.* 2000;**9**:1169-1175.

38. Wald NJ, Law MR. A strategy to reduce cardiovascular disease by more than 80%. *BMJ.* 2003;**326**:1419-1423.

Special Populations and Special Situations

SECTION CONTENTS

Hypertension in Pregnancy
Tiina Podymow and Phyllis August

Hypertensive disorders are the most common medical disorders during pregnancy and are a leading cause of maternal and perinatal morbidity and mortality worldwide. Hypertension complicates 6% to 10% of pregnancies.[1,2] Of 4 million women giving birth in the United States each year, an estimated 240,000 are affected by hypertension.[3] Hypertension during pregnancy can lead to serious maternal and fetal problems and accounts for approximately 15% of maternal deaths in the United States.

Although the obstetrician manages most cases of hypertension during pregnancy, the internist, cardiologist, or nephrologist may be consulted if hypertension precedes conception or when accelerated hypertension is present. In this chapter, a medical perspective is taken, with the focus on diagnostic and therapeutic issues that are nonobstetric.

CLASSIFICATION

The four major hypertensive disorders in pregnancy are as follows: (1) chronic hypertension; (2) preeclampsia, which is pregnancy-induced hypertension associated with proteinuria; (3) preeclampsia superimposed on chronic hypertension; and (4) gestational hypertension. All four types may lead to maternal and perinatal complications, although the syndrome of preeclampsia with severe hypertension is associated with the highest maternal and fetal risks.

Chronic Hypertension

Chronic hypertension is defined as blood pressure (BP) of 140/90 mm Hg or higher that either predates pregnancy or develops before 20 weeks. This condition complicates approximately 3% of pregnancies. Higher rates may be seen in older women, obese women, and African Americans. Chronic hypertension in pregnancy is classified as either mild or severe, with severe defined by diastolic readings of 110 mm Hg or higher.

Preeclampsia-Eclampsia

Preeclampsia-eclampsia is a pregnancy-specific syndrome that develops in the latter half of pregnancy (after 20 weeks). The syndrome is characterized by increased BP ($\geq$140/90 mm Hg) and proteinuria (>0.3 g/day) in a woman who was normotensive before 20 weeks.[4] It occurs in 5% to 6% of pregnancies. A severe variant of preeclampsia features *h*emolysis, *e*levated *l*iver enzymes, and *l*ow *p*latelet count (HELLP syndrome), which occurs in 1 in 1000 pregnancies. Eclampsia complicates approximately 3% of cases of preeclampsia and is the occurrence of seizures that cannot be attributed to other causes. Risk factors for preeclampsia are shown in Table 36-1.

Preeclampsia Superimposed on Chronic Hypertension

Women with chronic hypertension are at increased risk for the development of superimposed preeclampsia, which complicates 25% of chronic hypertensive pregnancies (versus 5% of nonhypertensive pregnancies). The diagnosis of superimposed preeclampsia is made in women with chronic hypertension if proteinuria develops for the first time in the latter half of pregnancy, in association with an increase in BP. In women with both hypertension and proteinuria before 20 weeks' gestation, superimposed preeclampsia is diagnosed (1) when a sudden increase in proteinuria or a sudden increase in BP occurs in the latter half of pregnancy in a woman whose hypertension had previously been well controlled or (2) as part of the HELLP syndrome when the patient has new-onset thrombocytopenia with hemolysis and elevated levels of alanine aminotransferase or aspartate aminotransferase.[5]

Gestational Hypertension

Gestational hypertension, seen in 6% of pregnancies, is hypertension developing in the latter half of pregnancy and not associated with the systemic features of preeclampsia (e.g., proteinuria). Some women may ultimately develop signs of preeclampsia, so the final diagnosis can be made only post partum.

CHRONIC HYPERTENSION DURING PREGNANCY

The prevalence of hypertension in premenopausal women is close to 25% in whites and 30% in blacks, and it increases with age. Approximately 2% to 5% of pregnancies are complicated by chronic hypertension.

Differential Diagnosis

If hypertension was clearly documented before conception, then the diagnosis of chronic hypertension in pregnancy is straightforward (Fig. 36-1). Chronic hypertension is also the most likely diagnosis when hypertension (and no proteinuria) is present before 20 weeks of gestation. BP normally falls in early pregnancy; systolic pressure changes little, whereas diastolic BP falls by approximately 10 mm Hg by 13 to 20 weeks, with a nadir at 24 weeks, and then rises again to prepregnancy levels in the third trimester (weeks 28 to 40). This physiologic fall may be more exaggerated in women with chronic hypertension, and difficulties in diagnosis arise when these women are seen for the first time in the second trimester, during the

Table 36-1   Risk Factors for Preeclampsia

Nulliparity
Multiple gestation
Family history of preeclampsia
Chronic hypertension
Diabetes
Renal disease
History of early (<34 wk) preeclampsia in a previous
    pregnancy
History of HELLP syndrome
Obesity
Hydatidiform mole

HELLP, *hemolysis, elevated liver enzymes, low platelet count.*

expected physiologic decrease in BP. In this circumstance, women may be presumed normotensive and later erroneously diagnosed with gestational hypertension or preeclampsia when BP rises in the third trimester. In such cases, the diagnosis of preeclampsia can be ruled out by the absence of proteinuria and other classic laboratory abnormalities of preeclampsia or HELLP syndrome, such as elevated serum uric acid, liver function tests, and decreased platelets.

White-coat hypertension (elevated office BP with normal BP outside the medical setting) may be seen in up to 29% of women without preexisting hypertension. A noninvasive 24-hour BP monitor can distinguish white-coat hypertension from true hypertension in the pregnant patient.[6] White-coat hypertension does not appear to predispose patients to preeclampsia.

Women who present with hypertension before 20 weeks' gestation likely have chronic hypertension. Young women are somewhat more likely to have secondary hypertension (e.g., intrinsic renal disease, renovascular hypertension, primary aldosteronism, Cushing's syndrome, pheochromocytoma). When this condition is suspected, noninvasive evaluation may

be appropriate (Fig. 36-2). For example, if proteinuria is documented in early pregnancy, then noninvasive evaluation for renal disease is indicated. This may include 24-hour urinary protein excretion, creatinine clearance, renal ultrasound, and serologic testing to rule out systemic lupus erythematosus, if symptoms are suggestive. Another form of secondary hypertension that should be considered is caused by pheochromocytoma, which although rare is associated with high morbidity and mortality rates during pregnancy, particularly if it is undiagnosed.[7] This lesion should be considered in pregnant women with severe hypertension, especially when it is associated with headache, palpitations, pallor, and sweats.

Routine laboratory tests including uric acid, platelets, liver function tests, urea, creatinine, and 24-hour urine for protein should be performed in women with hypertension in early pregnancy as a baseline to determine the clinical significance of any later changes in BP or laboratory tests.

The distinction between chronic hypertension (first noted in pregnancy) and gestational hypertension is not possible until after delivery. In some instances, women with undocumented hypertension before pregnancy have normal BP throughout the entire pregnancy, then return to prepregnancy hypertensive levels in the postpartum period, thus accounting for the mysterious cases of isolated postpartum hypertension.

Maternal Risks

Approximately 25% of women with chronic hypertension in pregnancy develop superimposed preeclampsia, which carries higher morbidity and mortality rates (both maternal and fetal) than all other forms of pregnancy hypertension.[8,9] The risk of abruptio placentae is increased threefold in women with chronic hypertension, and this complication can lead to life-threatening maternal hemorrhage. Other risks include accelerated hypertension with potential target organ damage and cerebrovascular catastrophes.[1] Preeclampsia also confers increased risk of fatal intracerebral hemorrhage. Indeed, although maternal mortality rates are reduced considerably in

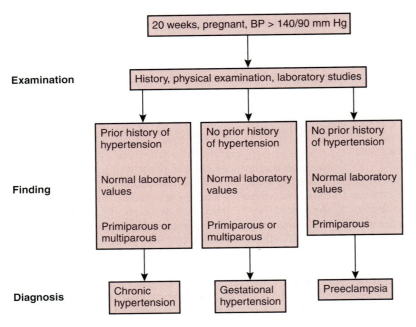

Figure 36-1   Algorithm for diagnostic evaluation of pregnant women with hypertension. BP, blood pressure.

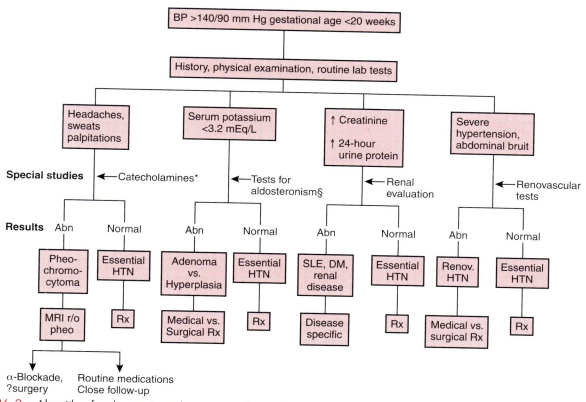

Figure 36–2   Algorithm for diagnosis and treatment of secondary hypertension in pregnancy. *Serum and urine. §Renin, urine aldosterone, urine potassium; difficult to interpret in pregnancy. Renal evaluation: serologic evaluation, 24-hour urine, renal ultrasound. Renovascular tests: renin (normally elevated in pregnancy), Doppler ultrasound of renal arteries. Abn, abnormal; BP, blood pressure; DM, diabetes mellitus; HTN, hypertension; MRI, magnetic resonance imaging; pheo, pheochromocytoma; r/o, rule out; Rx, treatment; SLE systemic lupus erythematosus.

developed compared with developing nations, hypertension still accounts for 15% of maternal deaths, most resulting from cerebral hemorrhage.[10]

Women with renal disease and collagen vascular disease may experience irreversible deterioration in either renal function or multiorgan system morbidity, regardless of the development of superimposed preeclampsia.[11] If significant azotemia is present (serum creatinine >1.9 mg/dL, or 168 μmol/L), the maternal and fetal outcomes are poor, with worsened azotemia, proteinuria, and hypertension commonly seen in the mother and growth restriction in the fetus.[11] Finally, pregnancies in women with uncomplicated chronic hypertension are usually successful, but such women are more likely to undergo cesarean delivery and be hospitalized for high BP.

Fetal Risks

Perinatal death rates are higher in pregnancies of women with chronic hypertension than in those of normotensive women, and superimposed preeclampsia confers an even greater risk. Maternal chronic hypertension is a risk factor for intrauterine growth restriction (defined as birth weight <10th percentile), which is seen in 5% to 13% of pregnancies of chronically hypertensive women. When superimposed preeclampsia develops, delivery resulting in prematurity occurs in 13% to 54% of cases, and fetal death is the outcome in less than 1%.[12]

The incidence of intrauterine growth restriction is reported at 35% in women with superimposed preeclampsia and at 10.5% in women with uncomplicated chronic hypertension.[13] Thus, chronic hypertension is associated with increased risk of perinatal death, intrauterine growth restriction, and premature delivery, which are considerably magnified by superimposed preeclampsia.

GENERAL MANAGEMENT PRINCIPLES

Preconception Management

Management of the pregnant woman with chronic hypertension begins before conception, to establish the diagnosis and to rule out secondary hypertension. Patients who have had hypertension for longer than 5 years should be evaluated for target organ damage, such as left ventricular hypertrophy, funduscopic changes, and azotemia. Medications with deleterious fetal effects, such as angiotensin-converting enzyme (ACE) inhibitors and angiotensin II receptor blockers should be addressed (see the later discussion of medications). Preconception is also the appropriate time to discuss the risks of hypertension in pregnancy: a high likelihood of a favorable outcome with risks nonetheless of superimposed preeclampsia and fetal complications. Compliance with appointment keeping is essential, because frequent visits will increase the likelihood of detecting preeclampsia and other complications before they become life-threatening. Finally, in complicated conditions such as kidney transplantation or diabetes with renal disease, a multidisciplinary team consisting of obstetricians and internists familiar with the care of pregnant women can optimize the chances of a successful outcome.[14]

Nonpharmacologic Management

The approach to hypertension in the gravid patient represents a departure from accepted guidelines for nonpregnant hypertensive patients. Pregnant patients are advised not to exercise vigorously to avoid decreasing uteroplacental blood flow. Women who work outside the home have both higher BP and an increased risk of preeclampsia.[15] Decreased work hours and more rest may theoretically increase placental blood flow and decrease BP.

Excessive weight loss during pregnancy is not advisable, even in obese women. Salt restriction is not recommended during pregnancy because of concerns that the normal physiologic plasma volume expansion will not occur. In women adhering to a low-sodium diet before conception, it is reasonable to continue. Calcium supplementation in excess of the recommended dietary allowance has not been shown to reduce the incidence of superimposed preeclampsia, though evidence from the developing world indicates that in women with low dietary calcium intake, calcium supplementation may prevent preeclampsia.

Pharmacologic Management

In nonpregnant adults, BP control can decrease the long-term incidence of cardiovascular disease and mortality. During the 9 months of pregnancy, however, untreated mild to moderate hypertension is unlikely to lead to unfavorable outcomes, and antihypertensive drugs in this setting are used primarily to protect the mother from cardiovascular or cerebrovascular complications.

An important issue for women with chronic hypertension is the prevention of preeclampsia. There is little evidence that the treatment of hypertension early in pregnancy reduces the incidence of superimposed preeclampsia, and several reviews concluded that data are insufficient to determine the benefits and risks of antihypertensive therapy for mild to moderate hypertension.[16-18]

Because most women with chronic hypertension in pregnancy have modest elevations in BP, it is often possible to manage their hypertension without medication. No large clinical trial has addressed the appropriate level of BP in a pregnant woman with hypertension. Guidelines vary, with recommendations to treat ranging from thresholds of 140/90, 160/90, to 160/105 mm Hg or higher in Canada, Australia, and the United States, respectively.[1,19,20] Our recommendations are in accord with those of the National High Blood Pressure Education Program (NHBPEP) Working Group on High Blood Pressure in Pregnancy.[1] When maternal BP reaches levels equal to or greater than 150/90 to 100 mm Hg, treatment should be instituted to avoid hypertensive vascular damage. Most physicians prescribe more aggressive treatment in women with renal disease or with a history of target organ damage.

Because BP normally falls in early pregnancy, even in women with chronic hypertension, if the patient has no known target organ damage, clinicians can consider discontinuing antihypertensive drugs and monitoring BP. Therapy can then be initiated at a BP of 150/90 to 100 mm Hg, regardless of the type of hypertension.[21] Various agents are available for use (Table 36-2). Orally administered antihypertensive agents should be used in standard doses in pregnancy. The U.S. Food and Drug Administration's (FDA's) classification of drugs in pregnancy designates most antihypertensive drugs as category C, stating that the drug should be given only if potential benefits justify potential risks to the fetus.[22] This category cannot be interpreted as having no risk and is so broad as to preclude its usefulness in clinical practice. The most recent evidence assessing risks and benefits for the drugs to treat hypertension in pregnancy is reviewed later. These medications have the longest history of safe use in pregnancy, although some are rarely used in the nonpregnant population because of side effects or inconvenient dosing schedules (see Table 36-2).

Central Adrenergic Agonists

Methyldopa
Methyldopa remains the drug of first choice for treatment of hypertension in pregnancy. It has been found to be nonteratogenic during a 40-year history of use. In trials, methyldopa has compared favorably with placebo or alternative agents in decreasing the occurrence of severe hypertension in pregnancy, as well as of hospital admissions, compared with untreated patients. The drug has no known adverse uteroplacental or fetal effects. Birth weight and development in the first year were similar in children exposed in utero to methyldopa compared with placebo, as was neurocognitive development up to the age of 7 years. The adverse effects of methyldopa are primarily the result of its action at the brainstem and include decreased mental alertness, drowsiness, impaired sleep, and decreased salivation. It causes elevated liver enzymes in 5% of patients, with hepatitis or hepatic necrosis rarely reported, and it has been associated with Coombs positivity, with (or more commonly without) associated hemolytic anemia.

Clonidine
Clonidine is another α_2-adrenergic agonist comparable to methyldopa with respect to safety and efficacy. Of some concern is a reported excess of sleep disturbance in exposed infants. Clonidine should be avoided in early pregnancy because of suspected embryopathy; there is little justification for its use in preference to methyldopa, given the proven safety of the latter. The potential for rebound hypertension exists when clonidine is abruptly discontinued, so this drug is reserved for patients who develop rash or liver dysfunction from methyldopa.

β-Adrenoceptor Blockers

β-Blockers have been studied extensively in pregnancy, and none of them have been associated with teratogenicity, although fetal safety remains a concern. Atenolol in one study resulted in clinically significant fetal growth restriction compared with placebo.[23] Oral and parenteral β-blockade has been associated with neonatal bradycardia; rarely, effects related to parenteral therapy required intervention.[17,24]

Table 36-2   Drugs* for Chronic Hypertension in Pregnancy[†]

Drug (FDA Risk[‡])	Dose	Concerns or Comments
Preferred Agent		
Methyldopa (B)	0.5-3.0 g/day in 2-3 divided doses	Drug of choice according to National High Blood Pressure Education Program Working Group; safety after first trimester well documented, including 7-year follow-up of children
Second-Line Agents[§]		
Labetalol (C)	200-1200 mg/day in 2-3 divided doses	May be associated with fetal growth restriction and neonatal bradycardia
Nifedipine (C)	30-90 mg/day of a slow-release preparation	May inhibit labor and have a synergistic interaction with magnesium sulfate
Hydralazine (C)	50-300 mg/day in 2-4 divided doses	Few controlled trials, but long experience with few adverse events documented; useful only in combination with sympatholytic agent; may cause neonatal thrombocytopenia
β-Receptor blockers (C)	Depends on specific agent	May cause fetal bradycardia and decrease uteroplacental blood flow; this effect may be less for agents with partial agonist activity; may impair fetal response to hypoxic stress; risk of growth restriction when started in first or second trimester (especially atenolol)
Hydrochlorothiazide (C)	25 mg/day	Majority of controlled studies in normotensive pregnant women rather than hypertensive patients; can cause volume depletion and electrolyte disorders; may be useful in combination with methyldopa and vasodilator to mitigate compensatory fluid retention
Contraindicated		
Angiotensin-converting enzyme inhibitors and angiotensin I receptor antagonists (D[¶])	—	Lead to fetal loss in animals; human use in second and third trimesters associated with fetopathy, oligohydramnios, growth restriction, and neonatal anuric renal failure, which may be fatal

*No antihypertensive has been proven safe for use during the first trimester.
[†]Drug therapy is indicated for uncomplicated chronic hypertension when diastolic blood pressure ≥100 mm Hg (using Korotkoff V phase for diastolic measurement). Treatment at lower levels may be indicated for patients with diabetes mellitus, renal disease, or target organ damage.
[‡]U.S. Food and Drug Administration (FDA) classification.
[§]Some agents are omitted (e.g., clonidine, α-blockers) because of limited data on use for long-term hypertension in pregnancy.
[¶]We would classify them in category X during the second and third trimesters.
B, Fetal risk not demonstrated in animal or human studies, but data are insufficient. C, Animal studies demonstrated risk; human fetal risk unknown or no adequate studies; should only be given if the potential benefits justify the risk to the fetus. D, Evidence of human fetal risk.

Reassurance is derived from a 1-year follow-up study, which showed normal development of infants exposed to β-blockers in utero.[25]

Maternal outcomes improve with the use of β-blockers, which control maternal BP and decrease both the incidence of severe hypertension and the rate of admission to hospital before delivery.[17] β-Blockers have been compared with, and found equivalent to, methyldopa in 15 trials. Adverse effects of β-blockade include fatigue, lethargy, exercise intolerance, sleep disturbance, and bronchoconstriction.

Labetalol, a nonselective β-blocker with vascular α_1-receptor blocking capabilities, has gained wide acceptance in pregnancy, and it is as safe and effective as methyldopa. Labetalol was associated with fetal growth restriction in one placebo-controlled study. It is used parenterally to treat severe hypertension, and it has been associated with a lower incidence of maternal hypotension and other side effects compared with hydralazine.[26]

α-Adrenergic Blockers

α-Blockers are indicated during pregnancy in the management of pheochromocytoma. Both prazosin and phenoxybenzamine have been used, along with β-blockers as adjunctive agents. Because experience with these agents in pregnancy is limited, their routine use is not advocated.

Calcium Channel Blockers

Calcium channel blockers have been used to treat chronic hypertension, mild preeclampsia presenting late in gestation, and urgent hypertension in preeclampsia. Orally administered nifedipine and verapamil do not appear to pose teratogenic risks to fetuses exposed in the first trimester.[27] Although the numbers of treated patients are small, these data are reassuring, because women with hypertension associated with kidney disease or transplantation may be difficult to manage during pregnancy without calcium channel blockers. Maternal side effects include tachycardia, palpitations, peripheral edema, headaches, and facial flushing. Most investigators have focused on nifedipine, although there are at least case reports regarding nicardipine, isradipine, felodipine, and verapamil; amlodipine has not been studied in pregnancy. Long-acting nifedipine does not cause a detectable decrease in uterine blood flow and is commonly used in pregnancy. Short-acting nifedipine is not recommended, because it has been associated with an increased incidence of myocardial infarction and death in hypertensive (nonpregnant) patients with coronary artery disease. At least one emergency cesarean section has been required in a gravid patient following a dose of short-acting nifedipine. Administration of nifedipine capsules has been associated with maternal hypotension and fetal distress. Short-acting nifedipine capsules have been withdrawn in several countries, thus limiting choices for oral treatment of hypertension, particularly by midwives. One study has shown efficacy and increased safety in pregnant patients using long-acting oral nifedipine tablets instead of the short-acting formulations.[28] One concern about the use of calcium antagonists for BP control in preeclampsia is the concomitant use of magnesium sulfate to prevent seizures. Drug interactions between nifedipine and magnesium sulfate have been reported to cause neuromuscular blockade, myocardial depression, and circulatory collapse in some cases, although in practice these medications are commonly used together, and the absolute risk appears to be low.

Diuretics

Although diuretics are widely used in the treatment of nonpregnant hypertensive patients, obstetricians are reluctant to use diuretics, because of concern that they will interfere with the physiologic volume expansion of normal pregnancy. However, a meta-analysis of trials involving more than 7000 subjects suggested that diuretics prevented preeclampsia.[29] Although volume contraction could be expected to limit fetal growth, outcome data do not support these concerns. Diuretics are commonly prescribed in essential hypertension before conception, and, given the apparent safety of these drugs, NHBPEP concluded that they may be continued through gestation or used in combination with other agents.[1] Hydrochlorothiazide is used in low doses, no more than 25 mg daily, to minimize the side effects of impaired glucose tolerance and hypokalemia.[21] Triamterene and amiloride are not teratogenic, based on small numbers of case reports.[21] Spironolactone is not recommended, because of theoretical antiandrogenic effects during fetal development, although this was not borne out in an isolated case report. Mild volume contraction with diuretics may lead to hyperuricemia, and in so doing may invalidate serum uric acid levels as a laboratory marker for superimposed preeclampsia.

Direct Vasodilators

Hydralazine is effective orally, intramuscularly, or intravenously; parenteral administration is useful for rapid control of severe hypertension. Adverse effects are mostly those resulting from excessive vasodilation or sympathetic activation and include headache, nausea, flushing, and palpitations. In rare cases, long-term use can lead to a polyneuropathy or to a drug-induced lupus syndrome (typically with high doses).

Hydralazine has been used in all trimesters of pregnancy and has not been associated with teratogenicity, although neonatal thrombocytopenia and lupus have been reported. It has been used for chronic hypertension in the second and third trimesters, but it has been largely supplanted by agents with more favorable side effect profiles.[30] For acute severe hypertension later in pregnancy, intravenous hydralazine has been associated with more adverse effects than intravenous labetalol or oral nifedipine.[26] These adverse effects include maternal hypotension, cesarean sections, placental abruptions, Apgar scores lower than 7, and oliguria. Furthermore, the common side effects (headache, nausea, and vomiting) of hydralazine mimic the symptoms of deteriorating preeclampsia. Effects on uteroplacental blood flow are unclear.[31,32]

Nitroprusside is seldom used in pregnancy; use is limited to cases of cases of life-threatening refractory hypertension associated with heart failure. Adverse effects include vasodilation and syncope in volume-depleted preeclamptic women. The risk of fetal cyanide intoxication is unknown, but it is a grave concern. Given the long experience with hydralazine, parenteral labetalol, and oral calcium channel blockers, nitroprusside is considered a last resort.

Isosorbide dinitrate was investigated in a small study of gestational hypertensive and preeclamptic pregnant patients. It was found to lower BP, but not cerebral perfusion, thus decreasing the risk for ischemia and infarction.

Serotonin$_2$-Receptor Blockers

Ketanserin is a selective S_2-receptor-blocking drug that decreases systolic and diastolic BP in nonpregnant patients with acute or chronic hypertension. Ketanserin has been found to be nonteratogenic in animals and humans, and it has been studied primarily in Australia and South Africa in small trials. These studies suggest that the drug may be safe and useful in treatment of chronic hypertension in pregnancy, preeclampsia, and HELLP syndrome.[33] Ketanserin has not been approved by the FDA in the United States.

Angiotensin-Converting Enzyme Inhibitors and Angiotensin Receptor Antagonists

ACE inhibitors and angiotensin receptor blockers (ARBs) are contraindicated in the second or third trimesters because of toxicity associated with reduced perfusion of the fetal kidneys. The use of these agents is associated with a fetopathy similar to that observed in Potter's syndrome (i.e., bilateral renal agenesis) including renal dysgenesis, oligohydramnios as a result of fetal oliguria, calvarial and pulmonary hypoplasia, intrauterine growth retardation, and neonatal anuric renal failure leading to death of the fetus. ARB use in pregnancy has also caused fetal demise, amid the same pathogenic features.

The available evidence on first trimester exposure to ACE inhibitors demonstrated increased risk for malformations of the cardiovascular and central nervous systems.[33a] Whether adverse outcomes are the result of a hemodynamic effect in the fetus or of specific (nonhemodynamic) requirements for angiotensin II as a fetal growth factor is unknown. As such, first trimester drug exposure should be avoided. Because exposure to ACE inhibitors during the first trimester cannot be considered safe, it may be best to counsel women to switch to alternate agents while attempting to conceive.

PREECLAMPSIA

Clinical Features and Diagnosis

Preeclampsia is the development of hypertension in association with new-onset proteinuria (>0.3 g/day), edema, and serum uric acid concentration greater than 5.5 mg/dL (325 μmol/L) after 20 weeks' gestation. Edema alone has been abandoned as a marker of preeclampsia, because it is present in too many physiologically normal pregnant women to be specific. The American College of Obstetrics and Gynecology and the NHBPEP distinguish mild from severe preeclampsia. Features of severe preeclampsia include severe hypertension (BP >160/110 mm Hg on two occasions), eclampsia, pulmonary edema, cortical blindness, proteinuria greater than 5 g/24 hours, renal failure or oliguria (<500 mL/24 hours), hepatocellular injury (serum transaminase levels twice normal values or higher), thrombocytopenia (<100,000 platelets/mm^3), coagulopathy, or HELLP syndrome.[1] Previously part of the diagnostic criteria, but now abandoned, was the magnitude of increase in BP (≥30 mm Hg systolic BP or 15 mm Hg diastolic BP).

It is important to recognize which women are at increased risk for preeclampsia and to follow them more closely during pregnancy. Women at increased risk include those with chronic hypertension, those with early (<34 weeks' gestation) or severe preeclampsia in a previous pregnancy, and women with diabetes, collagen vascular disease, renovascular disease, renal parenchymal disease, or a multifetal pregnancy or who themselves were the product of a pregnancy complicated by preeclampsia (see Table 36-1). Such women need a baseline laboratory evaluation early in gestation. Recommended tests to discriminate preeclampsia from chronic or transient hypertension later in pregnancy include hematocrit, hemoglobin, platelet count, serum creatinine, and liver function tests. If qualitative dipstick proteinuria is documented, a 24-hour urine collection should be performed for protein content and creatinine clearance. An extensive literature describes clinical signs and laboratory tests to predict preeclampsia, but none of them are considered sensitive or specific enough to warrant widespread clinical application.

Prevention and Management

Strategies to prevent preeclampsia, including sodium restriction, diuretics, high-protein diets, fish oil, magnesium, low-dose aspirin, calcium supplementation, and antihypertensive medication, have all been unsuccessful. Aspirin is thought to reverse the imbalance between prostacyclin and thromboxane possibly responsible for some of the manifestations of the disease. A Cochrane analysis as well as a recently conducted single-patient meta-analysis (the PARIS collaboration) demonstrate a small but consistent benefit with the use of aspirin to prevent adverse maternal and fetal outcomes.[34]

Pathophysiology and Implications for Treatment

The pathophysiology of preeclampsia has been divided into two stages: alterations in placental perfusion and the maternal syndrome. Abnormalities begin in the developing placenta and lead to the production of vasculogenic substances, which, on reaching the maternal circulation, produce the maternal clinical syndrome.

Placenta

In a placenta destined for preeclampsia, the uterine artery invasion into the placenta is shallow, blood flow is diminished, and the ensuing placental ischemia early in the second trimester is thought to trigger the release of placenta-derived factors causing the multisystemic maternal disorder. The incidence of preeclampsia is increased in women with medical conditions associated with microvascular disease such as hypertension, diabetes, and collagen vascular disease, and the impaired placental perfusion may be the common starting point of this disease.

Angiogenic proteins such as placental growth factor (PlGF) and vascular endothelial growth factor (VEGF) are required for normal angiogenesis and endothelial function in pregnancy, and these factors are reduced in women with preeclampsia. Recent studies reported elevated maternal serum levels of a protein that, in preeclampsia, appears to scavenge these factors and to induce endothelial dysfunction: a soluble *fms*-like tyrosine kinase 1 (sFlt1). This molecule is a modified VEGF receptor that circulates and neutralizes VEGF and PlGF (Fig. 36-3). In human studies, decreased urinary PlGF in the second trimester is associated with the subsequent early development of preeclampsia.[35]

Maternal Syndrome

Blood Pressure

BP in preeclampsia is characteristically labile. It is elevated as the result of a reversal of the vasodilatation of normal pregnancy that is replaced by a marked increase in peripheral vascular resistance.[36] Reversal of the normal circadian rhythm also occurs, with BPs often higher at night.[37] This change is mediated, at least in part, by an increase in sympathetic vasoconstrictor activity that reverts to normal after delivery, thus lending mechanistic support for the use of methyldopa. Investigations of gravid dogs, rats, and primates have demonstrated that acute reduction of uterine perfusion results in maternal hypertension.[38] As mentioned, compromised uteroplacental perfusion is believed to be of pathophysiologic significance in the preeclampsia syndrome. Bed rest often ameliorates hypertension in pregnancy (particularly twin pregnancies); the likely mechanism is improvement in uteroplacental perfusion.

Metabolic Disturbances

Obesity remains an important risk factor for preeclampsia, with a strong positive association between maternal prepregnancy body mass index and the risk of preeclampsia. Early-pregnancy dyslipidemia and gestational diabetes are also associated with a two- to threefold increased risk of preeclampsia. These conditions may be markers of endothelial dysfunction, or they may cause increased oxidative stress in preeclampsia.

Renal Changes

In preeclampsia, patients have a decrease in filtration fraction that is usually modest (~25%). Because renal function normally rises 35% to 50% during pregnancy, serum creatinine

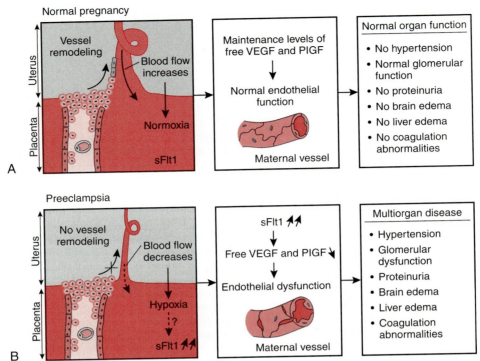

Figure 36–3   Hypothesis of the role of *fms*-like tyrosine kinase 1 (sFlt1) in preeclampsia. **A,** During normal pregnancy, the uterine spiral arteries are infiltrated and remodeled by endovascular invasive trophoblasts, thereby increasing blood flow significantly to meet the oxygen and nutrient demands of the fetus. **B,** In the placenta of preeclamptic women, trophoblast invasion does not occur and blood flow is reduced, resulting in placental hypoxia. In addition, increased amounts of soluble sFlt1 are produced by the placenta and scavenge vascular endothelial growth factor (VEGF) and placental growth factor (PlGF), thereby lowering circulating levels of unbound VEGF and PlGF. This altered balance causes generalized endothelial dysfunction and results in multiorgan disease. It remains unknown whether hypoxia is the trigger for stimulating sFlt1 secretion in the placenta of preeclamptic mothers and whether the higher sFlt1 levels interfere with trophoblast invasion and spiral artery remodeling. (From Serreze DV, Leiter EH. Tracking autoimmune T cells in diabetes. *J Clin Invest.* 2003;**111**:600-602.)

levels are usually still lower than the upper limits of normal. Fractional uric acid clearance decreases, often before overt disease is apparent, and a serum uric acid concentration greater than 5.5 mg/dL (327 μmol/L) is an important marker of preeclampsia, presumably because of decreased renal clearance and glomerular filtration. Proteinuria of less than 3 g/day (but in some cases in the nephrotic range, i.e., >3 g/day) is a hallmark. Rarely, renal insufficiency may result from acute tubular or cortical necrosis associated with eclampsia or preeclampsia.

Cardiac Function
Pulmonary artery catheterization studies of nulliparous gravid women with preeclampsia in the third trimester showed decreased cardiac output in preeclamptic patients compared with control subjects.[36,39] Peripheral vascular resistance is typically increased, and pulmonary capillary wedge pressure is in the low-normal range. Essentially, a normal ventricle contracts normally against a markedly increased afterload.[40] Peripartum heart failure can occur in this setting, although it is usually a complication of preexisting heart disease.

Plasma volume is increased in normal pregnancy. In preeclampsia, however, plasma volume is decreased, and the renin-angiotensin system is suppressed. Thus, the decreased plasma volume results from vasoconstriction and a "smaller" intravascular compartment.

Central Nervous System
Eclampsia, defined as seizures in preeclampsia that cannot be attributed another cause, is the most common central nervous system complication of pregnancy and is responsible for the greatest number of maternal deaths. Seizures may occur when the BP is only mildly elevated. These seizures are often preceded by headache (in ~64%) and visual changes (in ~32%) including blurred vision, scotomas, and reversible cortical blindness (from reversible posterior leukoencephalopathy).[41] In these cases, computed tomography and magnetic resonance imaging studies show extensive bilateral white matter abnormalities suggestive of vasogenic edema, without infarction, in the occipital and posterior parietal lobes of the cerebral hemispheres.

Treatment
One of the most difficult management issues in preeclampsia is the timing of delivery when fetal maturity is questionable. If preeclampsia occurs at a time remote from term (23 to 32 weeks' gestation), bed rest and close monitoring of the maternal and fetal conditions may allow prolongation of pregnancy and may improve maternal and fetal outcomes. There must be no evidence of fetal distress and no indication of serious maternal disease (headache, abdominal pain, signs of HELLP syndrome).[42,43] Most patients with preeclampsia,

however, present close to term and are managed by obstetricians with bed rest with or without hospitalization, use of antihypertensive medication, and urgent delivery, followed or preceded by seizure prophylaxis with magnesium sulfate. In the latter half of pregnancy, when early signs are detected in the office (new elevation of BP to ≥140/90 mm Hg, new dipstick proteinuria ≥1+), hospitalization should be considered, to permit close monitoring of the patient.

The primary role of the internal medicine consultant in the care of women with preeclampsia is to participate in decisions regarding antihypertensive therapy. Lowering BP does not cure preeclampsia, but it may permit prolongation of pregnancy, because uncontrolled hypertension is frequently an indication for delivery. Before delivery and even afterward, BP can remain dangerously high and be labile for days. The main reason to lower BP in a woman with preeclampsia is to prevent maternal cerebrovascular and cardiovascular complications of hypertension. The consensus is that severe hypertension, defined as BP greater than 160/110 mm Hg, requires treatment because these women are at increased risk of intracerebral hemorrhage, and lowering BP leads to a decrease in maternal death.[1,44] Women with hypertensive encephalopathy, hemorrhage, or eclampsia (seizures) require treatment with parenteral agents to lower mean arterial pressure (two thirds diastolic and one third systolic BP) by 25% over minutes to hours and then to lower BP further to 160/100 mm Hg or less over subsequent hours.[1] In women with preeclampsia, treatment of acute severe hypertension should be initiated at lower doses, because these patients may have intravascular volume contraction and are at increased risk for hypotension (Table 36-3). If delivery is not anticipated immediately (within 24 to 48 hours), antihypertensive therapy should be considered when diastolic BP reaches 105 mm Hg; in this instance, oral agents are appropriate.

Maternal factors that may signal the time for delivery in preeclampsia include gestational age greater than 38 weeks, platelet count lower than $100 \times 10^3/mm^3$, progressive deterioration in liver or renal function, suspected abruptio placentae, and uncontrolled severe hypertension, despite medication. Fetal factors include fetal growth restriction, nonreassuring fetal testing results, and oligohydramnios.

Renal function in preeclampsia is usually well preserved, and oliguria is usually a manifestation of renal vasoconstriction, rather than impaired glomerular filtration rate. It is not advisable to "push fluids" to increase urine output, because aggressive hydration of women with preeclampsia may result in acute pulmonary edema. Appropriate hydration should be maintained (100 to 150 mL/hour), however. In the setting of hypertension, when the serum creatinine level is close to normal, decreased urinary output will usually resolve within 24 hours of delivery and will not be associated with acute tubular necrosis.

In the postpartum period, edema may worsen because of administration of intravenous fluids during surgery or delivery. Moreover, hypertension may be worse in the first postpartum week, and it tends to peak by the fifth postpartum day. On occasion, it may be necessary to administer small doses of diuretics when edema becomes marked. Antihypertensive therapy should be combined with intravenous magnesium sulfate in the postpartum period, because magnesium sulfate is the anticonvulsant of choice to prevent eclamptic seizures.

The HELLP syndrome is associated with a poor prognosis and is usually an indication for urgent delivery. Women with liver involvement may develop epigastric or right upper quadrant pain from hepatocellular necrosis, ischemia, or edema that stretches the Glisson capsule. Elevations in liver enzymes are noted. Hepatic rupture is a fatal complication of preeclampsia if it is not recognized early and treated aggressively with supportive therapy and surgery. The consultant should recognize the potential severity of the development of epigastric, chest, or abdominal pain in a woman with preeclampsia.

Table 36-3   Drugs for Urgent Control of Severe Hypertension in Pregnancy[*]

Drug (FDA Risk[†])	Dose and Route	Concerns or Comments[‡]
Labetalol (C)	20 mg IV, then 20-80 mg every 20-30 min, up to maximum of 300 mg; or constant infusion of 1-2 mg/min	Less risk of tachycardia and arrhythmia than with other vasodilators
Hydralazine (C)	5 mg IV or IM, then 5-10 mg every 20-40 min; or constant infusion of 0.5-10 mg/hr	Long experience of safety and efficacy
Nifedipine (C)	Tablets recommended only: 10-30 mg PO	No longer thought to interact synergistically with magnesium sulfate
Relatively Contraindicated		
Nitroprusside (C[§])	Constant infusion of 0.5-10 µg/kg/min	Possible cyanide toxicity; agent of last resort

[*]Indicated for acute elevation of diastolic blood pressure ≥105 mm Hg; the goal is gradual reduction to 90-100 mm Hg.
[†]U.S. Food and Drug Administration (FDA) classification. C indicates that studies in animals revealed adverse effects on the fetus (teratogenic, embryocidal, or other), no controlled studies were conducted in women, or studies in women and animals are not available. Drugs should be given only if the potential benefits justify the potential risk to the fetus.
[‡]Adverse effects for all agents, except as noted, may include headache flushing, nausea, and tachycardia (primarily from precipitous hypotension and reflex sympathetic activation).
[§]We would classify this in category D. There is positive evidence of human fetal risk, but the benefits of use in pregnant women may be acceptable despite the risk (e.g., if the drug is needed in a life-threatening situation or for a serious disease for which safer drugs cannot be used or are ineffective).
IM, intramuscularly; IV, intravenously; PO, per os, orally.

POSTPARTUM COUNSELING AND FOLLOW-UP

Hypertension frequently persists after delivery in women with antenatal hypertension or preeclampsia, and BP may be labile in the days post partum. BP may increase even more if patients are treated with nonsteroidal anti-inflammatory drugs. The goal of treatment is to prevent severe hypertension, and oral antihypertensive treatment given antenatally should be reordered post partum and then discontinued in days to weeks, after the BP normalizes. If BP was normal before conception, then normalization is likely after 2 to 8 weeks. Hypertension that persists beyond 12 weeks post partum may represent previously undiagnosed chronic hypertension or secondary hypertension, which should be evaluated, followed, and treated (as appropriate) (see Fig. 36-2).

Evaluation should also be considered post partum for patients with preeclampsia who developed the condition early (<34 weeks' gestation), who had severe or recurrent preeclampsia, or who have persistent proteinuria. In these cases, renal disease, secondary hypertension, and thrombophilias (e.g., factor V Leiden) may be considered.

Counseling for future pregnancies requires consideration of different recurrence rates for preeclampsia, depending on the pathogenesis and population characteristics. The earlier in gestation that preeclampsia occurred, the higher the risk of recurrence is; before week 30, recurrence rates may be as high as 40%.[45] If preeclampsia has developed in a nulliparous woman close to term (i.e., >36 weeks), the risk of recurrence is thought to be about 10%. Women who have had preeclampsia are also at increased risk for hypertension in future pregnancies.[46] Patients who had HELLP syndrome have a high risk of subsequent obstetric complications, with preeclampsia occurring in 55%, although the rate of recurrent HELLP appears to be low, at only 6%.[43]

Hypertensive diseases of pregnancy have been associated with an elevated risk of hypertension and stroke later in life. In one study, gestational hypertension was associated with a relative risk of 3.72 for subsequent hypertension, and preeclampsia was associated with a relative risk of 3.98 for subsequent hypertension and of 3.59 for stroke.[30] When studied retrospectively, preeclampsia is also a risk factor for coronary disease.[47] These associations may serve to increase awareness of the need to monitor for future hypertensive and cardiovascular disorders.

Antihypertensive Medications and Lactation

In general, drugs that are bound to plasma proteins are not transferred to breast milk. Lipid-soluble drugs may achieve higher concentrations than water-soluble drugs. Neonatal exposures to methyldopa, labetalol, captopril, and nifedipine through nursing are low, and these medications are considered safe during breast-feeding.[48] Atenolol and metoprolol are concentrated in breast milk, possibly to levels that could affect the infant, and they are not recommended. Finally, although the concentration of diuretics in breast milk is low, these agents may reduce milk production because of mild volume contraction and may interfere with the ability to breast-feed successfully.

SUMMARY

Hypertensive disorders in pregnancy are associated with increased maternal and perinatal risks. Preeclampsia-eclampsia (regardless of BP level) and severe hypertension (regardless of type) are associated with the greatest risks. Although it is clear that severe hypertension must be treated to avoid cerebrovascular catastrophes in the mother, the benefits and risks of treating mild to moderate hypertension are less clearly supported. Large studies are required to determine the best BP targets for prevention of preeclampsia in this population. Until more data are available, mild to moderate hypertension may be treated at levels 150/90 mm Hg or higher with various agents that are safe in pregnancy. The ACE inhibitors and ARBs are contraindicated in late pregnancy because of adverse fetal effects. Severe hypertension exceeding 160/110 mm Hg in the setting of preeclampsia may require parenteral therapy, and treatment with intravenous labetalol has supplanted the use of hydralazine. Early or severe preeclampsia warrants an evaluation for secondary causes of hypertension. Women may remain hypertensive post partum and may require treatment for a short interval. Pregnancy-induced hypertension and preeclampsia are emerging as risk factors for future cardiovascular disease.

References

1. Report of the National High Blood Pressure Education Program Working Group on High Blood Pressure in Pregnancy. *Am J Obstet Gynecol.* 2000;**183**:S1-S22.
2. Samadi AR, Mayberry RM, Zaidi AA, et al. Maternal hypertension and associated pregnancy complications among African-American and other women in the United States. *Obstet Gynecol.* 1996;**87**:557-563.
3. Sibai BM. Antihypertensive drugs during pregnancy. *Semin Perinatol.* 2001;**25**:159-164.
4. Higgins JR, de Swiet M. Blood-pressure measurement and classification in pregnancy. *Lancet.* 2001;**357**:131-135.
5. Sibai BM. Diagnosis, controversies, and management of the syndrome of hemolysis, elevated liver enzymes, and low platelet count. *Obstet Gynecol.* 2004;**103**:981-991.
6. Bellomo G, Narducci PL, Rondoni F, et al. Prognostic value of 24-hour blood pressure in pregnancy. *JAMA.* 1999;**282**: 1447-1452.
7. Schenker JG, Chowers I. Pheochromocytoma and pregnancy: Review of 89 cases. *Obstet Gynecol Surv.* 1971;**26**:739-747.
8. Rey E, Couturier A. The prognosis of pregnancy in women with chronic hypertension. *Am J Obstet Gynecol.* 1994;**171**: 410-416.
9. Dunlop JC. Chronic hypertension and perinatal mortality. *Proc R Soc Med.* 1966;**59**:838-841.
10. Chang J, Elam-Evans LD, Berg CJ, et al. Pregnancy-related mortality surveillance: United States, 1991-1999. *MMWR CDC Surveill Summ.* 2003;**52**:1-8.
11. Jones DC, Hayslett JP. Outcome of pregnancy in women with moderate or severe renal insufficiency. *N Engl J Med.* 1996;**335**:226-232.
12. Brown MA, Buddle ML. Hypertension in pregnancy: Maternal and fetal outcomes according to laboratory and clinical features. *Med J Aust.* 1996;**165**:360-365.
13. Mabie WC, Pernoll ML, Biswas MK. Chronic hypertension in pregnancy. *Obstet Gynecol.* 1986;**67**:197-205.
14. Podymow T, August P. Pregnancy and gender issues in the renal transplant recipient. *In:* Weir M (ed.) Medical Management of

Kidney Transplantation. Philadelphia: Lippincott Williams & Wilkins, 2005 pp.238-243.

15. Higgins JR, Walshe JJ, Conroy RM, Darling MR. The relation between maternal work, ambulatory blood pressure, and pregnancy hypertension. *J Epidemiol Commun Health.* 2002;**56**:389-393.

16. Abalos E, Duley L, Steyn DW, Henderson-Smart DJ. Antihypertensive drug therapy for mild to moderate hypertension during pregnancy. *Cochrane Database Syst Rev.* 2001:CD002252.

17. Magee LA, Ornstein MP, von Dadelszen P. Fortnightly review: Management of hypertension in pregnancy. *BMJ.* 1999;**318**:1332-1336.

18. von Dadelszen P, Ornstein MP, Bull SB, et al. Fall in mean arterial pressure and fetal growth restriction in pregnancy hypertension: A meta-analysis. *Lancet.* 2000;**355**:87-92.

19. Helewa ME, Burrows RF, Smith J, et al. Report of the Canadian Hypertension Society Consensus Conference: Part 1. Definitions, evaluation and classification of hypertensive disorders in pregnancy. *Can Med Assoc J.* 1997;**157**:715-725.

20. Brown MA, Hague WM, Higgins J, et al. The detection, investigation and management of hypertension in pregnancy: Full consensus statement. *Aust N Z J Obstet Gynaecol.* 2000;**40**:139-155.

21. Magee LA. Drugs in pregnancy: Antihypertensives. *Best Pract Res Clin Obstet Gynaecol.* 2001;**15**:827-845.

22. Teratology Society Public Affairs Committee. FDA classification of drugs for teratogenic risk. *Teratology.* 1994;**49**:446-447.

23. Lip GY, Beevers M, Churchill D, et al. Effect of atenolol on birth weight. *Am J Cardiol.* 1997;**79**:1436-1438.

24. Magee LA, Elran E, Bull SB, et al. Risks and benefits of beta-receptor blockers for pregnancy hypertension: Overview of the randomized trials. *Eur J Obstet Gynecol Reprod Biol.* 2000;**88**:15-26.

25. Reynolds B, Butters L, Evans J, et al. First year of life after the use of atenolol in pregnancy associated hypertension. *Arch Dis Child* 1984;**59**:1061-1063.

26. Magee LA, Cham C, Waterman EJ, et al. Hydralazine for treatment of severe hypertension in pregnancy: Meta-analysis. *BMJ.* 2003;**327**:955-960.

27. Magee LA, Schick B, Donnenfeld AE, et al. The safety of calcium channel blockers in human pregnancy: A prospective, multicenter cohort study. *Am J Obstet Gynecol.* 1996;**174**:823-828.

28. Brown MA, Buddle ML, Farrell T, Davis GK. Efficacy and safety of nifedipine tablets for the acute treatment of severe hypertension in pregnancy. *Am J Obstet Gynecol.* 2002;**187**:1046-1050.

29. Collins R, Yusuf S, Peto R. Overview of randomised trials of diuretics in pregnancy. *BMJ Clin Res Ed.* 1985;**290**:17-23.

30. Wilson BJ, Watson MS, Prescott GJ, et al. Hypertensive diseases of pregnancy and risk of hypertension and stroke in later life: Results from cohort study. *BMJ.* 2003;**326**:845.

31. Fenakel K, Fenakel G, Appelman Z, et al. Nifedipine in the treatment of severe preeclampsia. *Obstet Gynecol.* 1991;**77**:331-337.

32. Vink GJ, Moodley J, Philpott RH. Effect of dihydralazine on the fetus in the treatment of maternal hypertension. *Obstet Gynecol.* 1980;**55**:519-522.

33. Bolte AC, van Geijn HP, Dekker GA. Pharmacological treatment of severe hypertension in pregnancy and the role of serotonin(2)-receptor blockers. *Eur J Obstet Gynecol Reprod Biol.* 2001;**95**:22-36.

33a. Cooper WO, Hernandez-Diaz S, Arbogast PG, et al. Major congenital malformations after first-trimester exposure to ACE inhibitors. *N Engl J Med.* 2006;**354**:2443-2451.

34. Duley L, Henderson-Smart DJ, Knight M, King JF. Antiplatelet agents for preventing pre-eclampsia and its complications. *Cochrane Database Syst Rev.* 2004:CD004659.

35. Levine RJ, Thadhani R, Qian C, et al. Urinary placental growth factor and risk of preeclampsia. *JAMA.* 2005;**293**:77-85.

36. Visser W, Wallenburg HC. Central hemodynamic observations in untreated preeclamptic patients. *Hypertension.* 1991;**17**:1072-1077.

37. Ayala DE, Hermida RC, Mojon A, et al. Circadian blood pressure variability in healthy and complicated pregnancies. *Hypertension.* 1997;**30**:603-610.

38. Venuto T, Lindheimer M. Animal models. *In:* Lindheimer M, Roberts J, Cunningham F (eds). Chesley's Hypertensive Disorders in Pregnancy. Stamford, Conn: Appleton & Lange, 1999, pp 487-517.

39. Groenendijk R, Trimbos JB, Wallenburg HC. Hemodynamic measurements in preeclampsia: Preliminary observations. *Am J Obstet Gynecol.* 1984;**150**:232-236.

40. Lang RM, Pridjian G, Feldman T, et al. Left ventricular mechanics in preeclampsia. *Am Heart J.* 1991;**121**:1768-1775.

41. Katz VL, Farmer R, Kuller JA. Preeclampsia into eclampsia: Toward a new paradigm. *Am J Obstet Gynecol.* 2000;**182**:1389-1396.

42. Sibai BM, Mercer BM, Schiff E, Friedman SA. Aggressive versus expectant management of severe preeclampsia at 28 to 32 weeks' gestation: A randomized controlled trial. *Am J Obstet Gynecol.* 1994;**171**:818-822.

43. Chames MC, Haddad B, Barton JR, et al. Subsequent pregnancy outcome in women with a history of HELLP syndrome at < or = 28 weeks of gestation. *Am J Obstet Gynecol.* 2003;**188**:1504-1508.

44. Rey E, LeLorier J, Burgess E, et al. Report of the Canadian Hypertension Society Consensus Conference: Part 3. Pharmacologic treatment of hypertensive disorders in pregnancy. *Can Med Assoc J.* 1997;**157**:1245-1254.

45. Sibai BM, Mercer B, Sarinoglu C. Severe preeclampsia in the second trimester: Recurrence risk and long-term prognosis. *Am J Obstet Gynecol.* 1991;**165**:1408-1412.

46. Chesley L. Hypertensive Disorders in Pregnancy. New York: Appleton-Century-Crofts, 1978.

47. Haukkamaa L, Salminen M, Laivuori H, et al. Risk for subsequent coronary artery disease after preeclampsia. *Am J Cardiol.* 2004;**93**:805-808.

48. Beardmore KS, Morris JM, Gallery ED. Excretion of antihypertensive medication into human breast milk: A systematic review. *Hypertens Pregnancy.* 2002;**21**:85-95.

Chapter 37

Hypertension in Children and Adolescents

Bonita Falkner

Hypertension may occur at any phase of childhood, from the newborn period through adolescence. The earlier understanding of hypertension in the pediatric age range was that hypertension was rare, usually caused by underlying renal disease. However, this perspective is now changing. The cardiovascular literature generally regards hypertension in children and adolescents as a "special population" problem that should be approached as a unique issue. Compared with hypertension in adults, childhood hypertension is defined differently and occurs less frequently. The diagnosis of hypertension requires blood pressure (BP) measurements, systolic and diastolic, that are consistently equal to or higher than the 95th percentile for age, sex, and height.[1] With this statistical definition, it is expected that the prevalence of hypertension would be 1% to 5%. As more attention is given to evaluating the BP level in children during routine health care visits, and as a result of the rising rates of childhood obesity, more cases of hypertension in the young are being identified. Secondary causes of hypertension are detected more frequently in children than in adults, a finding indicating a different approach in evaluation of the hypertension. Nonetheless, childhood hypertension has some striking similarities to hypertension in adults. Severe untreated hypertension in children has as poor an outcome as it does in adults.[2] Children with essential hypertension can express the same risk factors for cardiovascular disease as adults, and children with hypertension can benefit from interventions to control BP. An important aspect in the management of high BP in the young is to determine when elevated BP is a sign of an underlying disease, as with secondary hypertension, and when elevated BP in childhood is an early expression of primary (essential) hypertension.

DEFINITION OF HYPERTENSION IN CHILDHOOD

The definition of hypertension in adults is based on the level of BP that is linked with an increase in risk for cardiovascular events. Although the risk for cardiovascular events increases as systolic BP rises to more than 120 mm Hg,[3] hypertension continues to be defined as BP that equals or exceeds 140/90 mm Hg, regardless of adult age or gender. However, in children, with the exception of extreme hypertension noted earlier, data do not yet link a particular level of BP with subsequent cardiovascular events. In the absence of such data, hypertension is defined statistically. The results of several large epidemiologic studies that measured BP in healthy children[1,4-8] provide data from which the normal distribution of BP in children and adolescents in the United States has been established.[5] An analysis of BP data from healthy children in Europe describes a very similar BP distribution pattern in childhood.[9,10]

A progressive rise in the BP level occurs with increasing age throughout childhood. The increase in BP level with increasing age is concurrent with the normal age-related increase in height and weight throughout childhood. Thus, there is a consistent relationship of BP with body size in childhood, as well as a normal upward shift in BP with growth. A gender difference in BP distribution emerges in adolescence that is concurrent with a gender difference in height.

The current definition of hypertension in children and adolescents is systolic or diastolic BP that, on repeated measurement, is equal to or greater than the 95th percentile for age, sex, and height.[1,4,6] The severity of hypertension is now staged. Stage 1 hypertension is systolic or diastolic BP that is between the 95th percentile and 5 mm Hg higher than the 99th percentile. Stage 2 hypertension is average systolic or diastolic BP that is greater than 5 mm Hg higher than the 99th percentile for age, sex, and height. Prehypertension in children is defined as systolic or diastolic BP that is between the 90th and 95th percentile for age, sex, and height. Because the BP level at the 90th percentile is greater than 120/80 mm Hg in some taller adolescents, a BP level that is greater than 120/80 mm Hg but less than the 95th percentile is considered prehypertension in adolescents. Normal BP is systolic and diastolic BP that is less than the 90th percentile for age, sex, and height. Table 37-1 provides the level of BP for the 90th, 95th, and 99th percentiles for age, sex, and height percentile for boys, and Table 37-2 provides the same percentile levels for girls.[1] In each table, the 50th percentile for systolic and diastolic BP is also provided to denote the midpoint of the BP distribution.

Hypertension can also occur in newborn infants. Data on normal levels of BP in newborns and very young infants are limited.[7,8,11] When daily BP measurements in healthy newborns are examined, a rapid and consistent increase in BP occurs from the day of birth through the first 5 days of life.[12] This upward shift in BP over a few days reflects the normal hemodynamic transition from intrauterine to extrauterine life. Similar observations were made in a larger study on newborn infants that included a broad range of birth weights and gestational ages.[13] There is a direct relationship of BP with both birth weight and gestational age at birth. Regardless of birth weight or gestational age at birth, a transition occurs, reflected by a progressive increase in BP that occurs during the first 5 days of postnatal life. Subsequently, BP is directly related to body weight and age, in terms of gestation or postconceptional age. The upper 95% confidence limit (CL) for a term infant (40 weeks postconceptional age) is 90 mm Hg for systolic BP. BP levels that exceed 90 mm Hg are considered to be hypertensive in a term infant, and by 4 to 6 weeks of age (44 to 46 weeks postconceptional age), systolic BP that exceeds 100 mm Hg is hypertension.

MEASUREMENT OF BLOOD PRESSURE IN THE YOUNG

Measurement of BP in children and adolescents should be performed in a standardized manner that is similar to the methods used in the development of the BP tables. In an ambulatory clinic setting, the preferred method for BP measurement in children is by auscultation with a standard sphygmomanometer.

Correct BP measurement in children requires the use of a cuff that is appropriate for the size of the child's upper arm.[14] A technique that can be used to select a BP cuff of appropriate size is to select a cuff that has a bladder width that is approximately 40% of the arm circumference midway between the olecranon and the acromion. This will usually be a cuff bladder that covers 80% to 100% of the circumference of the arm. Most manufacturers of BP cuffs provide lines on the cuff that are useful in choosing the correct cuff size for a given child. The equipment necessary to measure BP in children 3 years of age through adolescence includes three pediatric cuffs of different sizes, as well as a standard adult cuff, an oversized cuff, and a thigh cuff for leg BP measurements. The latter two cuffs may be needed for obese adolescents.

BP measurement in children should be conducted in a quiet and comfortable environment after 3 to 5 minutes of rest. With the exception of acute illness, BP should be measured with the child in the seated position with the cubital fossa supported at heart level. It is preferable that the child has her or his feet on the floor while the BP is measured, rather than having the feet dangling from an examination table. Overinflation of the cuff should be avoided because of discomfort, particularly in younger children. The BP should be measured and recorded at least twice on each measurement occasion.

Systolic BP is determined by the onset of the auscultated pulsation or first Korotkoff sound. The disappearance of Korotkoff sounds or fifth Korotkoff sound (K_5) is the definition of diastolic pressure in adults. In children, particularly preadolescents, a difference of several millimeters of mercury is frequently present between the fourth Korotkoff sound, the muffling of Korotkoff sounds (K_4), and K_5.[15] A substantial body of normative BP data in children indicates that K_5 can be used as the measure of diastolic BP in children as well as in adults.

The measured BP level in a child is interpreted by comparing the child's BP with the BP tables. Precise interpretation requires plotting the BP according to the child's height percentile as well as to age and sex. The child's height is measured and plotted on the standard child growth curves. The height percentile is used in the tables, wherein the BP level for the 90th and 95th percentile at the child's age, sex, and height percentile are compared with the child's measured BP.

Elevated BP measurements in a child or adolescent must be confirmed on repeated visits before the patient is characterized as having hypertension. A more accurate characterization of an individual's BP level is an average of multiple BP measurements taken for weeks or months. A notable exception to this general guideline for asymptomatic, generally well children would be situations in which the child is symptomatic or has profoundly elevated BP. There continues to be an increase in the use of automated devices to measure BP in children. Situations in which use of an automated devices is acceptable include BP measurement in newborn and young infants in whom auscultation is difficult, as well as in an intensive care setting, where frequent BP measurement is necessary. The reliability of these instruments in an ambulatory clinical setting is less clear because of the need for frequent calibration of the instruments and the current lack of established reference standards.

Ambulatory BP monitoring (ABPM) for 24 hours has become increasingly used in the evaluation of adults with hypertension.[16] Some population standards for ambulatory BP values in children and adolescents are now available,[17] and in some situations this information can be quite helpful.[18] The devices for 24-hour ABPM can be used in older children and adolescents in the evaluation of hypertension. ABPM can be used to detect white-coat hypertension, to determine the need for pharmacologic therapy, and to assess the effectiveness of therapeutic interventions. When ABPM is used in children or adolescents, the appropriate cuff size should be used, and the appropriate childhood BP cut-points should be used for interpretation of the results.

CAUSES OF HYPERTENSION IN THE YOUNG

Secondary Hypertension

Underlying causes of hypertension, or secondary hypertension resulting from underlying renal or endocrine disorders, occur more frequently during childhood than in adults. Before the development of normative data on BP levels in children, BP was measured infrequently. When elevated BP was detected in children, the hypertension was, by current standards, quite severe. Because secondary hypertension is generally characterized by marked BP elevation, this led to the belief that hypertension in children was *always* secondary. This concept has now changed, largely because of better understanding of normal levels of BP in the young and the practice of measuring the BP regularly in children as part of health assessment and health maintenance. The prevalence of secondary hypertension in the young varies according to the age and severity of hypertension. Hanna and colleagues identified a secondary cause of hypertensive in 90% of children who were less than 10 years of age, and only 10% of these young children were considered to have essential hypertension.[19] A report on a series that included both children and adolescents with hypertension describes secondary hypertension in 65% of the adolescents and essential hypertension in 35% of the adolescents.[20]

Young children, less than 12 years of age, with sustained hypertension are more likely to have a secondary cause for the hypertension. The degree of hypertension is also an important clue, because severe BP elevation in a young child is most likely to result from an underlying abnormality. Children and adolescents with stage 2 hypertension should have a careful evaluation for a possible cause of the hypertension and also for evidence of target organ damage from the hypertension. Although the list of conditions that can cause hypertension in the young is quite long, most of the identifiable causes of hypertension in the young are related to renal disorders. Table 37-3 provides a list of underlying causes for chronic

text continued on page 446.

Table 37-1 Blood Pressure Levels for Boys by Age and Height Percentile

Age (Year)	BP Percentile →	Systolic BP (mm Hg) ← Percentile of Height →							Diastolic BP (mm Hg) ← Percentile of Height →						
		5th	10th	25th	50th	75th	90th	95th	5th	10th	25th	50th	75th	90th	95th
1	50th	80	81	83	85	87	88	89	34	35	36	37	38	39	39
	90th	94	95	97	99	100	102	103	49	50	51	52	53	53	54
	95th	98	99	101	103	104	106	106	54	54	55	56	57	58	58
	99th	105	106	108	110	112	113	114	61	62	63	64	65	66	66
2	50th	84	85	87	88	90	92	92	39	40	41	42	43	44	44
	90th	97	99	100	102	104	105	106	54	55	56	57	58	58	59
	95th	101	102	104	106	108	109	110	59	59	60	61	62	63	63
	99th	109	110	111	113	115	117	117	66	67	68	69	70	71	71
3	50th	86	87	89	91	93	94	95	44	44	45	46	47	48	48
	90th	100	101	103	105	107	108	109	59	59	60	61	62	63	63
	95th	104	105	107	109	110	112	113	63	63	64	65	66	67	67
	99th	111	112	114	116	118	119	120	71	71	72	73	74	75	75
4	50th	88	89	91	93	95	96	97	47	48	49	50	51	51	52
	90th	102	103	105	107	109	110	111	62	63	64	65	66	66	67
	95th	106	107	109	111	112	114	115	66	67	68	69	70	71	71
	99th	113	114	116	118	120	121	122	74	75	76	77	78	78	79
5	50th	90	91	93	95	96	98	98	50	51	52	53	54	55	55
	90th	104	105	106	108	110	111	112	65	66	67	68	69	69	70
	95th	108	109	110	112	114	115	116	69	70	71	72	73	74	74
	99th	115	116	118	120	121	123	123	77	78	79	80	81	81	82
6	50th	91	92	94	96	98	99	100	53	53	54	55	56	57	57
	90th	105	106	108	110	111	113	113	68	68	69	70	71	72	72
	95th	109	110	112	114	115	117	117	72	72	73	74	75	76	76
	99th	116	117	119	121	123	124	125	80	80	81	82	83	84	84
7	50th	92	94	95	97	99	100	101	55	55	56	57	58	59	59
	90th	106	107	109	111	113	114	115	70	70	71	72	73	74	74
	95th	110	111	113	115	117	118	119	74	74	75	76	77	78	78
	99th	117	118	120	122	124	125	126	82	82	83	84	85	86	86
8	50th	94	95	97	99	100	102	102	56	57	58	59	60	60	61
	90th	107	109	110	112	114	115	116	71	72	72	73	74	75	76
	95th	111	112	114	116	118	119	120	75	76	77	78	79	79	80
	99th	119	120	122	123	125	127	127	83	84	85	86	87	87	88
9	50th	95	96	98	100	102	103	104	57	58	59	60	61	61	62
	90th	109	110	112	114	115	117	118	72	73	74	75	76	76	77
	95th	113	114	116	118	119	121	121	76	77	78	79	80	81	81
	99th	120	121	123	125	127	128	129	84	85	86	87	88	88	89
10	50th	97	98	100	102	103	105	106	58	59	60	61	61	62	63
	90th	111	112	114	115	117	119	119	73	73	74	75	76	77	78
	95th	115	116	117	119	121	122	123	77	78	79	80	81	81	82
	99th	122	123	125	127	128	130	130	85	86	86	88	88	89	90

Table 37-1 Blood Pressure Levels for Boys by Age and Height Percentile—cont'd

Age (Year)	BP Percentile	Systolic BP (mm Hg) ← Percentile of Height →							Diastolic BP (mm Hg) ← Percentile of Height →						
		5th	10th	25th	50th	75th	90th	95th	5th	10th	25th	50th	75th	90th	95th
11	50th	99	100	102	104	105	107	107	59	59	60	61	62	63	63
	90th	113	114	115	117	119	120	121	74	74	75	76	77	78	78
	95th	117	118	119	121	123	124	125	78	78	79	80	81	82	82
	99th	124	125	127	129	130	132	132	86	86	87	88	89	90	90
12	50th	101	102	104	106	108	109	110	59	60	61	62	63	63	64
	90th	115	116	118	120	121	123	123	74	75	75	76	77	78	79
	95th	119	120	122	123	125	127	127	78	79	80	81	82	82	83
	99th	126	127	129	131	133	134	135	86	87	88	89	90	90	91
13	50th	104	105	106	108	110	111	112	60	60	61	62	63	64	64
	90th	117	118	120	122	124	125	126	75	75	76	77	78	79	79
	95th	121	122	124	126	128	129	130	79	79	80	81	82	83	83
	99th	128	130	131	133	135	136	137	87	87	88	89	90	91	91
14	50th	106	107	109	111	113	114	115	60	61	62	63	64	65	65
	90th	120	121	123	125	126	128	128	75	76	77	78	79	79	80
	95th	124	125	127	128	130	132	132	80	80	81	82	83	84	84
	99th	131	132	134	136	138	139	140	87	88	89	90	91	92	92
15	50th	109	110	112	113	115	117	117	61	62	63	64	65	66	66
	90th	122	124	125	127	129	130	131	76	77	78	79	80	80	81
	95th	126	127	129	131	133	134	135	81	81	82	83	84	85	85
	99th	134	135	136	138	140	142	142	88	89	90	91	92	93	93
16	50th	111	112	114	116	118	119	120	63	63	64	65	66	67	67
	90th	125	126	128	130	131	133	134	78	78	79	80	81	82	82
	95th	129	130	132	134	135	137	137	82	83	83	84	85	86	87
	99th	136	137	139	141	143	144	145	90	90	91	92	93	94	94
17	50th	114	115	116	118	120	121	122	65	66	66	67	68	69	70
	90th	127	128	130	132	134	135	136	80	80	81	82	83	84	84
	95th	131	132	134	136	138	139	140	84	85	86	87	87	88	89
	99th	139	140	141	143	145	146	147	92	93	93	94	95	96	97

BP, blood pressure.
From Fourth Report on the Diagnosis, Evaluation, and Treatment of High Blood Pressure in Children and Adolescents. US Department of Health and Human Services, National Institutes of Health, National Heart, Lung, and Blood Institute. NIH Publication No. 95-5267, originally printed September 1996 (96-3790), revised May 2005.

Table 37-2 Blood Pressure Levels for Girls by Age and Height Percentile

Age (Year)	BP Percentile	Systolic BP (mm Hg) ← Percentile of Height →							Diastolic BP (mm Hg) ← Percentile of Height →						
		5th	10th	25th	50th	75th	90th	95th	5th	10th	25th	50th	75th	90th	95th
1	50th	83	84	85	86	88	89	90	38	39	39	40	41	41	42
	90th	97	97	98	100	101	102	103	52	53	53	54	55	55	56
	95th	100	101	102	104	105	106	107	56	57	57	58	59	59	60
	99th	108	108	109	111	112	113	114	64	64	65	65	66	67	67
2	50th	85	85	87	88	89	91	91	43	44	44	45	46	46	47
	90th	98	99	100	101	103	104	105	57	58	58	59	60	61	61
	95th	102	103	104	105	107	108	109	61	62	62	63	64	65	65
	99th	109	110	111	112	114	115	116	69	69	70	70	71	72	72
3	50th	86	87	88	89	91	92	93	47	48	48	49	50	50	51
	90th	100	100	102	103	104	106	106	61	62	62	63	64	64	65
	95th	104	104	105	107	108	109	110	65	66	66	67	68	68	69
	99th	111	111	113	114	115	116	117	73	73	74	74	75	76	76
4	50th	88	88	90	91	92	94	94	50	50	51	52	52	53	54
	90th	101	102	103	104	106	107	108	64	64	65	66	67	67	68
	95th	105	106	107	108	110	111	112	68	68	69	70	71	71	72
	99th	112	113	114	115	117	118	119	76	76	76	77	78	79	79
5	50th	89	90	91	93	94	95	96	52	53	53	54	55	55	56
	90th	103	103	105	106	107	109	109	66	67	67	68	69	69	70
	95th	107	107	108	110	111	112	113	70	71	71	72	73	73	74
	99th	114	114	116	117	118	120	120	78	78	79	79	80	81	81
6	50th	91	92	93	94	96	97	98	54	54	55	56	56	57	58
	90th	104	105	106	108	109	110	111	68	68	69	70	70	71	72
	95th	108	109	110	111	113	114	115	72	72	73	74	74	75	76
	99th	115	116	117	119	120	121	122	80	80	80	81	82	83	83
7	50th	93	93	95	96	97	99	99	55	56	56	57	58	58	59
	90th	106	107	108	109	111	112	113	69	70	70	71	72	72	73
	95th	110	111	112	113	115	116	116	73	74	74	75	76	76	77
	99th	117	118	119	120	122	123	124	81	81	82	82	83	84	84
8	50th	95	95	96	98	99	100	101	57	57	57	58	59	60	60
	90th	108	109	110	111	113	114	114	71	71	71	72	74	74	74
	95th	112	112	114	115	116	118	118	75	75	75	76	78	78	78
	99th	119	120	121	122	123	125	125	82	82	83	83	84	86	86
9	50th	96	97	98	100	101	102	103	58	58	58	59	60	61	61
	90th	110	110	112	113	114	116	116	72	72	72	73	74	75	75
	95th	114	114	115	117	118	119	120	76	76	76	77	78	79	79
	99th	121	121	123	124	125	127	127	83	83	84	84	85	86	87
10	50th	98	99	100	102	103	104	105	59	59	59	60	61	61	62
	90th	112	112	114	115	116	118	118	73	73	73	74	75	75	75
	95th	116	116	117	119	120	121	122	77	77	77	78	79	79	80
	99th	123	123	125	126	127	129	129	84	84	85	86	86	87	88

Table 37-2 Blood Pressure Levels for Girls by Age and Height Percentile—cont'd

Age (Year)	BP Percentile →	Systolic BP (mm Hg) ← Percentile of Height →							Diastolic BP (mm Hg) ← Percentile of Height →						
		5th	10th	25th	50th	75th	90th	95th	5th	10th	25th	50th	75th	90th	95th
11	50th	100	101	102	103	105	106	107	60	60	60	61	62	63	63
	90th	114	114	116	117	118	119	120	74	74	74	75	76	77	77
	95th	118	118	119	121	122	123	124	78	78	78	79	80	81	81
	99th	125	125	126	128	129	130	131	85	85	86	87	87	88	89
12	50th	102	103	104	105	107	108	109	61	61	61	62	63	64	64
	90th	116	116	117	119	120	121	122	75	75	75	76	77	78	78
	95th	119	120	121	123	124	125	126	79	79	79	80	81	82	82
	99th	127	127	128	130	131	132	133	86	86	87	88	88	89	90
13	50th	104	105	106	107	109	110	110	62	62	62	63	64	65	65
	90th	117	118	119	121	122	123	124	76	76	76	77	78	79	79
	95th	121	122	123	124	126	127	128	80	80	80	81	82	83	83
	99th	128	129	130	132	133	134	135	87	87	88	89	89	90	91
14	50th	106	106	107	109	110	111	112	63	63	63	64	65	66	66
	90th	119	120	121	122	124	125	125	77	77	77	78	79	80	80
	95th	123	123	125	126	127	129	129	81	81	81	82	83	84	84
	99th	130	131	132	133	135	136	136	88	88	88	89	90	91	92
15	50th	107	108	109	110	111	113	113	64	64	64	65	66	67	67
	90th	120	121	122	123	125	126	127	78	78	78	79	80	81	81
	95th	124	125	126	127	129	130	131	82	82	82	83	84	85	85
	99th	131	132	133	134	136	137	138	89	89	90	91	91	92	93
16	50th	108	108	110	111	112	114	114	64	64	65	66	66	67	68
	90th	121	122	123	124	126	127	128	78	78	79	80	81	81	82
	95th	125	126	127	128	130	131	132	82	82	83	84	85	85	86
	99th	132	133	134	135	137	138	139	90	90	90	91	92	93	93
17	50th	108	109	110	111	113	114	115	64	65	65	66	67	67	68
	90th	122	122	123	125	126	127	128	78	79	79	80	81	81	82
	95th	125	126	127	129	130	131	132	82	82	83	84	85	85	86
	99th	133	133	134	136	137	138	139	90	90	91	91	92	93	93

BP, blood pressure.
From Fourth Report on the Diagnosis, Evaluation, and Treatment of High Blood Pressure in Children and Adolescents. US Department of Health and Human Services, National Institutes of Health, National Heart, Lung, and Blood Institute. NIH Publication No. 95-5267, originally printed September 1996 (96-3790), revised May 2005.

Table 37-3 Secondary Causes of Hypertension

Chronic Hypertension

Renal Disorders
Chronic glomerulonephritis
Interstitial nephritis
Collagen vascular diseases
Reflux nephropathy
Polycystic kidney disease
Medullary cystic disease
Hydronephrosis
Hypoplastic/dysplastic kidney

Cardiac and Vascular Disorders
Coarctation of the aorta
Renal artery stenosis
Takayasu's arteritis

Endocrine Disorders
Hyperthyroidism
Pheochromocytoma
Primary aldosteronism

Drugs
Corticosteroids
Alcohol
Appetite suppressants
Anabolic steroids
Oral contraceptive
Nicotine

Syndromes
Alport's syndrome
Williams' syndrome (renovascular lesions)
Turner's syndrome (coarctation or renovascular)
Tuberous sclerosis (cystic renal)
Neurofibromatosis (renovascular)
Adrenogenital syndromes
Little's syndrome

Acute Hypertension

Renal Disorders
Post infectious glomerulonephritis
Schönlein-Henoch purpura
Hemolytic uremic syndrome
Acute tubular necrosis

Vascular Disorders
Renal or renal vascular trauma

Neurogenic Disorders
Increased intracranial pressure
Guillain-Barré syndrome

Drugs
Cocaine
Phencyclidine
Amphetamines
Jimson weed

Miscellaneous Causes
Burns
Orthopedic surgery
Urologic surgery

hypertension in the young, as well as the conditions associated with acute hypertension in this age group.

Hypertension is uncommon in healthy newborn infants. However, certain infants have conditions that increase the risk for hypertension. Some newborn infants require treatment in intensive care units where umbilical artery catheterization may be required for vascular access. Umbilical artery catheters carry a risk for thromboembolic events.[21,22] Low birth weight infants, with respiratory distress syndrome, can progress to bronchopulmonary dysplasia and can develop sodium retention from long-term steroid therapy.[23] The most commonly identified causes of hypertension in the newborn infant are renal artery thrombosis, renal artery stenosis, congenital renal malformations, coarctation of the aorta, and bronchopulmonary dysplasia.[5] In some critically ill newborn infants with hypertension, an underlying cause may not be identified. Regardless of whether a cause for the hypertension is determined, BP control and monitoring in these infants are important.

For children up to 10 years of age, the leading causes of hypertension are renal parenchymal diseases, coarctation of the aorta, and renal artery stenosis. Coarctation of the aorta, a congenital cardiac anomaly that can be missed in infants and toddlers, should be considered in a hypertensive child.[24-26] In later childhood, essential hypertension can also be detected. The disorders that cause acute hypertension include post-infectious glomerulonephritis and hemolytic uremic syn-

drome. Some conditions such as hemolytic uremic syndrome may cause permanent renal scarring that results in chronic hypertension.

During the adolescent years, the most common cause of hypertension is essential hypertension. The secondary causes of hypertension that are detected most frequently in adolescents are renal parenchymal diseases, such as chronic pyelonephritis, focal segmental glomerulosclerosis, and other types of chronic glomerulonephritis. Adolescent behaviors that may contribute to high BP are illicit substance use, especially use of cocaine and amphetamine-related compounds.[27,28] Other substances that have been associated with high BP in adolescents include appetite suppressants (both prescription and over-the-counter remedies), oral contraceptives, excessive alcohol intake, and anabolic steroids used for body building.[29]

Essential Hypertension

Essential hypertension has classically been considered a disorder of older adults. The concept that essential hypertension has its roots in childhood can be inferred from BP tracking data, which demonstrate that children with elevated BPs will continue to have elevated BPs as adults.[6] Classic risk factors for hypertension such as overweight and a positive family history of hypertension or cardiovascular disease may be present in childhood. The combination of higher BP and typical risk factors had been indicative of risk for future hypertension. More recent reports indicate, however, that this condition is more than a risk for future problems. Using echocardiography, and appropriate childhood reference values for cardiac structure, left ventricular hypertrophy has been reported in 30% to 40% of children and adolescents with hypertension.[30,31] Longitudinal data are now becoming available that demonstrate a direct link between risk factors in childhood, including BP levels, with evidence of target organ injury, including greater intima-media thickness of carotid arteries.[30,32,33] Essential hypertension in childhood should be considered an early phase of a chronic disease.

Children and adolescents with essential hypertension generally demonstrate several clinical characteristics or associated risk factors. The degree of BP elevation is generally mild, approximating the 95th percentile, and one often sees considerable variability in BP over time. Laboratory and observational studies have demonstrated a marked cardiovascular response to stress, characterized by large heart rate and BP responses to stimuli.[34-37] A consistent clinical observation in children exhibiting mild essential hypertension is a positive history of hypertension in parents or grandparents.[34,38,39]

In both children and adults, greater body weight and increases in body weight correlate with higher BP.[40,41] Essential hypertension in children is frequently associated with obesity, which appears to be a contributory factor because even a modest reduction in excess adiposity is associated with a reduction in BP.[42,43] The cluster of mild BP elevation, a positive family history of hypertension, and obesity is a typical pattern in children and adolescents with essential hypertension.[44]

Currently, the prevalence of childhood obesity is increasing,[45] and it has more than doubled since the mid-1980s.[46] An analysis of two separate sets of data from the National Health and Nutrition Examination Survey also demonstrated a small but statistically significant increase in childhood BP levels. The increase in BPs is largely the result of the concurrent increase in obesity.[47] Obesity has an adverse effect on risk for cardiovascular disease and warrants attention for prevention and health promotion. In a study by Daniels and colleagues, all adolescents with echocardiographic criteria for left ventricular hypertrophy who had mild BP elevations were obese.[31] Rocchini and associates demonstrated augmented BP sensitivity to sodium intake in obese adolescents and a significant dampening in the BP response to sodium following weight reduction.[42,43]

Since the mid-1980s, the literature on hypertension and cardiovascular disease in adults has focused on the overlap of hypertension, non–insulin-dependent diabetes mellitus, atherosclerosis, and obesity. This constellation within individuals and within populations has been described as the insulin resistance syndrome or the metabolic syndrome.[48-50] Children as well as adults may exhibit characteristics of the metabolic syndrome.[43,51-53] Some investigators have detected the metabolic syndrome in nonobese children of hypertensive parents,[54,55] a finding indicating an hereditary component to the syndrome. The characteristics of the metabolic syndrome are also congruent with a strong family history of hypertension or early heart disease in the overweight child. These children often have high BP.[56] Although these children are not at risk for immediate adverse effects of the higher than normal BP, they should be considered at risk for future cardiovascular

disease.[57] These children can benefit from health behavior changes that improve insulin action, including an increase in physical activity, diet modifications, and control of excess adiposity.

The cause of essential hypertension is believed to be multifactorial and the outcome of an interplay of genetic and environmental factors. Barker and colleagues proposed an alternative cause of hypertension based on observations of an association of hypertension and ischemic heart disease in adults with a low recorded birth weight.[58] These investigators proposed that lower birth weight reflects alteration in the intrauterine nutritional environment. Impaired fetal growth affects an alteration in organ structure and impairment in organ function in later life.[58,59] Higher BP is the putative link between compromised intrauterine growth and the long-term risk for cardiovascular disease.[58] Despite such reports, based on retrospective data, which support the low birth weight–high BP hypothesis,[58-61] this concept is in conflict with the body of data in childhood, as well as adulthood, that consistently demonstrates a direct relationship between body weight and BP,[62-65] as well as BP tracking in childhood.[38,66-71] Several clinical studies' cohorts have not detected a significant correlation.[64,65,72] When the body of reports on the association of birth weight with future BP is examined, the effect of birth weight on future BP is in the range of 2 to 3 mm Hg systolic BP reduction for each 1-kg increase in birth weight. When the current child or adult weight is taken into consideration, the birth weight effect is minimal.[73] Although the birth weight hypothesis has some appeal, clinical investigations have not yet firmly demonstrated that birth weight has a substantial effect on future BP.

EVALUATION

When sustained hypertension is established in a child by repeated BP measurements that are at or above the 95th percentile, additional evaluation is needed. The extent of the diagnostic evaluation is determined by the type of hypertension that is suspected. When a secondary cause is considered, a more extensive evaluation may be necessary. On the other hand, when the patient's elevated BP is more likely to be an early expression of essential hypertension, a few diagnostic screening studies may be sufficient. Children or adolescents with severe hypertension, in particular very young children, generally have an identifiable underlying cause. As noted previously, the higher the BP and the younger the child, the more likely a secondary cause is present. Currently, the recommendations for evaluation of hypertension in children include (1) evaluation for an identifiable cause, (2) evaluation for co-morbidity, and (3) evaluation for target organ damage.[1]

The medical history and physical examination are keys in determining whether the characteristics of a patient's presentation indicate essential hypertension or reflect a secondary, potentially correctable, cause. A particular symptom complex revealed in the history or findings on physical examination may also prompt a thorough investigation. In these patients, the direction of the evaluation is dictated by the particular symptom or physical examination findings. Any pediatric patient who is hypertensive and is not growing normally should also undergo an evaluation for secondary causes. A sudden onset of elevated BP in a previously normotensive child should always prompt a search for secondary causes. Absence of a positive family history of hypertension should increase the level of suspicion for an underlying disorder.

Another set of findings characterizes children and adolescents with essential hypertension. These characteristics include slight to mild elevations in BP, a strong family history of essential hypertension, elevated resting heart rate, variable BP readings on repeated measurement, and obesity. If no other abnormalities are found on history or physical examination, these children will require less extensive evaluation for an underlying disorder than those in whom secondary causes are suspected. Alternatively, it is the children with early expression of essential hypertension who may have associated co-morbidities, particularly children who are obese. The associated co-morbidities include dyslipidemia, sleep apnea, and impaired fasting glucose.

Medical History

The medical history and physical examination are used to detect clues to determine whether the BP elevation is secondary or essential. It is also helpful to determine whether the hypertension is long standing or of acute onset. The family history is particularly important. In both first- and second-degree relatives, the family history of essential hypertension, myocardial infarction, stroke, renal disease, diabetes, and obesity should be obtained. It can be relevant to the diagnosis in a hypertensive child if relatives had an onset at an early age of any of the foregoing conditions. Parents should also be asked about conditions in family members that are inheritable and have hypertension as a component (e.g., polycystic kidney disease, neurofibromatosis, pheochromocytoma). Another familial type of hypertension is glucocorticoid-remediable aldosteronism, an autosomal dominant condition, which should be considered when multiple family members have early-onset hypertension associated with hypokalemia or stroke.[74,75]

It is important to obtain details about previous health problems such as history of urinary tract infections, because the patient may have associated reflux nephropathy, renal scarring, and resultant hypertension. A history of medications and over-the-counter products used also can be helpful.[76,77] Information should be obtained about health-related behaviors such as usual diet, amount of physical activity, and athletic participation. Other adverse adolescent lifestyles to consider are use of "street" drugs, smokeless tobacco, oral contraceptive pills, cigarettes, diet aids, ethanol, and anabolic steroids.

Physical Examination

The physical examination for a hypertensive child should be comprehensive. An assessment of the child's general growth rate and growth pattern should be done. Weight, height, and body mass index should be plotted according to age and sex on the child growth charts. Abnormalities in growth that are associated with hypertension can be seen in chronic renal disease, hyperthyroidism (causing primarily systolic hypertension), pheochromocytoma, adrenal disorders, and certain genetic abnormalities such as Turner's syndrome.

To rule out coarctation of the aorta, the evaluation of every child for hypertension should include upper and lower extremity BP measurements taken with appropriately sized cuffs. Normally, the leg BP levels are slightly higher than the arm BP levels. A child with coarctation will have systolic hypertension in an upper extremity, sometimes absent or decreased femoral pulses, and a BP differential greater than 10 mm Hg between the upper and lower extremities.[24,26]

Other physical examination clues may suggest a secondary cause of a child's hypertension.[78] Abnormal facies or dysmorphic features may suggest a specific syndrome, some of which are associated with specific lesions causing hypertension. For example, both Turner's and Williams syndromes are associated with renovascular or cardiac lesions that cause hypertension. Renovascular lesions may sometimes have an audible abdominal bruit detectable by auscultation of the abdomen. Skin lesions are sometimes the first manifestations of disorders such as tuberous sclerosis and systemic lupus erythematosus. Acanthosis nigricans in overweight children may be a sign of abnormal glucose tolerance.

Diagnostic Testing

When the history and physical examination provide clues to a specific underlying cause for the hypertension, such as an endocrine or cardiac disorder, testing should be directed to the area of clinical suspicion. Other important historical information such as a history of urinary tract infections may dictate studies to evaluate vesicoureteral reflux and renal scarring. In the absence of clues, however, renal parenchymal disease should be considered likely because this diagnosis is the most frequent cause of secondary hypertension in the pediatric population. The initial studies to screen for renal abnormalities include a full urinalysis, electrolytes, creatinine, complete blood count, urine culture, and renal ultrasound. An evaluation for the presence of co-morbidity includes fasting plasma lipids for dyslipidemia, a sleep history to screen for sleep apnea, and, if there is a positive family history of diabetes, possibly additional testing of glucose tolerance.

The other component of the evaluation includes an assessment of target organ injury. The presence of target organ injury provides a measure of chronicity and severity (characteristics sometimes difficult to ascertain from the history) and will aid in deciding whether pharmacologic therapy should be instituted. Echocardiography is a sensitive means to detect interventricular septal and posterior ventricular wall thickening.[79-82] In children, the echocardiographic measurements of left ventricular mass should be indexed to height (in meters) to the 2.7 power ($m^{2.7}$). Left ventricular hypertrophy is left ventricular mass/$m^{2.7}$ greater than 50 g.[1] Chest radiographs and electrocardiograms are much less sensitive measures of left ventricular hypertrophy in children. An ophthalmologic examination can also be helpful. In a study of 97 children and adolescents with essential hypertension, Daniels and associates found that 51% displayed retinal abnormalities.[83] The usefulness of microalbuminuria, sometimes recommended as a marker for renal injury or inflammation in adults,[84] has not been determined for children. The remainder of the evaluation should be directed by specific findings on history and physical examination, as well as results of initial screening studies.

An algorithm for the evaluation of hypertension in the young is provided in Figure 37-1. The algorithm indicates steps to be taken in the evaluation and management of hyper-

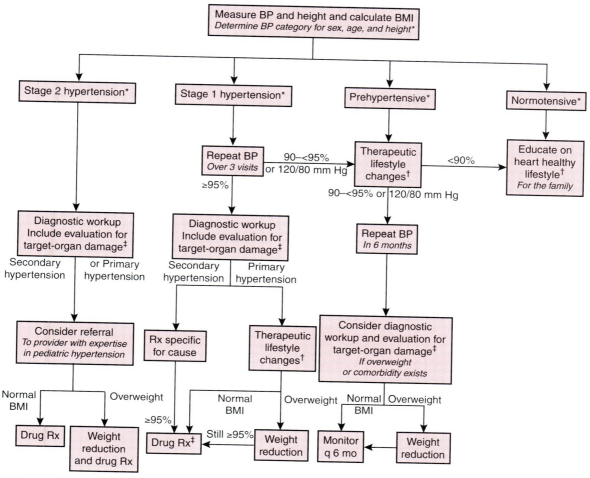

Figure 37-1 An algorithm is provided to guide the evaluation and management of prehypertension, stage 1 hypertension, and stage 2 hypertension. Children and adolescents with stage 1 and stage 2 hypertension should receive an echocardiogram to evaluate for target organ damage. BP, blood pressure; BMI, body mass index; Rx, treatment. *See Tables 37-1 and 37-2; †Diet and physical activity change; ‡Especially if very young and no risk factors.

tension in children according to the severity of the hypertension and the presence or absence of obesity.

TREATMENT

Health-related behavior changes in diet, physical activity, and weight control improve BP control in adults. Children may also benefit from these lifestyle changes. Children and adolescents with stage 1 or mild elevation of BP, and without target organ damage, should begin treatment with nonpharmacologic interventions including weight reduction or control, exercise, and diet modifications.

Obesity is often associated with mild hypertension in childhood, and weight reduction has benefit in obese children. Using a program of both behavior modification and parental involvement, Brownell and colleagues showed that weight loss in obese adolescents was associated with a significant decrease in BP.[85] Exercise training also lowers BP in both school aged children and adolescents.[86-88] Rocchini and colleagues showed that a program that included both caloric restriction and exercise produced a decrease in BP, as well as a reversal of structural changes in forearm resistance vessels.[42] Weight reduction

can be extremely difficult and generally requires multiple strategies that include the input of a nutritionist, dietary education, emotional support, information about exercise, and family involvement. Power weight lifting should be discouraged in hypertensive adolescents because of its potential to induce marked BP elevation. Participation in other sports should be encouraged as long as BP is under reasonable control, regular monitoring of BP occurs, and a thorough examination has been conducted to exclude cardiac conditions.[29]

The guidelines for dietary modifications in the pediatric population are less clear than in adults. Information on the effects of salt on BP in children is not as definitive as in adults. There does seem to be a subset of adolescents, particularly those who are obese, who demonstrate BP sensitivity to salt as well as other risk factors for hypertension.[43] Because the usual dietary intake of sodium for most children and adolescents in the United States far exceeds nutrient requirements, it is reasonable to restrict sodium intake to less than 4 g/day by decreasing fast-food consumption and refraining from adding salt to cooked foods.[89]

Current information on the effects of potassium and calcium intake on BP in children is even less definitive. Some reports suggest that a diet high in potassium and calcium may help to lower BP,[90] yet no study has definitively shown this effect in children or adolescents. The dietary intervention clinical trial, Dietary Approaches to Stop Hypertension (DASH), reported results that could be relevant to diet benefits in children. This study, which enrolled 459 adults with mild BP elevation (<160 mm Hg systolic, 80 to 95 mm Hg diastolic), demonstrated a significant reduction in both systolic and diastolic BP in subjects consuming a diet high in fruits, vegetables, and low-fat dairy products, compared with subjects consuming the usual diet. These results indicate that a benefit on BP occurs from diets that are high in potassium, calcium, magnesium, and other vitamins.[91] A similar approach may be of benefit for children, and investigations to examine this issue would be appropriate.

Pharmacologic therapy is indicated if nonpharmacologic approaches are unsuccessful or when a child is symptomatic, has severe hypertension, or target organ damage. Children with diabetes mellitus or chronic kidney disease may achieve renal protective benefits from BP reduction. For children with these disorders, it is reasonable to use pharmacologic therapy to lower BP to a level that is less than the 90th percentile for age, sex, and height.

Most of the medications used for adults can be used for children. However, efficacy data, as well as long-term safety data, are limited for the pediatric population. The choice of antihypertensive medication must be individualized and depends on the child's age, the cause of the hypertension, the degree of BP elevation, adverse effects, and concomitant medical conditions. In most patients, therapy is begun with a single agent. The dose is titrated upward until control of the BP is attained. BP control, in most instances, is defined as maintaining systolic and diastolic pressure lower than the 90th percentile. If control cannot be achieved using the maximum dose of a single agent, a second medication can be added, or, alternatively, another agent from a different class can be selected. The more commonly used medications for chronic antihypertensive therapy in children are listed in Table 37-4, and those for use in acute, hypertensive emergencies are shown in Table 37-5.[1] Currently, the dosage recommendations for children have been largely based on practitioners' experience, not on large, multicenter trials. Some clinical trial work is now being conducted on the medications that are already approved and prescribed for hypertension in adults. This information, as it becomes available, will provide more information on efficacy, safety, and dosage in children.

β-Adrenergic blockers, such as propranolol, metoprolol, and atenolol, are good choices in some nonasthmatic children, but these drugs may not be well tolerated by athletes in whom exercise capacity could be decreased. More frequently, first-line medications are either angiotensin-converting enzyme (ACE) inhibitors or calcium channel blockers (calcium antagonists or CCBs). ACE inhibitors rarely cause side effects (e.g., cough, rash, neutropenia) in children and are usually well tolerated, and many formulations have the advantage of once-a-day dosing. Not only are these agents effective in controlling BP, but they may also have beneficial effects on renal function, peripheral vasculature, and cardiac function.[92] Importantly, children with diabetes and those with chronic kidney disease may be at special risk for progressive renal deterioration and may benefit from ACE inhibitors.[93,94] Because of their vasodilator effects on the efferent arteriole, ACE inhibitors can severely reduce glomerular filtration and

should therefore be used with caution in patients with renal artery stenosis, a solitary kidney, or a transplanted kidney.[95] ACE inhibitors are contraindicated during pregnancy because of possible teratogenic effects on the lungs, kidneys, and brain of the fetus.[96] Therefore, these agents should be used with special caution in adolescent female patients who are or may be sexually active. Angiotensin receptor blockers (ARBs) also interact with the renin-angiotensin system and have benefits similar to those of ACE inhibitors. Some experience is now being developed with these agents in treatment of children with hypertension.

Several of the CCBs are used in children. In this age group, CCBs can be used as initial therapy or as the second or third medication when more than one drug is needed to control BP. As with most of the oral antihypertensive preparations, the appropriate dose for small children is often lower than the strength of available tablets, thus making initial dose determinations challenging. Both short-acting and longer-acting forms are available. Use of short-acting CCBs should be limited to children with acute hypertension, such as occurs in acute glomerulonephritis. When CCBs are needed for BP control in chronic hypertension, long-acting preparations are preferred, provided the correct dosage preparation can be used.

Diuretics are generally recommended as initial drug therapy for uncomplicated hypertension in adults, based on a vast amount of clinical trial data. No such information is available to guide recommendations for pharmacologic management of hypertension in children and adolescents. Unless clinical evidence indicates fluid retention in a hypertensive child, such as may occur when the elevated BP is related to long-term steroid use, diuretics are usually not the preferred first step in drug treatment. Although some hypertensive children achieve adequate BP control with a thiazide diuretic alone, most do not. Children receiving thiazide diuretics often develop hypokalemia and require potassium supplements. In addition, for children, taking the potassium supplements is extremely unpleasant. The necessity to take potassium supplements can lead to problems with adherence to the regimen. Although not favored as initial drugs to treat hypertension in children, low-dose diuretics can be very useful as second or third drugs in those children who require multiple drugs to achieve BP control.

SUMMARY

Essential, or primary, hypertension can occur in childhood. Because of the rising rates of childhood obesity, the expression of essential hypertension in childhood will increase. Despite this trend, the possibility of secondary hypertension should be considered in a child with documented hypertension. Children with suspected secondary hypertension may require a more extensive evaluation compared with children and adolescents expressing characteristics of essential hypertension. Whether the hypertension is determined to be secondary or essential, these children require careful monitoring, interventions to control the BP, and long-term follow up. Considering the long-term morbidity and mortality associated with essential hypertension, interventions, including preventive interventions, are needed that focus on BP control beginning in youth. Essential hypertension may encompass several distinct

Table 37-4 Antihypertensive Drugs for Outpatient Management of Hypertension in Children 1 to 17 Years Old*

Class	Drug	Dose†	Dosing Interval	Evidence‡	FDA labeling§	Comments¶
ACE inhibitor	Benazepril	Initial: 0.2 mg/kg/day up to 10 mg/day Maximum: 0.6 mg/kg/day up to 40 mg/day	qd	RCT	Yes	1. All ACE inhibitors are contraindicated in pregnancy—female patients of childbearing age should use reliable contraception.
	Captopril	Initial: 0.3-0.5 mg/kg/dose Maximum: 6 mg/kg/day	tid	RCT, CS	No	2. Check serum potassium and creatinine periodically to monitor for hyperkalemia and azotemia.
	Enalapril	Initial: 0.08 mg/kg/day up to 5 mg/day Maximum: 0.6 mg/kg/day up to 40 mg/day	qd-bid	RCT	Yes	3. Cough and angioedema are reportedly less common with newer members of this class than with captopril.
	Fosinopril	Children >50 kg: Initial: 5-10 mg/day Maximum: 40 mg/day	qd	RCT	Yes	4. Benazepril, enalapril, and lisinopril labels contain information on the preparation of a suspension; captopril may also be compounded into a suspension.
	Lisinopril	Initial: 0.07 mg/kg/day up to 5 mg/day Maximum: 0.6 mg/kg/day up to 40 mg/day	qd	RCT	Yes	5. FDA approval for ACE inhibitors with pediatric labeling is limited to children ≥6 yr of age and to children with creatinine clearance ≥30 mL/min/1.73m².
	Quinapril	Initial: 5-10 mg/day Maximum: 80 mg/day	qd	RCT, EO	No	
Angiotensin receptor blocker	Irbesartan	6-12 yr: 75-150 mg/day ≥13 yr: 150-300 mg/day	qd	CS	Yes	1. All ARBs are contraindicated in pregnancy—female patients of childbearing age should use reliable contraception.
	Losartan	Initial: 0.7 mg/kg/day up to 50 mg/day Maximum: 1.4 mg/kg/day up to 100 mg/day	qd	RCT	Yes	2. Check serum potassium, creatinine periodically to monitor for hyperkalemia and azotemia. 3. Losartan label contains information on the preparation of a suspension. 4. FDA approval for ARBs is limited to children ≥6 yr of age and to children with creatinine clearance ≥30 mL/min/1.73m².
α- and β-Blocker	Labetalol	Initial: 1-3 mg/kg/day Maximum: 10-12 mg/kg/day up to 1,200 mg/day	bid	CS, EO	No	1. Asthma and overt heart failure are contraindications. 2. Heart rate is dose-limiting. 3. May impair athletic performance. 4. Should not be used in insulin-dependent diabetic patients.

continued

Table 37-4 Antihypertensive Drugs for Outpatient Management of Hypertension in Children 1 to 17 Years Old*—cont'd

Class	Drug	Dose[†]	Dosing Interval	Evidence[‡]	FDA labeling[§]	Comments[¶]
β-Blocker	Atenolol	Initial: 0.5-1 mg/kg/day Maximum: 2 mg/kg/day up to 100 mg/day	qd-bid	CS	No	1. Noncardioselective agents (propranolol) are contraindicated in asthma and heart failure. 2. Heart rate is dose-limiting. 3. May impair athletic performance. 4. Should not be used in insulin-dependent diabetic patients. 5. A sustained-release formulation of propranolol is available that is given once daily.
	Bisoprolol/HCTZ	Initial: 2.5/6.25 mg/day Maximum: 10/6.25 mg/day	qd	RCT	No	
	Metoprolol	Initial: 1-2 mg/kg/day Maximum: 6 mg/kg/day up to 200 mg/day	bid	CS	No	
	Propranolol	Initial: 1-2 mg/kg/day Maximum: 4 mg/kg/day up to 640 mg/day	bid-tid	RCT, EO	Yes	
Calcium channel blocker	Amlodipine	Children 6-17 yr: 2.5-5 mg once daily	qd	RCT	Yes	1. Amlodipine and isradipine can be compounded into stable extemporaneous suspensions. 2. Felodipine and extended-release nifedipine tablets must be swallowed whole. 3. Isradipine is available in both immediate-release and sustained-release formulations; the sustained-release form is given qd or bid. 4. It may cause tachycardia.
	Felodipine	Initial: 2.5 mg/day Maximum: 10 mg/day	qd	RCT, EO	No	
	Isradipine	Initial: 0.15-0.2 mg/kg/day Maximum: 0.8 mg/kg/day up to 20 mg/day	tid-qid	CS, EO	No	
	Extended-release nifedipine	Initial: 0.25-0.5 mg/kg/day Maximum: 3 mg/kg/day up to 120 mg/day	qd-bid	CS, EO	No	
Central α-agonist	Clonidine	Children ≥12 yr: Initial: 0.2 mg/day Maximum: 2.4 mg/day	bid	EO	Yes	1. May cause dry mouth and/or sedation. 2. Transdermal preparation also available. 3. Sudden cessation of therapy can lead to severe rebound hypertension.
Diuretic	HCTZ	Initial: 1 mg/kg/day Maximum: 3 mg/kg/day up to 50 mg/day	qd	EO	Yes	1. All patients treated with diuretics should have electrolytes monitored shortly after initiating therapy and periodically thereafter. 2. Useful as add-on therapy in patients being treated with drugs from other drug classes. 3. Potassium-sparing diuretics (spironolactone, triamterene,
	Chlorthalidone	Initial: 0.3 mg/kg/day Maximum: 2 mg/kg/day up to 50 mg/day	qd	EO	No	

Table 37-4   Antihypertensive Drugs for Outpatient Management of Hypertension in Children 1 to 17 Years Old*—cont'd

Class	Drug	Dose†	Dosing Interval	Evidence‡	FDA labeling§	Comments¶
Diuretic —cont'd	Furosemide	Initial: 0.5-2.0 mg/kg/dose Maximum: 6 mg/kg/day	qd-bid	EO	No	amiloride) may cause severe hyperkalemia, especially if given with ACE inhibitor or ARB.
	Spironolactone	Initial: 1 mg/kg/day Maximum: 3.3 mg/kg/day up to 100 mg/day	qd-bid	EO	No	4. Furosemide is labeled only for treatment of edema but may be useful as add-on therapy in children with resistant hypertension, particularly in children with renal disease.
	Triamterene	Initial: 1-2 mg/kg/day Maximum: 3-4 mg/kg/day up to 300 mg/day	bid	EO	No	5. Chlorthalidone may precipitate azotemia in patients with renal diseases and should be used with caution in those with severe renal impairment.
	Amiloride	Initial: 0.4-0.625 mg/kg/day Maximum: 20 mg/day	qd	EO	No	
Peripheral α-antagonist	Doxazosin	Initial: 1 mg/day Maximum: 4 mg/day	qd	EO	No	May cause hypotension and syncope, especially after the first dose.
	Prazosin	Initial: 0.05-0.1 mg/kg/day Maximum: 0.5 mg/kg/day	tid	EO	No	
	Terazosin	Initial: 1 mg/day Maximum: 20 mg/day	qd	EO	No	
Vasodilator	Hydralazine	Initial: 0.75 mg/kg/day Maximum: 7.5 mg/kg/day up to 200 mg/day	qid	EO	Yes	1. Tachycardia and fluid retention are common side effects.
	Minoxidil	Children <12 yr: Initial: 0.2 mg/kg/day Maximum: 50 mg/day Children ≥12 yr: Initial: 5 mg/day Maximum: 100 mg/day	qd-tid	CS, EO	Yes	2. Hydralazine can cause a lupus-like syndrome in slow acetylators. 3. Prolonged use of minoxidil can cause hypertrichosis. 4. Minoxidil is usually reserved for patients with hypertension resistant to multiple drugs.

*Includes drugs with prior pediatric experience or recently completed clinical trials.
†The maximum recommended adult dose should not be exceeded in routine clinical practice.
‡Level of evidence on which dosing recommendations are based (CS, case series; EO, expert opinion; RCT, randomized controlled trial).
§Food and Drug Administration (FDA)–approved pediatric labeling information is available. Recommended doses for agents with FDA-approved pediatric labels are the doses contained in the approved labels. Even when pediatric labeling information is not available, the FDA-approved label should be consulted for additional safety information.
¶Comments apply to all members of each drug class except where otherwise stated.
ACE, angiotensin-converting enzyme; ARB, angiotensin-receptor blocker; bid, twice daily; HCTZ, hydrochlorothiazide; qd, once daily; qid, four times daily; tid, three times daily.
From Fourth Report on the Diagnosis, Evaluation, and Treatment of High Blood Pressure in Children and Adolescents. US Department of Health and Human Services, National Institutes of Health, National Heart, Lung, and Blood Institute. NIH Publication No. 95-5267, originally printed September 1996 (96-3790), revised May 2005.

Table 37-5 Antihypertensive Drugs for Management of Severe Hypertension in Children 1 to 17 Years Old

Most Useful*				
Drug	Class	Dose[†]	Route	Comments
Esmolol	β-Blocker	100-500 μg/kg/min	IV infusion	Very short acting—constant infusion preferred. May cause profound bradycardia. Produced modest reductions in BP in a pediatric clinical trial.
Hydralazine	Vasodilator	0.2-0.6 mg/kg/dose	IV, IM	Should be given every 4 hr when given by IV bolus. Recommended dose is lower than FDA label.
Labetalol	α- and β-Blocker	Bolus: 0.2-1.0 mg/kg/dose up to 40 mg/dose Infusion: 0.25-3.0 mg/kg/hr	IV bolus or infusion	Asthma and overt heart failure are relative contraindications.
Nicardipine	Calcium channel blocker	1-3 μg/kg/min	IV infusion	May cause reflex tachycardia.
Sodium nitroprusside	Vasodilator	0.53-10 μg/kg/min	IV infusion	Monitor cyanide levels with prolonged (>72 hr) use or in renal failure; or co-administer with sodium thiosulfate.

Occasionally Useful[‡]				
Drug	Class	Dose[†]	Route	Comments
Clonidine	Central α-agonist	0.05-0.1 mg/dose, may be repeated up to 0.8 mg total dose	PO	Side effects include dry mouth and sedation.
Enalaprilat	ACE inhibitor	0.05-0.1 mg/kg/dose up to 1.25 mg/dose	IV bolus	May cause prolonged hypotension and acute renal failure, especially in neonates.
Fenoldopam	Dopamine receptor agonist	0.2-0.8 μg/kg/min	IV infusion	Produced modest reductions in BP in a pediatric clinical trial in patients ≤12 yr.
Isradipine	Calcium channel blocker	0.05-0.1 mg/kg/dose	PO	Stable suspension can be compounded.
Minoxidil	Vasodilator	0.1-0.2 mg/kg/dose	PO	The most potent oral vasodilator; it is long acting.

*Useful for hypertensive emergencies and some hypertensive urgencies.
[†]All dosing recommendations are based on expert opinion or case series data except as otherwise noted.
[‡]Useful for hypertensive urgencies and some hypertensive emergencies.
ACE, angiotensin-converting enzyme; BP, blood pressure; FDA, Food and Drug Administration; IM, intramuscular; IV, intravenous; PO, oral.
From Fourth Report on the Diagnosis, Evaluation, and Treatment of High Blood Pressure in Children and Adolescents. US Department of Health and Human Services, National Institutes of Health, National Heart, Lung, and Blood Institute. NIH Publication No. 95-5267, originally printed September 1996 (96-3790), revised May 2005.

pathophysiologic entities, each with its own genetic basis and management approach. As new information develops, improved management strategies can be created for hypertension in young patients as well as in adults.

References

1. National High Blood Pressure Education Program Working Group on High Blood Pressure in Children and Adolescents. The Fourth Report on the Diagnosis, Evaluation and Treatment of High Blood Pressure in Children and Adolescents. *Pediatrics.* 2004;**114**:555-576.
2. Still JL, Cottom D. Severe hypertension in childhood. *Arch Dis Child.* 1967;**42**:34-39.
3. Chobanian AV, Bakris GL, Black HR, et al., and the National High Blood Pressure Education Program Coordinating Committee on Prevention, Detection, Evaluation and Treatment of High Blood Pressure. The Seventh Report of the Joint National Committee on Prevention, Detection, Evaluation, and Treatment of High Blood Pressure: The JNC 7 Report. *JAMA.* 2003;**289**:2560-2572.
4. National Heart, Lung, and Blood Institute. Report of the Task Force on Blood Pressure Control in Children. *Pediatrics.* 1977;**59**:797-820.
5. Task Force on Blood Pressure Control in Children. Report of the Second Task Force on Blood Pressure Control in Children, 1988. *Pediatrics.* 1987;**79**:1-25.
6. National High Blood Pressure Education Program Working Group Report on Hypertension Control in Children and Adolescents. The update on the 1987 Task Force Report on High Blood Pressure in Children and Adolescents: A Working Group Report from the National High Blood Pressure Education Program. *Pediatrics.* 1996;**98**:649-658.
7. de Swiet M, Fayers P, Shinebourne EA. Blood pressure survey in a population of newborn infants. *BMJ.* 1976;**2**:9-11.
8. Schachter J, Kuller LH, Perfetti C. Blood pressure during the first five years of life: Relation to ethnic group (black or white) and to parental hypertension. *Am J Epidemiol.* 1984;**119**:541-553.

9. Menghetti E, Virdis R, Strambi M, et al., on behalf of the Study Group on Hypertension of the Italian Society of Pediatrics. Blood pressure in childhood and adolescence: The Italian normal standards. *J Hypertens.* 1999;**17**:1363-1372.

10. Pall D, Katona E, Fulesdi B, et al. Blood pressure distribution in a Hungarian adolescent population: Comparison with normal values in the USA. *J Hypertens.* 2003;**21**:41-47.

11. Zinner SH, Rosner B, Oh WO. Significance of blood pressure in infancy. *Hypertension.* 1985;**7**:411-416.

12. Hulman S, Edwards R, Chen Y, et al. Blood pressure patterns in the first three days of life. *J Perinatol.* 1991;**11**:231-234.

13. Zubrow AB, Hulman S, Kushner H, Falkner B. Determinants of blood pressure in infants admitted to neonatal intensive care units: A prospective multicenter study. *J Perinatol.* 1995;**15**:470-479.

14. Prineas RJ, Elkwiry ZM. Epidemiology and measurement of high blood pressure in children and adolescents. *In:* Loggie JMH (ed): Pediatric and Adolescent Hypertension. Boston: Blackwell Scientific Publications, 1992, pp 91-103.

15. Sinaiko AR, Gomez-Martin O, Prineas RJ. Diastolic fourth and fifth phase blood pressure in 10-15 year old children: The Children and Adolescent Blood Pressure Program. *Am J Epidemiol.* 1990;**132**:647-655.

16. Townsend RR, Ford V. Ambulatory blood pressure monitoring: Coming of age in nephrology. *J Am Soc Nephrol.* 1996;**7**:2279-2287.

17. Soergel M, Kirschstein M, Busch C, et al. Oscillometric 24-hour ambulatory blood pressure values in healthy children and adolescents: A multicenter trial including 1141 subjects. *J Pediatr.* 1997;**130**:178-184.

18. Harshfield GA, Alpert BS, Pulliam DA, et al. Ambulatory blood pressure recordings in children and adolescents. *Pediatrics.* 1994;**94**:180-184.

19. Hanna JD, Chan JCM, Gill JR Jr. Hypertension and the kidney. *J Pediatr.* 1991;**118**:327-340.

20. Arar MY, Hogg RJ, Arant BS Jr, Seikaly MG. Etiology of sustained hypertension in children in the southwestern United States. *Pediatr Nephrol.* 1994;**8**:186-189.

21. Plumer LB, Kaplan GW, Mendoza SA. Hypertension in infants: A complication of umbilical arterial catheterization. *J Pediatr.* 1976;**89**:802-805.

22. Vailas GN, Brouillette RT, Scott JP, et al. Neonatal aortic thrombosis: Recent experience. *J Pediatr.* 1986;**109**:101-108.

23. Abman SH, Warady BA, Lum GM, Koops BL. Systemic hypertension in infants with bronchopulmonary dysplasia. *J Pediatr.* 1984;**104**:928-931.

24. Ing FF, Starc TJ, Griffiths SP, Gersony WM. Early diagnosis of coarctation of the aorta in children: A continuing dilemma. *Pediatrics.* 1996;**98**:378-382.

25. Stafford MA, Griffiths SP, Gersony WM. Coarctation of the aorta: A study in delayed detection. *Pediatrics.* 1982;**69**:159-163.

26. Thoele DG, Muster AJ, Paul MH. Recognition of coarctation of the aorta. *Am J Dis Child.* 1987;**141**:1201-1204.

27. Adelman RD. Smokeless tobacco and hypertension in an adolescent. *Pediatrics.* 1987;**79**:837-838.

28. Blachley JD, Knochel JP. Tobacco chewer's hypokalemia: Licorice revisited. *N Engl J Med.* 1980;**302**:784-785.

29. Committee on Sports Medicine and Fitness. Athletic participation by children and adolescents who have systemic hypertension. *Pediatrics.* 1997;**99**:637-638.

30. Sorof JM, Alexandrov AV, Dardwell G, Portman JR. Carotid artery intimal-medial thickness and left ventricular hypertrophy in children with elevated blood pressure. *Pediatrics.* 2003;**111**:61-66.

31. Daniels SR, Loggie JM, Hhoury P, Kimball TR. Left ventricular geometry and severe left ventricular hypertrophy in children and adolescents with essential hypertension. *Circulation.* 1998;**97**:1907-1911.

32. Li S, Chen W, Srinivasan SR, et al. Childhood cardiovascular risk factors and carotid vascular changes in adulthood: The Bogalusa Heart Study. *JAMA.* 2003;**290**:2271-2276.

33. Raitakari OT, Juonala M, Kahonen M, et al. Cardiovascular risk factors in childhood and carotid artery intima-media thickness in adulthood: The Cardiovascular Risk in Young Finns Study. *JAMA.* 2003;**290**:2277-2283.

34. Falkner B, Onesti G, Angelakos ET, et al. Cardiovascular response to mental stress in normal adolescents with hypertensive parents. *Hypertension.* 1979;**1**:23-30.

35. Warren P, Fischbein C. Identification of labile hypertension in children and hypertensive parents. *Conn Med.* 1980;**44**:77-79.

36. Matthews KA, Manuck SB, Saab PG. Cardiovascular responses of adolescents during a naturally occurring stressor and their behavioral and psychophysiological predictors. *Psychophysiology.* 1984;**23**:198-209.

37. Falkner B, Kushner H. Racial differences in stress induced reactivity in young adults. *Health Psychol.* 1989;**8**:613-617.

38. Shear CL, Burke GL, Freedman DS, Berenson GS. Value of childhood blood pressure measurements and family history in predicting future blood pressure status: Results from 8 years of follow-up in the Bogalusa Heart Study. *Pediatrics.* 1986;**77**:862-869.

39. Munger R, Prineas R, Gornez-Marin O. Persistent elevation of blood pressure among children with a family history of hypertension: The Minneapolis children's blood pressure study. *J Hypertens.* 1988;**6**:647-653.

40. Himes JH, Dietz WH. Guidelines for overweight in adolescent preventive services: Recommendations from an expert committee. *Am J Clin Nutr.* 1994;**59**:307-316.

41. Havlik R, Hubert H, Fabsity R, Feinleib M. Weight and hypertension. *Ann Intern Med.* 1983;**98** 855-859.

42. Rocchini AP, Katch V, Anderson J, et al. Blood pressure in obese adolescents: Effect of weight loss. *Pediatrics.* 1988;**82**:16-23.

43. Rocchini AP, Key J, Bondie D, et al. The effect of weight loss on the sensitivity of blood pressure to sodium in obese adolescents. *N Engl J Med.* 1989;**321**:580-585.

44. Sinaiko AR. Hypertension in children. *N Engl J Med.* 1996;**35**:1968-1973.

45. Troiano RP, Flegal KM, Kuczmarski RJ et al. Overweight prevalence and trends for children and adolescents. *Arch Pediatr Adolesc Med.* 1995;**149**:1085-1091.

46. Ogden CL, Flegal KM, Carroll MD, Johnson CL. Prevalence and trends in overweight among US children and adolescents, 1999-2000. *JAMA.* 2002;**288**:1728-1732.

47. Munter P, He J, Cutler JA, et al. Trends in blood pressure among children and adolescents. *JAMA.* 2004;**291**:2107-2113.

48. DeFronzo R, Tobin J, Andres R. Glucose clamp technique: A method for quantifying insulin secretion and resistance. *Am J Physiol.* 1979;**237**:E214-E223.

49. Ferrannini E, Buzzigoli G, Bonadonna R, et al. Insulin resistance in essential hypertension. *N Engl J Med.* 1987;**317**:350-357.

50. Reaven GM. Role of insulin resistance in human disease. *Diabetes.* 1988;**37**:1595-1607.

51. Berenson GS, Wattigney WA, Bao W, et al. Epidemiology of early primary hypertension and implication for prevention: The Bogalusa Heart Study. *J Hum Hypertens.* **8**:303-311.

52. Falkner B, Hulman S, Tannenbaum J, Kushner H. Insulin resistance and blood pressure in young Black men. *Hypertension.* 1990;**16**:706-711.

53. Cruz ML, Huang TTK, Johnson MS, et al. Insulin sensitivity and blood pressure in black and white children. *Hypertension.* 2002;**40**:18-22.

54. Ferrari P, Weidmann P, Shaw S, et al. Altered insulin sensitivity, hyperinsulinemia, and dyslipidemia in individuals with a hypertensive parent. *Am J Med.* 1991;**91**:589-596.

55. Grunfeld B, Balzareti M, Romo M, et al. Hyperinsulinemia in normotensive offspring of hypertensive parents. *Hypertension.* 1994;**23 (Suppl 1)**:12-15.

56. Sorof J, Daniels S. Obesity hypertension in children. *Hypertension.* 2002;**40**:441-455.

57. Bao W, Srinivasan SR, Wattigney WA, Berenson GS. Persistence of multiple cardiovascular risk clustering related to syndrome X from childhood to young adulthood. *Arch Intern Med.* 1994;**154**:1842-1847.

58. Barker DJP, Osmond C, Golding J, et al. Growth in utero, blood pressure in childhood and adult life, and mortality from cardiovascular disease. *BMJ.* 1989;**298**:564-567.

59. Law CM, Shiell AW. Is blood pressure inversely related to birth weight? The strength of evidence from a systematic review of the literature. *J Hypertens.* 1996;**14**:935-941.

60. Barker DJP, Gluckman PD, Godfrey KM, et al. Fetal nutrition and cardiovascular disease in adult life. *Lancet.* 1993;**341**: 938-941.

61. Osmond C, Barker DJP, Winter PD, et al. Early growth and death from cardiovascular disease in women. *BMJ.* 1993;**307**:1519-1524.

62. Harlan WR, Cornoni Huntley J, Leaverton PE. Blood pressure in childhood: National Health Examination Survey. *Hypertension.* 1979;**1**:566-571.

63. Katz SH, Hediger MC, Schall HI, et al. Blood pressure, growth and maturation from childhood to adolescence. *Hypertension.* 1980;**2 (Suppl 1)**:55-69.

64. Falkner B, Hulman S, Kushner H. Birth weight vs childhood growth as determinants of adult blood pressure. *Hypertension.* 1998;**31**:145-150.

65. Hulman S, Kushner H, Katz S, Falkner B. Can cardiovascular risk be predicted by newborn, childhood, and adolescent body size? An examination of longitudinal data in urban African Americans. *J Pediatr.* 1988;**132**:90-97.

66. Lauer RM, Clarke WR, Beaglehole R. Level, trend, and variability of blood pressure during childhood: The Muscatine Study. *Circulation.* 1984;**69**:242-249.

67. Michels V, Bergstralh E, Hoverman V, et al. Tracking and prediction of blood pressure in children. *Mayo Clin Proc.* 1987;**62**:875-881.

68. Julius S, Jamerson K, Mejia A, et al. The association of borderline hypertension with target organ changes and higher coronary risk: Tecumseh Blood Pressure Study. *JAMA.* 1990;**264**:354-358.

69. Mahoney LT, Clarke WR, Burns TL, Lauer RM. Childhood predictors of high blood pressure. *Am J Hypertens.* 1991;**4**: 608S-610S.

70. Nelson M, Ragland D, Syme S. Longitudinal prediction of adult blood pressure from juvenile blood pressure levels. *Am J Epidemiol.* 1992;**136**:633-645.

71. Lauer RM, Clarke WR, Maloney LT, Witt J. Childhood predictors for high adult blood pressure: The Muscatine Study. *Pediatr Clin North Am.* 1993;**40**:23-40.

72. Huxley R, Neil A, Collins R. Unraveling the fetal origins hypothesis: Is there really an inverse association between birthweight and subsequent blood pressure? *Lancet.* 2002;**360**:659-665.

73. Falkner B, Hulman, S, Kushner H. Effect of birth weight on blood pressure and body size in early adolescence. *Hypertension.* 2004;**43**:203-207.

74. Rich GM, Ulick S, Cook S, et al. Glucocorticoid-remediable aldosteronism in a large kindred: Clinical spectrum and diagnosis using a characteristic biochemical phenotype. *Ann Intern Med.* 1992;**116**:813-820.

75. Lifton RP, Dluhy RG, Powers M, et al. Hereditary hypertension caused by chimeric gene duplications and ectopic expression of aldosterone synthase. *Nat Genet.* 1992;**2**:66-74.

76. Kroenke K, Omori DM, Simmons JO, et al. The safety of phenylpropanolamine in patients with stable hypertension. *Ann Intern Med.* 1989;**111**:1043-1044.

77. Lake CR, Gallant S, Masson E, Miller P. Adverse drug effects attributed to phenylpropanolamine: A review of 142 case reports. *Am J Med.* 1990;**89**:195-208.

78. Hurley JK. A pediatrician's approach to the evaluation of hypertension. *Pediatr Ann.* 1989;**18**:542, 544-546, 548-549.

79. Laird WP, Fixler DE. Left ventricular hypertrophy in adolescents with elevated blood pressure: Assessment by chest roentgenography, electrocardiography and echocardiography. *Pediatrics.* 1981;**67**.255-259.

80. Shieken RM, Clark WR, Lauer RM. Left ventricular hypertrophy in children with blood pressures in the upper quintile of the distribution: The Muscatine Study. *Hypertension.* 1981;**3**:669-675.

81. Zahka KG, Neill CA, Kidd L, et al. Cardiac involvement in adolescent hypertension. *Hypertension.* 1981;**3**:664-668.

82. Culpepper WS, Sodt PC, Messerli FH, et al. Cardiac status in juvenile borderline hypertension. *Ann Intern Med.* 1983;**98**:1-7.

83. Daniels SR, Lipman MJ, Burke MJ, Loggie JM. The prevalence of retinal vascular abnormalities in children and adolescents with essential hypertension. *Am J Ophthalmol.* 1991;**111**: 205-208.

84. Yudkin JS, Forrest RD, Jackson CA. Microalbuminuria as predictor of vascular disease in non-diabetic subjects. *Lancet.* 1988;**2**:530-533.

85. Brownell KD, Kelman JH, Stunkard AJ. Treatment of obese children with and without their mothers: Changes in weight and blood pressure. *Pediatrics.* 1983;**71**.515-523.

86. Hagberg JM, Goldring D, Ehsani AA, et al. Effect of exercise training on the blood pressure and hemodynamic features of hypertensive adolescents. *Am J Cardiol.* 1983;**52**:763-768, 1983.

87. Hansen HS, Froberg K, Hyldebrandt N, Nielson JR. A controlled study of eight months of physical training and reduction of blood pressure in children: The Odense Schoolchild Study. *BMJ.* 1991;**303**:682-685.

88. Shea S, Basch CE, Gutin B, et al. The rate of increase in blood pressure in children 5 years of age is related to changes in aerobic fitness and body mass index. *Pediatrics.* 1994;**94**: 465-470.

89. Falkner B, Michel S. Blood pressure response to sodium in children and adolescents. *Am J Clin Nutr.* 1997;**65 (Suppl)**:618S-621S.

90. Sinaiko AR, Gomez-Marin O, Prineas RJ. Effect of low sodium diet or potassium supplementation on adolescent blood pressure. *Hypertension.* 1993;**21**:989-994.

91. Appel LJ, Moore TJ, Obarzanek B, et al., for the DASH Collaborative Research Group. A clinical trial of the effects of dietary patterns on blood pressure. *N Engl J Med.* 1997;**336**:1117-1124.

92. Doyle AK. Angiotensin-converting enzyme (ACE) inhibition: Benefits beyond blood pressure control. *Am J Med.* 1992;**92 (Suppl 4B)**:1S-107S.

93. Krolewski AS, Canessa M, Warram JH, et al. Predisposition to hypertension and susceptibility to renal disease in insulin-dependent diabetes mellitus. *N Engl J Med.* 1988;**318**:140-145.

94. National High Blood Pressure Education Program. Working Group Report on Hypertension and Diabetes. *Hypertension.* 1994;**23**:145-158.

95. Hricik DE, Dunn MJ. Angiotensin-converting enzyme inhibitor-induced renal failure: Causes, consequences, and diagnostic uses. *J Am Soc Nephrol.* 1990;**1**:845-858.

96. Pryde PG, Sedman AB, Nugent CE, Barr M. Angiotensin-converting enzyme inhibitor fetopathy. *J Am Soc Nephrol.* 1993;**3**:1575-1582.

Chapter 38

Hypertension in the Elderly

Michael J. Bloch and Jan N. Basile

EPIDEMIOLOGY

Elderly patients comprise the most rapidly growing segment of the U.S. population and account for the largest share of health care expenditures. In 1990, 13% of people in the United States were more than 65 years of age, and by the year 2040 that number is expected to grow to 20%.[1] Between 1999 and 2050, the number of people in the United States who are more than 85 years old is expected to increase from 8.5 million to 16 million.[2] This rapid demographic change can be expected to have far-reaching implications for the management of cardiovascular disease (CVD) and for the allocation of health care dollars. Already, hypertension is the most common primary office diagnosis in the United States, with more than 35 million visits to physician offices each year. Because the incidence of hypertension increases dramatically with age, this number will certainly increase with the aging of the U.S. population.

Hypertension is clearly a powerful independent risk factor for heart failure, stroke, atherosclerotic CVD, renal failure, and death. Importantly for older persons, some studies have also shown that the risk of dementia, both Alzheimer's and vascular types, may be associated with elevated blood pressure (BP).[3] As described in the Seventh Report of the Joint National Committee on Prevention, Detection, Evaluation, and Treatment of High Blood Pressure (JNC 7), the association between CVD events and hypertension is linear, graded, and continuous; the higher the BP, the higher the risk.[4]

Age is also a major risk factor for CVD; however, unlike hypertension, it is not modifiable. As discussed in JNC 7, CVD risk rises with increasing BP, and given the same BP, CVD risk rises with increasing age. Thus, epidemiologic evidence suggests that an individual 60 to 69 years old who has an average systolic BP (SBP) of 160 mm Hg has a similar risk of stroke and ischemic heart disease mortality as a 70- to 79-year-old person with an SBP of 130 mm Hg. In general, high BP in elderly persons confers a three- to fourfold increase in risk for CVD compared with the same BP in younger individuals.[4]

Both the prevalence and the incidence of hypertension in elderly persons increased significantly between 1988 and 2000.[5] Approximately 60% of people in the United States who are more than 65 years old have hypertension, with higher rates among those of African-American and Mexican-American descent. In all, more than 27 million people older than 65 years and more than 14 million people older than 75 years of age have hypertension. Observational data from the Framingham Heart Study suggest that the lifetime risk of developing hypertension is more than 90% for a U.S. resident 55 to 65 years of age.[6]

Although overall BP control rates in the United States have improved modestly since the mid 1990s, still only 27% of elderly hypertensive patients had their BP controlled in 1999 to 2000, a lower rate than in the general hypertensive population.[7] In elderly patients, it is virtually always the SBP rather than the diastolic BP (DBP) that is poorly controlled.

Isolated Systolic Hypertension

Whereas both SBP and DBP are independently predictive of CVD risk in persons less than 50 years of age, SBP is a stronger predictor of risk and DBP is inversely associated with risk for those 50 years of age and older.[8] Although this observation was originally made more than 3 decades ago, it was not included in U.S. guidelines until 1993, when the Fifth Report of the Joint National Committee on Detection, Evaluation, and Treatment of High Blood Pressure (JNC V) recognized isolated systolic hypertension (ISH) as an important marker of CVD risk.[9,10] In JNC 7, ISH is defined as SBP of 140 mm Hg or more and DBP lower than 90 mm Hg. Stage 1 ISH refers to SBP of 140 to 159 mm Hg and DBP lower than 90 mm Hg. Stage 2 ISH is defined as SBP of 160 mm Hg or higher and DBP lower than 90 mm Hg.[4] The staging of hypertension in elderly subjects is usually closely related to SBP. In an analysis of the Framingham Heart Study, knowledge of only the SBP correctly classified the stage of hypertension in 99% of subjects who were more than 60 years of age.[11]

The prevalence of ISH increases with age, and it is the most common form of hypertension in elderly persons.[12] ISH is also the most common form of uncontrolled hypertension in this age group. In the Third National Health and Nutrition Examination Survey (NHANES III), more than 90% of subjects who were older than 70 years and who had uncontrolled hypertension had ISH. In contrast, in subjects less than 40 years of age who had uncontrolled hypertension, only 22% had ISH.[13]

The frequent development of ISH in elderly patients is the result of age-related loss of distensibility of the larger arteries, especially the aorta.[14] In young people, the distensibility of the aorta acts as a cushion during systole to minimize the rise in SBP. With advancing age, the aorta progressively stiffens, thus decreasing this cushioning effect. The decreased distensibility of the aorta and the resulting decrease in arterial compliance cause an increase in pulse wave velocity such that, when cuff measurement occurs at the level of the brachial artery, the pulse wave reflected from the peripheral resistance arteries augments measured SBP. This elevation in SBP and the tendency for DBP to remain normal or to decrease with age contribute to a higher pulse pressure (SBP-DBP), which increases left ventricular load and may compromise coronary blood flow. These physiologic changes help to explain why SBP and pulse pressure are stronger predictors of CVD risk than is DBP in older individuals with hypertension.[15]

Despite the observation that pulse pressure may be the strongest predictor of CVD risk in elderly persons, considerable controversy exists over the clinical use of this parameter. In the Multiple Risk Factor Intervention Trial (MRFIT) screenees, the highest rates of coronary heart disease mortality were found in subjects with SBP higher than 160 mm Hg and DBP lower than 70 mm Hg.[16] In other studies, however, pulse pressure lost much of its predictive value after correction for SBP.[17] Because most intervention trials enrolled subjects based on either SBP or DBP and because antihypertensive treatment generally decreases pulse pressure concomitantly with SBP, current guidelines suggest that SBP, rather than pulse pressure, be used for risk stratification and to establish appropriate goals of therapy.[4] The recent analysis by Lewington and colleagues also found that SBP was more informative than pulse pressure in 61 observational studies including more than 1 million people.[18]

CLINICAL EVALUATION

As in all patients with hypertension, a thorough history and physical examination should be performed in elderly patients with suspected hypertension. Patients should be specifically questioned about the duration and severity of past BP elevations, the tolerability and efficacy of previously used antihypertensive medications, and any history of CVD. Most elderly patients with hypertension are asymptomatic, but symptoms of high BP such as headache, fatigue, and confusion should be explored.

Elderly patients may be taking multiple medications for other medical conditions, and many of these drugs can increase BP. Patients should specifically be questioned about their use of nonsteroidal anti-inflammatory drugs, decongestants, corticosteroids, hormone replacement therapy (HRT), and ephedrine-containing supplements. Because more elderly patients with hypertension have salt-sensitive hypertension, they may be more susceptible to the BP-elevating effects of nonsteroidal anti-inflammatory drugs or corticosteroids than younger individuals with hypertension. To determine the overall risk of CVD, appropriate laboratory studies should be ordered to evaluate for the presence of dyslipidemia, diabetes mellitus, and chronic kidney disease. In addition, a family history and a smoking history should be obtained. The presence of end-organ damage should be assessed through a complete physical examination that includes a careful funduscopic examination and an abdominal examination to look for a widened abdominal aortic pulsation that could suggest abdominal aortic aneurysm. An electrocardiogram to evaluate for the presence of left ventricular hypertrophy, a urinalysis to assess for heavy proteinuria, and a specific test for microalbuminuria should also be performed.

As in the younger patient, the diagnosis of hypertension in older patients should be based on the average of at least two standardized measurements taken over separate office visits. This approach is extremely important in elderly patients because SBP is more variable than in younger individuals with hypertension. Use of an appropriate cuff size is also important as well, because a small cuff may cause an overestimation of actual BP. Given that postural hypotension is more common in elderly persons, orthostatic changes must be assessed with BP measured while the patient is supine, sitting, and standing, at least on the first visit and anytime the patient complains of lightheadedness or dizziness.

Home BP monitoring in elderly subjects followed over 3 years was shown to be more predictive of future CVD events than office BP.[19] However, the appropriate interpretation of home and ambulatory BP monitoring to diagnose and to follow elderly patients with hypertension remains unresolved. Both the American Society of Hypertension and the American Heart Association (AHA) issued recent guidelines promoting the use of more out-of-office BP measurements.[20]

Secondary or reversible causes of hypertension are uncommon in the general population; therefore, it is neither cost-effective nor rewarding to perform an extensive workup for every elderly patient with hypertension. However, when an elderly patient presents with new-onset or severe hypertension, the sudden deterioration of what was previously well controlled hypertension, or clinical clues suggestive of a particular form of secondary hypertension, reversible causes should be considered.

The evaluation and management of secondary hypertension are often more complicated in elderly patients. For example, although it is not uncommon to find evidence of atherosclerotic renal artery stenosis in older patients, it is often difficult to determine whether an identified atherosclerotic lesion in the renal artery is an incidental finding or is responsible for renovascular hypertension. Percutaneous or surgical intervention for renovascular hypertension may be less efficacious, and possibly more risky, in older individuals. Sleep apnea is an often unrecognized but relatively common cause of increased BP in elderly patients. This disorder should be considered in overweight individuals and in those who complain of daytime hypersomnolence or whose spouse notes excessive snoring or irregular breathing during sleep. Chronic renal insufficiency, obstructive uropathy, and thyroid disease are other potential secondary causes of hypertension in elderly persons. Evaluation of serum creatinine alone may underestimate the loss of renal function in older patients. Instead, available formulas that incorporate age and race to estimate the glomerular filtration rate should be used.[21] Rarely, obstructive uropathy can raise BP through sympathetic nervous system stimulation; catheterization may lead to improvement in BP.

One final situation to consider in the elderly individual with hypertension is the presence of pseudohypertension. Pseudohypertension occurs when the brachial artery is calcified and hardened so a BP cuff cannot easily compress it. In these patients, auscultatory BP measurement may overestimate actual intra-arterial pressure. Pseudohypertension should be suspected in those individuals with persistently high BP who have no evidence of target-organ damage or when antihypertensive medication causes hypotensive symptoms in elderly patients with continually elevated cuff-determined BP. Although it is a difficult procedure to perform repeatedly, intra-arterial BP measurement can confirm the diagnosis of pseudohypertension.

ANTIHYPERTENSIVE THERAPY

Benefits of Lifestyle Modifications

Lifestyle changes are beneficial in controlling BP and should be an integral part of therapy for all elderly patients with hypertension. Lifestyle modifications recommended by JNC 7

Table 38-1   Recommendations of the Joint National Committee on Prevention, Detection, Evaluation, and Treatment of High Blood Pressure for Lifestyle Modifications in Patients with Hypertension

Modification	Approximate Range of Reduction in Systolic Blood Pressure (mm Hg)
Weight reduction	5-20/each 10 kg weight lost
DASH eating plan	8-14
Sodium restriction	2-8
Increase in physical activity	4-9
Moderation in alcohol consumption	2-4

DASH, Dietary Approaches to Stop Hypertension.
Modified from Chobanian AV, Bakris GL, Black HR, et al., and the National High Blood Pressure Education Program Coordinating Committee. The Seventh Report of the Joint National Committee on Prevention, Detection, Evaluation, and Treatment of High Blood Pressure: The JNC 7 Report. *JAMA*. 2003;**289**:2560-2572.

Table 38-2   Results of Placebo-Controlled Trials of Mixed Systolic-Diastolic Hypertension in the Elderly

Study	Percentage of Reduction in Events			
	Stroke	CAD	HF	All CVD
Australian	33	18	—	31
EWPHE	36	20	22	29*
HDFP	44*	15*	—	16*
MRC	25*	19	—	17*
STOP	47*	13[†]	51*	40*
HYVET	47*	—	—	—

*Statistically significant.
[†]Myocardial infarction only.
Australian, Australian National Blood Pressure trial;
CAD, coronary artery disease; CVD, cardiovascular disease;
EWPHE, European Working Party on Hypertension in the Elderly; HDFP, Hypertension Detection and Follow-up Program;
HF, heart failure; HYVET, Hypertension in the Very Elderly Trial;
MRC, Medical Research Council trial;
STOP, Swedish Trial in Old Patients.

are shown in Table 38-1.[4] Weight reduction is the most effective lifestyle intervention for lowering BP, especially in patients who are overweight. Because older patients with hypertension are more likely to have salt-sensitive hypertension, sodium restriction is more likely to reduce BP in older than in younger individuals with hypertension. The Trial of Nonpharmacologic Interventions in the Elderly (TONE) found that restricting salt to 80 mmol (2 g)/day reduced SBP by 4.3 mm Hg and DBP by 2 mm Hg after 30 months of follow-up. When used together, the combination of weight loss and salt restriction enabled almost half of the elderly participants to avoid antihypertensive drug therapy altogether.[22]

Additional lifestyle changes include adopting the Dietary Approaches to Stop Hypertension (DASH) eating program. This diet, which is low in fat but rich in fruits, vegetables, and low-fat dairy products, has been successful in reducing BP, especially SBP, in older patients with hypertension, even when they consume an average salt intake.[23] Restriction of salt intake leads to an additional reduction in BP. No elderly subjects were included in the DASH trial, so the value of this approach has not been demonstrated conclusively in older hypertensive patients. Reducing alcohol intake and increasing physical activity may also lower BP in elderly patients with hypertension. Although lifestyle interventions have been shown to reduce BP, no clinical trial has been performed in older individuals to determine whether these interventions lead to a decrease in CVD events.

Benefits of Pharmacologic Treatment: Combined Systolic-Diastolic Hypertension

Since the 1980s, several well-designed prospective clinical trials have demonstrated the benefits of treating elderly patients with hypertension (Table 38-2). Although entry in these trials was often based on DBP, the majority of subjects had elevations in both SBP and DBP. These studies demonstrated significant decreases in the rates of stroke, heart failure, myocardial infarction (MI), and all CVD events.

Although all classes of antihypertensive agents effectively lower both SBP and DBP elevation in the elderly, early outcome-based trials mostly compared diuretics, with or without the addition of β-blocker therapy, with placebo. More recently, trials comparing different antihypertensive agents as initial therapy in older subjects with both systolic and diastolic forms of hypertension have been performed. The open-label Swedish Trial in Old Patients with Hypertension-2 (STOP-2) compared three initial strategies to control BP: an angiotensin converting-enzyme (ACE) inhibitor, a calcium antagonist (or calcium channel blocker, CCB), or a thiazide-type diuretic with or without add-on β-blocker therapy, in 6628 subjects 70 to 84 years of age.[24] With similar BP reductions achieved in all three treatment groups, no difference was noted in CVD mortality, the primary outcome. Similarly, the double-blind International Nifedipine Study: Intervention as a Goal in Hypertension Treatment (INSIGHT) trial enrolled men and women 55 to 80 years of age, 75% of whom were more than 60 years old. In this trial, initial treatment with nifedipine GITS (gastrointestinal therapeutic system) or with a thiazide-type diuretic had similar overall rates of subsequent CVD events.[25]

The Antihypertensive and Lipid-Lowering Treatment to Prevent Heart Attack Trial (ALLHAT) was the largest outcome trial of antihypertensive therapy ever performed. It was designed to determine whether in high-risk patients with hypertension, the incidence of the primary outcome, fatal coronary heart disease (CHD) or nonfatal MI, was reduced when these patients were treated with a dihydropyridine CCB (amlodipine) or an ACE inhibitor (lisinopril), each compared with a long-acting thiazide-like diuretic (chlorthalidone).[26] The third active comparator arm with an α-blocker (doxazosin) was stopped early because of a 25% greater overall CVD event rate, compared with the diuretic. This decision was mostly driven by a twofold greater risk of heart failure in the α-blocker group.[27]

In the remaining three arms of the trial, ALLHAT enrolled 33,357 men and women aged 55 or older with at least one other risk factor for CVD. After a mean 4.9 years of treatment, 2956 subjects experienced a primary outcome event, with no difference noted among the treatment groups. Neither amlodipine nor lisinopril was superior to chlorthalidone in preventing major coronary events or in improving overall survival.[26]

Although not specifically designed as a trial of hypertension in elderly patients, the mean age in ALLHAT was 67 years, and the large sample size allowed for meaningful subgroup analyses. Patients older than 65 years of age were a prespecified subgroup. After 36 months of therapy, older age was associated with a lower chance of having BP under control and a higher chance of requiring two or more antihypertensive medications. In patients who were more than 65 years of age, there was no difference in the primary endpoint or total mortality among the three treatment groups. The trend was toward fewer strokes, combined CVD events, and heart failure events in subjects randomized to chlorthalidone compared with lisinopril. The investigators also reported fewer heart failure events in subjects randomized to chlorthalidone compared with amlodipine, without significant differences in other endpoints.[26] Whether these differences in secondary outcomes can be explained by the small differences in BP seen early and sustained throughout the trial, by the choice of add-on medications, or by the doses and choice of the representative agent used for each drug class is unknown. What is clear is that the thiazide-like diuretic chlorthalidone improved outcomes and reduced BP to a greater degree in older high-risk patients with hypertension.

Benefits of Pharmacologic Treatment: Isolated Systolic Hypertension

As shown in Table 38-3, several prospective randomized placebo-controlled trials have demonstrated that pharmacologic treatment of ISH can reduce CVD events and stroke. The landmark Systolic Hypertension in the Elderly Program (SHEP), published in 1991, included 4736 subjects 60 years of age and older with SBP of 160 mm Hg or higher and DBP lower than 90 mm Hg. Subjects were randomized to placebo treatment or to active treatment with the thiazide-like diuretic chlorthalidone (12.5 to 25 mg/day), with the possible addition of the β-blocker atenolol or reserpine. Mean BP at baseline was 170/77 mm Hg. After a mean 4.5 years of treatment, active drug therapy reduced first stroke by 36% and CVD events by 27%. No significant difference in total mortality was noted.[28] Heart failure was reduced by 49%, with an 81% reduction in patients with either a history of MI or evidence of a prior MI on the electrocardiogram.[29] That these favorable effects were demonstrated is even more impressive, because

up to 44% of patients randomized to placebo ended up taking active antihypertensive medications.[28] In the 583 SHEP patients with type 2 diabetes, major CVD events were reduced by 34%, similar to the overall cohort.[30] The benefits of active drug therapy were lost in the 7% of subjects whose serum potassium fell to less than 3.5 mg/dL.[31] In long-term follow-up of the SHEP subjects, the benefits of active therapy were sustained; after 14.3 years of follow-up, there remained a 19% reduction in CVD-related mortality.[32]

The Systolic Hypertension in Europe (Syst-Eur) trial included 4695 patients 60 years of age or older with SBP of 160 to 219 mm Hg and DBP lower than 95 mm Hg. Subjects were randomized to active treatment with the dihydropyridine CCB nitrendipine (10 to 40 mg/day), with the addition of the ACE inhibitor enalapril and a thiazide-type diuretic as necessary, or matching placebo, titrated to reduce SBP by at least 20 mm Hg and to less than 150 mm Hg. The trial was terminated early after a median of 2 years of follow-up. Active treatment reduced the incidence of the primary endpoint, fatal and nonfatal stroke, by 42%. A composite of all cardiac endpoints was reduced 26%, with all CVD endpoints reduced by 32%. Based on these results, treating 1000 patients for 5 years would prevent 29 fatal and nonfatal strokes. Even greater benefits were noted among subjects with diabetes at baseline, with a 73% reduction in stroke and a 55% reduction in overall mortality.[33] Subsequent post hoc analyses demonstrated that the incidence of new-onset renal dysfunction and proteinuria also decreased by 64% and 33%, respectively.[34]

The Systolic Hypertension in China (Syst-China) trial used inclusion criteria and treatment regimens identical to those used in Syst-Eur, except captopril was substituted for enalapril. After a mean 2 years of follow-up, the 1253 patients randomized to active treatment had 38% fewer fatal and nonfatal strokes. All CVD events were reduced by 37%, and total mortality was reduced by 39%. Similar to the findings of Syst-Eur, subjects with diabetes at baseline showed even more dramatic benefits.[35]

A meta-analysis of eight placebo-controlled trials of elderly patients with ISH, which included 15,693 patients 60 years of age and older who were followed for an average of 3.8 years, found that active treatment reduced coronary events by 23%, fatal and nonfatal stroke by 30%, CVD mortality by 18%, and total mortality by 13%.[36] In patients older than 70 years of age, the absolute benefit was particularly high; treating 19 patients for 5 years prevented one major fatal or nonfatal CVD event.

Whereas the aforementioned trials were placebo controlled, data comparing different classes of antihypertensive agents are much less common. One such trial, the Losartan

Table 38-3 Clinical Results of Major Placebo-Controlled Trials of Isolated Systolic Hypertension in the Elderly

Reductions in Clinical Events	SHEP	Syst-Eur	Syst-China	Meta-analysis
Stroke (%)	33	42	38	30
CAD (%)	27	30	27	23
HF (%)	55	29	—	—
All CVD (%)	32	31	25	26

CAD, coronary artery disease; CVD, cardiovascular disease; HF, heart failure; SHEP, Systolic Hypertension in the Elderly Program; Syst-China, Systolic Hypertension in China trial; Syst-Eur, Systolic Hypertension in Europe trial.

Intervention for Endpoint Reduction in Hypertension (LIFE), randomized 9193 subjects with electrocardiographic evidence of left ventricular hypertrophy to initial treatment with the angiotensin receptor blocker (ARB) losartan or the β-blocker atenolol. Additional medications, including a thiazide-type diuretic and a CCB, were added in both groups, as necessary, to achieve the goal BP. In a prespecified subgroup analysis of the 14% of subjects with ISH during placebo run-in, losartan-based therapy led to a 25% reduction in the combined end-point of CVD death, acute MI, and stroke over a mean 4.7 years of follow-up.[37]

In summary, for study subjects with ISH, initial therapy with a thiazide-like diuretic or a dihydropyridine CCB reduced CVD endpoints. In those with electrocardiographic evidence of left ventricular hypertrophy, initial therapy with an ARB was more effective than initial therapy with a β-blocker. Because fewer than 60% of elderly patients with ISH have their BP controlled by a single agent, most patients require additional antihypertensive medications to reach their BP goal.

Benefits of Pharmacologic Treatment: Choice of Initial Antihypertensive Agent

No overwhelming evidence indicates that one particular anti-hypertensive class dramatically improves outcome over another antihypertensive class in elderly patients with either combined systolic-diastolic hypertension or ISH. Substantial data from outcome studies support the use of diuretics, β-blockers, ACE inhibitors, CCBs, or ARBs as initial therapy, although the effectiveness of β-blocker use as initial therapy in elderly hypertensive patients has been questioned.[38] In addition, based on the results of ALLHAT, α-blockers should not be used as initial monotherapy for treatment of hypertension, although these agents do remain reasonable add-on medications, especially in patients with benign prostatic hypertrophy.

Without clear differences in outcomes, issues of tolerability, cost, compatibility with other medications, other compelling conditions, and patient preference may dictate the choice of an initial antihypertensive agent. Taking all these issues into consideration, the use of thiazide-type diuretics as initial therapy for most elderly hypertensive patients with either systolic-diastolic hypertension or ISH seems reasonable.[4] Other antihypertensive classes as initial therapy should be considered when a compelling indication exists for their

use. Compelling indications from JNC 7 are shown in Table 38-4. Thiazide-type diuretics should be used with caution in patients prone to hypokalemia or gout. Data from ALLHAT also suggest that the incidence of new-onset diabetes mellitus may be greater in patients treated with thiazide-like diuretics than in patients treated with ACE inhibitors or CCBs.[26] Although the choice of preferred initial antihypertensive agent in elderly patients is controversial, a recent meta-analysis found that for cardiovascular outcomes, the initial agent chosen is less important than the achieved BP reduction.[39] Most elderly patients with hypertension require two or more medications to control their BP.[4]

Goals of Therapy

The primary reason for treating hypertension in the elderly is to decrease the risk of CVD morbidity and mortality. A consensus statement from the National High Blood Pressure Education Program calls for treating SBP to a goal of less than 140 mm Hg in older individuals with ISH.[12] In addition, JNC 7 calls for a goal SBP lower than 140 mm Hg (and DBP <90 mm Hg) in all patients with hypertension, including the elderly. JNC 7 sets a more aggressive SBP goal of less than 130 mm Hg (and DBP <80 mm Hg) for patients with diabetes or renal disease.[4] Although these recommendations are widely promulgated, the evidence on which they are based is limited in older people.

Recommendations to achieve a specific target BP in patients with ISH come from epidemiologic observations or post hoc analyses of clinical trial data. In a post hoc analysis of SHEP, published almost 10 years after the original results were released, the risk of stroke was calculated according to on-treatment BP during follow-up. Treated subjects who achieved an SBP lower than 160 mm Hg and at least a 20 mm Hg reduction in SBP from baseline sustained a 33% reduction in stroke. The subjects who achieved an SBP lower than 150 mm Hg did even better, with a 38% reduction in stroke. The group that achieved an SBP lower than 140 mm Hg had a 22% reduction in stroke risk, which did not reach statistical significance because of the smaller numbers of participants who achieved this lower BP.[40] None of the major trials of hypertension in the elderly achieved a mean SBP lower than 140 mm Hg in the active treatment group. As shown in Table 38-5, both SHEP and Syst-Eur called for a reduction in SBP of at least 20 mm Hg from baseline and to less than

Table 38-4 Compelling Indications for Use of Specific Classes of Antihypertensive Medications According to the Seventh Report of the Joint National Committee on Prevention, Detection, Evaluation, and Treatment of High Blood Pressure

Heart Failure	Post–Myocardial Infarction Status	High CAD Risk	Diabetes Mellitus	Chronic Kidney Disease	Recurrent Stroke Prevention
β-Blockers ACE inhibitors ARBs Aldo antag Thiazides	β-Blockers ACE inhibitors Aldo antag	Thiazides ACE inhibitors ARBs CCBs	Thiazides ACE inhibitors ARBs β-Blockers CCBs	ACE inhibitors ARBs	Thiazides ACE inhibitors

ACE, angiotensin-converting enzyme; Aldo antag, aldosterone antagonists; ARBs, angiotensin receptor blockers; CAD, coronary artery disease; CCBs, calcium channel blockers; thiazides, thiazide or thiazide-type diuretics.
Modified from Chobanian AV, Bakris GL, Black HR, et al., and the National High Blood Pressure Education Program Coordinating Committee. The Seventh Report of the Joint National Committee on Prevention, Detection, Evaluation, and Treatment of High Blood Pressure: The JNC 7 Report. JAMA. 2003;**289**:2560-2572.

Table 38-5 Design and Blood Pressure Results of Selected Placebo-Controlled Trials of Isolated Systolic Hypertension in the Elderly

	SHEP	Syst-Eur
Number of subjects	4,736	4,695
Inclusion BP criteria (mm Hg)	160-219/<90	160-219/<95
Mean baseline BP (mm Hg)	170/77	174/86
Active treatment	Chlorthalidone with or without atenolol	Nitrendipine with or without enalapril and HCTZ
Goal systolic BP reduction (mm Hg)	20 and/or <160	20 and to at least <150
BP reduction achieved with active treatment compared with baseline (mm Hg)	27/9	23/7
BP reduction achieved with active treatment compared with placebo	12/4	10/5
Achieved BP with active treatment (mm Hg)	143/68	151/79
Mean follow-up (yr)	4.5	2.0

BP, blood pressure; HCTZ, hydrochlorothiazide; SHEP, Systolic Hypertension in the Elderly Program; Syst-Eur, Systolic Hypertension in Europe trial.

160 mm Hg (SHEP) or less than 150 mm Hg (Syst-Eur). Mean achieved SBP in the treatment groups was 143 and 151 mm Hg, respectively (~10 mm Hg lower than the placebo groups).[28,33]

The only large-scale prospective study that included a significant number of elderly individuals and randomized subjects to different BP targets was the Hypertension Optimal Treatment (HOT) trial; however, targets were used only for DBP. In this study, 18,790 subjects aged 50 to 84 years (mean age, 61.5 years) with diastolic hypertension were randomized to three different DBPs: 90 mm Hg or less, 85 mm Hg or less, or 80 mm Hg or less. After an average of 3.8 years, no differences were found in outcomes for the DBP goal of 80 mm Hg or less versus 90 mm Hg or less.[41] In a subgroup analysis of subjects 65 years of age or older on entry, no difference in event rates was seen among the three groups. Although SBP was not a specific target of treatment in this study, the achieved SBPs were 147, 145, and 143 mm Hg, corresponding to the DBP of up to 90, 85, and 80 mm Hg, respectively.[41]

These and other data suggest that in patients with stage 2 ISH (SBP >160 mm Hg), a reduction of at least 20 mm Hg, even if not to the currently recommended goal of less than 140 mm Hg, improves clinical outcomes.[42] Epidemiologic data suggest that perhaps lower targets may lead to even better outcomes; however, this approach needs to be proven in a prospective clinical trial. Although the CVD risk associated with stage 1 ISH (140 to 159 mm Hg) is well established and current guidelines call for pharmacologic treatment of these patients, no clinical trial has tested whether treatment in this large patient population is beneficial.

J-Curve Hypothesis

The *J-curve hypothesis* refers to the concern that lowering DBP to less than a certain critical value, often while attempting to reduce SBP, increases the risk of CVD-related death. Prospective data validating this hypothesis are limited. In fact, the bulk of the evidence available to support this hypothesis is from retrospective and observational trials, which may be associated with inherent bias.[43] Because an increased occurrence of ischemic events has been prospectively observed in both placebo-treated and actively treated patients, a low DBP is thought to serve more as a marker for, rather than a cause of, CVD events in patients with underlying coronary disease.[44,45]

The HOT trial found no increased CVD risk in patients achieving the DBP goal of less than 80 mm Hg versus less than 90 mm Hg.[41] Although few elderly subjects in the intervention trials achieved a low DBP, a retrospective analysis of the SHEP trial found that in those patients whose DBP was less than 55 mm Hg during therapy, there was no benefit in outcome.[46] Although investigators continue to disagree about whether there should be a lower limit for achieved DBP, current evidence suggests exercising caution when lowering DBP to less than 55 mm Hg.

Postural Hypotension and Nocturnal Dipping

Many major intervention trials of hypertension, including those in elderly patients, have used seated BP to diagnose and evaluate response of BP to therapy. Because elderly persons are especially prone to postural hypotension, concerns about falls are common and often limit the ability to control SBP.[47] In 1994, the National High Blood Pressure Education Working Group suggested that the standing BP should also be measured and used to evaluate treatment goals in elderly patients.[48] This approach may be especially important in the very old, who are particularly prone to developing postural hypertension during treatment. In the pilot study of the Hypertension in the Very Elderly Trial (HYVET) involving 1283 subjects 80 years of age or older who had SBP higher than 160 mm Hg, 7.7 % of participants developed a postural fall in SBP of 20 mm Hg or more at the initial screening.[49] Accordingly, the initial dose of antihypertensive medication used in elderly patients should be approximately one half that used in younger individuals. This approach reduces the risk of orthostatic symptoms and takes into account the lower renal or hepatic drug metabolism that often occurs in elderly persons. The initial dose should be slowly increased until the maximum BP reduction occurs at the dose with the fewest side effects. Additional agents should be added until the BP goal is attained. Postural hypotension may limit up-titration of medications and, when present, should cause one to consider reducing the dose. Whether certain agents or combinations of agents lead to a greater risk of postural hypotension in elderly patients is unclear. Although JNC 7 calls for "consideration of" initiating two-drug combination therapy in persons with stage 2 hypertension,[4] this should generally be done with caution in older hypertensive patients, given the risk of postural hypotension.

Because BP is routinely measured during waking hours, there has been a concern that elderly patients who are taking antihypertensive therapy may have extreme nocturnal "dipping" of BP leading to cerebral hypoperfusion. In an ambulatory BP monitoring substudy of Syst-Eur, the benefit seen in the treatment group was confined to those subjects who maintained an average nighttime SBP of at least 130 mm Hg.[50] In another ambulatory BP monitoring study performed in Japan, elderly hypertensive subjects with chronic ischemic cerebrovascular disease who exhibited a more pronounced nocturnal BP "dip" during therapy were more likely to have stroke recurrence and new silent ischemic lesions on cerebral imaging when compared with patients whose BP did not dip at night.[51] Future clinical trials using 24-hour ambulatory BP monitoring are required to clarify this issue further.

OTHER IMPORTANT ISSUES IN ELDERLY HYPERTENSIVE PATIENTS

Cognitive Impairment

Observational studies, often associated with significant bias, have found an association between high BP and the risk of cognitive impairment.[3] Moreover, post hoc analyses of clinical trials in treated hypertensive patients suggest that these patients may be at decreased risk of cognitive decline.[52,53] Cognitive impairment has been included as a prespecified outcome in several trials of antihypertensive treatment in elderly patients (Table 38-6). In a sample of 2584 elderly subjects with hypertension in the Medical Research Council (MRC) trial who were treated with a diuretic, a β-blocker, or placebo over a mean of 54 months, no significant difference in cognitive decline was found between active treatment and placebo groups.[54] In a subgroup of 2034 patients in SHEP, no significant difference in the results of cognitive function tests was seen between treatment and control groups at approximately 5 years.[55] Similarly, in the Perindopril Protection against Recurrent Stroke Study (PROGRESS), although the incidence of recurrent stroke was decreased by treatment with a combination of an ACE inhibitor and a diuretic, no significant effect on the incidence of dementia or cognitive decline was noted in subjects with established cerebrovascular disease and no benefit was seen for the ACE inhibitor alone.[56]

A beneficial effect was found in the Vascular Dementia Project, a substudy nested within Syst-Eur. This study was undertaken in 1418 Syst-Eur participants who had no evidence of dementia at baseline. Cognitive function was assessed on entry and at study conclusion with the Mini-Mental State Examination (MMSE). Median follow-up was limited to 2 years because of the early termination of the original study. Despite the short follow-up period, active treatment (with a dihydropyridine CCB plus an add-on ACE inhibitor or diuretic as needed) reduced the incidence of dementia by 50% compared with placebo, from 7.7 to 3.7 cases per 1000 patient-years. Identified cases of dementia were further evaluated with cerebral imaging; the incidence of both Alzheimer's disease and vascular-type dementia was reduced with active therapy.[57] In an open-label follow-up to Syst-Eur that extended the observation period by approximately 4 years, the incidence of dementia was reduced by 55% with active treatment.[58] In the Study on Cognition and Prognosis in the Elderly (SCOPE) trial, 4964 patients were randomized to the ARB candesartan or placebo. In SCOPE, many patients in the placebo group were also given add-on antihypertensive therapy, resulting in little difference in achieved BP at the end of the study. In patients with mild cognitive impairment at baseline, as evidenced by MMSE scores of 24 to 28, active treatment over 5 years of follow-up with an ARB protected against the further deterioration in MMSE scores seen in the placebo group. There was no difference in change in MMSE score in patients with a score higher than 28 at baseline.[59]

The results of the Vascular Dementia Project and SCOPE suggest that antihypertensive treatment in elderly patients may decrease the likelihood of developing cognitive impairment or its progression once already established. Whether the specific agents used in these trials, including dihydropyridine

Table 38-6 Findings of Major Antihypertensive Trials That Assessed Effects on Cognitive Function

Trial	Intervention	Major Findings
MRC	Diuretic, β-blocker, or placebo	No significant difference in rate of cognitive decline
SHEP	Diuretic with β-blocker as needed or placebo	No significant difference in cognitive function
Syst-Eur	CCB with or without diuretic or ACE inhibitor vs. placebo	Reduction in incidence of dementia in active treatment group
SCOPE	ARB vs. placebo with add-on medications in both groups	No difference in cognitive decline in subjects with no cognitive decline at baseline
		Reduction in progression of cognitive decline in subjects with mild cognitive decline at baseline
PROGRESS	ACE inhibitor with or without diuretic vs. placebo	No difference in rate of cognitive decline

ACE, angiotensin-converting enzyme; ARB, angiotensin receptor blocker; CCB, calcium channel blocker; MRC, Medical Research Council; PROGRESS, Perindopril Protection against Recurrent Stroke Study; SCOPE, Study on Cognition and Prognosis in the Elderly; SHEP, Systolic Hypertension in the Elderly Program; Syst-Eur, Systolic Hypertension in Europe trial.

CCBs or ARBs, confer any benefit over other classes of anti-hypertensive agents remains unclear. Although long-term treatment of hypertension may allow cognitive function to be maintained in elderly patients, initiating therapy in middle age may ultimately allow greater benefit to be realized.

The Very Old

As in younger subjects, hypertension in the very old, usually defined as those persons who are more than 80 years of age, is associated with significant target organ damage, often in multiple organ systems. A recent study found that 24-hour ambulatory BP values were more closely associated with target organ damage in this age group than were values recorded by casual measurement of BP taken in the office.[60] Even though there has been enormous interest in determining whether the benefits of antihypertensive therapy extend to the very old, few subjects older than 80 years have been included in the major trials of antihypertensive therapy. A meta-analysis evaluating the effects of antihypertensive therapy in very old participants enrolled in randomized controlled trials found that in the subgroup of 1640 subjects 80 to 99 years of age, antihypertensive therapy significantly reduced the incidence of stroke and of fatal and nonfatal CVD events, but not total mortality.[61]

The ongoing HYVET trial aims to determine prospectively whether hypertensive subjects who are more than 80 years old derive benefit from pharmacologic treatment of their high BP. In a pilot study of the same trial, HYVET-PILOT, 1253 hypertensive subjects 80 years of age or older with SBP of at least 160 mm Hg were randomized to one of three treatments: a thiazide-type diuretic-based regimen, an ACE inhibitor–based regimen, or a placebo-based regimen, with a nondihydropyridine CCB as add-on therapy. Target BP was less than 150/80 mm Hg, and follow-up lasted an average of 13 months. The combined-treatment groups had a 53% reduction in the incidence of stroke and a 43% reduction in the incidence of fatal stroke compared with the placebo group. This finding was countered, however, by an unexplained increase in overall mortality.[62] Pending the results of the main HYVET trial, it seems reasonable to extrapolate the findings for subjects older than 60 years of age to these very elderly patients and to use similar guidelines to determine their need for treatment and goals for BP reduction. If a patient 80 years of age or older has hypertension, a reasonable quality of life, and a life expectancy of 2 years or longer, he or she should be treated with antihypertensive therapy using the same guidelines as for a patient in the 60- to 80-year range.[63]

Hormone Replacement Therapy and Hypertension

The effect of HRT on BP and CVD risk in older women has long been a matter of debate. After years of observational studies supporting the use of HRT in postmenopausal women for prevention of CVD, more recently published controlled clinical trials provided no evidence for cardiovascular benefit and have noted the occurrence of serious adverse effects for women taking HRT.

The Heart and Estrogen/Progestin Replacement Study (HERS) followed 2763 postmenopausal women with known CHD who were randomized to estrogen and progestin or placebo. The investigators found an increased incidence of recurrent CHD for those women given HRT in the first year of follow-up and a reduction of CHD in years 3 to 5. No overall benefit in preventing CVD events could be identified.[64] To determine whether the later risk reduction for CHD seen during years 3 though 5 in the HERS trial persisted, HERS II followed women from the original study for a total duration of 6.8 years. No significant decrease in CVD events was seen during this extended follow-up. The authors of this study therefore do not recommend HRT to reduce CHD risk in postmenopausal women.[65]

Subsequent analysis of HERS data identified poorly controlled hypertension as a risk factor for future CVD events, but controlled hypertension was not associated with an increase in risk.[66] Both antihypertensive and lipid-lowering therapies were underutilized in HERS subjects, all of whom had established CHD at baseline. Inadequate secondary prevention measures have also been observed in other studies of older patients, especially women.[67-69]

The Women's Health Initiative (WHI) included a randomized, double-blind clinical trial that compared a combination of 0.625 mg equine estrogens and 2.5 mg medroxyprogesterone acetate (E + P) with placebo in more than 16,000 apparently healthy women 50 to 79 years of age without known CVD at baseline.[70] The trial was stopped early after a mean follow-up of 5.2 years because of an increased incidence of adverse outcomes, including breast cancer, in the group receiving E + P. The numbers of cases of CHD (CHD deaths plus nonfatal MIs), stroke, pulmonary embolism, and venous thromboembolic disease were all increased in those women randomized to E + P. In addition, E + P was associated with a 44% increased risk of ischemic stroke in women with and without hypertension.[71]

In the WHI, a slight increase in SBP was noted in the E + P treatment group; SBP was 1 mm Hg higher after 1 year and increased to 1.5 mm Hg higher at 2 years. Analysis of baseline BP data at the time of enrollment in the trial revealed that current postmenopausal hormone use was associated with a 25% greater likelihood of developing hypertension than nonuse when adjusted for other co-morbidities. Not surprisingly, the prevalence of hypertension was higher in women 70 to 79 years of age than in younger women. As shown in Table 38-7, even though women with hypertension who were 70 to 79 years of age were as likely to be receiving antihypertensive treatment as the younger, 50- to 69-year-old participants with hypertension, a significantly lower percentage of the older age group had adequate BP control. Almost two thirds of the women who were 70 to 79 years old had BP higher than 140/90 mm Hg, even though they had often seen a health care provider in the past year.[69]

Among women with baseline hypertension in the WHI observational trial, the baseline use of CCB monotherapy and combination therapy with CCB in addition to a thiazide or thiazide-type diuretic was associated with an increased risk of CVD-related mortality as compared with monotherapy with other agents or different combinations of agents, respectively. This association held even after adjustment for certain potential cofounders. This finding is provocative; however, because this was a nonrandomized observational analysis, it should be considered hypothesis generating only at this point. Perhaps more importantly, the same analysis demonstrated that despite receiving antihypertensive medication, only 57.9% of

Table 38-7   Prevalence of Hypertension and Rates of Treatment and Control at Baseline in the Women's Health Initiative Stratified by Age

Age Range (yr)	Hypertension Prevalence (%)	Hypertension Treated (%)	Hypertension Controlled (%)
50-59	27	64	41
60-69	41	65	37
70-79	53	63	29

Modified from Wassertheil-Smoller S, Garnet A, Psaty B, et al. Hypertension and its treatment in postmenopausal women. *Hypertension.* 2000;**36**:780-789.

these women with hypertension had a baseline reading lower than 140 mm Hg, and among women with diabetes and hypertension, only 21.1% had a baseline BP of less than 130/80 mm Hg.[72]

In contrast to the modest BP increase seen with HRT in WHI, other studies have found little or no increase in BP with HRT. The Postmenopausal Estrogen/Progestin Intervention (PEPI) trial, which studied younger postmenopausal women, all of whom were normotensive on entry, found no difference in BP after 3 years of follow-up between any of four HRT treatment groups and placebo.[73] Similarly, in the 226 healthy postmenopausal women followed an average of 5.7 years in the Baltimore Longitudinal Study on Aging, SBP increased 3 mm Hg more in the two thirds of participants receiving placebo compared with those who received HRT, with no change in DBP.[74]

Elderly women with hypertension should have their BP monitored closely both on initiation of HRT therapy and at 6-month intervals. No clear consensus exists about the effects of HRT on BP, but any HRT-related changes in BP that do occur are generally modest and should not preclude the use of HRT in most postmenopausal women. In rare cases, the hypertensive effect may be more robust, and discontinuation of HRT should be considered. Because of the adverse CVD outcomes seen in both HERS and WHI, HRT should not be given to prevent adverse CVD outcomes in postmenopausal women regardless of the baseline BP.[64,71]

CONCLUSIONS

Hypertension is common in elderly persons and confers considerable morbidity and mortality. Older adults with hypertension experience CVD events at a rate two to three times greater than younger patients with the same SBP and DBP. As the elderly population continues to grow, physicians will see more elderly patients with hypertension. Given the increased incidence of CVD events in this age group, the absolute benefit of antihypertensive therapy in elderly patients exceeds that seen in younger patients. Even persons 80 years of age and older appear to benefit, although more data are needed in the very old. ISH remains the most common form of hypertension in elderly patients and the most difficult to treat. Substantial evidence supports the value of treating ISH as well as combined SBP and DBP elevation. Therapy in older individuals with hypertension should include lifestyle modifications, including weight loss and salt restriction. When antihypertensive therapy is indicated, the starting dose of medication should often be one half of that used in younger patients, and BP should be reduced more gradually

in elderly patients. When there is no compelling indication for another agent, a thiazide-type diuretic is recommended as initial therapy, although other classes of antihypertensive agents are safe and effective. In patients with ISH, initial treatment with a thiazide-type diuretic or a dihydropyridine CCB has been shown to improve outcomes. α-Blocker therapy can be added to existing therapy but should not be used as monotherapy. Compelling indications exist for specific classes of antihypertensive agents and are similar to recommendations for younger patients. Few patients have their BP controlled with initial monotherapy, and combination therapy is often required.

The minimum recommended BP target for elderly patients with hypertension is less than 140/90 mm Hg, whereas in patients with diabetes and renal disease, the goal is less than 130/80 mm Hg. Patients with ISH should be treated to an SBP lower than 140 mm Hg, although more data on those with a baseline SBP of 140 to 159 mm Hg are needed. When treating ISH, one should exercise caution in lowering DBP to less than 55 mm Hg. Some data suggest that cognitive decline can be prevented with antihypertensive therapy, but this area needs further study. Although the effects of HRT on BP are usually small, BP should be monitored closely in women who are prescribed HRT, and HRT should not be used for CVD prevention.

References

1. U.S. Census Bureau. Persons 65 Years Old and Over—Characteristics by Sex: 1980 to 2000. Statistical Abstracts of the United States: 2002. Washington, DC: U.S. Census Bureau, 2001.
2. American Heart Association. Heart and Stroke Statistical Update, 2005. Dallas, Tex: American Heart Association, 2004.
3. Launer LJ, Ross GW, Perovitch H, et al. Midlife blood pressure and dementia: The Honolulu-Asia aging study. *Neurobiol Aging.* 2000;**21**:49-55.
4. Chobanian AV, Bakris GL, Black HR, et al., and the National High Blood Pressure Education Program Coordinating Committee. The Seventh Report of the Joint National Committee on Prevention, Detection, Evaluation, and Treatment of High Blood Pressure: The JNC 7 Report. *JAMA.* 2003;**289**:2560-2572.
5. Fields LE, Burt VL, Cutler JA, et al. The burden of hypertension in the United States 1999-2000: A rising tide. *Circulation.* 2004;**44**:398-404.
6. Vasan R, Beiser A, Seshadri S, et al. Residual lifetime risk for developing hypertension in middle-aged women and men: The Framingham Heart Study. *JAMA.* 2002;**287**:1003-1010.
7. Hajjar I, Kotchen T. Trends in prevalence, awareness, treatment, and control of hypertension in the United States, 1988-2000. *JAMA.* 2003;**290**:199-206.

8. Franklin SS, Larson MG, Khan SA, et al. Does the relation of blood pressure to coronary heart disease risk change with aging? The Framingham Heart Study. *Circulation.* 2001;**103**:1245-1249.

9. Kannel WB, Schwartz MJ, McNamara PM. Blood pressure and risk of coronary heart disease: The Framingham Study. *Dis Chest.* 1969;**56**:43-62.

10. Fifth Report of the Joint National Committee on Detection, Evaluation, and Treatment of High Blood Pressure (JNC V). *Arch Intern Med.* 1993;**153**:154-183.

11. Lloyd-Jones DM, Evans JC, Larson MG, et al. Differential impact of systolic and diastolic blood pressure level on JNC-VI staging. *Hypertension.* 1999;**34**:381-385.

12. Izzo JL Jr, Levy D, Black HR. Importance of systolic blood pressure in older Americans. *Hypertension.* 2000;**35**:1021-1024.

13. Franklin S, Jacobs M, Wong N, et al. Predominance of isolated systolic hypertension among middle-aged and elderly USA hypertensives: Analysis based on National Health and Nutrition Examination Survey (NHANES III). *Hypertension.* 2001;**37**: 869-874.

14. Tonkin A, Wing L. Management of isolated systolic hypertension. *Drugs.* 1996;**51**:738-749.

15. Madhaven S, Ooi H, Cohen H, et al. Relation of pulse pressure and blood pressure reduction to the incidence of myocardial infarction. *Hypertension.* 1994;**23**:395-401.

16. Neaton JD, Wentworth D. Serum cholesterol, blood pressure, cigarette smoking, and death from coronary heart disease: Overall findings and differences by age for 316,099 white men. *Arch Intern Med.* 1992;**152**:56-64.

17. Franklin S, Khan S, Wong D, et al. Is pulse pressure useful in predicting risk for coronary heart disease? The Framingham Heart Study. *Circulation.* 1999;**100**:354-360.

18. Lewington S, Clarke R, Quizilbash N. Age-specific relevance of usual blood pressure to vascular mortality: A meta-analysis of individual data for one million adults in 61 prospective studies. *Lancet.* 2003;**360**:1903-1913.

19. Bobrie G, Chatellier G, Genes N, et al. Cardiovascular prognosis of "masked hypertension" detected by blood pressure self-measurement in elderly treated hypertensive subjects. *JAMA.* 2004;**291**:1342-1349.

20. Pickering TG, Hall JE, Appel LJ, et al. Recommendations for blood pressure measurement in humans and experimental animals: Part 1. Blood pressure measurement in humans: A statement for professionals from the Sub-committee of Professional and Public Education of the American Heart Association Council on High Blood Pressure Research. *Hypertension.* 2005;**45**:142-161.

21. Stevens LA, Levey AS. Clinical implications of estimating equations for glomerular filtration rate. *Ann Intern Med.* 2004;**141**:959-961.

22. Whelton PK, Appel LJ, Espeland MA, et al. Sodium restriction and weight loss in the treatment of hypertension on older persons: A randomized controlled Trial of Nonpharmacologic Interventions in the Elderly (TONE). Tone Collaborative Research Group. *JAMA.* 1998;**279**:839-846.

23. Appel L, Moore T, Obarzanek E, et al. The effect of dietary patterns on blood pressure: Results from the Dietary Approaches to Stop Hypertension (DASH) randomized clinical trial. *N Engl J Med.* 1997;**336**:1117-1124.

24. Hansson L, Lindholm LH, Ekbom T, et al., for the STOP-Hypertension-2 Study Group. Randomized trial of old and new antihypertensive drugs in elderly patients: Cardiovascular mortality and morbidity in the Swedish Trial in Old Patients with Hypertension-2 (STOP-2) study. *Lancet.* 1999;**354**: 1751-1756.

25. Brown MJ, Palmer CR, Castaigne A, et al. Morbidity and mortality in patients randomised to double-blind treatment with a long-acting calcium-channel blocker or diuretic in the International Nifedipine Study Intervention as a Goal in Hypertension Treatment (INSIGHT). *Lancet.* 2000;**356**:366-372.

26 Antihypertensive and Lipid-Lowering Treatment to Prevent Heart Attack Trial (ALLHAT). Major outcomes in high-risk hypertensive patients randomized to angiotensin-converting enzyme inhibitor or calcium channel blocker vs. diuretic. *JAMA.* 2002;**288**:2981-2997.

27. ALLHAT Officers and Coordinators for the ALLHAT Collaborative Research Group. Major cardiovascular events in hypertensive patients randomized to doxazosin vs. chlorthalidone: The Antihypertensive and Lipid-Lowering Treatment to Prevent Heart Attack Trial (ALLHAT). *JAMA.* 2000;**283**:1967-1975.

28. SHEP Cooperative Research Group. Prevention of stroke by antihypertensive drug treatment in older persons with isolated systolic hypertension. *JAMA.* 1996;**265**:3255-3264.

29. Kostis JB, Davis BR, Cutler JA, et al., for the SHEP Cooperative Research Group. Prevention of heart failure by antihypertensive drug treatment in older persons with isolated systolic hypertension. *JAMA.* 1997;**278**:212-216.

30. Curb JD, Pressel SL, Cutler JA, et al. Effect of diuretic-based antihypertensive treatment on cardiovascular disease risk in older diabetic patients with isolated systolic hypertension. *JAMA.* 1996;**276**:1886-1892.

31. Franse LV, Pahor M, Di Bari M, et al. Hypokalemia associated with diuretic use and cardiovascular events in the Systolic Hypertension in the Elderly Program. *Hypertension.* 2000;**35**:1025-1030.

32. Kostis JB, Wilson AC, Freudenberger AS, et al. Long term effect of diuretic based therapy on fatal outcomes in subjects with isolated systolic hypertension with and without diabetes. *Am J Cardiol.* 2005; **95**:29-35.

33. Staessen JA, Fagard R, Thijs L, et al. Randomised double blind comparison of placebo and active treatment for older patients with isolated systolic hypertension: The Systolic Hypertension in Europe (Syst-Eur) trial investigators. *Lancet.* 1997;**350**:757-764.

34. Voyak SM, Staessen JA, Thijs L, et al. Follow-up of renal function in treated and untreated older patients with systolic hypertension. *J Hypertens.* 2001;**19**:511-519.

35. Wang JG, Staessen JA, Gong I, et al. Chinese trial on isolated systolic hypertension in the elderly. *Arch Intern Med.* 2000;**160**:211-220.

36. Staessen JA, Gasowski J, Wang JG, et al. Risk of untreated and treated isolated systolic hypertension in the elderly: Meta-analysis of outcome trials. *Lancet.* 2000;**355**:865-872.

37. Kjeldsen S, Dahlof B, Devereux R, et al. Effects of losartan on cardiovascular morbidity and mortality in patients with isolated systolic hypertension and left ventricular hypertrophy: A Losartan Intervention for Endpoint Reduction (LIFE) substudy. *JAMA.* 2002;**288**:1491-1498.

38. Messerli FH, Grossman E, Goldbourt U. Are beta-blockers efficacious as first-line therapy for hypertension in the elderly? *JAMA.* 1998;**279**:1903-1907.

39. Blood Pressure Lowering Treatment Trialists Collaboration. Effects of different blood-pressure-lowering regimens on major cardiovascular events: Results of prospectively-designed overviews of randomized trials. *Lancet.* 2003;**362**:1527-1535.

40. Perry HM Jr, Davis BR, Price TR, et al. Effect of treating isolated systolic hypertension on the risk of developing various types and subtypes of stroke: The Systolic Hypertension in the Elderly Program (SHEP). *JAMA.* 2000;**284**:465-471.

41. Hansson L, Zanchetti A, Carruthers SG, et al. Effects of intensive blood-pressure lowering and low-dose aspirin in patients with hypertension: Principal results of the Hypertension Optimal Treatment (HOT) randomized trial. *Lancet.* 1998;**351**:1755-1762.

42. Kjeldsen SE, Kolloch RE, Leonetti G, et al. Influence of gender and age on preventing cardiovascular disease by

antihypertensive treatment and acetylsalicylic acid: The HOT study. *J Hypertens.* 2000;**18**:629-642.

43. Farnett L, Mulrow CD, Linn WD, et al. The J-curve phenomenon and the treatment of hypertension: Is there a point beyond which blood pressure reduction is dangerous? *JAMA.* 1991;**265**:489-495.

44. Coope J, Warrender TS. Randomized trial of treatment of hypertension in elderly patients in primary care. *BMJ.* 1986;**293**:1145-1151.

45. Staessen J, Bulpitt C, Clement D, et al. Relation between mortality and treated blood pressure in elderly patients with hypertension: Report of the European Working Party on High Blood Pressure in the Elderly. *BMJ.* 1989;**298**:1552-1556.

46. Somes GW, Pahor M, Schorr RI, et al. The role of diastolic blood pressure when treating isolated systolic hypertension. *Arch Intern Med.* 1999;**159**:2004-2009.

47. Tinetti ME, Speechley M. Prevention of falls among the elderly. *N Engl J Med.* 1989;**320**:1055-1059.

48. National High Blood Pressure Working Group. Report on hypertension in the elderly. *Hypertension.* 1994;**23**:275-285.

49. Beckett NS, Connor M, Sadler JD, et al. Orthostatic fall in blood pressure in the very elderly hypertensive: Results from the Hypertension in the Very Elderly Trial pilot (HYVET). *J Hum Hypertens.* 1999;**13**:839-840.

50. Staessen J, Thijs L, Fagard R, et al. Predicting cardiovascular risk using conventional vs. ambulatory blood pressure in older patients with systolic hypertension: Systolic Hypertension in Europe trial investigators *JAMA.* 1999;**282**:539-546.

51. Nakamura K, Oita J, Yamaguchi T. Nocturnal blood pressure and silent cerebrovascular lesions in elderly Japanese. *Stroke.* 1996;**26**:1373-1378.

52. Tzourio C, Dufouil C, Ducimetiere P, et al. Cognitive decline in individuals with high blood pressure. *Neurology.* 1999;**53**:1948-1952.

53. Guo Z, Fratiglioni L, Zhu L, et al. Occurrence and progression of dementia in a community population aged 75 years and older: Relationship of antihypertensive medication use. *Arch Neurol.* 1999;**65**:991-996.

54. Prince MJ, Bird AS, Blizzard RA, et al. Is the cognitive function of older patients affected by antihypertensive treatment? Results from 54 months of the Medical Research Council's treatment trial of hypertension in older adults. *BMJ.* 1996;**312**:801-805.

55. Applegate WB, Pressel S, Wittes J, et al. Impact of the treatment of isolated systolic hypertension on behavioral variables: Results from the Systolic Hypertension in the Elderly Program. *Arch Intern Med.* 1994;**154**:2154-2160.

56. Tzourio C, Anderson C, Champman N, et al. Effects of blood pressure lowering with perindopril and indapamide therapy on dementia and cognitive decline in patients with cerebrovascular disease. *Arch Intern Med.* 2003;**163**:1069-1075.

57. Forette F, Seux MI, Staessen JA, et al. Prevention of dementia in randomized double blind placebo controlled Systolic Hypertension in Europe (Syst-Eur) trial. *Lancet.* 1998;**352**:1347-1351.

58. Rigaud AS, Olde-Rikkert MGM, Hanon O, et al. Antihypertensive drugs and cognitive function. *Curr Hypertens Rep.* 2002;**4**:211-215.

59. Lithell H, Hansson L, Skoog I, et al. The Study on Cognition and Prognosis in the Elderly (SCOPE): Principal results of randomized double blind intervention trial. *J Hypertens.* 2003;**21**:875-876.

60. O'Sullivan CO, Duggan J, Lyons S, et al. Hypertensive target organ damage in the very elderly. *Hypertension.* 2003;**42**:130-135.

61. Gueyffier F, Bulpitt C, Boissel JP, et al. Antihypertensive drugs in very old people: A subgroup meta-analysis of randomized controlled trials. *Lancet.* 1999;**353**:793-796.

62. Bulpitt CJ, Beckett NS, Cooke J, et al. Results of the Pilot Study for the Hypertension in the Very Elderly Trial (HYVET-PILOT). *J Hypertens.* 2003;**21**:2409-2417.

63. Elliott WJ. Management of hypertension in the very elderly patient. *Hypertension.* 2004;**44**:800-804.

64. Hulley S, Grady D, Bush T, et al. Randomized trial of estrogen plus progestin for secondary prevention of coronary heart disease in postmenopausal women. *JAMA.* 1998;**280**:605-613.

65. Grady D, Herrington D, Bittner V, et al. Cardiovascular disease outcomes during 6.8 years of hormone therapy. *JAMA.* 2002;**288**:49-57.

66. Vittinghof E, Shilpak MG, Varosy PD, et al. Risk factors and secondary prevention in women with heart disease: The Heart and Estrogen/Progestin Replacement Study. *Ann Intern Med.* 2003;**138**:81-89.

67. Giugliano R, Camargo CA, Lloyd-Jones DM, et al. Elderly patients receive less aggressive medical and invasive management of unstable angina. *Arch Intern Med.* 1998;**158**:1113-1120.

68. Hyman DJ, Pavlik VN. Characteristics of patients with uncontrolled hypertension in the United States. *N Engl J Med.* 2001;**345**:479-486.

69. Wassertheil-Smoller S, Garnet A, Psaty B, et al. Hypertension and its treatment in postmenopausal women. *Hypertension.* 2000;**36**:780-789.

70. Writing Group for the Women's Health Initiative Investigators. Risks and benefits of estrogen plus progestin in healthy postmenopausal women. *JAMA.* 2002;**288**:321-333.

71. Wassertheil-Smoller S, Hendrix S, Limacher M, et al. Effect of estrogen plus progestin on stroke in post-menopausal Women: The Women's Health Initiative. A randomized trial. *JAMA.* 2003;**289**:2673-2684.

72. Wassertheil-Smoller S, Psaty B, Greenland P, et al. Association between cardiovascular outcomes and antihypertensive drug treatment in older women. *JAMA.* 2004;**292**:2849-2859.

73. Writing Group for the PEPI trial. Effects of estrogen or estrogen/progestin regimens on heart disease risk factors in postmenopausal women. *JAMA.* 1995;**273**:199-208.

74. Scuteri A, Bos A, Brant LJ, et al. Hormone replacement therapy and longitudinal changes in blood pressure in postmenopausal women. *Ann Intern Med.* 2001;**135**:229-238.

Chapter 39

Hypertension in African Americans

John M. Flack, Tariq Shafi, Shalini Chandra, Jason Ramos, Samar A. Nasser, and Errol D. Crook

Hypertension in African Americans has long been considered a distinct and intriguing entity and will likely continue to be viewed this way. Differences have been observed among African Americans, whites, and other race-ethnicity groups in the burden of hypertension, at the *group* level. Specific racial and ethnic differences have also been documented in national probability population samples for age of onset, prevalence of pressure-related target organ injury, coexisting cardiovascular conditions, and the burden of risk factors for hypertension.[1-3]

Most of the speculation about the genetic underpinnings of hypertension in African Americans is derived from observations in nonprobability, convenience samples that compared African American and white hypertensive patients (and sometimes normotensive persons) in terms of physiologic and biochemical characteristics as well as blood pressure (BP) responsiveness to antihypertensive drugs (Fig. 39-1). Most of these BP response studies typically, although not exclusively, were crude (unadjusted for confounders) nonrandomized comparisons of single-drug responses between racial groups. Accordingly, the racial cohorts often differed on key pretreatment characteristics that almost assuredly distorted racial BP response differences.[4,5] Rather than providing insight into the racial determinants of BP response, these studies instead often led to broad recommendations about the best *single-drug* choice for African Americans. The greater BP lowering seen in African Americans with diuretic or calcium antagonist monotherapy, relative to an angiotensin-converting enzyme (ACE) inhibitor, angiotensin receptor blocker (ARB), or β-blocker, provided tantalizing mechanistic clues about factors influencing pharmacologic BP responses. Relatively modest shifts in the BP response distribution to single drugs between racial groups were overinterpreted as the optimal pharmacologic choice for *individuals* of both races. This chapter summarizes factors that contribute to hypertension and its sequelae in African Americans, highlights pivotal clinical trials, and then provides a framework for understanding hypertension and its consequences in this high-risk population.

EPIDEMIOLOGY

Hypertension is on the rise in the U.S. population, a finding that has been linked to both obesity and aging.[1-3] In the National Health and Nutrition Examination Surveys (NHANES) of 1999 to 2002, the age-adjusted prevalence of hypertension in the U.S. population aged 18 years and older was 28.6%.[1] However, non-Hispanic blacks had the highest prevalence at 40.5%, followed by non-Hispanic whites at 27.4% and Mexican Americans at 25.1%.[1] The increase in prevalence of hypertension between 1988 to 1991 and 1999 to 2000 was greatest in non-Hispanic blacks (4.6%), followed by Mexican Americans (3.6%) and non-Hispanic whites (3.1%).[3] The racial disparity in prevalence of hypertension between non-Hispanic blacks and whites was less for men (30.9% versus 27.7%) than for women (35.8% versus 30.2%).[3] Among women, the rates of increase in hypertension prevalence in non-Hispanic blacks, whites, and Mexican Americans were 7.2%, 5.1%, and 4.2%, respectively. In men, the rates of increase in hypertension prevalence were lower and were more similar for non-Hispanic blacks, whites, and Mexican Americans, at 1.8%, 1.0%, and 2.7%, respectively. Hypertension prevalence is higher for African Americans residing in the southeastern U.S. than for those in other regions of the country.[6] In NHANES III (1988 to 1994), the prevalence of severe hypertension (>180/110 mm Hg) was 8.5% in non-Hispanic blacks, but it was slightly less than 1% in non-Hispanic whites.

The higher prevalence of hypertension in non-Hispanic blacks in the United States is not an invariable phenomenon in all persons of African descent. For example, the prevalence of hypertension in a probability-based sample in Cuba was 46% in blacks and 43% in whites (*P* = .19). After age and sex adjustment, a small excess remained among blacks, although the differential was significantly less than what has been observed in U.S. probability samples. However, in the United Kingdom, most epidemiologic studies corroborated previously reported data in the United States showing higher hypertension prevalence and mean levels of BP in persons of African descent compared with those of European descent.[7]

In Africa, hypertension prevalence rates are very low in less acculturated, rural Africans, as compared with city-dwelling Africans or with U.S. whites or Mexican Americans. The rural Natal Zulus have a hypertension prevalence of only 10% versus a prevalence of 25% for urban Zulus, 17.2% for urban whites, and 14.2% in urban South Asians. In Africa, average BP levels are lower, and less of an age-related (cross-sectional) rise in BP levels is seen in rural compared with urban adults. Hypertension prevalence increases from West Africa (16%) to the Caribbean (26%) to Maywood, Illinois (33%), findings that parallel the prevalence of obesity as well as dietary intakes of sodium and potassium.[8] The gradient in hypertension prevalence across age (adults ≥25 years old) was twice as steep in the United States as in Africa. These observations in geographically and genetically close populations suggest that both BP levels and the hypertension burden are higher in populations that are urban, more obese, and consume diets with higher sodium-to-potassium ratios.

Pressure-Related Target Organ Injury and Mortality

Compared with whites, African Americans have a higher prevalence of pressure-sensitive target organ injury, such as higher left ventricular mass index,[9] heart failure,[10] chronic kidney disease (CKD),[11] end-stage renal disease,[11] and stroke.[6] The reasons for these observations are multiple and controversial. The greater prevalence of hypertension, the earlier onset, and the higher BP burden throughout the day and night in African Americans likely account for some of the excess target organ injury. African Americans have a higher prevalence of other modifiable lifestyle factors, such as obesity and low-potassium, high-sodium diets, which are more common in African Americans residing in the southeastern U.S., where end-stage renal disease and stroke rates are especially high.

Speculation that a given level of BP per se has a more deleterious impact on pressure-sensitive target organs and death in African Americans than in whites was refuted by the NHANES I Epidemiological Follow-up Study.[12] Although the population attributable risk of death associated with systolic BP of 140 mm Hg or higher was greater in African Americans than in whites, the logistic regression coefficients were actually greater for white than for African American women and were not different for African American and white men.

Secondary Hypertension

Investigators have long thought that African Americans infrequently harbor critical renal artery stenosis (see Chapter 8). In the population-based Cardiovascular Health Study (CHS), the prevalence of critical renal artery stenosis, estimated by renal duplex sonography, in a cohort of 834 free-living older adults, was 6.9% and 6.7% in whites and African Americans, respectively.[13] BP reductions and improvements in renal function after renal artery revascularization procedures are quite similar for African Americans and for whites.

Although population-based data about the prevalence of primary hyperaldosteronism are not available, Calhoun and colleagues documented primary hyperaldosteronism in 20% of 88 patients with resistant hypertension. These investigators found no difference in prevalence between African Americans and whites.[14]

Although population-based studies are lacking, sleep-disordered breathing and obstructive sleep apnea are probably both more common in African Americans, perhaps independent of body mass index (BMI).[15] African Americans with obstructive sleep apnea, both children and adults, become more hypoxic than whites during apneic episodes; this finding correlates with an attenuated nocturnal fall in BP in a community-based sample.[16] Sleep-disordered breathing could account for the increased sympathetic nervous system (SNS) activity and decreased nocturnal fall in BP (discussed later) that are common in African American patients with hypertension.

PATHOPHYSIOLOGY OF HYPERTENSION IN AFRICAN AMERICANS: A DISTINCT ENTITY?

Some hemodynamic and physiologic tendencies observed in African Americans with hypertension are listed in Table 39-1. We purposely call these "tendencies," because none is found exclusively in African Americans. Most of the following studies were convenience samples of African Americans and whites. Thus, these racial cohorts may not have been

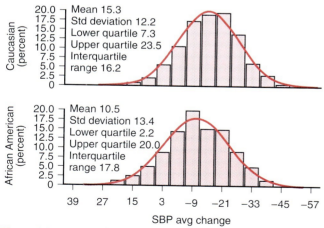

Figure 39–1   Systolic blood pressure (SBP) responses to monotherapy with quinapril, an angiotensin-converting enzyme inhibitor, in African Americans and whites with stage 1 to 2 hypertension. (From Mokwe E, Ohmit SE, Nasser SA, et al. Determinants of blood pressure response to quinapril in black and white hypertensive patients: The Quinapril Titration Interval Management Evaluation trial. *Hypertension.* 2004;**43**:1202-1207.)

Table 39-1   Hemodynamic and Physiologic Tendencies of Hypertensive African Americans

Hemodynamic Tendencies
Early onset, more severe hypertension
Attenuated nocturnal fall in blood pressure
Attenuated average blood pressure decrease after renin-angiotensin-system blockers
Salt sensitivity
Normal to increased peripheral vascular resistance
Abnormal endothelium dependent vascular function
Normal to increased plasma volume

Renin-Angiotensin System
Normal to decreased circulating plasma renin activity
Augmented local angiotensin II activity
Decreased urinary kallikrein
Decreased nitric oxide activity
Decreased urinary aldosterone excretion

Neurohumoral Tendencies
Normal to increased sympathetic nervous system activity
Increased α-adrenoreceptor sensitivity
Decreased β-adrenoreceptor sensitivity
Increased endothelin levels and activity
Increased transforming growth factor-β_1 levels and activity
Decreased urinary dopamine excretion

representative of the general population; these individuals may have had different environmental exposures that influenced the physiologic parameters of interest, or they may have been at a different point in the natural history of hypertension when they were studied. For a more detailed discussion of the pathophysiology of hypertension, see Chapter 3.

Diurnal Blood Pressure Variation

Compared with daytime values, BP normally falls at least 10% during sleep (see Chapter 7). Individuals with attenuated or absent nocturnal reductions in BP are called "nondippers," and they are more likely to have pressure-sensitive target organ damage. In many studies, young, presumably healthy African Americans, especially boys, are more likely to be nondippers than are girls, whites, or black South Africans.[17] However, many factors influence ambulatory BP patterns and confound racial contrasts. Physical activity, salt sensitivity, dietary electrolyte intake, gender, body size, socioeconomic status, nocturnal pulmonary respiratory mechanics, SNS activity, age or menopausal status, and psychological factors all influence the pattern of ambulatory BP variation.[18-20] All these are seldom accounted for in small studies that claim racial differences in ambulatory BP profiles.

In addition, body size and psychosocial stressors, coping strategies, and shift work all appear to affect the nocturnal decline in BP. A study of 69 African Americans with normal to mildly elevated BP showed that those reporting greater perceived racism had higher ambulatory daytime BP levels; perceived racism correlated with anger inhibition, which, in turn, was linked to a lesser fall in nocturnal diastolic BP and higher nocturnal BP levels.[21,22] Another report from a biracial cohort found that religious coping was linked to lower awake and sleep ambulatory BP readings in African American, but not white, adults.[23] Thus, the determinants of the nocturnal fall in BP are multiple, interactive, and underexplored. However, many of the known correlates of an attenuated nocturnal decline in BP are found disproportionately in African Americans, compared with whites.

Plasma Volume

In some studies, hypertensive African Americans have an expanded plasma volume and suppressed circulating plasma renin activity (PRA).[24] However, plasma volume expansion was not found in all studies of African American hypertensive patients, and even when greater plasma volume expansion was found in African Americans, the majority of African Americans had either normal or decreased intravascular volumes.[25] Thus, only a minority of African Americans or whites had plasma volume expansion; however, this percentage was greater in African Americans than in whites in some studies. In some African-American hypertensive patients, a close correlation did not appear to exist between plasma volume expansion and suppressed circulating renin activity.[25]

Sympathetic Nervous System Activity

The Coronary Artery Risk Development in Young Adults (CARDIA) study provided several important longitudinal observations linking psychosocial factors and the SNS to inci-

dent hypertension in mostly healthy young adults. High levels of time urgency or impatience and hostility in 18 to 30 years olds was associated with an increased 15-year risk of hypertension.[26] In young African American men and women, a higher systolic BP at 3 years of follow-up was found between systolic BP reactivity to star tracing and cold pressor stress; diastolic star tracing reactivity was also significantly associated with ambulatory BP in African American women.[27] A rise in BP on standing (≥5 mm Hg) predicted a higher 8-year risk of incident hypertension across all racial and gender subgroups.[28] These data implicate the SNS in the genesis of hypertension in both African American and white young adults.

The preponderance of the evidence regarding SNS activity favors heightened α-adrenergic responsiveness but diminished β-adrenergic responsiveness in African Americans, compared with whites.[29] Importantly, however, dietary and anthropometric factors modify SNS tone. For example, in a biracial cohort of normotensive and hypertensive persons, high dietary sodium intake (200 versus 10 mmol/day) heightened sensitivity to infused norepinephrine; among hypertensive patients only, whites down-regulated their sensitivity, whereas African Americans manifested even greater sensitivity to this α-adrenergic–mediated response.[30] Obesity, especially in African American women, has been linked to heightened SNS activity.[31] In lean African American normotensive men, SNS activity is comparable to levels observed in overweight African American women and is about the same as that in overweight white men and women.[31] Finally, although in several studies basal SNS tone has not always differed between African Americans and whites,[29] stress-induced increases in SNS activity and the impact of a given level of increased SNS activity on the rise in vascular resistance all appear to be greater in African Americans than in whites.[31]

Renin-Angiotensin System

Renin is the rate-limiting enzyme in the synthesis of angiotensin II. However, the control of circulating renin is complex and is influenced by SNS tone, intravascular volume status, dietary sodium and potassium intake, tissue angiotensin II activity, and baroreceptor mechanisms, among others. Accordingly, at higher levels of BP, circulating PRA is lower, although plasma angiotensin II levels and arteriovenous differences in angiotensin II are higher in hypertensive blacks than in whites.[32] Similarly, suppressed circulating renin activity is not always a marker for reduced activity of the local vascular renin-angiotensin system (RAS).[32,33]

Some investigators claim that the RAS system is less involved in the pathogenesis of hypertension in African Americans than in whites, because the former have both a tendency toward suppression of circulating renin levels and diminished average BP responses to RAS blocking drugs. In addition, normotensive African American children excrete approximately 40% less aldosterone, and less kallikrein, in their urine than do white children.[34] However, environmental factors, especially potassium intake, influence these levels,[34] and across the United States, African American children consume lower amounts of dietary potassium than do white children.[35]

The RAS does play an important role in BP regulation and vascular function in African Americans, a role that is perhaps more important than in whites. A series of elegant experiments by Price and co-workers supports this position. These investigators examined the interaction of the RAS system with dietary sodium intake on intrarenal hemodynamics in response to angiotensin II infusions and acute pharmacologic interruption of the angiotensin II effect in healthy African Americans and whites.[36,37] Thirty-two healthy African Americans and 82 whites with similar PRA levels were studied while subjects consumed a diet containing 200 mmol sodium and 100 mmol potassium.[36] Glomerular filtration rates (GFRs) were similar, but renal plasma flow (RPF) was lower in African Americans than in whites. After administration of captopril, African Americans had a sevenfold greater rise in RPF than whites; angiotensin II–induced reductions in RPF were blunted in African Americans compared with whites. These data were consistent with greater activation (or less suppression) of the local renal RAS system during high dietary sodium intake in African Americans than in whites. The relationship of dietary sodium and the racial differences in renal hemodynamics were then studied.[37] Despite the higher RPF in whites during consumption of the high-sodium diet, there was no racial difference in RPF during angiotensin II infusions during consumption of a low-sodium diet (10 mmol/day). These studies suggest a sodium-dependent activation (or inadequate suppression) of the renal RAS system as the underlying cause of the observed racial differences in intrarenal hemodynamics.

Another important study of dietary sodium loading in humans provides clear insight into the relationship of dietary salt intake with local RAS activation.[33] Changes in circulating PRA and vascular generation of angiotensin II were correlated with controlled variations in dietary sodium intake. As dietary sodium was increased from 108 to 400 mmol/day, circulating PRA was suppressed to less than baseline levels. However, there was greater fractional conversion of angiotensin I to angiotensin II, as well as an *increase* in the absolute amount of angiotensin II generation. Conversely, when dietary sodium was restricted to 20 mmol/day, PRA increased, but the fractional conversion of angiotensin I to angiotensin II and angiotensin II levels *fell*, the latter to undetectable levels. Although this experiment was not conducted in African Americans, it provides unambiguous evidence in humans that increases in dietary sodium intake of sufficient magnitude to suppress circulating plasma renin do not depress vascular RAS system activity, but, in fact, augment it. Other studies have shown that dietary sodium loading (~250 mmol/day) lowers nitric oxide (NO) metabolites in salt-sensitive and salt-resistant African Americans,[38] and intravenous saline loading worsens endothelium-dependent vascular function in response to administration of acetylcholine.[39] We believe that these observations are relevant to African Americans, a population characterized by high levels of dietary sodium intake and a tendency toward suppressed circulating renin levels. Thus, dietary sodium loading causes or worsens dysequilibrium (increased angiotensin II and reduced NO) of the RAS-kinin system in salt-sensitive African Americans. This RAS system dysequilibrium, in turn, is a likely contributor to the documented endothelial dysfunction that occurs in both normotensive and hypertensive African Americans. Dysequilibrium of the RAS system may also augment SNS tone, because NO tonically inhibits, whereas angiotensin II stimulates, SNS activity.

Endothelin

Endothelin (ET-1) is a very potent vasoconstrictor of endothelial cell origin. ET-1 receptors are overexpressed in the venous capacitance vessels of African Americans, compared with whites.[40] Circulating ET-1 levels are higher in African American hypertensive men than in either normotensive African American men or white men irrespective of hypertension status.[41] Similarly, normotensive African Americans have higher levels than do normotensive whites.[42] ET-1 has several physiologic effects that may be important in the pathogenesis of hypertension in African Americans. In addition to its potent vasoconstrictive properties, ET-1 augments SNS activity and has a natriuretic effect on the kidneys. ET-1 release is stimulated by dietary sodium intake or various stressors.[43,44] However, salt-sensitive individuals manifest a blunted ET-1 response during sodium loading.[43] The stress-induced rise in ET-1 levels and the simultaneous rise in diastolic BP and total peripheral resistance are more pronounced in African American than in white male adolescents.[44]

Other Natriuretic Hormones

African Americans have abnormalities in several natriuretic hormones other than urinary kallikrein and NO. For example, in normotensive and hypertensive salt-sensitive blacks, a deficit in urinary dopamine excretion after salt loading has been identified, possibly attributable to a reduction in the decarboxylation of 3,4-dihydroxyphenylalanine to dopamine.[45] Other studies have made similar observations. During high sodium intake, salt-sensitive African Americans manifest a paradoxical fall in atrial natriuretic peptide secretion.[38] Finally, deficits of prostaglandin E_2 in persons of African descent have also been reported.

Transforming Growth Factor-β

Transforming growth factor-β_1 (TGF-β_1) is a fibrogenic cytokine that is overexpressed in hypertensive patients relative to normotensive persons, both African American and white.[46] Normotensive African Americans have higher circulating levels of TGF-β_1 than do normotensive whites.

TGF-β_1 augments ET-1 release from endothelial cells, stimulates renin release from renal juxtaglomerular cells, and inhibits NO. TGF-β_1 causes hypertrophy of vascular smooth muscle cells and may have an important role in the pathogenesis of renal injury via augmented interstitial fibrosis and extracellular matrix accumulation. Both angiotensin II and sodium loading increase TGF-β_1 expression.

Salt Sensitivity

Operationally, salt sensitivity can be defined as a rise in BP when sodium is given, or a fall in BP when sodium is restricted, that exceeds the magnitude of directionally appropriate random BP fluctuations. Some studies have substituted intravenous saline infusion for dietary sodium and furosemide administration for salt restriction. The reason the BP rises after dietary sodium in salt-sensitive persons is not clear. However, the rise in BP in salt-sensitive persons may occur to augment renal pressure natriuresis, to eliminate enough sodium to maintain or restore intravascular volume homeostasis. The higher pressure is needed because factors linked to salt sensitivity (e.g., obesity, advanced age, activation of the renal RAS and SNS systems, NO/bradykinin deficits) have shifted the pressure-natriuresis curve to the right. In other words, natriuresis is accomplished at the expense of a higher systemic BP throughout the day or night. This may conceivably explain why salt sensitivity has been linked to an attenuated nocturnal decline in BP or the nondipper ambulatory BP phenotype.

Salt sensitivity for individuals has been defined using several arbitrary cutoff values for directionally appropriate variations in BP when dietary sodium exposure has been changed. Although salt sensitivity has been described as more common in African Americans than in whites, this finding is not universal.[47] Salt sensitivity is not unique to African Americans, because it has been documented in whites,[47] Japanese persons, Spanish persons,[48] and other populations. In addition, salt sensitivity has been described both in normotensive and hypertensive populations, although to a greater degree in the latter. Individual characteristics linked to salt sensitivity, most notably obesity,[49] diabetes mellitus, and reduced kidney function, are more prevalent among African Americans than among whites.

Vascular Function

Several studies suggested that normotensive African Americans have higher total peripheral vascular resistance. However, other comparative studies in hypertensive patients failed to show higher total peripheral vascular resistances in African Americans than in whites.[25] Provocative maneuvers that augment SNS activity, such as lower body negative pressure, result in greater increases in peripheral arterial resistance in African Americans than in whites.[29] Other studies documented reduced NO-mediated vasodilatory responses in resistance vessels, including after mental stress, as well as exaggerated vascular relaxation responses to L-arginine administration in African Americans compared with whites.[50] Similar observations have been made in relation to nitroglycerin-induced vascular dilatation.[51] In aggregate, these studies suggest abnormal vascular function in African Americans that includes diminished endothelium-dependent vascular relaxation in arterial resistance vessels. It is conceivable that these abnormalities may also exist in the microcirculation of pressure-sensitive organs such as the kidney, brain, and myocardium.

Preterm Birth and Low Birth Weight

Maternal obesity increases the risk of preexisting maternal hypertension, pregnancy-induced hypertension, preeclampsia, and eclampsia. All these conditions increase the likelihood of preterm delivery and poor intrauterine growth resulting in low birth weight (LBW <2500 g) infants.[52] The risk of delivering a LBW infant is very high among African American women. According to the 2003 Centers for Disease Control Pediatric Nutrition Surveillance System, the prevalence of LBW is higher for black infants (12.9%) than for white (8.5%), Asian or Pacific Islander (8.3%), Hispanic (7.3%), and American Indian or Alaskan Native (7.1%) infants.[53] As with hypertension and many of its sequelae, higher proportions of LBW babies are born in the southeastern United States, compared with other geographic regions.

In African American women, preterm births are also twofold higher in women with pregnancy-induced hypertension, 1.5-fold higher in women with chronic hypertension preceding pregnancy, and more than fourfold higher in pregnancy-induced hypertension. In New York City between 1988 and 1994, the period prevalence of LBW babies was two to four times higher in women with hypertension during pregnancy than in those with normal BP levels. African American women had more preterm live births (17.4%), a higher prevalence of hypertension during pregnancy (4.6%), and more LBW babies (24.4%) than did white women (7.8%, 2.5%, and 16.8%, respectively).[54] The estimated population-attributable risk of hypertension during pregnancy for LBW in African Americans was an impressive 557/100,000 births.[54] Almost 25% of obese mothers failed to gain adequate weight during pregnancy, thus leading to intrauterine growth retardation. Thus, the relation of obesity to birth weight later in life is nonlinear; LBW and premature babies as well as large for gestational age babies have an increased risk of obesity later in life.

Prematurity and LBW have been linked to central obesity and higher BMI later in life and a reduced number of nephrons. In a review of 80 studies with more than 444,000 subjects, systolic BP was 2 mm Hg lower for each extra kilogram of birth weight.[55] Similarly, in a renal biopsy series, both glomerular volume and number increased (by 257,426/kg birth weight) directly in proportion to birth weight.[56] Young healthy African Americans have higher glomerular volumes than their white counterparts, a finding suggestive of compensatory glomerular hypertrophy in response to a reduced number of glomeruli.[56] Approximately 60% of glomeruli form during the third trimester of pregnancy, with no further formation after 36 weeks, and this may be the link between LBW and future hypertension.[57] Moreover, the last glomeruli to form are the cortical glomeruli, which autoregulate their GFR (and thus transmission of systemic pressure) more efficiently than earlier-formed juxtamedullary nephrons. Thus, LBW and premature babies likely embark on life with fewer glomeruli that are more susceptible to hemodynamic injury because they autoregulate GFR less efficiently. Endothelial dysfunction occurs in LBW newborns with intrauterine growth retardation and contributes to the inability of the glomerular afferent arteriole to constrict adequately when BPs are elevated, thereby resulting in hemodynamic injury to glomeruli. Also contributing is the excessive vasodilation of the afferent, more so than the efferent, glomerular arteriole as a consequence of the reduced nephron number (Fig. 39-2).

Other Mechanisms of Pressure-Related Renal Injury

Premature delivery and LBW may set the stage for renal injury and hypertension later in life. However, obesity and other factors, including high dietary sodium intake, diabetes, dyslipidemia, smoking, and physical inactivity, that either cause endothelial dysfunction or raise BP are likely mediators of excess renal injury in African Americans.

Glomeruli protect themselves from hemodynamic injury by afferent arteriolar vasoconstriction when BP rises and by dilatation when BP falls to less than the lower limit of the renal autoregulatory curve. When high levels of sodium reach the macula densa in the distal nephron, the afferent arteriole constricts; conversely, when the amount of sodium reaching

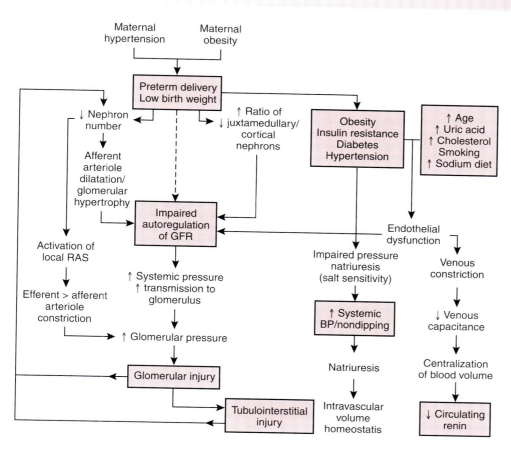

Figure 39–2   A unifying hypothesis to explain pressure-related renal injury in African Americans. RAS, renin-angiotensin system.

the macula densa falls, the afferent arteriole dilates. Dynamic autoregulation of GFR has been attributed to the myogenic reflex and to tubuloglomerular feedback. The myogenic reflex occurs rather rapidly in response to increased intraluminal pressure in the afferent arteriole, as a consequence of membrane depolarization leading to increased calcium transit intracellularly via voltage-gated L-type calcium channels.[57] *Tubuloglomerular feedback* refers to the sodium-linked changes in afferent arteriolar caliber, based on the load of sodium delivered to the macula densa. Both mechanisms provide an important buffer to the preglomerular circulation against hemodynamic injury. Chronic intermittent tubular hyperperfusion of the macula densa with sodium leads to a resetting of the tubuloglomerular feedback mechanism to higher levels of BP, thus increasing the risk of glomerular hyperfiltration and hemodynamic injury in African Americans.[58]

Hall and co-workers did pioneering work in linking obesity to renal injury (Fig. 39-3).[59] Compared with persons of normal weight, obese persons have higher BP levels during both day and night. The nondipping BP phenotype is also associated with obesity, particularly when sodium intake is high or potassium intake is low. However, because of activation of the RAS and SNS systems, obesity-mediated compression of renal tissues, and reductions in NO, the pressure-natriuresis curve is abnormally shifted rightward. When sodium intake is plentiful, the salt-sensitive phenotype emerges, because higher BPs are necessary to maintain steady-state sodium homeostasis and intravascular volume. However, because of the augmented sodium reabsorption in the proximal tubule, there

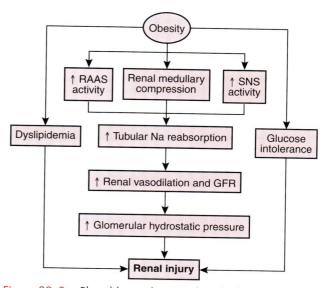

Figure 39–3   Plausible mechanisms by which obesity can either cause or facilitate renal injury. GFR, glomerular filtration rate; RAAS, renin-angiotensin-aldosterone system; SNS, sympathetic nervous system. (From Hall JE, Henegar JR, Dwyer TM, et al. Is obesity a major cause of chronic kidney disease? *Adv Ren Replace Ther.* 2004;**11**:41-54.)

is a reduction in delivery of sodium to the macula densa in the distal nephron. This occurs despite the higher GFR seen in obesity, because of powerful forces augmenting sodium reabsorption in the proximal tubule. This directly influences afferent arteriolar tone. The afferent arteriole dilates, even though BP may be high. Endothelial dysfunction, previously linked to obesity, dietary sodium intake, and obesity-related conditions such as diabetes and dyslipidemia, conspires to cause further dysfunction of the afferent arteriole. The net sum of this situation is to transmit increased hydrostatic pressure into the glomerulus, thus setting the stage for pressure-related renal injury.

As nephron number and GFR decline, local activation of the RAS system occurs, causing greater efferent arteriolar constriction and further afferent arteriolar dilatation. Thus, in an effort to compensate for the loss of nephrons, each remaining glomerulus now has a higher single nephron GFR that further facilitates renal hemodynamic injury. Finally, as nephron number and GFR fall, one notes a shift of the lower limits of renal autoregulation to higher levels of pressure and movement of the upper range to lower levels. This means that lesser BP elevations can disrupt autoregulation of GFR and may cause renal injury. The overall shape of the relation of GFR to systemic pressure transforms from the normal sigmoidal shape to one that is quasilinear in persons with hypertension and CKD.[60] Thus, significant numbers of African Americans are probably predisposed to pressure-mediated renal injury because of preterm delivery or LBW. Theoretically, this should make BP control even more important for prevention of renal disease and preservation of renal function. Finally, all factors related to endothelial dysfunction—dietary sodium intake, dyslipidemia, diabetes, smoking, physical inactivity—are all attractive targets to control both for the prevention of renal disease and for the preservation of kidney function once the GFR begins to fall.

IMPORTANT CLINICAL TRIALS INVOLVING HYPERTENSIVE AFRICAN AMERICANS

Clinical trials that are focused on BP responses and that also report clinical endpoints provide valuable information about the best strategies for lowering BP and preserving target organ function. Nevertheless, these trials must be viewed within the context of previously reported clinical trials, rather than in isolation. Moreover, the data from all trials must be interpreted with ample consideration of the strengths and weaknesses of their respective study designs.

Dietary Approaches to Stop Hypertension Study

The first Dietary Approaches to Stop Hypertension (DASH) feeding trial was a classic feeding study that enrolled adults with untreated systolic BP lower than 160 mm Hg and diastolic BP between 80 and 95 mm Hg. These subjects were randomized to one of three diets for 8 weeks: (1) a control diet, (2) a diet rich in fruits and vegetables, or (3) a combination diet rich in fruits and vegetables and reduced in saturated fat, total fat, and cholesterol. Each diet contained approximately 3 g of sodium/day. The combination diet lowered systolic BP in African Americans (−6.8 mm Hg) and whites (−3.0 mm Hg) and was particularly effective in hypertensive subjects, in whom it lowered systolic BP by −11.4 mm Hg. In the subsequent DASH-Sodium study, reduction in dietary sodium intake, even to levels lower than 100 mmol/day, lowered BP significantly, although more so with the control diet than with the DASH diet.[61] These studies were important because they showed impressive BP lowering with the diets in African Americans and hypertensive subjects independent of weight loss or dietary sodium intake. The magnitude of BP reductions in African Americans overall and in hypertensive patients was roughly equivalent to that attained with a single antihypertensive medication. There are, however, several important caveats. The DASH study was an expensive feeding study because 20 of 21 meals/week were prepared in a research kitchen, and the DASH study was also relatively short in duration.

The PREMIER trial was a 6-month multifaceted lifestyle intervention in 810 free-living individuals aged 25 years and older (average, 50 years) with a BMI of 18.5 to 45.0 kg/m^2 and a systolic BP 120 to 159 mm Hg and diastolic BP 80 to 95 mm Hg.[62] Persons taking BP medication or other medications affecting BP, patients with diabetes, or those with target organ injury were excluded. Three randomized interventions were administered: (1) behavioral intervention consisting of traditional lifestyle modifications (Est), (2) behavioral intervention plus the DASH diet (Est + DASH), or (3) advice only. The first two interventions sought to achieve weight loss of at least 15 lb (6.8 kg) at 6 months when BMI was 25 kg/m^2 or greater, 180 minutes/week of moderate intensity physical activity, no more than 100 mmol/day of dietary sodium, and no more than two alcoholic drinks/day in men and no more than one drink/day in women. The Est + DASH group was additionally counseled to achieve the following dietary goals: 9 to 12 servings/day of fruits and vegetables, 2 to 3 servings/day of low-fat dairy products, and intake of total fat and saturated fat of no more than 25% and 7%, respectively, of total calories. The advice-only comparison group received a single 30-minute counseling session at the time of randomization when these subjects were given verbal instructions and written materials on the DASH dietary pattern. The behavioral intervention and behavioral intervention plus DASH diet groups received 18 face-to-face intervention contacts administered by trained interventionists. Thirty-four percent of participants were African American; 74% of the African Americans were women.

The Est + DASH group in African Americans was superior to the advice-only and Est interventions in achieving the goals related to intake of fruits and vegetables and dairy intake (both men and women) and saturated fat intake (women only). The dietary sodium goal was similarly attained across all three groups in women and in significantly more men in the Est group, compared with either the Est + DASH group or the advice-only group. Weight loss was similar in the Est and Est + DASH groups (women) but was greater in the Est than Est + DASH or advice-only groups in men. At 6 months, African American women in the three groups had reductions in systolic BP of −6.2, −7.7, and −8.6 mm Hg, respectively; among African American men, reductions were −6.4, −11.5, and −10.2 mm Hg, respectively. Thus, the PREMIER trial, in part, a real-world test of the DASH diet, had less impressive results over a longer duration of follow-up than the DASH study.

Accupril Titration Interval Management Evaluation Trial

In the Accupril Titration Interval Management Evaluation (ATIME) trial, in an effort to examine the impact of race and other covariates on the BP response to monotherapy with quinapril, dose titration was performed on two different schedules: slow (every 6 weeks) and fast (every 2 weeks) to attain BP control at less than 140/90 mm Hg.[5,63] The 533 African American and 2046 white participants all had systolic BP between 140 and 169 mm Hg or diastolic BP between 90 and 104 mm Hg. Most of the African Americans were women, whereas the sexes were almost evenly split in the white participants. The crude fall in BP from baseline averaged −10.6/7.4 and −15.3/9.8 mm Hg, respectively, for African American and white study subjects, a difference of 4.7/2.4 mm Hg in favor of greater BP lowering in whites. However, despite this racial difference, many of the study participants of either race had BPs that remained higher than 140/90 mm Hg, and, importantly, both the systolic BP (see Fig. 39-1) and diastolic BP change distributions heavily overlapped. Accordingly, the interquartile range (BP boundaries of the middle 50% of the distribution) of systolic BP responses in both racial groups was almost fourfold larger than the between-racial group difference in responses. In addition, in multivariate linear regression models, after consideration of study design factors and other confounders such as age, gender, medication dose, baseline BP, randomized treatment group, and BMI, the racial differences in systolic BP and diastolic BP response differences were reduced 51% (to 2.3 mm Hg) and 19% (to 1.9 mm Hg), respectively. The conclusions were as follows: (1) modest BP differences with ACE inhibitor monotherapy represented shifts in the central tendencies of the BP change distributions that largely overlapped; (2) the greatest source of variability in BP response was within, not between, the racial groups; and (3) race was therefore a poor predictor of BP response, because the range of BP responses for the two races was very similar. Sehgal came to virtually identical conclusions regarding racial differences in BP responses to antihypertensive monotherapies using study-level data from 15 clinical trials involving 9370 white and 2902 black hypertensive subjects.[64]

Antihypertensive and Lipid-Lowering Treatment to Prevent Heart Attack Trial

The Antihypertensive and Lipid-Lowering Treatment to Prevent Heart Attack Trial (ALLHAT) was the largest hypertension clinical trial ever conducted. Even after premature termination of the doxazosin arm (containing 9067 participants), the final study report was on 33,357 high-risk subjects with stage 1 and 2 hypertension who were 55 years old and older and who had at least one other cardiovascular risk factor.[4,65] Blacks comprised 35% of study participants; most of these were African Americans. Eligible participants were randomized to chlorthalidone (12 to 25 mg/day), amlodipine (2.5 to 10 mg/day), or lisinopril (10 to 40 mg/day) in a ratio of 1.7:1:1 and were assigned a target BP of less than 140/90 mm Hg. Other antihypertensive medications (reserpine, clonidine, atenolol, and hydralazine) could be added if monotherapy failed to attain goal BPs. The primary outcome was the composite of fatal coronary heart disease (CHD) and

nonfatal myocardial infarction. The mean duration of follow-up was 4.9 years. In all three treatment arms, BP reductions in whites exceeded those of African Americans.[65] However, the racial BP response differential was largest in the chlorthalidone group compared with the lisinopril group. In African Americans relative to whites in the lisinopril group, the deficit in systolic BP response was −8.2, −6.8, and −4.9 mm Hg, respectively, at the end of study years 1, 2, and 4. BP control to less than 140/90 mm Hg was also more common in whites than in African Americans in all randomized treatment arms of the trial. Over the course of the trial, systolic BP in African Americans was lowered approximately 1.5 to 2 mm Hg more in the chlorthalidone treatment group compared with the amlodipine treatment group. The prevalence of controlled BP (<140/90 mm Hg) at baseline was 26% to 28% across the randomized arms of the trial, and it increased steadily during the trial. At year 4, control rates in the chlorthalidone, amlodipine, and lisinopril treatment arms were 63.4% versus 68.9%, 60.2% versus 68.6%, and 54.2% versus 67.4%, for blacks versus nonblacks, respectively. An interim analysis of the 3-year data showed that African Americans were less likely than whites to receive two or more antihypertensive medications, an indicator of less intensive treatment. In addition, female gender and residence in the southeastern United States also were linked, similarly to African American race, to a lower likelihood of receiving intensive treatment. Moreover, patient characteristics such as obesity, target organ damage, residence in the southeastern United States, and elevated serum creatinine—traits that are all typically more common in African American than in white hypertensives—were also independently linked to a lesser likelihood of BP control and treatment resistance.[66]

No significant differences were observed in the primary study endpoint or in any of the secondary outcomes among African American ALLHAT participants randomized to the chlorthalidone and amlodipine treatment arms of the trial. However, in the lisinopril group compared with the chlorthalidone group, African Americans experienced excess rates of stroke (+40%), combined cardiovascular disease (+19%), and combined CHD (+15%). Heart failure, a component of a secondary endpoint, occurred less commonly in African Americans and non–African Americans randomized to chlorthalidone than to either amlodipine or lisinopril. Angina, another component of both secondary endpoints, combined CHD and combined cardiovascular disease, occurred more commonly in African Americans given lisinopril than in those given chlorthalidone.

ALLHAT, which had the largest number of African Americans ever in a hypertension endpoint trial, provides important lessons. The lesser BP response of African Americans (and older patients) to the ACE inhibitor versus the diuretic does not invariably mean that these agents are uniformly ineffective and should not be used in these groups. Rather, these data, coupled with observations from many other studies, suggest different strategies for the use of ACE inhibitors, diuretics, and calcium antagonists in African Americans. In highly salt-sensitive groups such as African American and older hypertensive patients, ACE inhibitors should be combined with lifestyle modifications (especially sodium restriction), diuretics, or calcium antagonists to obtain optimal BP lowering. In ALLHAT, use of full-dose diuretics in any other treatment arm was actively discouraged by protocol, because it could confuse the results of the initial randomization.

Losartan Intervention for Endpoint Reduction in Hypertension Trial

The Losartan Intervention for Endpoint Reduction in Hypertension (LIFE) trial was an actively controlled clinical trial of 4.8 years' duration that randomized 9193 hypertensive patients (533 blacks, 523 of whom were African American) with left ventricular hypertrophy detected by electrocardiogram and seated BP of 160 to 200 mm Hg systolic or 95 to 115 diastolic (after 1 to 2 weeks of placebo) to blinded therapy with 50 mg/day of either losartan or atenolol.[67] Target BP was less than 140/90 mm Hg. Hydrochlorothiazide, 12.5 mg/day, was step 2 therapy, followed by increase of the initial randomized medication to 100 mg/day as step 3. Additional medications could be added as needed to achieve BP control. The primary study endpoint was the composite of cardiovascular mortality, stroke, or myocardial infarction. On-treatment BP reductions were similar in blacks and whites, as well as between treatment groups within racial groups. However, losartan was more effective than atenolol in regressing left ventricular hypertrophy as shown electrocardiographically. Forty-six of the 270 blacks taking losartan and 29 of 263 blacks taking atenolol experienced the primary endpoint. In nonblacks, the hazard ratio for losartan versus atenolol was 0.829 ($P = .003$); in blacks, the hazard ratio was 1.666 ($P = .033$). Adjustment for selected covariates did not change the results. The rates for the primary composite endpoint in African Americans were similar in the losartan and atenolol treatment groups in the first 2 years; however, after year 2, the rate of new events appeared to fall in the atenolol group. Tests performed for quantitative and qualitative interactions between ethnicity and treatment were significant.

Numerous pretreatment differences were noted between blacks and nonblacks in the LIFE trial. Black participants residing in the United States were more likely to be younger, female, smokers, diabetic, have higher uric acid levels, and excrete more urinary albumin, and they were more likely to have been treated previously with diuretics and calcium antagonists. Nonblack U.S. participants more often had prior CHD, slightly higher Framingham Heart Study risk scores, and prior prescription of RAS blocking drugs. The meaning of the different effect of the randomized treatments by ethnic group in LIFE is unclear, despite careful post hoc analyses examining a variety of potentially explanatory pretreatment and response variables. However, the relatively small number of events raises the question of the stability of the risk estimates and therefore may represent a chance finding. It is also possible that self-reported ethnicity was a marker for an unidentified cluster of pretreatment patient characteristics that differentially partitioned the groups and led to real differences in response to the randomized treatments. It is plausible that the study entry criteria requiring electrocardiographically documented left ventricular hypertrophy may have allowed distinctly different black and nonblack hypertensive populations into the study, because the prevalence of electrocardiographically documented left ventricular hypertrophy is much higher in blacks than in whites, whereas echocardiographic determinations typically show a smaller, if any, racial differential in the prevalence of left ventricular hypertrophy.

African American Study of Kidney Disease and Hypertension Trial

The African American Study of Kidney Disease and Hypertension (AASK) trial enrolled 1094 African Americans, aged 18 to 70 years with nondiabetic hypertensive kidney disease and directly measured GFRs of 20 to 65 mL/minute/1.73 m^2 (average, ~ 46 mL/minute/1.73 m^2), into a 3 × 2 factorial design study.[68,69] Eligible participants were randomized to amlodipine (5 to 10 mg/day), ramipril (2.5 to 10 mg/day), or metoprolol succinate (50 to 200 mg/day). The second randomization involved two BP targets: a low mean arterial pressure target (<92 mm Hg) or a usual BP target (92 to 107 mm Hg). Add-on drug therapy to attain target BP levels consisted of furosemide, doxazosin, clonidine, hydralazine, and/or minoxidil. BP averaged 151/96 mm Hg at baseline. The primary study outcome was the rate of change in GFR between 3 months and 3 years. The major secondary outcome was the composite of the reduction in GFR of greater than 50% or 25 mL/minute/1.73 m^2, end-stage renal disease, or death. In the overall AASK cohort, there was no difference over 3 years in the decline in GFR between the amlodipine and ramipril groups. However, in participants with a urinary protein-to-creatinine ratio greater than 0.22 (~300 mg/day of proteinuria), ramipril, the ACE inhibitor, slowed the loss of GFR by 36%. In addition, there was also a 48% lower composite endpoint rate over 3 years, compared with amlodipine, the dihydropyridine calcium antagonist. As a result, the amlodipine arm of the AASK trial was terminated early.

A second report from AASK examined the impact of the lower BP target on loss of kidney function and the composite clinical endpoint in participants followed up for 3 to 6.4 years.[69] Achieved BP in the low-BP target group was 128/78 mm Hg versus 141/85 mm Hg in the usual-BP target group. The low-BP target group did not experience less rapid loss of GFR or have less of the composite endpoint. No significant differences in GFR change were noted among the three active drug treatment groups. However, the ramipril group experienced less of the composite clinical endpoint than the metoprolol group and the amlodipine group, which, respectively, had 22% and 38% higher event rates. No statistically significant difference occurred between the amlodipine and metoprolol treatment groups regarding the occurrence of the secondary composite endpoint.

Multiple important lessons can be learned from the AASK trial. First, these findings were consistent with many other observations in non–African American populations with CKD. The major benefit of RAS blockade occurs in patients with heavy proteinuria, who typically experience a faster loss of kidney function over time than do hypertensive patients with CKD but lower levels of proteinuria. Second, African Americans with nondiabetic CKD should definitely have an ACE inhibitor included in the multidrug regimen that will be needed to attain BP control. Third, investigators noted a less than 2 mm Hg difference in systolic BP lowering between amlodipine and ramipril, largely because add-on therapy that included a diuretic markedly attenuated any racial disparity in BP response between these agents. Fourth, the relatively slow loss of GFR in the low-BP group (−2.21 mL/minute/1.73 m^2/year) was probably a function of the low prevalence of participants with proteinuria greater than 300 mg/day (approximately one third of the cohort).

Finally, the absence of a detectable renal benefit between the low-BP and usual-BP therapeutic target groups must be interpreted in the context of the relatively slow progression of GFR loss in all treatment groups (171 end-stage renal disease events in 1094 patients) and in terms of the finding that over the long term, the nonrenal risk for pressure-sensitive cardiovascular disease complications (e.g., stroke, heart failure, myocardial infarction) is high (29 cardiovascular deaths or hospitalizations). Accordingly, the goals of long-term antihypertensive treatment in persons with CKD should be not only to protect the kidneys but also to prevent *nonrenal* cardiovascular events.

THERAPEUTIC CONSIDERATIONS

Diet and Lifestyle Modifications

Although drug therapy is necessary to attain goal BP levels in the majority of hypertensive patients of any race or ethnic group, this treatment should be undertaken along with dietary and lifestyle modifications (see Chapter 17). The more diet and lifestyle modifications that can be adopted, the fewer antihypertensive drugs will be needed to attain goal BP levels. The following strategies should be implemented, to the degree possible, when either treating or attempting to prevent hypertension.

Diet: Focus on Sodium and Potassium

The consumption of a DASH-like diet that is relatively low in sodium, saturated fat, and calories, but high in potassium, calcium, and fiber, is very appropriate in persons either at risk for or who already have established hypertension. On average, in large populations, dietary sodium intake does not differ significantly between African Americans and whites. However, the consumption of dietary sodium in African Americans is not uniform. For example, in the Treatment of Mild Hypertension Study (TOMHS), higher-income and college-educated African Americans had lower urinary sodium excretion rates and lower sodium-to-potassium ratios than did individuals with lower income and less education; only African Americans with less education and lower incomes had higher urinary sodium-to-potassium ratios than whites.[70] Both African American and white TOMHS participants had higher urinary sodium-to-potassium ratios in the Birmingham, Alabama clinic compared with subjects in the Chicago clinic.[70] Reductions in dietary sodium lower BP in African Americans.[71,72] Increased dietary sodium limits the degree of BP reduction that can be achieved with virtually all antihypertensive drug therapies, particularly RAS blockers.[72]

The diets of African Americans contain less potassium than the diets of white Americans, on average. Dietary potassium supplementation lowers BP and restores the normal nocturnal decline in BP, even when daytime BPs remain unchanged.[73] Potassium supplementation also attenuates vasopressor responses to stress, an α-adrenoreceptor–mediated mechanism, in African Americans.[74] Conversely, in normotensive blacks but not in whites, reduced dietary intake of potassium reversibly enhances adrenergically mediated vasopressor responsiveness to stress. Thus, deficits in dietary potassium intake appear to be linked to hypertension through several physiologic abnormalities that affect African Americans.

Exercise

Most people (including most African Americans) do not get enough exercise. The lack of regular physical activity or a sedentary lifestyle is particularly problematic among African American women, children, and adolescents. In a meta-analysis of 54 randomized controlled trials, a decrease of 3.8/2.6 mm Hg was reported with at least 2 weeks of regular aerobic exercise.[75] In these studies, African Americans experienced the most impressive drops in BP (−11/−3.3 mm Hg). The effect was greater in hypertensive, middle-aged, obese women, although the benefit was present in all subjects. Both hypertensive and normotensive individuals had reductions in BP, although hypertensive subjects experienced greater reductions than did normotensive subjects. Regular aerobic exercise may lower BP by decreasing SNS activity, augmenting renal sodium excretion, improving insulin sensitivity, and reversing endothelial dysfunction.

Obesity and Weight Loss

The current epidemic of obesity is a major reason for the increase in prevalence of hypertension.[2,3] Increases in BMI contributed more than half (or 2%) of the 3.6% rise in the prevalence of hypertension between NHANES III and NHANES 1999 to 2000.[2] Obesity and hypertension overlap in 3.7 million (or 76%) of 4.9 million hypertensive African Americans.[76] The relationship between adiposity and hypertension has been confirmed in prospective studies of both African Americans and whites.[77] Many mechanisms have been implicated for the increase in BP related to obesity, including increased SNS tone, activation of the RAS, higher levels of oxidative stress, reduced production of NO and endothelial hyperpolarizing factor, and extracellular fluid volume expansion (especially in the central compartment). Obesity is a marker for resistance to antihypertensive drug therapy in both African Americans and whites. Finally and most importantly, weight loss is widely recognized to be the most effective lifestyle modification to lower BP, with a 5 to 20 mm Hg drop in systolic BP for every 10 kg lost.[71] Weight loss delays or prevents the return of hypertension in hypertensive patients in whom BP-lowering medications were discontinued. Thus, strategies aimed at achievement and maintenance of normal body weight are easily justified.

Hypertension Pharmacotherapy

In our opinion, no particular drug class or therapeutic approach can be reliably extrapolated and applied to African American hypertensive patients with the expectation of uniformly predictable BP responses. However, conditions linked to hypertension treatment resistance (obesity, proteinuria, target organ damage, female gender, and residence in the southeastern United States) are more commonly encountered in African Americans. Inordinate attention has been given to racial differences in BP responses to monotherapy with antihypertensive agents. Similarly, among African Americans with hypertension, considerable focus has been directed to the greater BP lowering of monotherapy with diuretics and calcium antagonists, compared with β-blockers, ACE inhibitors, and ARBs. We classify the attention given to the between- and within-race BP responses as excessive and misleading, for several reasons. First and foremost, the BP response attained with any monotherapy leaves the majority of treated hypertensive patients (irrespective of race) with BP levels higher than 140/90 mm Hg and much higher than the currently recommended lower treatment goal (<130/80 mm Hg) for persons with diabetes or CKD. Thus, many African American patients will have less than optimal protection against BP-related clinical sequelae when the focus is on the most effective *monotherapy* for any racial group. Second, most hypertensive patients require multiple drugs—not a single agent—to attain goal BP. Third, health habits, including diet and exercise, vary considerably within racial and ethnic groups, so universal recommendations about the "best" therapy for a population may not be applicable to a given individual.

Racial contrasts of BP responses are fraught with hazard for a variety of reasons. Clinical trial eligibility criteria have never been developed that led to highly comparable racial groups in any study. Typically, African Americans had higher baseline BP levels, and racial contrasts are only infrequently adjusted for confounders of BP responses that differ across races. Furthermore, BP responses for African Americans and whites to ACE inhibitors, although less overall for African Americans, are largely overlapping.[5,64] Thus, the racial difference is mostly a shift of the mean responses that cannot be used to predict BP responses for individuals of either race accurately. In addition, the variability in BP response is far greater within racial groups than between them.[5,64] We have proposed that the racial differences in BP response to treatment do not form a logical basis for a blanket policy of drug prescription or avoidance by race, but rather offer clues to the determinants of BP responses (e.g., baseline BP level, obesity, kidney function, dietary sodium intake, proteinuria, gender) that vary at the level of the individual, but may cluster more in one racial group than the other. In fact, gender and geographic place of residence in the United States are associated with similar or greater BP response differences than is race.[66,78]

Treatment Goals

According to JNC 7, no unique BP treatment targets exist for African Americans.[79] However, African Americans, more often than whites, have *individualized* lower BP targets because of CKD or diabetes mellitus. Application of the International Society on Hypertension in Blacks (ISHIB) guidelines results in low BP targets (<130/80 mm Hg) for even more African American than white hypertensive patients, because of recommendations for more aggressive therapy in high-risk patients with metabolic syndrome, CHD, prior stroke, heart failure, and known vascular disease.[80] Like all hypertensive patients, African Americans frequently require more than a single drug to attain goal BP.

Limiting Expansion of Intravascular Volume during Treatment

The largest BP responses to monotherapy in African American hypertensive patients have been with diuretics and calcium antagonists. We have postulated that either attenuating or preventing a rise in intravascular volume that often accompanies pharmacologic BP lowering helps to prevent the attenuation of the BP fall that occurs when free-living persons

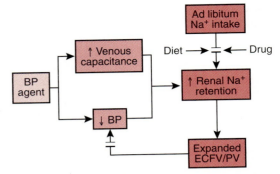

Figure 39–4 Putative mechanism to explain how dietary sodium (Na⁺) intake attenuates the blood pressure (BP)–lowering effect of antihypertensive drugs that expand venous capacitance. ECFV, extracellular fluid volume; PV, plasma volume.

consuming ad libitum amounts of dietary sodium take drugs that not only lower BP, but also expand venous capacitance (Fig. 39-4).[5] With the exception of diuretics, calcium antagonists, and β-blockers, most other commonly used antihypertensives expand venous capacitance, the site of approximately 80% of the circulating blood volume. This action decentralizes blood volume and, along with a drop in BP, sends signals to the kidney that lead to augmentation of the high pretreatment levels of renal sodium reabsorption. In addition, now that venous capacitance has expanded, the kidney attempts to retain enough sodium to "refill the tank." Diuretics attenuate the kidneys' capacity to expand intravascular volume when BP falls or venous capacitance is expanded. Calcium antagonists do not expand venous capacitance, but they have natriuretic properties. This likely explains why, in African American hypertensive patients, the BP-lowering effect of calcium antagonists is much less diminished than with ACE inhibitors (which expand venous capacitance) when dietary sodium intake is unrestricted. Thus, diuretics and calcium antagonists both make excellent "anchors" for multidrug regimens typically needed to attain goal BP.

Ample data show that both thiazide diuretics and aldosterone antagonists lower BP as monotherapy very effectively in African Americans with hypertension.[78] Moreover, we and others have shown that diuretics in combination with other drug classes, such as ACE inhibitors or ARBs, effectively augment the BP lowering obtained with either RAS blocker alone. We rarely attempt a treatment regimen comprising more than two drugs without including a diuretic that is appropriate to the patient's level of kidney function.

Attenuated Nocturnal Decline in Blood Pressure

The attenuated nocturnal decline in BP in African Americans seems like a justifiable therapeutic target. The higher nighttime BP readings appear linked to the need for greater pressure natriuresis and for the restoration and maintenance of intravascular homeostasis, and they likely contribute to greater pressure-sensitive target organ injury. The normal nocturnal decline in BP has been restored by at least one drug from each of the commonly used antihypertensive drug classes: thiazide diuretics,[81] ACE inhibitors,[82] ARBs,[83] and calcium antagonists.[84] The lack of nocturnal decline in BP would provide another reason to use antihypertensive drugs with long therapeutic half-lives and high BP-lowering trough-to-peak ratios. Excessive SNS activity has also been linked to abnormal diurnal variation in BP; however, the side effect profile of most drugs used to antagonize the SNS, except the α-blockers, limits their tolerability in routine clinical practice.

Optimal Use of Renin-Angiotensin System Antagonists

RAS antagonists should be used when indicated in African Americans for diabetes, CKD, and heart failure. However, several important issues assist in the optimal use of these medications. In a sodium-depleted environment, some African Americans manifest a suboptimal BP response to these agents, particularly at low doses. As discussed earlier, it is unlikely that the explanation for this is that the RAS system is unimportant for BP control. The addition of a diuretic or calcium antagonist to an RAS antagonist often nicely augments the reduction in BP. The diuretic probably augments RAS blocker monotherapy response by limiting the compensatory expansion in plasma volume that occurs when BP falls and blood volume is decentralized in a sodium-replete environment. Another concern with the use of ACE inhibitors in African Americans is the approximately threefold higher rate of angioedema in African Americans than in whites.[65] As always, the balance between these and other risks and the potential benefits of RAS blockers on BP,[65,69] CKD,[68,69] incident diabetes,[85] and cardiovascular events[65,69] must be assessed for each patient, African American or not.

SUMMARY

Hypertension in African Americans remains a substantial clinical and public health problem. The origin of hypertension in most African Americans is a calorie-rich, sodium-replete, and potassium-depleted diet, coupled with stress and inadequate levels of physical activity. Many of the physiologic tendencies described in African Americans with hypertension can be linked to diet and lifestyle influences. The optimal therapy of hypertension in African Americans should have as its primary goal control of BP by the implementation of as many favorable lifestyle changes as possible in addition to enough pharmacologic treatments to lower BP to the therapeutic goal over the long term. Multidrug therapy will be the rule if BP goals are to be attained. The role of race per se has been far overemphasized as a pivotal determinant for optimizing the selection of antihypertensive drugs for African American and white patients.

References

1. Glover MJ, Greenlund KJ, Ayala C, Croft JB. Racial/ethnic disparities in prevalence, treatment and control of hypertension: United States, 1999-2002. *MMWR Morb Mortal Wkly Rep*. 2005;**54**:7-9.
2. Hajjar I, Kotchen TA. Trends in prevalence, awareness, treatment, and control of hypertension in the United States, 1988-2000. *JAMA*. 2003;**290**:199-206.
3. Fields LE, Burt VL, Cutler JA, et al. The burden of adult hypertension in the United States 1999 to 2000: A rising tide. *Hypertension*. 2004;**44**:398-404.
4. ALLHAT Collaborative Research Group. Major cardiovascular events in hypertensive patients randomized to doxazosin vs. chlorthalidone: The Antihypertensive and Lipid-Lowering Treatment to Prevent Heart Attack Trial (ALLHAT). *JAMA*. 2000;**283**:1967-1975.
5. Mokwe E, Ohmit SE, Nasser SA, et al. Determinants of blood pressure response to quinapril in black and white hypertensive patients: The Quinapril Titration Interval Management Evaluation trial. *Hypertension*. 2004;**43**:1202-1207.
6. Mensah GA, Mokdad AH, Ford ES, et al. State of disparities in cardiovascular health in the United States. *Circulation*. 2005;**111**:1233-1241.
7. Agyemang C, Bhopal R, Bruijnzeels M. Do variations in blood pressures of South Asian, African and Chinese descent children reflect those of the adult populations in the UK? A review of cross-sectional data. *J Hum Hypertens*. 2004;**18**:229-237.
8. Cooper R, Rotimi C, Ataman S, et al. The prevalence of hypertension in seven populations of west African origin. *Am J Public Health*. 1997;**87**:160-168.
9. Watkins LO. Perspectives on coronary heart disease in African Americans. *Rev Cardiovasc Med*. 2004;**5 (Suppl 3)**:S3-S13.
10. East MA, Peterson ED, Shaw LK, et al. Racial differences in the outcomes of patients with diastolic heart failure. *Am Heart J*. 2004;**148**:151-156.
11. Jamerson KA. Preventing chronic kidney disease in special populations. *Am J Hypertens*. 2005;**18 (4 Suppl)**:106-111.
12. Cooper RS, Liao Y, Rotimi C. Is hypertension more severe among U.S. blacks, or is severe hypertension more common? *Ann Epidemiol*. 1996;**6**:173-180.
13. Hansen KJ, Edwards MS, Craven TE, et al. Prevalence of renovascular disease in the elderly: A population-based study. *J Vasc Surg*. 2002;**36**:443-451.
14. Calhoun DA, Nishizaka MK, Zaman MA, et al. Hyperaldosteronism among black and white subjects with resistant hypertension. *Hypertension*. 2002;**40**:892-896.
15. Meetze K, Gillespie MB, Lee FS. Obstructive sleep apnea: A comparison of black and white subjects. *Laryngoscope*. 2002;**112**:1271-1274.
16. Stradling JR, Barbour C, Glennon J, et al. Prevalence of sleepiness and its relation to autonomic evidence of arousals and increased inspiratory effort in a community based population of men and women. *J Sleep Res*. 2000;**9**:381-388.
17. Fumo MT, Teeger S, Lang RM, et al. Diurnal blood pressure variation and cardiac mass in American blacks and whites and South African blacks. *Am J Hypertens*. 1992;**5**:111-116.
18. Stepnowsky CJ Jr, Nelesen RA, DeJardin D, Dimsdale JE. Socioeconomic status is associated with nocturnal blood pressure dipping. *Psychosom Med*. 2004;**66**:651-655.
19. Sherwood A, Thurston R, Steffen P, et al. Blunted nighttime blood pressure dipping in postmenopausal women. *Am J Hypertens*. 2001;**14**:749-754.
20. Wilson DK, Kliewer W, Teasley N, et al. Violence exposure, catecholamine excretion, and blood pressure nondipping status in African American male versus female adolescents. *Psychosom Med*. 2002;**64**:906-915.
21. Steffen PR, McNeilly M, Anderson N, Sherwood A. Effects of perceived racism and anger inhibition on ambulatory blood pressure in African Americans. *Psychosom Med*. 2003;**65**:746-750.
22. Thomas KS, Nelesen RA, Dimsdale JE. Relationships between hostility, anger expression, and blood pressure dipping in an ethnically diverse sample. *Psychosom Med*. 2004;**66**:298-304.
23. Steffen PR, Hinderliter AL, Blumenthal JA, Sherwood A. Religious coping, ethnicity, and ambulatory blood pressure. *Psychosom Med*. 2001;**63**:523-530.

24. Messerli FH, DeCarvalho JG, Christie B, Frohlich ED. Essential hypertension in black and white subjects: Hemodynamic findings and fluid volume state. *Am J Med.* 1979;**67**:27-31.

25. Chrysant SG, Danisa K, Kem DC, et al. Racial differences in pressure, volume and renin interrelationships in essential hypertension. *Hypertension.* 1979;**1**:136-141.

26. Yan LL, Liu K, Matthews KA, et al. Psychosocial factors and risk of hypertension: The Coronary Artery Risk Development in Young Adults (CARDIA) study. *JAMA.* 2003;**290**:2138-2148.

27. Knox SS, Hausdorff J, Markovitz JH. Coronary Artery Risk Development in Young Adults Study: Reactivity as a predictor of subsequent blood pressure. Racial differences in the Coronary Artery Risk Development in Young Adults (CARDIA) Study. *Hypertension.* 2002;**40**:914-919.

28. Thomas RJ, Liu K, Jacobs DR Jr, et al. Positional change in blood pressure and 8-year risk of hypertension: The CARDIA Study. *Mayo Clin Proc.* 2003;**78**:951-958.

29. Ray CA, Monahan KD. Sympathetic vascular transduction is augmented in young normotensive blacks. *J Appl Physiol.* 2002;**92**:651-656.

30. Johnson JA, Burlew BS, Stiles RN. Racial differences in beta-adrenoceptor–mediated responsiveness. *J Cardiovasc Pharmacol.* 1995;**25**:90-96.

31. Abate NI, Mansour YH, Tuncel M, et al. Overweight and sympathetic overactivity in black Americans. *Hypertension.* 2001;**38**:379-383.

32. He FJ, Markandu ND, Sagnella GA, MacGregor GA. Importance of the renin system in determining blood pressure fall with salt restriction in black and white hypertensives. *Hypertension.* 1998;**32**:820-824.

33. Boddi M, Poggesi L, Coppo M, et al. Human vascular renin-angiotensin system and its functional changes in relation to different sodium intakes. *Hypertension.* 1998;**31**:836-842.

34. Pratt JH, Jones JJ, Miller JZ, et al. Racial differences in aldosterone excretion and plasma aldosterone concentrations in children. *N Engl J Med.* 1989;**321**:1152-1157.

35. Ford ES. Race, education, and dietary cations: Findings from the Third National Health And Nutrition Examination Survey. *Ethn Dis.* 1998;**8**:10-20.

36. Price DA, Fisher ND, Osei SY, et al. Renal perfusion and function in healthy African Americans. *Kidney Int.* 2001;**59**:1037-1043.

37. Price DA, Fisher ND, Lansang MC, et al. Renal perfusion in blacks: Alterations caused by insuppressibility of intrarenal renin with salt. *Hypertension.* 2002;**40**:186-189.

38. Campese VM, Tawadrous M, Bigazzi R, et al. Salt intake and plasma atrial natriuretic peptide and nitric oxide in hypertension. *Hypertension.* 1996;**28**:335-340.

39. Cardillo C, Campia U, Kilcoyne CM, et al. Improved endothelium-dependent vasodilation after blockade of endothelin receptors in patients with essential hypertension. *Circulation.* 2002;**105**:452-456.

40. Grubbs AL, Anstadt MP, Ergul A. Saphenous vein endothelin system expression and activity in African American patients. *Arterioscler Thromb Vasc Biol.* 2002;**22**:1122-1127.

41. Ergul S, Parish DC, Puett D, Ergul A. Racial differences in plasma endothelin-1 concentrations in individuals with essential hypertension. *Hypertension.* 1996;**28**:652-655.

42. Evans RR, Phillips BG, Singh G, et al. Racial and gender differences in endothelin-1. *Am J Cardiol.* 1996;**78**:486-488.

43. Perez del Villar C, Garcia Alonso CJ, Feldstein CA, et al. Role of endothelin in the pathogenesis of hypertension. *Mayo Clin Proc.* 2005;**80**:84-96.

44. Treiber FA, Jackson RW, Davis H, et al. Racial differences in endothelin-1 at rest and in response to acute stress in adolescent males. *Hypertension.* 2000;**35**:722-725.

45. Damasceno A, Santos A, Serrao P, et al. Deficiency of renal dopaminergic-dependent natriuretic response to acute sodium load in black salt-sensitive subjects in contrast to salt-resistant subjects. *J Hypertens.* 1999;**17**:1995-2001.

46. Suthanthiran M, Li B, Song JO, et al. Transforming growth factor-beta 1 hyperexpression in African-American hypertensives: A novel mediator of hypertension and/or target organ damage. *Proc Natl Acad Sci U S A.* 2000;**97**:3479-3484.

47. Wright JT Jr, Rahman M, Scarpa A, et al. Determinants of salt sensitivity in black and white normotensive and hypertensive women. *Hypertension.* 2003;**42**:1087-1092.

48. Poch E, Gonzalez D, Giner V, et al. Molecular basis of salt sensitivity in human hypertension: Evaluation of renin-angiotensin-aldosterone system gene polymorphisms. *Hypertension.* 2001;**38**:1204-1209.

49. Flack JM, Grimm RH Jr, Staffileno BA, et al. New salt-sensitivity metrics: Variability-adjusted blood pressure change and the urinary sodium-to-creatinine ratio. *Ethn Dis.* 2002;**12**:10-19.

50. Houghton JL, Philbin EF, Strogatz DS, et al. The presence of African American race predicts improvement in coronary endothelial function after supplementary L-arginine. *J Am Coll Cardiol.* 2002;**39**:1314-1322.

51. Campia U, Choucair WK, Bryant MB, et al. Role of cyclooxygenase products in the regulation of vascular tone and in the endothelial vasodilator function of normal, hypertensive, and hypercholesterolemic humans. *Am J Cardiol.* 2002;**89**:286-290.

52. Castro LC, Avina RL. Maternal obesity and pregnancy outcomes. *Curr Opin Obstet Gynecol.* 2002;**14**:601-606.

53. Centers for Disease Control and Prevention. Pediatric Nutrition Surveillance System 2003. Atlanta, Ga: Division of Nutrition, National Center for Chronic Disease Prevention and Health Promotion, Centers for Disease Control and Prevention, 2004.

54. Samadi AR, Mayberry RM. Maternal hypertension and spontaneous preterm births among black women. *Obstet Gynecol.* 1998;**91**:899-904.

55. Huxley RR, Shiell AW, Law CM. The role of size at birth and postnatal catch-up growth in determining systolic blood pressure: A systematic review of the literature. *J Hypertens.* 2000;**18**:815-831.

56. Hoy WE, Douglas-Denton RN, Hughson MD, et al. A stereological study of glomerular number and volume: Preliminary findings in a multiracial study of kidneys at autopsy. *Kidney Int.* 2003;**63 (Suppl)**:S31-S37.

57. Palmer BF. Disturbances in renal autoregulation and the susceptibility to hypertension-induced chronic kidney disease. *Am J Med Sci.* 2004;**328**:330-343.

58. Aviv A, Hollenberg NK, Weder AB. Sodium glomerulopathy: Tubuloglomerular feedback and renal injury in African Americans. *Kidney Int.* 2004;**65**:361-368.

59. Hall JE, Henegar JR, Dwyer TM, et al. Is obesity a major cause of chronic kidney disease? *Adv Ren Replace Ther.* 2004;**11**:41-54.

60. Palmer BF. Renal dysfunction complicating the treatment of hypertension. *N Engl J Med.* 2002;**347**:1256-1261.

61. Sacks FM, Svetkey LP, Vollmer WM, et al. Effects on blood pressure of reduced dietary sodium and the Dietary Approaches to Stop Hypertension (DASH) diet: DASH-Sodium Collaborative Research Group. *N Engl J Med.* 2001;**344**:3-10.

62. Appel LJ, Champagne CM, Harsha DW, et al. Effects of comprehensive lifestyle modification on blood pressure control: Main results of the PREMIER clinical trial. *JAMA.* 2003;**289**:2089-2093.

63. Flack JM, Yunis C, Preisser J, et al. The rapidity of drug dose escalation influences blood pressure response and adverse effects burden in patients with hypertension: The Quinapril Titration Interval Management Evaluation (ATIME) Study. ATIME Research Group. *Arch Intern Med.* 2000;**160**:1842-1847.

64. Sehgal AR. Overlap between whites and blacks in response to antihypertensive drugs. *Hypertension.* 2004;**43**:566-572.

65. Wright JT Jr, Dunn JK, Cutler JA, et al. Outcomes in hypertensive black and nonblack patients treated with chlorthalidone, amlodipine, and lisinopril: ALLHAT Collaborative Research Group. *JAMA*. 2005;**293**:1595-1608.

66. Cushman WC, Reda DJ, Perry HM, et al. Regional and racial differences in response to antihypertensive medication use in a randomized controlled trial of men with hypertension in the United States: Department of Veterans Affairs Cooperative Study Group on Antihypertensive Agents. *Arch Intern Med*. 2000;**160**:825-831.

67. Dahlöf B, Devereux RB, Kjeldsen SE, et al. Cardiovascular morbidity and mortality in the Losartan Intervention for Endpoint Reduction in Hypertension study (LIFE): A randomised trial against atenolol. LIFE Study Group. *Lancet*. 2002;**359**:995-1003.

68. Agodoa LY, Appel L, Bakris GL, et al. Effect of ramipril vs. amlodipine on renal outcomes in hypertensive nephrosclerosis: A randomized controlled trial. African American Study of Kidney Disease and Hypertension (AASK) Study Group. *JAMA*. 2001;**285**:2719-2728.

69. Wright JT Jr, Bakris G, Greene T, et al. Effect of blood pressure lowering and antihypertensive drug class on progression of hypertensive kidney disease: Results from the AASK trial. African American Study of Kidney Disease and Hypertension Study Group. *JAMA*. 2002;**288**:2421-2431.

70. Ganguli MC, Grimm RH Jr, Svendsen KH, et al. Urinary sodium and potassium profile of blacks and whites in relation to education in two different geographic urban areas: TOMHS Research Group. Treatment of Mild Hypertension Study. *Am J Hypertens*. 1999;**12**:69-72.

71. Lopes AA, James SA, Port FK, et al. Meeting the challenge to improve the treatment of hypertension in blacks. *J Clin Hypertens*. 2003;**5**:393-401.

72. Milan A, Mulatero P, Rabbia F, Veglio F. Salt intake and hypertension therapy. *J Nephrol*. 2002;**15**:1-6.

73. Wilson DK, Sica DA, Miller SB. Effects of potassium on blood pressure in salt-sensitive and salt-resistant black adolescents. *Hypertension*. 1999;**34**:181-186.

74. Sudhir K, Forman A, Yi SL, et al. Reduced dietary potassium reversibly enhances vasopressor response to stress in African Americans. *Hypertension*.1997;**29**:1083-1090.

75. Whelton SP, Chin A, Xin X, He J. Effect of aerobic exercise on blood pressure: A meta-analysis of randomized, controlled trials. *Ann Intern Med*. 2002;**136**:493-503.

76. Collins R, Winkleby MA. African American women and men at high and low risk for hypertension: A signal detection analysis of NHANES III, 1988-1994. *Prev Med*. 2002;**35**:303-312.

77. Norman JE, Bild D, Lewis CE, et al. The impact of weight change on cardiovascular disease risk factors in young black and white adults: The CARDIA study. *Int J Obes Relat Metab Disord*. 2003;**27**:369-376.

78. Flack JM, Oparil S, Pratt JH, et al. Efficacy and tolerability of eplerenone and losartan in hypertensive black and white patients. *J Am Coll Cardiol*. 2003;**41**:1148-1155.

79. Chobanian AV, Bakris GL, Black HR, et al., and the National High Blood Pressure Education Program Coordinating Committee. The Seventh Report of the Joint National Committee on Prevention, Detection, Evaluation, and Treatment of High Blood Pressure: The JNC 7 report. *JAMA*. 2003;**289**:2560-3572.

80. Douglas JG, Bakris GL, Epstein M, et al., Hypertension in African Americans Working Group of the International Society on Hypertension in Blacks. Management of high blood pressure in African Americans: Consensus statement of the Hypertension in African Americans Working Group of the International Society on Hypertension in Blacks. *Arch Intern Med*. 2003;**163**:525-541.

81. Uzu T, Kimura G. Diuretics shift circadian rhythm of blood pressure from nondipper to dipper in essential hypertension. *Circulation*. 1999;**100**:1635-1638.

82. Czupryniak L, Wisniewska-Jaronsinska M, Drzewoski J. Trandolapril restores circadian blood pressure variation in normoalbuminuric normotensive type 1 diabetic patients. *J Diabetes Complications*. 2001;**15**:75-79.

83. Ivanova OV, Fomicheva OA, Sergakova LM, et al. [Angiotensin II receptor blocker telmisartan: Effect on 24-hour blood pressure profile and left ventricular hypertrophy in patients with hypertension.] (in Russian) *Kardiologiia*. 2002;**42**:45-49.

84. Portaluppi F, Vergnani L, Manfredini R, et al. Time-dependent effect of isradipine on the nocturnal hypertension in chronic renal failure. *Am J Hypertens*. 1995;**8**:719-726.

85. Scheen AJ. Prevention of type 2 diabetes mellitus through inhibition of the renin-angiotensin system. *Drugs*. 2004;**64**:2537-2565.

Chapter 40

Hypertension in Hispanics

David J. Hyman, Carlos Vallbona, Paul Pisarik, and Valory N. Pavlik

By 2010, Hispanics will comprise the largest minority group in the United States.[1] For this reason, clinicians and health care planners need to be aware of any special considerations that may apply in evaluating the risk of hypertension among Hispanics and in implementing effective treatment plans.

DEFINITION OF HISPANIC

First, it is useful to review the historical background of the current ethnic group designation of Hispanic. The definitions of race and ethnicity in the United States have undergone constant evolution since the first census survey was conducted in 1740.[2,3] Until 1930, race was classified primarily on the basis of country or tribe of origin (e.g., Celtic, Italian, Jewish). Accordingly, the 1930 census classified Mexicans as a separate race, but in 1940 and 1950, the classification was based on having Spanish as one's native language or on having a Spanish surname. After complaints from Hispanic groups that these definitions were unsatisfactory, population surveys in the 1960s and 1970s classified Hispanics as white.

The concept of using ethnicity to denote identifiable population subgroups was introduced in the 1970s. Ethnicity focused on cultural, behavioral, and environmental attributes, whereas racial classification schemes had traditionally implied biologic differences. In response to social and political debate, the Office of Management and Budget attempted to standardize the manner in which racial and ethnic identification is carried out across all government agencies. Beginning in 1978,[4,5] the term *Hispanic* was used to define a person from a Mexican, Puerto Rican, Cuban, Central or South American, or other Spanish culture or origin, regardless of race. The designation Hispanic referred to the individual's ethnic identification. After self-identifying as Hispanic or non-Hispanic, individuals then classify themselves into any of several racial groups, including white, black, Asian, Pacific Islander, Native American, or other. Consequently, individuals whose ethnicity is Hispanic may be classified as white, black, or of some other race.

Despite attempts to standardize the definition of Hispanic, considerable controversy exists about the usefulness of a single rubric for the genetically and culturally diverse population groups that it encompasses. Genetic admixture studies in samples of Hispanics in the western and southwestern United States reflect a trihybrid model consisting of European (ranging from 46% to 67% selected alleles), Native American (34% to 68% of alleles), and African (0% to 13% of alleles) origins.[6] Hispanics in the eastern United States conform more closely to a dihybrid model, with European ancestry predominating and with the African genetic contribution ranging from 6% to 17%. Although some population samples on the Eastern Seaboard evidence some Native American ancestry,[6,7] this contribution is not as predominant as it is in populations residing in the southwestern and western states. In addition to this documented genetic heterogeneity, current federal standards for racial and ethnic classification rely primarily on self-identification. Studies reveal high variability among Hispanics in their racial self-identification, and this variability complicates efforts to discern racial correlates of health status measures and outcomes and makes those efforts exceedingly difficult.[8] In our review of data on prevalence, awareness, treatment, and control of hypertension in Hispanics, we identify, whenever possible, the Hispanic subgroups to which the data apply and mention any limitations on the generalizability of the data to all persons classified as Hispanic.

PREVALENCE OF HYPERTENSION IN HISPANICS IN THE UNITED STATES

The most robust and widely cited source of data on the prevalence, awareness, treatment, and control of hypertension in the United States is the Centers for Disease Control and Prevention through its National Health and Nutrition Examination Survey (NHANES) studies. The NHANES studies collect information on a national probability sample of noninstitutionalized persons by means of both personal interviews and physical examinations. Mexican Americans have been oversampled in recent surveys to provide reliable estimates of health parameters in the largest Hispanic subgroup in the United States. The NHANES results for Hispanics apply only to individuals of Mexican origin. The NHANES studies were conducted episodically until 1999, at which time the surveys became an ongoing process with additional subjects accrued every year. Detailed analyses of hypertension trends through 1999 to 2000 have been published,[9] and limited summary data are available through 2002.[10]

According to the most recent NHANES data, the prevalence of hypertension in Mexican Americans is 25.1% (95% confidence interval [CI], 23.1% to 27.1%), as compared with 27.4% (95% CI, 25.3% to 29.5%) in non-Hispanic whites and 40.5% (95% C.I, 38.2% to 48.2%) in blacks.[10] The prevalence of hypertension is relatively similar in men and women and increases significantly with age, from levels as low as 7.2% in persons 18 to 39 years of age to as high as 65.4% in persons more than 60 years of age.[9] A comparison of data from the NHANES studies conducted in 1988 to 1991 and in 1999 to 2000 shows a 3.5% increase in the age-adjusted prevalence rate for Hispanics. A similar increase also occurred among non-Hispanic whites and among African Americans.[9]

Given the documented high prevalence of risk factors for hypertension (obesity, diabetes, and low socioeconomic status) in Hispanics (especially Mexican Americans), the low prevalence of hypertension among Hispanics in the NHANES studies is unexpected. Studies conducted in San Antonio, Texas, and in other communities, however, also showed that the prevalence and incidence of hypertension in Mexican Americans are similar to or lower than in non-Hispanic whites.[11-14] When sociodemographic factors were considered, the prevalence of hypertension in Hispanics living in California was not significantly different from that of non-Hispanic whites.[15] A recent study of racial-ethnic differences in hypertension based on data of the Multi-Ethnic Study of Atherosclerosis (MESA) also revealed that the prevalence of hypertension in Hispanics did not differ significantly from that of non-Hispanic whites.[16]

The apparent advantage of being Hispanic in relation to hypertension risk is also observed in the age-adjusted mortality rates for heart diseases and, to a lesser extent, for cerebrovascular diseases. The age-adjusted (to year 2000) mortality rate per 100,000 for the overall U.S. population in 2002 was 240.8 for heart diseases and 56.2 for cerebrovascular diseases. In contrast, the age-adjusted mortality rate for Hispanics was 180.5, for non-Hispanic whites it was 236.7, and for African Americans it was 308.4; the corresponding age-adjusted mortality rates (per 100,000) for cerebrovascular diseases were 41.3, 54.2, and 76.3, respectively.[17] The discrepancy in age-adjusted cardiovascular mortality, which has been pointed out for many years,[18,19] and has been referred to as the "Hispanic hypertension paradox,"[20] has been contradicted in recent studies conducted among Mexican Americans in San Antonio.[21-23]

The heterogeneity of the Hispanic population in the United States is also reflected in differences in prevalence of hypertension among specific Hispanic subgroups. This heterogeneity has been documented in several studies conducted in Hispanic communities with a high proportion of individuals from a given subgroup. In the Hispanic Health and Nutrition Examination Survey (HANES) study of 1982 to 1984, the subgroup of Mexican Americans had a slightly higher prevalence of hypertension than did Cuban Americans or Puerto Ricans.[24] In the Northern Manhattan Stroke Study,[25] Hispanic Caribbean Americans, mostly Dominicans, had a prevalence of hyperten-

sion of 58%, significantly higher than in non-Hispanic whites (43%) and similar to rates in African Americans (62%).[24]

Results regarding the role of acculturation in the development of hypertension among Hispanics are conflicting. In one study, acculturation seemed to be a stronger predictor of hypertension in elderly Mexican Americans than was socioeconomic status,[26] although other studies of Mexican Americans of varying ages showed that the process of acculturation was not a major predictor.[27] In summary, the prevalence of hypertension in Hispanic Americans in the United States is currently lower than that of non-Hispanic whites and of African Americans. The current low prevalence of hypertension among Hispanics may not be sustained, however, given the increasing prevalence of diabetes and obesity in this ethnic subgroup.

AWARENESS, TREATMENT, AND CONTROL OF HYPERTENSION IN HISPANICS

National data suggest that, despite a similar or lower prevalence of hypertension, disparities exist in the detection and treatment of hypertension in Hispanics when compared with African Americans and non-Hispanic whites. The most representative and commonly cited data on hypertension awareness, treatment, and control come from the NHANES studies. The most recent NHANES study data (1999 to 2002) are shown in Table 40-1. There appears to be a much larger fraction of Mexican Americans who are unaware of having hypertension than are blacks or non-Hispanic whites, a lower percentage of Mexican Americans who are being treated for hypertension than are blacks or non-Hispanic whites, and a lower overall control rate of hypertension among Mexican Americans than among blacks or whites. The percentage of Mexican Americans who are aware of their hypertension and are being treated for it (70%) is also lower when compared with 77% and 79% in whites and blacks, respectively. The percentage of Mexican Americans whose hypertension is controlled if treated also appears to be lower, 50%, as compared with 59% in blacks and 61% in whites.

Another recent description of hypertension control in Hispanics comes from MESA.[16] In this study, 6814 adults

Table 40-1   Percentage of Noninstitutionalized United States Adults with Hypertension* 1999 to 2002

	Aware[†] Percentage (95% CI)	Under Treatment[‡] Percentage (95% CI)	Controlled[§] Percentage (95% CI)
White, non-Hispanic	62.9 (25.3-29.5)	48.6 (44.1-53.1)	29.8 (25.7-34.0)
Black, non-Hispanic	70.3 (64.9-75.8)	55.4 (51.2-59.6)	29.8 (25.2-34.5)
Mexican American	49.8 (40.4-59.2)	34.9 (27.5-42.3)	17.3 (10.7-23.8)[¶]

*Adults who had systolic blood pressure ≥140 mm Hg or diastolic blood pressure ≥90 mm Hg or who were taking antihypertensive medication.
[†]Told by a health care professional that their blood pressure was high.
[‡]Were taking antihypertensive medication.
[§]Systolic blood pressure <140 mm Hg and a diastolic blood pressure <90 mm Hg.
[¶]Estimates should be used with caution; relative standard error is 20% to 29%.
CI, confidence interval.
From Centers for Disease Control and Prevention. Racial/ethnic disparities in prevalence, treatment, and control of hypertension: United States, 1999-2002. *MMWR Morb Mortal Wkly Rep.* 2004;**54**:7-9.

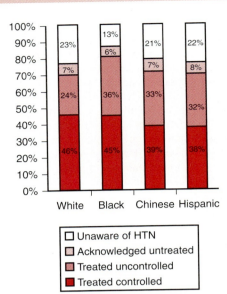

Figure 40–1   The results of hypertension (HTN) awareness, treatment, and control in the Multi-Ethnic Study of Atherosclerosis. (Data from Kramer H, Han C, Post W, et al. Racial/ethnic differences in hypertension and hypertension treatment and control in the Multi-Ethnic Study of Atherosclerosis (MESA). *Am J Hypertens.* 2004;**17**:963-970.)

between the ages of 45 and 84 years were recruited from six metropolitan areas of the United States from 2000 to 2002. The sample included 1494 Hispanics who resided in the Minneapolis–St. Paul metroplex, in northern Manhattan Island, or in Los Angeles.[28] The results from this study for hypertension awareness, treatment, and control are shown in Figure 40-1. These results suggested that although the Hispanic participants who had hypertension were aware of their disease and were being treated for it in similar proportions to non-Hispanic whites, their hypertension was less likely to be controlled. The Hispanics in this study were more likely to be treated with angiotensin-converting enzyme (ACE) inhibitors than were the other racial and ethnic groups. Contrary to what was found in African Americans, the "excess" of treated but uncontrolled hypertension decreased to statistical nonsignificance in Hispanics when data were analyzed by the MESA investigators in logistic regression models adjusted for education, income, and financial strain. Even in this large study, there were not enough subjects to comment on possible differences among Hispanic subgroups.

A study of unionized health workers with insurance in New York City found that Hispanic workers with hypertension were more likely to be untreated than were others.[29] A study of a public clinic system in Texas, where access issues across racial and ethnic groups should be fairly constant, showed worse control among blacks and Hispanics treated for hypertension.[30] An examination of the National Ambulatory Medical Care Survey and the National Hospital Ambulatory Medical Care Survey, both of which are national probability samples that examine standardized information from outpatient visits, found that Hispanics were actually more likely than whites to receive nutritional counseling or exercise counseling.[31] Although the Hispanics in this study tended to receive fewer antihypertensive drugs and fewer combination antihypertensive drugs than did blacks or whites,

these comparisons did not reach statistical significance. This data set did not include measured blood pressure and, consequently, has limited usefulness in elucidating treatment and control patterns in racial and ethnic subgroups.

The only national survey that included the three major Hispanic subgroups in the United States—Mexican Americans, Cubans, and Puerto Ricans—was the Hispanic HANES study conducted in 1981 to 1983, immediately following NHANES II.[32-34] Unfortunately, the methodology and the interpretation of the study results have been controversial, and the results themselves are now dated.

Evidence Regarding Optimal Treatment Regimens in Hispanics

The major randomized trials with morbidity or mortality outcomes provide little information regarding optimal hypertension treatment regimens for Hispanics. Only the recent Antihypertensive and Lipid-Lowering Treatment to Prevent Heart Attack Trial (ALLHAT; $N = 3876$)[35] and the Controlled Onset Verapamil Investigation of Cardiovascular End Points (CONVINCE; $N = 1178$)[36] included more than 100 persons identified as Hispanic. Subgroup analyses of the data in these trials have not yet been reported, and such analyses can be expected only to generate hypotheses. Limited numbers of pharmaceutical trials have targeted United States Hispanics or have been conducted in Latin American countries from which the U.S. immigrant populations originate. Long-acting ACE inhibitors and calcium antagonists were compared with placebo in studies with small samples of Mexican nationals or Mexican Americans and seemed to perform in a range similar to that in non-Hispanic white populations,[37] as did two ACE inhibitors (i.e., enalapril and perindopril) when compared in a trial against each other.[38] In small, short-term, non–double-blinded studies in Mexico, high-dose (80 mg/day) telmisartan, an angiotensin receptor blocker (ARB), was superior to 50 mg/day of atenolol or 20 mg/day of enalapril in controlling blood pressure.[39,40] However, data from these studies are not convincing enough to justify a recommendation for using ARBs as first-line agents. The putative role of ACE inhibitors and ARBs in diabetes prevention may theoretically make them an attractive option in subpopulations such as Mexican Americans, who are at high risk for diabetes, but any actual benefit has not been proven.

As discussed earlier, some Hispanic populations have gene pools with substantial admixture of African genes, and others do not. One would expect that drug selection issues that pertain to African Americans would also pertain to Hispanics with African genetic admixture. In a study conducted in New York City, 69 Caribbean Hispanics, a group sometimes referred to as Afro-Caribbean, were profiled.[41] These patients had participated in several general antihypertensive drug studies previously, and 62% of the subjects had been diagnosed with low-renin hypertension. Calcium antagonists, hydrochlorothiazide, and a combined regimen of an ACE inhibitor and hydrochlorothiazide were more effective than placebo, whereas monotherapy with an ACE inhibitor or a β-blocker was not.[41] This finding is what one would expect to see in African Americans.

Trials directly comparing renin-angiotensin blocking drugs with other agents are sparse in Hispanics. One multicenter trial compared an ARB with a calcium antagonist in self-declared African American, white, and "other" racial and ethnic groups, of whom more than half (54 of 80) of the individuals in the last category were Hispanic.[42] The probable genetic admixture of the Hispanics who participated in the study was not described. The investigators found the blood pressure–lowering response rates to ARB to be lower both in blacks and in the individuals in the other racial and ethnic group. A Brazilian study found the combination of an ARB and hydrochlorothiazide to be as effective as a calcium antagonist in lowering blood pressure.[43] A Venezuelan study found the efficacy of amlodipine, a calcium antagonist, and captopril, an ACE inhibitor, to be comparable.[44]

Sociocultural Issues

Because of the heterogeneity of the population groups defined as Hispanic, broad generalizations regarding the role of sociocultural factors in achieving optimal blood pressure control must be made with caution. Drs. Perez-Stable and Salazar provided a recent summary of cultural factors that may influence adherence to hypertension treatment in Hispanics.[42] These authors pointed out that engaging the family and forming a personal bond with the patient may be congruent to the cultural expectations of Hispanics. Their cultural beliefs about smooth and harmonious relationships with authority figures may lead physicians to believe that patients agree with a hypertension treatment plan when they do not understand it or accept it. Fatalism, a belief that there is little one can do to alter one's fate, is common in many cultures, including Hispanic cultures. No published reports are available on the effect of this construct on preventive cardiovascular behaviors. The use of complementary and alternative medicine (CAM) is widespread among most racial and ethnic groups in the United States, and many traditional CAM practitioners operate in Hispanic communities. It is not known whether Hispanics with hypertension are any more or less likely to use CAM therapies than are other persons with hypertension who belong to different racial and ethnic groups. As with all patients, it is important to ask Hispanic patients about their use of CAM and to make efforts to ensure that CAM therapies do not displace effective antihypertensive treatments.

SUMMARY

Improving hypertension diagnosis and control in many Hispanic communities will likely require special efforts. Public screening may be necessary to reach individuals who make infrequent contact with the health care system. Lack of insurance and inadequate financial and other resources are the major barriers to health care for many persons.[45] Drug costs may be a major issue for immigrant and other low-wage workers who are unlikely to be insured or to have prescription drug coverage. Physicians and health planners should also be prepared to deal with language barriers.

In considering how well hypertension is controlled among Hispanics, we must recognize that many whites and blacks in the United States have been exposed to public education about hypertension—known to them by its pseudonym, the "silent killer"—for more than 30 years. We must also recognize that whites and blacks in this country have embraced the once-radical idea that people should take pills for years when they feel good to prevent something serious from happening in the future. Many members of the Hispanic community have likely had much less exposure to this paradigm and will probably need more convincing.

Acknowledgments

We are grateful to Pamela Paradis Tice, ELS(D), and to Patricia Parra-Arevalo for their expert contributions to the preparation of this chapter.

References

1. Bureau of the Census. Population Projections for States, by Age, Sex, Race, and Hispanic Origin: 1992-2020. Current Population Reports. Report No. P25-1111.Washington, DC: U.S. Department of Commerce, Bureau of the Census, 1994.
2. Oppenheimer GM. Paradigm lost: Race, ethnicity, and the search for a new population taxonomy. *Am J Public Health.* 2001;**91**:1049-1055.
3. Borak J, Fiellin M, Chemerynski S. Who is Hispanic? Implications for epidemiologic research in the United States. *Epidemiology.* 2004;**15**:240-244.
4. Hahn RA, Stroup DF. Race and ethnicity in public health surveillance: Criteria for the scientific use of social categories. *Public Health Rep.* 1994;**109**:7-15.
5. Office of Management and Budget. Standards for the classification of federal data on race and ethnicity. *Fed Reg.* 1994;**59**:29831-29899.
6. Bertoni B, Budowle B, Sans M, et al. Admixture in Hispanics: Distribution of ancestral population contributions in the continental United States. *Hum Biol.* 2003;**75**:1-11.
7. Bonilla C, Shriver MD, Parra EJ, et al. Ancestral proportions and their association with skin pigmentation and bone mineral density in Puerto Rican women from New York City. *Hum Genet.* 2004;**115**:57-68.
8. Amaro H, Zambrana RE. Criollo, mestizo, mulatto, LatiNegro, indigena, white, or black? The US Hispanic/Latino population and multiple responses in the 2000 census. *Am J Public Health.* 2000;**90**:1724-1727.
9. Hajjar I, Kotchen TA. Trends in prevalence, awareness, treatment, and control of hypertension in the United States, 1988-2000. *JAMA.* 2003;**290**:199-203.
10. Centers for Disease Control and Prevention. Racial/ethnic disparities in prevalence, treatment, and control of hypertension: United States, 1999-2002. *MMWR Morb Mortal Wkly Rep.* 2004;**54**:7-9.
11. Franco LJ, Stern MP, Rosenthal M, et al. Prevalence, detection, and control of hypertension in a biethnic community: The San Antonio Heart Study. *Am J Epidemiol.* 1985;**121**:684-696.
12. Haffner S, Gonzalez Villalpando C, Valdez R, et al. Prevalence of hypertension in Mexico City and San Antonio, Texas. *Circulation.* 1994;**90**:1542-1549.
13. Haffner SM. Hypertension in the San Antonio Heart Study and the Mexico City Diabetes Study: Clinical and metabolic correlates. *Public Health Rep.* 1996;**111** (**Suppl 2**):11-14.
14. Shetterly SM, Rewers M, Hamman RF, Marshall JA. Patterns and predictors of hypertension incidence among Hispanics and non-Hispanic whites: The San Luis Valley Diabetes Study. *J Hypertens.* 1994;**12**:1095-1102.
15. Winkleby MA, Kraemer H, Lin J, et al. Sociodemographic influences on Hispanic-white differences in blood pressure. *Public Health Rep.* 1996;**111** (**Suppl 2**):30-32.
16. Kramer H, Han C, Post W, et al. Racial/ethnic differences in hypertension and hypertension treatment and control in the

Multi-Ethnic Study of Atherosclerosis (MESA). *Am J Hypertens.* 2004;**17**:963-970.

17. National Center for Health Statistics. Health, USA, 2004 with Chartbook on Trends in the Health of Americans. Hyattsville, Md, National Center for Health Statistics, 2004.

18. Sorlie PD, Backlund E, Johnson NJ, Rogot E. Mortality by Hispanic status in the United States. *JAMA.* 1993;**270**: 2464-2468.

19. Liao Y, Cooper RS, Cao G, et al. Mortality from coronary heart disease and cardiovascular disease among adult U.S. Hispanics: Findings from the National Health Interview Survey (1986 to 1994). *J Am Coll Cardiol.* 1997;**30**:1200-1205.

20. Pickering TG. Hypertension in Hispanics. *J Clin Hypertens.* 2004;**6**:279-282.

21. Wei M, Valdez RA, Mitchell BD, et al. Migration status, socioeconomic status, and mortality rates in Mexican Americans and non-Hispanic whites: The San Antonio Heart Study. *Ann Epidemiol.* 1996;**6**:307-313.

22. Stern MP, Wei M. Do Mexican Americans really have low rates of cardiovascular disease? *Prev Med.* 1999;**29**:S90-S95.

23. Hunt KJ, Resendez RG, Williams K, et al. All-cause and cardiovascular mortality among Mexican-American and non-Hispanic white older participants in the San Antonio Heart Study: Evidence against the "Hispanic paradox." *Am J Epidemiol.* 2003;**158**:1048-1057.

24. Crespo CJ, Loria CM, Burt VL. Hypertension and other cardiovascular disease risk factors among Mexican Americans, Cuban Americans, and Puerto Ricans from the Hispanic Health and Nutrition Examination Survey. *Public Health Rep.* 1996;**111** (**Suppl 2**):7-10.

25. Sacco RL, Boden-Albala B, Abel G, et al. Race-ethnic disparities in the impact of stroke risk factors: The Northern Manhattan Stroke Study. *Stroke.* 2001;**32**:1725-1731.

26. Espino DV, Maldonado D. Hypertension and acculturation in elderly Mexican Americans: Results from 1982-84 Hispanic HANES. *J Gerontol.* 1990;**45**:M209-M213.

27. Markides KS, Lee DJ, Ray LA. Acculturation and hypertension in Mexican Americans. *Ethn Dis.* 1993;**3**:70-74.

28. Bild DE, Bluemke DA, Burke GL, et al. Multi-Ethnic Study of Atherosclerosis: Objectives and design. *Am J Epidemiol.* 2002;**156**:871-881.

29. Stockwell DH, Madhavan S, Cohen H, et al. The determinants of hypertension awareness, treatment, and control in an insured population. *Am J Public Health.* 1994;**84**:1768-1774.

30. Pavlik V, Hyman D, Vallbona C. Hypertension control in multi-ethnic primary care clinics. *J Hum Hypertens.* 1996;**10** (**Suppl 3**):S19-S23.

31. Bonds DE, Palla S, Bertoni AG, et al. Hypertension treatment in the ambulatory setting: Comparison by race and gender in a national survey. *J Clin Hypertens (Greenwich).* 2004;**6**:223-228.

32. Pappas G, Gergen PJ, Carroll M. Hypertension prevalence and the status of awareness, treatment, and control in the Hispanic Health and Nutrition Examination Survey (HHANES), 1982-84. *Am J Public Health.* 1990;**80**:1431-1436.

33. Geronimus AT, Neidert LJ, Bound J. A note on the measurement of hypertension in HHANES. *Am J Public Health.* 1990;**80**:1437-1442.

34. Murphy RS. At last—a view of Hispanic health and nutritional status. *Am J Public Health.* 1990;**80**:1429-1430.

35. ALLHAT Officers and Coordinators for the ALLHAT Collaborative Research Group. Major outcomes in high-risk hypertensive patients randomized to angiotensin-converting enzyme inhibitor or calcium channel blocker vs. diuretic: The Antihypertensive and Lipid-Lowering Treatment to Prevent Heart Attack Trial (ALLHAT). *JAMA.* 2002;**288**:2981-2997.

36. Black HR, Elliott WJ, Grandits G, et al. Principal results of the Controlled Onset Verapamil Investigation of Cardiovascular End Points (CONVINCE) trial. *JAMA.* 2003;**289**:2073-2082.

37. Herrera CR, Lewin A, Fiddes R, et al. Long-acting diltiazem CD is safe and effective in a hypertensive Mexican-American population. *Pharmacotherapy.* 1997;**17**:1254-1259.

38. Alcocer L, Campos C, Bahena JH, et al. Clinical acceptability of ACE inhibitor therapy in mild to moderate hypertension: A comparison between perindopril and enalapril. *Cardiovasc Drugs Ther.* 1995;**9**:431-436.

39. Alcocer L, Fernandez-Bonetti P, Campos E, et al. Clinical efficacy and safety of telmisartan 80 mg once daily vs. atenolol 50 mg once daily in patients with mild-to-moderate hypertension. *Int J Clin Pract Suppl.* 2004;**145**:35-39.

40. Alcocer L, Fernandez-Bonetti P, Campos E, et al. Clinical efficacy and safety of telmisartan 80 mg once daily compared with enalapril 20 mg once daily in patients with mild-to-moderate hypertension: Results of a multicentre study. *Int J Clin Pract Suppl.* 2004;**145**:23-28.

41. Laffer CL, Elijovich F. Essential hypertension of Caribbean Hispanics: Sodium, renin, and response to therapy. *J Clin Hypertens (Greenwich).* 2002;**4**:266-273.

42. Perez-Stable EJ, Salazar R. Issues in achieving compliance with antihypertensive treatment in the Latino population. *Clin Cornerstone.* 2004;**6**:49-64.

43. Franco RJ, Goldflus S, McQuitty M, Oigman W. Efficacy and tolerability of the combination valsartan/hydrochlorothiazide compared with amlodipine in a mild-to-moderately hypertensive Brazilian population. *Blood Press.* 2003; **2** (**Suppl**):41-47.

44. Velasco M, Hernandez R, Urbina A, et al. A double-blind, parallel, comparative evaluation of amlodipine against captopril in the monotherapeutic treatment of mild and moderate essential hypertension: Interim results. *Postgrad Med J.* 1991; **67** (**Suppl 5**):S32-S34.

45. Schur CL, Albers LA, Berk ML. Health care use by Hispanic adults: Financial vs. non-financial determinants. *Health Care Financ Rev.* 1995;**17**:71-88.

Chapter 41

Hypertension in East Asians and Pacific Islanders

Nathan D. Wong

- The prevalence of hypertension has increased in developing Asian nations, is significant among the Native Hawaiian population, and varies dramatically among Asian ethnic subgroups.
- Pharmacologic therapy shown effective in white populations appears efficacious in East Asian populations in clinical trials.
- Side effects may be greater among certain Asian ethnic subgroups, and consideration should be given to careful dosage titration and combination therapeutic approaches to maximize tolerability.

Hypertension has become increasingly prevalent both in developing East Asian populations and among immigrant East Asian and Pacific Islander populations living in the United States (Table 41-1). Hypertension is a major contributor to cardiovascular disease morbidity and mortality, and it has been noted among some Asian immigrants to the United States to be higher than among their white counterparts.[1]

CHINESE POPULATIONS

In large surveys carried out in 13 regions of China between 1992-1994 ($n = 18,746$) and 1998 ($n = 13,504$), the prevalence of hypertension among those aged 35 to 59 years increased from 21.7% to 24.0%, with higher prevalences in men and in people living in urban areas.[2] Hypertension is less common among those living in southern China, particularly in rural areas, where dietary and exercise patterns are substantially different from those in northern or urban areas.[3,4] The most recent survey (2000 to 2001) included 15,838 nationally representative adults aged 35 to 74 years from 13 populations in China. These data showed a higher prevalence of hypertension (27.2% overall, representing 130 million hypertensive persons nationwide), with prevalences by age decade from 35 to 44 years to 65 to 74 years ranging from 10.7% to 50.2% for women and 17.4% to 47.3% for men. Among those persons who were hypertensive, 44.7% were aware of the diagnosis, and 28.2% were taking medication, but only 8.1% had their blood pressure (BP) controlled (to <140/90 mm Hg). These numbers represent relative increases of 86%, 93%, and 145% in awareness, treatment, and control, respectively, compared with a similar survey done in 1991.[5] Awareness, treatment, and control rates increased with age and were highest in urban areas and in women.[6] Controlled hypertension in a large Chinese population was more common among those who had more recently had their BP measured, those aware that they had hypertension, and those who undertaken lifestyle modifications.[7] In an investigation into the significant increase in mortality from coronary heart disease (50% in men and 27% in women) from 1984 to 1999 in Beijing, most of this increase was attributed to increases in cholesterol levels, some was attributed to increases in diabetes and obesity, contrary to observed decreases in BP during this period. One fourth (24%) of the deaths that were prevented or postponed, however, were attributed to treatment of hypertension.[8]

The prevalence of hypertension in 346 Chinese persons 60 years old or older who were living in the United States was 29.7% for men and 33.5% for women.[9] Older surveys of Chinese Americans reported lower prevalence rates, but the investigators noted a low level of awareness and understanding of the potentially serious implications of hypertension.[10,11] More recently, the population-based National Institutes of Health–sponsored Multi-Ethnic Study of Atherosclerosis (MESA) reported the unadjusted prevalence of hypertension in Chinese adults living in the United States to be 39%, not significantly different from the prevalence of 38% in whites. However, after adjustment for risk factors, Chinese ethnicity was associated with a significantly greater likelihood (odds ratio, 1.30; 95% confidence interval, 1.07 to 1.56) of hypertension compared with whites. In addition, among those patients treated, the proportion with uncontrolled hypertension was higher in Chinese patients (33%) than in whites (24%, $P = .003$) and diuretic use was lowest in Chinese persons (22% versus 47% for whites with hypertension).[12]

JAPANESE POPULATIONS

Among native Japanese persons, a national survey of 12 rural communities involving 11,302 subjects (mean age, 55 years) showed a prevalence of hypertension of 37% for men and 33% for women. Only 7% of the hypertensive patients, however, had their BP controlled to less than 140 mm Hg systolic and less than 90 mm Hg diastolic.[13] In contrast, among 907 treated hypertensive patients who were followed by cardiologists in 2000, 41.5% achieved a target BP of less than 140/90 mm Hg.[14] In 419 Japanese persons who were 60 years old or older and who were enrolled in the National Intervention Cooperative Study in Elderly Hypertensives, the prevalence of hypertension at baseline was 53%, and more than one third of these patients had isolated systolic hypertension.[15] After 14 years of follow-up in the National Survey on Cardiovascular Diseases, hypertension was associated with a 130% excess mortality among men and 42% among women, although BP levels themselves were related only to heart disease mortality among men.[16] More recently, the substantial increase in the prevalence of overweight and its

Table 41-1 Prevalence of Hypertension among East Asians and Native Hawaiians

Group	Prevalence (%) in Men	Prevalence (%) in Women	Author, Year, Reference
Chinese, People's Republic of China, ages 35-74 yr	17.4% (35-44 yr) 28.2% (45-54 yr) 40.7% (55-64 yr) 47.3% (65-74 yr)	10.7% (35-44 yr) 26.8% (45-54 yr) 38.9% (55-64 yr) 50.2% (65-74 yr)	Gu et al., 2003[5]
Chinese American, age ≥60 yr	29.7%	33.5%	Choi, 1990[9]
Japanese, mean age 55 yr	37%	33%	Asai et al., 2001[13]
Japanese American, men ages 60-81 yr	53% (60-64 yr) 67% (75-81 yr)		Curb et al., 1996[20]
Japanese American, ages 34-75 yr	41.5%	33.8%	Fujimoto et al., 1996[22]
Korean, ages 35-59 yr	28.9%	15.9%	Jee et al., 1998[25]
Korean, ages 18-92 yr	41.5%	24.5%	Jo et al., 2001[26]
Native Hawaiian, ages 20-54 yr	6% (20-24 yr) 37% (45-54 yr)	8% (20-24 yr) 41% (50-54 yr)	Curb et al., 1996[20]

relation to incident hypertension among Japanese persons was investigated. During the 4-year period between 1992 and 1996, 11.7% of men and 8.9% of women developed hypertension, and the increase in body mass index was significantly associated with the incidence of hypertension.[17] Moreover, the increasing prevalence of the metabolic syndrome can also be demonstrated among Japanese persons with increasing severity of BP by the criteria of the Seventh Report of the Joint National Committee on Prevention, Detection, Evaluation, and Treatment of High Blood Pressure (JNC 7), from 9.9% in normotensive persons, to 19.2% in those with prehypertension, and 35.5% in hypertensive patients.[18]

Among Japanese Americans, systolic and diastolic BPs have been shown to be the most important independent predictors of total, cardiovascular, coronary heart disease, and stroke mortality.[19] In the Honolulu Heart Study, the prevalence of hypertension increased in men from 53% to 67% as age increased from 60 to 64 years to 75 to 81 years.[20] Those who had isolated systolic hypertension, isolated diastolic hypertension, and systolic-diastolic hypertension at baseline, compared with normotensive subjects, were 4.8, 1.4, and 4.3 times, respectively, more likely to suffer a stroke over the next 20 years.[21] Among second- and third-generation Japanese Americans aged 34 to 75 years and living in King County, Washington, 41.5% of men and 33.8% of women were hypertensive; three fourths were aware of their hypertension, more than half were receiving treatment, and of those treated, more than 40% had their BP controlled.[22] In 1979, the prevalence of hypertension among Japanese Americans in California was only 14%, but awareness, treatment, and control rates were poor.[10,11]

KOREAN POPULATIONS

A large meta-analysis estimates that, for Koreans, hypertension is associated with a 4.1-fold increase in risk for all stroke, with a 6.6-fold increase for hemorrhagic stroke, and with a 3.3-fold increase for ischemic stroke.[23] A Korean national BP survey among 21,242 persons who were more than 30 years old showed 20% with hypertension, but only 25% were aware of it, 16% were treated, and 5% had their BP controlled.[24]

Among more than 180,000 Korean workers 35 to 59 years old who attended insurance examinations, a prevalence of hypertension of 28.9% in men and 15.9% in women was noted.[25] Another urban survey conducted among 2278 men and 1948 women aged 18 to 92 years showed 41.5% of men and 24.5% of women to have hypertension. Although only 24.6% of these persons were aware that they had hypertension, of these, 78% were receiving treatment, and 24% had their BP under control.[26] Recently, in a survey of 53,477 Korean adults, important predictors of high BP included insulin resistance, body mass index, and waist circumference; those in the highest quintile of insulin resistance had a 1.6-fold greater likelihood of hypertension.[27] The prevalence of metabolic syndrome among an urban Korean population was 16% in men and 10.7% in women 30 to 80 years old, although if modified waist circumference cut-points more appropriate for an Asian Pacific population are used (90 cm in men and 80 cm in women), this prevalence increases to 29% and 16.8%, respectively.[28]

NATIVE HAWAIIANS

Prevalence data for hypertension in Native Hawaiians are limited to one survey conducted among patients 20 to 59 years old in the Molokai Heart Study. Rates ranged from 6% in men and 8% in women 20 to 24 years old to 37% of men and 41% of women 45 to 54 years old.[20] The degree of Hawaiian ancestry has been linked to hypertension, with a 23% prevalence of hypertension among those with less than 25% Hawaiian ancestry to a 52% prevalence among those with 75% to 99% Hawaiian ancestry.[29] Because hypertension is a major component of the metabolic syndrome, along with abdominal obesity and glucose intolerance or diabetes, all of which are common among the Native Hawaiian population,[30] increased efforts aimed at detection and management of hypertension and associated risk factors are critically needed in this group.

TREATMENT CONSIDERATIONS

Some ethnic differences in response to antihypertensive agents have long been recognized, but only recently have data become available in East Asian populations. Comparative efficacy and tolerability data are still lacking among Native Hawaiian and Pacific Islander populations, however.

Documenting the efficacy of Western therapeutic approaches in East Asian populations, the Systolic Hypertension in China (Syst-China) trial was conducted in 2394 older patients with isolated systolic hypertension (average BP, 170/86 mm Hg), who were assigned to either active therapy (with nitrendipine, with addition of either captopril or hydrochlorothiazide if needed) or placebo. Active therapy (assigned originally to 1253 patients) reduced BP by 9.1/3.1 mm Hg compared with those originally assigned placebo and led to an impressive 38% reduction in strokes and other benefits, as discussed later.[31] Among 7443 Japanese patients treated and followed for 5 years, reduced cardiovascular event risk was seen with the use of diuretics and β-blockers, but increased risk was noted with calcium channel blockers (CCBs).[32] An increased cardiovascular risk with CCBs has also been seen in several epidemiologic studies (but not in large randomized trials) of non-Asian patients and has been attributed to "indication bias" (nonrandom assignment of a specific drug therapy to individuals with a higher baseline risk).

A review of hypertension management in 200 Asian patients and 196 white patients showed the preferred therapy to be monotherapy with either CCBs or angiotensin-converting enzyme (ACE) inhibitors for both groups. However, medication changes, dose reduction, and side effects were all significantly more commonly recorded in Asian patients.[33] Among 6289 Japanese patients who were receiving antihypertensive treatment, CCBs were most often prescribed, followed by ACE inhibitors, β-blockers, and diuretics. Hypertension control was similar regardless of class of agent, and of those patients whose BP was controlled, 49% reported at least one side effect, compared with 61% of patients with poorly controlled hypertension (who also had the worst adherence rates).[34] Among Chinese patients (in Hong Kong[35] and Taiwan[36]), similar effectiveness and tolerability of commonly used medications (amlodipine, atenolol, felodipine, and isradipine) have been observed, but with some reports of higher side effect rates in patients taking felodipine.[36]

Studies of ACE inhibitors in Chinese patients show efficacy similar to that in white patients, but Asians especially (and perhaps Chinese patients more than other Asians) experience more cough (see later) from this class of medications, although differences among the ACE inhibitors studied could possibly explain some of this difference.[37] Other investigators have documented greater efficacy of amlodipine over enalapril in Chinese patients with hypertension.[38] In Chinese patients with mild to moderate essential hypertension, the combination of losartan and hydrochlorothiazide was also shown to be more efficacious, despite similar tolerability, compared with losartan alone.[39] Among more than 900 treated patients with hypertension in Japan in 2000, CCBs were the most frequent class of medications utilized (73% of patients were taking at least one of these drugs), followed by ACE inhibitors (31.3%), angiotensin receptor blockers (18.9%), β-blockers (16.2%), and diuretics (10.1%).[14]

A relatively large body of evidence shows increased cough in Asians as a result of treatment with ACE inhibitors.[40-48] It is *no* coincidence that the first reports of ACE inhibitor–related cough came from Japan.[40] Two studies involving nearly 300 Japanese patients who were taking various ACE inhibitors

showed incidence rates of cough to vary from approximately 12% to 17%.[41,42] Studies in Hong Kong Chinese patients, however, tend to show higher incidences of cough of 48% (29 of 50 subjects) during treatment with lisinopril,[43] 46% with captopril, and 42% with enalapril (among 191 patients taking captopril or enalapril, in contrast to 382 controls in whom the rate of cough was only 11%). Other adverse reactions were similar, however, and the complication of cough was not related significantly to age, sex, underlying disease, dose, or smoking status.[44]

Some evidence indicates that Chinese (and other Asian-based) herbal therapeutic approaches, generally involving an orally administered mixture of multiple herbs and other ingredients that are designed to act synergistically, may reduce BP. Among 50 well-matched patients with mild to moderate hypertension, reductions in BP were greater among those assigned to the Western therapy including hydrochlorothiazide and atenolol.[49] However, patients assigned to the Chinese mixture of nine herbs still showed a statistically significant ($P < .01$) reduction in mean systolic and diastolic BP from 168/96 to 146/81 mm Hg.[49] Such therapy, however, has not shown to be sufficient to control more advanced forms of hypertension.[50] Additional clinical trials conducted in a standardized fashion are needed to confirm reported benefits of herbal therapies,[51] transcendental meditation,[52,53] and other alternative and complementary approaches for the control of BP and cardiovascular disease.[54]

OUTCOMES STUDIES

In addition to studies of the BP-lowering efficacy of antihypertensive drugs, several long-term clinical trials have included large numbers of Asians. The first clinical study of a CCB or placebo in hypertension was carried out at the Shanghai Institute of Hypertension. After a 4-week placebo treatment, hypertensive patients between 60 and 79 years of age were allocated to either nifedipine or placebo; 74 patients originally assigned to placebo were given nifedipine instead, according to local custom (for safety reasons). After 30 months of follow-up, 77 clinical events occurred in those patients originally assigned to placebo, compared with only 32 events in the original nifedipine group.[55] Only 16 strokes occurred in the group originally given nifedipine, as compared with 36 in the original placebo group. These data are seldom included in Western literature summaries and meta-analyses because of the lack of randomization and the reallocation of 74 subjects to active therapy. Nonetheless, the rather impressive 57% reduction in strokes and 59% reduction in cardiovascular events with a dihydropyridine CCB were early evidence in favor of a beneficial effect of this class of drugs on stroke and all cardiovascular events.

The clinical trial involving Asian hypertensive patients that is most widely accepted in the West is the Syst-China study, the design of which is discussed earlier.[31] After an average of 3 years of follow-up, those patients originally assigned to active treatment had a 38% reduction in stroke, the primary endpoint. This relative risk reduction was almost identical to the reduction in stroke seen in a similar U.S. study (Systolic Hypertension in the Elderly Program [SHEP]; see Chapters 14 and 38) of 36% and in a nearly identical European study (Systolic Hypertension in Europe [Syst-Eur]) of 42%. In addition to the significant reduction in stroke, patients assigned to active drug in Syst-China also enjoyed reductions in all-cause mortality (39%, $P = .003$), cardiovascular mortality (39%, $P = .03$), stroke mortality (58%, $P = .02$), and all cardiovascular endpoints (37%, $P = .004$). The major differences between Syst-China and other well-accepted clinical trials were the lack of randomization and the paucity of myocardial infarctions (which is also true in the Chinese population in general, as compared with Western populations).[56]

The National Intervention Cooperative Study in Elderly Hypertensives randomized 419 elderly hypertensive patients to therapy with either a CCB or a diuretic. Perhaps because of the small sample size, the investigators noted no significant differences in cardiovascular events (8 versus 10, respectively) or strokes (6 versus 8, respectively) after an average of 4 years of follow-up.[57] Another small trial of 1748 older hypertensive patients in Japan who were randomized to treatment for 1 year with either a dihydropyridine CCB or a diuretic showed no significant differences in stroke (2.2% versus 2.0%).[58]

A very important randomized clinical trial of nearly maximal doses of ACE inhibitor versus angiotensin receptor blocker versus their combination was conducted in 263 Japanese hypertensive patients with nondiabetic chronic kidney disease. This study, which has not yet been repeated in non-Asian patients, showed a significant prolongation of time to doubling of serum creatinine level or end-stage renal disease and a significant reduction in proteinuria in the 88 patients randomized to dual blockade of the angiotensin system, despite no difference in BPs over the 3 years of follow-up.[59]

The Post-stroke Antihypertensive Treatment Study (PATS) was a randomized, double-blind, placebo-controlled clinical trial comparing the incidence of fatal or nonfatal stroke in 5665 Chinese patients with a prior neurologic event. After an average of 2 years of therapy, the indapamide group had a slightly lower BP (149/89 versus 144/87 mm Hg) and a 29% reduction in the risk of a secondary stroke ($P = .0009$).[60] This was the first clinical trial in Asian patients to show a significant benefit of antihypertensive therapy on stroke.

The Perindopril Protection against Recurrent Stroke Study (PROGRESS) was a randomized clinical trial that enrolled 6105 patients with a prior history of cerebrovascular disease (84% with a stroke, 16% with a transient ischemic attack in the past 5 years), and randomized them to perindopril with or without indapamide or placebo with or without placebo. The clinician was asked to choose whether he or she wished the subject to receive either perindopril alone or both drugs before randomization. The majority (57%) selected the two-drug regimen. Fifty percent of these patients were hypertensive; 25% were Chinese, 13% were Japanese, and 62% were white. After approximately 4 years of follow-up, patients receiving active antihypertensive therapy had a 9/4 mm Hg lower BP, a highly significant 28% reduction in recurrent stroke, and a 26% reduction in cardiovascular events.[61] All the benefit was observed in those patients who received both drugs. In a multivariate model, Asian patients derived significantly greater benefits (in terms of stroke reduction) than did non-Asian patients.

Taken together, these clinical data show that, even when evaluated rigorously in clinical trials, Asian patients derive substantial benefit from antihypertensive drug therapy. The relative risk reduction in stroke is especially important, because stroke has traditionally been a greater public health problem for Asians than has heart disease.

CONCLUSIONS

Hypertension is an important contributor to morbidity and mortality from cardiovascular diseases in East Asians and Pacific Islanders. As these populations, particularly those residing in China, Japan, and Korea, undergo continuing acculturation to the Western lifestyle, hypertension will increase in prevalence, and increased efforts at detection, evaluation, and management will be needed. In addition, the Native Hawaiian population, with its particularly high rates of hypertension, obesity, diabetes, and cardiovascular disease, represents a significant need for greater efforts at detection and management. Recent studies have demonstrated similar efficacy of treatment with conventional classes of antihypertensive therapy, but health care providers need to have a better understanding of how best to minimize side effects (e.g., lower doses of combination therapy) that tend to be more prevalent in certain Asian populations. Finally, provider sensitivity to cultural barriers (e.g., difficulty navigating the health care system and beliefs regarding traditional, including herbal, therapies) that may affect adherence to Western therapies is needed. The use of proven Western therapeutic approaches, including established consensus treatment guidelines, needs to be the focus of hypertension management in East Asian and Pacific Islander populations as in any population. However, integrative medical approaches that combine proven Western therapies with traditional beliefs and treatment modalities should be considered, once they are backed with a rigorous research evidence base.

References

1. Hoyert DL, Kung H-C, Smith BL. Deaths: Preliminary data for 2003. *Natl Vital Stat Rep*. 2005;**53**:1-48.
2. Wang Z, Wu Y, Zhao L, et al. Trends in prevalence, awareness, treatment, and control of hypertension in the middle-aged population of China, 1992-1998. *Hypertens Res*. 2004;**27**:703-709.
3. Huang ZD, Wu XG, Stamler J, et al. A North-South comparison of blood pressure and factors related to blood pressure in the People's Republic of China: A report from the PRC-USA Collaborative Study of Cardiovascular Epidemiology. *J Hypertens*. 1994;**12**:1103-1112.
4. Wu XG, Huang ZD, Stamler J, et al. Changes in average blood pressure and incidence of high blood pressure 1983-1984 to 1987-1988 in four population cohorts in the People's Republic of China. *J Hypertens*. 1996;**14**:1267-1274.
5. Gu DF, Jiang H, Wu XG, et al. [Prevalence, awareness, treatment, and control of hypertension in Chinese adults.] *Zhonghua Yu Fang Yi Zue Za Zhi*. 2003;**37**:84-89.
6. Wang ZW, Wu YF, Zhao LC, et al. [Trends in prevalence, awareness, treatment and control of hypertension in middle-aged Chinese population.] *Zhonghua Liu Xing Bing Zue Za Zhi*. 2004;**25**:407-411.
7. Muntner P, Gu D, Wu X, et al. Factors associated with hypertension awareness, treatment, and control in a representative sample of the Chinese population. *Hypertension*. 2004;**43**:578-585.
8. Critchley J, Liu J, Zhao D, et al. Explaining the increase in coronary heart disease mortality in Beijing between 1984 and 1999. *Circulation*. 2004;**110**:1236-1244.

9. Choi E. The prevalence of cardiovascular risk factors among elderly Chinese Americans. *Arch Intern Med.* 1990;**150**:413-418.

10. Stavig G, Igra A, Leonard AR. Hypertension among Asians and Pacific Islanders in California. *Am J Epidemiol.* 1984;**119**:677-691.

11. Stavig G, Igra A, Leonard AR. Hypertension and related health issues among Asians and Pacific Islanders in California. *Public Health Rep.* 1988;**103**:28-37.

12. Kramer H, Han C, Post W, et al. Racial/ethnic differences in hypertension and hypertension treatment and control in the Multi-ethnic Study of Atherosclerosis (MESA). *Am J Hypertens.* 2004;**17**:963-970.

13. Asai Y, Ishikawa S, Kayaba K, et al. [Prevalence, awareness, treatment, and control of hypertension in Japanese rural communities.] *Nippon Koshu Eisei Zasshi.* 2001;**48**:827-836.

14. Yamamoto Y, Sonoyama K, Matsubara K, et al. The status of hypertension management in Japan in 2000. *Hypertens Res.* 2002;**25**:717-725.

15. Kuramoto K. Treatment of elderly hypertensives in Japan: National Intervention Cooperative Study in Elderly Hypertensives. The National Intervention Cooperative Study Group. *J Hypertens.* 1994;**12 (Suppl)**:S35-S40.

16. Lida M, Ueda K, Okayama A, et al. Impact of elevated blood pressure on mortality from all causes, cardiovascular diseases, heart disease and stroke among Japanese: 14 year follow-up of randomly selected population from Japanese-Nippon data 80. *J Hum Hypertens.* 2003;**17**:851-857.

17. Lee JS, Kawakubo K, Kashihara H, Mori K. Effect of long-term body weight change on the incidence of hypertension in Japanese men and women. *Int J Obes Relat Metab Disord.* 2004;**28**:391-395.

18. Kanauchi M, Kanauchi K, Hasimoto T, Saito Y. Metabolic syndrome and new category 'pre-hypertension' in a Japanese population. *Curr Med Res Opin.* 2004;**20**:1365-1370.

19. Yano K, McGee D, Reed DM. The impact of elevated blood pressure among 10-year mortality and Japanese men in Hawaii: The Honolulu Heart Program. *J Chronic Dis.* 1983;**36**:569-579.

20. Curb JD, Aluli NE, Huang BJ. Hypertension in elderly Japanese Americans and adult Native Hawaiians. *Pub Health Rep.* 1996;**111 (Suppl 2)**:53-55.

21. Petrovitch H, Curb JD, Bloom-Marcus E. Isolated systolic hypertension and risk for stroke in Japanese-American men. *Stroke.* 1995;**26**:25-29.

22. Fujimoto W, Boyko EJ, Leonetti DL, et al. Hypertension in Japanese Americans: The Seattle Japanese-American Community Diabetes Study. *Pub Health Rep.* 1996;**111 (Suppl 2)**:56-58.

23. Park JK, Kim CB, Kim KS, et al. Meta-analysis of hypertension as a risk factor for cerebrovascular disorders in Koreans. *J Korean Med Sci.* 2001;**16**:2-8.

24. Jones DW, Kim JS, Kim SJ, Hong YP. Hypertension awareness, treatment and control rates for an Asian population: Results from a national survey in Korea. *Ethn Health.* 1996;**1**:269-273.

25. Jee SH, Appel LJ, Suh I, et al. Prevalence of cardiovascular risk factors in South Korean adults: Results from the Korea Medical Insurance Corporation (KMIC) Study. *Ann Epidemiol.* 1998;**8**:1-2.

26. Jo I, Ahn Y, Lee J, et al. Prevalence, awareness, treatment, control and risk factors of hypertension in Korea: The Ansan study. *J Hypertens.* 2001;**19**:1523-1532.

27. Sung KC, Rhu SH. Insulin resistance, body mass index, waist circumference are independent risk factor for high blood pressure. *Clin Exp Hypertens.* 2004;**26**:547-556.

28. Oh JY, Hong YS, Sung YA, Barrett-Connor E. Prevalence and factor analysis of metabolic syndrome in an urban Korean population. *Diabetes Care.* 2004;**27**:2027-2032.

29. Grandinetti A, Chen R, Kaholokula JK, et al. Relationship of blood pressure with degree of Hawaiian ancestry. *Ethn Dis.* 2002;**12**:221-228.

30. Mau MK, Grandinetti A, Arakaki RF, et al. The insulin resistance syndrome in native Hawaiians. Native Hawaiian Health Research (NHHR) Project. *Diabetes Care.* 1997;**20**:1376-1380.

31. Liu L, Wang JG, Gong L, et al. Comparison of active treatment and placebo in older Chinese patients with isolated systolic hypertension. Systolic Hypertension in China (Syst-China) Collaborative Group. *J Hypertens.* 1998;**16**:1823-1829.

32. Uchiyama M, Kondo T, Tsuzuki Y, et al. Difference in occurrence of cardiovascular events according to class of antihypertensive agent, based on a follow-up study of Japanese hypertension patients. *Jpn Heart J.* 2001;**42**:585-595.

33. Hui KK, Pasic J. Outcome of hypertension management in Asian Americans. *Arch Intern Med.* 1997;**157**:1345-1348.

34. Toyoshima H, Takahashi K, Akera T. The impact of side effects on hypertension management: A Japanese survey. *Clin Ther.* 1998;**20**:373-374.

35. Cheung BM, Lau CP, Wu BZ. Amlodipine, felodipine, and isradipine in the treatment of Chinese patients with mild-to-moderate hypertension. *Clin Ther.* 1998;**20**:1159-1169.

36. Chern MS, Lin FC, Wu D. [Comparison of clinical efficacy and adverse effects between extended-release felodipine and atenolol in patients with mild and moderate essential hypertension.] *Changeng Yi Zue Za Zhi.* 1997;**20**:86-93.

37. Ding PY, Hu OY, Pool PE, Liao W. Does Chinese ethnicity affect the pharmacokinetics and pharmacodynamics of angiotensin-converting enzyme inhibitors? *J Hum Hypertens.* 2000;**14**:163-170.

38. Tomlinson B, Woo J, Thomas GN, et al. Randomized, controlled, parallel-group comparison of ambulatory and clinic blood pressure responses to amlodipine or enalapril during and after treatment in adult Chinese patients with hypertension. *Clin Ther.* 2004;**26**:1292-1304.

39. Li Y, Liu G, Jiang B, et al. A comparison of initial treatment with losartan/HCTZ versus losartan monotherapy in Chinese patients with mild to moderate essential hypertension. *Int J Clin Pract.* 2003;**57**:673-677.

40. Sesoko S, Kaneko Y. Cough associated with the use of captopril. *Arch Intern Med.* 1985;**145**:1524.

41. Fujimori K. [Angiotensin converting enzyme (ACE) inhibitor-induced cough in non-smoking hypertensive patients]. *Arerugi.* 1991;**40**:1327-1333.

42. Kaku T, Yamasaki H, Harada N, et al. [Dry cough in the elderly patients treated with angiotensin converting enzyme inhibitor.] *Nippon Ronen Igakkai Zasshi.* 1991;**28**:365-370.

43. Woo J, Chan TY. A high incidence of cough associated with combination therapy of hypertension with isradipine and lisinopril in Chinese subjects. *Br J Clin Pract.* 1991;**45**:178-180.

44. Woo KS, Nicholls MG. High prevalence of persistent cough with angiotensin converting enzyme inhibitors in Chinese. *Br J Clin Pharmacol.* 1995;**40**:141-144.

45. Chan WK, Chan TY, Luk WK, et al. A high incidence of cough in Chinese subjects treated with angiotensin converting enzyme inhibitors [letter]. *Eur J Clin Pharmacol.* 1993;**44**:299-300.

46. Woo KS, Norris RM, Nicholls G. Racial difference in incidence of cough with angiotensin-converting enzyme inhibitors (a tale of two cities). *Am J Cardiol.* 1995;**75**:967-968.

47. Furuya K, Yamaguchi E, Hirabayashi T, et al. Angiotensin-I-converting enzyme gene polymorphism and susceptibility to cough [letter]. *Lancet.* 1994;**343**:354.

48. Ogihara T, Mikami H, Katahira K, Otsuka A. Comparative study of the effects of three angiotensin converting enzyme inhibitors on the cough reflex. *Am J Hypertens.* 1991;**4 (Suppl 2)**:46S-51S.

49. Wong ND, Ming S, Zhou HY, Black HR. A comparison of Chinese traditional and Western medical approaches for the treatment of mild hypertension. *Yale J Biol Med.* 1991;**64**:79-87.

50. Black HR, Ming S, Poll DS, et al. A comparison of the treatment of hypertension with Chinese herbal and Western medication. *J Clin Hypertens (Greenwich)*. 1986;**2**:371-378.

51. Townsend RR. Common questions and answers in the management of hypertension: Everyday practice in hypertension. Herbal remedies for high blood pressure. *J Clin Hypertens (Greenwich)*. 2000;**2**:54-55.

52. Wenneberg SR, Schneider RH, Walton KG, et al. A controlled study of the effects of the transcendental meditation program on cardiovascular reactivity and ambulatory blood pressure. *Int J Neurosci*. 1997;**89**:15-28.

53. Zamarra JW, Schneider RH, Besseghini I, et al. Usefulness of the transcendental meditation program in the treatment of patients with coronary artery disease. *Am J Cardiol*. 1996;15:867-870.

54. Lin MC, Nahin R, Gershwin ME, et al. State of complementary and alternative medicine in cardiovascular, lung, and blood research: Executive summary of a workshop. *Circulation*. 2001;**103**:2038-2041.

55. Gong L, Zhang W, Zhu Y, et al. Shanghai trial of nifedipine in the elderly (STONE). *J Hypertens*. 1996;**14**:1237-1245.

56. Wang JG, Staessen JA, Gong L, Liu L. Chinese trial on isolated systolic hypertension in the elderly. Systolic Hypertension in China (Syst-China) Collaborative Group. *Arch Intern Med*. 2000;**160**:211-220.

57. National Intervention Cooperative Study in Elderly Hypertensives Study Group. Randomized double-blind comparison of a calcium antagonist and a diuretic in elderly hypertensives. *Hypertension*. 1999;**34**:1129-1133.

58. Ogihara T. Practitioner's trial on the efficacy of antihypertensive treatment in the elderly hypertension (the PATE-Hypertension Study) in Japan. *Am J Hypertens*. 2000;**13**:461-467.

59. Nakao N, Yoshimura A, Morita H, et al. Combination treatment of angiotensin-II receptor blocker and angiotensin-converting-enzyme inhibitor in non-diabetic renal disease (COOPERATE): A randomised controlled trial. *Lancet*. 2003;**361**:117-124.

60. Post-stroke Antihypertensive Treatment Study. A preliminary result: PATS Collaborating Group. *Chin Med J*. 1995;**108**:710-717.

61. PROGRESS Collaborative Group. Randomised trial of a perindopril-based blood-pressure-lowering regimen among 6105 individuals with previous stroke or transient ischaemic attack. *Lancet*. 2001;**358**:1033-1041.

Chapter 42

Hypertension in South Asians

Prakash C. Deedwania and Rajeev Gupta

Cardiovascular diseases caused 2.3 million deaths in India in 1990; by 2020, this number is projected to double. Hypertension is the attributable cause of 57% of stroke-related deaths and of 24% of coronary heart disease–related deaths in India. Indian urban population studies in the mid-1950s used older World Health Organization (WHO) guidelines for diagnosis (blood pressure [BP] ≥160 mm Hg systolic or ≥95 mm Hg diastolic) and reported a hypertension prevalence of only 1.2% to 4.0%. Subsequent studies reported a steadily increasing prevalence from 5% in the 1960s to 12% to 15% in the 1990s. Hypertension prevalence is lower in the rural Indian population, although this group has also seen a steady increase in the condition over time. Recent studies using current criteria (BP ≥140 mm Hg systolic or ≥90 mm Hg diastolic) have shown that hypertension is present in 25% of urban and 10% of rural subjects in India. At minimum, this translates to about 42 million hypertensive persons in rural areas and 45 million in urban areas. Approximately 70% of these persons have stage 1 hypertension (systolic BP 140 to 159 or diastolic BP 90 to 99 mm Hg). Population-based cost-effective hypertension control strategies should be developed for Indian and other South Asian populations.

GLOBAL BURDEN OF HYPERTENSION

Cardiovascular diseases account for a large proportion of all deaths and disability worldwide. The Global Burden of Disease study estimated that cardiovascular diseases were responsible for 5.2 million deaths in economically developed countries and 9.1 million deaths in developing countries in 1990.[1] In developed countries, about one fourth of cardiovascular disease–related deaths occurred in persons less than 70 years of age, but more than approximately half of these deaths in developing countries occurred in persons less than 70 years old.[2] By the year 2020, the global cardiovascular disease burden is predicted to increase by almost 75%. Almost all of this increase will occur in developing countries (Table 42-1).

The emerging burden of cardiovascular disease in India is more alarming. In 1990, cardiovascular diseases accounted for 25% of all deaths (2.3 of 9.4 million); coronary heart disease was responsible for 1.2 million deaths, and another 0.5 million deaths were attributed to stroke.[1] The Global Burden of Disease study estimated that, by 2020, cardiovascular disease deaths in India will increase by 111%, which is even more than the predicted 77% for China, 106% for other Asian countries and islands, and 15% for economically developed countries.[2] Downward revision of this predicted increase in cardiovascular disease will require modification of risk factors with two characteristics. First, the risk factors must have high attributable risk, high prevalence, or both. Second, reversal of most or all of the risks must be cost-effective. BP is a major risk factor

for several types of cardiovascular disease, and the association of BP with cardiovascular risk is continuous. Large proportions of most populations have nonoptimal BP values.[3] Moreover, most or all of the BP-related risk can be significantly reduced within a few years using relatively inexpensive interventions.

In India, 57% of all stroke-related deaths and 24% of all coronary heart disease–related deaths have been attributed to hypertension.[2] Current estimates predict that if a 2 mm Hg population-wide decrease in systolic BP were achieved in India, 151,000 stroke-related and 153,000 coronary heart disease-related deaths could be prevented.[2]

RECENT STUDIES OF THE PREVALENCE OF HYPERTENSION IN INDIA

Both urban and rural areas in India have been surveyed to estimate the prevalence of hypertension (Table 42-2).[3-5] In the mid-1950s, Indian urban population studies used the standardized WHO guidelines for the diagnosis of hypertension (known hypertension or BP ≥160 mm Hg systolic or ≥95 mm Hg diastolic) and reported a prevalence of hypertension of 1.2% to 4.0%. Subsequently, the prevalence of hypertension in Indian cities steadily increased: 4.35% in Agra (1963), 6.43% in Rohtak (1978), 15.52% in Bombay (1980), 14.08% in Ludhiana (1985), 10.99% in Jaipur (1995), 11.59% in Delhi (1997), and 13.11% in Chandigarh (1999). These time trends were significant, regardless of statistical methodology (nonparametric analysis; Mantel-Haenszel test, $P = .014$; or regression analysis, $r = .70$, $P = .026$).

Although rural populations in India generally had a lower prevalence of hypertension compared with urban areas, rural areas had a steady increase over time as well: 0.52% in Bombay (1959), 1.99% in Delhi (1959), 3.57% in Haryana (1977), 5.41% in Delhi (1983), 5.59% in Rajasthan (1984), 2.63% in Punjab (1985), 4.02% in Maharashtra (1993), 3.41% in Maharashtra (1993), 7.08% in Rajasthan (1994), and 3.58% in Delhi (1998) (χ^2 for trend = 2.75, $P = .097$). In South Indian rural subjects who are almost urbanized, the prevalence of hypertension was reported to be as high as 17.8% (1993) and 12.46% (1994). Overall, a significant increase in the prevalence of hypertension in rural areas has occurred, although the rise is not as steep as in urban populations ($r = 0.67$, $P = .025$). On average, from 1942 to 1995, urban Indian men aged 40 to 49 years had a significant increase in systolic BP ($r = 0.95$, $P < .001$), but not in diastolic BP ($r = 0.43$, $P > .2$). This finding is of obvious clinical importance in light of recent evidence that systolic BP is more closely linked to cardiovascular events and cardiac mortality.[6,7]

Systolic BP 140 mm Hg or higher or diastolic BP 90 mm Hg or higher is the currently accepted diagnostic threshold for hypertension, based on epidemiologic and intervention

Table 42-1   Cardiovascular Deaths by Region in the Years 1990 and 2020: Global Burden of Disease

	Cardiovascular Deaths, 1990			
	Number (Millions)	Related to Coronary Heart Disease (%)	Related to Stroke (%)	Predicted Increase by 2020 (%)
Established market economies	3.2	53	25	15
Former socialist economies	2.1	50	31	26
India	2.3	52	20	111
China	2.6	30	50	77
Other Asian countries and islands	1.3	34	29	106
Sub-Saharan Africa	0.8	26	47	114
Latin America and Caribbean	0.8	44	32	120
Middle Eastern Crescent	1.3	47	16	129

Data from Murray CJL, Lopez AD. Mortality by cause for eight regions of the world: Global Burden of Disease Study. *Lancet.* 1997;**349**:1269-1276; and Rodgers A, Lawes C, MacMahon S. Reducing the global burden of blood pressure related cardiovascular disease. *J Hypertens.* 2000;**18 (Suppl 1)**:S3-S6.

Table 42-2   Indian Hypertension Prevalence Studies (Blood Pressure >160/95 mm Hg)

First Author	Year	Age Group	Place	Sample Size	Prevalence (% ±SE)
Urban					
Dotto BB	1949	18-50	Calcutta	2,500	1.24±0.2
Dubey VD	1954	18-60	Kanpur	2,262	4.24±0.4
Sathe RV	1959	20-80	Bombay	4,120	3.03±0.3
Mathur KS	1963	20-80	Agra	1,634	4.35±0.5
Malhotra SL	1971	20-58	Railways	4,232	9.24±0.4
Gupta SP	1978	20-69	Rohtak	2,023	6.43±0.5
Dalal PM	1980	20-80	Bombay	5,723	15.52±0.5
Sharma BK	1985	20-75	Ludhiana	1,008	14.08±1.1
Gupta R	1995	20-80	Jaipur	2,212	10.99±0.7
Chadha SL	1998	25-69	Delhi	13,134	11.59±1.0
Thakur K	1999	30-80	Chandigarh	1,727	13.11±1.0
Rural					
Shah VV	1959	30-60	Bombay	5,996	0.52±0.1
Padmavati S	1959	20-75	Delhi	1,052	1.99±0.4
Gupta SP	1977	20-69	Haryana	2,045	3.57±0.4
Wasir HS	1983	20-69	Delhi	905	5.41±0.8
Baldwa VS	1984	21-60	Rajasthan	912	5.59±0.8
Sharma BK	1985	20-75	Punjab	3,340	2.63±0.3
Kumar V	1991	21-70	Rajasthan	6,840	3.83±0.2
Joshi PP	1993	16-60	Maharashtra	448	4.02±0.9
Jajoo UN	1993	20-69	Maharashtra	4,045	3.41±0.3
Gupta R	1994	20-80	Rajasthan	3,148	7.08±0.5
Chadha SL	1998	25-69	Delhi	1,732	3.58±0.5

From Gupta R, Al-Odat NA, Gupta VP. Hypertension epidemiology in India: Meta-analysis of fifty-year prevalence rates and blood pressure trends. *J Hum Hypertens.* 1996;**10**:465-472.

studies,[8] mostly conducted in the United States and Europe.[9,10] No prospective epidemiologic studies similar to the Framingham Heart Study or clinical trials exist among Indians. Therefore, the level of BP at which the risk of cardiovascular events begins to increase is not well defined. Most studies from developing countries show a lower mean population BP as compared with developed countries.[11-13] Therefore, the values above which high BP increases cardiovascular risk could be lower in these countries.[13] However, in the absence of prospective data and also because of the current recommendations of the WHO[8] and of many Indian Consensus Groups, the criterion of systolic BP 140 mm Hg or higher or diastolic BP 90 mm Hg of higher is accepted as the cut-off level for the diagnosis of hypertension.

The prevalence of hypertension, defined by 2005 WHO criteria, was reported among some urban Indian populations (Table 42-3).[14-20] Although fewer surveys used the threshold BP of 140/90 mm Hg or higher, and the time between the first and the last study was only 7 years, these data hint that hypertension is becoming more prevalent in Indian cities. In the

Table 42-3   Recent Indian Hypertension Prevalence Studies (Blood Pressure >140/90 mm Hg)

Reference	Year	Age Group (yr)	Place	Sample Size		Prevalence (%)	
				Men	Women	Men	Women
Urban							
Gupta et al.[14]	1995	20-75	Jaipur	1,415	797	29.5	33.5
Gupta et al.[15]	1999	18-60	Mumbai	40,067	59,522	43.8	44.5
Joseph et al.[16]	2000	20-89	Trivandrum	76	130	31.0	41.2
Anand[19]	2000	30-60	Mumbai	1,521	141	34.1*	
Mohan et al.[17]	2001	20-70	Chennai	518	657	14.0*	
Gupta et al.[18]	2002	20-75	Jaipur	550	573	36.4	37.5
Rural							
Gupta and Sharma[21]	1994	20-75	Rajasthan	1,982	1,166	23.7	16.9
Malhotra et al.[22]	1999	16-70	Haryana	2,559		3.0	5.8†

*Gender-specific data not available.
†Prevalence rates based on multiple examinations.

two surveys conducted by Gupta and colleagues (1995[14] and 2002[18]), both done in Jaipur, hypertension prevalence increased from 30% to 36% among men and from 34% to 38% among women 20 years old or older. When these prevalence rates are adjusted to an identical age distribution, however, the differences are not significant; the age-adjusted hypertension prevalence rates are 30% and 34% (for men and women, respectively). The prevalence of hypertension in India is similar to, if not greater than, the prevalence of this condition in the United States[20] or in other regions of Asia, where it has been reported that, at any one time, about half of all urbanized individuals have high BP.[2]

Among Indian rural populations, the prevalence of hypertension (using current diagnostic criteria) is lower than in urban areas (see Table 42-3). In a 1994 survey of 3148 men and women who were more than 19 years old and who lived in rural Rajasthan,[21] hypertension was present in 24% of men and in 17% of women. Using similar methodology in urban Jaipur,[14] the same authors found hypertension in 30% of 1415 men and in 34% of 797 women in 1995. The importance of population-based differences in risk factors for hypertension is highlighted by the data of Malhotra and colleagues.[22] In a survey of 2559 men and women aged 16 to 70 years, these investigators found hypertension in only 3.0% of men and 5.8% of women in rural Haryana, and they attributed the low prevalence to very low body mass index in this population. These observations highlight the need for prospective cohort studies in a larger Indian population to address differences in hypertension prevalence across time and regional subpopulations.

RISK FACTORS FOR HYPERTENSION IN INDIANS

Although the precise reasons for the increase in hypertension prevalence among Indians have not been established, several possibilities exist. BPs in so-called unindustrialized societies are generally lower, and they do not increase with age.[23] In unindustrialized and less-industrialized Indian rural populations, only a small increase in the prevalence in hypertension occurs as the population ages.[4] Conversely, in urban Indian populations exposed to the stress of acculturation and modernization, hypertension prevalence rates have more than doubled in the last 30 years.

Epidemiologic evidence indicates that population demographic changes in India have increased environmental risk factors for hypertension.[24] Life expectancy, urbanization, development, and affluence have all increased in India.[25] In 1901, only 11% of the population lived in an urban area; this proportion grew impressively over time: 17.6% in 1951, 18.3% in 1961, 20.2% in 1971, 23.7% in 1981, and 26.1% in 1991. A strong correlation exists between urbanization and the increase in hypertension prevalence ($r = 0.92$, $P < .01$). Affluence (as measured by evaluation of per capita net domestic product, growth of production, and human development index) has also increased sharply in India in recent years and correlates positively with the rise in the prevalence of hypertension. Tobacco production, a surrogate for its consumption, is increasing at a very high rate in India. Per capita fat and oil consumption has also risen since 1960. It was 5.79 kg/person/year in 1961, 5.85 in 1971, 6.48 in 1981, and 6.96 in 1987. Salt consumption was 10.7 g/person/day in 1971 and increased to 13.0 in 1981, 15.8 in 1991, and 16.9 in 1994. Taken together, these sociodemographic and lifestyle factors may be accelerating the hypertension epidemic currently sweeping India and other developing countries.

OTHER SOUTH ASIAN POPULATIONS

According to the WHO, in adults 40 to 55 years old, BP levels were highest among Indian men, as compared with men of 20 other developing countries.[8] Hypertension prevalence greater than 20% was found in 6 of the 12 communities studied in different parts of Asia and Latin America, according to the International Clinical Epidemiology Network study, which used current WHO diagnostic criteria.[26]

Population-based studies of hypertension prevalence among other South Asian countries are sparse. A study in

Nepal in the early 1980s reported hypertension in 10% of urban subjects.[27] In Bangladesh, hypertension was reported in fewer than 5% of rural subjects.[28]

Several reports indicate that South Asians who emigrate have high hypertension prevalence rates, perhaps even slightly higher than those who remain in their native countries. In Great Britain, a few population prevalence studies reported that hypertension prevalence in Indians is similar to that of native whites. Bhatnagar and associates reported that mean BP among emigrant South Asians as compared with their Indian siblings was 146 ± 23 mm Hg versus 132 ± 22 mm Hg in men and 143 ± 28 mm Hg versus 142 ± 23 mm Hg in women.[29] Williams analyzed various South Asian emigrant studies and commented that hypertension prevalence was not different in this group as compared with whites.[30] Bhopal and colleagues compared hypertension prevalence rates in Indians, Pakistanis, and Bangladeshis living in Britain and reported that the hypertension was more pronounced in Indians as compared with other South Asian groups.[31] In the Study of Health Assessment and Risk in Ethnic Groups (SHARE) study in Canada, the prevalence of self-reported hypertension in South Asians was 12.5%. This percentage was similar to that in Europeans (11.0%), but lower than in Chinese persons (15.9%).[32]

IMPLICATIONS OF EPIDEMIOLOGIC STUDIES FOR TREATMENT OF HYPERTENSION IN SOUTH ASIANS

Treatment of hypertension is associated with reductions in cardiovascular morbidity and mortality, but the number of events prevented is generally related to the absolute risk of the population treated. In high-risk populations (e.g., older individuals, diabetic patients, or those with very high BPs), many events can be prevented with relatively inexpensive drug treatment. However, with lower-risk patients, lifestyle modifications are sometimes recommended over drug therapy because these changes can be implemented in large populations and involve fewer direct costs. In the Treatment of Mild Hypertension Study (TOMHS),[33] lifestyle modifications *in addition to* drug treatment in individuals with only mildly raised BP (stage 1 hypertension, systolic 140 to 159 mm Hg or diastolic 90 to 95 mm Hg; average, 142/91 mm Hg) was associated with improved outcomes as compared with subjects who received placebo in addition to lifestyle modifications. In 1992, Stamler recommended an average population systolic BP of 110 mm Hg as a realistic goal.[34] In India, an estimate is required of the absolute numbers of patients with hypertension who would be eligible for treatment if WHO recommendations were followed.

Epidemiologic studies have shown that hypertension is present in 25% of urban and 10% of rural subjects in India. Because of a difference in the number of BP measurements (typically one in epidemiologic studies, at least two for a proper diagnosis in clinical studies), investigators have estimated that epidemiologic studies overdiagnose hypertension by 20% to 25%.[19] If we discount this proportion, 19% of adults in the urban areas and 7.5% in the rural areas of India would be eligible for antihypertensive therapies. Translating these proportions into numbers reveals a massive burden of this disease in India. According to the 2001 census, 600 million adults live in India, of whom 420 million are in rural areas and 180 million are in urban areas. The absolute number of hypertensive persons in India would therefore be 31.5 million in rural areas and 34 million in urban areas, for a total of 65.5 million persons with hypertension. An Indian epidemiologic study reported that 70% of all hypertensive persons had stage 1 hypertension (systolic BP 140 to 159 or diastolic BP 90 to 99 mm Hg).[35] Patients with stage 1 hypertension (or 45.5 million subjects) could be managed initially by lifestyle modifications. However, reports from the Seven Countries Study[36] and the Framingham Heart Study[37] showed that what was termed "high normal" BP (systolic BP 130 to 139 mm Hg or diastolic BP 85 to 89 mm Hg) and stage 1 hypertension carry a significant cardiovascular risk, and the need exists to reduce this BP level. Pharmacologic therapies for these individuals will be expensive and will require more studies, although TOMHS demonstrated that drug therapy reduces cardiovascular endpoints.[33] For BPs higher than stage 1 hypertension, multiple authorities recommend pharmacologic therapy, which translates into regular antihypertensive medications for 20 million persons in India. This recommendation carries a huge economic burden on an already overstressed Indian economy. Studies that examine cost-effective approaches to control BP optimally among Indians are needed.

Ethnic differences occur in therapeutic response to antihypertensive drug treatment.[38] African Americans respond less well to drugs that suppress the renin-angiotensin system (e.g., β-blockers and angiotensin-converting enzyme inhibitors) as compared with other drugs (diuretics and calcium channel blockers). No trials of efficacy of different antihypertensive agents are available in South Asians. However, because of the greater prevalence of diabetes, insulin resistance, and metabolic syndrome in this population,[39,40] drugs that improve insulin sensitivity and provide vasculoprotective effects such as angiotensin-converting enzyme inhibitors or angiotensin receptor blockers could be considered first-line options.

Hypertension carries a huge economic burden on already overstressed economies of South Asian countries as well as developing countries worldwide.[41,42] Poor control of high BP has been attributed to various socioeconomic factors, and studies that examine cost-effective approaches to control BP optimally among these persons are urgently required.

References

1. Murray CJL, Lopez AD. Mortality by cause for eight regions of the world: Global Burden of Disease study. *Lancet.* 1997;**349**:1269-1276.
2. Rodgers A, Lawes C, MacMahon S. Reducing the global burden of blood pressure related cardiovascular disease. *J Hypertens.* 2000;**18 (Suppl 1)**:S3-S6.
3. Deedwania P, Gupta R. Hypertension in South Asians, 3rd ed. *In:* Izzo JL, Black HR (eds). Hypertension Primer. Dallas, Tex: American Heart Association, 2003, pp 269-271.
4. Gupta R, Al-Odat NA, Gupta VP. Hypertension epidemiology in India: Meta-analysis of fifty-year prevalence rates and blood pressure trends. *J Hum Hypertens.* 1996;**10**:465-472.
5. Gupta R. Hypertension in India: Definition, prevalence and evaluation. *J Indian Med Assoc.* 1999;**97**:74-80.
6. Deedwania P. The changing face of hypertension: Is systolic blood pressure the final answer? *Arch Intern Med.* 2002;**162**:506-508.

7. Prospective Studies Collaborative. Age-specific relevance of usual blood pressure to vascular mortality: A meta-analysis of individual data for one million adults in 61 prospective studies. *Lancet.* 2002;**360**:1903-1913.

8. World Health Organization Expert Committee. Hypertension control. *World Health Organ Tech Rep Ser.* 1996;**862**:2-10.

9. Collins R, MacMahon S. Blood pressure, antihypertensive drug treatment and the risks of stroke and coronary heart disease. *Br Med Bull.* 1994;**50**:272-298.

10. Stamler J, Stamler R, Neaton JD. Blood pressure, systolic and diastolic, and cardiovascular risks: US population data. *Arch Intern Med.* 1993;**153**:598-615.

11. Nissinen A, Bothig S, Grenroth H, Lopez AD. Hypertension in developing countries. *World Health Stat Q.* 1988;**41**:141-154.

12. People's Republic of China–United States Cardiovascular and Cardiopulmonary Epidemiology Research Group. An epidemiological study of cardiovascular and cardiopulmonary disease risk factors in four populations in the People's Republic of China. *Circulation.* 1992;**85**:1083-1096.

13. Gupta R. Defining hypertension in the Indian population. *Natl Med J India.* 1997;**10**:139-143.

14. Gupta R, Guptha S, Gupta VP, Prakash H. Prevalence and determinants of hypertension in the urban population of Jaipur in Western India. *J Hypertens.* 1995;**13**:1193-1200.

15. Gupta PC, Gupta R. Hypertension prevalence and blood pressure trends among 99,589 subjects in Mumbai, India [abstract]. *Indian Heart J.* 1999;**51**:691.

16. Joseph A, Kutty VR, Soman CR. High risk for coronary heart disease in Thiruvananthapuram City: A study of serum lipids and other risk factors. *Indian Heart J.* 2000;**52**:29-35.

17. Mohan V, Deepa R, Rani SS, Premalatha G. Prevalence of coronary artery disease and its relationship to lipids in a selected population in South India. *J Am Coll Cardiol.* 2001;**38**:682-687.

18. Gupta R, Gupta VP, Sarna M, et al. Prevalence of coronary heart disease and risk factors in an urban Indian population: Jaipur Heart Watch-2. *Indian Heart J.* 2002;**54**:59-66.

19. Anand MP. Prevalence of hypertension amongst Mumbai executives. *J Assoc Physicians India.* 2000;**48**:1200-1201.

20. Hajjar I, Kotchen TA. Trends in prevalence, awareness, treatment, and control of hypertension in the United States, 1988-2000. *JAMA.* 2003;**290**:199-203.

21. Gupta R, Sharma AK. Prevalence of hypertension and subtypes in an Indian rural population: Clinical and electrocardiographic correlates. *J Hum Hypertension.* 1994;**8**:823-829.

22. Malhotra P, Kumari S, Kumar R, Sharma BK. Prevalence and determinants of hypertension in an unindustrialised rural population of North India. *J Hum Hypertens.* 1999;**13**:467-472.

23. Harrap SB. Hypertension: Genes versus environment. *Lancet.* 1994;**344**:169-171.

24. Yusuf S, Reddy S, Ounpuu S, Anand S. Global burden of cardiovascular diseases: Parts 1 and 2. *Circulation.* 2001;**104**:2746-2753; 2855-2864.

25. Gupta R, Singhal S. Coronary heart disease in India [letter]. *Circulation.* 1997;**96**:3785.

26. Body mass index and cardiovascular disease risk factors in seven Asian and five Latin American centers: Data from the International Clinical Epidemiology Network (INCLEN). *Obes Res.* 1996;**4**:221-228.

27. Umemura S, Kawasaki T, Ishigami T, et al. Angiotensin-converting enzyme gene polymorphism in Nepal. *J Hum Hypertens.* 1998;**12**:527-531.

28. Zaman MM, Rouf MA. Prevalence of hypertension in a Bangladeshi adult population. *J Hum Hypertens.* 1999;**13**:547-549.

29. Bhatnagar D, Anand IS, Durrington PN, et al. Coronary risk factors in people from the Indian subcontinent living in West London and their siblings in India. *Lancet.* 1995;**345**:405-409.

30. Williams B. Westernised Asians and cardiovascular disease: Nature or nurture? *Lancet.* 1995;**345**:401-402.

31. Bhopal R, Unwin R, White M, et al. Heterogeneity of coronary heart disease risk factors in Indian, Pakistani, Bangladeshi, and European origin populations: Cross sectional study. *BMJ.* 1999;**319**:215-220.

32. Anand SS, Yusuf S, Vuksan V, et al. Differences in risk factors, atherosclerosis and cardiovascular disease between ethnic groups in Canada: The Study of Health Assessment and Risk in Ethnic Groups (SHARE). *Lancet.* 2000;**356**:279-284.

33. Neaton JD, Grimm RH Jr, Prineas RJ, et al. Treatment of Mild Hypertension Study (TOMHS): Final results. *JAMA.* 1993;**270**:713-724.

34. Stamler R. The primary prevention of hypertension and the population blood pressure problem. *In:* Marmot MG, Elliot P (eds). Coronary Heart Disease Epidemiology. Oxford: Oxford University Press, 1992, pp 415-434.

35. Gupta R, Sharma AK, Kapoor A, Prakash H. Epidemiological studies and treatment of hypertension. *J Assoc Physicians India.* 1997;**45**:863-864.

36. van den Hoogen PCW, Feskens EJM, Nagelkere NJD, et al., for the Seven Countries Study Research Group. The relation between blood pressure and mortality due to coronary heart disease among men in different parts of the world. *N Engl J Med.* 2000;**342**:1-8.

37. Vasan RS, Larson MG, Leip EP, et al. Impact of high normal blood pressure on the risk of cardiovascular disease. *N Engl J Med.* 2001;**345**:1291-1297.

38. Wood AJJ, Zhou HH. Ethnic differences in drug disposition and responsiveness. *Clin Pharmacokinet.* 1991;**20**:350-373.

39. Misra A. Insulin resistance syndrome and obesity in Asian Indians: Evidence and implications. *Nutrition.* 2004;**20**:482-491.

40. Gupta R. Gupta R, Deedwania PC, et al. Prevalence of metabolic syndrome in an urban Indian population. *Int J Cardiol.* 2004;**97**:257-261.

41. Gupta R, Prakash H, Gupta RR. Economic issues in coronary heart disease prevention in India. *J Hum Hypertens.* 2005;**19**:655-657.

42. Kearney PM, Whelton M, Reynolds K, et al. Global burden of hypertension: Analysis of worldwide data. *Lancet.* 2005;**365**:217-223.

Resistant Hypertension

John F. Setaro

Before about 1997, the designation of resistant or refractory hypertension was applied to patients whose blood pressure (BP) exceeded 140/90 mm Hg (or 160/90 mm Hg for older patients), despite appropriate multidrug pharmacotherapy.[1] The current definition has evolved, with a downward revision in treatment goals, based on large clinical trials (<140/90 mm Hg for all patients, <130/80 mm Hg for diabetics and patients with renal disease),[2] even as hypertension prevalence has increased in an aging, more overweight, and less physically active population in the United States.[3,4] Nationally, only one third of known hypertensive patients meet the less strict pre-2003 treatment standards.[3] With lower goals in an enlarging population, resistant hypertension will pose an ever-greater management challenge in the future.

Patients with resistant hypertension require careful assessment and vigorous treatment, given their greater degree of target organ damage and adverse long-term cardiovascular (CV) risk.[5,6] This chapter focuses on resistant hypertension, including novel insights into secondary hypertension, medical management emphasizing volume control and systolic BP therapy in older patients, adherence to treatment, chemical substances that antagonize therapy, and the role of obesity and the metabolic syndrome.

CURRENT BLOOD PRESSURE TREATMENT GOALS

More stringent current guideline BP goals are founded on the favorable results for CV and renal outcomes in large clinical trials, particularly in older persons with systolic hypertension,[7,8] in diabetic patients,[9] and in patients with preexisting renal disease (serum creatinine >1.5 mg/dL or proteinuria >300 mg/24 hours).[10] The Prospective Studies Collaboration analyzed 120,000 deaths in 61 cohorts of nearly 1 million persons and reported that an increase of 15 to 20 mm Hg was associated with elevated morbidity and mortality and for each 20/10 mm Hg increment over 115/75 mm Hg, there is a twofold increase in the CV death rate.[11] The most common reason for resistant hypertension is systolic hypertension in older individuals,[7,12,13] in whom a favorable outcome has been linked to the degree of BP lowering, rather than to the drug type employed.[14] Prospective trials in diabetic patients revealed that each 10 mm Hg fall in systolic BP reduced diabetic or CV endpoints by 11% to 15%,[15] and tighter overall control generally translated into better CV outcomes. The Hypertension Optimal Treatment (HOT) trial (17,980 subjects, including 1501 with diabetes) reported that the diabetic subgroup randomized to goal diastolic BP of 80 mm Hg or less had 51% fewer CV events versus a subgroup randomized to 90 mm Hg or less.[16] Yet, as recently analyzed in a university

hypertension clinic, control to goal level is difficult to achieve in diabetic patients; only 52% met the outdated standard of less than 140/90 mm Hg, and fewer than 20% attained the contemporary goal of less than 130/80 mm Hg.[17]

DEFINITION AND PREVALENCE

Resistant hypertension is present when BP does not meet goal, despite a regimen containing three drugs with different mechanisms of action, including a diuretic, given at full doses for an adequate period (thiazide diuretics may require 3 to 6 weeks).[2] Patients with newly identified or untreated hypertension should not be considered to have resistant hypertension at the initial evaluation, irrespective of the severity of measured BP.

In the United States, 29% of adults (nearly 60 million persons) have hypertension, with a prevalence of 72% by age 80 years.[2,3] General BP control rates are inadequate, with the lowest rates among older patients, ethnic minorities, and diabetic patients. Many patients with suboptimally controlled BP may have resistant hypertension.[3] The true prevalence of resistant hypertension is unknown, varying from 3% to 18% between primary and tertiary settings.[1] In the HOT trial, despite 4 years of intensive and free multidrug therapy, 12% of patients randomized to a diastolic BP goal of less than 90 mm Hg failed to meet that target.[16]

Recent trials suggest a higher prevalence of resistance. In the Antihypertensive and Lipid-Lowering Treatment to Prevent Heart Attack Trial (ALLHAT) and the Controlled Onset Verapamil Investigation of Cardiovascular End Points (CONVINCE) trial, in which protocols mandated titration of BP medications to achieve goal BP, approximately 90% of subjects reached the diastolic goal of less than 90 mm Hg, and 60% met the systolic goal of less than 140 mm Hg, but only 60% achieved the combined goal of less than 140/90 mm Hg.[18,19] After 5 years, 34% of ALLHAT subjects had BP uncontrolled to the trial target, and 27% of all patients were receiving three or more drugs.[20] After 3 years, 33% of CONVINCE patients exceeded goal BPs, and 18% of all subjects required three or more agents.[19] The International Verapamil-Trandolapril Study (INVEST), which included patients with hypertension and coronary artery disease, reported that 29% of subjects were not at goal BP at 2 years, although 50% were receiving three or more medications.[21] In the Losartan Intervention for Endpoint Reduction in Hypertension (LIFE) study, a trial assessing hypertensive patients with left ventricular hypertrophy, 48% of subjects achieved systolic BP of less than 140 mm Hg after 5 years of intensive combination therapy.[22] In a university hypertension specialty clinic, only 59% of patients met the target of less than 140/90 mm Hg, despite vigorous drug titration; among older and black subjects, 56% achieved BP control.[17] These findings imply that nearly 40% of patients under the care of either generalists or specialists may exhibit treatment resistance.

ISSUES IN BLOOD PRESSURE MEASUREMENT

BP should be measured by a qualified observer, with the patient in a nonstressful setting, seated quietly for 5 minutes, arm supported at heart level, and with the use of a properly calibrated sphygmomanometer with an adequately sized cuff (the cuff bladder should encircle >80% of the arm).[23] Systolic BP is signaled by the first sound (phase 1), and diastolic BP is the point before the disappearance of all sounds (phase 5). Nicotine and beverages containing caffeine raise BP transiently but not permanently: measurement should be delayed until 30 minutes after ingestion. Measurement of BP is surveyed in detail in Chapter 5.

Pseudohypertension

In some patients, indirect BP measurement does not reflect true intra-arterial BP. Such patients, often older and without signs of true target organ injury, may have pseudohypertension, ascribable to poorly compliant sclerotic vessels. In this condition, the radial artery remains palpable, despite maximal inflated cuff pressure, a sign termed the *Osler maneuver*. In the Systolic Hypertension in the Elderly Program (SHEP), 7% of patients screened had pseudohypertension.[24] Yet the Osler maneuver is not consistently reliable for identifying pseudohypertension, and invasive measurement may be required. If pseudohypertension is unrecognized, the patient may have apparent resistance, with consequent symptoms of overtreatment (lightheadedness, confusion, fatigue, and cold extremities) when therapy is intensified.

Office or White-Coat Resistant Hypertension

Some patients may have white-coat or office resistant hypertension, with normal values at home, that may not require additional therapy. A 24-hour ambulatory BP monitor can distinguish office resistance from true resistance. Patients should be evaluated if they have consistent elevated office readings and are poorly responsive to medications, yet have no sign of target organ injury. As many as 35% of apparently resistant subjects may manifest average BPs lower than 130/85 mm Hg by 24-hour or home recordings. In a recent article analyzing 400 patients (39% of whom appeared resistant on a multidrug regimen), home self-measurement successfully identified a white-coat effect, a finding suggesting that home monitoring can complement ambulatory studies in defining true resistance.[25] *White-coat hypertension* is a term that should be reserved for hypertensive patients who are not receiving drug therapy, and *office resistance* is a term that should be applied to those receiving treatment whose BP is still elevated in the office. These topics are treated in Chapters 6 and 7.

DIFFERENTIAL DIAGNOSIS: SIX DOMAINS

Once the condition has been diagnosed, a search can begin for causes of resistant hypertension. A practical system of classification is modified from earlier criteria,[1] and it has been validated in two university hypertension referral clinics.[26,27] Most patients fall into one or more general domains, listed in Table 43-1. Resistant hypertension may be caused by (1) a specific identifiable disorder (secondary hypertension), (2) inappropriate or inadequate medical treatment by the clinician, (3) patient nonadherence to prescribed medications, (4) systolic hypertension in older patients, (5) exogenous substances that raise BP or antagonize antihypertensive agents, or (6) obesity and metabolic syndrome. Once the disorder has been classified, management can be optimized (Fig. 43-1), although formal studies of this process are few. Strategies are drawn from data gathered in university specialty clinics and suggest that systematic evaluation and treatment will permit normalization or improvement in BP in most cases.[1,26,27]

Specific Identifiable Disorder (Secondary Hypertension)

Secondary hypertension (Table 43-2), defined as high BP caused by a specific treatable organ system disorder, increases in prevalence with age. Therapy is often ineffective until the underlying cause is addressed (Table 43-3). The prevalence of secondary hypertension rises in older cohorts: among patients who are more than 60 years old and whose hypertension is difficult to manage, 17% have secondary hypertension.[28] When patients are referred to tertiary centers for resistant hypertension, 5% to 11% have secondary causes.[26,27] In 4429 patients evaluated over 18 years for difficult hypertension, full investigations for secondary causes yielded a prevalence of 10.2%.[28] Renovascular hypertension was present in 3.1%, primary aldosteronism in 1.4% (more recent studies indicate a higher prevalence of primary aldosteronism than previously recognized[29]), Cushing's syndrome in 0.5%, pheochromocytoma in 0.3%, primary hypothyroidism in 3.0%, and renal insufficiency (defined as serum creatinine >2.0 mg/dL) in 1.8% overall, although the prevalence in patients with resistant hypertension was 8.0% when widespread atherosclerosis was also present.[28] Because renal parenchymal disease is the most common form of secondary hypertension in the general population, such patients may not have been referred, thus accounting for the low frequency in this series.

Table 43-1   Classification of Resistant Hypertension: Six Domains

1. Specific identifiable disorder (secondary hypertension)
2. Inappropriate or inadequate medical treatment
3. Patient nonadherence to the prescribed program
4. Systolic hypertension in older patients
5. Exogenous interfering substances
6. Obesity and the metabolic syndrome

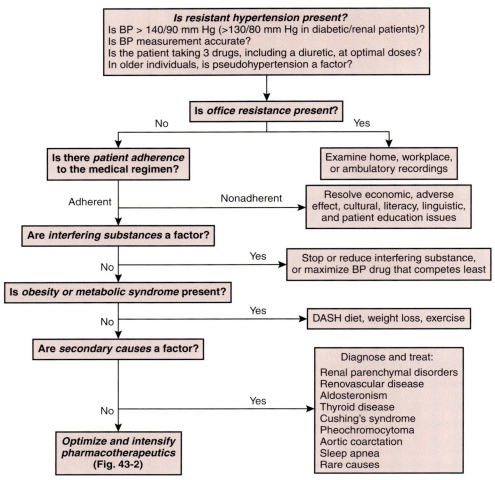

Figure 43–1 Approach to the management of resistant hypertension. BP, blood pressure; DASH, Dietary Approaches to Stop Hypertension.

Table 43-2 Causes of Secondary Hypertension

More Common Causes
Renal parenchymal disease
Renal vascular disorders
Thyroid disease
Mineralocorticoid excess
Glucocorticoid excess
Pheochromocytoma
Coarctation of the aorta
Sleep apnea

Rare Causes
Hypercalcemia of hyperparathyroidism
Central nervous system tumors
Autonomic dysreflexia associated with spinal cord lesion
Baroreflex failure
Porphyria
Carcinoid
Acromegaly
Anxiety or psychogenic conditions

Renal Parenchymal Disease

Typically manifested by edema, nocturia, active urine sediment, proteinuria, and elevated serum creatinine, chronic renal parenchymal disease constitutes the most widespread disease-related cause of secondary hypertension. Diabetic nephropathy and hypertensive nephrosclerosis are most common, followed by glomerular diseases, chronic interstitial nephritis, and pyelonephritis, as well as polycystic disease. Elevated creatinine may signal coexisting conditions such as renovascular disease. Volume regulation is critical to BP control, and loop diuretics as a part of multidrug therapy are necessary to lower BP to newer goals (<130/80 mm Hg). Inhibitors of the renin-angiotensin system can preserve renal function in hypertensive patients with nephropathy,[30,31] although a modest rise in serum creatinine (≤35%) may be noted after beginning treatment with an angiotensin-converting enzyme (ACE) inhibitor.

Renovascular Disease

Atherosclerotic renal artery disease may cause renovascular hypertension when previously controlled BP becomes resistant, especially in the context of tobacco use or obstruc-

Table 43-3 Approach to Secondary Causes of Resistant Hypertension

	Symptoms and Findings	Treatment
Renal parenchymal disease	Nocturia Edema Proteinuria with or without cells and casts Elevated serum creatinine	ACE inhibitor/ARB ACE inhibitor/ARB plus loop diuretic β-Blocker Calcium channel blocker
Renal artery disease	Recent onset in older patients Tobacco use Widespread vascular disease Multidrug resistance Severe hypertension in young patients Epigastric or flank bruit Disparity in kidney size Azotemia on ACE inhibitor/ARB Magnetic resonance angiography, Doppler, ACE inhibitor renogram, arteriogram	Angioplasty/stent in selected patients Balloon angioplasty for fibromuscular dysplasia ACE inhibitor/ARB with diuretic if disease is unilateral
Aldosteronism	Fatigue, hypokalemia May not respond to potassium supplementation May be more common than previously thought Abnormal aldosterone/renin levels Abnormal response to sodium loading Imaging (CT/MRI)	Aldosterone antagonists ACE inhibitor/ARB if hyperplasia Surgery for adenoma
Pheochromocytoma	Palpitations, headache, diaphoresis, paroxysms of hypertension Abnormal urinary catecholamines, plasma metanephrines, CT/MRI	α-Adrenergic inhibitors β-Blockers, surgical removal
Cushing's syndrome	Obesity, striae, muscle weakness, elevated glucose, fluid retention Elevated urinary cortisol (+) dexamethasone suppression CT/MRI	Surgical intervention
Hyper/hypothyroidism	Hyperthyroidism: increased systolic BP Hypothyroidism: increased diastolic BP	Treatment of underlying disorder Treatment of underlying disorder
Sleep apnea	Interrupted sleep Daytime somnolence Obesity	Weight loss Positive-pressure breathing
Coarctation of the aorta	Brachial/femoral pulse differential Echocardiogram CT/MRI	Surgery/balloon angioplasty

ACE, angiotensin-converting enzyme; ARB, angiotensin receptor blocker; BP, blood pressure; CT, computed tomography; MRI, magnetic resonance imaging.

tive arterial disease in other distributions. This topic is reviewed in detail in Chapter 8.

In a large series, renovascular hypertension was found in 3.1% of patients with resistant hypertension, with a prevalence of 9.5% when generalized atherosclerosis was present.[28] Given the increasing prevalence of atherosclerosis with age, renovascular hypertension is more common among older patients with resistant hypertension. Other clues consist of epigastric or flank bruit, severe retinopathy, disparity in kidney size, and azotemia while receiving an ACE inhibitor or an angiotensin receptor blocker (ARB). In the setting of reduced renal perfusion, glomerular filtration is maintained via activation of the renin-angiotensin system, consisting of angiotensin II–dependent constriction of the efferent arterioles, systemic sympathetic activation, and volume retention in advanced cases.

Nonatherosclerotic renovascular hypertension is rare, and causes include fibromuscular dysplasia, vasculitis, tuberculosis, and neurofibromatosis. Renal ischemia with consequent resistant hypertension may arise from a cyst, an arterial aneurysm, a spontaneous or post-traumatic hematoma, or post-traumatic compressive fibrosis.

Management of renal artery disease is evolving as a result of advances in imaging techniques, medical therapy, and catheter-based treatments, including endoluminal stenting. A search for remediable renovascular hypertension has become less critical with the introduction of blockers of the renin-angiotensin system that can overcome angiotensin II–dependent hypertension. Many cases in older patients likely remain undetected when renal function is stable and BP is adequately controlled. Prevention of progressive renal dysfunction when renal artery stenosis is present has become an important focus, although the subject is outside the scope of this discussion of resistant hypertension. Resistant hypertension is an accepted indication for renal artery revascularization if a lesion is found.

When clinical suspicion justifies testing, scintigraphic assessment of functional angiotensin II dependence and differential renal perfusion using the captopril renogram has a high negative predictive value for excluding significant (>75%) renal artery stenosis, and it predicts improvement following revascularization. However, the test is less useful in advanced renal impairment, in bilateral disease, or in the general clinical setting versus the research setting.

Doppler ultrasound is inexpensive and noninvasive, and the measurement of resistive indices may allow assessment of functional viability of the kidney. In obese patients, renal artery imaging by ultrasound may be technically difficult, if not impossible.

Magnetic resonance angiography with gadolinium contrast enhancement is non-nephrotoxic, provides excellent correlation with conventional angiography, and supplies functional information (nephrogram images defining filtration volume), but it is limited by cost and availability. Arterial anatomy, renal flow, and parenchymal volume measurements provide both anatomic and functional data and may permit prediction of response to revascularization.

Invasive angiography, often coupled with potential catheter-based intervention, is the conventional diagnostic test of choice, but it carries with it risks of radiocontrast nephrotoxicity, hemorrhage, and atheroembolization. Computed tomographic angiography has shown promise as a safer diagnostic technique.

For the patient who has resistant renovascular hypertension, treatment options include medical therapy and catheter-based balloon angioplasty with stenting. Medical therapy, including an ACE inhibitor or an ARB, a full-dose diuretic, calcium channel blockers (CCBs), which maintain blood flow and function by their action as preglomerular afferent arteriolar dilators, and β-blockers if necessary, may be effective for older patients in whom disease is unilateral, creatinine is stable, and the risks of catheter-based procedures are elevated (radiocontrast nephropathy, atheroembolization). However, BP in such patients often resists control. Renal function can worsen, with a consequent increase in medication requirement. ACE inhibitor or ARB treatment may lead to creatinine elevation, usually reversible, when such therapy is given to patients with severe bilateral disease or unilateral disease in a solitary kidney in whom glomerular filtration depends on angiotensin II. Such a rise in creatinine suggests the diagnosis in high-risk patients with resistant hypertension.

Three randomized trials addressed medication versus angioplasty in atherosclerotic disease, with mixed results. None of the three trials employed stenting, now considered the treatment of choice for ostial lesions, located at the aortic origin of the renal arteries, an anatomic site with a particularly high potential for vascular recoil and restenosis, and thus optimal for stenting rather than simple balloon angioplasty. Ideally, if a procedure is planned, the objective should be to intervene earlier, when creatinine is still normal or only slightly abnormal. No medication versus stenting trial has yet been published, although two studies are under way.

For patients with resistant hypertension who may have renal artery stenosis, summary recommendations include a general aim of screening those most at risk and treating invasively those who have most to gain. If clinical clues point toward renal artery stenosis, imaging should be performed, with magnetic resonance angiography likely the optimal contemporary alternative. If a functional evaluation, for instance, renal scintigraphy with captopril, shows symmetric bilateral blood flow, then medical therapy can be selected. If asymmetric flow or bilateral disease is observed, then revascularization is suggested, particularly if the serum creatinine is normal or is only mildly elevated. Balloon angioplasty with a high potential for cure should almost always be offered to patients with fibromuscular dysplasia. In patients with atherosclerotic renal artery stenosis, BP may improve by stenting with reduced medication requirements, yet cure is rare, especially if baseline creatinine is abnormal.[32] With stenting, the potential exists for preservation of renal function and avoidance of CV consequences. These questions form the focus of the upcoming Cardiovascular Outcomes in Renal Atherosclerotic Lesions (CORAL) study, a National Heart, Lung and Blood Institute–sponsored randomized trial of optimal medication versus stenting with optimal medication. Surgery is preferable if major aortic disease also exists.

Primary Aldosteronism

Several recent reports suggest that primary aldosteronism is a more common cause of resistant hypertension than previously believed.[29] In 600 hypertensive patients, the prevalence of aldosteronism rose with increasingly severe degrees of hypertension.[33] Earlier, patients were assessed only if they had hypokalemia. Currently, expanded screening has exposed a prevalence of 8% to 32% (primary versus tertiary centers), for example, 20% in one tertiary clinic with large numbers of patients with resistant hypertension who were equally distributed between white and African American subjects.[34] All subjects had high-salt-ingestion suppression testing for plasma renin and 24-hour urinary aldosterone measurements, confirmed by response to the mineralocorticoid receptor antagonist spironolactone, with subsequent imaging. However, not all patients underwent confirmatory adrenal vein sampling or surgery.[34]

Primary aldosteronism is often a subtle diagnosis, with some (but not all) patients manifesting hypokalemia (serum potassium <3.5 mmol/L), unresponsive to potassium supplementation or the use of potassium-sparing diuretics. Most patients with primary aldosteronism are referred for resistant hypertension, rather than hypokalemia. Because current therapies (ACE inhibitors, ARBs, CCBs, β-blockers) do not provoke potassium loss, hypokalemia is seen less often. Moreover, mild hyperaldosteronism and essential hypertension (formerly termed low-renin hypertension) may overlap, thus explaining the excellent BP response to aldosterone antagonists in a wide spectrum of patients.[35,36]

Serum aldosterone levels and plasma renin activity can be measured in outpatients. An elevated ratio of serum aldosterone to plasma renin activity (ARR) greater than 20:1 suggests the diagnosis, although patients with low-renin essential hypertension also can exhibit an elevated ARR. Low or low-normal serum potassium levels with elevated renin exclude the diagnosis. Previous evaluations required stopping all agents that affect renin levels (exempting only α-adrenergic blockers and centrally acting agents), but this approach was inconvenient and undesirable in multidrug-resistant patients. In a series of 90 patients with resistant hypertension, the ARR was a valid screening test for aldosteronism, without the need for cessation of antihypertensive therapy.[37] In this study, 15 of 90 patients had an elevated ARR greater than 100:1, with 15 cases of primary aldosteronism confirmed by computed tomography or magnetic resonance imaging and scintigraphy using 131-iodocholesterol.

Most patients have bilateral adrenal hyperplasia, rather than a solitary adenoma. Although operation may cure adenoma, longitudinal evidence supports the acceptability of medical therapy without CV, renal, or neoplastic consequences. However, a large (>2.5 cm) lesion suggests malignancy. For bilateral hyperplasia, long-term medical therapy is safe and feasible, although no prospective randomized trials have been reported. Clinical response to spironolactone is predicted by the ARR. BP improves modestly with CCBs and weaker potassium-sparing diuretics, such as amiloride or triamterene. The response to ACE inhibitors and ARBs is better if bilateral hyperplasia is present, rather than an adenoma.

If primary aldosteronism were indeed highly prevalent, a controversial option would be to offer all patients with resistant hypertension a trial of spironolactone to avoid a difficult and potentially hazardous diagnostic protocol. This strategy was evaluated in 76 patients with resistant hypertension, with and without aldosteronism, who were treated using 12.5 to 25 mg/day of spironolactone in addition to preexisting ACE inhibitor, ARB, and diuretic therapy. At 6 months, the average BP reduction was 25/12 mm Hg.[38] A second similar trial reported parallel favorable results.[39] Yet such an approach would forfeit the opportunity to excise an adenoma surgically and could entail significant drug side effects such as gynecomastia, mastodynia, hyperkalemia, and azotemia. In this situation, the newer competitive selective aldosterone receptor antagonist, eplerenone, may prove efficacious with fewer adverse effects. Chapter 9 contains a more complete discussion of hyperaldosteronism.

Pheochromocytoma

Pheochromocytoma produces headache, palpitations, diaphoresis, and pallor in individuals of light complexion, and it is frequently marked by paroxysms of BP that are difficult to regulate, especially in the absence of α-adrenergic blocking therapy. Diagnosis depends on a high index of clinical suspicion, verified by elevated 24-hour urine catecholamines (norepinephrine >80 μg/24 hours and vanillylmandelic acid >5 mg/24 hours). Reports suggest major diagnostic utility for assays of plasma free metanephrines, particularly in familial syndromes, although the test is relatively new and is not universally available.[40] Imaging of the abdomen or adrenal glands will usually localize the tumor before surgical treatment. If the results are negative, whole-body scintigraphic imaging using iodine-123–metaiodobenzylguanidine may locate unusual extra-abdominal tumors. Most masses are benign and respond well to surgical treatment. This diagnosis should be a strong consideration if resistant hypertension is encountered in patients who have multiple endocrine neoplasia or neurocutaneous syndromes, such as neurofibromatosis or von Hippel–Lindau disease. Chapter 10 offers a further discussion of pheochromocytoma and related diseases.

Sleep Disorders

Obstructive sleep apnea represents the newest addition to classic causes of secondary hypertension. This topic is addressed in greater depth in Chapter 11. Accumulating evidence links sleep apnea with diverse CV disorders including resistant hypertension,[41] likely on the basis of sympathetic overactivity. Obesity is a confounding factor, although a recent analysis found a correlation between sleep apnea and resistant hypertension, even after adjusting for body mass index (BMI).[41] A spouse or partner may provide a history of snoring and interrupted sleep. If resistant hypertension is associated with daytime somnolence, obesity, erythrocytosis, and arterial carbon dioxide retention, then a formal sleep study is advised. Positive-pressure breathing therapy at night may lower BP, although a controlled prospective trial in resistant hypertension is yet to be done.[41] Yet in hypertensive patients, therapeutic positive pressure has improved nocturnal as well as daytime BP.[42,43] A relationship between sleep apnea and aldosterone excess has been proposed, supported by use of aldosterone antagonists in this group of patients with resistant hypertension.[44]

Cushing's Syndrome

Glucocorticoid excess states, with heightened sensitivity to pressor stimuli, may be seen in resistant hypertension when the patients have weight gain, truncal obesity, moon facies, muscle weakness, abdominal striae, hirsutism, hyperglycemia, and fluid retention, with cortisol acting as a mineralocorticoid in the kidney. Cushing's syndrome is confirmed by (1) assay of 24-hour urinary free cortisol (abnormal >55 μg/24 hours by liquid chromatography with local variations in reference values), (2) low-dose dexamethasone suppression (failure of morning plasma cortisol to decrease to <3 μg/dL after 1 mg dexamethasone given the evening before), (3) subsequent plasma corticotropin testing (if required), and (4) imaging for adrenal or pituitary lesions in preparation for operative intervention. Chapter 12 presents a more extensive discussion of this topic.

Thyroid Disorders

Hyperthyroidism can increase cardiac output and can magnify sensitivity to catecholamine stimulation, consequently elevating systolic BP. Hyperthyroidism should always be considered in a younger person with elevated systolic BP and a wide pulse pressure. Hypothyroidism is linked with abnormal peripheral vascular resistance, leading to diastolic hypertension. The diagnosis is based on clinical suspicion in the setting of resistant hypertension, with laboratory confirmation. Either form typically responds well to correction of the underlying thyroid status. Chapter 12 contains a more extensive discussion of this topic.

Vascular Disorders

Occasional cases of aortic coarctation escape undetected into adulthood. These patients display severe and often resistant brachial hypertension, but with diminished lower extremity pulses. Takayasu's disease and Buerger's disease, both obliterative arteriopathies, may be associated with multidrug-resistant hypertension.

Rare Causes

Very rare causes of secondary hypertension are listed in Table 43-2. These causes include the following: hypercalcemia caused by hyperparathyroidism and manifested by polyuria, renal calculi, osteoporosis, and drug-resistant hypertension; tumors of the central nervous system; autonomic dysreflexia associated with spinal cord lesions; baroreflex failure; porphyria; carcinoid syndrome; acromegaly, in which excess growth hormone promotes vascular hypertrophy; and anxiety-related or psychogenic causes.[45]

Inappropriate or Inadequate Medical Treatment

Inappropriate therapy, insufficient doses, or inattention to the patient-specific BP goal (physician inertia) may explain resistance in up to 60% of patients who are eventually found to be receiving suboptimal pharmacotherapy.[27] Often volume overloaded, most such individuals (>50%) respond well to adding or adjusting diuretics.[1,26,27,46,47]

Medication-related resistance, in which the clinician does not prescribe or the patient cannot tolerate an effective program, constitutes the most common reason for resistant hypertension. Although treatment goals have evolved in the past decade, the distribution of causes for resistant hypertension has remained remarkably similar, with medication-related reasons forming the largest category.[26,27] In a 2005 analysis of 141 patients with resistant hypertension at a university center, 58% had resistant hypertension attributed to inappropriate or inadequate pharmacotherapy (Table 43-4).[27] Patient nonadherence to the regimen accounted for 16% of cases, psychological causes accounted for 9%, office resistance for 6%, secondary hypertension for 5%, and interfering substances for 1%.

The value of optimal medical therapy is underscored by the observation in large clinical trials that the progression from mild to severe hypertension was 15-fold more likely to occur in subjects administered placebo rather than active antihypertensive therapy.[48] Therefore, if resistance is to be prevented, early and intensive medical treatment for high BP is desirable. Table 43-5 lists lifestyle modification and nonpharmacologic approaches that can serve as therapeutic adjuncts in managing resistant hypertension.[2]

Importance of Diuretic Treatment in Resistant Hypertension

In an earlier series of patients with resistant hypertension, the most important therapeutic maneuver was the addition or increase in a diuretic or a change to a diuretic type more appropriate to the patient's renal function.[1,26] In a more recent series, intensified diuretic therapy was again discovered to be critical for optimized BP control.[27]

Several analyses suggest that patients with resistant hypertension are volume overloaded, in some cases because vasodilator therapy leads to reactive sodium and water retention, with consequent volume expansion. It has been understood for decades that that thiazides are more effective than loop diuretics in patients with normal renal function (serum creatinine <1.5 mg/dL), yet when the glomerular filtration rate is less than 30 to 50 mL/minute (or serum creatinine >1.5 mg/dL), thiazides are no longer effective at optimizing sodium excretion and plasma volume. At that stage of renal impairment, loop agents are needed. Loop diuretics also are preferred in states of overt volume overload with edema, heart failure, and concurrent therapy with direct vasodilators. Conversely, if short-acting loop diuretics (furosemide or bumetanide) are used in the setting of normal renal function, natriuresis leads to reactive sodium retention, mediated by the renin-angiotensin system, with failure to control BP. Longer-acting torsemide may assist as a once-a-day medication, or short-acting agents can be given more frequently. Volume is an important consideration in low-renin patients, such as African Americans, obese individuals, diabetic patients, and older persons; in these patients, thiazides are often indispensable for BP control.[48]

A prospective study of plasma volume in patients with resistant hypertension revealed elevated volume in a majority

Table 43-4 Reasons for Resistance in a University Hypertension Clinic (N = 128)

Medication related	58%
Patient nonadherence	16%
Secondary hypertension	5%
Psychological causes	9%
Interfering substances	1%
Office resistance	6%
Unknown	5%

From Garg JP, Elliott WJ, Folker A, et al. Resistant hypertension revisited: A comparison of two university-based cohorts. *Am J Hypertens.* 2005;**18**:619-626.

Table 43-5 Dietary and Lifestyle Approaches That May Improve Resistant Hypertension

Action	Anticipated Systolic Blood Pressure Response
Weight reduction	5-20 mm Hg/10 kg weight loss
Adoption of DASH plan	8-14 mm Hg
Sodium reduction	2-8 mm Hg
Physical activity	4-9 mm Hg
Alcohol limitation	2-4 mm Hg

DASH, Dietary Approaches to Stop Hypertension.
Modified from Chobanian AV, Bakris GL, Black HR, et al., and the National High Blood Pressure Education Program Coordinating Committee: The Seventh Report of the Joint National Committee on Prevention, Detection, Evaluation, and Treatment of High Blood Pressure: The JNC 7 Report. *JAMA.* 2003;**289**:2560-2572.

of patients devoid of any physical signs of congestion, such as elevation of neck veins, rales, or peripheral edema, with improved BP once adequate diuretics were properly administered.[46] Underutilization of useful medications, particularly thiazide diuretics, has been linked to concern for metabolic side effects, which have been overstated for many years and may be less problematic with currently used low doses. Rather, diuretics have served as an essential ingredient in most recent large clinical trials that showed benefit using ACE inhibitors and ARBs in diverse hypertensive populations, in which diuretics were necessary to attain goal BP in 50% to 60% of subjects.[22,30,31,49] In ALLHAT, BP was lowered to a greater degree in the cohort begun on a diuretic, which was not permitted by protocol as a second or third agent in other randomized arms of the trial.[18] Recent studies have confirmed the usefulness of aldosterone inhibitors in resistant hypertension, a finding underscoring both the importance of diuretic therapy and the potential overlap between essential hypertension and subtle forms of medically remediable hyperaldosteronism.[29,36]

Designing a Rational Multidrug Program in Resistant Hypertension

Evidence from large clinical trials indicates that multidrug combination therapy is necessary to reach goal BP, particularly in high-risk patients. In major trials in hypertensive patients with diabetes and renal impairment, attaining the strictest goals required using an average of 3.5 drugs. By the end of 5 years in ALLHAT, the average treatment program comprised 2.0 antihypertensive drugs/day for each patient, and 43% of the subjects randomized to the lisinopril treatment arm were receiving multiple agents.[20] In the HOT trial, 75% of subjects randomized to a diastolic goal BP of less than 80 mm Hg needed combination therapy.[16]

Combination therapy is based on physiologic mechanisms of action (Fig. 43-2). Arterial pressure is proportional to cardiac output and systemic vascular resistance; therefore, control of BP is attainable via simultaneous regulation of the following: (1) volume, with diuretics, such as thiazides, loop

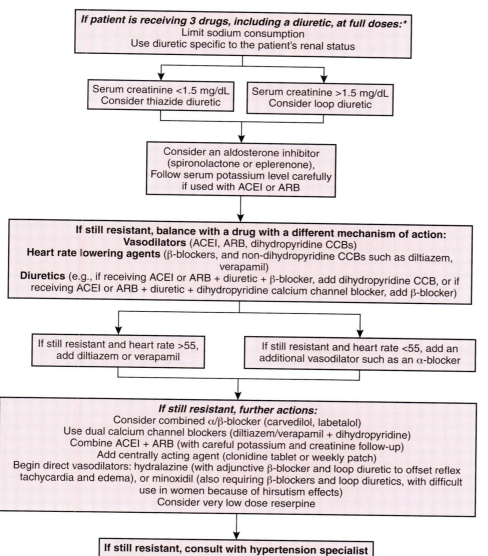

Figure 43–2 Approach to optimizing drug therapy in the patient with resistant hypertension. *For a full listing of maximal doses and available combinations, refer to reference 2. ACEI, angiotensin-converting enzyme inhibitor; ARB, angiotensin receptor blocker; CCB, calcium channel blocker.

diuretics, and aldosterone antagonists; (2) heart rate, with β-blockers, because of their negative inotropy and chronotropy and antirenin effects, and with verapamil and diltiazem, because of their negative inotropy and chronotropy and mild vasodilation; and (3) vascular resistance, with vasodilation by inhibition of the renin-angiotensin system (with ACE inhibitors and ARBs), smooth muscle relaxation (with dihydropyridine CCBs and α-adrenergic blockers), and direct vasodilation (with hydralazine and minoxidil). By addressing an alternate physiologic axis, a well-chosen second or third agent overcomes BP-elevating compensatory changes caused by the first, for example, stimulation of the renin-angiotensin system by diuretics, elevation of heart rate by vasodilating CCBs, or induction of volume retention by direct vasodilators. However, direct vasodilators (hydralazine, minoxidil) should be agents of final resort. These drugs possess significant side effects, are incapable of reversing cardiac hypertrophy, and produce reflex tachycardia and fluid retention, which would ultimately negate their antihypertensive properties if they were used as monotherapy. To avoid these consequences, they are most typically used with loop diuretics and β-blockers.

The management concept whereby compensatory changes are pharmacologically counteracted has been formalized as the *AB/CD or Cambridge rule,* in which a drug is initially chosen from between two classes of renin inhibitors (AB, or ACE inhibitors/ARBs, β-blockers). If the goal is not reached, then a second drug is added by choosing between two classes of drugs that either stimulate renin or at least do not inhibit products of the renin-angiotensin cascade (CD, or CCBs, diuretics).[50] Combination therapy tends to maximize benefit while limiting adverse effects by using several drugs at lower doses. In a meta-analysis of 354 randomized trials, all the major classes of drugs offered similar BP reductions. When multiple drugs at lower doses were used in combination versus single agents at standard doses, BP reduction was additive, but side effects were less than additive.[51] Specifically, the adverse effects of diuretics, β-blockers, and CCBs were dose related; ACE inhibitor–related cough (the most common side effect) was not dose related, and ARBs were not associated with excess adverse effects. Numerous combinations of two or three antihypertensive drugs are commercially available.

In some very difficult cases of resistant hypertension, unorthodox drug combinations may be tried (see Fig. 43-2). Few data address the question whether to delete some components of the program before adding others if multiple drugs are inadequate. Dual CCBs in combination, one a dihydropyridine and one a nondihydropyridine, effectively lower BP,[52] as do combinations of ACE inhibitors and ARBs,[53] and dual diuretic therapy with spironolactone added to previous thiazide or loop diuretics.[38] Combined α-/β-adrenergic blockers, such as labetalol and carvedilol, may prove useful in constructing a multidrug program for patients with resistant hypertension. Additional agents available for resistant cases include clonidine, α-adrenergic blockers,[54] and vasodilators such as hydralazine and minoxidil (see Fig. 43-2). In severe cases, low-dose reserpine (0.05 to 0.1 mg/day) may mitigate resistance. Other than for spironolactone[38] and α-adrenergic blockers,[54] few studies predict the magnitude of further BP lowering available by adding the foregoing medications, although, in our experience, a benefit of 5 to 10 mm Hg systolic may be anticipated.

Certain co-morbid conditions may disqualify some treatment choices, for instance, diuretics in patients with gout or β-blockers in asthmatic patients. Many side effects correspond to commonly observed situations, for instance, cough with ACE inhibitors or edema with dihydropyridine CCBs, a situation termed *objective medication intolerance.*

In other instances, anxiety may lead to *subjective medication intolerance,* in which perceived side effects do not correspond anatomically or physiologically to previously reported adverse effects of a given compound as quoted in the medical literature.[55] Such subjective intolerance frequently complicates treatment if patients attribute symptoms of anxiety to antihypertensive drugs, thereby ruling out the legitimate use of numerous drugs or drug classes. Recognition of the psychological factor is critical to providing optimal care.

The Resistant Physician

National surveys report that twice as many patients receive hypertension treatment as have their BP controlled during treatment. This finding suggests that clinicians may fail to intensify the regimen when BP is elevated, thus raising the prospect that the physician is resistant, rather than the patient's condition.[3] In a study conducted at Veterans Affairs medical centers in New England in the 1990s, physicians often failed to augment therapy in patients whose BP was found to be higher than goal values, even though cost, access, and cultural barriers were not at issue.[56] Other series showed that primary physicians did not increase the treatment program in 61% of patients whose BP was uncontrolled,[57] and 96% of patients with treated but uncontrolled BP had visited a physician within the previous 12 months.[13] The reasons for this reluctance to treat are unclear, but clinical inertia can be cited as an underlying factor.

A forced-titration protocol may be helpful in this regard. In a university-based specialist hypertension clinic, goal-oriented management without a specific algorithm proved greatly more successful than national survey data; 63% of patients were at systolic BP goal, 86% were at diastolic goal, 59% were at both, and 71% of all patients were receiving multidrug therapy.[3,17] Whatever the protocol employed, clinicians clearly need to add, change, and increase medications to attain modern BP goals, especially in high-risk patients.[17]

Patient Nonadherence to the Prescribed Program

Patient nonadherence to the prescribed program is typically listed as treatment resistance because it is difficult to recognize, verify, or exclude in an objective manner.[58] Clues to nonadherence are missed office visits and failure to show physiologic evidence of drug administration, for instance, reduced heart rate during therapy with β-blockers or diltiazem. Among patients with resistant hypertension in a tertiary setting, nonadherence may be as frequent as 16%,[27] although it may be more prevalent in the general setting because patients with known nonadherence are less likely to be referred for (or to attend) tertiary care.[1] However, in a study of 103 Swiss patients in whom adherence was defined as the self-administration of more than 80% of prescribed doses, as measured by an electronic monitoring system, nonadherence was no more prevalent in patients with treatment-resistant hypertension (82%) than in those patients with treatment-responsive hypertension (85%).[59]

Patient adherence is influenced by whether an incentive exists to continue medication. Although some hypertensive patients experience symptoms related to high BP, most patients are asymptomatic at lower ranges of abnormal BP, a predictor of lower treatment adherence in general.[60] Although many efforts at patient education have been made, ideal education materials are not yet readily available. Nonadherence may be related to issues of cost, a patient's level of literacy and education, linguistic, geographic, and cultural barriers, complexity of the regimen, and anticipated or actual side effects of the drugs. Nonadherence may be a risk factor for not achieving BP control, irrespective of patient's educational or economic background or professed understanding of the rationale for treatment. Nonetheless, several series have shown that lack of access to primary care in a socioeconomically disadvantaged population constitutes a major risk factor for severe uncontrolled hypertension.

Improving Adherence

One important predictor of adherence to a medication regimen is the use of less frequent doses. Several analyses demonstrate that hypertensive subjects showed significantly better adherence to doses taken once daily versus those taken twice or three times daily. However, most contemporary antihypertensive agents, with the exception of labetalol, carvedilol, and hydralazine, are given in once-daily doses, so the issue of once-daily administration may become less relevant. Technologic solutions could prove helpful. In a well-conceived study performed by Swiss investigators examining a group of patients with resistant hypertension, the institution of an electronic monitoring system that tracked pill use led to achievement of normal BP after 1 month in one third of patients, without alteration of the previously prescribed therapy. An additional 20% of patients were unmasked as nonadherent, thus raising the possibility that a relatively large percentage of study subjects were nonadherent at study entry.[58]

Other general advice to improve adherence includes the provision of both oral and written instructions, counseling about the regimen, manual or computer-based reminders, cuing of medication ingestion to daily events, reinforcement and praise, working to overcome cultural barriers to treatment, self-monitoring of BP at home with regular physician review, and involvement of family members.[60] With empathy and trust, the patient can develop an understanding of the hypertension problem, as well as its consequences and the merits of treatment.

Nonetheless, this is a particularly challenging area of contemporary medical practice, with low success rates for adherence to medication prescriptions, in which even the most effective interventions have modest effects. All the foregoing strategies are time and labor intensive. New ideas are clearly needed.[60,61]

Isolated Systolic Hypertension

In the Third National Health and Nutrition Examination Survey (NHANES III), among patients with uncontrolled hypertension, the most frequent characteristic was stage 1

isolated systolic hypertension.[12,13] Data from the Framingham Heart Study support this finding: 90% of patients with treated hypertension had BP regulated to the diastolic goal, yet only 49% had BP at the systolic target.[62] Clinicians may not appreciate the relatively greater importance of systolic versus diastolic BP, particularly in older patients. Isolated systolic hypertension may be difficult to treat because of reduced arterial compliance in the setting of a low renin, volume-overloaded state, often associated with vascular and ventricular hypertrophy, and elevated sympathetic tone. Thus, some patients are truly resistant because sclerotic arteries are refractory to vasodilation. CCBs, diuretics, and ARBs have been proven useful for BP reduction and modification of adverse outcomes.[7,8] Combination therapy is often needed, and a gradual multistage approach in older patients may be desirable, to allow baroreceptors adequate time to reset.

Interfering Exogenous Substances

Interfering or competing exogenous substances, also termed *antagonizing substances,* can elevate BP, aggravate existing hypertension, or inhibit the therapeutic effects of antihypertensive drugs (Table 43-6). These compounds may be illicit, available as legal dietary supplements, offered as over-the-counter medications, or prescribed by the clinician. The use of these agents is probably increasing, particularly herbal remedies, weight loss therapies, anabolic steroids for body building, and nonprescription nonsteroidal anti-inflammatory agents. If the interfering agent is a drug necessary to treat another

Table 43-6   Interfering Exogenous Substances

Amphetamines
Anabolic steroids
Anti-inflammatory agents
Appetite suppressants
Caffeine
Cocaine
Corticosteroids
Cyclooxygenase-2 inhibitors
Cyclosporine
Erythropoietin
Ephedra (ma huang)
Ethanol
Ginseng
Guarana
Licorice (natural licorice, herbal remedies, and chewing tobacco)
Monoamine oxidase inhibitors
Nicotine
Oral contraceptives
Phenylephrine
Phenylpropanolamine
Pseudoephedrine
Sibutramine
Sodium chloride
Sympathomimetic agents
Synephrine
Tacrolimus
Venlafaxine
Yohimbine

condition, the antihypertensive program may need to be changed or increased, or new BP-lowering drugs may need to be added. In general, the interfering substance should be used only for the minimum required time and dose needed.

Sympathomimetic compounds can raise BP, and these include phenylpropanolamine, ephedra (ma huang), pseudoephedrine, phenylephrine, decongestant nasal sprays, β-adrenergic nebulized bronchodilators, illicit substances such as cocaine, and amphetamine preparations such as methamphetamine and 3,4-methylenedioxymethamphetamine (MDMA or ecstasy).[63] In users of ephedra, hypertension was the single most frequently reported adverse event.[64] Based on reports of strokes and CV events, the U.S. government took regulatory actions against phenylpropanolamine and ephedra.

Apart from ephedra, other herbal preparations may contribute to resistance to BP treatment. Ginseng may elevate BP, and yohimbine increases central sympathetic outflow, thus opposing the beneficial properties of clonidine and other centrally acting BP-lowering agents.[65] Natural licorice, found in some herbal therapies and chewing tobaccos, has mineralocorticoid effects that produce a hyperaldosterone-like syndrome of hypertension with hypokalemia. In discussing herbal treatments with patients, it is essential that the clinician maintain communications by remaining nonjudgmental and sensitive to individual health beliefs.[66]

Nonsteroidal anti-inflammatory agents and cyclooxygenase-2 (COX-2) inhibitors impair sodium excretion and cause volume retention. They also counteract local renal vasodilatory prostaglandins on which ACE inhibitors, loop diuretics, and most other classes of BP-lowering agents (except CCBs) depend for their therapeutic actions.[67,68] Prostaglandins are also systemic vasodilators, as well as renal vasodilators and enhancers of renal sodium excretion. In a randomized 3-week study of hypertensive patients, an ibuprofen-treated group showed a mean BP rise of 7/6 mm Hg versus none for acetaminophen or placebo; a recent article analyzing both nonsteroidal agents and COX-2 inhibitors confirmed these findings.[69] If the analgesic cannot be changed, higher doses of antihypertensive medications, including CCBs, may overcome these BP-raising effects. No consistent prospective data define the degree of BP improvement available by stopping these agents, and there may be differences in this respect among various agents.[69] Nonsteroidal anti-inflammatory agents have been available without prescription for several years, and they, along with COX-2 inhibitors, are frequently used for arthritis and other ailments in the older population that is also most affected by hypertension. Patients who exhibit relatively greater dependence on prostaglandins for vasodilation and sodium excretion include older individuals, diabetic patients, and those with renal impairment or sodium overload, all of whom are more sensitive to prostaglandin inhibition. A recent retrospective analysis showed elevation in BP in older patients with rofecoxib therapy, and this effect may be part of the reason that this drug was associated with a higher risk of CV events and was removed from the worldwide market.[68] A meta-analysis of trials comparing BP effects of COX-2 inhibitors versus nonsteroidal anti-inflammatory agents and placebo suggests that some COX-2 inhibitors cause greater BP elevation than nonsteroidal anti-inflammatory agents or placebo, and rofecoxib exerts greater effects on both systolic and diastolic BP than does celecoxib.[70] Corticosteroids raise BP in a dose-dependent manner through salt and water retention, in part related to mineralocorticoid actions. Oral contraceptives are less problematic now that low-dose estrogen formulations are available. Sibutramine, an anorectic treatment for obesity, can elevate BP. Chlorpromazine and other psychotropic drugs can produce resistant hypertension by neutralizing the actions of sympatholytic antihypertensive agents.

Excessive alcohol use (more than four or five drinks/day) contributes to elevated BP in a dose-dependent fashion,[71] and it is linked to hypertension in several epidemiologic studies. In an older experience at a hypertension clinic in Scandinavia, 23% of patients who had abnormal hepatic enzymes reflecting heavy alcohol intake could not achieve BP control, versus 7% of subjects with normal enzymes, and among those patients admitting heavy alcohol consumption, 46% failed to attain BP goal. Reduced alcohol consumption is linked to BP lowering in a dose-response fashion,[71] with a prospective evaluation of alcohol cessation yielding an average 24-hour BP lowering of 7.2/6.6 mm Hg.

High sodium intake may underlie resistant hypertension, particularly in salt-sensitive patients such as older individuals, African Americans, obese patients, or those with renal impairment. Most antihypertensive agents including diuretics and combination preparations are more effective when dietary salt is restricted. Adherence to treatment can be proven by documenting urinary sodium excretion of less than 100 to 120 mmol/24 hours.

Nicotine may transiently raise BP, yet permanent hypertensive consequences have not been found. Caffeine has been exonerated in a similar fashion: a pooled analysis concluded that each cup of coffee raises BP on average 0.8/0.5 mm Hg.

Obesity and Metabolic Syndrome

In several series, more than 40% of patients with resistant hypertension were obese, a finding implying that obesity is a principal factor in resistance. At a university referral center, 43% of patients with resistant hypertension were obese, a tendency also observed in the primary care setting.[72] Among 141 patients with resistant hypertension evaluated at Rush University in Chicago, the average body BMI was in the obese range (mean BMI, 32 kg/m^2).[27] Subgroups of patients with resistant hypertension who are also obese may have glucose intolerance and hyperinsulinemia,[73] and they may require more intensive therapy, irrespective of BMI. Obesity is linked to a higher rate of uncontrolled hypertension and the use of higher medication doses to achieve similar BP effects compared with lean persons, even when one adjusts for variables such as gender, age, and upper arm circumference. Excess body fat is a principal contributing factor to hypertension worldwide, and 122 million adults in United States are now overweight or obese. Of particular concern is the potential progression from obesity to metabolic syndrome (consisting of at least three of the following: central adiposity, BP >130/85 mm Hg, glucose intolerance, low high-density lipoprotein cholesterol, and hypertriglyceridemia) to frank type 2 diabetes. In NHANES III, 80% of patients with the metabolic syndrome had high BP.[74] Increased BMI is independently correlated with higher rates of hypertension.[3] Compared with adults of normal weight, those with a BMI greater than 40 (class III obesity) have a more than sevenfold higher risk of hypertension.[4]

Several factors explain why obese patients or those with the metabolic syndrome may have hypertension that is difficult to manage. Physiologically, obese individuals have elevations in heart rate, cardiac output, and intravascular volume, which eventually may progress to end-organ injury such as ventricular hypertrophy, heart failure, and glomerular hyperfiltration with consequent microalbuminuria. The interaction of obesity, insulin resistance, and hyperinsulinemia may promote resistance through diverse mechanisms, including vasoconstriction and vascular hypertrophy, based on progrowth effects of insulin, with abdominal adiposity predicting vascular endothelial dysfunction.[73] Activation of the renin-angiotensin system contributes to hypertension, and angiotensinogen gene expression has been discovered in adipose tissue associated with abdominal fat distribution in obesity.[75] High circulating insulin levels may also exert sympathomimetic and sodium retentive effects.

Optimal treatment for obese patients with resistant hypertension is not well defined, and there is little trial evidence or guideline support concerning therapy. Weight reduction is a valuable adjunct to drug therapy, as are other lifestyle modifications (see Table 43-5).[76] ACE inhibitors, ARBs, and CCBs pose no negative metabolic issues. ACE inhibitors and ARBs can prevent nephropathy and the onset of new type 2 diabetes,[22,30,31,49] and CCBs may assist in natriuresis. However, volume expansion and elevated sodium intake suggest a strong role for diuretics, which are well tolerated metabolically when they are used in low to moderate doses. When diabetes is present, an even lower BP goal is sought (<130/80 mm Hg).[2]

PROGNOSIS AND FUTURE DIRECTIONS

Overall, the outlook is favorable for pharmacologic regulation of resistant hypertension in most, yet not all, patients who have resistant hypertension. In ALLHAT and CONVINCE, BP control to the standard of less than 140/90 mm/Hg eventually was achieved in nearly 70% of the study population, and diuretics were important elements in both protocols.[18,19] These findings compare favorably with the 34% BP control rate in NHANES.[3] In some cases, improved rather than ideal values may be acceptable. In older patients with severe systolic hypertension or advanced nephropathy, a goal of less than 130/80 mm Hg may not be attainable, even with a triple-drug regimen or greater. In a recent series, 53% of patients with resistant hypertension achieved BP control to less than 140/90 mm Hg, based on medication optimization and intensification, as well as use of proper diuretics; these patients required overall an average of 4.1 agents.[27] The most frequent changes included additions of CCBs, α-adrenergic blockers, ACE inhibitors, and diuretics. Patients whose resistant hypertension was medication based, or was related to secondary causes or interfering substances, had BP that was easier to control than those patients exhibiting nonadherence, psychological issues, or office resistance.[27] If medical management is particularly challenging, consultation with a hypertension specialist may be sought.

Numerous questions in the area of resistant hypertension remain for future investigation. Is the majority of resistance based on physician-related or patient-related factors? What percentage of patients with uncontrolled but treated hypertension will have true resistant hypertension? Are there cases of isolated systolic hypertension that simply cannot be treated successfully to goal, and how should they be approached? Which evaluations for secondary hypertension are cost-effective, particularly as prevalence and therapeutic options increase for primary aldosteronism and renal artery stenosis? What is the true prevalence of primary aldosteronism? What is the best way to manage renovascular hypertension on a long-term basis? Which patients are taking interfering exogenous substances? Can novel drugs and combinations address resistant hypertension with better success? How can clinical inertia be overcome? Will mechanical therapies, for instance, carotid baroreflex stimulators that serve to modulate central sympathetic outflow, successfully address severe drug-resistant hypertension? When should a patient with resistant hypertension be referred to a hypertension specialist? Will studies not yet published conclude that treatment goals should be even stricter and lower, especially for systolic hypertension, thereby once again enlarging the scope of resistant hypertension?

References

1. Setaro JF, Black HR. Refractory hypertension. *N Engl J Med*. 1992;**327**:543-547.
2. Chobanian AV, Bakris GL, Black HR, et al., and the National High Blood Pressure Education Program Coordinating Committee. The Seventh Report of the Joint National Committee on Prevention, Detection, Evaluation, and Treatment of High Blood Pressure: The JNC 7 Report. *JAMA*. 2003;**289**:2560-2572.
3. Hajjar I, Kotchen TA. Trends in prevalence, awareness, treatment, and control of hypertension in the United States, 1988-2000. *JAMA*. 2003;**290**:199-206.
4. Mokdad AH, Ford ES, Bowman BA, et al. Prevalence of obesity, diabetes, and obesity-related health risk factors, 2001. *JAMA*. 2003;**289**:76-79.
5. Isaksson H, Ostergrten J. Prognosis in therapy-resistant hypertension. *J Intern Med*. 1994;**236**:643-649.
6. Cuspidi C, Macca G, Sampieri L, et al. High prevalence of cardiac and extracardiac organ damage in refractory hypertension. *J Hypertens*. 2001;**19**:2063-2070.
7. Staessen JA, Gasowski J, Wang JG, et al. Risks of untreated and treated systolic hypertension in the elderly: Meta-analysis of outcome trials. *Lancet*. 2000;**355**:865-872.
8. Kjeldsen SE, Dahlof B, Devereux RB, et al. Effects of losartan on cardiovascular morbidity and mortality in patients with isolated systolic hypertension and left ventricular hypertrophy: A Losartan Intervention for Endpoint Reduction (LIFE) substudy. *JAMA*. 2002;**288**:1491-1498.
9. American Diabetes Association. Hypertension management in adults with diabetes. *Diabetes Care*. 2004;**27** (**Suppl 1**):S65-S67.
10. K/DOQI clinical practice guidelines on hypertension and antihypertensive agents in chronic kidney disease. *Am J Kidney Dis*. 2004;**43** (**5 Suppl 2**):1-290.
11. Lewington S, Clarke R, Qizilbash N, et al., for the Prospective Studies Collaboration. Age-specific relevance of usual blood pressure to vascular mortality: A meta-analysis of individual data for one million adults in 61 prospective studies. *Lancet*. 2002;**360**:1903-1913.
12. Franklin SS, Jacobs MJ, Wong ND, et al. Predominance of isolated systolic hypertension among middle-aged and elderly US hypertensives: Analysis based on National Health and Nutrition Examination Survey (NHANES) III. *Hypertension*. 2001;**37**:869-874.

13. Hyman DJ, Pavlik VN. Characteristics of patients with uncontrolled hypertension in the United States. *N Engl J Med.* 2001;**345**:479-486.

14. Staessen JA, Wang JG, Thijs L. Cardiovascular prevention and blood pressure reduction: A quantitative overview updated until 1 March 2003. *J Hypertens.* 2001;**21**:1055-1076.

15. Adler AI, Stratton IM, Neil HA, et al. Association of systolic blood pressure with macrovascular and microvascular complications in type 2 diabetes (UKPDS 36). *BMJ.* 2000;**321**:412-419.

16. Hansson L, Zanchetti A, Carruthers SG, et al., for the HOT Study Group. Effects of intensive blood pressure lowering and low dose aspirin in patients with hypertension: Principal results of the Hypertension Optimal Treatment (HOT) randomized trial. *Lancet.* 1998;**351**:1755-1762.

17. Singer GM, Izhar M, Black HR. Goal-oriented hypertension management: Translating clinical trials to practice. *Hypertension.* 2002;**40**:464-469.

18. ALLHAT Officers and Coordinators for the ALLHAT Collaborative Research Group. Major outcomes in high-risk hypertensive patients randomized to angiotensin-converting enzyme inhibitor or calcium channel blocker vs. diuretic: The Antihypertensive and Lipid-Lowering Treatment to Prevent Heart Attack Trial (ALLHAT). *JAMA.* 2002;**288**:2981-2997.

19. Black HR, Elliott WJ, Grandits G, et al., for the CONVINCE Research Group. Principal results of the Controlled Onset Verapamil Investigation of Cardiovascular End Points (CONVINCE) trial. *JAMA.* 2003;**289**:2073-2082.

20. Cushman WC, Ford CE, Cutler JA, et al. Success and predictors of blood pressure control in diverse North American settings: The Antihypertensive and Lipid-Lowering Treatment to Prevent Heart Attack Trial (ALLHAT). *J Clin Hypertens (Greenwich).* 2002;**4**:393-404.

21. Pepine CJ, Handberg EM, Cooper-DeHoff RM, et al. A calcium antagonist vs. a non-calcium antagonist hypertension treatment strategy for patients with coronary artery disease: The International Verapamil-Trandolapril Study (INVEST). A randomized controlled trial. *JAMA.* 2003;**290**:2805-2816.

22. Dahlof B, Devereux RB, Kjeldsen S, et al. Cardiovascular morbidity and mortality in the Losartan Intervention for Endpoint Reduction in Hypertension study (LIFE): A randomized trial against atenolol. *Lancet.* 2002;**359**:995-1003.

23. Pickering TG, Hall JE, Appel LJ, et al. Recommendations for Blood Pressure Measurement in Humans and Experimental Animals: Part 1. Blood Pressure Measurement in Humans: A Statement for Professionals From the Subcommittee of Professional and Public Education of the American Heart Association Council on High Blood Pressure Research. *Hypertension.* 2005;**45**:142-161.

24. Wright JC, Looney SW. Presence of positive Osler's maneuver in 3387 persons screened for the Systolic Hypertension in the Elderly Program (SHEP). *J Hum Hypertens.* 1997;**11**:285-829.

25. Staessen JA, Hond ED, Celis H, et al., for the Treatment of Hypertension Based on Home or Office Blood Pressure (THOP) Trial Investigators. Antihypertensive treatment based on blood pressure measurement at home or in the physician's office: A Randomized controlled trial. *JAMA.* 2004;**291**:955-964.

26. Yakovlevitch M, Black HR. Resistant hypertension in a tertiary care clinic. *Arch Intern Med.* 1991;**151**:1786-1792.

27. Garg JP, Elliott WJ, Folker A, et al. Resistant hypertension revisited: A comparison of two university-based cohorts. *Am J Hypertens.* 2005;**18**:619-626.

28. Anderson GH, Blakeman N, Streeten DHP. The effect of age on prevalence of secondary forms of hypertension in 4429 consecutively referred patients. *J Hypertens.* 1995;**12**:609-615.

29. Nishizaka MK, Calhoun DA. Use of aldosterone antagonists in resistant hypertension. *J Clin Hypertens (Greenwich).* 2004;**6**:458-460.

30. Agodoa L, Appel L, Bakris G, et al. Effect of ramipril versus amlodipine on renal outcomes in hypertensive nephrosclerosis: African American Study of Kidney Disease (AASK). A randomized controlled trial. *JAMA.* 2001;**285**:2719-2728.

31. Brenner BM, Cooper ME, DeZeeuw D, et al. Effects of losartan on renal and cardiovascular outcomes in patients with type 2 diabetes and nephropathy (RENAAL). *N Engl J Med.* 2001;**345**:861-869.

32. Safian RD, Textor SC. Renal-artery stenosis. *N Engl J Med.* 2001;**344**:431-442.

33. Mosso L, Carvajal C, Gonzalez A. Primary aldosteronism and hypertensive disease. *Hypertension.* 2003;**42**:161-165.

34. Calhoun DA, Nishizaka MK, Zaman MA, et al. Hyperaldosteronism among black and white subjects with resistant hypertension. *Hypertension.* 2002;**40**:892-896.

35. Lim PO, Jung RT, MacDonald TM. Is aldosterone the missing link in refractory hypertension? Aldosterone-to-renin ratio as a marker of inappropriate aldosterone activity. *J Hum Hypertens.* 2002;**16**:153-158.

36. Vasan RS, Evans JC, Larson MG, et al. Serum aldosterone and the incidence of hypertension in nonhypertensive persons. *N Engl J Med.* 2004;**351**:33-41.

37. Gallay BJ, Ahmad S, Xu L, et al. Screening for primary aldosteronism without discontinuing hypertensive medications: Plasma aldosterone-renin ratio. *Am J Kidney Dis.* 2001;**37**:699-705.

38. Nishizaka MK, Zaman MA, Calhoun DA. Efficacy of low-dose spironolactone in subjects with resistant hypertension. *Am J Hypertens.* 2003;**16**:925-930.

39. Ouzan J, Pérault C, Lincoff AM, et al. The role of spironolactone in the treatment of patients with refractory hypertension. *Am J Hypertens.* 2002;**15**:333-339.

40. Eisenhofer G. Biochemical diagnosis of pheochromocytoma. *In:* Pacak K (moderator). Recent advances in genetics, diagnosis, localization, and treatment of pheochromocytoma. *Ann Intern Med.* 2001;**134**:317-320.

41. Logan AG, Perlikowski SM, Mente A, et al. High prevalence of unrecognized sleep apnoea in drug-resistant hypertension. *J Hypertens.* 2001;**19**:2271-2277.

42. Pepperell JCT, Ramdassingh-Dow S, Costhwaite N, et al. Ambulatory blood pressure after therapeutic and subtherapeutic nasal continuous positive airway pressure for obstructive sleep apnea, a randomized parallel trial. *Lancet.* 2002;**359**:204-210.

43. Dhillon S, Chung SA, Fargher T, et al. Sleep apnea, hypertension, and the effects of continuous positive airway pressure. *Am J Hypertens.* 2005;**18**:594-600.

44. Goodfriend TL, Calhoun DA. Resistant hypertension, obesity, sleep apnea, and aldosterone: Theory and therapy. *Hypertension.* 2004;**43**:518-524.

45. Davies SJ, Ghahramani P, Jackson PR, et al. Panic disorder, anxiety and depression in resistant hypertension: A case control study. *J Hypertens.* 1997;**15**:1077-1082.

46. Graves JW, Bloomfild RL, Buckalew VM. Plasma volume in resistant hypertension: Guide to pathophysiology and therapy. *Am J Med Sci.* 1989;**298**:361-365.

47. Taler SJ, Textor SC, Augustine JE. Resistant hypertension: Comparing hemodynamic management to specialist care. *Hypertension.* 2002;**39**:982-988.

48. Moser M. Why are physicians not prescribing diuretics more frequently in the management of hypertension? *JAMA.* 1998;**279**:1813-1816.

49. Heart Outcome Prevention Evaluation (HOPE) Study Investigators. Effects of ramipril on cardiovascular and microvascular outcomes in people with diabetes mellitus: Results of the HOPE Study and the MICRO HOPE substudy. *Lancet.* 2000;**255**:253-259.

50. Dickerson JEC, Hingorani AD, Ashby MJ, et al. Optimisation of antihypertensive treatment by crossover rotation of four major classes. *Lancet.* 1999;**353**:2008-2013.

51. Law MR, Wald NJ, Morris JK, Jordan RE. Value of low dose combination treatment with blood pressure lowering drugs: Analysis of 354 randomised trials. *BMJ.* 2003;**326**:1427.

52. Saseen JJ, Carter BL, Brown TE, et al. Comparison of nifedipine alone and with diltiazem or verapamil in hypertension. *Hypertension.* 1996;**28**:109-114.

53. Mogensen CE, Neldam S, Tikkanen I, et al. Randomised controlled trial of dual blockade of renin-angiotensin system in patients with hypertension, microalbuminuria, and non-insulin dependent diabetes: The Candesartan and Lisinopril Microalbuminuria (CALM) study. *BMJ.* 2000;**321**:1440-1444.

54. Black HR, Sollins JS, Garofalo JL. The addition of doxazosin to the therapeutic regimen of hypertensive patients inadequately controlled with other antihypertensive medications: A randomized, placebo controlled study. *Am J Hypertens.* 2000;**13**:468-474.

55. Davies SJ, Jackson PR, Ramsay LE, Ghahramani P. Drug intolerance due to non-specific adverse effects related to psychiatric morbidity in hypertensive patients. *Arch Intern Med.* 2003;**163**:592-600.

56. Berlowitz DR, Ash AS, Hickey EC, et al. Inadequate management of blood pressure in a hypertensive population. *N Engl J Med.* 1998;**339**:1957-1963.

57. Oliveria SA, Lapuerta P, McCarthy BD, et al. Physician-related barriers to the effective management of uncontrolled hypertension. *Arch Intern Med.* 2002;**162**:413-420.

58. Burnier M, Schneider MP, Chioléro A, et al. Electronic compliance monitoring in resistant hypertension: The basis for rational therapeutic decisions. *J Hypertens.* 2001;**19**:335-341.

59. Nuesch R, Schroeder K, Dieterle T, et al. Relation between insufficient response to antihypertensive treatment and poor compliance with treatment: A prospective case-control study. *BMJ.* 2001;**323**:142-146.

60. Haynes RB, McDonald HP, Garg AX. Helping patients follow prescribed treatment: Clinical applications. *JAMA.* 2002;**288**:2880-2883.

61. McDonald HP, Garg AX, Haynes RB. Interventions to enhance patient adherence to medication prescriptions: Scientific review. *JAMA.* 2002;**288**:2868-2879.

62. Lloyd-Jones DM, Evans JC, Larson A. Differential control of systolic and diastolic blood pressure: Factors associated with lack of blood pressure control in the community. *Hypertension.* 2000;**36**:594-599.

63. Ferdinand KC. Substance abuse and hypertension. *J Clin Hypertens (Greenwich).* 2000;**2**:37-40.

64. Haller CA, Benowitz NL. Adverse cardiovascular and central nervous system events associated with dietary supplements containing ephedra alkaloids. *N Engl J Med.* 2000;**343**: 1833-1838.

65. Valli G, Giardina EGV. Benefits, adverse effects and drug interactions of herbal remedies with cardiovascular effects. *J Am Coll Cardiol.* 2002;**39**:1083-1095.

66. DeSmet PAGM. Herbal remedies. *N Engl J Med.* 2002;**347**: 2046-2056.

67. Whelton A, Fort JG, Puma JA, et al., for the SUCCESS VI Study Group. Cyclooxygenase-2–specific inhibitors and cardiorenal function: A randomized, controlled trial of celecoxib and rofecoxib in older hypertensive osteoarthritis patients. *Am J Ther.* 2001;**8**:85-95.

68. Cho J, Cooke CE, Proveaux W. A retrospective review of the effect of COX-2 inhibitors on blood pressure change. *Am J Ther.* 2003;**10**:311-317.

69. Sowers JR, White WB, Pitt B, et al., for the Celecoxib Rofecoxib Efficacy and Safety in Comorbidities Evaluation Trial (CRESECENT) Investigators. The effects of cyclooxygenase-2 inhibitors and nonsteroidal anti-inflammatory therapy on 24-hour blood pressure in patients with hypertension, osteoarthritis, and type 2 diabetes mellitus. *Arch Intern Med.* 2005;**165**:161-168.

70. Aw T-J, Haas SJ, Liew D, Krum H. Meta-analysis of cyclooxygenase-2 inhibitors and their effects on blood pressure. *Arch Intern Med.* 2005;**165**:490-496.

71. Xin X, He J, Frontini MG, et al. Effects of alcohol reduction on blood pressure: A meta-analysis of randomized controlled trials. *Hypertension.* 2001;**38**:1112-1117.

72. Bramlage P, Pittrow D, Wittchen HU, et al. Hypertension in overweight and obese primary care patients is highly prevalent and poorly controlled. *Am J Hypertens.* 2004;**17**:904-910.

73. Martell N, Rodgriguez-Cerillo M, Grobbee DE, et al. High prevalence of secondary hypertension and insulin resistance in patients with refractory hypertension. *Blood Press.* 2003;**12**: 149-154.

74. Wong ND, Pio JR, Franklin SS, et al. Preventing coronary events by optimal control of blood pressure and lipids in patients with the metabolic syndrome. *Am J Cardiol.* 2003;**91**:1421-1426.

75. Van Harmelen V, Elizalde M, Aripart P, et al. The association of human adipose angiotensinogen gene expression with abdominal fat distribution in obesity. *Int J Obes.* 2000;**24**: 673-678.

76. Appel LJ, Champagne CM, Harsha DW, et al., for the PREMIER Collaborative Research Group. Effects of comprehensive lifestyle modification on blood pressure control: Main results of the PREMIER clinical trial. *JAMA.* 2003;**289**:2083-2093.

Hypertension and the Perioperative Period

Robert L. Bard, Robert D. Brook, and Kim A. Eagle

Data concerning the cardiovascular (CV) risks of hypertension and the benefits of its treatment in the perioperative period are limited. Nevertheless, clinical practice guidelines consider an elevated blood pressure (BP) of greater than 180 mm Hg systolic or greater than 100 mm Hg diastolic as a "minor" clinical risk predictor of adverse CV events. We discuss the surgical risk in patients with hypertension and review the role of an elevated BP in perioperative complications. We conclude by offering a clinical management algorithm for the hypertensive patient who is undergoing surgery.

PERIOPERATIVE HYPERTENSION

High BP may occur in the perioperative period for two reasons: patients may present with a previous history of hypertension, or it may occur acutely during the perioperative period in response to several factors. Anxiety, pain, drug withdrawal (e.g., discontinued medications, alcohol), and stress-induced sympathetic nervous system activation can all increase BP and heart rate. Postoperative hypertension may be further induced by intravenous fluid administration, particularly in patients with chronic kidney disease or postoperative worsening of renal function. Studies that assess the effect of hypertension on operative outcomes have usually been limited to patients with chronic hypertension.

BP plays a relatively minor role in the risk assessment of CV complications in surgical candidates.[1] According to the current guidelines of the American College of Cardiology (ACC) and the American Heart Association (AHA), hypertension is only a "minor clinical predictor," even when systolic BP is greater than 180 mm Hg or diastolic BP is greater than 110 mm Hg. Lower BP values, even if within the hypertensive range, are not independent predictors of CV complications based on the results of a variety of studies.[1] However, several studies have shown that preoperative hypertension does raise the risk for increased intraoperative BP variability in patients with electrocardiographic evidence of ischemia.[1] Moreover, hypertension is frequently associated with other CV risk factors,[2] such as diabetes mellitus, an established independent risk factor for coronary artery disease (CAD)[3] and a more potent risk factor for perioperative complications.[1] As such, an elevated BP should cue clinicians to evaluate patients more thoroughly for intermediate (e.g., diabetes) or high-risk (e.g., class 3 angina) clinical predictors during the preoperative assessment (Table 44-1). The identification of hypertension during the preoperative risk assessment also offers an opportunity for a more complete evaluation of the patient's overall long-term CV risk, so health and risk modification efforts can be started at this time (e.g., lipid-lowering therapy, BP control) if appropriate.

MORBIDITY ASSOCIATED WITH HYPERTENSION IN THE PERIOPERATIVE PERIOD

Most studies of the risks of noncardiac surgery have been concerned with the incidence of adverse CV complications, such as myocardial infarction or death.[4-9] Most of these publications included the rates of complications related to several different risk predictors. We are not aware of any study that specifically sought to determine the role of hypertension alone in perioperative morbidity; however, elevated BP was a component of risk in many of these previous investigations.

In 1977, Goldman and colleagues published one of the first articles about the risks of cardiac complications of surgery.[4] Even though this study was limited by its small size (1001 patients), acutely high BP or a history of hypertension during preoperative assessment was not a significant predictor of perioperative cardiac complications.

Similarly, in noncardiac surgical patients, Lette and colleagues tested the ability of 23 different clinical descriptors, 7 different multivariable indices, and quantitative dipyridamole-thallium imaging to predict postoperative and long-term myocardial infarction and cardiac death.[5] After an average follow-up of 15 months, 303 patients had no cardiac event, and 43 patients had a cardiac event. The clinical descriptors, including hypertension, were not useful in predicting the outcome of individual patients. The authors concluded that quantitative indices reflecting the amount of jeopardized myocardium, and not clinical indicators, accurately identified high-risk patients who needed preoperative coronary angiography.

In a higher-risk cohort of patients, Raby and associates prospectively evaluated the correlation of preoperative ischemia with intraoperative and postoperative ischemia in 115 patients undergoing elective peripheral vascular surgery.[6] Ischemia was detected with ambulatory monitors for at least 24 hours preoperatively, throughout the intraoperative period, and for up to 72 hours postoperatively (96% of patients for ≥24 hours). Ischemia was present in 18% of patients intraoperatively and in 30% of patients postoperatively, but no correlation was noted between ischemia and hypertension. Postoperatively, hypertension was present in 66% of patients with ischemia and in 56% of patients without ischemia. Intraoperatively, hypertension was present in 62% of patients with ischemia and in 59% of patients without ischemia. Although this study was small and had few CV events, the authors reported that the risk of ischemia associated with hypertension nearly met statistical significance.

Ashton and colleagues evaluated the incidence of perioperative myocardial infarction in 835 men at risk for CV

Table 44-1 Clinical Predictors for Cardiovascular Complications in the Perioperative Period, According to Current Practice Guidelines of the American College of Cardiology and the American Heart Association

Minor	Intermediate	Major
Advanced age	Mild angina pectoris	Unstable coronary syndromes
Rhythm other than sinus	Prior myocardial infarction	Decompensated heart failure
Abnormal electrocardiogram	Compensated or prior heart failure	Significant arrhythmias
Low functional capacity	Diabetes mellitus	Severe valvular disease
History of stroke	Chronic kidney disease	
Uncontrolled systemic hypertension (>180/110 mm Hg)		

From Eagle KA, Berger PB, Calkins H, et al. ACC/AHA Guideline update for perioperative cardiovascular evaluation for noncardiac surgery: A report of the American College of Cardiology/American Heart Association task force on Practice Guidelines (Committee to Update the 1996 Guidelines on Perioperative cardiovascular evaluation for noncardiac surgery), 2002. Available on the internet at the American College of Cardiology Web site: http://www.acc.org/clinical/guidelines/perio/dirIndex.htm, accessed 31 JAN 05.

events who underwent noncardiac surgery.[7] There were 15 (1.8%) perioperative myocardial infarctions, but 7 of the 15 patients who had a myocardial infarction had a preoperative history of hypertension, which was also seen in 368 of the 820 who did not have a myocardial infarction (relative risk, 1.07; $P > .20$). Although the study was small and few events occurred, the authors reported that men who experienced intraoperative hypotension, rather than hypertension, were more likely to have a perioperative myocardial infarction.

In 1996, 3 years after publication of the article of Ashton and colleagues,[7] Mangano and associates published the results of a randomized, double-blind, clinical trial conducted to determine whether a simple and inexpensive risk reduction strategy could alter CV morbidity.[8] Two hundred patients were randomized to atenolol or placebo before noncardiac surgical procedures. All patients had, or were at risk for, CAD and were followed for 2 years postoperatively. The atenolol-treated patients who survived to hospital discharge had no cardiac events as compared with the placebo group, who had 12 events in the 6 months after surgery. After 8 months, no differences were noted in additional events between the two groups, but the early benefit of β-blockade allowed the 2-year follow-up survival analysis to maintain its statistical significance. The atenolol-treated group had more hypertensive patients than did the placebo group ($n = 71$ versus $n = 60$, $P = .08$), but hypertension itself did not influence cardiac events or mortality. The only significant independent predictors at 2 years of follow-up were a history of diabetes mellitus and β-blocker therapy. Atenolol improved survival in the 63 patients with diabetes by about 75%.

More recently, Poldermans and colleagues evaluated outcomes in high-risk patients with inducible ischemia on preoperative stress testing who were undergoing high-risk vascular surgery.[9] Patients were randomized to receive perioperative β-blockade with bisoprolol (5 to 10 mg, $n = 59$), for an average of 37 days preoperatively, or to standard care ($n = 53$). The primary endpoint (cardiac death or nonfatal myocardial infarction) was significantly reduced in the bisoprolol-treated group ($n = 2$, or 3.4%) compared with the group receiving standard care ($n = 18$, or 34%). The authors concluded that β-blockade (with heart rate control to an average of 66 beats/minute) is very effective in reducing CV complications in high-risk patients undergoing major vascular surgery. Once again, this study was not specifically designed to investigate the role of hypertension or perioperative BP control.

Although most of the evidence supports the CV benefit of β-blockade (with subsequent heart rate control) in high-risk patients undergoing major noncardiac surgery, the effect of hypertension per se (or the lowering of BP itself) remains unclear. To date, no studies have investigated CV risk associated with mild to moderate hypertension (140 to 179/90 to 109 mm Hg), measured in the immediate preoperative situation. Additionally, no clinical trials have been conducted to determine whether outcomes are improved by delaying surgery until adequate BP control has been achieved in hypertensive patients. Therefore, the national guidelines and the management algorithm provided in this chapter are based primarily on prudent caution against performing major surgery in patients with uncontrolled hypertension, rather than on clear clinical trial evidence.

Several methodologic issues should be considered when reviewing hypertension and the perioperative risk literature. Fleisher criticized the statistical design of studies and stated that most studies were underpowered to evaluate the primary endpoints of myocardial infarction and death appropriately, and this author was particularly critical of trials that used surrogate markers.[10] For example, some studies use electrocardiographic changes to suggest ischemia as a surrogate for myocardial infarction and death, but suppressing myocardial ischemia alone does not necessarily correlate with a reduced incidence of myocardial infarction or death. The methodology of perioperative BP studies may be inherently flawed or limited because the perioperative environment that influences BP cannot be replicated during follow-up. Anxiety, pain, and sympathetic nervous system activation can increase both the BP and heart rate, and these states may not be present during follow-up evaluations in the clinic. Postoperative hypertension may be influenced by intravenous fluid administration, particularly in patients with chronic kidney disease. Finally, proper measurement of consecutive, resting, seated BPs may not have been obtained, or may have been impossible to obtain, during the preoperative evaluation.

EFFECT OF VARIOUS ANTIHYPERTENSIVE MEDICATIONS

Among specific antihypertensive medications used perioperatively, β-blockers have traditionally been the first choice of therapy for several reasons. If surgery is urgent, β-blockers can lower BP rapidly, prevent fluctuations in BP, reduce heart rate, and prevent myocardial ischemia.[10] Preoperative β-blocker administration has been reported to decrease the incidence of atrial fibrillation,[1] mortality,[8] and CV complications,[8] both in patients with CAD and in patients at risk for CAD. β-Blockers have been judged to be "probably beneficial" during any high-risk surgical procedure in patients with chronic kidney disease and even in patients with poor functional status whose limitations may suggest CAD or heart failure.[1,10] Therefore, the American College of Physicians,[11] the AHA, and the ACC recommended perioperative β-blockers for patients who have or are at risk for CAD when they undergo noncardiac surgical procedures, regardless of their history of hypertension. However, most (but not all[8]) of the studies that reported reduced events with β-blockers were performed only in very high-risk patients with adequate heart rate control (~60 beats/minute) for at least several days preoperatively.[9]

At present, there is still considerable debate,[12,13] as well as poor compliance,[14] with the perioperative β-blocker recommendations. Commentaries have criticized task forces for basing decisions on evidence from small, mostly single-center, observational studies.[12,15] To heighten the debate, the results of a 2006 randomized trial did not confirm the benefit of β-blockers.[16] Before noncardiac operations (including orthopedic, gynecologic, and neurologic procedures), 921 patients with type 2 diabetes who were not previously taking β-blockers were randomized to 100 mg/day of metoprolol versus placebo for a maximum of 8 days preceding surgery.[17] The mean duration of treatment was 5 days preoperatively in each group. The primary outcome was a composite score of all-cause mortality, acute myocardial infarction, unstable angina, or heart failure. Although the heart rate was significantly lower in the group receiving a β-blocker (71 ± 13 versus 84 ±1 4 beats/minute, $P < .001$) no difference in the primary outcome was noted after a median follow-up of 18 months (99 versus 93 patients, or 21% versus 20%; hazard ratio, 1.10; 95% confidence interval, 0.82 to 1.46; $P = .53$). The results of this study suggest that the presence of diabetes alone does not support an indication for the perioperative addition of β-blocker therapy. This study differs from previous studies that demonstrated a benefit, because both the patients and the type of surgery may have been lower risk.[16] In addition, the less than adequate degree of heart rate control and moderate β-blocker dose may have influenced the results. These findings cannot be generalized to all patients, especially to higher-risk patients with myocardial ischemia on stress testing who are candidates for major vascular surgery. It is possible that the benefit of β-blockade will be more definitively answered by the ongoing Perioperative Ischemic Evaluation (POISE) trial of approximately 10,000 patients randomized to controlled-release metoprolol, 200 mg/day for 30 days, versus placebo.[12] Yet again, the effect of treatment of hypertension itself (or the BP level per se) is not under investigation.

Other antihypertensive medications are not as well studied as β-blockers. However, evidence indicates that perioperative use of either an angiotensin-converting enzyme (ACE) inhibitor or an angiotensin receptor blocker (ARB) is more likely to cause severe hypotension. Coriat and associates investigated the incidence of hypotension in 51 hypertensive patients who used ACE inhibitors on a long-term basis and

who were referred for peripheral vascular surgery.[18] These investigators compared four different treatment regimens: two different ACE inhibitors (enalapril or captopril) that were either continued until the day of surgery or were withdrawn the day before surgery. Patients had significantly greater rates of hypotension, defined as a systolic BP lower than 90 mm Hg and the need for ephedrine, in the continued-treatment groups than in the withdrawn-treatment groups. Every patient ($n = 7$) who continued taking enalapril experienced hypotension, whereas only 2 of 11 patients (18%) who discontinued enalapril experienced hypotension. Likewise, 9 of the 14 patients (64%) who continued taking captopril experienced hypotension, whereas only 4 of 19 (21%) who discontinued captopril experienced hypotension. Regardless of the ACE inhibitor, stopping the medication the evening before surgery resulted in lower rates of hypotension.

ARBs have been tested in similar fashion.[19] Patients with hypertension ($n = 37$) receiving ARB therapy were randomized either to discontinue the ARB the day before surgery or to take the ARB 1 hour before anesthesia. The incidence of hypotension and the administration of both intravenous fluids and vasoconstrictors were noted until the time of incision. Patients given an ARB on the surgical day experienced more episodes of hypotension than patients who discontinued the ARB (19 versus 12, $P < .01$). Furthermore, the hypotensive episodes were of statistically longer duration in patients given an ARB than in those in whom the drug was discontinued (8 ± 7 versus 3 ± 4 minutes, $P < .001$). The authors concluded that blockade of the renin-angiotensin system increases the potential hypotensive effect of anesthetic induction. They hypothesized that because several anesthetics are sympatholytic, adequate perioperative BP is primarily maintained by a functioning renin-angiotensin system. Patients taking either an ACE inhibitor or an ARB may be prone to severe hypotension because of blockade of the remaining physiologically important mechanism to maintain BP following anesthesia induction. Contrary to the general advice regarding antihypertensive medications, in particular β-blockers, it may be prudent to hold the morning dose of either an ACE inhibitor or an ARB on the day of surgery.

ALGORITHM FOR THE MANAGEMENT OF THE HYPERTENSIVE PATIENT UNDERGOING SURGERY

The primary factors to consider in the preoperative evaluation of patients with a history of hypertension are (1) the level of BP and (2) intermediate or major clinical risk predictors as defined by the ACC/AHA.[1] If BP is higher than 180 systolic or 110 mm Hg, then surgery should be delayed, if possible, to achieve adequate BP control.[1] Patients with more significant risk predictors (e.g., diabetes) who have lower BP should undergo further evaluation. For most of these patients, stress testing is indicated.

Figure 44-1 summarizes our recommendations in the preoperative evaluation of hypertensive patients based ACC/AHA guidelines.[1] BP measurement should be performed in the least anxiety-provoking environment, if possible, while using appropriate clinical techniques.[20] Such procedures include ensuring that the patient is seated for at least 5 minutes, the brachial artery is at heart level (midsternum),

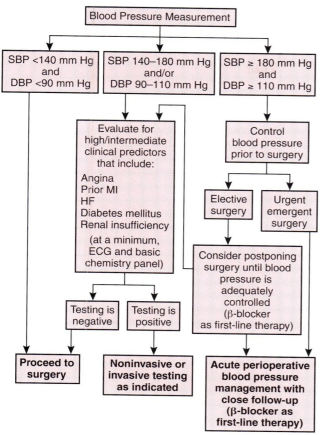

Figure 44–1 Recommendations for the preoperative evaluation of hypertensive patients. DBP, diastolic blood pressure; ECG, electrocardiogram; HF, heart failure; MI, myocardial infarction; SBP, systolic blood pressure.

the appropriate cuff size is used, and the average of three measurements is recorded. Further office measurements, home measurements, or ambulatory BP measurement may be necessary in some patients in whom white-coat hypertension is suspected.

Figure 44-1 shows that patients whose BP is less than 140 mm Hg systolic or 90 mm Hg diastolic in the absence of other higher risk predictors may proceed to surgery, with the expectation of safety. In patients with stage 1 or with lower levels of stage 2 hypertension (<180/110 mm Hg), perioperative risk may be greater because of the tendency for other diseases to be present. Therefore, the primary clinical concern is to exclude the presence of other intermediate- or high-risk predictors (see Table 44-1).

Initially, noninvasive testing is warranted during preoperative evaluations in medically stable patients with hypertension and predictors of intermediate risk who are undergoing high-risk surgery (e.g., major vascular surgery). Patients with predictors of high risk should not undergo surgery unless absolutely necessary. A detailed medical history, a physical examination, an electrocardiogram, and a basic chemistry panel should be performed first. If any of these evaluations reveals an abnormality, then the clinician may order additional noninvasive or invasive stress tests to determine the patient's surgical risk more definitively, per ACC/AHA guidelines.[1]

As in any clinical situation, the benefits of the surgery should clearly outweigh the risks associated with the surgery and its anesthesia. Therefore, the clinical recommendations for a patient who presents with BP of 180 mm Hg or higher systolic or 110 mm Hg or higher diastolic rely on each patient's situation. If the surgical procedure is considered urgent and necessary, then it may be performed, provided the patient has sufficient cardiac reserve to tolerate anesthesia. Acute BP reduction can be achieved perioperatively in such patients with intravenous medications (e.g., β-blockade). Clinicians must avoid lowering the BP to a relatively hypotensive level that may itself precipitate adverse CV events. If the patient's situation is not urgent, then the surgical procedure may be postponed until BP is adequately controlled on an outpatient basis. Additionally, postponing surgery may be beneficial to the patient, because it can allow for closer risk evaluation and normalization of BP, which will likely reduce both the surgical risk and the long-term CV risk.

In the perioperative period, patients should try to maintain optimal BP control, and they should take their antihypertensive medications before and throughout the perioperative period, including the morning of surgery. The possible exception to this rule may be an ACE inhibitor or an ARB, which could be omitted on the day of surgery only. β-Blockers are the first line of therapy both for patients previously not taking other BP medications and who require BP control and for hypertensive patients (taking or not taking other BP medications) with intermediate risk predictors (particularly with ischemia on stress testing).[1] Cardioselective β-blockers, such as metoprolol, may be introduced at a dose of 25 to 50 mg twice daily and gradually titrated to levels at which patients' heart rates are approximately 60 beats/minute.[10,21]

CONCLUSIONS

Little clinical trial evidence is available to guide therapy of hypertension in the perioperative period. To date, most studies suggest that β-blockade, with adequate heart rate control in high-risk patients undergoing major surgery, reduces CV events. However, more recent studies suggest that β-blockade may not be helpful in relatively lower-risk patients, such as those with diabetes only, who are undergoing lower-risk surgeries. Ongoing studies will help to clarify the role for perioperative β-blockade further. Because hypertension is frequently accompanied by other CV risk factors, elevated preoperative BP should alert clinicians to the need to undertake a more thorough evaluation and to consider methods to reduce long-term CV risk. No data are available to substantiate recommendations regarding surgical risk and the treatment of patients with BP of up to 180 mm Hg systolic or up to 110 mm Hg diastolic.

References

1. Eagle KA, Berger PB, Calkins H, et al. ACC/AHA Guideline update for perioperative cardiovascular evaluation for noncardiac surgery: A report of the American Collage of Cardiology/ American Heart Association task force on Practice Guidelines (Committee to Update the 1996 Guidelines on Perioperative cardiovascular evaluation for noncardiac surgery), 2002. Available on the internet at the American College of

Cardiology Web site: http://www.acc.org/clinical/guidelines/perio/dirIndex.htm, accessed 31 JAN 05.

2. Kannel WB. Risk stratification in hypertension: New insights from the Framingham Study. *Am J Hypertens.* 2000;**13**:3S-10S.

3. Chobanian AV, Bakris GL, Black HR, et al., for the National High Blood Pressure Education Program Coordinating Committee. Seventh Report of the Joint National Committee on Prevention, Detection, Evaluation, and Treatment of High Blood Pressure. *Hypertension.* 2003;**42**:1206-1252.

4. Goldman L, Caldera DL, Nussbaum SR, et al. Multifactorial index of cardiac risk in noncardiac surgical procedures. *N Engl J Med.* 1977;**297**:845-850.

5. Lette J, Waters D, Bernier H, et al. Preoperative and long-term cardiac risk assessment. Predictive value of 23 clinical descriptors, 7 multivariate scoring systems, and quantitative dipyridamole imaging in 360 patients. *Ann Surg.* 1992;**216**:192-204.

6. Raby KE, Barry J, Creager MA, et al. Detection and significance of intraoperative and postoperative myocardial ischemia in peripheral vascular surgery. *JAMA.* 1992;**268**:222-227.

7. Ashton CM, Petersen NJ, Wray NP, et al. The incidence of perioperative myocardial infarction in men undergoing noncardiac surgery. *Ann Intern Med.* 1993;**118**:504-510.

8. Mangano DT, Layug EL, Wallace A, Tateo I. Effect of atenolol on mortality and cardiovascular morbidity after noncardiac surgery: Multicenter Study of Perioperative Ischemia Research Group. *N Engl J Med.* 1996;**335**:1713-1720.

9. Poldermans D, Boersma E, Bax JJ, et al. The effect of bisoprolol on perioperative mortality and myocardial infarction in high-risk patients undergoing vascular surgery. *N Engl J Med.* 1999;**341**:1789-1794.

10. Fleisher LA. Preoperative evaluation of the patient with hypertension. *JAMA.* 2002;**287**:2043-2046.

11. American College of Physicians. Guidelines for assessing and managing the perioperative risk from coronary artery disease associated with major noncardiac surgery. *Ann Intern Med.* 1997;**127**:309-312.

12. Devereaux PJ, Leslie K, Yang H. The effect of perioperative beta blockers on patients undergoing noncardiac surgery: Is the answer in? *Can J Anaesth.* 2004;**51**:749-755.

13. Devereaux PJ, Yusuf S, Yang H, et al. Are the recommendations to use perioperative beta blocker therapy in patients undergoing noncardiac surgery based on reliable evidence? *Can Med Assoc J.* 2004;**171**:245-247.

14. Siddiqui AK, Ahmed S, Delbeau H, et al. Lack of physician concordance with guidelines on the perioperative use of beta blockers. *Arch Intern Med.* 2004;**164**:664-667.

15. Casadei B, Abuzeid H. Is there a strong rationale for deferring elective surgery in patients with poorly controlled hypertension? *J Hypertens.* 2005;**23**:19-22.

16. Juul AB, Wetterslev J, Gluud C, et al. Effect of perioperative β-blockade in patients with diabetes undergoing major noncardiac surgery: Randomised placebo controlled, blinded multicentre trial. *BMJ.* 2006;**332**:1482.

17. Juul AB, Wetterslev J, Kofoed-Enevoldsen A, et al. The Diabetic Postoperative Mortality and Morbidity (DIPOM) trial: Rationale and design of a multicenter, randomized, placebo-controlled, clinical trial of metoprolol for patients with diabetes mellitus who are undergoing major noncardiac surgery. *Am Heart J.* 2004;**147**:677-683.

18. Coriat P, Richer C, Douraki T, et al. Influence of chronic angiotensin-converting enzyme inhibition on anesthetic induction. *Anesthesiology.* 1994;**81**:299-307.

19. Bertrand M, Godet G, Meersschaert K, et al. Should the angiotensin II antagonists be discontinued before surgery? *Anesth Analg.* 2001;**92**:26-30.

20. Pickering TG, and the Subcommittee of Professional and Public Education of the American Heart Association Council on High Blood Pressure Research. Recommendations for blood pressure measurement in humans and experimental animals: Part 1. Blood pressure measurement in humans: A statement for professionals from the Subcommittee of Professional and Public Education of the American Heart Association Council on High Blood Pressure Research. *Hypertension.* 2005;**45**:142-161.

21. Fleisher LA, Eagle KA. Lowering cardiac risk in noncardiac surgery. *N Engl J Med.* 2001;**345**:1677-1682.

Chapter 45

Hypertensive Emergencies and Urgencies

Shakaib U. Rehman, Jan N. Basile, and Donald G. Vidt

Hypertension is one of the most undertreated cardiovascular conditions in the United States. Twenty-nine percent of U.S. residents (58.4 million) have hypertension, yet only 31% of these persons have their BP adequately controlled (systolic BP [SBP] <140 mm Hg and diastolic BP [DBP] <90 mm Hg).[1] Although hypertensive crises represent only about 1% of patients who present for evaluation of hypertension,[2,3] these crises account for up to one fourth of all emergency department visits.[4,5] The clinical outcome for untreated patients with a hypertensive emergency is extremely poor: the 1-year mortality rate is 70% to 90%, and the 5-year mortality rate is nearly 100%.[6] In 1939, the 1-year survival rate in patients with papilledema was only 17%.[7] In that series, renal failure accounted for 40% of deaths, followed by stroke (24%), myocardial infarction (11%), and heart failure (10%). The availability of improved antihypertensive therapy and dialysis improved 1-year and 5-year survival rates to 75% and 50%, respectively, with adequate BP control in two large series reported in the 1990s.[8,9]

Traditionally, hypertensive crises have been divided into emergencies and urgencies.[10] A *hypertensive emergency* combines a severe elevation in BP with acute, ongoing target organ damage, and it is a true medical emergency requiring prompt BP reduction (although not necessarily into the normal range). In contrast, *hypertensive urgencies* (except for perioperative hypertension, discussed later) may be better termed severe elevations in BP without acute target organ damage. Most of these patients are not adherent to drug therapy or have inadequately treated hypertension, and they often present to the emergency department for other reasons. These patients require neither hospital admission nor acute lowering of BP, and they can safely be treated in the outpatient setting with oral medications. The correct differentiation of these two forms of hypertensive crises presents the greatest challenge to the physician. In this chapter, we discuss the clinical presentation and appropriate evaluation and treatment of the patient with hypertensive crises, and we also construct an algorithm for triage of patients with severe elevations of BP to in-hospital treatment or outpatient therapy.

DEFINITIONS

Hypertensive Emergency

A hypertensive emergency is associated with severe and often sudden elevation in BP, accompanied by progressive target organ dysfunction. It can present as an acute cerebrovascular event or disordered cerebral function, acute coronary syndrome with ischemia or infarction, acute pulmonary edema, or acute renal dysfunction.[2-5,10] Although the level of BP on presentation is often very high (SBP usually >180 mm Hg or DBP >120 mm Hg), it is not the degree of BP elevation, but the clinical status of the patient that defines it as an emergency.[4,5,10] Rarely, patients with only moderate elevations of BP may also present as an emergency. For example, a BP of 160/110 mm Hg in a 65-year-old man with an acute aortic dissection and a woman in her third trimester of pregnancy with eclampsia represent true hypertensive emergencies. Patients with hypertensive emergencies almost always need to be treated with parenteral medications in the intensive care unit or a monitored hospital bed. Table 45-1 lists clinical situations that are typical hypertensive emergencies. Low socioeconomic status with poor access to health care, nonadherence to antihypertensive drug therapy (including sudden withdrawal from an antihypertensive medicine, e.g., clonidine), drug (particularly cocaine) and alcohol abuse, oral contraceptive use, and cigarette smoking all increase one's risk of a hypertensive emergency.[11]

Severe Blood Pressure Elevation (Hypertensive Urgency)

According to the Seventh Report of the Joint National Committee on Prevention, Detection, Evaluation and Treatment of High Blood Pressure,[10] "hypertensive urgencies are those situations associated with severe elevations in BP without progressive target organ dysfunction. Examples include upper level of stage II hypertension associated with severe headache, shortness of breath, epistaxis, or severe anxiety." Other sources define a hypertensive urgency as a patient with DBP higher than 115 to 120 mm Hg or SBP higher than 180 mm Hg.[3,12-14] Even though these patients may have signs of chronic target organ damage, such as grade II hypertensive retinopathy, left ventricular hypertrophy, or chronic kidney disease with stable proteinuria, the absence of progressively worsening hypertensive target organ damage differentiates these patients from those with hypertensive emergencies. Despite the very high BP, these patients have a low risk of cardiovascular events over the first few months (even if they are left untreated), as shown by the first Veterans' Administration Cooperative Study on Antihypertensive Agents, in which 70 patients with DBP between 115 and 129 mm Hg who were randomized to placebo had no (95% confidence interval, 0% to 5%) major adverse events over the next 2 months.[15] Currently, no evidence shows any benefit of acutely lowering BP in asymptomatic patients with severe hypertension.[10,12,16] Unfortunately, the term *urgency* has led to overly aggressive treatment of these patients in the emergency department with one or more parenteral medications to normalize BP rapidly, sometimes with net harm to the patient.[17-21] Even oral loading doses of antihypertensive agents can have cumulative effects, including hypotension, sometimes following discharge from the emergency department.[10]

Table 45-1 Clinical Situations That Are Usually Hypertensive Emergencies

Hypertensive encephalopathy
Malignant hypertension: elevated blood pressure with papilledema or acute retinal hemorrhages or exudates
Intracranial hemorrhage (intracerebral or subarachnoid) or acute atherothrombotic brain infarction
Acute coronary syndromes (unstable angina or myocardial infarction)
Acute left ventricular failure with pulmonary edema
Acute aortic dissection
Rapidly progressive renal failure (e.g., systemic vasculitis), including scleroderma crisis
Eclampsia
Life-threatening arterial bleeding[10]
Head trauma[10]
Less common situations:
    Pheochromocytoma crisis
    Tyramine interaction with monoamine oxidase inhibitors
    Overdose with sympathomimetic drugs (e.g., phencyclidine, lysergic acid diethylamide [LSD], cocaine, or phenylpropanolamines)
    Rebound hypertension following the sudden withdrawal of antihypertensive agents (e.g., clonidine or β-blockers)[49,54]

One study found no difference at 24 hours in BP control between groups of patients who had or had not received clonidine loading before initiation of maintenance therapy.[18] We believe that the traditional classification of hypertensive urgency needs to be updated and simplified, and more diagnostic importance should be placed on presenting signs and symptoms, and not on the BP level. We suggest replacing the term *hypertensive urgencies* with *severe BP elevation without ongoing target organ damage*.

EVALUATION

Early triage of hypertensive emergency versus severe BP elevation without ongoing target organ damage should limit the expenditure of scarce health care resources to those patients who truly need hospitalization, and it should also reduce morbidity and mortality.[22] The evaluation of patients presenting with hypertensive crises should include a targeted history, a focused physical examination, and a limited laboratory examination to differentiate these two conditions. The main purpose of the diagnostic exercise is to assess whether target organ damage is acute and progressive.

The clinical presentation of hypertensive emergencies is most easily classified based on the target organ involved. These emergencies include cerebral infarction (24%), pulmonary edema (22%), hypertensive encephalopathy (16%), heart failure (14%), acute coronary syndrome (12%), intracerebral or subarachnoid hemorrhage (4%), eclampsia (4%), and aortic dissection (2%).[5] A focused history should be obtained, especially regarding headaches, seizures, mental status changes, chest pain, shortness of breath, change in urination, and development of edema. BP should be measured in both arms using a standard sphygmomanometer with an appropriately sized cuff, because automated BP monitoring devices may not be accurate at very high BPs. All patients should have a funduscopic examination by an experienced clinician, who looks carefully for hemorrhages, exudates, and papilledema. A cardiovascular examination should document radial, femoral, and carotid pulses. Pulse deficits should raise the suspicion of aortic dissection. A thorough neurologic examination, including mental status, should be conducted.

Few studies have looked at the prognostic value of abnormal laboratory findings in patients with severe asymptomatic hypertension,[12,23] but this is a valuable method of documenting acute target organ damage. The laboratory evaluation should include a complete blood count, including peripheral smear, to look for schistocytes (indicative of microangiopathic hemolytic anemia), a metabolic profile (blood urea nitrogen, serum creatinine, electrolytes), and a urinalysis. The urinalysis may show an increase in proteinuria, red blood cells, or red blood cell casts, which are typical of acute glomerular or tubular injury. An electrocardiogram and portable chest radiograph should be performed in patients with chest pain or dyspnea, but obtaining a routine chest radiograph in asymptomatic hypertensive patients is not beneficial.[24,25] For patients with an acute change in mental status or acute neurologic signs and symptoms suggestive of cerebral encephalopathy, ischemia, or hemorrhage, a computed tomographic scan of the head should be done. Therapy may need to be initiated before all test results are obtained or before the underlying cause of the emergency becomes known.

Laragh and colleagues have described their therapeutic approach for treating hypertensive emergencies.[26-29] Hypertensive patients are divided according to the baseline plasma renin activity and are then treated accordingly. High plasma renin activity (>0.65 ng/mL/hour, or direct renin >5 μU/mL), defines patients as renin dependent (so-called R-hypertensives), who may be treated with angiotensin-converting enzyme inhibitors, β-blockers, or angiotensin receptor blockers. Patients with low plasma renin activity (<0.65 ng/mL/hour, or direct renin <5 μU/mL) are volume-sodium dependent (so-called V-hypertensives), who may be treated with diuretics or calcium antagonists. In most hospitals, the laboratory turnaround time is much too long for this strategy to be useful. This classification and treatment scheme needs to be prospectively evaluated before it can be widely accepted. Until then, empirical treatment for patients presenting with a hypertensive emergency will remain the standard of care.

MANAGEMENT

Because no long-term randomized clinical trials of different drugs in hypertensive emergencies have been conducted, the data come from long-term cohort studies, comparative trials of acute BP-lowering agents, and expert opinion.[3,10,12,30-33] All authorities agree that therapeutic decisions should be based on the presence of acute and progressive target organ damage and not solely on the level of BP. The first priority should be diagnosis in each patient who presents with very high BP, as shown in Figure 45-1.

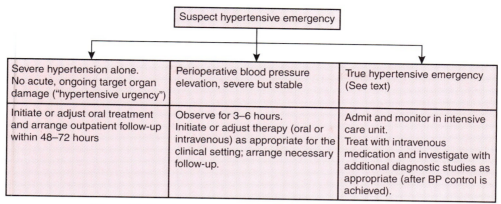

Suspect hypertensive emergency		
Severe hypertension alone. No acute, ongoing target organ damage ("hypertensive urgency")	Perioperative blood pressure elevation, severe but stable	True hypertensive emergency (See text)
Initiate or adjust oral treatment and arrange outpatient follow-up within 48–72 hours	Observe for 3–6 hours. Initiate or adjust therapy (oral or intravenous) as appropriate for the clinical setting; arrange necessary follow-up.	Admit and monitor in intensive care unit. Treat with intravenous medication and investigate with additional diagnostic studies as appropriate (after BP control is achieved).

Figure 45–1   Triage of suspected hypertensive emergencies.

Hypertensive Emergencies

When a hypertensive emergency has been diagnosed, therapy should be initiated immediately. This often occurs before the results of all laboratory studies are available. Once the patient is more clinically stable, investigation into the cause of the presentation should be performed.

The primary goal in treating the hypertensive emergency is to limit target organ damage. These patients require immediate admission to an intensive care unit or monitored hospital bed for parenteral therapy and continuous monitoring.[34] Although lowering the BP is necessary, BP should not be rapidly lowered into the "normal" range (BP <120/80 mm Hg),[10] because this may cause acute deterioration in renal function or precipitate cardiac or cerebral events.[10] The initial goal of therapy is to reduce mean arterial BP to no more than 25% lower than pretreatment levels within the first 2 hours after presentation. Over the next 2 to 6 hours, BP should be reduced slowly toward 160/100 mm Hg. If this level of BP is well tolerated and the patient is clinically stable, further gradual reductions toward normal BP can be implemented in the next 24 to 48 hours. The most notable exceptions to these general principles (see later) are with acute aortic dissection (SBP target: <120 mm Hg over 20 minutes) and acute stroke in evolution (for which no BP lowering is generally recommended). Drugs used in the management of hypertensive emergencies are listed in Table 45-2. Because of the lack of large, comparative randomized controlled trials, it is unclear whether any of these drugs is superior to another.[12,33] All authorities agree that parenteral agents should be used initially, simply because they are easier to titrate and to stop (if necessary).[10] Once BP has been lowered into the target range, oral agents can be started as the parenteral agent is tapered, thus avoiding rebound hypertension. Typically, patients with hypertensive emergencies are volume depleted, so loop diuretics are not recommended unless there is evidence of volume overload.[10,31] The judicious use of diuretics may be necessary after many (typically >12) hours of intravenous vasodilator therapy, because (with the exception of fenoldopam) the use of these agents is accompanied by sodium and volume retention and resistance to further BP reduction (so-called tachyphylaxis).[31]

Special Situations

Aortic Dissection

The initial aim of medical therapy in patients with acute aortic dissection is to decrease both the systemic BP and the shear stress on the torn aorta (by decreasing cardiac contractility). Short-acting, titratable β-blockers, such as esmolol and labetalol, are most commonly recommended. If a β-blocker is contraindicated, a ganglionic blocker or diltiazem can be used. Although no clinical trial data exist to prove it, most authorities recommend that patients presenting with acute aortic dissection should have their SBP lowered to less than 120 mm Hg over about 20 minutes, if tolerated.[10] Nitroprusside can be used (along with the β-blocker, to block reflex tachycardia) to achieve this very low target. Direct vasodilators such as diazoxide, hydralazine, and minoxidil should not be used alone, because these drugs cause reflex sympathetic activity, worsen myocardial ischemia, and increase shear stress on the aorta. Surgical consultation should be obtained as soon as possible.

Myocardial Infarction

BP lowering in this setting can be accomplished with a variety of medications and should not retard efforts to open the offending artery. Intravenous β-blockers and nitroglycerin are both useful.[31,35] Direct vasodilators should be avoided, because they may cause reflex tachycardia and increase myocardial oxygen demand.

Pulmonary Edema or Heart Failure

Intravenous nitroglycerin or sodium nitroprusside may be used to lower BP.[31] Angiotensin-converting enzyme inhibitors have been used extensively because of beneficial effects on both preload and afterload,[36] but these drugs can lower BP precipitously and should be used with caution, if at all. Diuretics should be used as needed for volume control, but they may exacerbate pressure natriuresis and may further stimulate the renin-angiotensin axis.[37,38] Although intravenous nesiritide has a modest antihypertensive effect and is

Table 45-2   Parenteral Drugs for Treatment of Hypertensive Emergencies

Drug (and Reference)	Dose	Onset of Action	Duration of Action	Adverse Effects	Special Indication	Special Caution
Sodium nitroprusside[55,56]	0.25-10 µg/kg/min infusion IV	~20 sec	1-2 min	Nausea, vomiting, muscle spasm, sweating, thiocyanate and cyanide intoxication; extended use for periods >3 days may result in thiocyanate toxicity	Most hypertensive emergencies	Raised intracranial pressure: cerebral blood flow may decrease in a dose-dependent manner; in azotemia, toxic metabolites may accumulate; contraindicated in pregnancy; special equipment: requires shielding from light
Nitroglycerin	5-100 µg/min infusion IV	2-5 min	5-10 min	Headache, vomiting, methemoglobinemia, tolerance with prolonged use	Coronary ischemia, acute left ventricular failure, postoperative hypertension	Not first-line therapy in other situations owing to unpredictable antihypertensive effects and development of tolerance
Fenoldopam mesylate[6,57-61]	0.1-1.5 µg/kg/min infusion IV	<5 min	20 min	Reflex tachycardia, hypokalemia, headache, flushing, nausea, increased intraocular pressure and electrocardiographic changes	Most hypertensive emergencies, comparable to nitroprusside; may not require intra-arterial monitoring; may be the drug of choice in those with chronic kidney disease	Never administer as bolus IV; acutely improves several measures of renal function; caution with glaucoma
Esmolol	250-500 µg/kg/min bolus IV, then 50-100 µg/kg/min by infusion; may repeat	1-2 min	10-30 min	Hypotension, nausea, asthma, first-degree heart block, heart failure	Especially useful in aortic dissection, myocardial infarction, thyrotoxicosis, and patients undergoing coronary artery bypass grafting[61]	Avoid in cocaine-induced hypertension
Enalaprilat[62]	1.25-5 mg every 6 hr IV	15-30 min	6-12 hr	Precipitous fall in pressure in high-renin states; variable response	Acute left ventricular failure; drug of choice in scleroderma renal crisis	Contraindicated in bilateral renal artery stenosis or pregnancy; avoid in acute myocardial infarction
Labetalol[63]	20-80 mg bolus IV every 10 min; 0.5-2 mg/min infusion IV	5-10 min	3-6 hr	Asthma, vomiting, scalp tingling, burning sensation in throat, dizziness, nausea, heart block, orthostasis	Most hypertensive emergencies; particularly useful in eclampsia; may be used for pheochromocytoma and states of excess catecholamines	Contraindicated in heart block, bradycardia or bronchospasm; avoid in acute heart failure

Table 45-2 Parenteral Drugs for Treatment of Hypertensive Emergencies—cont'd

Drug (and Reference)	Dose	Onset of Action	Duration of Action	Adverse Effects	Special Indication	Special Caution
Nicardipine[64,65]	5-15 mg/hr IV	5-10 min	1-4 hr	Tachycardia, flushing, headache, local phlebitis	Most hypertensive emergencies; comparable to nitroprusside; reduces both cardiac and cerebral ischemia; dosage not dependent on weight	Avoid in acute heart failure; caution with coronary ischemia
Hydralazine	10-20 mg IV 10-40 mg IM	10-20 min IV 20-30 min IM	1-4 hr IV 4-6 hr IM	Tachycardia flushing, headache, vomiting, aggravation of angina	Eclampsia	Contraindicated in coronary artery disease or aortic dissection
Diazoxide	50-100 mg bolus IV or IM repeated at 5-15 min interval, or 15-30 mg/min infusion IV	2-4 min	6-12 hr	Nausea, vomiting	Now obsolete; used when no intensive monitoring is available	Salt and water retention, hyperglycemia, hyperuricemia; contraindicated in aortic dissection or myocardial infarction
Phentolamine	5-15 mg IV	1-2 min	3-10 min	Tachycardia, flushing, headache	Catecholamine excess, cocaine and amphetamine overdose, monoamine oxidase inhibitor crisis	Contraindicated in preexisting coronary artery disease

IM, intramuscularly; IV, intravenously.
Modified from Chobanian AV, Bakris GL, Black HR, et al., and the National High Blood Pressure Education Program Coordinating Committee. The Seventh Report of the Joint National Committee on Prevention, Detection, Evaluation, and Treatment of High Blood Pressure: The JNC 7 Report. JAMA. 2003;**289**:2560-2571.

expensive, it improves hemodynamic function in patients with decompensated heart failure.[39]

Ischemic Stroke

Lowering BP in the setting of an acute ischemic stroke in evolution is, in general, not currently recommended. Although hypertension is very common in this setting, the elevated BP may be a physiologic compensatory response to increase cerebral perfusion to ischemic brain tissue.[10] Lowering BP (especially if the decrease is rapid or great) can acutely worsen ischemia and can expand the ischemic penumbra.[5,13,40] Judicious use of short-acting antihypertensive therapy was not associated with worse outcomes at 3 months in the National Institute of Neurological Disorders and Stroke Recombinant Tissue Plasminogen Activator (NINDS rt-PA) stroke trial.[41] Similarly, low-dose candesartan was associated with improved 12-month survival in the Acute Candesartan Cilexetil Evaluation in Stroke Survivors (ACCESS) trial.[42] The most recent American Heart Association (AHA) and American Stroke Association guidelines recommend cautious reduction of BP by about 10% to 15% *only* when SBP is higher than 220 mm Hg or DBP is 120 to 140 mm Hg, along with careful monitoring of patients for neurologic deterioration.[10,43,44] Sodium nitroprusside, esmolol, and labetalol have been recommended, primarily because they are very short acting.[40] Calcium channel blockers may increase intracranial pressure and therefore are generally avoided in patients with acute ischemic stroke.[12]

Hemorrhagic Stroke

With the exception of nicardipine in subarachnoid hemorrhage, there is little evidence that antihypertensive drug treatment benefits patients with hemorrhagic stroke. Current AHA guidelines for hemorrhagic stroke recommend lowering BP only when SBP is higher than 220 mm Hg.[45] Although nimodipine is a very short-acting and relatively weak antihypertensive agent, its use decreases cerebral arterial spasm and rebleeding after subarachnoid hemorrhage.[40]

Preeclampsia

Apart from magnesium infusion and delivery of the fetus,[10,46] methyldopa, hydralazine, and labetalol have been the drugs of choice for the treatment of preeclampsia.[31,47] Intravenous hydralazine is still favored by obstetricians because it does not inhibit uterine contractions and only minimally crosses the placental barrier. Hydralazine may cause reflex tachycardia and should be monitored closely. Angiotensin-converting enzyme inhibitors, angiotensin receptor blockers, and nitroprusside are contraindicated during pregnancy.

Catecholamine Crisis

Pheochromocytoma is a very rare cause of hypertensive crises, usually accompanied by headache and sweating. Patients with severe hypertension caused by pheochromocytoma are commonly successfully treated with the nonselective α-blocker, phentolamine, administered intravenously. A β-blocker can be added, if needed to control tachycardia. Administration of a β-blocker alone leaves the α-receptors unblocked and can abruptly increase BP. Treatment failures have been reported with either a selective α_1-blocker (e.g., doxazosin) or with labetalol, an α,β-blocker.

Sympathomimetic drugs, such as phenylephrine, cocaine, and methamphetamine, can also cause hypertensive crises. Phentolamine, labetalol, and nitroprusside have each been successfully used in this situation.

Perioperative Hypertension

BP elevation during the perioperative period can result from adrenergic stimulation of the surgical event, changes in intravascular volume, or postoperative pain or anxiety. To minimize perioperative BP problems, patients should continue their usual outpatient oral antihypertensive regimen until surgery, and the pharmacotherapy should be resumed as soon as possible thereafter. If oral therapy is not possible, other routes of administration (e.g., intravenous nitroprusside, labetalol, metoprolol, or transdermal clonidine) can be substituted temporarily. Patients with BP levels of 180/110 mm Hg or higher either before or immediately after surgery have a greater risk for cardiac events,[6,10] and they should have their BP lowered over the next 6 to 24 hours with either intravenous or oral agents.

Miscellaneous Situations

In other clinical situations in which severe BP elevation is accompanied by gross hematuria, epistaxis, mental status changes, agitation, or severe anxiety, intravenous therapy may be appropriate. Both clonidine and methyldopa should be avoided in hypertensive encephalopathy because of their potential for adverse central nervous system effects, which make it difficult to judge whether the primary process is progressing or whether the deterioration in the patient's mental status is the result of the drugs.

Severe Elevation in Blood Pressure (Hypertensive Urgency)

After ruling out a true hypertensive emergency, a more thorough history should address the duration and severity of hypertension. The patient's medication profile should be reviewed, with a focus on antihypertensive agents, but including other prescription, alternative, over-the-counter, and recreational drugs (especially cocaine). Intoxication with either alcohol or illicit drugs can elevate BP. Acute withdrawal from some antihypertensive drugs (especially clonidine) may cause rebound BP elevation. Sympathomimetic medications such as decongestants, anticholinergics, amphetamines, and cocaine may acutely elevate BP.[30] Most patients presenting with a hypertensive urgency have a previous diagnosis, but they are nonadherent to a medication regimen, extremely anxious, in acute pain, or inadequately treated.

Even though some emergency department staff may be alarmed by the severity of the BP elevation, there is little reason to normalize the patient's BP before discharge. Some degree of BP reduction typically occurs spontaneously during observation, without pharmacologic intervention.[48] In the absence of acute, ongoing target organ damage, the very elevated BP itself confers very little short-term cardiovascular risk.[10,12,32] Sometimes, antihypertensive drug treatment carries an even greater risk. Short-acting nifedipine capsules,[3,19,49,50] whether given by mouth or sublingually, can cause precipitous and unpredictable hypotension, thus leading to acute ischemic stroke or myocardial infarction. For these reasons, nifedipine capsules are seldom used and rarely, if ever, indicated.[51] Most patients with severe elevations in BP but without acute target organ damage should be treated with oral agents, with the intent to decrease the BP over the next 24 to 48 hours. According to the Seventh Report of the Joint National Committee on Prevention, Detection, Evaluation, and Treatment of High Blood Pressure, two antihypertensive agents, one of which usually is a diuretic, may be started simultaneously in patients with stage 2 hypertension.[10] Resuming a previously well-tolerated regimen is an acceptable alternative. Patients may leave the emergency department with elevated BP as long as there is a definite plan for follow-up with a primary care physician during the next 48 to 72 hours for reevaluation and long-term management. Follow-up is very important for all patients with substantial BP elevations, because some patients mistake treatment provided in the emergency situation for a "cure" and do not understand the benefit of long-term BP control. Patients therefore require close clinical follow-up to monitor their adherence to medications and lifestyle modifications, such as tobacco avoidance, physical activity, dietary management, and weight loss. This opportunity to improve long-term BP control should not be lost.[52]

On occasion, patients present with severely elevated BPs that can be attributed either to pain or to anxiety and fear, as in a panic attack. These patients should be treated with analgesics or anxiolytics, respectively, before antihypertensive agents are considered.[53]

CONCLUSION

A hypertensive emergency is a severe elevation in BP accompanied by progressive, acute target organ damage, such as acute coronary or cerebral ischemia, pulmonary edema, renal failure, aortic dissection, or eclampsia. This condition, if untreated, carries a very high mortality, and patients should be promptly treated with intravenous medication in an intensive care unit or a monitored bed. Although BP should be reduced within minutes to hours, the initial mean arterial pressure reduction should be no more than 20% to 25% of baseline BP, to avoid hypoperfusion of vital organs. Once stable, patients should be investigated more thoroughly for a remediable cause of hypertension. Proper education and appropriate follow-up should be arranged to ensure continued and optimal management of hypertension as well as of the other cardiovascular risk factors usually present.

Often the result of inadequate treatment of preexisting hypertension, a hypertensive urgency is a severe elevation in BP without evidence of progressive, acute target organ damage. Such patients should be treated as outpatients with oral medications to achieve BP control over several days. Close follow-up in an ambulatory setting to achieve BP control and proper education to avoid future urgent presentations are recommended. The major feature distinguishing a true hypertensive emergency from a hypertensive urgency is the presence of ongoing acute target organ damage, not the degree of BP elevation itself.

References

1. Hajjar IM, Kotchen TA. Trends in prevalence, awareness, treatment, and control of hypertension in the United States, 1988-2000. *JAMA.* 2003;**290**:199-206.
2. Varon J, Fromm RE. Hypertensive crises. *Postgrad Med.* 1996;**99**:189-203.
3. Calhoun DA, Oparil S. Treatment of hypertensive crisis. *N Engl J Med.* 1990;**323**:1177-1183.
4. Kitiyakara C, Guzman NJ. Malignant hypertension and hypertensive emergencies. *J Am Soc Nephrol.* 1998;**9**:133-142.
5. Zampaglione B, Pascale C, Marchisio M, et al. Hypertensive urgencies and emergencies: Prevalence and clinical presentation. *Hypertension.* 1996;**27**:144-147.
6. Oparil S, Aronson S, Deeb GM, et al. Fenoldopam: A new parenteral antihypertensive. Consensus roundtable on the management of perioperative hypertension and hypertensive crises. *Am J Hypertens.* 1999;**12**:653-664.
7. Keith NM, Wagener HP, Barker NW. Some different types of essential hypertension: Their course and prognosis. *Am J Med Sci.* 1939;**197**:332-343.
8. Webster J. Petrie JC. Jeffers TA, et al. Accelerated hypertension: Patterns of mortality and clinical factors affecting outcome in treated patients. *Q J Med.* 1993;**86**:485-493.
9. Lip GY, Beevers M, Beevers DG. Complication and survival of 315 patients with malignant-phase hypertension. *J Hypertens.* 1995;**13**:915-924.
10. Chobanian AV, Bakris GL, Black HR, et al., and the National High Blood Pressure Education Program Coordinating Committee. The Seventh Report of the Joint National Committee on Prevention, Detection, Evaluation, and Treatment of High Blood Pressure: The JNC 7 Report. *JAMA.* 2003;**289**:2560-2571.
11. Shea S, Misra D, Ehrlich MH, et al. Predisposing factors for severe, uncontrolled hypertension in an inner-city minority population. *N Engl J Med.* 1991;**327**:776-778.
12. Shayne PH, Pitts SR. Severely increased blood pressure in the emergency department. *Ann Emerg Med.* 2003;**41**:513-529.
13. Murphy C. Hypertensive emergencies. *Emerg Med Clin North Am.* 1995;**13**:973-1007.
14. Kaplan NM. Hypertensive crises. *In:* Kaplan NM (ed). Clinical Hypertension, 7th ed. Baltimore: Williams & Wilkins, 1998, pp 265-266.
15. Veterans' Administration Cooperative Study Group on Antihypertensive Agents. Effects of treatment on morbidity in hypertension: Results in patients with diastolic blood pressures averaging 115 through 129 mm Hg. *JAMA.* 1967;**202**:1028-1034.
16. Fagan TC. Acute reduction of blood pressure in asymptomatic patients with severe hypertension: An idea whose time has come and gone. *Arch Intern Med.* 1989;**149**:2169-2170.
17. Vidt DG. Management of hypertensive emergencies and urgencies. *In:* Izzo JL Jr, Black HR (eds). Hypertension Primer: The Essentials of High Blood Pressure. Dallas, Tex: American Heart Association, 1999, pp 437-440.
18. Zeller KR, Von Kuhnert L, Mathews C. Rapid reduction of severe asymptomatic hypertension: A prospective, controlled trial. *Arch Intern Med.* 1989;**149**:2186-2189.
19. Gifford RW. Management of hypertensive crises. *JAMA.* 1991;**266**:829-835.
20. O'Mailia JJ, Sander GE, Giles TD. Nifedipine-associated myocardial ischemia or infarction in the treatment of hypertensive urgencies. *Ann Intern Med.* 1987;**107**:185-186.
21. Grossman E, Messerli FH, Grodzicki T, et al. Should a moratorium be placed on sublingual nifedipine capsules given for hypertensive emergencies and pseudoemergencies? *JAMA.* 1996;**276**:1328-1331.
22. Vidt DG. Emergency room management of hypertensive urgencies and emergencies. *J Clin Hypertens (Greenwich).* 2001;**3**:158-164.
23. Peters H, Baldwin M, Clarke M. The utility of laboratory data in the evaluation of the aysmptomatic hypertensive patient [abstract]. *Ann Emerg Med.* 2002;**40**:S48.
24. Bartha GW, Nugent CA. Routine chest roentgenograms and electrocardiograms: Usefulness in the hypertensive workup. *Arch Intern Med.* 1978;**138**:1211-1213.
25. Dimmitt SB, West JN, Littler WA. Limited value of chest radiography in uncomplicated hypertension [letter]. *Lancet.* 1989;**2**:104.
26. Blumenfeld JD, Laragh JH. Management of hypertensive crises: The scientific basis for treatment decisions. *Am J Hypertens.* 2001;**14**:1154-1167.
27. Laragh JH, Ulick S, Januszewicz V, et al. Electrolyte metabolism and aldosterone secretion in benign and malignant hypertension. *Ann Intern Med.* 1960;**53**:259-272.
28. Laragh JH. Vasoconstriction-volume analysis for understanding and treating hypertension: The use of renin and aldosterone profiles. *Am J Med.* 1973;**55**:261-274.
29. Laragh JH. Renin profiling for diagnosis, risk assessment, and treatment of hypertension. *Kidney Int.* 1993;**44**:1163-1175.
30. Grossman E, Messerli FH. High blood pressure: A side effect of drugs, poisons, and food. *Arch Intern Med* 1995;**155**:450-460.
31. Vaughan CJ, Delanty N. Hypertensive emergencies. *Lancet.* 2000;**356**:411-417.
32. Gallagher EJ. Hypertensive urgencies: Treating the mercury? *Ann Emerg Med.* 2003;**41**:530-531.
33. Cherney D, Strauss S. Management of patients with hypertensive urgencies and emergencies: A systematic review of the literature. *J Gen Intern Med.* 2002;**19**:937-945.
34. Prisant LM, Carr AA, Hawkins DW. Treating hypertensive emergencies: Controlled reduction of blood pressure and protection of target organs. *Postgrad Med.* 1993;**93**:92-110.
35. First International Study of Infarct Survival Collaborative Group. Randomised trial of intravenous atenolol among 16 027 cases of suspected acute myocardial infarction: ISIS-1. *Lancet.* 1986;**328**:57-66.
36. Hamilton RJ, Carter WA, Gallagher EJ. Rapid improvement of acute pulmonary edema with sublingual captopril. *Acad Emerg Med.* 1996;**3**:205-212.
37. Francis GS, Siegel RM, Goldsmith SR, et al. Acute vasoconstrictor response to intravenous furosemide in patients with chronic congestive heart failure: Activation of the neurohumoral axis. *Ann Intern Med.* 1985;**103**:1-6.

38. Hoffman JR, Reynolds S. Comparison of nitroglycerin, morphine and furosemide in treatment of presumed pre-hospital pulmonary edema. *Chest.* 1987;**92**:586-593.

39. Publication Committee for the Vasodilatation in the Management of Acute Congestive Heart Failure Investigators. Intravenous nesiritide vs. nitroglycerin for treatment of decompensated congestive heart failure: A randomized controlled trial. *JAMA.* 2002;**287**:1531-1540.

40. Tietjen CS, Hurn PD, Ulatowski JA, et al. Treatment modalities for hypertensive patients with intracranial pathology: Options and risks. *Crit Care Med.* 1996;**24**:311-322.

41. Brott T, Lu M, Kothari R, et al. Hypertension and its treatment in the NINDS rt-PA stroke trial. *Stroke.* 1998;**29**:1504-1509.

42. Schrader J, Luders S, Kulschewski A, et al. The ACCESS study: Evaluation of acute candesartan cilexetil therapy in stroke survivors. *Stroke.* 2003;**34**:1699-1703.

43. Adams HP, Brott TG, Crowell RM, et al. Guidelines for the management of patients with acute ischemic stroke: A statement for healthcare professionals from a special writing group of the Stroke Council, American Heart Association. *Stroke.* 1994;**25**:1901-1914.

44. Adams HP Jr, Adams RJ, Brott T, et al. Guidelines for the early management of patients with ischemic stroke: A scientific statement from the Stroke Council of the American Stroke Association. *Stroke.* 2003;**34**:1056-1083.

45. Broderick JP, Adams HP Jr, Barsan W, et al. Guidelines for the management of spontaneous intracerebral hemorrhage: A statement for healthcare professionals from a special writing group of the Stroke Council, American Heart Association. *Stroke.* 1999;**30**:905-915.

46. Lucas MJ, Leveno KJ, Cunningham FG. A comparison of magnesium sulfate with phenytoin for prevention of eclampsia. *N Engl J Med.* 1995;**333**:201-205.

47. Mabie WC, Gonzalez AR, Sibai BM, et al. A comparative trial of labetalol and hydralazine in the acute management of severe hypertension complicating pregnancy. *Obstet Gynecol.* 1987;**70**:328-333.

48. Pitts SR, Adams RP. Emergency department hypertension and regression to the mean. *Ann Emerg Med.* 1998;**31**:214-218.

49. Reuler JB, Margarian GJ. Hypertensive emergencies and urgencies: Definition, recognition, and management. *J Gen Intern Med.* 1988;**3**:64-67.

50. Bertel O, Conen LD. Treatment of hypertensive emergencies with the calcium channel blocker nifedipine. *Am J Med.* 1985; **79 (Suppl 4A)**:31-35.

51. Jaker M, Atkin S, Soto M, et al. Oral nifedipine vs oral clonidine in the treatment of urgent hypertension. *Arch Intern Med.* 1989;**149**:260-265.

52. MacMahon S, Peto R, Cutler J, et al. Blood pressure, stroke, and coronary heart disease: Part 1. Prolonged differences in blood pressure: Prospective observational studies corrected for the regression dilution bias. *Lancet.* 1990;**335**:765-774.

53. White WB, Baker LH. Ambulatory blood pressure monitoring in patients with panic disorder. *Arch Intern Med.* 1987;**147**:1973-1975.

54. Stumpf JL. Drug therapy of hypertensive crisis. *Clin Pharm.* 1998;**7**:582-591.

55. Hirschl MM, Binder M, Bur A, et al. Safety and efficacy of urapidil and sodium nitroprusside in the treatment of hypertensive emergencies. *Intensive Care Med.* 1997;**23**:885-888.

56. Franklin C, Nightengale S, Mambani B. A randomized comparison of nifedipine and sodium nitroprusside in severe hypertension. *Chest.* 1993;**90**:500-503.

57. Panacek EA, Bednarczyk EM, Dunbar LM, et al. Randomized, prospective trial of fenoldopam vs. sodium nitroprusside in the treatment of acute severe hypertension. *Acad Emerg Med.* 1995;**2**:959-965.

58. Pilmer BL, Green JA, Panacek EA, et al. Fenoldopam mesylate versus sodium nitroprusside in the acute management of severe systemic hypertension. *J Clin Pharmacol.* 1993;**33**:549-553.

59. Reisin E, Huth M. Intravenous fenoldopam versus sodium nitroprusside in patients with severe hypertension. *Hypertension.* 1990;**15 (Suppl I)**:159-162.

60. Brogden RN; Markham A. Fenoldopam: A review of its pharmacodynamic and pharmacokinetic properties and intravenous clinical potential in the management of hypertensive urgencies and emergencies. *Drugs.* 1999;**54**:634-650.

61. Murphy MB, Murray C, Shorten GD. Fenoldopam: A selective peripheral dopamine-receptor agonist for the treatment of severe hypertension. *N Engl J Med.* 2001;**345**:1548-1555.

62. Rutledge J, Ayers C, Davidson R, et al. Effect of intravenous enalaprilat in moderate and severe hypertension. *Am J Cardiol.* 1988;**62**:1062-1067.

63. Gonzales ER, Peterson MA, Racht EM, et al. Dose response evaluation of oral labetalol in patients presenting to the emergency department with accelerated hypertension. *Ann Emerg Med.* 1991;**20**:333-338.

64. Wallin JD, Fletcher E, Ram CV, et al. Intravenous nicardipine for the treatment of severe hypertension: A double blind, placebo-controlled, multicenter trial. *Arch Intern Med.* 1989;**149**:2662-2669.

65. Habib GB, Dunbar LM, Rodrigues R, et al. Evaluation of the efficacy and safety of oral nicardipine in the treatment of urgent hypertension: A multicenter, randomized, double-blind, parallel, placebo-controlled trial. *Am Heart J.* 1995;**129**:917-923.

Hypertension Treatment in the Future

SECTION CONTENTS

Hypertension Disease Management Services

Barry L. Carter

Blood pressure (BP) in the United States is currently controlled in only 31% of hypertensive patients, in spite of the goal of 50% recommended by Healthy People 2000 and 2010.[1] BP control is more difficult to achieve in patients with diabetes or chronic kidney disease, for which the BP goal is lower.[2] Some investigators have bluntly stated that treatment of hypertension has been a failure worldwide, and there is an urgent need of improvement everywhere.[3-5]

Controlled clinical trials (efficacy studies) have found that BP can be controlled in 60% to 70% of patients when close follow-up and forced drug titration are used.[6-9] The National Committee for Quality Assurance (NCQA) accredits managed care organizations (MCOs) and evaluates BP control rates using the Health Plan Employer Data and Information Set (HEDIS). BP control rates reported by MCOs increased from 52% in 2000 to 62% in 2003, compared with 49% nationally.[10] If the entire U.S. population achieved BP control at the level of the 90th percentile of care reported by the best MCOs, an estimated 15,000 to 26,000 deaths, $463 million in health care costs, and 21.4 million sick days could be prevented annually.

These HEDIS BP estimates are likely overly generous, and the number of preventable events is too low for several reasons.[2] First, the NCQA criteria require only BP lower than or equal to 140/90 mm Hg, whereas guidelines specify this target only for uncomplicated hypertension. In addition, the HEDIS standard does not differentiate the need for lower BP goals of less than 130/80 mm Hg for patients with diabetes or chronic kidney disease. Thus, many patients with diabetes or kidney disease whose BP is considered controlled by HEDIS are far from their goal BP. One study evaluated BP control rates in a hypertension specialty clinic and found that BP was controlled in 66% of patients based on HEDIS 2001 standards (≤140/90 mm Hg) but in only 59% if the criterion was BP lower than 140/90 mm Hg.[2] When these investigators examined only patients with diabetes in 1999 to 2001, the patients had BP control rates of 52% based on a BP of less than 140/90 mm Hg, but only 15% had controlled BP based on current JNC 7 or American Diabetes Association guidelines. Nonetheless, HEDIS has been a major force to increase BP control rates for patients in MCOs that seek accreditation voluntarily through the NCQA. Some of these health plans have developed unique systems of care and disease state management techniques that may be adaptable to other practices.

It has been commonly believed that poor BP control is the result of limited access to care or poor patient adherence.[11,12] Although these are important problems for some populations, it is increasingly clear that poor patient adherence and inadequate access to care are uncommon reasons for poor BP control.[13] Hyman and Pavlik found that most cases of uncontrolled BP occur in patients who are more than 65 years of age, who have access to health care, and who have frequent contact with physicians.[14] Two other studies confirmed that BP remained poorly controlled despite up to six visits to physicians per year.[15,16] These findings suggested that access to care and frequency of visits are not the primary reasons for poor BP control, and they led to a major overhaul of the Department of Veterans Affairs Medical Centers (VAMCs), to ensure better BP recording and management.

Oliveria and co-workers found that patient factors (adherence, patient acceptance, regimen complexity) were uncommon (9%) barriers cited by physicians or patients.[16] The primary barrier (91% of patient visits) was related to physicians who were satisfied with poorly controlled BPs. The physicians cited lack of time in only 1% of visits. These findings may be explained by physicians' lack of awareness of the guidelines or their disagreement with the guidelines or with BP goals. Another study recently examined patients with "resistant" hypertension who were referred to a specialized hypertension center at Rush University Medical Center in Chicago.[13] The most common reasons for resistance were drug-related causes (61%, including suboptimal regimens), patient nonadherence (13%), secondary hypertension (7%), and other factors (18%).

Many studies indicate that physicians do not adhere to hypertension guidelines.[17] Numerous factors can negatively influence physician adherence to guidelines.[18] Physicians have to treat patients with multiple complex problems in a short amount of clinic time. BP can become a secondary priority when caring for patients with uncontrolled diabetes or psychiatric conditions such as depression. Patients also have personal or social factors that can affect care. A physician may be reluctant, for example, to increase the intensity of the medication regimen for a patient who takes medications inconsistently or who lacks sufficient financial resources. Lack of time and the absence of payment mechanisms can decrease physicians' use of important educational activities known to improve BP control. Finally, several situations can lead to physicians' acceptance of poor BP control, including patients' resistance to adding another medication, the presence of a stressor in a patient that could explain an isolated elevated BP, improvement in BP from baseline, or a BP that is close to goal. Although understandable, these influences can lead to physicians' complacency and failure to achieve goal BP in a timely manner. To overcome these challenges, disease state management programs have been developed by individual practitioners and by health systems to overcome barriers to achieving good BP control.

DISEASE STATE MANAGEMENT

The challenges of managing chronic conditions have led to strategies to provide case management or disease state management. Disease state management programs often focus on a given condition, in this case hypertension. Comprehensive programs may manage several diseases such as diabetes, dyslipidemia, hypertension, smoking cessation, and weight management in an attempt to provide cardiac risk reduction. Large health systems or MCOs may provide population-based strategies to target these patients, to identify gaps in care, and to guide these patients to programs that improve care. Smaller offices or clinics identify individual patients who require improvements in care. In either case, the most effective strategies rely on changing the delivery of care and utilizing a multidisciplinary approach to improve care. The remainder of this chapter highlights changes in care processes with a focus on the chronic care model (CCM), describes studies that have demonstrated improved BP control with either nurse case management or pharmacist-managed hypertension care (alone or in combination), and concludes with a proposed integrated model for improving the care of patients with hypertension.

Chronic Care Model

In recent years, the CCM has been proposed as a method to improve the care of patients with chronic medical conditions.[19-29] The CCM has utilized nurses and pharmacists as care managers to assist with care delivery. The CCM is a conceptual model for organizing the delivery of care. It does not focus on a given patient-physician interaction, but rather on the organization of care delivery within a system and community. The complete CCM includes six elements: (1) health care delivery is linked to community resources; (2) the organization's structure, process, and goals have an impact on improvements in care; (3) organizations provide for patient self-management support with tools to improve patients' knowledge and skills; (4) the delivery system must be redesigned from an acute, episodic care model to one that can identify and support chronic conditions and establish a support role for nonphysician providers; (5) decision support is provided; and (6) clinical information is provided using evidence-based guidelines. When the CCM is effectively implemented, the model leads to an informed, activated patient who interacts with a prepared, proactive care team, with resulting improvements in quality of care and outcomes. Implementation of the model has been shown to improve the management of several chronic medical conditions, and the model is now used in numerous health care organizations.[19,20,24,25,28,29]

Many disease state management programs incorporate some, but usually not all, components of the CCM. The likely reasons are the significant time and resources required to implement such a program and the lack of payment for such services in many locales and practices. The CCM is also an intensive approach that requires good communication and coordination between physicians and nonphysician providers. Strategies are discussed later to deal with these challenges. First, individual components of the model are discussed, including nurse case management, physician-pharmacist collaborative models, and, finally, comprehensive and integrated programs to improve BP control. Several components of the CCM are reviewed so practicing physicians can determine which components can best be incorporated into their practices or health systems.

Nurse Case Management

The use of nurses to provide case management of hypertension has been well described since the 1970s and has included mobile clinics, home visits, work-based programs, and clinic settings.[30-32] One long-established model was developed at the Mayo Clinic in Rochester, Minnesota, and continues to be used to improve BP control.[33] This model uses physician hypertension specialists, nurses, dietitians, and nurse educators to care for patients with hypertension in a tertiary center. The physician reviews the patient's progress during regular visits, and nurses provide interim education and hypertension management. Nurses are the primary caregivers for the long-term management of patients with hypertension, and they see patients from once a week to every 6 months, depending on patient needs. For these patients, nurses also provide monitoring of anticoagulation, assessment of adverse reactions and medication adherence, teaching of home BP monitoring, triage of telephone calls, and rescheduling of missed appointments.

A now-classic study enrolled 457 hypertensive patients and randomized half to a worksite-based nurse-run clinic, at which drug therapy was prescribed and changed by nurses with weekly chart review by physicians.[32] The control group had their BPs managed by their usual physician outside the workplace. After 6 months of follow-up, nurse-managed patients were more likely to receive a new (95% versus 63%, $P < .001$) or two antihypertensive drugs (44% versus 18%, $P < .001$), to adhere to the medication regimen (68% versus 49%, $P < .005$), and to achieve goal BP (49% versus 28%, $P < .001$).

Rudd and colleagues studied nurse case management of hypertension in a randomized controlled trial, in which 76 subjects were managed by their usual physician, and 74 received nurse-based care.[34] At baseline, nurse case managers provided education regarding use of an automated BP device, strategies to improve medication adherence, and identification of adverse drug events. The nurses then conducted telephone interviews at 1 week and at 1, 2, and 4 months, for an average of 10 minutes per telephone call. The nurse independently made medication dosage increases but contacted the physician before initiating new BP medication. The results may have been confounded because only patients randomized to nurse case management received portable BP monitors, which could have improved BP control independent of nurse functions. Nonetheless, systolic BP declined by 14.2 mm Hg in the intervention group compared with only 5.7 mm Hg in the control group ($P < .01$) after 6 months, when significantly more medications were taken and significantly more medication changes (223 versus 52, $P < .01$) had been made in the intervention group than the control group. Medication adherence at 6 months was 81% in the intervention group and 69% in the control group ($P = .03$).

In contrast to these studies, Guerra-Riccio and associates evaluated more frequent nurse visits for BP follow-up (every 15 days) versus regular physician visits (every 3 months) and found no effect on the number of antihypertensive agents taken or on medication adherence between groups.[30] The major effect was that more frequent nurse visits reduced the white-coat effect or the difference between clinic and 24-hour BP measurements.

Few comparisons have been made of the care provided by nurse practitioners and by physicians. One large study evaluated primary care delivered by nurse practitioners compared with physicians.[35] Patients could have any condition, but those with diabetes, asthma, and hypertension were oversampled. Most patients were Hispanic immigrants, and all patients were enrolled after an emergency department or urgent care visit. Patients were then randomized to either a nurse practitioner ($n = 806$) or a physician ($n = 510$). The nurse practitioners and physicians had the same roles and responsibilities for prescribing medications, consulting, referring, or admitting patients. The primary outcome was quality of life, and this was equivalent in the two groups. Care provided by nurse practitioners was equivalent to that given by physicians for control of diabetes and asthma, and it was slightly better for BP (137/82 versus 139/85 mm Hg, $P = .28$ for systolic and $P = .04$ for diastolic BP). This was the first study to demonstrate similar quality of care provided by physicians and nurse practitioners in primary care.

Thus, some studies found that nurse management can lead to improved BP control, whereas others found that BP was similar to that in patients receiving usual care or care provided by physicians. These seemingly diverse findings are likely explained by important principles indicating the benefits of focused care. Nurse practitioners with a broad scope of practice and who care for a wide variety of patients achieve similar BP control rates as physicians.[35] However, when nurse case managers are carefully integrated into a practice setting, are focused on hypertension, and are given responsibility for achieving BP goals and making medication modifications, BP control rates can be improved.[32]

Use of Pharmacists in Disease State Management

Pharmacists now practice in many different settings in addition to traditional community pharmacies. Clinical pharmacists are located within physician office practices, academic primary care clinics, and VAMCs, which now often house pharmacist-managed hypertension clinics.[36-38] Pharmacists in all these environments have assisted physicians with managing patients with hypertension. Most pharmacists who engage in these activities have had specialized training in addition to a Doctor of Pharmacy degree (Pharm.D.), including residency or fellowship experience, formalized disease state management programs, or board certification (e.g., Board Certified Pharmacotherapy Specialists). More than 75% of U.S. states have enacted legislation or rules that allow pharmacist disease state management following the development of collaborative practice agreements with physicians.[39] Some states have specific rules and requirements for these agreements. Each unique environment and health system structure affects how physicians may utilize pharmacists in disease state management. Therefore, several examples that physicians may consider as strategies to assist with the care of their patients are discussed. In the past, it was difficult for an office or group practice to hire a clinical pharmacist unless the position was co-funded with a college of pharmacy.[40] However, changes in state and federal law, especially the new Medicare prescription drug benefit, have established mechanisms by which pharmacists can bill for disease management services.[41-43] These changes may well increase the ability of a group practice to hire clinical pharmacists to assist with managing patients with hypertension. Many examples of disease state management by phar-

macists for anticoagulation, dyslipidemia, heart failure, or diabetes have been published.[36,44-50] However, this chapter focuses on disease state management specifically developed for hypertension.

Community Pharmacy

Community pharmacists can assist physicians with hypertension management in numerous ways, including screening and referral, education on lifestyle modifications, and monitoring medication adherence. The primary goal of these programs is to assist the physician with monitoring of BP in the patient's community environment. This engagement of community resources is one important factor in the CCM.[21-24,26,27] Collaboration between physicians and community pharmacists can be challenging because of the distance between providers and the limited accessibility of data from medical records to community pharmacists. However, these barriers can be overcome if the physician and pharmacist agree to collaborate and jointly establish policies and procedures regarding patient treatment. These policies and procedures should include goals of therapy, physician preference for the initiation of care plans, including whether the pharmacist can initiate new therapies or change dosages, whether medication changes are according to a specific protocol or with physician consent, and when to triage or refer patients back to the physician, especially those patients with urgent needs (e.g., new onset of symptoms that may result from cardiovascular complications).

For pharmacists to provide disease management for hypertension, they should have access to diagnoses, coexisting conditions, diagnostic information, and laboratory results. The issue of patient information transfer can be handled several ways. In some cases, patients simply sign a release of medical information, and this document is sent to the patient's physician. In other cases, the pharmacist may visit the physician's office to review the patient's medical record. In either case, the patient should sign a typical Health Insurance Portability and Accountability Act (HIPAA) waiver to allow access to medical record information. This mechanism is similar to, and can be handled the same way as, information transfer between two physicians or between a physician and another provider. Pharmacists then frequently communicate with the physician by facsimile and with written notes and recommendations mailed to the physician.[41,51]

Another classic study of disease management was published in 1973.[52] This study was a controlled trial, and 50 patients were randomized to traditional pharmacy services or to an intervention group. The community pharmacist evaluated patients in the intervention group who had poor BP control, poor medication adherence, or adverse events. The pharmacist worked closely with two physicians in an urban health center in Detroit, visited the physicians' office to review medical records, and made recommendations for changes in therapy. Patients in the intervention group were seen monthly for 5 months by appointment with the pharmacist in one of three community pharmacies participating in the study. BP in the physician's office deteriorated in the control group (163/93 versus 166/101 mm Hg) but improved in the intervention group (157/99 versus 146/90 mm Hg). The difference between the two groups was significant ($P < .001$). Significant improvements were also reported in medication adherence and patient knowledge of hypertension in the intervention group but not in the control group. Once the intervention was discontinued, BP control and adherence declined in the intervention group.

Park and colleagues conducted a similar study in two chain community pharmacies.[53] At each of four visits, 27 intervention-group patients had their BP measured and were provided with comprehensive education (including lifestyle modifications) and monitoring for hypertension. BPs, interim histories (including adverse reactions), and recommendations for medication modifications were communicated to the physician, usually by facsimile. Twenty-six patients in the control group received only traditional dispensing pharmacy services. BP declined significantly in the intervention group, but not the control group. The physicians accepted 53% of the pharmacists' recommendations for medication modifications.

Carter and associates conducted a similar study that utilized a clinic pharmacy located within a private, rural medical practice.[54] In this setting, the pharmacists reviewed medical records and were able to make face-to-face recommendations to the physicians in the practice. At 6 months, systolic BP was significantly reduced in the intervention group ($n = 25$, 146/83 to 135/75 mm Hg, $P < .001$ for SBP) but not in the control group ($n = 26$, 147/82 to 142/82 mm Hg). A blinded peer review panel rated appropriateness of the BP regimen and dose ($P < .01$), patient assessment for adverse reactions ($P < .001$), and potential benefit of the regimen ($P < .05$) significantly better after the intervention compared with baseline. Several quality of life measures were significantly improved in the intervention group but not in the control group.

Although still uncommon, collaborative disease management programs can be found in community pharmacies throughout the country. These programs rely on high levels of communication and trust between collaborating pharmacists and physicians to be successful.

Pharmacist-Managed Clinics

Pharmacist-managed hypertension clinics are found in specific settings such as VAMCs or academic health sciences centers. In fact, a survey found that 56% of hypertension clinics in 50 VAMCs had clinical pharmacists in them, and 33% of the clinics were pharmacist managed.[55] I practiced in the pharmacist-managed Hypertension Clinic in the West Side VAMC in Chicago. In this setting, pharmacists provided all the patient follow-up and medication changes, but any changes were "staffed" with an internist. In other settings with specific protocols and scope of practice descriptions for pharmacists in a VAMC, pharmacists modify medications independently. One study used blinded judges to evaluate medication selection by pharmacists compared with physicians for patients with hypertension.[56] The judges evaluated 169 patients managed by pharmacists and 157 managed by physicians. The pharmacists scored better than the physicians on choosing drugs most appropriate for hypertension ($P < .01$) and overall when considering absence of drug interactions, proper quantity, dose, and directions ($P < .05$). More patients in the pharmacist group had controlled BP than in the physician group (97% versus 78%, $P < .05$) as determined by the blinded judges. Another study found better medication adherence in a pharmacist-managed group of 349 patients and similar BP control when compared with 280 patients

managed by physicians.[57] This latter study was conducted in an indigent, largely Hispanic population in San Antonio, Texas. Although pharmacist-managed hypertension clinics could be established in environments other than VAMCs,[42] pharmacist-managed anticoagulation clinics are currently more common in private and other group practices, as well as in the VAMC setting.[40,50]

Physician-Pharmacist Collaborative Models

Most disease state management services for hypertension provided by pharmacists are performed in group practices and in close collaboration with physicians.[37,39,43,58-60] One study evaluated the effect of a pharmacist working closely with physicians in a medical resident teaching clinic to improve BP control.[60] Patients with uncontrolled hypertension were randomized to either a control group ($n = 46$) or an intervention group ($n = 49$). Systolic BP decreased 23 mm Hg in the intervention group versus 11 mm Hg in the control group ($P < .001$). BP control at the end of the study was 55% in the intervention versus 20% in the control group ($P < .001$). The pharmacist made 162 recommendations for changes in medications or dosages, for discontinuing medications, or for laboratory monitoring. Physicians accepted 93% of the pharmacist's recommendations. Mean medication charges decreased $6.80 per month in the intervention group but increased by $6.50 per month in the control group. No differences in physician visits, referrals, emergency department visits, or hospitalizations were observed.

Borenstein reported on the effect of physician-pharmacist co-management of hypertension in an integrated health system in California.[58] Patients were randomized to either usual care ($n = 99$) or a co-managed group ($n = 98$), who attended a hypertension clinic run by pharmacists. The pharmacists saw patients every 2 to 4 weeks and assessed patients for adherence, adverse reactions, and lifestyle modifications. The pharmacist then contacted the patient's physician with an assessment and recommendations based on a previously designed evidence-based algorithm. Physicians decided whether to implement treatment changes. BP was reduced significantly more in the co-managed group than in the usual care group ($P < .01$) at 6, 9, and 12 months (22 versus 9 mm Hg, 25 versus 10 mm Hg, and 22 versus 11 mm Hg, respectively). Significantly more patients in the co-managed group (60%) achieved BP control than in the usual care group (43%, $P = .02$). Other, smaller studies conducted in physician offices have also found significant reductions in BP when clinical pharmacists assisted with hypertension disease state management.[37,61]

Another study evaluated the effect of a clinical pharmacist in a family practice office.[62] The pharmacist used home BP monitoring to assist with medication management and made recommendations for changes to the family physician. Compared with baseline, office systolic BP was reduced 17 mm Hg in the intervention group ($n = 18$, $P < .0001$) but only 7 mm Hg in the control group ($n = 18$, $P = .12$).

Nurse-Pharmacist Models

Few studies describe outcomes following a nurse-pharmacist model for providing disease state management of hypertension. One study conducted in a VAMC was designed to investigate the impact of a clinical pharmacist on physician prescribing, medication documentation, and patient compliance.[63] The pharmacist attended the rheumatology and renal clinic during all clinic hours. The study included 75 control and 98 study group patients. Following the intervention, medication adherence was 72% in the intervention group and only 20% in the control group ($P < .001$). BP was controlled in 69% of the intervention group but in only 29% of the control group. Documentation of prescriptions in the medical record was seen with 66% of prescriptions in the control group and 100% in the study group ($P < .02$). The pharmacist reduced medication cost and duplicate medications. Because of this positive experience, the investigators attempted to determine whether the effect could be sustained and whether disease control could be improved after 4.75 years of follow-up.[64] However, during the follow-up period, a nurse clinician supplemented the clinical pharmacist, because they had different training and educational backgrounds. The nurse and pharmacist had the same responsibilities, and their roles were equal and interchangeable. In the study group, 75% of patients were adherent to all medications compared with 20% in the control group ($P < .001$). In the study group, BP control was 90%, as compared with 20% in the control group ($P < .01$). The investigators concluded: "Utilization of a clinical pharmacist and a nurse clinician improves drug documentation, compliance, and disease control. Our intervention model also shows potential savings that would more than offset the investment in personnel involved."

In the aforementioned study by Guerra-Riccio and colleagues, a pharmacist initially supplied the patient with medications and instructions for their proper use and potential side effects.[30] The nurse then saw patients every 15 days. This study found a reduction in the white-coat effect (clinic BPs) following more frequent nurse visits but no major effect on 24-hour ambulatory BPs. These limited findings perhaps were related to the modest intervention. Medication regimens did not change during the study, and they were similar in the intervention and the control group when the study was concluded.

AN INTEGRATED MODEL TO PROVIDE DISEASE STATE MANAGEMENT

It is likely that benchmarking measures such as HEDIS and compensation for outcome performance will become increasingly common.[10] Not only are MCOs implementing these strategies, but so too is the Center for Medicare & Medicaid Services (CMS). These measures often lead health systems better to integrate care through the use of teams to provide disease management to improve performance.

The studies discussed earlier suggest that disease state management provided by either nurses or pharmacists can improve BP control. Whether a nurse, pharmacist, or both are utilized to assist the physician is largely determined by the size and structure of the clinic, office, or health system. The foregoing studies, however, do not help physicians or administrators determine how to utilize most efficiently the blend of professionals required to optimize BP control in large populations cared for by a clinic, health system, or MCO.

One of the best-performing MCOs in the United States is Kaiser Permanente of Colorado. It rates in the top 10 on national HEDIS effectiveness care measures including hypertension management.[10] Hypertension management in the Kaiser Permanente Colorado region is an integrated approach among physicians, clinical pharmacy specialists, nurse practitioners, nurses, and ancillary support staff. The specific mechanism by which each medical office manages its hypertensive population is left to the discretion of the medical office physicians and health care team. Efforts to determine the "best practices" are currently being undertaken. Eleven of the 15 medical offices have developed hypertension clinics. Models fall into one of two categories: group visits or individual patient appointments in which care is typically managed by a nurse-pharmacist team in consultation with a physician, if needed. Clinics are typically held two to four times per month for 2 to 3 hours.

Group models of care are most often held in a large room and involve a variety of disciplines, including a medical assistant, nurse, a clinical pharmacy specialist, a nurse practitioner, a physician, and sometimes a dietitian. Roles for each practitioner are clearly defined: medical assistants and dietitians check each patient in and weigh the patient. The nurse practitioner, nurse, and clinical pharmacy specialist review history, obtain vital signs, review and order laboratory tests as needed, and develop a plan to adjust or alter medications if needed. Patients with complicated medication regimens are typically assigned to the clinical pharmacy specialist. The physician is available to review new prescription requests and to care for patients with issues that fall outside the scope of practice of the other practitioners.

Models that utilize individual patient appointments differ from usual care in that they are at specified, regular times, and a specific support structure is in place to make decisions about the patient's therapy. For example, a nurse will see the patient, take vital signs, and gather history. If the BP is higher than goal, the nurse will consult with the clinical pharmacy specialist to determine whether a change in medication therapy is needed, and the clinical pharmacy specialist will develop a therapeutic plan if needed, based on national hypertension guidelines. An interdisciplinary approach to caring for patients with hypertension has been the basis for some very innovative care models within the Kaiser Permanente managed care system and may be the reason for its high HEDIS performance measures.

Reorganizing the Structure and Process of Care Delivery

The following proposed models require that BP is properly measured and classified as discussed in Chapters 4 to 7. In addition, the proposed models here closely parallel the CCM that has been studied for other conditions.[21-24,26,27] Perhaps the most important aspect of achieving success is for the clinic or health system to have a goal-oriented approach to treating hypertension. Everyone involved with the care of patients with hypertension must understand and have a commitment to their responsibility to achieve goal BP in each patient. Achieving optimal control rates will likely require a complete change in the structure and process of delivering care. The clinic must move from an acute care model to a model for managing chronic conditions proactively. For instance, staff members who schedule patients must understand the requirement for continuity with the hypertension disease state management team. The clinic must institute processes to track patients, remind them of their upcoming office visit, and contact them when they do not show up for an appointment.

Decision-support tools and evidence-based approaches to managing hypertension that effectively support physicians and other providers are critical to the success of disease management programs. These approaches do not necessarily require computerized medical records and can be accomplished by the use of teams responsible for providing these data to providers. Many large clinics rely on a clinical pharmacist and physician committee to provide evidence-based support to providers.

The patient should be engaged in treatment decisions and management, including home monitoring. The average patient visits the pharmacy at least monthly to retrieve multiple prescriptions that are refilled at different times, or he or she visits the pharmacy to obtain other products. Therefore, the clinic may selectively engage community pharmacies that provide more advanced services to help with monitoring BP, assessing BP control, and monitoring for adverse reactions or drug interactions. The pharmacist will be able to assist with more cost-effective medication regimens.

Proposed Responsibilities of Team Members

The physician will be responsible for properly diagnosing and evaluating hypertension for potential secondary causes, additional risk factors, and target organ damage. The nurse may provide education and counseling for patients with uncomplicated hypertension who are not taking any antihypertensive medication. This education would include thorough discussions about all lifestyle modifications, including smoking cessation, and how to empower the patient to implement these strategies. If the office or health system includes a dietitian or nutritionist, this person may provide the patient with in-depth counseling about diet and weight loss strategies. If these professionals are not available, the nurse who specializes in hypertension management can provide this education. The nurse can then see patients for follow-up at appropriate intervals to evaluate progress. If medication has been prescribed, the nurse may be given responsibility to modify medications and adjust dosages. If the clinic employs a pharmacist to assist with disease management, the pharmacist could assist with designing a specific drug and monitoring regimen, especially for patients with coexisting conditions or who may experience important drug-drug interactions. The pharmacist could also counsel patients about proper medication use, administration, storage, and possible adverse reactions.

Efficiency can be greatly improved by the use of telephone follow-up by the nurse to evaluate medication and diet adherence.[19] Monitoring and patient involvement can be further strengthened by the use of home BP monitoring so long as the patient is properly trained and reliably and accurately reports BP values. It is also critical that the patient and team understand the importance of lower goals for home BP (e.g., <135/85 mm Hg) compared with clinic pressures (<140/90 mm Hg). Again, community monitoring may be facilitated by engaging community pharmacists.

An effective disease management program must have a mechanism to remind patients of office visits and to call patients who do not appear for office visits, and perhaps it should include an individual to serve as an initial point of contact when the patient needs assistance. This individual need not be a highly trained professional and, if fact, could be a lay person.[65] Some models include this individual in a care role that includes providing telephone reminders, follow-up scheduling coordination, and initially greeting the patient and placing them in the examination room as a strategy to improve continuity.

The physician should also see the patient at proper intervals to conduct periodic physical examinations and follow-up assessments for target organ damage. The physician should coordinate the care provided to the patient. If at any point new signs or symptoms develop, the physician should evaluate the patient.

Many patients with hypertension have coexisting conditions, complications, or other drug therapy that may make treatment decisions more difficult. The model described earlier would generally be effective for these patients with these complicated cases, with a few modifications. First, the physician likely would need to see the patient more frequently. In addition, it may be appropriate to engage the clinical pharmacist more fully for such patients, as in the Kaiser model discussed earlier. In this model, the pharmacist would perform a thorough assessment of medications and dosages and evaluate laboratory parameters, adverse reactions, drug-drug interactions, drug-disease interactions, and costs. Depending on the health system, the pharmacist may be delegated responsibility to make medication modifications or dosage adjustments to improve BP control or the control of other conditions such as

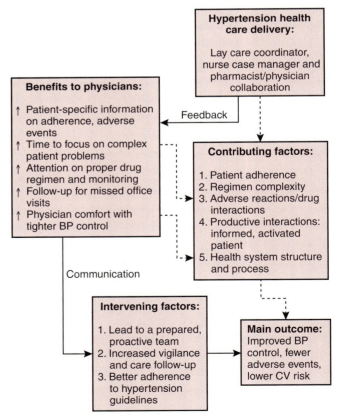

Figure 46–1 Comprehensive chronic care model for hypertension. BP, blood pressure; CV, cardiovascular.

diabetes or dyslipidemia. In other settings, the pharmacist would make specific recommendations for changes to the physician. The nurse would continue to see the patient for follow-up visits, but the pharmacist could also see the patient to assist with more complex medication modifications. This comprehensive model is conceptually shown in Figure 46-1.

This proposed model would obviously require a great deal of communication among the primary care physician, clinical pharmacist, nurse, and any other providers involved with the care of the patient. Accurate and complete medical record documentation is critical. In addition, it would be ideal to establish protocols, policies, and procedures for communication, triage, and referral back to the physician, so information transfers are coordinated and complete.

SUMMARY

Goal-oriented disease management for patients with hypertension can be provided by physicians, pharmacists, nurses, and perhaps other professionals. However, coordinated and collaborative models that include interdisciplinary management have been superior to care provided by individuals. To provide chronic care for patients with hypertension optimally, the entire delivery system needs to be structured to focus on a CCM. Instead of waiting for patients to present to the office or expecting them to come to each scheduled visit, strategies must be implemented to ensure adherence to office visits through reminders and telephone calls for missed appointments. Care needs to be provided at times that are convenient for the patient with minimal waits before being seen. Care and office visits may be coordinated by a lay person who ensures that the patient has been reminded of the visit and helps to guide the patient through the visit with a personal touch. In settings where this interdisciplinary model has been implemented, BP control rates have been markedly improved. Health systems and physician offices should determine how they can incorporate these concepts into the care of patients with chronic conditions, especially patients with hypertension.

References

1. Chobanian AV, Bakris GL, Black HR, et al., and the National High Blood Pressure Education Program Coordinating Committee. The Seventh Report of the Joint National Committee on Prevention, Detection, Evaluation, and Treatment of High Blood Pressure: The JNC 7 Report. *JAMA.* 2003;**289**:2560-2572.
2. Singer GM, Izhar M, Black HR. Guidelines for hypertension: Are quality-assurance measures on target? *Hypertension.* 2004;**43**:198-202.
3. Meissner I, Whisnant JP, Sheps SG, et al. Detection and control of high blood pressure in the community: Do we need a wake-up call? *Hypertension.* 1999;**34**:466-471.
4. Trilling JS, Froom J. The urgent need to improve hypertension care. *Arch Fam Med.* 2000;**9**:794-801.
5. Laragh JH. Treatment of hypertension is a worldwide failure. *Am J Hypertens.* 2001;**14**:84-89.
6. Carter BL, Frohlich ED, Elliott WJ, et al. Selected factors that influence responses to antihypertensives: Choosing therapy for the uncomplicated patient. *Arch Fam Med.* 1994;**3**:528-536.
7. Hansson L, Zanchetti A, Carruthers SG, et al. Effects of intensive blood-pressure lowering and low-dose aspirin in patients with hypertension: Principal results of the Hypertension Optimal Treatment (HOT) randomised trial. HOT Study Group. *Lancet.* 1998;**351**:1755-1762.
8. Black HR, Elliott WJ, Neaton JD, et al. Baseline characteristics and early blood pressure control in the CONVINCE trial. *Hypertension.* 2001;**37**:12-18.
9. Grimm RH Jr., Margolis KL, Papademetriou VV, et al. Baseline characteristics of participants in the Antihypertensive and Lipid-Lowering Treatment to Prevent Heart Attack Trial (ALLHAT). *Hypertension.* 2001;**37**:19-27.
10. The National Committee for Quality Assurance. The State of Health Care Quality 2004. Washington, DC: National Committee for Quality Assurance. Available at: http://www.ncqa.org. Accessed 12 NOV 04.
11. The Sixth Report of the Joint National Committee on Prevention, Detection, Evaluation, and Treatment of High Blood Pressure. *Arch Intern Med.* 1997;**157**:2413-2446.
12. Miller NH, Hill M, Kottke T, Ockene IS. The multilevel compliance challenge: Recommendations for a call to action. A statement for healthcare professionals. *Circulation.* 1997;**95**:1085-1090.
13. Garg JP, Elliott WJ, Folker AC, et al. Resistant hypertension revisited: A comparison of two university-based cohorts. *Am J Hypertens.* 2005;**18**:619-626.
14. Hyman DJ, Pavlik VN. Characteristics of patients with uncontrolled hypertension in the United States. *N Engl J Med.* 2001;**345**:479-486.
15. Berlowitz DR, Ash AS, Hickey EC, et al. Inadequate management of blood pressure in a hypertensive population. *N Engl J Med.* 1998;**339**:1957-1963.
16. Oliveria SA, Lapuerta P, McCarthy BD, et al. Physician-related barriers to the effective management of uncontrolled hypertension. *Arch Intern Med.* 2002;**162**:413-420.
17. Milchak JL, Carter BL, James PA, Ardery G. Measuring adherence to practice guidelines for the management of hypertension: An evaluation of the literature. *Hypertension.* 2004;**44**:602-608.
18. Cabana MD, Rand CS, Powe NR, et al. Why don't physicians follow clinical practice guidelines? A framework for improvement. *JAMA.* 1999;**282**:1458-1465.
19. Simon GE, Von Korff M, Rutter C, Wagner E. Randomised trial of monitoring, feedback, and management of care by telephone to improve treatment of depression in primary care. *BMJ.* 2000;**320**:550-554.
20. Wagner EH, LaCroix AZ, Grothaus L, et al. Preventing disability and falls in older adults: A population-based randomized trial. *Am J Public Health.* 1994;**84**:1800-1806.
21. Wagner EH, Austin BT, Von Korff M. Organizing care for patients with chronic illness. *Milbank Q.* 1996;**74**:511-544.
22. Wagner EH. Chronic disease management: What will it take to improve care for chronic illness? *Eff Clin Pract.* 1998;**1**:2-4.
23. Wagner EH, Austin BT, Davis C, et al. Improving chronic illness care: Translating evidence into action. *Health Aff (Millwood).* 2001;**20**:64-78.
24. Wagner EH, Glasgow RE, Davis C, et al. Quality improvement in chronic illness care: A collaborative approach. *Jt Comm J Qual Improv.* 2001;**27**:63-80.
25. Coleman EA, Grothaus LC, Sandhu N, Wagner EH. Chronic care clinics: A randomized controlled trial of a new model of primary care for frail older adults. *J Am Geriatr Soc.* 1999;**47**:775-783.
26. Bodenheimer T, Wagner EH, Grumbach K. Improving primary care for patients with chronic illness. *JAMA.* 2002;**288**:1775-1779.
27. Bodenheimer T, Wagner EH, Grumbach K. Improving primary care for patients with chronic illness: The chronic care model. Part 2. *JAMA.* 2002;**288**:1909-1914.

28. McCulloch DK, Price MJ, Hindmarsh M, Wagner EH. A population-based approach to diabetes management in a primary care setting: Early results and lessons learned. *Eff Clin Pract*. 1998;**1**:12-22.

29. Feifer C, Ornstein SM, Nietert PJ, Jenkins RG. System supports for chronic illness care and their relationship to clinical outcomes. *Top Health Inf Manage*. 2001;**22**:65-72.

30. Guerra-Riccio GM, Artigas Giorgi DM, Consolin-Colombo FM, et al. Frequent nurse visits decrease white coat effect in stage III hypertension. *Am J Hypertens*. 2004;**17**:523-528.

31. Hill MN, Han HR, Dennison CR, et al. Hypertension care and control in underserved urban African American men: Behavioral and physiologic outcomes at 36 months. *Am J Hypertens*. 2003;**16**:906-913.

32. Logan AG, Milne BJ, Achber C, et al. Work-site treatment of hypertension by specially trained nurses: A controlled trial. *Lancet*. 1979;**2**:1175-1178.

33. Schultz JF, Sheps SG. Management of patients with hypertension: A hypertension clinic model. *Mayo Clin Proc*. 1994;**69**:997-999.

34. Rudd P, Miller NH, Kaufman J, et al. Nurse management for hypertension: A systems approach. *Am J Hypertens*. 2004;**17**:921-927.

35. Mundinger MO, Kane RL, Lenz ER, et al. Primary care outcomes in patients treated by nurse practitioners or physicians: A randomized trial. *JAMA*. 2000;**283**:59-68.

36. Carter BL, Helling DK. Ambulatory care pharmacy services: Has the agenda changed? *Ann Pharmacother*. 2000;**34**:772-787.

37. Carter BL, Zillich AJ, Elliott WJ. How pharmacists can assist physicians with controlling blood pressure. *J Clin Hypertens*. 2003;**5**:31-37.

38. Lipton HL, Byrns PJ, Soumerai SB, Chrischilles EA. Pharmacists as agents of change for rational drug therapy. *Int J Technol Assess Health Care*. 1995;**11**:485-508.

39. Hammond RW, Schwartz AH, Campbell MJ, et al. Collaborative drug therapy management by pharmacists: 2003. *Pharmacotherapy*. 2003;**23**:1210-1225.

40. Ernst ME, Brandt KB. Evaluation of 4 years of clinical pharmacist anticoagulation case management in a rural, private physician office. *J Am Pharm Assoc (Wash DC)*. 2003;**43**: 630-636.

41. Chrischilles EA, Carter BL, Lund BC, et al. Evaluation of the Iowa Medicaid pharmaceutical case management program. *J Am Pharm Assoc (Wash DC)*. 2004;**44**:337-349.

42. Snella KA, Sachdev GP. A primer for developing pharmacist-managed clinics in the outpatient setting. *Pharmacotherapy*. 2003;**23**:1153-1166.

43. Kuo GM, Buckley TE, Fitzsimmons DS, Steinbauer JR. Collaborative drug therapy management services and reimbursement in a family medicine clinic. *Am J Health Syst Pharm*. 2004;**61**:343-354.

44. Chiquette E, Amato MG, Bussey HI. Comparison of an anticoagulation clinic with usual medical care: Anticoagulation control, patient outcomes, and health care costs. *Arch Intern Med*. 1998;**158**:1641-1647.

45. Garabedian-Ruffalo SM, Gray DR, Sax MJ, Ruffalo RL. Retrospective evaluation of a pharmacist-managed warfarin anticoagulation clinic. *Am J Hosp Pharm*. 1985;**42**:304-308.

46. Gattis WA, Hasselblad V, Whellan DJ, O'Connor CM. Reduction in heart failure events by the addition of a clinical pharmacist to the heart failure management team: Results of the Pharmacist in Heart Failure Assessment Recommendation and Monitoring (PHARM) study. *Arch Intern Med*. 1999;**159**: 1939-1945.

47. Hanlon JT, Weinberger M, Samsa GP, et al. A randomized, controlled trial of a clinical pharmacist intervention to improve inappropriate prescribing in elderly outpatients with polypharmacy. *Am J Med*. 1996;**100**:428-437.

48. Rothman R, Weinberger M. The role of pharmacists in clinical care: Where do we go from here? *Eff Clin Pract*. 2002;**5**:91-94.

49. Tillman DJ, Charland SL, Witt DM. Effectiveness and economic impact associated with a program for outpatient management of acute deep vein thrombosis in a group model health maintenance organization. *Arch Intern Med*. 2000;**160**:2926-2932.

50. Wilt VM, Gums JG, Ahmed OI, Moore LM. Outcome analysis of a pharmacist-managed anticoagulation service. *Pharmacotherapy*. 1995;**15**:732-739.

51. Carter BL, Chrischilles EA, Scholz D, et al. Extent of services provided by pharmacists in the Iowa Medicaid Pharmaceutical Case Management program. *J Am Pharm Assoc*. 2003;**43**:24-33.

52. McKenney JM, Slining JM, Henderson HR, et al. The effect of clinical pharmacy services on patients with essential hypertension. *Circulation*. 1973;**48**:1104-1111.

53. Park JJ, Kelly P, Carter BL, Burgess PP. Comprehensive pharmaceutical care in the chain (pharmacy) setting. *J Am Pharm Assoc*. 1996;**NS36**:443-451.

54. Carter BL, Barnette DJ, Chrischilles E, et al. Evaluation of hypertensive patients after care provided by community pharmacists in a rural setting. *Pharmacotherapy*. 1997;**17**: 1274-1285.

55. Alsuwaidan S, Malone DC, Billups SJ, Carter BL. Characteristics of ambulatory care clinics and pharmacists in Veterans Affairs medical centers: IMPROVE investigators. Impact of Managed Pharmaceutical Care on Resource Utilization and Outcomes in Veterans Affairs Medical Centers. *Am J Health Syst Pharm*. 1998;**55**:68-72.

56. McGhan WF, Stimmel GL, Hall TG, Gilman TM. A comparison of pharmacists and physicians on the quality of prescribing for ambulatory hypertensive patients. *Med Care*. 1983;**21**:435-444.

57. Hawkins DW, Fiedler FP, Douglas HL, Eschbach RC. Evaluation of a clinical pharmacist in caring for hypertensive and diabetic patients. *Am J Hosp Pharm*. 1979;**36**:1321-1325.

58. Borenstein JE, Graber G, Saltiel E, et al. Physician-pharmacist comanagement of hypertension: A randomized, comparative trial. *Pharmacotherapy*. 2003;**23**:209-216.

59. Bogden PE, Koontz LM, Williamson P, Abbott RD. The physician and pharmacist team: An effective approach to cholesterol reduction. *J Gen Intern Med*. 1997;**12**:158-164.

60. Bogden PE, Abbott RD, Williamson P, et al. Comparing standard care with a physician and pharmacist team approach for uncontrolled hypertension. *J Gen Intern Med*. 1998;**13**: 740-745.

61. Erickson SR, Slaughter R, Halapy H. Pharmacists' ability to influence outcomes of hypertension therapy. *Pharmacotherapy*. 1997;**17**:140-147.

62. Mehos BM, Saseen JJ, MacLaughlin EJ. Effect of pharmacist intervention and initiation of home blood pressure monitoring in patients with uncontrolled hypertension. *Pharmacotherapy*. 2000;**20**:1384-1389.

63. Monson R, Bond CA, Schuna A. Role of the clinical pharmacist in improving drug therapy: Clinical pharmacists in outpatient therapy. *Arch Intern Med*. 1981;**141**:1441-1444.

64. Bond CA, Monson R. Sustained improvement in drug documentation, compliance, and disease control: A four-year analysis of an ambulatory care model. *Arch Intern Med*. 1984;**144**:1159-1162.

65. Sackett DL, Haynes RB, Gibson ES, et al. Randomised clinical trial of strategies for improving medication compliance in primary hypertension. *Lancet*. 1975;**1**:1205-1207.

Antihypertensive Drug Development: A Regulatory Perspective

Mehul G. Desai, Norman Stockbridge, Douglas C. Throckmorton, and Robert Temple

Antihypertensive drugs have been one of the most intensely studied therapies in clinical medicine. This is not surprising considering that hypertension affects more than 50 million people in the United States alone and requires lifelong treatment. It affects individuals of both sexes and is not restricted to any particular age or ethnic group. Over the past few decades, numerous antihypertensive agents representing a variety of pharmacologic classes have been studied and approved, including diuretics, α-adrenergic receptor blockers, β-adrenergic receptor blockers, central α-agonists, direct vasodilators, angiotensin-converting enzyme (ACE) inhibitors, calcium channel blockers (CCBs), angiotensin receptor blockers (ARBs), and others. Within each class of antihypertensives, numerous products have been developed and approved. An important aspect of the search for new antihypertensive agents is the quest for drugs that are well tolerated and can be added to existing treatments.

To gain regulatory approval by the U.S. Food and Drug Administration (FDA or the Agency), an antihypertensive drug, like any therapeutic agent, must demonstrate effectiveness. Effectiveness for an antihypertensive drug is established by showing that the drug lowers blood pressure (BP). BP is a *surrogate endpoint*. A surrogate "endpoint, or 'marker,' is a laboratory measurement or physical sign used in therapeutic trials as a substitute for a clinically meaningful endpoint that is a direct measure of how a patient feels, functions, or survives."[1] The effect of the drug or intervention on the surrogate is expected to predict a clinical benefit of the therapy. The effect on the surrogate endpoint is not itself noticeable by the patient and is of value only if it leads to the desired clinical benefit.

The law and regulations do not stipulate whether or not effectiveness must be demonstrated as an actual clinical benefit (e.g., fewer strokes, fewer myocardial infarctions, or symptomatic improvement) or as an effect on a validated surrogate endpoint for such benefit (e.g., decreased BP or decreased serum cholesterol). The law calls for evidence that the drug will do what its labeling claims it will do. However, the effect must be clinically meaningful. BP is considered a validated surrogate endpoint. An effect on BP is well supported as a predictor of clinical benefit, based on epidemiologic data, animal models, and, most importantly, numerous placebo-controlled studies. Epidemiologic evidence clearly shows that the risk of cardiovascular and cerebrovascular events increases with increases in BP. Many, large, randomized, placebo-controlled outcome trials involving a variety of antihypertensive drug classes (e.g., diuretics, reserpine, β-adrenergic receptor blockers, CCBs, ACE inhibitors) have shown that lowering elevated BP leads to a decreased risk of cardiovascular events, notably strokes, myocardial infarctions, and death from vascular causes.[2-5] This does not mean that all antihypertensive drugs will affect all outcomes similarly. For example, possible differences exist in the effects of different agents on heart failure,[6] an important consequence of hypertension. It also does not mean that drugs could not differ in effects on stroke and myocardial infarction, because these disorders are influenced by factors other than BP. The possibility of such differences is regularly examined,[7-10] and it is of great interest. These possible differences, however, do not undermine the observation that benefits of BP lowering have been seen in essentially all adequately sized, placebo-controlled studies with a variety of pharmacologically dissimilar agents.

Because BP is a validated surrogate, approval of antihypertensive drugs continues to be based on a demonstration that a drug can produce a sustained decrease in BP with an acceptable safety profile. This greatly simplifies the development of new agents. An effect on BP is an objective, noninvasive, reproducible, titratable, and rapidly demonstrated endpoint that can be studied in placebo-controlled trials. Demonstrating that a drug is an effective antihypertensive can be accomplished using a relatively small number of patients treated for a few weeks, with longer-term open or active-control follow-up and a randomized withdrawal study to confirm long-term effectiveness. Long-term outcome studies in hypertension could no longer ethically use a placebo group, but instead would require an active-control, noninferiority design, a type of study that is often difficult to interpret.[11,12]

The aim of this chapter is to discuss regulatory aspects of drug approval of antihypertensive drugs intended for long-term use. The development of an antihypertensive new molecular entity (NME) is discussed with a focus on the steps involved in drug development from the original submission of an Investigational New Drug (IND) application to submission of a New Drug Application (NDA). An NME is a drug whose active moiety, the part of the molecule responsible for its activity (irrespective of the particular salt or ester), has not been previously marketed. The chapter also addresses the quantity and quality of evidence necessary for approval of an NME, with attention to clinical trial design and analysis. Development of combination antihypertensives is also considered, as are the issues of outcome and comparative claims for antihypertensive drugs.

OVERVIEW OF DRUG DEVELOPMENT

Clinical drug development ordinarily proceeds in a systematic manner through "phases," as described in the Code of Federal Regulations (CFR; 21CFR312.21). Each step or phase in drug development builds on data acquired during earlier steps and in general exposes larger numbers of patients for longer periods of time. The goal of drug development is the acquisition of data that will provide the evidence needed for drug approval described in Section 505(b)(1) of the Food, Drug and Cosmetic (FD&C) Act. The law requires a showing, through adequate and well-controlled investigations, of "substantial evidence that the drug will have the effect it purports or is represented to have under the conditions of use prescribed, recommended, or suggested in the proposed labeling" (Section 505[d], 21USC355). The available data must also enable the applicant to provide "adequate directions for use" of the drug (Section 502[f], 21USC352). The FDA not only monitors the development process to ensure patient safety, but also interacts with the sponsor to help ensure that the studies, if successful, will provide the data needed for approval by discussing, among other things, specific study designs, study endpoints, and adequacy of planned safety databases.

In the United States, the study of any NME in humans requires that an IND (notice of claimed investigational exemption for a new drug, generally called an IND application) be filed with the FDA. The submission goes to the appropriate review division within the Center for Drug Evaluation and Research (CDER), which, in the case of antihypertensive drugs, is the Division of Cardiovascular and Renal Products. An initial IND submission (1) alerts the Agency to a sponsor's intent to initiate clinical studies in the United States, (2) provides the preliminary animal data needed to assess potential targets of toxicity and to ensure that it is reasonably safe to begin drug administration to humans, (3) provides information about the manufacturing process and chemistry of the new drug, (4) describes the initial clinical study to be conducted with a focus on safety measures, and (5) provides assurance that an Institutional Review Board (IRB) will approve the study before it is initiated. If the Agency identifies no major safety issues that result in the study's being put on "hold," the sponsor can begin the initial clinical study of the investigational drug 30 days after submission of the IND. Often, before submitting an IND, a sponsor will meet with Agency staff for a pre-IND meeting, during which preliminary development plans are discussed. For antihypertensive drugs, sponsors often forgo such meetings, probably because the development path is relatively straightforward. After IND submission, all subsequent clinical study protocols must also be submitted to the FDA but are not subject to a 30-day waiting period. These protocols can be initiated on the day of submission to the Agency.

As part of the IND submission process, the sponsor completes FDA form 1571, which describes what a typical IND application should contain. A link to the form is shown in Table 47-1. Every investigator participating in the study must also sign FDA form 1572, which, among other items, contains a list of the qualifications of the investigator, the location of the research facility where the investigation will be conducted, the name of the IRB responsible for review and approval of the protocol, and a list of certain commitments from the investigator related to the conduct of the clinical study, stating that the investigator intends (1) to conduct the study in accordance with the current protocol, (2) to conduct or supervise the described investigation personally, (3) to inform potential subjects that the drugs are being used for investigational pur-

Table 47-1 Useful Web Addresses

Web Address	Information Contained at That Web Address
http://www.fda.gov/	Main FDA Web site with links to many valuable informational and educational resources
http://www.fda.gov/cder/guidance/guidance.htm	Center for Drug Evaluation and Research guidances
http://www.ich.org/UrlGrpServer.jser?@_ID=276&@_TEMPLATE=254	International Conference on Harmonization guidances
http://www.fda.gov/opacom/morechoices/fdaforms/cder.html	FDA forms 1571 and 1572 containing the Investigational New Drug application and investigator statement
http://www.accessdata.fda.gov/scripts/cdrh/cfdocs/cfcfr/cfrsearch.cfm	Code of Federal Regulations Database. If a specific Code of Federal Regulations reference is known, a detailed description of that regulation can be obtained.
http://www.fda.gov/oc/advisory/accalendar/2005/default.htm	FDA Advisory Committee Calendar
http://www.fda.gov/medwatch/index.html	MedWatch Web page containing links to recent Safety Alerts for Drugs, Biologics, Devices, etc. It also contains links to the adverse event reporting forms 3500 and 3500A.
http://www.fda.gov/cder/foi/nda/index.htm	Center for Drug Evaluation and Research, Freedom of Information New Drug Approval Packages (includes approval letters and posted reviews)
http://www.fda.gov/CDER/drug/drugInteractions/default.htm	List of drug-metabolizing enzymes and their substrates, inhibitors, and inducers

FDA, Food and Drug Administration.

poses, and (4) to report to the sponsor adverse events that occur in the course of the investigation (21CFR312.53). These forms are retained by the IND's sponsor.

Substantial resources are expended by sponsors even before an IND is submitted to the FDA. Apart from the discovery process, the sponsor will have performed standard toxicology studies, animal pharmacology studies, and absorption/distribution/metabolism/excretion (ADME) studies in animals before initial exposure of humans to the investigational drug. These types of studies may provide clues to possible safety problems in humans and can influence the kind of monitoring that may be needed during future clinical studies. The IND and the clinical studies proposed in the IND are reviewed by a team of scientists at the FDA consisting of a pharmacologist/toxicologist, a chemist, a clinical pharmacologist, a statistician, and a medical/clinical reviewer. Certain disciplines are more actively involved than others at various stages of drug development. One of the main concerns of FDA reviewers during the initial 30-day IND review period is the appropriateness of the initial dose and duration of exposure. Usually, the human starting dose is chosen by identifying the no-observed-adverse-effect level (NOAEL) dose in two animal species, a rodent and a nonrodent, and then dividing that dose by a "safety factor" of about 10 to 100, to obtain the recommended starting dose in humans. Because the initial human study is usually a single-dose or limited repeat-dose study, animal studies of relatively short duration of exposure (e.g., 2 weeks) are sufficient to support initiation of human studies. Completion of animal studies with longer durations will be needed to support initiation of clinical studies of longer duration. Generally, the duration of animal studies will be similar to the duration of the planned human study, up to 6 months. Animal studies of 6 to 12 months' duration will support longer human studies.[13] In addition, for drugs used on a long-term basis such as antihypertensives, carcinogenicity studies in rats and mice, as well as reproductive toxicity studies in rats and rabbits, are needed before marketing approval.[14,15]

The pharmacology/toxicology reviewer is usually the most active member of the review team during the initial IND submission for an NME, with principal responsibility for evaluating the extensive body of nonclinical data submitted to support initial human use. The chemistry reviewer is also critical, in evaluating the manufacturing process to ensure that the NME is a stable, reproducible compound and in assessing the drug's formulation for impurities. The medical reviewer evaluates the initial phase 1 study primarily to ensure that adequate safety assessments are in place, including laboratory and electrocardiographic monitoring, that appropriate contraceptive measures are taken for women of childbearing potential, that provisions have been made for adequate subject follow-up, and that the initial dose chosen for human use is appropriate. Under the regulations, protocols for phase 1 studies may be less detailed relative to protocols for phase 2 or 3 studies, although phase 1 protocols should specify in detail only elements that are critical to safety (21CFR312.23). The Agency actively encourages the inclusion of women in the earliest clinical studies, and in fact for a study of a serious or life-threatening condition that affects both men and women, may put on hold a trial that excludes women because of their reproductive potential (21CFR312.42). The initial and subsequent phase 1 studies should provide enough information about the drug's tolerability, pharmacokinetics (PK), and

pharmacologic effects to permit the design of well-controlled phase 2 studies. The clinical pharmacology reviewer is involved in the early IND submissions to characterize the PK profile of single and repeated doses of drug and to consider in vitro and later in vivo studies of drug-drug interactions. Later in development, it will be important to consider details of drug metabolism and excretion and the effects of impaired renal and hepatic function. PK/pharmacodynamic (PK/PD) modeling can inform the choice of doses in controlled studies. The role of the statistician is limited in the early studies submitted for the IND, but it becomes far greater in later stages of drug development, generally beginning with the end-of-phase-2 (EOP2) meetings, when discussion focuses on issues related to the statistical analysis of clinical endpoints. Better design of early (phase 2) studies, however, may be possible with the help of PK/PD modeling, use of enrichment designs,[16] and more attention to studying a full range of doses.

Once clinical studies are initiated, sponsors of INDs have certain obligations defined in the regulations. Some of these obligations include selecting qualified investigators, monitoring all clinical investigations being conducted under the IND, keeping investigators informed of new findings or observations related to the safe use of the new drug, submitting annual reports that update the progress of an IND, and submitting reports of serious and unexpected adverse events to all investigators and the FDA within 15 days.

A critical task of the medical reviewer during the IND stage is the review of reports of serious and unexpected adverse events associated with use of the drug. Sponsors of INDs are required to submit to the Agency reports of all serious and unexpected adverse events (those adverse events not described in the investigator's brochure) "associated with" the use of a drug (generally meaning at least possibly related to the study drug), in a timely manner on a MedWatch 3500A form (Web link available in Table 47-1), with appropriate follow-up as additional information becomes available. As experience with the NME grows, the sponsor is responsible for cautious monitoring of adverse effects and for taking any necessary steps to deal with them, including increasing safety monitoring, modifying the dose, conducting additional evaluations, and, when problems merit this, stopping the trial. The FDA regularly reviews safety reports and discusses them with sponsors as necessary.

After completion of phase 1 studies and the subsequent phase 2 studies (i.e., the first studies of effectiveness), an EOP2 meeting is often held between the Agency and the IND sponsor. A critical issue is the design of phase 3 studies, the definitive, well-controlled studies of effectiveness that will serve, if successful, as the basis for marketing approval. Issues considered during such meetings include the design of the trials, the number of trials needed, the population (and demographics of the population) to be studied, the endpoints to be evaluated, the doses to be evaluated, and the total safety exposure that will be adequate. The Agency also considers any special safety evaluations that are needed. In addition to the pharmacology/toxicology, chemistry, medical, clinical pharmacology, and biostatistics reviewers, these later meetings may also include representatives from the FDA's Office of Drug Safety.

On completion of the phase 3 studies, and if the results are satisfactory, the sponsor submits an NDA to the Agency. The Agency currently recommends and eventually may require that an NDA be submitted in the Common Technical Document (CTD) format.[17] The CTD represents an effort by the International Conference of Harmonization (ICH) to create a core information package that can be sent to any of the three ICH regions (the United States, the European Union, and Japan) to support marketing authorization and includes a well-constructed overview of the application. The Agency's data requirements for establishing efficacy or safety have not been changed by the CTD. The CTD leaves room for specific FDA requirements, notably the case report tabulations, case report forms, integrated summaries of safety and efficacy, and complete study reports that are outlined in the CFR (21CFR314.50). There is also an FDA guidance on integrated summaries.[18] The CTD can be submitted electronically and is reviewed by an FDA review team that consists of the same disciplines that were involved in the review of the IND.

Drugs that would be a significant improvement, compared with marketed products, are considered "priority" (P) applications. Details of what constitutes a "significant improvement" can be found in an FDA document called an MaPP (Manual of Policies and Procedures).[19] Under agreements reached at the time of the Prescription Drug User Fee Act (PDUFA) of 1992 and its subsequent renewals, priority applications will be reviewed by 6 months after the time the application is received by the Agency. Other applications are "standard" (S) and will be reviewed within 10 months. Because of the extensive armamentarium of antihypertensive drugs currently available for use, most NDAs for antihypertensive drugs fall into the standard review category.

Sometimes, during the FDA review process, NMEs that raise public health or other scientific issues may be brought before the Cardiovascular and Renal Drugs Advisory Committee (a committee of external advisors) for discussion at a meeting open to the general public. The Committee addresses specific questions posed by the FDA, often including whether there is substantial evidence of effectiveness and whether safety has been adequately assessed and shows the drug to be safe for its intended use. The Committee's recommendations are advisory, and the Agency is not bound to accept its recommendations.

After completion of the Agency's reviews, a decision regarding approvability is conveyed to the NDA applicant or sponsor in the form of an "action letter." Currently, there are three types of action letters: (1) approval, (2) approvable, and (3) not approvable. When a sponsor is granted an "approval" letter, the drug can be marketed as of the date of the letter, with the labeling identified in the approval letter. Following an approval action, the primary reviews of the various disciplines as well as secondary reviews are made available to the public (link available in Table 47-1). Approvable and not-approvable actions both indicate that something further needs to be done before a drug can be approved. In that sense, they are both indicators of a deficiency in the application. The deficiency can range from a need to revise labeling to a need to conduct additional studies of effectiveness or safety. At present, the Agency sends the sponsor an "approvable" letter if the application meets most of the requirements listed for marketing approval and can be approved if "specific additional information or material is submitted or specific conditions (for example, certain changes in labeling) are agreed to by the [sponsor]" or if additional information is provided, such as additional data analyses or even an additional study

(21CFR314.110). A "not-approvable" letter is issued if the Agency believes that the drug application is insufficient to justify approval because effectiveness is not supported or safety problems appear serious. The sponsor may undertake to correct any deficiencies noted by the FDA and file a resubmission. The Agency was asked in the FDA Modernization Act (FDAMA) to develop a single "complete response" letter (to replace the approvable and not-approvable letters) that would detail deficiencies when the drug cannot yet be approved.

At the time of approval, the agency may conclude that safety concerns require a risk management effort that could include further postmarketing studies, educational efforts, or specific labeling.[20-22] Sponsors may also agree to carry out postmarketing (phase 4) studies, such as studies of larger doses or of combinations with other antihypertensive drugs.

CLINICAL PHARMACOLOGY

Pharmacokinetics

The PK of a drug comprises descriptions of the fate of the drug and its metabolites in the body, including its absorption, distribution, metabolism, and excretion. These parameters are often described by analyzing the measurement of blood and urine concentrations of the drug and its metabolites over time, including certain important parameters including the highest concentration achieved after dosing (C_{max}), the time of peak concentrations (T_{max}), the trough concentration before the next dose (C_{min}), and area under the curve or the integration of time and concentration, representing a measure of drug exposure (AUC). Information about PK is obtained from single- and multiple-dose studies conducted in healthy subjects or in the patient population in whom the drug is intended. Areas of particular interest are those that make PK less predictable than expected (e.g., PK differences among people or nonlinearities of PK with changes in dose). For example, one expects blood levels of a drug to be proportional to the administered dose, and inversely related to body size, weight, or body surface area. It is thus of great interest when there is a nonlinear relationship such that drug levels do not change in direct proportion to the administered dose, or when substantial sex differences exist. Similarly, it is critical to know how impaired renal or hepatic function and other co-variates (e.g., age and sex) or the presence of concomitantly administered drugs affect PK. Deviations from linearity or substantial intersubject variation are particularly important for drugs with a narrow therapeutic index (drugs for which the difference between effective exposures and toxic exposures is small), and in the most extreme cases they may indicate the need for therapeutic drug monitoring.

Interpretation of PK findings also requires knowledge of the activity of major metabolites. Although many useful PK findings may emerge from special studies (e.g., of drug interactions, dose-response, or people with renal or hepatic impairment) using an intensive sampling protocol, it is often of value to conduct population PK analyses using sparse sampling in studies to detect unexpected causes of nonlinearity or individuals with unusually high drug exposure. Knowledge of the PK of a drug and its active metabolites can guide both how often to administer a particular compound in later studies and the timing of certain safety data that are to be collected (e.g., electrocardiograms to assess Q-T intervals, measurements of BP or heart rate). Finally, knowing how the PK of a drug changes in a particular population, or with a co-administered drug, can be useful in determining how to modify dosage regimens to optimize use of the drug.

Metabolism and Drug-Drug Interactions

The route by which a drug is metabolized or eliminated from the body is an important determinant of interindividual PK variability. Although the importance of metabolic pathways and their potential for creating individual differences in response and drug-drug interactions are now widely recognized, experience with an antihypertensive agent was an important early source of this recognition. Debrisoquine, an adrenergic blocking agent, was developed in the 1970s for the treatment of hypertension. Studies with this agent showed a positive correlation between BP lowering and the amount of unchanged drug excreted in the urine; this finding reflecting the fact that the parent compound, debrisoquine, is pharmacologically active, whereas its metabolite is not.[23] The enzyme responsible for the conversion of debrisoquine to its metabolite was originally called debrisoquine hydroxylase, but it is now recognized as cytochrome P-450 2D6 (CYP2D6), one of several important oxidizing enzymes in the liver. Cytochrome P-450 2D6 is polymorphic in humans, and approximately 5% to 10% of whites have a genetic deficiency of this enzyme (often referred to as poor metabolizers). They therefore experience exaggerated responses to drugs such as debrisoquine or tricyclic antidepressants,[24] as a result of greatly increased (sometimes 10-fold) drug exposure. Probably more important, because it can occur in people who have been receiving the drug and tolerating it, is that even in subjects without a genetic deficiency of CYP2D6, concomitant use of a drug that inhibits this enzyme can mimic the genetic deficiency and can lead to abrupt excess parent drug concentrations and potential toxicity. Inhibitors of CYP2D6 include fluoxetine, paroxetine, and quinidine. Inhibitors of cytochrome P-450 enzymes and other metabolic and transport systems are important, even for systems that are not genetically polymorphic such as CYP2D6. References to enzymes involved in drug disposition, their substrates, inhibitors, and inducers can be found at the links provided in Table 47-1.

Terfenadine, cisapride, and astemizole, all now removed from the market, were drugs that were metabolized by CYP3A and became far more toxic when their metabolism was blocked, thus leading to Q-T prolongation and torsades de pointes arrhythmias. Routine and early evaluation of the substrate, inhibitor, and inducer status of NMEs should be conducted, and these matters are considered at length in FDA guidances.[25,26]

One recently approved, then subsequently withdrawn, antihypertensive illustrates the importance of metabolic inhibition. Mibefradil was a CCB antihypertensive drug approved in 1997 for the treatment of hypertension and angina. In vitro and in vivo studies clearly showed that the drug was a potent inhibitor of CYP3A, an enzyme responsible for metabolizing a variety of medications, including several 3-hydroxy-3-methylglutaryl–coenzyme A (HMG-CoA) reductase inhibitors or statins, as well as astemizole and cisapride. The drug was labeled to describe these interactions, but mibefradil was linked to cases of torsades de pointes–type

arrhythmias when it was given, despite labeling, to patients receiving astemizole and cisapride (substrates for the enzyme CYP3A). More surprising was the extent of serious interactions with certain statin drugs. Although other CYP3A inhibitors were associated with rare cases of rhabdomyolysis when these drugs were taken with statins, mibefradil use quickly resulted in numerous reports of rhabdomyolysis when it was co-administered with simvastatin. In retrospect, it was probably the use of mibefradil for cardiovascular conditions that made its use with statins so common. Other potent CYP3A inhibitors (e.g., antifungals, such as ketoconazole) were less likely to be used concomitantly with statins. Because of its metabolic liability, mibefradil was soon withdrawn from the market.

Special Populations

Studies to characterize the PK of a drug in special populations, such as male and female patients, the elderly, and patients with renal or hepatic impairment (depending on how the drug is metabolized and excreted), should be carried out during drug development.[27-31] Factors such as sex, age, renal or hepatic impairment, and others are important determinants of interindividual differences in drug exposure and may identify a population at risk of drug-related adverse events. Nearly all ACE inhibitors undergo predominantly renal elimination. Labeling of these drugs therefore suggests a starting dose at the low end of the dosage range in patients with renal impairment (or elderly patients, who often have a degree of renal impairment), with titration to higher doses as needed. This is intended primarily to avoid dose-related adverse events such as hypotension.

Food Effects and Absorption

Food intake concomitant with oral drug administration can have marked effects on drug bioavailability, particularly for drugs with large first-pass effects or drugs in controlled-release forms. A controlled-release formulation of nisoldipine is an example of an antihypertensive whose PK profile is significantly altered in the setting of concomitant food intake. Administration of nisoldipine with a high-fat meal increases the peak plasma concentration by up to threefold, whereas the total exposure is reduced by about 25%.[32] This phenomenon, referred to as *dose dumping*, in effect converts the extended-release formulation into an immediate-release formulation, thus eliminating the 24-hour antihypertensive coverage of nisoldipine while exposing the patient to the risks of an acutely exaggerated hypotensive response. A similar phenomenon can occur when controlled-release formulations of nifedipine are taken with high-fat meals. Studying food effects of drugs should be a routine part of most new drug development programs,[33] unless the drug is an immediate-release, rapidly dissolving product that is not significantly metabolized.

Pharmacodynamics

The approval of antihypertensive drugs is based on their PD effect, that is, lowering BP. Many currently approved antihypertensive agents have additional effects (e.g., diuretics to treat edema, β-blockers or CCBs to treat angina), and, in many cases, an earlier PD effect represents the drug's mechanism of BP lowering (e.g., ACE inhibition for an ACE inhibitor). Evaluating the PD effects of antihypertensives other than their effects on BP may be of interest and can be used to suggest a therapeutic dose range for the other effects or to anticipate adverse effects. Studies of the drug's mechanism-based biomarkers (e.g., exercise-induced heart rate for β-blockers, urinary sodium excretion for diuretics, ACE activity or plasma renin activity for ACE inhibitors, and angiotensin II activity for ARBs) can be useful in selecting dose ranges for later controlled BP trials, although they are not a substitute for those clinical dose-response studies. The dose-response and duration of these effects can be initially characterized in healthy subjects, but eventually they should be assessed in the target population. It is often useful to relate PD effects to plasma concentrations through a PK/PD model or an exposure-response model. A wide range of doses should be studied to characterize these relationships adequately.

Exposure response data can sometimes facilitate development of new formulations. The immediate-release formulation of metoprolol was originally approved as a twice-daily treatment for hypertension and angina. Subsequently, a once-daily extended-release formulation was developed and approved, based on PK/PD studies in a relatively small number of healthy volunteers showing that the effects of the immediate-release and controlled-release products on exercise heart rate were similar (e.g., maximal reduction in exercise heart rate [E_{max}], plasma concentration of metaprolol that produces 50% E_{max} [EC_{50}]).[34] It was also shown that the plasma concentrations with the extended-release formulation remained higher than a level that produced clinically relevant reductions in exercise-induced tachycardia for the duration of the dosing interval, a finding indicating that this drug could be expected to provide 24-hour antihypertensive effectiveness.

CLINICAL EFFICACY

General Principles

The evidence needed to support the effectiveness of a new antihypertensive agent is based on the general requirements set forth in the FD&C Act as amended in 1962. The amended law required "substantial evidence of effectiveness," which it defined as evidence from "adequate and well-controlled investigations." The plural of investigations was intended. More recently, the FDAMA of 1997 amended the definition of substantial evidence to state that the Agency may determine that "data from *one* adequate and well-controlled clinical investigation and confirmatory evidence" to represent substantial evidence (Section 505[d], 21USC355). The law also requires that a drug label provide adequate directions for use. In practical terms, data from at least two studies, usually more, are needed and expected, considering what needs to be known about how to use antihypertensive drugs appropriately, including a good dose-response assessment and use with other antihypertensive drugs.

Study Design

The CFR describes criteria for an adequate and well-controlled study (21CFR314.126). The CFR identifies five kinds of control groups that can be used: placebo, no treatment, dose-response, active/positive, and historical. The choice among these control groups is discussed in much more detail in an ICH guidance document.[12] Until recently, with the advent of ambulatory BP monitoring (ABPM), only a placebo-controlled study, a dose-response study, or an active-controlled study showing superiority of the test drug would have been considered satisfactory evidence of effectiveness of an antihypertensive agent. Active-controlled non-inferiority studies would be difficult to interpret, given the substantial early "placebo response" in most hypertension trials.[11,12] Although the reasons for placebo response in hypertension studies are not fully documented, it is thought that the response can be attributed, at least in part, to digit preference, a tendency to read high at entry, when BP must be greater than some entry value, and then reading appropriately or low once treatment begins. In a placebo-controlled trial, this effect is simply subtracted, because the effect measured is the drug-placebo difference. In an active-controlled trial, however, this is not possible, and it is not uncommon for active-controlled trials to show changes from baseline of 20/15 mm Hg, a difference far larger than the difference between drug and placebo seen in placebo-controlled trials. An active-controlled noninferiority study would have to base its analysis on a noninferiority margin (the actual effect of the control drug in the study) of typically 4 to 5 mm Hg. Attempting to show that, for example, a difference of half that (e.g., 2 mm Hg) had been ruled out when the change from baseline is, for example 20/15 mm Hg, would be a significant challenge. As discussed in more detail later, ABPM, unlike manual cuff pressure measurements, appears to show little or no fall in BP in the placebo group, thus making active-controlled trials potentially feasible.

Placebo-controlled studies in hypertension commonly include more than one dose of the study drug (Fig. 47-1A). This is a very informative design, capable not only of providing unequivocal evidence of effectiveness, either by pairwise comparison with placebo or demonstration of a slope, but also of relating efficacy and adverse effects to dose. With a group of such studies, pooled data usually allow analyses of dose-response for relevant population subsets, including demographic subsets and BP severity subsets. A potential concern with a placebo-controlled design is denial of known effective treatment to patients enrolled in such a study. Although it is recognized that long-term placebo-controlled studies in hypertension cannot be ethically conducted, short-term (e.g., duration of 8 to 12 weeks) placebo-controlled studies appear acceptable. A meta-analysis of 25 randomized short-term placebo-controlled studies in more than 6400 patients demonstrated no increased risk of death, stroke, myocardial infarction, or heart failure in patients randomized to placebo.[35] The FDA also conducted a meta-analysis of short-term hypertension studies, referred to as the Placebo in Hypertension Adverse Reaction Meta-analysis (PHARM) project.[36] It also showed no significant increase in the risk of irreversible morbidity or harm in patients treated with placebo. Nonetheless, because the effects of most antihypertensives are fully developed within a few days to a couple of weeks, it appears prudent to limit studies to relatively short durations.

New antihypertensive agents are commonly studied for their additive effects on top of standard agents, although this has not been explicitly required (see Fig. 47-1B). A common

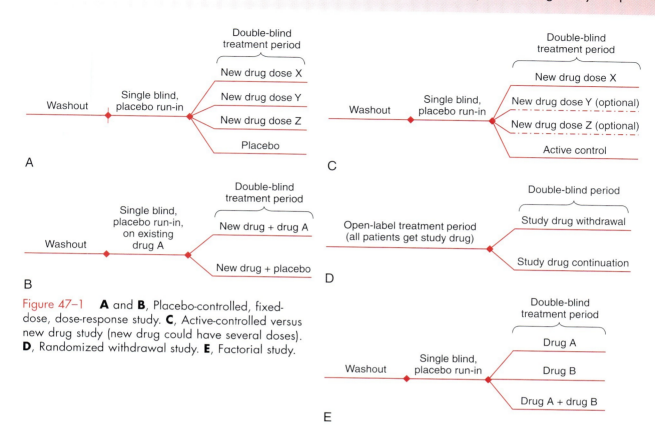

Figure 47–1   **A** and **B**, Placebo-controlled, fixed-dose, dose-response study. **C**, Active-controlled versus new drug study (new drug could have several doses). **D**, Randomized withdrawal study. **E**, Factorial study.

example of such a study is a comparison of the study drug and placebo, each added to a fixed dose of a diuretic. This is a placebo-controlled study and supports the effectiveness of the new agent, just as does a study that does not include the diuretic.[37] In long-term extension studies, other drugs are added to attain adequate BP control, thus allowing informal observation of other concomitant use. Later in this chapter, studies in support of a fixed-dose combination antihypertensive are discussed in more detail.

An active-controlled study (see Fig. 47-1C) showing superiority of the study drug over an active-control agent with respect to BP lowering can also be used to demonstrate effectiveness of the new drug. It could also support a labeling claim of superiority if the control drug is used properly, at its highest dose, and in an optimal regimen.[12,38] However, such a study provides neither a good estimate of effect size of the new drug relative to placebo nor a good assessment of the actual adverse effect rate (i.e., drug rate minus placebo rate). A labeling claim of greater effectiveness, based on BP lowering, is most credible for drugs of the same pharmacologic class, because differences in efficacy among classes are more difficult to interpret in full, given differences in side effects. In contrast, studies that compare drugs for effects on clinically relevant outcomes (e.g., mortality, stroke, and coronary heart disease), when they are used at equieffective doses, are of great interest, and convincing results could appear in labeling. Outcome claims in hypertension are discussed in more detail later in this chapter.

As discussed earlier, a dose-response study can be informative about both effectiveness and dose response. In a randomized, fixed-dose, dose-response study, the design

described in the 21CFR314.126 and identified in ICH E4[39] as optimal, patients are randomized to two or more fixed doses in a parallel group study. The fixed doses can be reached in steps. Such a study design may or may not incorporate a placebo and could include an active control as well. Doses should be spaced adequately (e.g., threefold increments) to increase the likelihood of seeing differences in BP response. Although a dose-response study with a nonzero slope is sufficient to demonstrate a drug effect even without a placebo, conducting such a study (in the absence of a placebo group) is ill advised. In the absence of a slope for the active treatments, the study is entirely uninformative, even if all doses would have been superior to placebo, had one been included. It is not uncommon in hypertension studies for all doses to have effect sizes close to each other. Including a placebo arm ensures that a study will have assay sensitivity, but, in addition, it allows dose-placebo pairwise comparisons that provide information on the particular doses, including the lower doses, that are effective. A dose-response study with a nonzero slope, in the absence of a placebo group, may need further evaluation to determine whether the lower doses are actually useful.

Recognition of the limitations of titration designs and acceptance of the randomized fixed dose-response study (ICH E4) have obscured the potential value of titration designs, properly analyzed.[40] Sheiner and colleagues used such a design, combined with analysis of individual dose-response curves that, if accompanied by a placebo group, could provide an initial estimate of the dose-response curve for effectiveness, as well as unequivocal evidence of effectiveness.[41] Such a titration design would be very useful as an initial controlled study that would ensure titration to an adequate dose and guide subsequent dose-response studies.

As their name implies, dose-response studies describe dose response but do not themselves indicate what the starting or maximal doses should be, because these are matters of judgment. When a drug is well tolerated, starting doses are usually chosen to give a substantial fraction of the drug's full effect. Only if there are dose-related toxicity concerns (e.g., α-blockers and hypotension, diuretics and hypokalemia) will a much lower starting dose be recommended in general or for certain patients.

A study design that can be used to help demonstrate efficacy and that is important to proper demonstration of the durability of effect after long-term use is the randomized withdrawal study (see Fig. 47-1D). In a randomized withdrawal study, all patients initially receive therapy with the study drug for some period of time (e.g., 6 months to 1 year or more, depending on how long an effect duration is to be evaluated) as part of a single-arm, open-label safety study or as part of an active-controlled comparison. At the end of the open-label study period, patients are randomized in a blinded manner either to continued use of study drug or to placebo (withdrawal of study drug, which can be down-titrated if there is concern about withdrawal effects). After a relatively short period (e.g., 2 weeks), BP effects between the two groups can be reassessed. Alternatively, patients can be monitored closely and discontinued from the study as soon as their BP rises to a predetermined level. In both cases, a withdrawal-type study that shows increased BP in the placebo-controlled group demonstrates that the study drug was continuing to have an effect. This durability of effect would otherwise be difficult to establish, because a long-term placebo-controlled study in hypertension would be ethically unacceptable.

Study Population

Patients enrolled in an antihypertensive efficacy study should be representative of the population for which the therapy may be targeted. Although regulations and guidances (except for ICH E7,[42] which suggests 100 people >65 years old) do not specifically state the percentage of subjects in a clinical study that should be of a particular subgroup (e.g., age ≥65 years, female, or black), a draft guidance urges reasonable participation of each group.[43] Moreover, the legal requirement (Section 502[f], 21USC352) to provide adequate directions for use in labeling suggests that the population studied ought to be representative of those that will receive the drug. There are several examples in which a particular subgroup has not had the same BP response as that of the whole group. The smaller antihypertensive effect of drugs directly affecting the renin-angiotensin system (β-blockers, ACE inhibitors, and ARBs) in black subjects is well recognized. In the Losartan Intervention for Endpoint Reduction in Hypertension (LIFE) study, a randomized, blinded, active-controlled study comparing losartan with atenolol in hypertensive patients with electrocardiographically documented left ventricular hypertrophy, statistical heterogeneity was observed in the primary endpoint with respect to race.[44] In this study, black patients responded more favorably to atenolol, whereas white patients responded more favorably to losartan in terms of a reduction in the composite primary endpoint of cardiovascular death, nonfatal stroke, or nonfatal myocardial infarction.

Dose Selection, Dosing Interval, and Dose Titration

Studying a relatively wide range of doses should be routine practice in hypertension drug development. As explained in ICH E4,[39] it is critical to describe the dose-response curve of a drug for favorable and unfavorable effects. With this information, it is possible to choose an appropriate starting dose and a dose beyond which there appears to be no further important benefit (this is a more accurate description of the goals of a dose-response study than seeking the so-called maximum effective dose and minimum effective dose). Some major historical errors in dose finding have occurred. Hydrochlorothiazide (HCTZ) and chlorthalidone were used at daily doses of 100 mg in major outcome studies in the 1960s and 1970s.[45-47] In retrospect, the selection of a high diuretic dose in these outcome studies was clearly an error, because subsequent dose-response studies of chlorthalidone revealed that BP lowering was maximal at a dose of 25 mg once daily,[48] and no additional BP lowering was observed with titration of chlorthalidone to doses as high as 200 mg once daily.[49] However, dose-dependent decreases in serum potassium and dose-dependent increases in blood glucose and uric acid occurred at the higher doses. These effects appear to have been consequences of the use of excessive doses. The findings from these studies and from subsequent confirmatory studies led to a revision in the product labeling, thus leading to lower starting doses and lower recommended doses. The excess doses and resulting hypokalemia, in all probability, led to a decrease in the cardiovascular benefit in the early outcome trials using thiazide diuretics.[2,10,40,50]

Demonstrating that an antihypertensive drug or drug regimen is effective requires demonstrating that BP is lowered meaningfully throughout the time period between one administered dose and the next, sometimes referred to as the *interdosing interval*. Showing that BP is reduced at "trough" (usually the time just before the next dose) is thus part of establishing antihypertensive efficacy for the proposed regimen. If an antihypertensive drug does not produce an effect of this duration, it is being administered too infrequently. Captopril, an ACE inhibitor approved for the treatment of hypertension in a dosing regimen twice daily or three times daily, was evaluated by the Agency for potential approval in a once-daily dosing regimen. That regimen was ultimately not approved by the Agency, however, because there was only a clinically trivial reduction in sitting diastolic BP at trough. Some short-acting dihydropyridine CCBs have also failed to retain an adequate trough effect when they are given once daily, a problem resolved for felodipine by development of a controlled-release dosage form. As a general matter, although no specific rule or guidance exists, it has been expected that the effect at trough should be at least 50% to 70% of the peak effect (with both effects measured as placebo-subtracted values).

It is also important to characterize the appropriate titration interval between dose increments. Although BP effects during a dosing interval generally depend on plasma concentrations of the drug, the full antihypertensive effects of a drug are often delayed, and may increase over time, even though plasma concentrations are stable. The reasons for this are not clear. Consequently, during a study, BP measurements should be assessed serially (e.g., weekly after study drug initiation) to determine when a plateau or steady state effect with respect to BP is reached relative to the initiation of therapy.

Endpoints

The Agency has not defined a minimum magnitude of BP lowering that must be attained by a drug for it to be approved. In theory, an antihypertensive that reduced mean BP on average by as little as 2 mm Hg could be considered approvable if the drug had no significant safety issues, although most antihypertensive drugs currently approved produce substantially greater mean BP reductions, and it is difficult to imagine that such a drug would be considered very useful. If used, such a drug could also create a delay for patients to receive other, more effective antihypertensives. Approval of such a drug would make most sense if the drug provided a novel mechanism, so it could be added to maximal medical therapy in a patient not at goal BP. A more interesting possibility, however, is that a drug could have a small effect in the general population, but a sizeable effect in some patients, possibly, but not necessarily, a genetically or proteomically definable subset of the population. Even if that subset were only a small fraction of the population, such a drug, if properly targeted, could be useful for the responsive subset.

In general, mean BP change in a population, rather than the response rate (i.e., percentage of the population that reaches a prespecified goal BP or has a change of a specified magnitude), has been used as the metric to evaluate antihypertensive efficacy. Although the response rate, relative to comparator, generally tracks mean BP changes, it depends on the starting BP and the non–drug-related component of response (i.e., digit preference), and thus it may be misleading. Moreover, the management of hypertension involves the addition of antihypertensive drugs in a sequential manner until adequate BP lowering is achieved, often requiring two or more medications, because single agents frequently will not enable a patient to achieve a desired goal. All antihypertensive agents are labeled for use alone or in combination to lower BP. How low a BP to target is determined by the treating physician based on a patient's co-morbidities and other factors. In contrast, in some cases it could be useful to examine the distribution of responses rather than simply the mean response, for example, when there are responder and nonresponder subsets, as would be the case for low-renin and high-renin patients in responding to ACE inhibitors, ARBs, or β-blockers. In those cases, mean responses and the distribution of responses have shown a larger effect of these drugs in whites. It would also be important to look at the combined effects of drugs. Despite the smaller response of blacks to monotherapy with drugs that work through the renin-angiotensin system, the response of blacks and whites to combinations of diuretics and ACE inhibitors, ARBs, and β-blockers is the same.[51]

Diastolic BP at trough has been the primary outcome measure in hypertension trials, but this no longer seems sensible. Changes in systolic BP are of at least equal interest and importance. Lowering systolic BP has been shown to improve cardiovascular morbidity and mortality in elderly patients.[3,4] In practice, every agent shown to reduce diastolic BP has also reduced systolic BP. Nonetheless, it is possible that drugs could differ in their effects on systolic and diastolic BP, and it is of interest to evaluate this possibility routinely.

AMBULATORY BLOOD PRESSURE MONITORING

BPs obtained in an office setting, using a mercury (cuff) sphygmomanometer, have been the basis of the epidemiologic evidence establishing the risks associated with an elevated BP and the measurement tool used in outcome studies that have demonstrated the benefits of lowering BP. ABPM is an alternative way to obtain BP measurements in both clinical and research settings, and it may have important advantages, including an ability to examine different patterns of BP control. ABPM has opened several new design possibilities in the study of antihypertensive drugs. ABPM provides a characterization of the time course of BP effects throughout the dosing interval, in contrast to the "sparse sampling" of BPs that is the best one can do with clinic cuff pressure measurements. There also appears to be essentially no change in BP in placebo-treated patients, thus leading to the possibility that a separate placebo group would not be needed for the purposes of demonstrating efficacy.[52] By obtaining BPs unaccompanied by the presence or interpretation of medical personnel, ABPM also appears to avoid the "white-coat effect" and digit preference effect, thus decreasing the likelihood of enrolling pseudohypertensive subjects into clinical trials.

Although BP measurements averaged over the last few hours of the interdosing interval (or trough) and the first few hours (for peak) appear most relevant for demonstrating efficacy (a drug with no effect during the morning hours would not seem desirable, even if it had a substantial mean effect over the day), it remains possible that drugs with similar trough and peak effects could have differential 24-hour effects, and some patterns could potentially prove more advantageous. Even though hypertension studies utilizing ABPM do not need a placebo-control arm, it remains advisable to include an active control in an ABPM study of a new antihypertensive drug, to help characterize the population being studied and to determine the BP-lowering ability of the new agent relative to a familiar control agent. An antihypertensive development program for an NME would not ordinarily be able to rely exclusively on ABPM active-control data, because the safety database needs controlled (preferably placebo-controlled) observations to assess adverse event rates. It seems possible, however, that comparison of a drug with multiple well-characterized, active controls could serve this purpose, certainly for longer-term safety observations.

OUTCOME LABELING CLAIMS FOR ANTIHYPERTENSIVES

As noted earlier, approval of antihypertensives is based on an effect on BP. With few exceptions, and for several reasons, antihypertensive labeling makes no reference to outcome claims, even though an effect on outcome is the reason for the use of these drugs. First, antihypertensive outcome studies do not evaluate the effect of a single drug. Rather, although they may start with an antihypertensive of particular interest, the addition of other drugs, usually in a planned sequence, is needed to reach a prespecified goal BP. How much of the benefit observed can be attributed to the single starting agent is invariably a complex question. It is, in contrast, relatively easy to conclude that the observed effects on outcomes with a wide variety of interventions compared with placebo are evidence of the benefit of lowering BP per se. Comparisons of individual drugs or classes, or of "old" versus "new," are at present of great interest, both through individual studies[7,8] and overviews,[9,10] but results are not consistent, and differences are clearly small except when agents differ in effects on particular conditions, such as heart failure or diabetic nephropathy.

A second problem is that most newer drugs, for which there could be commercial interest in outcome claims, have not been the subject of placebo-controlled trials, because these trials can no longer be ethically conducted. Interpreting the noninferiority studies in hypertension that can be conducted may initially seem simple, given the many historical placebo-controlled studies, but, in fact, such comparisons are not straightforward. The effect size may have been modified by many new effective treatments for hypertension-related comorbidities, such as lipid-lowering treatments, postinfarction treatment with β-blockers and ACE inhibitors, effective treatment of heart failure, aspirin, thrombolytics, and revascularization procedures (e.g., angioplasty, bypass). These therapies would generally not have been available during the placebo-controlled studies that form the basis for establishing a noninferiority margin.[11,12]

For these reasons, outcome claims in labeling of antihypertensive drugs are few. The claim for the reduction in the risk of stroke with losartan in patients with hypertension and left ventricular hypertrophy was based on a comparison of losartan and atenolol that significantly favored the former. Although the Agency did not allow a superiority claim relative to atenolol, it did conclude that losartan had clearly been shown to reduce the risk of stroke.

There is considerable irony in the present situation. Treatment of BP is recognized as critical because of well-documented effects in clinical trials on stroke, myocardial infarction, mortality, and other adverse cardiovascular outcomes, yet labeling usually remains silent about these benefits for the reasons given previously. Discussion at a recent Cardiovascular and Renal Drugs Advisory Committee led to support of an attempt to develop a general statement for inclusion in labeling for all antihypertensive drugs regarding the effect of BP lowering on these outcomes.[53]

FIXED-COMBINATION ANTIHYPERTENSIVE DRUG DEVELOPMENT

The underlying goal of combination drug product development is to make drug intake more convenient and thereby to improve patient adherence, although such improvement has never been demonstrated. Two active drugs can be combined when "each component makes a contribution to the claimed effects and the dosage of each component (amount, frequency, duration) is such that the combination is safe and effective for a significant patient population requiring such concurrent therapy as defined in the labeling for the drug" (21CFR300.50).

There are several ways to demonstrate the contribution of antihypertensive components to the BP effect, and the Agency has not expressed a particular preference for one or another. Most common is a factorial design study, in which the two

monotherapies are compared with the combination product (see Fig. 47-1E). Years ago, this was typically accomplished in a single three-arm study using relatively high doses, often the maximum labeled dose of each agent. This study design documented the contribution of each component when the agents were from different pharmacologic classes (one would not want to combine half doses of two ACE inhibitors or diuretics), but the design did not reveal anything about lower-dose combinations. This was not a major problem, however, because, in general, single drugs were used at full doses before a second drug was added ("stepped care"), and the appropriate combination product could be substituted for the titrated doses. More recently, effectiveness of antihypertensive drug combinations has been evaluated in a multidose factorial study design that compares several doses of each component and their combinations (Fig. 47-2). This design can detect shifts in the dose-response curve of the individual drugs and can support the value of lower-dose combinations, given that practice has moved from stepped care to considerations of side effect minimization by use of submaximal doses of two agents, at least partly because of the recognition that full doses of diuretics posed problems. As noted later, in some cases this has led to recommended use of combinations as initial therapy.

An alternative to the factorial study is the performance of two add-on studies (see Fig. 47-1B), each conducted in patients not responding adequately to an optimal regimen of one component. For example, patients whose BP is not adequately controlled on an optimal regimen of drug A would be randomized to A and B versus A alone. Similarly, patients whose BP is not adequately controlled on an optimal regimen of drug B would be randomized to A and B versus B alone. For either study, it would be possible to randomize subjects to one or more doses of the add-on agent.

Combination drug products should not distort the use of the components by forcing use of inappropriate doses. A full range of fixed-dose combinations should therefore be made available, including the lowest and highest doses of each com-

		Drug B			
		Placebo	Low dose	Medium dose	High dose
Drug A	Placebo	X	X		X
	Low dose	X			X
	Medium dose				
	High dose	X	X		X

Figure 47–2 Example of 4 × 4 factorial design involving three doses of drugs A and B in addition to placebo. In developing a combination antihypertensive, it is critical to know that the blood pressure–lowering effects of drugs A and B are additive when both drugs are used at their maximal or near maximal labeled doses. Additional cells within the factorial table should also be studied to characterize the surface response of blood pressure lowering and to ensure that the dose-response curve of the initial or starting drug is not affected by the add-on drug. The cells marked by "X" represent cells that, if studied, could help to demonstrate that a combination antihypertensive product was effective.

ponent, and all or most combinations of doses in between. Most combination antihypertensives are indicated for the treatment of hypertension with the labeling stating that the fixed-dose combination is not indicated for initial therapy, but rather for patients who have been titrated to the doses in the combination to be used. However, three exceptions to this labeling exist.

The first example is a combination of the β_1-selective adrenergic blocker, bisoprolol, and a thiazide diuretic, HCTZ. A 12-cell (placebo and three doses of bisoprolol; placebo and two doses of HCTZ) factorial design study demonstrated that each component of the combination contributed to the antihypertensive effect.[54] Of particular interest was the low-dose combination of 2.5 mg bisoprolol and 6.25 mg HCTZ. This combination lowered BP better than 25 mg HCTZ and had an effect similar to that of 40 mg bisoprolol. The low-dose combination, however, avoided dose-related bisoprolol adverse events, including somnolence, dyspepsia, diarrhea, and asthenia, as well as the dose-related HCTZ adverse effect of hypokalemia. Labeling therefore identified the low-dose combination as a reasonable initial therapy.

A second combination antihypertensive drug product approved for first-line use is the recently approved combination of losartan and HCTZ for administration in patients with more severe hypertension in whom the need for faster BP control outweighs the risks of initiating treatment with combination therapy. A randomized, double-blind study comparing the combination with losartan monotherapy was conducted in patients with sitting diastolic BPs higher than 110 mm Hg.[55] The primary endpoint in this study was the percentage of patients who reached the goal BP of less than 140/90 mm Hg. Slightly less than 10% of the patients in the losartan monotherapy arm reached the goal, whereas twice as many reached the goal in the combination arm of the study, a statistically significant difference. In this particular population of hypertensive patients, the benefit of reaching BP goal in a relatively short time was judged to outweigh the risk of exposing only approximately 10% of patients to an unnecessary second drug. The initial treatment indication was not extended to patients with lower BPs, because the number of patients in the monotherapy arm to reach the goal would be much greater than 10%, with less reason therefore to give a potentially unnecessary drug. There was no evidence from the studies conducted that initiating treatment with the combination product led to an increased risk of adverse events such as syncope or symptomatic hypotension, although the number of such events that occurred was small.

In the third case, the fixed-dose combination of captopril and HCTZ was approved for first-line use because it permitted once-daily use of captopril, whereas captopril monotherapy required administration twice or three times daily to give acceptable BP control at trough.

In some combination drug products that include an antihypertensive agent, the endpoint targeted by each component is different, such as the combination of amlodipine, a dihydropyridine CCB that lowers BP, and atorvastatin, an HMG-CoA reductase inhibitor that lowers cholesterol. In developing a fixed-dose combination of these two drugs, it was not necessary to show that each component had an effect on both endpoints because such an effect was neither anticipated nor needed. A possible PK interaction should be assessed, and it may be necessary, depending on the information available, to show that there is no PD interaction, for example, that the BP-lowering effect of amlodipine was not decreased in the presence of atorvastatin, and that the cholesterol-lowering effect of atorvastatin was not decreased in the presence of amlodipine. There are, moreover, considerable data showing that statin outcome effects are similar in patients who are, and who are not, receiving antihypertensives and a variety of other drugs, such as aspirin, so PD studies may not be necessary.

SAFETY

As a rule, it does not take very many patients to document and characterize the BP effects of a new antihypertensive agent, including dose-response and interactions with other drugs. The absence of a serious adverse event in a database of a few hundred patients treated for a few weeks, however, would provide very limited reassurance as to safety. Given the availability of many antihypertensives, as well as the potentially large treatment population, the Agency needs to be reasonably sure that the new agent does not have unacceptable toxicity. The ICH E1 guidance suggests approximately 1500 patient exposures for a new drug that is intended for long-term use, with at least 600 patients treated for 6 months.[56] Between 1998 and 2002, three approved antihypertensive NDAs evaluated between 2800 and 3400 patients (Internal FDA data).[57] The database for an unfamiliar class of drugs would probably be larger than the database for another member of a familiar class. Any suggestion of a safety problem would lead to the need for larger databases.

The safety assessment typical of all new drugs, including clinical observations over time, with special attention to deaths (rare in short-term hypertension studies) and other serious adverse events, and laboratory observations (hematology, chemistry, urinalysis, electrocardiograms) are expected of antihypertensive drugs. Assessments of effects on the Q-T interval would also be expected, because these predict an ability to cause torsades de pointes–type ventricular arrhythmias, which have been seen with antihypertensive and antianginal agents such as sotalol and bepridil. Understanding the drug's metabolism, the potential for drug-drug interactions, and drug-disease interactions is also expected. One safety assessment relatively specific for antihypertensive drugs is an evaluation of orthostatic hypotension. Experiences with certain antihypertensives, including β-blockers and central α-agonists, suggest a need to look for withdrawal and rebound effects.

Given the abundance of therapeutic options available for the treatment of hypertension, a new antihypertensive with clinically significant adverse events (e.g., Q-T prolongation, hepatotoxicity) will face difficulties during the approval process. If the drug is a member of a familiar class, such toxicity is likely to render it not approvable. Dilevalol, a β-blocker (with other properties), and tasosartan, an ARB, were not approved because of concerns about hepatotoxicity, an adverse effect not shared by other members of their respective therapeutic classes. Demonstrating an advantage over available therapy, however, could possibly have overcome such concerns. A recent example is omapatrilat, the first member of a new class of antihypertensive agents that simultaneously inhibits both ACE and neutral endopeptidase (NEP). Based on its pharmacologic properties, angioedema, an adverse effect characteristic of all ACE inhibitors, was not an unexpected finding with omapatrilat. However, this drug appeared to cause angioedema at an unacceptably higher rate than other ACE inhibitors and perhaps with greater severity. The sponsor of omapatrilat conducted a large study to show that the increased rate of angioedema with a lower dose of omapatrilat was not more than twice that of enalapril, but the 25,000-patient study showed a risk of angioedema that was 3.2-fold that of enalapril, with some severe cases requiring hospitalization.[57] These findings were not considered acceptable to the Cardiovascular and Renal Drugs Advisory Committee and the Agency in the absence of some documented advantage. The risk, however, could possibly be acceptable if omapatrilat were able to lower BP meaningfully in a patient population resistant to multiple other antihypertensives. Minoxidil is approved for such patients despite substantial toxicity.

ANTIHYPERTENSIVE THERAPY AND PEDIATRICS

The FDAMA of 1997 and the Best Pharmaceuticals for Children Act (BPCA) of 2002 allow the FDA to seek studies of drugs in the pediatric population, with the incentive of an additional 6 months of marketing exclusivity for completion of the requested studies. The Pediatric Research Equity Act of 2003 allows the FDA to require pediatric studies before approval, but the FDA usually defers such requirements until some postmarketing data are available, and then it usually makes the request for studies under the BPCA. These requests, referred to as "written requests," ask sponsors to show an effect on BP, as well as dose-response information, pediatric PK information, and longer-term safety information. Because several classes of antihypertensive agents, when used as monotherapy, have much smaller effects in the black population than they do in whites, a high priority is placed on evaluating the effects of race in studies of these drugs in children. Therefore, written requests for antihypertensive drugs call for 40% to 60% of the population to be black.

To qualify for exclusivity, the study must either show an effect on its prespecified primary endpoint (regardless of the effect size) or rule out a clinically meaningful effect. This latter requirement is implemented by having the observed variance be small enough that it would have been possible to exclude, with 95% confidence, an effect as large as 3 mm Hg had the true mean effect been nil. If no placebo group is used, and no dose response is seen, a randomized withdrawal study can be used to establish whether the drug had an effect.

CONCLUSION

Hypertension is one of the most data-rich therapeutic areas within the FDA. This chapter describes some of the main aspects of antihypertensive drug regulation and discusses evidence needed by the Agency to make an informed decision with respect to benefit and risk.

A future challenge to the Agency will be developing labeling for antihypertensives that describes the established outcome benefits of BP lowering. At a recent meeting of the Cardiovascular and Renal Drugs Advisory Committee,[53] members acknowledged that lowering BP is a very well-established surrogate endpoint, and incorporating outcome data from trials into antihypertensive drug labels would be a worthwhile endeavor.

Finally, because it is unethical to conduct long-term placebo-controlled trials in hypertension, future studies evaluating clinical outcomes can be expected to use active-controlled noninferiority designs. Such studies pose challenging medical and statistical issues, including the choice of a noninferiority margin and the applicability or relevance of evidence in the setting of a constantly changing standard of care.

References

1. Temple R. Are surrogate markers adequate to assess cardiovascular disease drugs? *JAMA.* 1999;**282**:790-795.
2. Collins R, Peto R, MacMahon S, et al. Blood pressure, stroke, and coronary heart disease: Part 2. Short-term reductions in blood pressure: Overview of randomized drug trials in their epidemiologic context. *Lancet.* 1990;**335**:827-838.
3. Staessen J, Fagard R, Thijs L, et al. Randomized double-blind comparison of placebo and active treatment for older patients with isolated systolic hypertension. *Lancet.* 1997;**350**:757-764.
4. SHEP Cooperative Research Group. Prevention of stroke by antihypertensive drug treatment in older persons with isolated systolic hypertension: Final results of the Systolic Hypertension in the Elderly Program (SHEP). *JAMA.* 1991;**265**:3255-3364.
5. Heart Outcomes Prevention Evaluation (HOPE) Study Investigators. Effects of an angiotensin-converting enzyme inhibitor, ramipril, on cardiovascular events in high-risk patients. *N Engl J Med.* 2000;**342**:145-153.
6. ALLHAT Collaborative Research Group. Major cardiovascular events in hypertensive patients randomized to doxazosin vs chlorthalidone: The Antihypertensive and Lipid-Lowering Treatment to Prevent Heart Attack Trial (ALLHAT). *JAMA.* 2000;**283**;1967-1975.
7. ALLHAT Officers and Coordinators for the ALLHAT Collaborative Research Group. Major outcomes in high risk hypertensive patients randomized to angiotensin-converting enzyme inhibitor or calcium channel blocker vs diuretic: The Antihypertensive and Lipid-Lowering Treatment to Prevent Heart Attack Trial (ALLHAT). *JAMA.* 2002;**288**;2981-2997.
8. Wing LMH, Reid CM, Ryan P, et al. A comparison of outcomes with angiotensin-converting-enzyme inhibitors and diuretics for hypertension in the elderly: Second Australian National Blood Pressure Study Group. *N Engl J Med.* 2003;**348**:583-592.
9. Blood Pressure Lowering Treatment Trialists' Collaboration. Effects of different blood pressure–lowering regimens on major cardiovascular events in individuals with and without diabetes mellitus. *Arch Intern Med.* 2005;**165**:1410-1419.
10. Psaty B, Lumley T, Furberg C, et al. Health outcomes associated with various antihypertensive therapies used as first-line agents: A network meta-analysis. *JAMA.* 2003;**289**:2534-2544.
11. Temple R, Ellenberg S. Placebo-controlled trials and active-control trials in the evaluation of new treatments: Part 1. Ethical and scientific issues. *Ann Intern Med.* 2000;**133**:455-463.
12. International Conference of Harmonization. ICH E10 Guidance: Choice of Control Group and Related Issues in Clinical Trials. July 2000. Available at: http://www.ich.org/cache/compo/475-272-1.html#E10 (Accessed August 9, 2006).
13. International Conference of Harmonization. ICH M3 Guidance: Maintenance of the ICH Guideline on Non-Clinical Safety Studies for the Conduct of Human Clinical Trials for Pharmaceuticals. November 2000. Available at: http://www.ich.org/cache/compo/2196-272-1.html#M3 (Accessed August 9, 2006).

14. International Conference of Harmonization. ICH S1A Guidance: Guideline on the Need for Carcinogenicity Studies of Pharmaceuticals. Adopted November 1995. Available at: http://www.ich.org/cache/compo/502-272-1.html#S1A (Accessed August 9, 2006).

15. International Conference of Harmonization. ICH S5 Guidance: Detection of Toxicity to Reproduction for Medicinal Products & Toxicity to Male Fertility. Adopted June 1993. Available at: http://www.ich.org/cache/compo/502-272-1.html#S5A (Accessed August 9, 2006).

16. Temple R. Special study designs: Early escape, enrichment studies in non-responders. *Comm Stat Theory Methods.* 1994;**23**:499-531.

17. International Conference of Harmonization. ICH M4 Guidance: Organization of the Common Technical Document for the Registration of Pharmaceuticals for Human Use. Adopted November 2000. Available at: http://www.ich.org/cache/compo/2196-272-1.html#M4 (Accessed August 9, 2006).

18. Food and Drug Administration/Center for Drug Evaluation and Research. FDA/CDER Guidance: Guideline for the Format and Content of the Clinical and Statistical Sections of an Application. July 1988. Available at: http://www.fda.gov/cder/guidance/statnda.pdf. Accessed November 22, 2005.

19. Center for Drug Evaluation and Research. CDER MaPP 6020.3: Priority Review Policy. April 1996. Available at: http://www.fda.gov/cder/mapp/6020-3.pdf. Accessed November 22, 2005.

20. Food and Drug Administration. FDA Guidance for Industry: Premarketing Risk Assessment. March 2005. Available at: http://www.fda.gov/cder/guidance/6357fnl.htm. Accessed November 22, 2005.

21. Food and Drug Administration. FDA Guidance for Industry: Development and Use of Risk Minimization Action Plans. March 2005. Available at: http://www.fda.gov/cder/guidance/6358fnl.htm. Accessed November 22, 2005.

22. Food and Drug Administration. FDA Guidance for Industry: Good Pharmacovigilance Practices and Pharmacoepidemiologic Assessment. March 2005. Available at: http://www.fda.gov/cder/guidance/6359OCC.htm. Accessed November 22, 2005.

23. Angel M, Dring LG, Lancaster R, et al. Proceedings: A correlation between the response to debrisoquine and the amount of unchanged drug excreted in the urine. *Br J Pharmacol.* 1975;**55**:264P.

24. Sjoqvist F, Bertilsson L. Slow hydroxylation of tricyclic antidepressants: Relationship to polymorphic drug oxidation. *Prog Clin Biol Res.* 1986;**214**:169-88.

25. Food and Drug Administration. FDA Guidance for Industry: Drug Metabolism/Drug Interactions Studies in the Drug Development Process—Studies in Vitro. April 1997. Available at: http://www.fda.gov/cder/guidance/clin3.pdf. Accessed November 22, 2005.

26. Food and Drug Administration. FDA Guidance for Industry: In Vivo Drug Metabolism/Drug Interaction Studies—Study Design, Data Analysis, and Recommendations for Dosing and Labeling. November 1999. Available at: http://www.fda.gov/cder/guidance/2635fnl.pdf. Accessed November 22, 2005.

27. Food and Drug Administration. FDA Guidance for Industry: Guideline for the study and evaluation of Gender Differences in the clinical evaluation of Drugs—Notice. July 1993. Available at: http://www.fda.gov/cder/guidance/old036fn.pdf. Accessed November 22, 2005

28. International Conference of Harmonization. ICH E7 Guidance: Studies in Support of Special Populations—Geriatrics. Adopted June 1993. Available at: http://www.ich.org/cache/compo/475-272-1.html#E7 (Accessed August 9, 2006).

29. Food and Drug Administration. FDA Guidance for Industry: Guideline for the Study of Drugs Likely to Be Used in the Elderly. November 1989. Available at: http://www.fda.gov/cder/guidance/old040fn.pdf. Accessed November 22, 2005.

30. Food and Drug Administration. FDA Guidance for Industry: Pharmacokinetics in Patients with Impaired Renal Function—Study Design, Data Analysis, and Impact on Dosing and Labeling. May 1998. Available at: http://www.fda.gov/cder/guidance/1449fnl.pdf. Accessed November 22, 2005.

31. Food and Drug Administration. FDA Guidance for Industry: Pharmacokinetics in Patients with Impaired Hepatic Function—Study Design, Data Analysis, and Impact on Dosing and Labeling. May 2003. Available at: http://www.fda.gov/cder/guidance/3625fnl.pdf. Accessed November 22, 2005.

32. Sular (nisoldipine) product label. Physicians' Desk Reference, 59th ed. Montvale, NJ: Medical Economics Press, 2005, pp 1260-1262.

33. Food and Drug Administration. FDA Guidance for Industry: Food-Effect Bioavailability and Fed Bioequivalence Studies. December 2002. Available at: http://www.fda.gov/cder/guidance/5194fnl.pdf. Accessed November 22, 2005.

34. Abrahamsson B, Lucker P, Olofsson B, et al. The relationship between metoprolol plasma concentration and beta 1-blockage in healthy subjects: A study on conventional metoprolol and metoprolol CR/ZOK formulations. *J Clin Pharmacol.* 1990; **30(2 Suppl)**:S46-S54.

35. Al-Khatib S, Califf R, Hasselblad V, et al. Placebo-controls in short-term clinical trials of hypertension. *Science.* 2001;**292**: 2013-2015.

36. Food and Drug Administration. PHARM Project (manuscript in preparation). Available at: http://www.fda.gov/ohrms/dockets/ac/06/slides/2006-4215S2-02-index.htm (Accessed August 9, 2006).

37. Food and Drug Administration. FDA Guidance for Industry: Providing Clinical Evidence of Effectiveness for Human Drug and Biologic Products. May 1998. Available at: http://www.fda.gov/cder/guidance/1397fnl.pdf. Accessed November 22, 2005.

38. Cardiovascular and Renal Drugs Advisory Committee meeting, June 2002. Transcript available at: http://www.fda.gov/ohrms/dockets/ac/02/transcripts/3877T1_01.pdf. Accessed November 22, 2005.

39. International Conference of Harmonization. ICH E4 Guidance: Dose-Response Information to Support Drug Registration. March 1994. Available at: http://www.ich.org/cache/compo/475-272-1.html#E4 (Accessed August 9, 2006).

40. Temple R. Dose-response and registration of new drugs. *In:* Lasagna L, Erill S, Naranjo C (eds). Dose-Response Relationships in Clinical Pharmacology. New York: Elsevier, 1989, pp 145-167.

41. Sheiner LB, Beal SL, Sambol NC. Study designs for dose-ranging. *Clin Pharmacol Ther.* 1989;**46**:63-77.

42. International Conference of Harmonization. ICH E7 Guidance: Studies in Support of Special Populations—Geriatrics. June 1993. Available at: http://www.ich.org/cache/compo/475-272-1.html#E7 (Accessed August 9, 2006).

43. Food and Drug Administration. FDA Guidance for Industry Clinical Studies Section of Labeling for Prescription Drugs and Biologics: Content and Format. July 2001. Available at: http://www.fda.gov/cder/guidance/1890dft.htm. Accessed November 22, 2005.

44. Dahlöf B, Devereux B, Kjeldsen S, et al. Cardiovascular morbidity and mortality in the Losartan Intervention for Endpoint Reduction in Hypertension study (LIFE): A randomized trial against atenolol. *Lancet.* 2002;**359**: 995-1003.

45. Veterans Administration Cooperative Study Group on Antihypertensive Agents. Effects of treatment on morbidity in hypertension: Results in patients with diastolic blood pressure averaging 115 through 129 mm Hg. *JAMA*. 1967;**202**: 1028-1034.

46. Veterans Administration Cooperative Study Group on Antihypertensive Agents. Effects of treatment on morbidity in hypertension: II. Results in patients with diastolic blood pressure averaging 90 through 114 mm Hg. *JAMA*. 1970;**213**: 1143-1152.

47. Hypertension Detection and Follow-up Program Cooperative Research Group. Mortality findings for stepped-care and referred-care participants in the Hypertension Detection and Follow-up Program, stratified by other risk factors. *Prev Med*. 1985;**14**:312-335

48. Materson B, Oster J, Michael U, et al. Dose response to chlorthalidone in patients with mild hypertension: Efficacy of a lower dose. *Clin Pharmacol Ther*. 1978;**24**:192-198.

49. Tweeddale M, Ogilvie R, Ruedy J. Antihypertensive and biochemical effects of chlorthalidone. *Clin Pharmacol Ther*. 1977;**22**:519-527.

50. Psaty BM, Furberg CD. Meta-analysis of health outcomes of chlorthalidone-based vs nonchlorthalidone-based low dose diuretic therapies. *JAMA*. 2004;**292**:43-44.

51. Fries ED. Veterans Administration cooperative study on nadolol as monotherapy and in combination with a diuretic. *Am Heart J*. 1984;**108**:1087-1091.

52. Smith D, Neutel J, Lacourciere Y, Kempthorne-Rawson J. Prospective, randomized, open-label, blinded-endpoint (PROBE) designed trials yield the same results as double-blind, placebo-controlled trials with respect to ABPM measurements. *J Hypertens*. 2003;**21**:1237-1239.

53. Cardiovascular and Renal Drugs Advisory Committee meeting, June 2005. Transcript available at: http://www.fda.gov/ohrms/dockets/ac/05/transcripts/2005-4145T1.pdf. Accessed November 22, 2005.

54. Frishman WH, Bryzinski BS, Coulson LR, et al. A multifactorial trial design to assess combination therapy in hypertension: Treatment with bisoprolol and hydrochlorothiazide. *Arch Intern Med*. 1994;**154**:1461-1468.

55. Salerno CM, Demopoulos L, Mukherjee R, Gradman AH. Combination angiotensin receptor blocker/hydrochlorothiazide as initial therapy in the treatment of patients with severe hypertension. *J Clin Hypertens*. 2004;**6**:614-620.

56. International Conference of Harmonization. ICH E1 Guidance: The Extent of Population Exposure to Assess Clinical Safety for Drugs Intended for Long-Term Treatment of Non–Life Threatening Conditions. October 1994. Available at: http://www.ich.org/cache/compo/475-272-1.html E1 (Accessed August 9, 2006).

57. Kostis JB, Packer M, Black HR, et al. Omapatrilat and enalapril in patients with hypertension: the Omapatrilat Cardiovascular Treatment vs. Enalapril (OCTAVE) trial. *Am J Hypertens*. 2004;**17**:103-111.

SECTION 9

Guidelines

U.S. and Canadian Guidelines for Hypertension

Larry E. Fields

Hypertension-focused clinical practice guidelines (CPGs) are the result of important and sustained collaborative efforts that provide evidence-based recommendations for effective prevention and control of high blood pressure (BP) while recognizing that the responsible clinician's judgment remains paramount.[1,2] Evidence-based medicine has the following components: *evidence-based CPGs*, developed by panels of experts for populations and programs; *evidence-based individual decision making* by the physician, tailored to the individual patient; and *other evidence-based health policies and procedures*, developed, implemented, or ensured by others, including health care providers, public health workers, and administrators, for populations as well as individuals.[3] The importance of guideline-based hypertension prevention and control is underscored by the substantial burden of hypertension in the United States and Canada, the 90% lifetime risk of hypertension in a 55-year-old adult, and the phenomenon in hypertensive adults whereby even a modest reduction in BP is typically associated with a moderate or greater decline in cardiovascular or stroke risk over a wide range of BPs.[4-6] This phenomenon is the result of the exponential relationship between BP and risk in adults whose BP is at least 115/75 mm Hg.[7,8] The ultimate impact of CPGs is typically measured in terms of secular trends for hypertension prevalence, awareness, treatment, control, and downstream outcomes. The main goal is to improve BP control rates among hypertensive individuals while reducing the incidence of hypertension in the general population. Success depends on the scientific soundness, clarity, practicality, and adaptability of the consensus recommendations themselves, as well as on successful adoption and implementation of the recommendations at multiple levels, including clinicians and health care team members, patients, health system and health plan administrators and staff, health care policy makers, public health professionals, and others. Accordingly, the pathway for translation of well-written and well-communicated CPGs into high-quality health policy, medical practice, and public health practice is complex and is emblematic of the scientific and artistic nature of effective practice of medicine.[9-11] This chapter includes a review of the U.S. and Canadian historical context, the most recent CPGs, challenges to effective translation into routine practice, and principal considerations for the future.

Challenges are what make life interesting; overcoming them is what makes life meaningful.

—*Joshua J. Marine*[12]

HISTORICAL PERSPECTIVE

In 1708 and 1714, Stephen Hales and his assistant conducted the first direct measurements of arterial BP in animals, the results of which were submitted to the Royal Society of London in 1725 and published in 1733.[13,14] In 1856, J. Faivre reported direct arterial BP measurement in humans.[15] In 1880, Samuel S. K. R. von Basch introduced clinical sphygmomanometry using a water- (later air-) filled bulb and a mercury column or an aneroid pressure gauge.[16] In 1896, Scipione Riva-Rocci reported use of a mercury sphygmomanometer, and the palpatory method for BP measurement.[17] In 1901, Harvey Cushing received a Riva-Rocci device as a gift while in Italy and is reported to be the first to introduce the palpatory method to North American physicians.[18,19] In 1904, Theodore Janeway published guidance on use of the sphygmomanometer.[20] Physicians did not readily adopt the palpatory method. Concerns included a misperceived inferiority of the new quantitative methodology to the well-established qualitative practice of pulse palpation, considerations regarding whether to simplify this technique for use by nonphysicians, and questions regarding whether to promote its standardization for use in individual physician practices.[21]

In 1905, Nicolai S. Korotkoff (also spelled Korotkow or Korotkov) reported an auscultatory method for BP determination.[22-24] The auscultatory technique was more readily accepted into medical practice in the early 1900s.[25-29] In 1917, George W. Norris presented a case definition of hypertension in the third edition of his textbook:

A systolic pressure constantly above 160 mm, or a diastolic pressure constantly above 100 mm Hg, is definitely pathologic at any age. The younger the subject with such a pressure the more abnormal it must be considered. Before middle life 145 mm [systolic] should not be exceeded.—A constant diastolic pressure of or above 100 mm indicates hypertension, regardless of whether the systolic pressure be 180 or 140 mm.[30]

The need for standardization of both practice and devices was formally articulated in 1917 by the Metropolitan Life Insurance Company and in 1927 by the U.S. Department of Commerce's Bureau of Standards.[31-33]

Between 1939 and 2005, the American Heart Association (AHA) published consensus guidelines on standardization of BP measurement.[34-40] The first report was the result of collaboration with an analogous committee representing Great Britain and Ireland. The series soon became the BP measurement standard for interested parties, including health care providers, health policy makers and administrators, investigators, and manufacturers.

The National High Blood Pressure Education Program (NHBPEP) was established in 1972 and is coordinated by the U.S. Department of Health and Human Services' (HHS) National Institutes of Health's (NIH) National Heart, Lung, and Blood Institute (NHLBI). The NHBEP Coordinating Committee is composed of representatives of 39 nonfederal and 8 federal U.S. organizations or agencies (Table 48-1). Since 1976, the NHBPEP Joint National Committee (JNC) on Prevention (added in 1997), Detection, Evaluation, and Treatment of High Blood Pressure has published and periodically updated the principal consensus U.S. hypertension CPGs for adults and for hypertension in pregnancy.[1,41-48] The JNC VI report included the 1993 AHA standards for BP measurement. Since 1977, another NHBPEP group, formerly called the Task Force on Blood Pressure Control in Children, and later named the Working Group on High Blood Pressure in Children and Adolescents (WGTF), has provided four U.S. BP guidelines for children and adolescents (Table 48-2).[49-52]

The U.S. Preventive Services Task Force (USPSTF) of the Agency for Healthcare Research and Quality (AHRQ) published and updated a reinforcing recommendation for hypertension screening, counseling, detection of related risk factors, and other clinical interventions in adults in 1996 and 2003.[53,54] In their latest report, the USPSTF recommendation for children was changed from B (recommends) to I (insufficient evidence). The AHRQ also funds 13 Evidence-based Practice Centers, for the promotion of evidence-based practice in everyday care, and it sponsors the National Guideline Clearing House, a Web-based database of CPGs and related information.[55] The National Guideline Clearing House is the result of a partnership among the AHRQ, the American Medical Association (AMA), and America's Health Insurance Plans (AHIP; formerly the American Association of Health Plans). In 2002, the AHA's Science Advisory and Coordinating Committee published reinforcing consensus guidelines for primary prevention of cardiovascular disease and stroke in adults by means of interventions that include BP control.[56] Additional reinforcing guidelines have been published by several U.S. organizations, including the American Academy of Family Physicians, American College of Obstetricians and Gynecologists, American Academy of Pediatrics, National Center for Education in Maternal and Child Health, American Society of Hypertension, and the AMA.[57-63]

The most recent published set of Canadian guidelines for hypertension was issued in 2006,[64-67] but it has a long history.[68] In 1977, a Health and Welfare Canada committee reported the first national Canadian recommendations on the clinical management of hypertension.[68] The Canadian Hypertension Society (CHS), established in 1979, sponsored development of recommendations in 1984,[69] 1985 (elderly focused), and 1989.[70] The CHS and the Canadian Coalition for High Blood Pressure Prevention and Control (CCHBPPC, established in 1985) co-sponsored recommendations in 1990[71,72] (updated by the CHS in 1993[73-77]) and 1999 (lifestyle focused).[78] The CHS and the Society of Obstetrics and Gynecology of Canada co-sponsored the 1997 recommendations on management of hypertension in pregnancy. The broader 1999 update of 1993 hypertension management

Table 48-1 Organizations Represented on the National High Blood Pressure Education Program's Coordinating Committee in 2006

Nonfederal Organizations

American Academy of Family Physicians
American Academy of Insurance Medicine
American Academy of Neurology
American Academy of Ophthalmology
American Academy of Physician Assistants
American Association of Occupational Health Nurses
American College of Cardiology
American College of Chest Physicians
American College of Occupational and Environmental Medicine
American College of Physicians—ASIM
American College of Preventive Medicine
American Dental Association
American Diabetes Association
American Dietetic Association
American Heart Association
American Hospital Association
American Medical Association
American Nurses Association
American Optometric Association
American Osteopathic Association
American Pharmaceutical Association
American Podiatric Medical Association
American Public Health Association
American Red Cross
American Society of Health-System Pharmacists
American Society of Hypertension
American Society of Nephrology
Association of Black Cardiologists
Citizens for Public Action on High Blood Pressure and Cholesterol, Inc.
Hypertension Education Foundation
International Society on Hypertension in Blacks
National Black Nurses' Association, Inc.
National Hypertension Association, Inc.
National Kidney Foundation, Inc.
National Medical Association
National Optometric Association
National Stroke Association
Society for Nutrition Education
Society of Geriatric Cardiology

Federal Agencies of the U.S. Department of Health and Human Services

Agency for Healthcare Research and Quality
Centers for Medicare & Medicaid Services
Department of Veterans Affairs
Health Resources and Services Administration
National Center for Health Statistics, Centers for Disease Control and Prevention
National Heart, Lung, and Blood Institute
National Heart, Lung, and Blood Institute Ad Hoc Committee on Minority Populations
National Institute of Diabetes and Digestive and Kidney Diseases

Table 48-2   Institutions Represented on the National High Blood Pressure Education Program's Working Group on High Blood Pressure in Children and Adolescents in 2004

Nonfederal Organizations
Children's Hospital of Philadelphia
Cincinnati Children's Hospital Medical Center
DuPont Hospital for Children
Harvard School of Public Health
MassGeneral Hospital for Children
Mayo Clinic
Montefiore Medical Center
Thomas Jefferson University
University of Iowa
University of Michigan
University of Minnesota Medical School
University of Texas Health Science Center
Wake Forest University School of Medicine

Federal Agencies of the U.S. Department of Health and Human Services
National Heart, Lung, and Blood Institute

Table 48-3   Institutions Represented on the Canadian Hypertension Education Program's Hypertension Guidelines Initiative*

Canadian Hypertension Education Program Core Sponsor Organizations (2006)
Blood Pressure Canada
Canadian Council of Cardiovascular Nurses
Canadian Hypertension Society
Canadian Pharmacists Association
College of Family Physicians of Canada
Heart and Stroke Foundation of Canada
Public Health Agency of Canada

Canadian Hypertension Education Program Evidence-Based Recommendations Task Force (Other Represented Institutions) (2005)
Hôtel-Dieu de Quebec
Hôtel-Dieu Health Sciences Hospital
Institut de recherches cliniques de Montréal
Jewish General Hospital
Memorial University of Newfoundland
McMaster University
Mount Sinai Hospital
Sunnybrook & Women's Health Sciences Centre
Université de Montréal
Université Laval
University of Alberta
University of British Columbia
University of Calgary
University of Western Ontario
York University

Canadian Hypertension Education Program Industry Sponsors (2005)
AstraZeneca Canada, Inc.
Bayer, Inc.
Biovail Pharmaceuticals Canada
Boehringer Ingelheim (Canada), Inc.
Bristol-Myers Squibb Canada, Inc.
Merck Frosst Canada & Company
Novartis Pharmaceuticals Canada, Inc.
Pfizer Canada, Inc.
Sanofi Synthelabo Canada, Inc.
Servier Canada, Inc.
Solvay Pharma, Inc.

*Includes an Executive Committee and Implementation and Outcomes Research Task Forces.

recommendations was co-sponsored by the CHS and a wide group of collaborators.[79] The Canadian Hypertension Education Program (CHEP) was formally initiated in 2000 to promote the 1999 recommendations. Since then, the CHEP Evidence-Based Recommendations Task Force has generated the primary Canadian guidelines with annual updates.[2,80-83] CHEP is composed of five core member organizations and is sponsored by 11 pharmaceutical companies (Table 48-3).

U.S. GUIDELINES FOR ADULTS

The Seventh Report of the JNC (JNC 7) provided CPGs for adults that were developed by the chair and members of the NHBPEP Coordinating Committee, based on patient-oriented scientific evidence, graded according to the potential to warrant changes in U.S. medical practice (Table 48-4).[1,41] Disease-oriented evidence was used when patient-oriented evidence was not available. Thirty-three external national hypertension leaders also provided comments.

JNC 7 guidelines recommend assessment and management of all major cardiovascular risk factors (CVRFs). This recommendation reflects the importance of CVRFs. Accordingly, clinical practice success rates are a function of BP control rates as well as rates of control of the other major CVRFs. These include not only hypertension, but also cigarette smoking, obesity (body mass index [BMI] ≥ 30 kg/m^2), physical inactivity, dyslipidemia, diabetes, microalbuminuria or estimated glomerular filtration rate (GFR) less than 60 mL/minute, age greater than 55 years for men and greater than 65 years for women, and a family history of premature cardiovascular disease (i.e., occurrence of a cardiovascular event at <55 years of age in a male or <65 years of age in a female first-degree family member).

JNC 7 guidelines recommend that BP be properly measured in accordance with the established standards for clinical practice.[40] Individuals measuring BP should be properly trained and regularly retrained, and equipment should be regularly

inspected and calibrated, at least semiannually. BP should be measured using the auscultatory method after the patient has been seated quietly for at least 5 minutes and using an appropriately sized cuff with the bladder covering at least 80% of the upper arm circumference. Diastolic BP (DBP) is defined by disappearance of the fifth Korotkoff sound, or by the fourth sound if the fifth sound is persistent. Avoidance of foods and drugs that significantly increase BP is recommended. When standing or palpatory BP measurements are indicated, the appropriate protocol should be followed. The average of at least two BP measurements made during each

Table 48-4 Guidance of the Seventh Report of the Joint National Committee on Prevention, Detection, Evaluation, and Treatment of High Blood Pressure for Adult Blood Pressure Classification, Clinical Follow-up, and Management (>18 Years of Age, Nonpregnant, without Acute End-Organ Damage, Not Hypotensive and Not Taking Antihypertensive Drugs)*

BP Classification	Systolic BP (mm Hg)	Diastolic BP (mm Hg)	Recommended Initial Follow-up	Lifestyle Changes	Initial Therapy Compelling Indications Absent	Initial Therapy Compelling Indications Present	BP Goal (mm Hg) Compelling Indications Absent	BP Goal (mm Hg) Compelling Indications Present
Normal	<120	and <80	Recheck in 2 yr	Encouraged	No antihypertensive drugs indicated	Drugs for compelling indications	<120/80	<120/80
Prehypertension	120-139	or 80-89	Recheck in 1 yr	Recommended: control BP and CVRFs to goal		As above and other antihypertensive drugs as needed (see below); control BP and CVRFs to goal	<140/90	<130/80
Stage 1 hypertension	140-159	or 90-99	Recheck in 2 mo; if confirmed, then evaluate or refer to care	Recommended: control BP and CVRFs to goal	A thiazide diuretic for most; may also consider ACE inhibitor, ARB, BB, CCB, or combination; control BP and CVRFs to goal	Drugs for compelling indications; other antihypertensive drugs as needed (diuretic, ACE inhibitor, ARB, BB, or CCB); control BP and CVRFs to goal	<140/90	<130/80
Stage 2 hypertension	>160	or >100	If BP <180/110 mm Hg, then evaluate or refer to care in <1 mo; if BP >180/110 mm Hg, then initiate evaluation and treatment immediately or in <1wk, depending on clinical assessment	Recommended: control BP and CVRFs to goal	Two-drug combination for most (usually a thiazide diuretic and ACE inhibitor or ARB or BB or CCB); control BP and CVRFs to goal		<140/90	<130/80

*Therapy is determined by the highest BP category. Initial combined therapy should be used cautiously in persons at-risk for hypotension. Compelling indications are heart failure, prior myocardial infarction, diabetes, chronic kidney disease, prior stroke, and high risk of coronary disease.
ACE, angiotensin-converting enzyme; ARB, angiotensin receptor blocker; BB, β-blocker; BP, blood pressure; CCB, calcium channel blocker; CVRF, cardiovascular risk factor.
Modified from Chobanian AV, Bakris GL, Black HR, et al., and the National High Blood Pressure Education Program Coordinating Committee. The Seventh Report of the Joint National Committee on Prevention, Detection, Evaluation, and Treatment of High Blood Pressure: The JNC 7 Report. JAMA. 2003;**289:**2560-2572.

of at least two office visits should be used for classification. All patients should be provided verbal and written documentation of their office visit BP numbers, including a specific BP goal.

JNC 7 guidelines recommend ambulatory BP monitoring (ABPM) for evaluation of adults with suspected white-coat hypertension and no target organ damage (TOD), episodic hypertension, apparent drug resistance, hypotensive symptoms when taking antihypertensive drugs, and autonomic dysfunction. This is at least in part because there are so many more individual measurements available compared with the conventional approach. ABPM is more strongly correlated with TOD than is BP measured during an office visit. In untreated hypertensive adults, an ABPM reading is typically greater than 135/85 mm Hg while the patient is awake or greater than 120/75 mm Hg during sleep.

JNC 7 guidelines note that home/self BP measurement (HSBPM) may be beneficial. HSBPM may be useful in evaluation of white-coat hypertension and response to antihypertensive drugs, and may improve therapeutic adherence. Untreated hypertensive adults typically report HSBPM readings higher than 135/85 mm Hg.

JNC 7 guidelines recommend the use of four categories for classification of BP in adults: normal, prehypertension, stage 1 hypertension, and stage 2 hypertension. This guidance is for nonpregnant U.S. adults who are at least 18 years of age, who are not taking antihypertensive medications, and who are not are not acutely hypotensive. The prior three JNC VI "optimal-normal-borderline" classifications were reduced to two categories, and the three JNC VI stages of hypertension were reduced to two stages. The rationale for these changes includes the findings that (1) the risk of death from ischemic heart disease and stroke rises or falls exponentially as BP rises or falls to more than 115/75 mm Hg, (2) the relative risk of cardiovascular disease is approximately twofold higher in adults whose BP is 130 to 139/85 to 89 mm Hg compared with adults whose BP is less than 120/80 mm Hg, and (3) the management of adults whose BP is 160 to 179/100 to 109 mm Hg is similar to that for those whose BP exceeds 180/100 mm Hg (the prior JNC VI stages 2 and 3 hypertension). Isolated systolic hypertension, defined as systolic BP (SBP) of 140 mm Hg or higher and DBP of less than 90 mm Hg, fits within the four-category JNC 7 framework.

JNC 7 guidelines recommend that adults who have normal BP and who lack a compelling indication for initial drug therapy be encouraged to make appropriate lifestyle changes to reduce cardiovascular risk and to lower the chances of developing hypertension. Prior JNC VI stratification of individuals according to their risk factor status and TOD status was not used in JNC 7. A *compelling indication* is defined as the presence of heart failure, a prior myocardial infarction, diabetes, chronic kidney disease (CKD), or an otherwise high risk of cardiovascular disease (Table 48-5). *CKD* is defined as a GFR lower than 60 mL/minute/1.73 m², more than 300 mg of albuminuria/day, or more than 200 mg albuminuria/1 g creatinine. *Lifestyle changes* include weight reduction in adults with excess weight (overweight or obese), adoption of the Dietary Approaches to Stop Hypertension (DASH) diet, dietary sodium reduction, regular physical activity, and moderation of alcohol consumption. Effective implementation of lifestyle changes in adults can be associated with measurable reductions in SBP such as 5 to 20 mm Hg/10 kg weight loss, 8 to 14 mm Hg with the

DASH diet plan, 2 to 8 mm Hg with dietary sodium reduction, 4 to 9 mm Hg with regular physical activity, and 2 to 4 mm Hg with moderation of alcohol consumption. A regular medical checkup and a BP check at least every 2 years are recommended by the USPSTF.[54]

JNC 7 guidelines recommend that adults who have normal BP and who have at least one compelling indication for initial drug therapy be encouraged to make appropriate lifestyle changes to reduce cardiovascular risk and to lower the chances of developing hypertension, be treated to control the compelling indications, and maintain normal BP. Therapy for a compelling indication is recommended and may include aspirin or management of dyslipidemia or diabetes (see Table 48-5).

JNC 7 guidelines recommend that adults who have prehypertension and who lack a compelling indication for initial drug therapy make appropriate lifestyle changes to reduce cardiovascular risk and to lower the chances of developing hypertension and maintain BP at less than 140/90 mm Hg. Antihypertensive treatment is not indicated for individuals in this category. The prehypertension category is new in JNC 7 and is included to underscore the importance of initiating lifestyle changes early, rather than after the development of hypertension, and to call attention to the increased risk in individuals with this level of BP. The JNC VI classification of "high-normal and normal" did not result in any significant increase in attention to providing unambiguous advice to those with BPs in this range, and so the JNC 7 authors felt the need to highlight the risk in these individuals.

JNC 7 guidelines recommend that adults who have prehypertension and who have at least one compelling indication for initial drug therapy that includes CKD or diabetes make appropriate lifestyle changes to reduce cardiovascular risk and to lower the chances of developing hypertension, be treated to control the compelling indications, and maintain BP lower than 130/80 mm Hg.

JNC 7 guidelines recommend further clinical evaluation of adults with hypertension to identify specific causes, CVRFs including lifestyle, and evidence of TOD or cardiovascular disease. Clinical evaluation should be performed in accordance with accepted standards and should include a high-quality medical history (including a CVRF assessment), physical examination (including assessment of BMI, BP, optic fundi, thyroid, cardiovascular, renal, and neurologic status), routine laboratory tests (including electrocardiogram, urinalysis, hematocrit, blood glucose, serum potassium, creatinine or other estimate of GFR, calcium, and lipid profile), and necessary diagnostic procedures. Additional testing is generally recommended only if BP control is not achieved. TOD is evidenced by the presence of left ventricular hypertrophy, prior myocardial infarction, angina, prior coronary revascularization, heart failure, prior stroke or transient ischemic attack, CKD, peripheral vascular disease, or retinopathy.[84] Identifiable conditions that cause hypertension include sleep apnea, drug-induced or -related causes such as long-term steroid therapy, CKD, primary aldosteronism, renovascular disease, non–drug-associated Cushing's syndrome, pheochromocytoma, coarctation of the aorta, and thyroid and parathyroid diseases. A wide range of drugs can be associated with development of or exacerbation of hypertension. They include nonsteroidal anti-inflammatory agents as well as cyclooxygenase-2 inhibitors (e.g., celecoxib), amphetamines,

Table 48-5   Drug Choices Recommended in the Seventh Report of the Joint National Committee on Prevention, Detection, Evaluation, and Treatment of High Blood Pressure for Adults with Compelling Indications

	ACE Inhibitor	Diuretic	BB	ARB	CCB	Aldosterone Antagonist	Comments
Heart failure	√	√	√	√	—	√	ACE inhibitor and BB if asymptomatic, addition of a loop diuretic along with other agents if symptomatic
Diabetes	√	√	√	√	√	—	Two or more drugs typically needed to achieve BP goal; ACE inhibitors and ARBs reduce albuminuria and slow nephropathy
High coronary disease risk	√	√	√	—	√	—	BB first-line therapy for stable angina, BB and ACE inhibitor first-line therapy for acute coronary syndrome; aspirin and intensive lipid management also indicated
Prior myocardial infarction	√	—	√	—	—	√	Aspirin and intensive lipid management also indicated
Chronic kidney disease	√	—	—	√	—	—	Three or more drugs and added doses of a loop diuretic are often required to reach BP goal, ACE inhibitors and ARBs reduce albuminuria and slow nephropathy
Prior stroke	√	√	—	—	—	—	Risk-to-benefit ratio of acutely lowering BP during a stroke remains unclear

ACE, angiotensin-converting enzyme; ARB, angiotensin receptor blocker; BB, β-blocker; BP, blood pressure; CCB, calcium channel blocker.
Modified from Chobanian AV, Bakris GL, Black HR, et al., and the National High Blood Pressure Education Program Coordinating Committee. The Seventh Report of the Joint National Committee on Prevention, Detection, Evaluation, and Treatment of High Blood Pressure: The JNC 7 Report. *JAMA.* 2003;**289**:2560-2572.

cocaine and other illicit drugs, sympathomimetics (e.g., decongestants or anorectics), oral contraceptives, corticosteroids, cyclosporine and tacrolimus, erythropoietin, high-quality and usually imported licorice (which may also be found in some chewing tobacco), and certain over-the-counter drugs and dietary supplements (ephedra, also known as Ma huang, which was banned by the U.S. government in 2004, or bitter orange; Table 18 in the full report).

JNC 7 guidelines recommend that adults who have stage 1 hypertension and who lack a compelling indication for initial drug therapy make appropriate lifestyle changes to reduce cardiovascular risk and to lower the chances of developing hypertension and receive antihypertensive drug therapy to lower BP to less than 140/90 mm Hg. A thiazide-type diuretic is typically appropriate as initial antihypertensive drug therapy for most adults with stage 1 hypertension who lack a compelling indication. Additional antihypertensive drugs include an

angiotensin-converting enzyme (ACE) inhibitor, an angiotensin receptor blocker (ARB), a β-blocker (BB), a calcium channel blocker (CCB), or a combination. The BP goal can be achieved in most hypertensive adults. The stepped-care model should be used in which drug therapy begins at the lowest dose, followed by a stepwise increase until the BP goal is achieved or until the development of side effects necessitates addition or substitution of another class of drug.

JNC 7 guidelines recommend that adults who have stage 1 hypertension and who have at least one compelling indication for initial drug therapy make appropriate lifestyle changes to reduce cardiovascular risk and to lower the chances of developing hypertension and be treated to control the compelling indications and to lower BP to less than 140/90 mm Hg. Antihypertensive drugs may include a thiazide-type diuretic, an ACE inhibitor, an ARB, a BB, or a CCB as needed. The recommended first-line drug for hypertensive adults with stable angina is a BB, and a CCB is an alternative. Initial therapy with a BB and an ACE inhibitor is recommended for hypertensive adults with recent acute coronary syndrome.

JNC 7 guidelines recommend that adults who have stage 2 hypertension and who lack a compelling indication for initial drug therapy make appropriate lifestyle changes to reduce cardiovascular risk and to lower the chances of developing hypertension and receive antihypertensive drug therapy to lower BP to less than 140/90 mm Hg. Two classes of antihypertensive drugs are typically required as initial drug therapy for most adults with stage 2 hypertension who lack a compelling indication, one of which is a thiazide-type diuretic for most people. The other classes of antihypertensive drugs include an ACE inhibitor, an ARB, a BB, or a CCB.

JNC 7 guidelines recommend that adults who have stage 2 hypertension and who have at least one compelling indication for initial drug therapy make appropriate lifestyle changes to reduce cardiovascular risk and to lower the chances of developing hypertension and be treated to control the compelling indications and to lower BP to less than 140/90 mm Hg. Other antihypertensive drugs include a diuretic, an ACE inhibitor, an ARB, a BB, or a CCB as needed.

JNC 7 guidelines recommend a thiazide diuretic as the initial therapy for most hypertensive adults, either alone or in combination with another class of antihypertensive drug, toward reaching the designated BP goal. JNC 7 continues to base pharmacologic treatment on the stepped-care model (Fig. 48-1).

JNC 7 guidelines note that diuretics continue to be underutilized in the treatment of hypertensive adults, either alone or in combination with another class of antihypertensive drug. Use of diuretics is usually associated with achievement of BP control when this class of drugs is used alone or in combination, it enhances the efficacy of multidrug antihypertensive regimens, and it typically costs significantly less to purchase than any other antihypertensive drug.

JNC 7 guidelines recommend that adults with a hypertension emergency be treated using intravenous antihypertensive drugs. A hypertensive emergency requires immediate medical care. A hypertensive emergency is the presence of hypertension (typically >180/120 mm Hg, but occasionally with lower readings in a previously healthy and normotensive person) accompanied by symptoms or signs of severe or ongoing TOD, including encephalopathy, intracranial hemorrhage, acute myocardial infarction, acute coronary syndrome, dissecting aortic aneurysm, and eclampsia. Therapy should be carefully titrated to achieve a controlled reduction of mean arterial BP, typically up to 10% to 25% over the first 2 to 4 hours after presentation and then gradually more toward normal levels over 24 to 48 hours. Exceptions include adults with ischemic stroke, for whom immediate BP reduction is generally not required or recommended, aortic dissection (for which the goal BP is an SBP <120 mm Hg), and those patients in whom BP is lowered to facilitate use of thrombolytic agents.

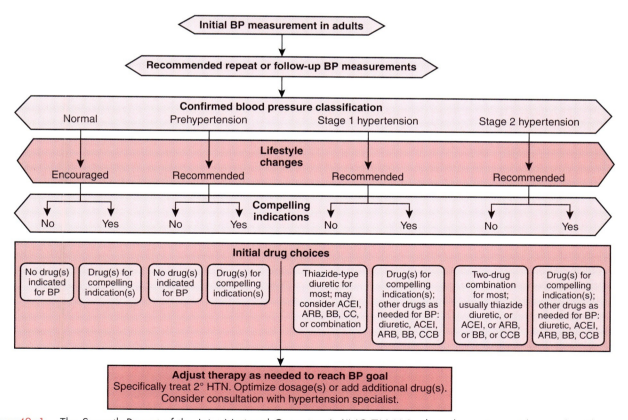

Figure 48-1   The Seventh Report of the Joint National Committee's (JNC 7's) U.S. clinical practice guidance algorithm for therapy of hypertension in adults. 2° HTN, secondary hypertension; ACEI, angiotensin-converting enzyme inhibitor; ARB, angiotensin receptor blocker; BB, β-blocker; BP, blood pressure; CCB, calcium channel blocker. (Data from reference 1.)

U.S. GUIDELINES FOR CHILDREN AND ADOLESCENTS

In 2004, the NHBPEP WGTF published the Fourth Report on the Diagnosis, Evaluation, and Treatment of High Blood Pressure in Children and Adolescents (WGTF 4; Table 48-6).[49] The overall WGTF 4 framework is consistent with that of JNC 7. WGTF 4 is based on patient-oriented scientific evidence, disease-oriented evidence, and consensus expert opinion when evidence was not available.

WGTF 4 guidelines recommend that all children who are more than 3 years of age have their BP measured at least once while in a medical setting, in accordance with the WGTF 4–recommended standard for clinical practice. Pending adoption of a universal standard for children and adolescents that is analogous to that for adults, WGTF 4 makes detailed recommendations for measuring BP. Only appropriately trained personnel who are regularly trained and retrained should perform BP measurements. Equipment should be inspected and calibrated at least semiannually. WGTF 4 recommends use of a well-calibrated aneroid manometer when a mercury column is not available. The auscultatory method is recommended as the preferred technique, because the BP tables are based on this technique. As with adults, WGTF 4 recommends avoidance of foods and drugs that significantly increase BP, having the patient be seated for at least 5 minutes, preferential use of the right arm, and use of an appropriately sized cuff, the bladder of which covers at least 80% of the arm circumference. The WGTF 4 guidelines recommend use of standard BP cuff bladder sizes, based on the arm circumference and a 1:2 bladder width-to-length ratio. As with adults, WGTF 4 recommends that DBP be defined as loss of the fifth Korotkoff sound. The fourth Korotkoff sound is used only when the fifth sound persists or is too low. If SBP or DBP is at the 90th percentile or higher or if an adolescent's BP is higher than 120/80 mm Hg, then measurement should be repeated during the same session. WGTF 4 recommends that in the absence of severe hypertension, an average of multiple BP measurements taken over weeks to months be used for BP classification in children and adolescents. Once hypertension is confirmed, BP should be measured in both arms and a leg to ascertain the presence or absence of coarctation of the aorta.

WGTF 4 guidelines recommend that selected children who are less than 3 years of age and who have specific conditions have their BP measured at least once while in a medical setting in accordance with the WGTF 4–recommended standard for clinical practice. The WGTF 4 guidelines recommend BP measurement in children less than 3 years of age who have specific conditions. Such conditions include neonatal complications requiring intensive care, including prematurity or low birth weight, treated or untreated congenital heart disease, renal disease or urologic malformations or recurrent urinary tract infection or hematuria or proteinuria, a family history of congenital renal disease, a solid organ transplant, malignancy or a bone marrow transplant, treatment with drugs known to increase BP, increased intracranial pressure, or the presence of a systemic illness typically associated with hypertension such as neurofibromatosis or tuberous sclerosis. WGTF 4 recommends use of a well-calibrated automated (oscillometric) BP measuring device for newborns, young infants, and children in the intensive care setting. WGTF 4 recommends confirmation of elevated oscillometric BP readings using the auscultatory method.

WFTF 4 guidelines recommend ABPM in children and adolescents for evaluation of white-coat hypertension, cardiovascular risk, and apparent antihypertensive drug resistance or associated hypotensive episodes. ABPM should be used by pediatric hypertension experts, experienced in its proper use and interpretation.

WGTF 4 guidelines recommend the use of the four categories for classification of BP in children and adolescents: normal, prehypertension, stage 1 hypertension, and stage 2 hypertension (see Table 48-6). Recommended standard BP tables for children and adolescents 1 to 17 years of age account for variability related to gender, age, and height.[49] SBP is used to define hypertension in children less than 1 year of age.[50] The use of four categories for BP classification results from use of the JNC 7 framework for consistency. The 50th and 99th percentiles are new relative to WGTF 3 to facilitate clinical decision making.

WGTF 4 guidelines recommend that children and adolescents who have normal BP and who lack a compelling indication for initial drug therapy be encouraged, along with their parents, to make appropriate lifestyle changes to reduce cardiovascular risk and to lower the chances of developing hypertension (Fig. 48-2). A *compelling indication* is defined as the presence of heart failure, diabetes, CKD, or left ventricular hypertrophy. Recommended lifestyle changes include adoption and use of the DASH diet (parents and children or adolescents may initially benefit from consultation with a registered or licensed nutritionist), appropriate sleep, and regular physical activity.

WGTF 4 guidelines recommend that children and adolescents who have normal BP and who have at least one compelling indication for initial drug therapy be encouraged to make appropriate lifestyle changes to reduce cardiovascular risk and to lower the chances of developing hypertension and be treated to control the compelling indications.

WGTF 4 guidelines recommend that children and adolescents who have prehypertension and who lack a compelling indication for initial drug therapy make appropriate lifestyle changes to reduce cardiovascular risk and to lower the chances of developing hypertension and maintain a BP at less than the 95th percentile or, for adolescents, lower than 120/80 mm Hg. Addition of the prehypertension category by WGTF 4 is consistent with JNC 7 and emphasizes the importance of initiating lifestyle changes early. Lifestyle changes in this and subsequent categories include losing excess weight, maintaining a healthy eating plan, and obtaining regular physical activity. A loss of excess weight (~10% decrease in BMI) can be associated with an 8 to 12 mm Hg fall in BP in adolescents. Reduced dietary sodium consumption by children and adolescents can be associated with 1 to 3 mm Hg reductions in BP. Weight reduction is better achieved when regular physical activity and a healthy eating plan are combined.

WGTF 4 guidelines recommend that children and adolescents who have prehypertension and who have at least one compelling indication for initial drug therapy that includes CKD or diabetes make appropriate lifestyle changes to reduce cardiovascular risk and lower the chances of developing hypertension, be treated to control the compelling indications, and maintain a BP at less than the 95th percentile or, for adolescents, lower than 120/80 mm Hg.

WGTF 4 guidelines recommend clinical evaluation of children and adolescents with hypertension (BP >95th percentile)

Table 48-6 Guidance of the Working Group on High Blood Pressure in Children and Adolescents, Fourth Report, for Child and Adolescent Blood Pressure Classification, Clinical Follow-up, and Management (1 to 18 Years of Age, Nonpregnant, without Acute End-Organ Damage, Not Hypotensive, and Not Taking Antihypertensive Drugs)*

BP Classification	Systolic or Diastolic BP (Percentile, mm Hg)	Recommended Initial Follow-up	Lifestyle Changes	Initial Therapy — Compelling Indications		BP Goal (Percentile, mm Hg) — Compelling Indications	
				Absent	Present	Absent	Present
Normal	<90th	Recheck at next physical examination	Encouraged: healthy diet, sleep, and physical activity	None	Treat compelling indications	<90th	<90th
Prehypertension	90th-<95th or BP >120/80 mm Hg (even if BP <90th)	Recheck in 6 mo	Recommended: loss of excess weight, healthy diet, and physical activity	None	Treat compelling indications	<95th or BP <120/80 mm Hg	<95th or BP <120/80 mm Hg
Stage 1 hypertension	95th-99th (+ 5 mm Hg)	Confirm in 1-2 wk or in <1 wk if symptomatic; if BP elevated on a total of three occasions, evaluate or refer to care in <1 mo	Recommended: loss of excess weight, healthy diet, and physical activity; control to goal	Initiate therapy if symptomatic or in presence of secondary hypertension, hypertensive target organ damage, diabetes, or if lifestyle changes alone are ineffective; control to goal	Treat compelling indications; initiate antihypertensive drug therapy as needed and control to goal	<95th or BP <120/80 mm Hg	<95th or BP <120/80 mm Hg
Stage 2 hypertension	>(99th + 5 mm Hg)	Confirm, evaluate, and refer immediately if symptomatic; otherwise, if BP elevated on a total of three occasions, evaluate or refer to care in <1 wk	Recommended: loss of excess weight, healthy diet, and physical activity; control to goal	Initiate therapy and control to goal	Treat compelling indications; initiate antihypertensive drug therapy as needed and control to goal	<95th or BP <120/80 mm Hg	<95th or BP <120/80 mm Hg

*Excess weight means overweight or obese. Therapy is determined by the highest blood pressure category and may require more than one drug. Compelling indications are heart failure, diabetes, chronic kidney disease, and left ventricular hypertrophy.
BP, blood pressure.
Modified from National High Blood Pressure Education Program Working Group on High Blood Pressure in Children and Adolescents. The Fourth Report on the diagnosis, evaluation, and treatment of high blood pressure in children and adolescents. *Pediatrics.* 2004;**114 (2 Suppl)**:555-576.

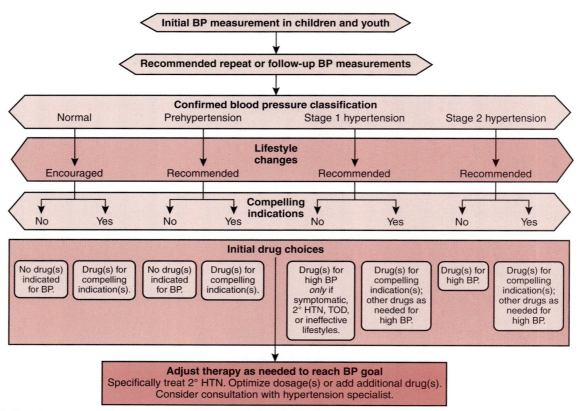

Figure 48–2   The Working Group (formerly Task Force) on High Blood Pressure in Children and Adolescents, Fourth Report's (WGTF 4's) U.S. clinical practice guidance algorithm for therapy of hypertension in children and adolescents. 2° HTN, secondary hypertension; BP, blood pressure; TOD, target organ damage.

to identify potential causes, CVRFs including lifestyle, and evidence of TOD or co-morbidity. Clinical evaluation should be performed in all hypertensive children and adolescents in accordance with accepted standards and should include a high-quality medical history (including sleep patterns, relevant family conditions, CVRF and lifestyle assessment, and symptoms of TOD), physical examination (including BMI and signs of TOD), routine laboratory tests (including electrolytes, complete blood count, blood urea nitrogen, serum creatinine, urinalysis, urine culture, and renal ultrasound; a lipid profile and fasting glucose for all hypertensive patients as well as for prehypertensive persons with excess weight, a family history of hypertension or cardiovascular disease, or CKD; an echocardiogram and retinal examination for all hypertensive patients as well as for prehypertensive persons with comorbidity including diabetes or CKD), and other diagnostic procedures as indicated. Additional testing may be indicated in specific circumstances, including the following: a drug screen or polysomnography if the history suggests substance or drug use or sleep disorder; ABPM for suspected white-coat hypertension or for other informational needs; and plasma renin, plasma and urine catecholamines, and steroid levels in young children with stage 1 hypertension or in children or adolescents with stage 2 hypertension. Plasma renin levels may also be indicated in children or adolescents with a family history of severe hypertension. Renovascular imaging may be indicated to identify renovascular disease in young children with stage 1 hypertension, or in children or adolescents with stage 2 hypertension.

WGTF 4 guidelines recommend that children and adolescents who have stage 1 hypertension and who lack a compelling indication for initial drug therapy make appropriate lifestyle changes to reduce cardiovascular risk and to lower the chances of developing hypertension, and, if indicated, receive antihypertensive drug therapy to lower BP to less than the 95th percentile or, in adolescents, to less than 120/80 mm Hg. Antihypertensive drug therapy is indicated for children and adolescents who are symptomatic, who have secondary hypertension or hypertensive TOD or diabetes, or who lack a desired response to lifestyle changes alone. Management decisions about hypertension in children and adolescents should be based on the degree or severity of BP elevation. The responsible physician makes the choice of drug for initial antihypertensive therapy. The stepped-care model is also recommended for children: begin with the lowest recommended dose of antihypertensive drug and increase it in stepwise fashion until BP control is achieved or until side effects dictate use of a second class of drug to facilitate avoidance of doses that are associated with development of side effects. Specific classes of antihypertensive drugs are recommended for children or adolescents with certain medical conditions such as use of an ACE inhibitor or ARB in individuals with diabetes and microalbuminuria or proteinuric CKD and the use of a BB or CCB in hypertensive children with migraine headaches. It may be appropriate to consider step-down therapy, an attempt to gradually reduce drug dose, in selected patients in whom BP has been controlled for an extended period of time. Individuals with hypertension who lack TOD or other complications, and those with excess weight who successfully lower their weight, are the best candidates for step-down therapy.

WGTF 4 guidelines recommend that children and adolescents who have stage 1 or 2 hypertension and who have at least one compelling indication for initial drug therapy make appropriate lifestyle changes to reduce cardiovascular risk and to lower the chances of developing hypertension, be treated to control the compelling indications, and to lower BP to less than the 95th percentile or, in adolescents, to less than 120/80 mm Hg. A definite indication for initiation of antihypertensive drug therapy in children or adolescents should be ascertained before beginning drug treatment (see earlier).

WGTF 4 guidelines recommend that children and adolescents who have stage 2 hypertension and who lack a compelling indication for initial drug therapy make appropriate lifestyle changes to reduce cardiovascular risk and to lower the chances of developing hypertension and receive antihypertensive drug therapy to lower BP to less than the 95th percentile or, in adolescents, to less than 120/80 mm Hg. Participation in competitive sports should be limited only in the presence of uncontrolled stage 2 hypertension. A definite indication for initiation of antihypertensive drug therapy in children or adolescents should be ascertained before beginning drug treatment (see earlier).

WGTF 4 guidelines recommend that children and adolescents who have stage 2 hypertension and who have at least one compelling indication for initial drug therapy make appropriate lifestyle changes to reduce cardiovascular risk and to lower the chances of developing hypertension and be treated to control the compelling indications and to lower BP to less than the 95th percentile or, in adolescents, to less than 120/80 mm Hg. A definite indication for initiation of antihypertensive drug therapy in children or adolescents should be ascertained before beginning drug treatment (see earlier). Participation in competitive sports should be limited only in the presence of uncontrolled stage 2 hypertension.

WGTF 4 guidelines recommend that children and adolescents with a hypertension emergency be treated using intravenous antihypertensive drugs. A hypertensive emergency requires immediate medical care. A hypertensive emergency is the presence of hypertension accompanied by symptoms or signs of encephalopathy, typically seizures. Therapy is carefully titrated to achieve a controlled reduction of mean arterial BP, typically less than 10% to 25% over the first 8 hours after presentation and then gradually more toward normal levels over 26 to 48 hours.

CANADIAN GUIDELINES FOR ADULTS

The 2006 CHEP Evidence-Based Recommendations Task Force adult hypertension guidelines are based on the most significant scientific evidence available (CHEP 7; Table 48-7). As before, recommendations are graded from A to D to reflect the strength of the evidence base.[68] Grade A indicates an evidence base consisting of studies with a high level of internal validity, statistical precision, clinical relevance, and applicability of the information to patients. Grades B and C are intermediate. Grade D indicates a basis composed primarily of expert opinion. Following discussions at consensus conferences, Canadian Hypertension Working Group members vote to accept or reject updated recommendations. The 2006 Canadian guidelines emphasize improved medication adher-

ence and continuity, expedited diagnosis of hypertension, the use of office or APBM or HSBPM to diagnose hypertension, and the significantly higher importance of achieving BP control to reduce risk than in choosing which first-line antihypertensive drug to use.

CHEP 7 guidelines continue to recommend assessment and management of the adult's global cardiovascular risk, including significant risk factors other than hypertension. Hypertension management recommendations including target BPs reflect the importance of CVRFs. Accordingly, BP control rates, as well as rates of control of other significant CVRFs, are important in evaluating the success of hypertension-related clinical practice.

CHEP 7 guidelines recommend that specifically trained health care professionals measure BP in adults at all appropriate visits using standardized techniques for sphygmomanometry. All BP measurement devices (mercury, aneroid, or oscillometric) should be calibrated at least annually and may be used to diagnose hypertension.[2,64] The individual should be comfortably and quietly seated for 5 minutes with legs uncrossed. BP should be measured at least once in each arm (at heart level), with an appropriately sized cuff, and using the arm with the higher pressure thereafter. Digit preference (rounding) should be avoided. If the initial reading is elevated, at least two measurements should be taken in the same arm and position. BP measurement after standing 2 minutes is recommended, and supine determinations may also be helpful. DBP is defined by disappearance of the fifth Korotkoff sound, or by the fourth sound if the fifth sound is persistent. The average of more than the usual number of BP measurements may be needed in persons with an arrhythmia.

CHEP 7 guidelines recommend the use of office- or clinic-based BP readings, ABPM, or HSBPM to expedite the diagnosis of hypertension further. This recommendation is based on accumulating evidence indicating significant variation in the accuracy of office-based measurements and similar or better effectiveness of ABPM or HSBPM, compared with the office- or clinic-based approach. All responsible parties should be properly trained, and devices should be regularly calibrated. ABPM-diagnosed hypertension is defined as awake SBP of 135 mm Hg or higher or awake DBP of 85 mm Hg higher or 24-hour SBP of 130 mm Hg or higher or 24-hour DBP of 80 mm Hg or higher. HSBPM-diagnosed hypertension is defined as SBP of 135 mm Hg or higher or DBP of 85 mm Hg or higher.

CHEP 7 guidelines recommend the use of the seven World Health Organization/International Society of Hypertension (WHO/ISH) categories for classification of BP in adults: optimal, normal, high normal, and grade 1, grade 2, grade 3, and isolated systolic hypertension (see Table 48-7).[85] Borderline hypertension and borderline isolated systolic hypertension comprise two classification subgroups (140 to 159/90 to 94 mm Hg and 140 to 159/<90 mm Hg, respectively).

CHEP 7 guidelines recommend expedited diagnosis of hypertension in adults. Diagnosis, evaluation, and management of a hypertensive emergency or urgency can be done during the initial encounter. Diagnosis can be made at the second encounter in adults with TOD, CKD, diabetes, or a BP of 180/110 mm Hg or more. Diagnosis can be made at the third encounter in the remaining adults with SBP of at least 160 but less than 180 mm Hg or DBP of at least 100 but less than 110 mm Hg. At visit 4 or 5 the diagnosis depends on an SBP of at least 140 or a DBP of at least 90 mm Hg.

Table 48-7 Guidance of the Seventh Report of the Canadian Hypertension Education Program for Adult Blood Pressure Classification, Clinical Follow-up, and Management (Patients Older than 18 Years of Age, Nonpregnant, without Acute End-Organ Damage, Not Hypotensive, and Not Taking Antihypertensive Drugs)*

BP Classification	Systolic BP (mm Hg)	Diastolic BP (mm Hg)	Lifestyle Changes	Recommended Initial Follow-up	Initial Therapy — Compelling Indications		BP Goal (mm Hg) — Compelling Indications	
					Absent	Present	Absent	Present
Optimal	<120	<80	Recommended achieve CVRF goal	Recheck in <2 yr	No antihypertensive drug(s) indicated	Drugs for CIs	<120/80	<120/80
Normal	<130	<85	Recommended control BP and other CVRFs to goal	Recheck in <2 yr		As above and other antihypertensive drugs as needed (see below); control BP and CVRFs to goal	<130/85	<130/80; if proteinuria >1 g/hr then <125/75
High-normal BP	130-139	85-89	Recommended control BP and other CVRFs to goal	Recheck in <1 yr			<140/90	<130/80; if proteinuria >1 g/hr then <125/75
Grade 1 hypertension	140-159	90-99	Recommended control BP and other CVRFs to goal	Recheck in <1 mo; if TOD, DM, CKD, or BP >180/110 mm Hg, then Dx is HTN; otherwise, recheck in <1 mo; if BP <160/100 mm Hg, then recheck in <1 mo; if BP >140/90 mm Hg, then Dx is HTN	Monotherapy (thiazide diuretic, ACE inhibitor, ARB, BB, or CCB); then combination therapy (e.g., thiazide diuretic or CCB plus ACE inhibitor or ARB or BB); then other classes of antihypertensive drugs including nonthiazide diuretic, α-blocker, centrally acting agent, or nondihydropyridine CCB; control BP and CVRFs to goal	Drugs for CIs; other antihypertensive drugs as needed (initially a diuretic, ACE inhibitor, ARB, BB, or CCB; then steps as noted in the left column); control BP and other CVRFs to goal	<140/90	<130/80; if proteinuria >1 g/hr then <125/75

Table 48-7 Guidance of the Seventh Report of the Canadian Hypertension Education Program for Adult Blood Pressure Classification, Clinical Follow-up, and Management (Patients Older than 18 Years of Age, Nonpregnant, without Acute End-Organ Damage, Not Hypotensive, and Not Taking Antihypertensive Drugs)*—cont'd

BP Classification	Systolic BP (mm Hg)	Diastolic BP (mm Hg)	Recommended Initial Follow-up	Initial Therapy Lifestyle Changes	Compelling Indications Absent	Compelling Indications Present	BP Goal (mm Hg) Absent	BP Goal (mm Hg) Present
Grade 2 hypertension	160-179	100-109	Recheck in <1 mo; if TOD, DM, CKD, or BP >180/110 mm Hg, then Dx is HTN; otherwise, recheck in <1 mo; if BP >160/100 mm Hg, then Dx is HTN	Recommended control BP and other CVRFs to goal			<140/90	<130/80; if proteinuria >1 g/hr then <125/75
Grade 3 hypertension	>180	>110	If symptomatic, then Dx is HTN; otherwise, recheck in <1 mo; if BP >180/110 mm Hg, then Dx is HTN	Recommended control BP and other CVRFs to goal			<140/90	<130/80; if proteinuria >1 g/hr then <125/75

*Ambulatory blood pressure measurement or home/self blood pressure measurement may be substituted for office-based measurements for diagnosis of hypertension, determined by the highest blood pressure category. Initial combined therapy should be used cautiously in persons at-risk for hypotension. Compelling indications are diabetes mellitus or chronic kidney disease. Isolated systolic hypertension is systolic blood pressure greater than 140 mm Hg and diastolic blood pressure less than 90 mm Hg, the goal is less than 140 mm Hg, and initial drug therapy includes a thiazide diuretic, calcium channel blocker, or angiotensin receptor blocker; other drug classes are added or substituted, or combination therapy is used as needed. Assess urinary albumin excretion in diabetic adults. First-line use of BB recommended only for appropriate adults younger than 60 years.

ACE, angiotensin-converting enzyme; ARB, angiotensin receptor blocker; BB, β-blocker; BP, blood pressure; CCB, calcium channel blocker; CI, compelling indication; CKD, chronic kidney disease; CVRF, cardiovascular risk factor; DM, diabetes mellitus; Dx, diagnosis; HTN, hypertension; TOD, target organ damage;
Modified from references 64 and 65.

CHEP 7 guidelines emphasize that the actual extent of BP lowering achieved is more important in reducing hypertension-related complications than is the specific first-line drug class used.

CHEP 7 guidelines recommend that adults with optimal, normal, or high-normal BP and who lack a compelling indication make appropriate lifestyle changes. These individuals do not require antihypertensive drugs (Tables 48-7 and 48-8; Fig. 48-3). Lifestyle changes (modifications) are important and continue to be the cornerstone of antihypertensive or antiatherosclerotic therapy. Lifestyles are mainly determined by a person's environment. Lifestyle interventions include *regular dynamic physical exercise* (30 to 60 minutes at moderate intensity, 4 to 7 days/week); *control of BMI and waist circumference* (to 18.5 to 24.9 kg/m² or <102 cm or 88 cm for men or women, respectively); *moderate alcohol consumption* for healthy adults who drink up to 2 drinks/day, not exceeding 14/week in men and 9/week in women (1 drink = 360 mL of 5% beer, 150 mL of 12% wine, or 45 mL of 40% spirits [80 proof]); *consumption of a DASH diet,* with *reduced salt intake* (for hypertensive adults or salt-sensitive populations including Canadians of African descent, adults >45 years of age or with diabetes or impaired renal function; 65 to 100 mmol/day sodium); *adequate intake of potassium, calcium, and magnesium* (supplementation is not recommended for prevention or treatment of hypertension); and *consideration of stress management* for hypertensive adults in whom stress is deemed to be a contributing factor. Most hypertensive adults require a combination of lifestyle changes and drug therapy to achieve adequate BP control.

CHEP 7 guidelines recommend that adults with optimal BP and who have at least one compelling indication make appro-

Table 48-8 Drug Choices Recommended by the Seventh Report of the Canadian Hypertension Education Program for Adults with Specific Comorbidities*

	ACE Inhibitor	Diuretic	β-Blocker	ARB	CCB	Aldosterone Antagonist	Comments
Heart failure	1	1	1	2	—	1	Spironolactone (1), thiazide or loop diuretic (2), hydralazine (2), isosorbide dinitrate (2)
Diabetes	1	1	2	1	2	—	Thiazide diuretic (1), combinations of first-line drugs (2), loop diuretic for serum creatinine >150 μmol/L
Diabetes and nephropathy	1	2	2	1	2	—	Add thiazide diuretic (2), ACE inhibitor/ARB combination (2)
Prior myocardial infarction	1	—	1	—	—	—	Combinations of additional agents (2)
Renal disease	1	2	—	—	—	—	Diuretic as additive therapy (2), combinations of additional agents (2), avoid ACE inhibitor in bilateral renal stenosis
Prior stroke or transient ischemic attack	1	1	—	—	—	—	ACE inhibitor/diuretic combinations preferred
Angina	—	—	1	—	2	—	Strongly consider adding ACE inhibitor (1), avoid short-acting nifedipine
Left ventricular hypertrophy	1	1	—	1	1	—	β-Blocker if <55 yr of age (1)
Peripheral artery disease	—	—	—	—	—	—	Does not affect initial treatment recommendations; avoid ACE inhibitor in bilateral renal stenosis
Dyslipidemia	—	—	—	—	—	—	Does not affect initial treatment recommendations

*Diabetes and chronic kidney disease are compelling indications.
1, first-line therapy; 2, second-line therapy; ACE, angiotensin-converting enzyme; ARB, angiotensin receptor blocker; CCB, calcium channel blocker. First-line use of β-blocker recommended only for appropriate adults younger than 60 years.
Modified from references 64 and 65.

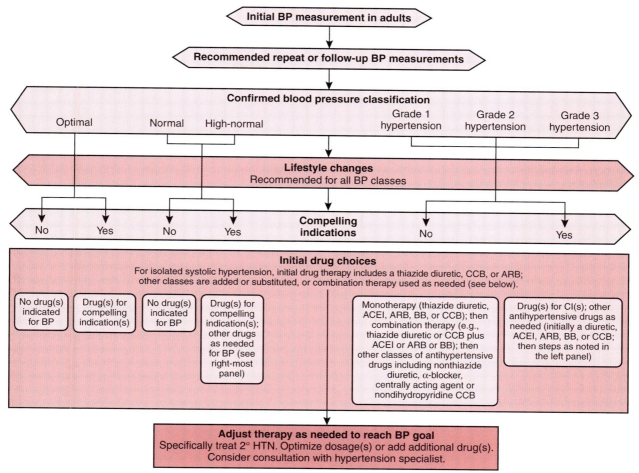

Figure 48–3　The Seventh Report of the Canadian Hypertension Education Program's (CHEP 7) clinical practice guidance algorithm for therapy of hypertension in adults. 2° HTN, secondary hypertension; ACEI, angiotensin-converting enzyme inhibitor; ARB, angiotensin receptor blocker; BB, β-blocker (age younger than 60 years); BP, blood pressure; CCB, calcium channel blocker.

priate lifestyle changes and receive therapy for the compelling indications. Treatment with antihypertensive drugs is not necessarily indicated for this population, but if the compelling indication requires treatment with an antihypertensive agent, it should be given. Drug therapy for a compelling indication may include aspirin or statins.

CHEP 7 guidelines recommend that adults with normal or high-normal BP and who have at least one compelling indication make appropriate lifestyle changes and receive therapy for compelling indications as well as antihypertensive therapy to achieve the recommended BP goal. The BP goal is less than 140/90 mm Hg for most patients without diabetes or CKD and less than 130/80 mm Hg for patients with diabetes or CKD (without significant proteinuria) and less than 125/75 mm Hg for patients with proteinuria exceeding 1g/day. Any one of the five antihypertensive drug classes may be used as first-line monotherapy in hypertensive adults, including a thiazide-like diuretic, a BB, an ACE inhibitor, an ARB, or a CCB (see Table 48-7 and Fig. 48-3). α-Blockers are not recommended as initial therapy. BB use is not recommended as initial therapy in adults more than 60 years of age. ACE inhibitor use is not recommended in blacks. If first-line therapy is not effective, then addition of other classes of anti-

hypertensive drugs is recommended. Hypokalemia should be avoided by using potassium-sparing agents in adults who are prescribed diuretics.

CHEP 7 guidelines recommend that adults with hypertension and without a compelling indication make appropriate lifestyle changes and receive antihypertensive drug therapy to lower BP to goal. Recommended initial therapy for isolated systolic hypertension is a thiazide diuretic, an ARB, or a CCB. Second-line therapy consists of combinations of first-line drugs.

CHEP 7 guidelines recommend that adults with hypertension and at least one compelling indication make appropriate lifestyle changes and receive therapy for compelling indications as well as antihypertensive drug therapy to reach the BP goal.

CHEP 7 guidelines emphasize the importance of actually achieving adaptation of individuals to a new, healthier lifestyle and to drug therapy (adherence). Adherence should be assessed at each visit and augmented by simplification of medical regimens (once-daily administration preferred), use of electronic medication compliance aids, tailoring the dose regimen to the individual's daily routine, encouraging greater individual responsibility and autonomy in BP monitoring and dose adjustment, coordination with worksite health care providers, and educating patients and their family members.

DISCUSSIONS RELATING TO GUIDELINES

The ultimate role of guidelines in clinical practice continues to be debated.[86-88] Discussants note that guidelines are only intended to serve as a framework for diagnosis and therapy and recognize that clinical judgment is the main clinical tool for counseling and managing individual patients. This approach merges the art and science of medicine at the bedside.

The perceived impracticality of one-size-fits-all clinical practice algorithms could lead some clinicians to delay or avoid adoption of guidelines. For example, although adult guidelines recommend nonpharmacologic treatment of a man or woman with a confirmed BP of 126/80 mm Hg, it seems impractical to advise lifestyle changes for a 42-year-old marathoner with a family history of coronary artery but who does not smoke or drink and who has a BMI of 23 kg/m^2 and a resting heart rate of 48 beats/minute.[89] A full consideration of guideline recommendations is intended to lead the clinician to confirm that this individual also lacks additional CVRFs or compelling indications, such as diabetes or dyslipidemia, consumes a DASH diet with modest amounts of sodium and adequate amounts of potassium, calcium, and magnesium, and, if relevant, manages stress well.

This example also highlights the discussion about use of the term prehypertension. The 42-year-old marathoner would be designated as having prehypertension, according to JNC 7 guidelines. Creation of this new category for BP was intended to call attention to an adult population at higher risk of cardiovascular disease and future development of hypertension, while underscoring the importance of lifestyle changes in lowering the risk of hypertension.[1] Some discussants note that the term prehypertension can be confusing when it is misperceived as a requirement for pharmacologic therapy, which it clearly was not. They also note that there may be negative actuarial, social, and psychological implications for persons designated prehypertensive. Additionally, for adults without diabetes, the evidence base demonstrating the benefit of intervention relative to the modest level of cardiovascular risk is small, but the risk of lifestyle modification, which is what JNC 7 recommends, is also small.

The approach to first-line drug therapy differs significantly in that U.S. guidelines emphasize use of a thiazide-like diuretic in most individuals, and Canadian guidelines leave open the choice from among five classes of antihypertensive agents, thus underscoring the importance of achieving BP control over the particular class of drugs used. Some discussants are calling for more rigorous studies comparing drug interventions with the lifestyle interventions recommended in hypertension-related guidelines.[89,90] Others call for a shift from single-factor guidelines to multifactorial or global risk guidelines.[91] This approach bases clinical management decisions on an individual's combined or global cardiovascular risk instead of on a single risk factor such as BP.

Both U.S. and Canadian guidelines are evidence-based recommendations. The U.S. classification of hypertension was further simplified with the JNC 7 framework, whereas the Canadian, European, and WHO classifications continue to be based on the JNC VI framework. Canadian guidelines place less emphasis on cost-effectiveness or pharmacoeconomic considerations, in view of the relatively small body of such evidence for chronic hypertension.[92] Making necessary assumptions about variables such as cost of laboratory monitoring or drug-related morbidity and mortality can be challenging, even for an antihypertensive drug with a low average wholesale price. Additional considerations include the costs of not adequately treating and controlling high BP, that is, the costs of hypertension-related morbidity and mortality. Comparisons of control rates among different countries and other geographic regions indicate significant variation and will foster further discussion about potential determinants.[93]

EFFECTIVENESS OF GUIDELINES

Treatment goals recommended by guideline committees are often used in the clinical practice setting as part of the quality assurance process.[1,94,95] Ultimately, the effectiveness of the application of CPGs in the clinical practice setting is evidenced by the rate of control of elevated BP in the population of individuals with diagnosed hypertension, that is, the percentage of hypertensive individuals whose BP is at or lower than the treatment goal. The importance of this metric has been recognized for decades and has relevance for all hypertensive populations, whether part of an independent or staff practice model or a managed care or alternative model. The extent of the application of CPGs in the clinical practice setting also affects the effectiveness of screening for and detecting individuals with hypertension or who are at a higher risk of developing hypertension or a hypertension-related complication.

The National Committee for Quality Assurance (NCQA) evaluates and accredits health plans or managed care organizations in the United States. Using BP JNC VI treatment goals, the NCQA added "controlling high BP" of adult enrollees 45 to 84 years of age who are members for at least 12 months to its Health Employer Data and Information Set (HEDIS) quality assessment standards in 2000 (<140 mm Hg SBP and <90 mm Hg DBP).[96] The most recent HEDIS measures use a less stringent standard (≤140 mm Hg SBP and ≤90 mm Hg DBP).[97]

In the Canadian Heart Health Survey (CHHS) of 10 provinces, more than four fifths of hypertensive Canadian adults were not at goal (<140/90 mm Hg; 1986 to 1992).[2] In the National Health and Nutrition Examination Surveys (NHANES), more than two thirds of hypertensive U.S. adults were not at goal (<140/90 mm Hg for 1999 to 2002), although hypertension control rates are higher than in the past.[1,98] A random sampling of the medical records of hypertensive patients in 12 U.S. metropolitan areas indicated that participants received only 55% of recommended general care, 57% received optimal antihypertensive care, and 42% were at BP goal (<140/90 mm Hg; 1998 to 2000).[99,100] Results from two large clinical trials and a study of an outpatient hypertension specialist clinic demonstrate the ability to achieve an SBP goal in 63% to 65% of patients and a DBP goal in 86% to 90% of hypertensive individuals (SBP <140 mm Hg and DBP <90 mm Hg).[94,101,102] Using less stringent criteria in 2003, hypertension control rates were 62%, 61%, and 59% for commercial, Medicare, and Medicaid health plans, respectively (≤140/90 mm Hg; 2003).[97] Evaluation of adherence to CPGs by clinicians contracting with a third-party payer indicates that only 38%, 29%, 34%, and 36% of members with hypertension-alone were prescribed a diuretic, a BB, a CCB or an ACE inhibitor, respectively, and approximately 50% of hypertensive members with certain comorbidities received non–first-line interventions.[95] BP control in patients with compelling indications offers additional challenges because of even lower treatment goals (e.g., <130/85 or <130/80 mm Hg).[103]

Determination of the cause of the suboptimal levels of hypertension control or quality of antihypertensive care evidenced earlier and the implementation of interventions designed to achieve better results or outcomes are extremely important.[104-106] Adherence to hypertension-related CPGs by health professionals and patients is feasible.[94] The extent of adherence to therapeutic guidelines by clinicians as well as patients continues to be important, although it is challenging to measure rigorously enough to permit generation of valid and meaningful conclusions.[107] Investigators have called for consensus methodology for evaluation of adherence to CPGs. Other potential determinants of achieving treatment goals include the following: the reasonableness, practicality, and communicability of guidelines; physician awareness of or agreement with guidelines; the adequacy of dosage, appropriateness of the drug combination, or simplicity of the treatment regimen; provider-specific or patient-specific characteristics; access to care, healthy options, healthful environments, or pharmaceuticals; and the presence of systemic policies, prompters, tracking systems, and feedback tools for providers and patients.[108-110] Irrespective of the predominant cause, the opportunity for greater effectiveness in the translation of evidence-based CPGs into high-quality practice regarding prevention, detection, and control of elevated BP is clear and significant.

FUTURE DIRECTIONS

Achievement of optimal BP control in individuals with elevated BP continues to be problematic, in spite of the proven efficacy and effectiveness of lifestyle changes, the presence of effective pharmacotherapies (including the approval of Aliskiren, an oral renin inhibitor), and the demonstrated feasibility of achieving BP goals in the clinical setting. Accordingly, an enhanced understanding of the causes of suboptimal outcomes, consistency in the definition of elevated BP, consensus about methodologies and measures of adherence to guidelines, greater commitment to population-based interventions as well as individual-centered interventions, and allocation of sufficient resources to the problem of hypertension locally, nationally, and internationally will continue to be important—far into the future.

Acknowledgments

I thank Dr. Ross Feldman for making available a draft copy of the 2005 CHEP summary and for comments, Dr. Norm Campbell for historical information, Dr. Jeffrey Cutler for comments, and LaForest Dupree and Health Services Research Library staff for kind assistance.

References

1. Chobanian AV, Bakris GL, Black HR, et al., and the National High Blood Pressure Education Program Coordinating Committee. The Seventh Report of the Joint National Committee on Prevention, Detection, Evaluation, and Treatment of High Blood Pressure: The JNC 7 Report. *JAMA*. 2003;**289**:2560-2572.
2. Feldman R, for the Canadian Hypertension Education Program. 2005 Canadian Hypertension Education Program recommendations: What are the new messages? *Perspect Cardiol*. 2005;**21**:30-34.
3. Eddy DM. Evidence-based medicine: A unified approach. *Health Aff (Millwood)*. 2005;**24**:9-17.
4. Joffres MR, Hamet P, MacLean DR, et al. Distribution of blood pressure and hypertension in Canada and the United States. *Am J Hypertens*. 2001;**14**:1099-1105.
5. Fields LE, Burt VL, Cutler JA, et al. The burden of adult hypertension in the United States 1999 to 2000: A rising tide. *Hypertension*. 2004;**44**:398-404.
6. Kearney PM, Whelton M, Reynolds K, et al. Global burden of hypertension: Analysis of worldwide data. *Lancet*. 2005;**365**: 217-223.
7. Lewington S, Clarke R, Qizilbash N, et al. Age-specific relevance of usual blood pressure to vascular mortality: A meta-analysis of individual data for one million adults in 61 prospective studies. Prospective Studies Collaboration. *Lancet*. 2002;**360**:1903-1913.
8. Fields LE. Mortality from stroke and ischemic heart disease increases exponentially with blood pressure. *Hypertension*. 2004;**43**:e28.
9. Lenfant C. Shattuck lecture: Clinical research to clinical practice—lost in translation? *N Engl J Med*. 2003;**349**: 868-874.
10. McAlister FA, Campbell NR, Zarnke K, et al. The management of hypertension in Canada: A review of current guidelines, their shortcomings and implications for the future. *CMAJ*. 2001;**164**:517-522.
11. Andrade SE, Gurwitz JH, Field TS, et al. Hypertension management: The care gap between clinical guidelines and clinical practice. *Am J Manag Care*. 2004;**10**:481-486.
12. Marine JJ. http://www.worldofquotes.com/author/Joshua-J.-Marine/1/. Accessed January 10, 2005.
13. Hales S. Statistical Essays: Containing Hoemastaticks; or, an account of some Hydraulick and Hydrostatical Experiments made on the Blood and Blood-Vessels of Animals. London: W. Innys and R. Manby, 1733.
14. Hall WD. Stephen Hales: Theologian, botanist, physiologist, discoverer of hemodynamics. *Clin Cardiol*. 1987;**10**:487-489.
15. Faivre J. Études expérimentales sur les lésions organiques du coeur. *Gaz Med Paris*. 1856;**11**:712-726.
16. von Basch SK. Ueber die Messung des Blutdrucks am Menschen. *Z Klin Med*. 1880;**2**:79.
17. Rica-Rocci S. Un nuovo sfigmomanometro. *Gaz Med Torino*. 1896; **50**:981-996, 1001-1017.
18. Cushing H. On routine determinations of arterial tension in operating room and clinic. *Boston Med Surg J*. 1903;**148**: 250-252.
19. Segall HN. Clinical measurement of arterial blood pressure. *In*: Pioneers of Cardiology in Canada, 1820-1970: The Genesis of Canadian Cardiology. Willowdale, Ontario, Canada: Hounslow Press, 1988, pp 53-58.
20. Janeway TC. The Clinical Study of Blood Pressure: A Guide to the Use of the Sphygmomanometer in Medical, Surgical, and Obstetrical Practice, with a Summary of the Experimental and Clinical Facts Relating to the Blood-Pressure in Health and Disease. New York: D. Appleton, 1904.

21. Crenner CW. Introduction of the blood pressure cuff into U.S. medical practice: Technology and skilled practice. *Ann Intern Med*. 1998;**128**:488-493.

22. Korotkoff NC. On methods of studying blood pressure. *Izvest Voennomed Akad*. 1905;**11**:365-367.

23. Cantwell JD. Profiles in cardiology: Nicolai S. Korotkoff (1874-1920). *Clin Cardiol*. 1989;**12**:233-235.

24. Segall HN. History of Medicine: How Korotkoff, the surgeon, discovered the auscultatory method of measuring arterial pressure. *Ann Intern Med*. 1975;**83**:561-562.

25. Schrumpf P, Zabel B. Ueber die auskultatorische Blutdruckmessung. *Munchen Med Wochenschr*. 1909;**56**:704-708.

26. Gittings JC. Auscultatory blood-pressure determinations. *Arch Intern Med*. 1910;**6**:196-204.

27. Goodman EH, Howell AA. Clinical studies in the auscultatory method of determining blood-pressure. *Univ Penna Bull*. 1910-11;**23**:469-475.

28. Cabot RC. Physical Diagnosis, 5th ed. New York: William Wood; 1913, p 111.

29. Goodman EH, Howell AA. Further clinical studies in the auscultatory method of determining blood pressure. *Am J Med Sci*. 1911;**142**:334-352.

30. Norris GW. Arterial hypertensive cardiovascular disease, nephritis, etc. *In:* Norris GW. Blood-Pressure: Its Clinical Applications, 3rd ed., rev. Philadelphia: Lea & Febiger, 1917, p 274.

31. Metropolitan Life Insurance Company. Instructions to Medical Examiners. New York: Metropolitan Life Insurance Company. 1917.

32. Bureau of Standards, U.S. Department of Commerce. Use and testing of sphygmomanometers. *Technol Papers Bureau Standards*. 1927;**21**:729-764.

33. Thulin T, Andersson G, Schersten B. Measurement of blood-pressure: A routine test in need of standardization. *Postgrad Med J*. 1975;**51**:390-395.

34. Committee for Standardization of Blood Pressure Readings of the American Heart Association and Committee for Standardization of Blood Pressure Readings of the Cardiac Society of Great Britain and Ireland. *JAMA*. 1939;**113**:294-297.

35. Bordley J III, Conner CAR, Hamilton WF, et al. Recommendations for human blood pressure determinations by sphygmomanometers. *Circulation*. 1951;**4**:503-509.

36. Kirkendall WM, Burton AC, Epstein FH, et al. Recommendations for human blood pressure determination by sphygmomanometers. *Circulation*. 1967;**36**:980-988.

37. Kirkendall WM, Feinleib M, Freis ED, et al. Recommendations for human blood pressure determination by sphygmomanometers: Subcommittee of the AHA Postgraduate Education Committee. *Circulation*. 1980;**62**:1146A-1155A.

38. Frolich ED, Grim C, Labarthe DR, et al. Recommendations for human blood pressure determination by sphygmomanometers. *Circulation*. 1988;**77**:501A-514A.

39. Perloff D, Grim C, Flack J, et al. Human blood pressure determination by sphygmomanometry. *Circulation*. 1993;**88**:2460-2470.

40. Pickering TG, Hall JE, Appel LJ, et al., Subcommittee of Professional and Public Education of the American Heart Association Council on High Blood Pressure Research. Recommendations for blood pressure measurement in humans and experimental animals: Part 1. Blood pressure measurement in humans: A statement for professionals from the Subcommittee of Professional and Public Education of the American Heart Association Council on High Blood Pressure Research. *Hypertension*. 2005;**45**:142-161.

41. Chobanian AV, Bakris GL, Black HR, et al., Joint National Committee on Prevention, Detection, Evaluation, and Treatment of High Blood Pressure, National Heart, Lung, and Blood Institute, National High Blood Pressure Education Program Coordinating Committee. Seventh Report of the Joint National Committee on Prevention, Detection, Evaluation, and Treatment of High Blood Pressure (full report). *Hypertension*. 2003;**42**:1206-1252.

42. Zamorski MA, Green LA. NHBPEP report on high blood pressure in pregnancy: A summary for family physicians. *Am Fam Physician*. 2001;**64**:263-270, 216.

43. The Sixth Report of the Joint National Committee on prevention, detection, evaluation, and treatment of high blood pressure. *Arch Intern Med*. 1997;**157**:2413-2446.

44. The Fifth Report of the Joint National Committee on Detection, Evaluation, and Treatment of High Blood Pressure (JNC V). *Arch Intern Med*. 1993;**153**:154-183.

45. Joint National Committee. Report of the Joint National Committee on Detection, Evaluation, and Treatment of High Blood Pressure (JNC IV). *Arch Intern Med*. 1988;**148**:1023-1038.

46. Joint National Committee. Report of the Joint National Committee on Detection, Evaluation, and Treatment of High Blood Pressure. *Arch Intern Med*. 1984;**144**:1045-1057.

47. Joint National Committee. The 1980 report of the Joint National Committee on Detection, Evaluation, and Treatment of High Blood Pressure. *Arch Intern Med*. 1980;**140**:1280-1285.

48. Joint National Committee. Report of the Joint National Committee on Detection, Evaluation, and Treatment of High Blood Pressure: A cooperative study. *JAMA*. 1977;**237**:255-261.

49. National High Blood Pressure Education Program Working Group on High Blood Pressure in Children and Adolescents. The Fourth Report on the diagnosis, evaluation, and treatment of high blood pressure in children and adolescents. *Pediatrics*. 2004;**114 (2 Suppl)**:555-576.

50. Task Force on High Blood Pressure in Children and Adolescents. Update on the Task Force (1987) on High Blood Pressure in Children and Adolescents: A working group from the National High Blood Pressure Education Program. *Pediatrics*. 1996;**98**:649-658.

51. Task Force on Blood Pressure Control in Children. Report of the Second Task Force on Blood Pressure Control in Children: 1987. *Pediatrics*. 1987;**79**:1-25.

52. National Heart, Lung, and Blood Institute's Task Force on Blood Pressure Control in Children. Report of the Task Force on Blood Pressure Control in Children: 1977. *Pediatrics*. 1977;**59 (Suppl)**:797-820.

53. U.S. Preventive Services Task Force of the Agency for Healthcare Quality and Research of the U.S. Department of Health and Human Services. Screening for high blood pressure: Recommendations and rationale. *Am J Prev Med*. 2003;**25**:159-164.

54. U.S. Preventive Services Task Force of the Agency for Healthcare Quality and Research of the U.S. Department of Health and Human Services. Screening for high blood pressure. *In:* Guide to Clinical Preventive Services: A report of the U.S. Preventive Services Task Force, 2nd ed. Baltimore: Williams & Wilkins, 1996, pp 39-51.

55. U.S. Department of Health and Human Services, Agency for Healthcare Research and Quality. Evidence-Based Practice Centers. Available at: http://www.ahrq.gov/clinic/epc. The National Guideline Clearing House. http://www.ahrq.gov/clinic/ngcfact.htm. Accessed January 18, 2005.

56. Pearson TA, Blair SN, Daniels SR, et al. AHA Guidelines for Primary Prevention of Cardiovascular Disease and Stroke: 2002 Update. Consensus Panel Guide to Comprehensive Risk Reduction for Adult Patients Without Coronary or Other Atherosclerotic Vascular Diseases: American Heart Association Science Advisory and Coordinating Committee. *Circulation*. 2002;**106**:388-391.

57. American Academy of Family Physicians. Age Charts for Periodic Health Examinations and Recommended Immunization Schedules for Children and Adults: Based on the American Academy of Family Physicians Summary of Policy Recommendations for Periodic Health Examinations, November 1996, Revisions 5.4 (August 2003), 5.5 (July 2004), and 5.6 (August 2004). Available at: http://www.aafp.org/PreBuilt/AgeChartsRev5_4-0604.pdf. http://www.aafp.org/x24996.xml. Accessed January 20, 2005.

58. American College of Obstetricians and Gynecologists. Guidelines for Women's Health Care, 2nd ed. Washington, DC: American College of Obstetricians and Gynecologists, 2002.

59. American Academy of Pediatrics. Committee on Practice and Ambulatory Medicine: Recommendations for Preventative Pediatric Health Care. Pediatrics. 2000;105:645-646.

60. American Heart Association. AHA Recommendation: High Blood Pressure in Children. Available at: http://www.americanheart.org/presenter.jhtml?identifier=460. Accessed January 20, 2005.

61. Green M, Palfrey J. Bright Futures: Guidelines for Health Supervision of Infants, Children, and Adolescents, revised 2nd ed. Arlington, VA: National Center for Education in Maternal and Child Health, Georgetown University, 2002.

62. American Society of Hypertension. Recommendations for routine blood pressure measurement by indirect cuff sphygmomanometry: American Society of Hypertension. Am J Hypertens. 1992;5:207-209.

63. Fleming M, Elster AB, Klein JD, Anderson SM. Lessons Learned: National Development to Local Implementation, Guidelines for Adolescent Preventive Services (GAPS). Chicago: American Medical Association, 2001.

64. Hemmelgarn BR, McAlister FA, Grover S, et al. The 2006 Canadian Hypertension Education Program recommendations for the management of hypertension: Part I—Blood pressure measurement, diagnosis and assessment of risk. Can J Cardiol. 2006;22:573-581.

65. Khan NA, McAlister FA, Rabkin SW, et al. The 2006 Canadian Hypertension Education Program recommendations for the management of hypertension: Part II—Therapy. Can J Cardiol. 2006;22:583-593.

66. Hemmelgarn BR, Zarnke KB, Campbell NR, et al., Canadian Hypertension Education Program, Evidence-Based Recommendations Task Force. The 2004 Canadian Hypertension Education Program recommendations for the management of hypertension: Part I. Blood pressure measurement, diagnosis and assessment of risk. Can J Cardiol. 2004;20:31-40.

67. Khan NA, McAlister FA, Campbell NR, et al., Canadian Hypertension Education Program. The 2004 Canadian recommendations for the management of hypertension: Part II. Therapy. Can J Cardiol. 2004;20:41-54.

68. Campbell NRC, Drouin D, Feldman R. A brief history of Canadian hypertension recommendations. Hypertens Canada. 2005;82:1-8.

69. Logan AG. Report of the Canadian Hypertension Society's consensus conference on the management of mild hypertension. CMAJ. 1984;131:1053-1057.

70. Myers MG, Carruthers SG, Leenen FH, et al. Recommendations from the Canadian Hypertension Society consensus conference on the pharmacologic treatment of hypertension. CMAJ. 1989;140:1141-1146.

71. Chockalingam A, Abbott D, Bass M, Battista R, et al. Recommendations of the Canadian Consensus conference on non-pharmacological approaches to the management of high blood pressure, Mar. 21-23, 1989, Halifax, Nova Scotia. CMAJ. 1990;142:1397-1409;

72. Fodor JG, Chockalingam A. The Canadian consensus report on non-pharmacological approaches to the management of high blood pressure. Clin Exp Hypertens A. 1990;12:729-743.

73. Carruthers SG, Larochelle P, Haynes RB, et al. Report of the Canadian Hypertension Society consensus conference: 1. Introduction. CMAJ. 1993;149:289-293.

74. Haynes RB, Lacourciere Y, Rabkin SW, et al. Report of the Canadian Hypertension Society consensus conference: 2. Diagnosis of hypertension in adults. CMAJ. 1993;149:409-418.

75. Ogilvie RI, Burgess ED, Cusson JR, et al. Report of the Canadian Hypertension Society consensus conference: 3. Pharmacologic treatment of essential hypertension. CMAJ. 1993;149:575-584.

76. Reeves RA, Fodor JG, Gryfe CI, et al. Report of the Canadian Hypertension Society consensus conference: 4. Hypertension in the elderly. CMAJ. 1993;149:815-820.

77. Dawson KG, McKenzie JK, Ross SA, et al. Report of the Canadian Hypertension Society consensus conference: 5. Hypertension and diabetes. CMAJ. 1993;149:821-826.

78. Campbell NR, Burgess E, Taylor G, et al. Lifestyle changes to prevent and control hypertension: Do they work? A summary of the Canadian consensus conference. CMAJ. 1999;160:1341-1343

79. Feldman RD. The 1999 Canadian recommendations for the management of hypertension: On behalf of the Task Force for the Development of the 1999 Canadian Recommendations for the Management of Hypertension. Can J Cardiol. 1999;15 (Suppl G):57G-64G.

80. McAlister FA, Levine M, Zarnke KB, et al., Canadian Hypertension Recommendations Working Group. The 2000 Canadian recommendations for the management of hypertension: Part one. Therapy. Can J Cardiol. 2001;17:543-559.

81. Zarnke KB, Levine M, McAlister FA, et al., Canadian Hypertension Recommendations Working Group. The 2000 Canadian recommendations for the management of hypertension: Part two. Diagnosis and assessment of people with high blood pressure. Can J Cardiol. 2001;17:1249-1263.

82. Zarnke KB, McAlister FA, Campbell NR, et al., Canadian Hypertension Recommendations Working Group. The 2001 Canadian recommendations for the management of hypertension: Part one. Assessment for diagnosis, cardiovascular risk, causes and lifestyle modification. Can J Cardiol. 2002;18:604-624.

83. McAlister FA, Zarnke KB, Campbell NR, et al., Canadian Hypertension Recommendations Working Group. The 2001 Canadian recommendations for the management of hypertension: Part two. Therapy. Can J Cardiol. 2002;18:625-641.

84. Wong TY, Mitchell P. Hypertensive retinopathy. N Engl J Med. 2004;351:2310-2317.

85. Whitworth JA, World Health Organization, International Society of Hypertension Writing Group. 2003 World Health Organization (WHO)/International Society of Hypertension (ISH) statement on management of hypertension. J Hypertens. 2003;21:1983-1992.

86. Moser M, Papademetriou V, Pickering TG, et al. Hypertension treatment guidelines. J Clin Hypertens (Greenwich). 2004;6:452-457.

87. Stergiou GS, Salgami EV, World Health Organization–International Society of Hypertension (WHO-ISH), USA Joint National Committee on Prevention, Detection, Evaluation, and Treatment of High Blood Pressure (JNC-7), European Society of Hypertension–European Society of Cardiology (ESH-ESC). New European, American and International guidelines for hypertension management: Agreement and disagreement. Expert Rev Cardiovasc Ther. 2004;2:359-368.

88. Landro L. The informed patient: Are treatment guidelines reliable? Wall Street Journal, p D4, January 26, 2005.

89. Nicolson DJ, Dickinson HO, Campbell F, et al. Lifestyle interventions or drugs for patients with essential hypertension: A systematic review. *J Hypertens*. 2004;**22**:2043-2048.

90. Gueyffier F. Are guidelines right to promote lifestyle interventions against hypertension? *J Hypertens*. 2004;**22**:2055-2056.

91. Jackson R, Lawes CMM, Bennett DA, et al. Treatment with drugs to lower blood pressure and blood cholesterol based on an individual's absolute cardiovascular risk. *Lancet*. 2005;**365**:434-441.

92. Khan NA, Campbell NR. Thiazide diuretics in the management of hypertension. *Can J Clin Pharmacol*. 2004;**11**:e41-e44.

93. Wolf-Maier K, Cooper RS, Kramer H, et al. Hypertension treatment and control in five European countries, Canada, and the United States. *Hypertension*. 2004;**43**:10-17.

94. Singer GM, Izhar M, Black HR. Guidelines for hypertension: Are quality-assurance measures on target? *Hypertension*. 2004;**43**:198-202.

95. Holmes JS, Shevrin M, Goldman B, et al. Translating research into practice: Are physicians following evidence-based guidelines in the treatment of hypertension? *Med Care Res Rev*. 2004;**61**:453-473.

96. Sennett C. Implementing the new HEDIS hypertension performance measure. *Manag Care*. 2000;**9 (4 Suppl)**:2-21.

97. National Committee for Quality Assurance. The State of Health Care Quality: 2004. Washington, DC: National Committee for Quality Assurance, p 33. Available at: http://www.ncqa.org/communications/SOMC/SOHC2004.pdf. Accessed January, 2005.

98. Glover MJ, Greenlund KJ, Ayala C, et al. Racial/ethnic disparities in prevalence, treatment, and control of hypertension: United States, 1999-2002. *MMWR Morb Mortal Wkly Rep*. 2005;**54**:7-9.

99. McGlynn EA, Asch SM, Adams J, et al. The quality of health care delivered to adults in the United States. *N Engl J Med*. 2003;**348**:2635-2645.

100. Asch SM, McGlynn EA, Hiatt L, et al. Comparison of quality of care for patients in the Veterans Health Administration and patients in a national sample. *Ann Intern Med*. 2004;**141**:938-945.

101. Black HR, Elliott WJ, Grandits G, et al. CONVINCE Research Group: Principal results of the Controlled Onset Verapamil Investigation of Cardiovascular Endpoints (CONVINCE) trial. *JAMA*. 2003;**289**:2073-2082.

102. Cushman WC, Ford CE, Cutler JA, et al., ALLHAT Collaborative Research Group. Success and predictors of blood pressure control in diverse North American settings: The Antihypertensive and Lipid-Lowering Treatment to Prevent Heart Attack Trial (ALLHAT). *J Clin Hypertens (Greenwich)*. 2002;**4**:393-404.

103. DiTusa L, Luzier AB, Jarosz DE, Snyder BD, Izzo JL Jr. Treatment of hypertension in a managed care setting. *Am J Manag Care*. 2001;**7**:520-524.

104. Lenfant C. High blood pressure control: Put the champagne away. *J Clin Hypertens (Greenwich)*. 2002;**4**:391-392.

105. Hyman DJ, Pavlik VN. Characteristics of patients with uncontrolled hypertension in the United States. *N Engl J Med*. 2001;**345**:479-486.

106. Timmermans S, Mauck A. The promises and pitfalls of evidence-based medicine. *Health Aff (Millwood)*. 2005;**24**:18-28.

107. Milchak JL, Carter BL, James PA, et al. Measuring adherence to practice guidelines for the management of hypertension: An evaluation of the literature. *Hypertension*. 2004;**44**:602-608.

108. Steinman MA, Fischer MA, Shlipak MG, et al. Clinician awareness of adherence to hypertension guidelines. *Am J Med*. 2004;**117**:747-754.

109. Canzanello VJ, Jensen PL, Schwartz LL, et al. Improved blood pressure control with a physician-nurse team and home blood pressure measurement. *Mayo Clin Proc*. 2005;**80**:31-36.

110. McAlister FA, Campbell NR, Zarnke K, et al. The management of hypertension in Canada: A review of current guidelines, their shortcomings and implications for the future. *CMAJ*. 2001;**164**:517-522.

European, American, and British Guidelines: Similarities and Differences

Giuseppe Mancia and Guido Grassi

In 2003, several important guidelines on hypertension were published: the guidelines of the European Society of Hypertension and the European Society of Cardiology (ESH/ESC),[1] the Seventh Report of the Joint National Committee on Prevention, Detection, Evaluation, and Treatment of High Blood Pressure (JNC 7),[2] the World Health Organization (WHO) and International Society of Hypertension (ISH) Guidelines,[3] and the Recommendations of the Task Force of the European Medical Societies.[4] Although all addressed overall cardiovascular prevention, each included a section on the management of hypertension. This chapter does not review these guidelines in detail, but it summarizes their points of agreement and discusses their major differences. A similar approach is taken with regard to the hypertension guidelines issued by the British Hypertension Society, published in 2004.[5] Guidelines of other national hypertension societies are not considered because in most instances they echo international guidelines, with only small differences based on local situations.

MAJOR AGREEMENTS

These guidelines have major areas of agreement on the diagnosis and treatment of hypertension (Table 49-1). All guidelines, for example, agree that evaluation for secondary hypertension is not generally required for all hypertensive patients. All agree that the complex, expensive, and sometimes risky examinations involved in diagnosis of secondary hypertension should be limited to the patients in whom the clinical suspicion of related conditions is strong, given the overall rarity of these conditions, the difficulty of proving their contribution to the blood pressure (BP) elevation, and the uncertainty regarding reversibility. The guidelines agree on the way BP should be measured during office visits and on the importance of measurements performed by the physician during screening, diagnosis, and follow-up of hypertensive patients.

Although the guidelines agree that self-measurements of BP at home and 24-hour ambulatory BP monitoring usually play only complementary roles, these alternative methods of measuring BPs can be important. Self-measurement of BP may increase a patient's long-term adherence to prescribed treatment regimens, thereby solving a major problem in hypertension treatment that limits BP control. Furthermore, both home and ambulatory BP measurements may provide useful information on conditions that depart from the norm in hypertensive patients (Table 49-2), the main example being isolated office or white-coat hypertension, in which BP is persistently elevated when it is measured in the office, but normal at home or over 24 hours. Finally, guidelines share the view that, compared with office BPs, home or 24-hour ambulatory BPs are definitely lower,[6] and thus using traditional office values (<140/90 mm Hg) to assess patients' home or ambulatory BPs may lead to an underestimation of the prevalence of hypertension or of the number of patients with inadequate BP control.

Guidelines also show substantial agreement on major important aspects of antihypertensive treatment. First, the guidelines concur that treatment is accompanied by a beneficial effect on virtually all hypertensive-related diseases and endpoints, with a substantial reduction in cardiovascular morbidity and mortality (Fig. 49-1).[7] Second, this is the case in both genders and at all ages, although the evidence is still inconclusive for patients who are more than 80 years of age.[8] Third, lifestyle changes are universally recommended (with complete agreement on which changes to advise), but all the guidelines recognize that antihypertensive drugs are frequently needed. Fourth, all recommend using drugs with a 24-hour duration of action and once-daily administration, because a simpler treatment schedule may increase a patient's acceptance of the treatment regimen. Fifth, all guidelines recognize that to control BP, a single drug is frequently ineffective, and combinations of two or more drugs are often necessary. Sixth, these guidelines all suggest that drugs to be combined should have complementary mechanisms of action, with a BP-lowering effect greater than that produced by the individual combination components. Finally, all guidelines now agree that low-dose drug combinations should be considered for initial treatment in hypertensive patients with BPs that are much higher than the goal, Under this circumstance, the large BP change that is required makes the use of two or more antihypertensive drugs almost inevitable, and the risk of a cardiovascular morbid or fatal event associated with delayed BP control may be greater than previously recognized.[9]

Most importantly, all current guidelines agree on the BP threshold at which to start treatment and the BP target treatment goals. Nonpharmacologic treatment and, if necessary, drug treatment should be implemented for all individuals in whom BP is persistently equal 140 mm Hg systolic or higher or 90 mm Hg diastolic or higher. In all patients, BP should be reduced to less than these values, and lower targets (<130/80 mm Hg) should be reached in patients with diabetes with or without concomitant nephropathy. Patients should be seen frequently to adapt treatment strategies to changing clinical patterns and to maintain a good patient-physician relationship, thus helping with adherence to treatment. With very few exceptions, treatment should be continued indefinitely, although a cautious downward titration may be attempted after persistent long-term BP control.

DIFFERENCES

The two European guidelines are largely similar. Both show certain differences with the JNC 7 guidelines (Table 49-3), and these differences are discussed in the following sections.

Table 49-1 Major Agreements between 2003 Guidelines from the European Society of Hypertension–European Society of Cardiology and the Joint National Committee on Prevention, Detection, Evaluation, and Treatment of High Blood Pressure

Routine avoidance of complex laboratory examinations
Blood pressure measuring procedures
Value and use of ambulatory blood pressure monitoring and home blood pressure measurements
Benefits of antihypertensive treatment
Lifestyle changes and their implementation as first-step treatment
Blood pressure thresholds and targets for treatment
Value of long-acting antihypertensive drugs
Importance of combination treatment, even as a first choice for some patients
Value of fixed-dose combinations
Use of additional antiplatelet and lipid-lowering treatments
Conditions requiring use of specific drugs and drug regimens
Importance of careful assessment of side effects
Follow-up visits and strategies

From Chobanian AV, Bakris GL, Black HR, et al., and the National High Blood Pressure Education Program Coordinating Committee. The Seventh Report of the Joint National Committee on Prevention, Detection, Evaluation and Treatment of High Blood Pressure: The JNC 7 Report. *JAMA*. 2003;**289**: 2560-2572.

Prehypertension

The European guidelines maintain the classification of BP values employed in the previous WHO/ISH guidelines.[10] In this classification, hypertensive subjects are divided into three groups according to the degree of BP elevation. Even among individuals within the normotensive range, however, data from the Framingham Heart Study and from other epidemiologic studies show a graded increase in cardiovascular risk among those with optimal (<120/80 mm Hg), normal (120 to 129/80 to 84 mm Hg), and high-normal (130 to 139/85 to 89 mm Hg) BPs, the classification used in the Sixth Report of the Joint National Committee on Prevention, Detection, Evaluation, and Treatment of High Blood Pressure (JNC VI).[11-13] The JNC 7 guidelines, conversely, simplify this classification by reducing to two groups the number of grades of hypertension and by joining into a single category anyone with BP between 120 and 139 mm Hg systolic or 80 and 89 mm Hg diastolic.[2] These persons are termed *prehypertensive*, and all are advised to adopt lifestyle changes to reduce BP.

The foregoing classification has generated considerable controversy. Its defenders maintain that simplification is

Table 49-2 Indications for 24-Hour Ambulatory Blood Pressure Monitoring According to Guidelines from the European Society of Hypertension–European Society of Cardiology

Considerable office blood pressure variability over the same and different visits
High office blood pressure in subjects at low global cardiovascular risk
Sustained discrepancy between office and home blood pressure
Resistance to drug treatment
Research studies

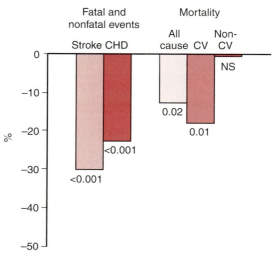

Figure 49–1   Effects of antihypertensive treatment on cardiovascular morbidity and mortality in systolic-diastolic and isolated systolic hypertension. CHD, coronary heart disease; CV, cardiovascular. (From Practice Guidelines Writing Committee. Practice guidelines for primary care physicians: 2003 ESH/ESC hypertension guidelines. *J Hypertens*. 2003;**21**:1779-1786.)

Table 49-3   Major Differences between 2003 Guidelines from the European Society of Hypertension–European Society of Cardiology and the Joint National Committee on Prevention, Detection, Evaluation and Treatment of High Blood Pressure

Greater emphasis on educational rather than prescriptive use of guidelines

Recommendation for assessment of total cardiovascular risk

Term "prehypertension" not used/life style changes not recommended in "prehypertension" category if risk not high or very high

Flexibility about need or timing of drug administration in stage 1 hypertension for patients at low risk

No preference for diuretics as first-choice drug treatment/five drug classes considered equally valid for treatment initiation and maintenance

Mention of central agents and α-blockers for combination treatment

Subclinical target organ damage included as intermediate endpoints in risk assessment and goal of treatment

No preference for data from the Antihypertensive and Lipid-Lowering Treatment to Prevent Heart Attack Trial versus data from other trials

Disclosure of "institutional" conflicts of interest

advantageous. Furthermore, they emphasize that persons with BPs in the range of 120 to 129/80 to 89 mm Hg have a much greater risk of becoming hypertensive than do persons with BPs lower than 120/80 mm Hg,[14] a finding that justifies both the term prehypertension and the effort to prevent this transformation. Opponents of this view emphasize the following: (1) rather than addressing population health strategies, guidelines should aim to help physicians in the management of individual patients; (2) the prehypertension category is highly differentiated because whereas persons in whom the overall cardiovascular risk is high (e.g., those with a history of cardiovascular disease or diabetes) need immediate drug treatment, those in whom no other risk factor is present hardly need active intervention for their BP; and (3) because hypertension has an ominous significance to the layperson, the designation prehypertension may increase requests for office visits or laboratory examinations, thereby precipitating a substantial increase in health care costs. In other words, it may create a considerable number of anxiety-driven patients.

Total Cardiovascular Risk

At variance with the JNC 7 guidelines,[2] the European guidelines emphasize the importance of quantifying the global or total cardiovascular risk in hypertensive patients, because in patients at high or very high cardiovascular risk (i.e., in whom the risk of a cardiovascular morbid or fatal event within 10 years is ≥20%), treatment should be more aggressive than in patients at lower risk.[1,4] For these high-risk patients, lifestyle changes should be implemented more strictly, if necessary, with the intervention of health care professionals other than physicians. Drug treatment should start at BPs lower than 140/90 mm Hg, with the aim of reaching values lower than 130/80 mm Hg. Combinations of two drugs should be considered as the initial steps to attain BP targets without

excessive delay. In the absence of specific contraindications, low-dose aspirin (or other antiplatelet treatments) should be added to the antihypertensive drug regimen.[15] Lipid-lowering interventions (typically a statin) should be implemented, regardless of the presence or the absence of an elevated serum total cholesterol level.[16] Antihypertensive drugs that have specific organ protective properties should be included in the antihypertensive multidrug treatment, because this may delay or reverse target organ damage in these patients, over and above the protection afforded by BP lowering alone. For example, drugs acting against the renin-angiotensin system (angiotensin-converting enzyme [ACE] inhibitors and angiotensin II receptor blockers) have specific renal protective effects in type 1 and type 2 diabetes.[17]

The two European guidelines differ in the methods employed for quantification of total cardiovascular risk.[1,4] The guidelines for cardiovascular prevention of the European Medical Societies use a continuous scale for risk quantification, based on traditional cardiovascular risk factors (gender, age, systolic BP, total serum cholesterol, smoking, diabetes) and data on cardiovascular mortality collected in several European populations.[4] The ESH/ESC guidelines[1] remain faithful to the former WHO/ISH approach,[10] regarding the subdivision of total cardiovascular risk into four categories (i.e., low, medium, high, and very high risk), which correspond to a progressive increase in the 10-year chance of cardiovascular morbidity and mortality from less than 15% to more than 30%. This risk classification is less precise than quantification on a continuous scale. However, it offers greater simplicity and includes subclinical target organ damage such as echocardiographic or electrocardiographic left ventricular hypertrophy, ultrasonographic carotid arterial wall thickening or plaques, modest elevations in serum creatinine (≥1.4 or 1.5 mg/dL), and microalbuminuria with or without diabetes mellitus. Any one of these four types of target organ damage boosts an individual into the high-risk category, because each is associated with an adverse prognosis.[18] The presence of these conditions in the hypertensive population is much more common than hitherto believed.[19] The identification and inclusion of these types of target organ damage as risk factor components may thus allow treatment and protection of a larger number of patients. The need to quantify total cardiovascular risk is also emphasized by the WHO/ISH guidelines,[3] which further simplify the risk categorization by lumping together high-risk and very-high-risk patients, based on the evidence that treatment decisions do not substantially differ between these two groups. Given that current data indicate that total cardiovascular risk is rarely assessed by physicians,[20] largely because of its complexity, simplifications should be worthwhile.

First-Choice Drugs

The JNC 7 guidelines recommend starting treatment with a thiazide diuretic in "most" patients and to consider other drugs only when "compelling" indications exist for their use.[2] This recommendation, shared by the WHO/ISH guidelines, which advise thiazide diuretics to be initially used at a "low" dose,[3] stems largely from the conclusion of the Antihypertensive and Lipid-Lowering Treatment to Prevent Heart Attack Trial (ALLHAT) that thiazide diuretics are more protective than other drugs in certain cardiovascular diseases and they have the additional advantage of lower cost.[21] The European guidelines,[1,4] conversely, maintain the following: (1) ALLHAT is open to methodologic criticism, and its results did not show an overall superiority of diuretic over the other two drugs (an ACE inhibitor and a calcium antagonist); (2) no trial has used a low-dose diuretic as monotherapy throughout the trial; (3) β-blockers, ACE inhibitors, calcium antagonists, and angiotensin II receptor antagonists have also been shown to protect hypertensive patients when these drugs are tested against placebo without substantial differences in cardiovascular morbidity and mortality among different drug classes[22,23]; and (4) thiazide diuretics are inexpensive to purchase, but at doses that lower BP as monotherapy, they frequently cause hypokalemia and dyslipidemia and are associated with an increased incidence of impaired fasting glucose, metabolic syndrome, and diabetes.[24-26]

The ESH/ESC guidelines list the criteria on which physicians should select the initial antihypertensive drug.[1] Mention is made of a patient's preference and a patient's experience with any given drug, although with the caveat that cost considerations should not take precedence over a patient's well-being. These guidelines suggest that drugs can be selected on the basis of patients' cardiovascular risk factors and subclinical organ damage, because antihypertensive drug classes can differentially affect metabolic risk factors and can variably regress left ventricular hypertrophy, large artery wall abnormalities, and urinary excretion of protein (Figs. 49-2 and 49-3).

Too much emphasis on a first-choice drug is regarded as unjustified, however, because of the need to use two or more drugs to control BP to goal in at least 67% of patients. Both the European and the JNC 7 guidelines regard a diuretic as an important drug class for combination treatment because its BP-lowering effect is manifest at low doses when it is combined with virtually all other drug classes.[1,2]

Specific Indications

Agreement is substantial between JNC 7 and European guidelines on the conditions that require use of specific drugs,

termed *compelling indications* by the former, and *conditions favoring use* by the latter.[1,2] However, European guidelines include in these conditions the regression or the lack of progression of target organ damage, such as left ventricular hypertrophy, carotid arterial wall thickening, and microalbuminuria, because these conditions have prognostic significance (see earlier).[1] Furthermore, regression or lack of progression of target organ damage represents the goal of treatment in certain patients (e.g., middle-aged patients and those with a low or medium cardiovascular risk) in whom reducing BP does not aim at decreasing the remote chance of a cardiovascular event in the next few years, but instead attempts to prevent or delay the progression of organ damage, which may lead to an event many years later. The recent demonstration that therapeutic-dependent improvement of target organ damage is associated with, and in part responsible for, a reduction in cardiovascular morbidity supports this recommendation.[27]

Other Issues

The European and JNC 7 guidelines have other differences mainly regarding the emphasis placed on an issue.[1,2] For example, the ESH/ESC guidelines emphasize that their aim is educational rather than prescriptive, because recommendations based on average results from large studies cannot force decisions on individual patients, who vary markedly in terms of their demographic, ethnic, clinical, and environmental characteristics.[1,4] These guidelines also emphasize that evidence about treatment of hypertension originates from observational and pathophysiologic studies, as well as from morbidity and mortality trials. Although these trials are important, they have limitations, especially regarding their limited duration, as compared with the life expectancy of many patients. The JNC 7 guidelines[2] emphasize lifestyle modifications based on the results from the Dietary Approaches to Stop Hypertension (DASH) trial,[28] the short duration and lack of prognostic data of which appealed less to the writers of the ESH/ESC guidelines. In contrast, both set of

MONOTHERAPY VERSUS COMBINATION THERAPY

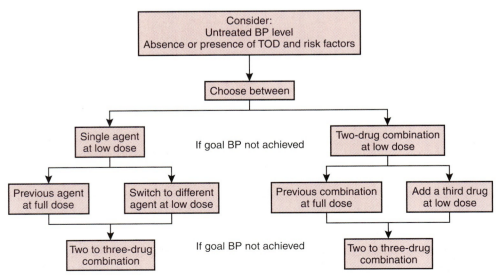

Figure 49–2 Flow chart guiding the choice between monotherapy and combination therapy. BP, blood pressure; TOD, target organ damage. (From European Society of Hypertension–European Society of Cardiology Guidelines Committee. 2003 European Society of Hypertension–European Society of Cardiology guidelines for the management of arterial hypertension. *J Hypertens.* 2003;**21**:1011-1059.)

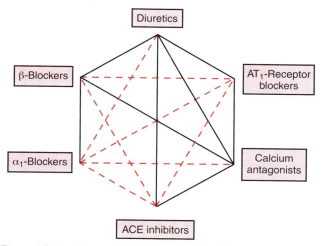

Figure 49–3 Possible combinations of different classes of antihypertensive drugs. The most rational combinations are represented as thick lines. ACE, angiotensin-converting enzyme; AT_1, angiotensin II, subtype 1. (From European Society of Hypertension–European Society of Cardiology Guidelines Committee. 2003 European Society of Hypertension–European Society of Cardiology guidelines for the management of arterial hypertension. *J Hypertens.* 2003;**21**:1011-1059.)

Table 49-4 Specific Features of British Guidelines

Blood pressure thresholds for drug treatment:
≥160 systolic or ≥90 mm Hg diastolic
≥140 systolic or ≥90 mm Hg diastolic in diabetes*
    Cardiovascular disease
    Target organ damage
    10-year cardiovascular risk ≥20%
Blood pressure targets for treatment:
<140/85 mm Hg optimal
<150/90 mm Hg acceptable
<130/80 mm Hg in diabetes
β-Blockers not included as first-choice drugs, but considered only for combination and in specific conditions
First-choice drugs indicated by the AB/CD rule, also recommended for selection of second-step therapy

*Drug treatment considered.

guidelines acknowledge that a major problem remains in the small percentage of patients in whom BP is not effectively controlled by treatment as a result of poor adherence to treatment regimens. These guidelines both strongly advocate the adoption of procedures that can improve adherence to treatment, as follows: (1) provision of information on the importance of hypertension as a risk factor, as well as on the benefit obtained by persistently reducing BP; (2) use of drugs that lower BP over 24 hours with once-daily administration, as well as a fixed combination of two drugs to simplify the treatment schedule; (3) frequent follow-up visits to establish and maintain an optimal physician-patient relationship; and (4) careful assessment of side effects of treatment, because of the primary importance of side effects in patients' withdrawal from prescribed drugs. As stated in the ESH/ESC guidelines, "Particular attention should be given to adverse events, even primarily subjective disturbances, because they may be an important cause of non-compliance. Patients should always be advised about adverse effects and doses or drugs changed accordingly."[1]

British Guidelines

The most recent British guidelines on hypertension are largely in line with the recommendations of other international guidelines.[5] A few specific features are worthy of mention, however (Table 49-4). First, British guidelines consider 160 mm Hg to be the threshold for administration of antihypertensive drugs, on the basis that trials showing the benefit of antihypertensive treatment have recruited patients only with BPs at or higher than this value, rather than at 140 mm Hg. A lower threshold (≥140/90 mm Hg) is recommended only when a patient's cardiovascular risk is high (e.g., diabetes, target organ damage, history of cardiovascular disease, or an

absolute 10-year risk of a cardiovascular event ≥20%). This is a more conservative position than that of the European guidelines,[1] which recommend starting drug treatment for high-risk patients at high-normal BP values (130 to 139/85 to 89 mm Hg). Second, British guidelines are, in contrast, no more conservative with regard to goal BPs, which are less than 140/85 mm Hg (rather than <140/90 mm Hg) in the general hypertensive population. This recommendation is based on the observation that when systolic BP is reduced to less than 140 mm Hg, diastolic values are usually in the low 80 mm Hg range. Third, target values lower than 150/90 mm Hg are regarded as "acceptable" by the British guidelines, because the investigators realistically acknowledged that achieving systolic BPs lower than 140 mm Hg is difficult. Fourth, British guidelines agree with the ESH/ESC guidelines that in the initial treatment of hypertension, one should consider several drug classes. Except for specific conditions (heart failure, angina pectoris after myocardial infarction), these drug classes do not include β-blockers, however, because the protective effects of these drugs are less convincingly demonstrated than are those of other drug classes. Moreover, β-blockers have more side effects, including worsening of the metabolic profile. Finally, British guidelines recommend that within the four drug classes available for first-step treatment, the choice makes use of the AB/CD rule,[29] which states that ACE inhibitors or angiotensin II receptor antagonists should be preferentially given to nonblack patients who are less than 55 years old, whereas diuretics or calcium antagonists should be given to blacks or to patients who are more than 55 years old. This last recommendation has been criticized, however, because the study on which the AB/CD rule is based has a very small number of enrolled patients. Furthermore, large-scale trials have shown ACE inhibitors and calcium antagonists to reduce BP effectively and to protect the cardiovascular system in elderly patients, as well as in younger patients.

References

1. European Society of Hypertension–European Society of Cardiology Guidelines Committee. 2003 European Society of Hypertension–European Society of Cardiology guidelines for the management of arterial hypertension. *J Hypertens.* 2003;**21**:1011-1059.

2. Chobanian AV, Bakris GL, Black HR, et al., and the National High Blood Pressure Education Program Coordinating Committee. The Seventh Report of the Joint National Committee on Prevention, Detection, Evaluation, and Treatment of High Blood Pressure: The JNC 7 Report. *JAMA*. 2003;**289**:2560-2572.

3. Whitworth JA, for the World Health Organization, International Society of Hypertension Writing Group. 2003 World Health Organization (WHO)/International Society of Hypertension (ISH) statement on management of hypertension. *J Hypertens*. 2003;**21**:1983-1992.

4. De Backer G, Ambrosioni E, Borch-Johnsen K, et al. European Guidelines on cardiovascular disease prevention in clinical practice: Third Joint Task Force of European and other societies on cardiovascular disease prevention in clinical practice (constituted by representatives of eight societies and by invited experts). *Eur J Cardiovasc Prev Rehabil*. 2003;**10**:S1-S10.

5. Williams B, Poulter NR, Brown MJ, et al. British Hypertension Society guidelines for hypertension management 2004 (BHS-IV): Summary. *BMJ*. 2004;**328**:634-640.

6. Mancia G, Sega R, Bravi C, et al. Ambulatory blood pressure normalities: Results from the PAMELA Study. *J Hypertens*. 1995;**13**:1377-1390.

7. Practice Guidelines Writing Committee. Practice Guidelines for primary care physicians: 2003 ESH/ESC hypertension guidelines. *J Hypertens*. 2003;**21**:1779-1786.

8. Gueyffier F, Bulpitt C, Boissel JP, et al. Antihypertensive drugs in very old people: A subgroup meta-analysis of randomised controlled trials. *Lancet*. 1999;**353**:793-796.

9. Weber MA, Julius S, Kjeldsen SE, et al. Blood pressure dependent and independent effects of antihypertensive treatment on clinical events in the VALUE Trial. *Lancet*. 2004;**363**:2049-2051.

10. Guidelines Sub-Committee. 1999 World Health Organization–International Society of Hypertension guidelines for the management of hypertension. *J Hypertens*. 1999;**17**:151-185.

11. Vasan RS, Larson MG, Leip EP, et al. Impact of high-normal blood pressure on the risk of cardiovascular disease. *N Engl J Med*. 2001;**345**:1291-1297.

12. Lewington S, Clarke R, Qizilbash N, for the Prospective Studies Collaboration. Age-specific relevance of usual blood pressure to vascular mortality: A meta-analysis of individual data for one million adults in 61 prospective studies. *Lancet*. 2002;**360**:1903-1913.

13. Psaty BM, Furberg CD, Kuller LH, et al. Association between blood pressure level and the risk of myocardial infarction, stroke, and total mortality: The Cardiovascular Health Study. *Arch Intern Med*. 2001;**161**:1183-1192.

14. Vasan RS, Larson MG, Leip EP, et al. Assessment of frequency of progression to hypertension in non-hypertensive participants in the Framingham Heart Study: A cohort study. *Lancet*. 2001;**360**:1682-1686.

15. Zanchetti A, Hansson L, Dahlof B, et al., for the HOT Study Group. Benefit and harm of low-dose aspirin in well-treated hypertensives at different baseline cardiovascular risk. *J Hypertens*. 2002;**20**:2301-2307.

16. Sever PS, Dahlof B, Poulter NR, et al., for the ASCOT investigators. Prevention of coronary and stroke events with atorvastatin in hypertensive patients who have average or lower-than-average cholesterol concentrations, in the Anglo-Scandinavian Cardiac Outcomes Trial-Lipid Lowering Arm (ASCOT-LLA): A multicentre randomised controlled trial. *Lancet*. 2003;**361**:1149-1158.

17. Lewis EJ, Hunsicker LG, Clarke WR, et al. Renoprotective effects of the angiotensin-receptors antagonists irbesartan in patients with nephropathy due to type II diabetes. *N Engl J Med*. 2001;**345**:851-860.

18. Kario K, Pickering TG: Special measures of end-organ damage. *In:* Mancia G, Chalmers J, Julius S, et al. (eds). Manual of Hypertension. New York: Churchill Livingstone, 2002, pp 284-304.

19. Cuspidi C, Ambrosioni E, Mancia G, et al., for the APROS Investigators. Role of echocardiography and carotid ultrasonography in stratifying risk in patients with essential hypertension: The Assessment of Prognostic Risk Observational Survey. *J Hypertens*. 2002;**20**:1307-1314.

20. Mancia G, Pessina AC, Trimarco B, et al. Blood pressure control according to new guidelines targets in low- to high-risk hypertensives managed in specialist practice. *J Hypertens*. 2004;**22**:2387-2396.

21. ALLHAT Officers and Coordinators for the ALLHAT Collaborative Research Group. Major outcomes in high-risk hypertensive patients randomized to angiotensin-converting enzyme inhibitor or calcium channel blocker vs. diuretic: The Antihypertensive and Lipid-Lowering Treatment to Prevent Heart Attack Trial (ALLHAT). *JAMA*. 2002;**288**:2981-2997.

22. Collins R, MacMahon S. Blood pressure, antihypertensive drug treatment and the risks of stroke and of coronary heart disease. *Br Med Bull*. 1994;**50**:272-298.

23. Blood Pressure Lowering Treatment Trialists' Collaboration. Effects of different blood-pressure-lowering regimens on major cardiovascular events: Results of prospectively-designed overviews of randomised trials. *Lancet*. 2003;**362**:1527-1535.

24. Grobbee DE, Hoes AW. Non–potassium-sparing diuretics and risk of sudden cardiac death. *J Hypertens*. 1995;**13**:1539-1545.

25. Franse LV, Pahor M, Di Bari M, et al. Hypokalemia associated with diuretic use and cardiovascular events in the Systolic Hypertension in the Elderly Program. *Hypertension*. 2000;**35**:1025-1030.

26. Lindholm LH, Persson M, Alaupovic P, et al. Metabolic outcomes during 1 year in newly detected hypertensives: Results of the Antihypertensive Treatment and Lipid Profile in a North of Sweden Efficacy Evaluation (ALPINE Study). *J Hypertens*. 2003;**21**:1563-1574.

27. Kannel WB, Vasan RS. Assessment of cardiovascular risk and choice of antihypertensive therapy. *Curr Hypertens Rep*. 2004;**6**:346-351.

28. Moore TJ, Vollmer WM, Appel LJ, et al. Effect of dietary patterns on ambulatory blood pressure: Results from the Dietary Approaches to Stop Hypertension (DASH) trial. *Hypertension*. 1999;**34**:472-477.

29. Brown MJ, Cruickshank JK, Dominiczak AF, et al., Executive Committee, British Hypertension Society. Better blood pressure control: How to combine drugs. *J Hum Hypertens*. 2003;**17**:81-86.

Index

Note: Page numbers followed by the letter f refer to figures and those followed by t refer to tables.

SHARE (Study of Health Assessment and Risk in Ethnic Groups), 496
SHELL study, 272t, 319t
SHEP. *See* Systolic Hypertension in the Elderly Program (SHEP) trial.
SHR (spontaneously hypertensive rat), sympathetic nervous system of, 31, 32
Sibutramine
 blood pressure response to, 377–378
 hypertension related to, 145–146
Shanghai Trial of Nifedipine in the Elderly (STONE), 161f, 272t